THE ANTIMICROBIAL DRUGS

THE
ANTIMICROBIAL DRUGS

SECOND EDITION

Eric M. Scholar
William B. Pratt

OXFORD
UNIVERSITY PRESS

2000

OXFORD
UNIVERSITY PRESS

Oxford   New York
Athens   Auckland   Bangkok   Bogotá   Buenos Aires   Calcutta
Cape Town   Chennai   Dar es Salaam   Delhi   Florence   Hong Kong   Istanbul
Karachi   Kuala Lumpur   Madrid   Melbourne   Mexico City   Mumbai
Nairobi   Paris   São Paulo   Singapore   Taipei   Tokyo   Toronto   Warsaw

and associated companies in
Berlin   Ibadan

Library of Congress Cataloging-in-Publication Data
Scholar, Eric M. (Eric Michael), 1939–
The antimicrobial drugs / Eric M. Scholar, William B. Pratt.—2nd ed.
p. ; cm.   Includes bibliographical references and index.
ISBN 0-19-512528-2 (cloth)—ISBN 0-19-512529-0 (pbk.)
1. Anti-infective agents.   2. Communicable diseases—Chemotherapy.
I. Pratt, William B., 1938–   II. Title.
[DNLM: 1. Anti-Infective Agents.   2. Communicable Diseases—drug therapy.
QV 250   S368a 2000]   RM267.S356 2000   616.9'0461—dc21   99-047277

Since this page cannot legibly accomodate all the copyright notes, the pages
following constitute an extension of the copyright page.

2 4 6 8 9 7 5 3 1

Printed in the United States of America
on acid-free paper

We would like to thank the authors, journals, and publishers for their permission
to reprint the following figures and tables in this text:

Fig. 1–2: E. Jawetz, *Annu. Rev. Pharmacol.* 1968; 8:151. Reproduced with permission from *Annual Review of Pharmacology.* Vol. 8. Copyright © 1968 by Annual Reviews, Inc. All rights reserved.

Fig. 2–2: S. Mitsuhashi, in *R Factor Drug Resistance Plasmid,* ed. S. Mitsuhashi. University Park Press, 1977.

Figs. 3–4, 3–5, 3–6: J. L. Strominger et al., *Fed. Proc.* 1967; 26:9. Federation of American Societies for Experimental Biology.

Fig. 3–7: D. J. Tipper and J. L. Strominger, *Proc. Natl. Acad. Sci.* 1965; 54:1133. National Academy of Sciences.

Fig. 3–9: D. Ayusawa et al., *J. Bacteriol.* 1975; 124:459. American Society for Microbiology.

Fig. 3–10: J. W. Costerton and K.-J. Chang, *J. Antimicrob. Chemother.* 1975; 1:363; H. Nikaido and T. Nakae, *Adv. Microb. Physiol.* 1979; 20:163.

Fig. 4–5: B. B. Levine, *J. Exp. Med.* 1960; 112:1131. The Rockefeller University Press.

Fig. 4–6: B. B. Levine and Z. Ovary, *J. Exp. Med.* 1961; 114:875. The Rockefeller University Press.

Fig. 5–5: R. C. Moellering, *Med. J. Aust.* 1977; 2(Special Suppl.):4. Australasian Medical Publishing Company.

Fig. 5–6: R. C. Moellering and A. N. Weinberg. *J. Clin. Invest.* 1971; 50:2580. The American Society for Clinical Investigation, Inc.

Fig. 5–7: R. A. Chan et al., *Ann. Intern. Med.* 1972; 76:773. American College of Physicians.

Fig. 6–1: C. L. Wisseman et al., *J. Bacteriol.* 1954; 67:662. American Society of Microbiology.

Fig. 6–2: S. Pestka, *Proc. Natl. Acad. Sci. U.S.A.* 1969; 64:709. National Academy of Sciences.

Fig. 6–3: C. F. Weiss et al., *N. Engl. J. Med.* 1960; 262:787. The Massachusetts Medical Society.

Fig. 6–4: W. R. Best, *JAMA* 1967; 201:99. The American Medical Association.

Figs. 7–1, 7–2: D. D. Woods, The biochemical mode of action of the sulfonamides. *J. Gen. Microbiol.* 1962; 29:687. Cambridge University Press.

Fig. 10–2: N. R. Cozzarelli, *Science* 1980; 207:953. American Association for the Advancement of Science.

Fig. 11–1: H. Tiitinen, *Scand. J. Respir. Dis.* 1969; 50:110. Munksgaard International Publishers Ltd.

Fig. 11–2: J. R. Mitchell et al., *Ann. Intern. Med.* 1976; 84:181. American College of Physicians; G. A. Ellard and P. T. Gammon, *J. Pharmacokinet. Biopharm.* 1976; 4:83.

Fig. 12–1: T. E. Andreoli, *Ann. N.Y. Acad. Sci.* 1974; 235:448. New York Academy of Science.

Fig. 12–2: A. Marty and A. Finkelstein, *J. Gen. Physiol.* 1975; 65:515.

Fig. 12–4: With permission from R. J. Langenbach, P. V. Danenberg, and C. Heidelberger, *Biochemistry* 1974; 13:471. Copyright 1974 by American Chemical Society.

Fig. 12–5: J. Bryan, *Fed. Proc.* 1974; 33:152. Reprinted from *Federation Proceedings* 1974; 33:152–157. Federation of American Societies for Experimental Biology.

Fig. 13–1: L. T. Coggeshall, in *Textbook of Medicine,* ed. P. B. Beeson and W. McDermott. W. B. Saunders Co., pp. 383–389, 1963.

Fig. 13–3: J. R. Zucker and C. C. Campbell, *Infect. Dis. Clin. North Am.* 1993; 7:547. W. B. Saunders Co.

Fig. 13–5: E. Beutler, *J. Lab. Clin. Med.* 1957; 49:84. D. V. Mosby Co.

Fig. 13–9: I. M. Rollo, *Br. J. Pharmacol.* 1955; 10:208. The Macmillan Co.

Fig. 14–2: B. B. Beaulieu et al., *Antimicrob. Agents Chemother.* 1981; 20:410. American Society for Microbiology.

Fig. 15–1: O. D. Standen, *Prog. Drug Res.* 1975; 19:158. Birkhäuser Verlag.

Fig. 15–2: S. Norton and E. J. deBeer. *Am. J. Trop. Med. Hyg.* 1957; 6:898. American Society of Tropical Medicine and Hygiene.

Fig. 16–2: K. C. Duff and R. H. Ashley, *Virology* 1992; 190:485. Academic Press.

Figs. 16–3, 16–4: G. B. Elion, *Am. J. Med.* 1982; 73(1A):7. Copyright by Technical Publishers.

Fig. 17–1: M. S. Hirsch and R. J. D'Aquila, *N. Engl. J. Med.* 1993; 328:1686. The Massachusetts Medical Society.

Fig. 17–3: C. Flexner and C. Hendrix, in *AIDS Biology, Diagnosis, Treatment and Prevention,* ed. by V. T. DeVita, S. Hellman, and S. A. Rosenberg. Lippincott-Raven, 1997, pp. 479–493.

Fig. 17–5: C. Flexner, *N. Engl. J. Med.* 1998; 338:1281. The Massachusetts Medical Society.

Fig. 17–6: J. P. Vacca and J. H. Condra, *Drug Discovery Today* 1997; 2:261. Elsevier Science.

Table 1–3: *The Medical Letter* 1996; 38:25. Published by The Medical Letter, Inc.

Table 1–4: W. L. Hewitt and M. C. HcHenry, *Med. Clin. North Am.* 1978; 62:1119.

Table 2–1: J. Davies, Nature 1996; 383:219.

Table 2–2: R. Moellering, *Am. J. Med.* 1995; 99(Suppl. 6A):6A.

Table 2–4: T. Watanabe, *Bacteriol. Rev.* 1963; 27:87. American Society for Microbiology.

Table 2–5: K. B. Linton et al., *J. Med Microbiol.* 1974; 7:91. The Pathological Society of Great Britain and Ireland.

Table 3–1: J. S. Anderson et al., *Proc. Natl. Acad. Sci. U.S.A.* 1965; 53:881. National Academy of Sciences.

Table 3–2: B. G. Spratt, *Proc. Natl. Acad. Sci. U.S.A.* 1975; 72:2999. National Academy of Sciences.

Table 3–3: C. G. Mayhall et al., *Antimicrob. Agents Chemother.* 1976; 10:707. American Society for Microbiology.

Table 3–4: J. Pitout et al., *Am. J. Med.* 1997; 103:51. Excerpta Medica.

Table 3–5: R. B. Sykes and M. Mathew, *J. Antimicrob. Chemother.* 1976; 2:115.

Table 3–6: R. P. Novik, *Biochem. J.* 1962; 83:229. The Biochemical Society.

Table 3–7: M. H. Richmond and S. Wotton, *Antimicrob. Agents Chemother.* 1976; 10:219. American Society for Microbiology.

Table 3–8: C. Reading and M. Cole, *Antimicrob. Agents Chemother.* 1977; 11:852.

Table 3–9: F. F. Barrett et al., *N. Engl. J. Med.* 1968; 279:441. The Massachusetts Medical Society.

Tables 4–2, 4–3: W. M. Bennett et al., *Ann. Intern. Med.* 1977; 86:754. American College of Physicians.

Table 4–4: B. B. Levine et al., *Ann N.Y. Acad. Sci.* 1967; 145:298. New York Academy of Science.

Table 4–5: L. D. Petz, *J. Infect. Dis.* 1978; 137(Suppl.):S74. The University of Chicago.

Table 4–9: S. R. Norrby, *Med. Clin. North Am.* 1995; 79:745. W. B. Saunders, Co.

Table 4–10: D. H. Johnson and B. Cunha, *Med. Clin. North Am.* 1995; 79:733. W. B. Saunders Co.

Table 4–11: J. W. Sensakovic and L. G. Smith, *Med. Clin. North Am.* 1995; 79:695. W. B. Saunders Co.

Table 5–1: J. E. Davies, *Proc. Natl. Acad. Sci. U.S.A.* 1964; 51:659. National Academy of Sciences.

Tables 5–2, 5–3: M. Ozaki et al., *Nature* 1969; 222:333. The Macmillan Co.

Table 6–1: D. Vazquez, *Nature* 1964; 203:257. The Macmillan Co.

Table 6–2: A. G. So and E. W. Davie, *Biochemistry* 1963; 2:132. American Chemical Society. Copyright by the American Chemical Society.

Table 6–3: A. S. Dajani and R. E. Kaufmann, *Pediatr. Clin. North Am.* 1981; 28:195.

Table 6–4: A. A. Yunis and G. R. Bloomberg, *Prog. Hematol.* 1964; 4:138. Grune & Stratton, Inc.

Table 6–6: D. A. Leigh, *J. Antimicrob. Chemother.* 1981; 7(Suppl. A):3. The British Society for Antimicrobial Chemotherapy.

Table 6–7: I. Suzuka et al., *Proc. Natl. Acad. Sci. U.S.A.* 1966; 55:1483. National Academy of Sciences.

Table 6–8: S. Sarkar and R. E. Thach, *Proc. Natl. Acad. Sci. U.S.A.* 1968; 60:1481. National Academy of Sciences.

Table 7–1: B. Wolf and R. D. Hotchkiss, *Biochemistry* 1963; 2:145. American Chemical Society. Copyright by the American Chemical Society.

Table 7–3: L. Weinstein, in *The Pharmacological Basis of Therapeutics,* ed. by L. S. Goodman and A. Gilman. Macmillan Co., 1970, p. 1197.

Table 7–4: J. J. Burchall and G. H. Hitchings, *Mol. Pharmacol.* 1965; 1:126. Academic Press.

Table 7–5: S. R. M. Bushby, *J. Infect. Dis.* 1973; 128(Suppl.):S422. The University of Chicago Press.

Table 7–6: G. P. Wormser and G. T. Keusch, *Ann. Intern. Med.* 1979; 91:420.

Table 7–7: M. C. Bach et al., *J. Infect. Dis.* 1973; 128(Suppl.):S508. The University of Chicago.

Table 9–2: R. E. Chamberlain, *J. Antimicrob. Chemother.* 1976; 2:325. The British Society for Antimicrobial Chemotherapy.

Table 9–3: J. Koch-Weser et al., *Arch. Intern. Med.* 1971; 128:399. American Medical Association.

Table 10–3: T. Bergan, in *The Quinolones,* ed. by V. T. Andriole. Academic Press, 1998, pp. 143–182.

Table 10–5: R. Stahlmann and H. Lode, in *The Quinolones,* ed. by V. T. Andriole. Academic Press, 1998, pp. 369–415.

Table 10–6: W. Christ and B. Esch, *Infect. Dis. Clin. Pract.* 1994; 3(Suppl. 3):S168. Lippincott, Williams and Wilkins.

Table 11–2: *The Medical Letter* 1998, pp. 60–66; W. C. Bailey et al., *Am. Rev. Respir. Dis.* 1977; 115:185.

Table 11–4: A. Heil and W. Zillig, *FEBS Lett.* 1970; 11:165. North-Holland Publishing Co. Copyright by the Federation of European Biochemical Societies.

Table 11–6: M. J. Colston et al., *Lepr. Rev.* 1978; 49:115. British Leprosy Relief Association.

Table 12–1: S. C. Kinsky, *Proc. Natl. Acad. Sci. U.S.A.* 1962; 48:1049. National Academy of Sciences.

Table 12–2: D. S. Feinbold, *Biochem. Biophys. Res. Commun.* 1965; 19:261. Academic Press.

Table 12–3: J. W. Rippon, in *Medical Mycology. The Pathogenic Fungi and the Pathogenic Actinomycetes,* 2nd ed. W. B. Saunders Co., 1982, p. 728.

Table 16–1: S. E. Luria, J. E. Darnell, D. Baltimore, and A. Campbell, in *General Virology,* 3rd ed. Wiley, 1978, Table 1–1.

Table 16–2: A. W. Galbraith et al., *Lancet* 1969; 2:1026.

Table 16–3: F. Hayden, in *Goodman and Gilman's Pharmacological Basis of Therapeutics,* 9th ed., ed. by J. G. Hardman, L. E. Limbird, P. Molinoff, R. Ruddon, and A. G. Gilman. McGraw-Hill, 1996, pp. 1191–1223.

Tables 16–5, 16–6: J. Vilcek and G. C. Sen, in *Fields Virology,* 3rd ed., ed. by B. N. Fields and D. M. Knipe. Lippincott, Williams and Wilkins, 1996, pp. 375–399.

Table 16–7: R. T. Dorr, *Drugs* 1993; 45:177.

Table 17–1: C. Flexner and C. Hendrix, in *AIDS Biology, Diagnosis, Treatment and Prevention,* ed. by V. T. DeVita, S. Hellman, and S. A. Rosenberg. Lippincott-Raven, 1997, pp. 479–493.

Table 17–2: K. Brinkman et al., *AIDS* 1998; 12:1735. Lippincott-Raven.

Table 17–3: J. Sahai, *AIDS* 1996; 10(Suppl. 1):S21. Lippincott-Raven.

Tables 17–5, 17–6, 17–7: C. Flexner, *N. Engl. J. Med.* 1998; 338:1281.

Preface

The field of chemotherapy has several different sources of information—the clinical sciences, pharmacology, biochemistry, molecular biology, and microbiology (including virology, bacteriology, mycology, parasitology, and immunology). It is the goal of this book to integrate information from all of these areas in describing the drugs used to treat infectious diseases. Our aim has been to make the book both comprehensive and concise.

This textbook provides the details of the action, pharmacology, and the adverse effects of the antibacterial, antifungal, antiparasitic, and antiviral drugs. A basic aim of previous versions (*Fundamentals of Chemotherapy*, 1973; *Chemotherapy of Infection*, 1977; *The Antimicrobial Drugs*, 1986) was to present the mechanisms by which the drugs act on microorganisms and the biochemical and pathophysiological basis for the drug toxicities, side effects, and hypersensitivity reactions. This edition continues with that tradition while adding additional sections on drug interactions for most of the antimicrobial agents. Our goal is to provide a text that is useful both to students in the health sciences who are learning infectious disease chemotherapy and to practicing physicians who need an in-depth treatment of these drugs. To achieve the first goal, we have presented integrated discussions of mechanisms that build on the student's knowledge of the basic sciences. To make the book a convenient source of information for the clinician we have included numerous charts and tables that summarize the pharmacokinetic properties of the drugs in each class and present appropriate regimens of therapy. The book is focused on understanding the properties of the antimicrobial drugs and their use; that is, on the drug and not on the pathogenesis, diagnosis, and clinical management of infectious diseases. We have described each drug concisely but without sacrificing the values of scholarship. Thus, for readers who wish to have even more detailed information we have provided a direct entry into the literature by citing several thousand references to other texts, reviews, and primary research papers.

The Antimicrobial Drugs is divided into five parts. The first part consists of two chapters which present the principles of antimicrobial therapy. Chapter 1 discusses those properties of the bacterium that determine whether the response to antimicrobial therapy will be successful. There are some concepts, such as selective toxicity and superinfection, that must be learned before chemotherapy can be really understood. These concepts are discussed in Chapter 1; specific examples appear throughout the text. This chapter also introduces how infecting organisms are identified and how their drug susceptibility is determined. It then discusses what the drugs of choice are for empiric therapy and how a variety of host factors, such as the patient's age, renal or hepatic function, pregnancy, and genetic and metabolic abnormalities modify the physician's choice of an antibiotic. The chapter concludes with the principles of prophylactic antibiotic administration during surgery and the use of antibiotic combinations in therapy. Chapter 2 discusses antibiotic resistance, including the causes, mechanisms, and possible ways it can be avoided.

The second part of the text consists of eight chapters which present the drugs used to treat bacterial infections. The first three chapters cover the major groups of bactericidal antibiotics: Chapters 3 and 4, the penicillins, cephalosporins, and other inhibitors of cell wall synthesis; Chapter 5, the aminoglycosides, which act by inhibiting bacterial protein synthesis. The discussion of biological mechanisms in Chapter 3 will help readers understand both how the penicillins and cephalosporins work and how the extended-spectrum penicillins (e.g., piperacillin, mezlocillin) and the third-generation cephalosporins are different from the old drugs of each class. Chapter 4 gives a detailed account of the pharmacology and side effects of the penicillins and cephalosporins. The aminoglycosides are among the most difficult drugs to administer; the detailed discussion of their pharmacologic and toxic properties in Chapter 5 is designed to provide physicians with a rational basis for administering these drugs. In organizing the presentation of the other antibacterial drugs, we have continued to group them, as far as possible, by their biochemical mechanism of action. Thus, Chapter 6 covers the common bacteriostatic inhibitors of protein synthesis (e.g., chloramphenicol, the lincomycins, erythromycin, the tetracyclines); Chapter 7, the antimetabolites (e.g., the sulfonamides, trimethoprim); Chapter 8, some less commonly used antibiotics that act on the permeability of cell membranes (e.g., the polymyxins). Chapter 9 deals with drugs used to treat urinary tract infections. The fluoroquinolones were developed from the quinolone group of urinary tract antiseptics, and Chapter 10 presents this important class of gram-negative antimicrobials, which act by inhibiting bacterial DNA synthesis. The final chapter in this section presents several drugs that are used to treat infections caused by mycobacteria (e.g., tuberculosis, leprosy).

Parts 3, 4, and 5 cover the drugs used to treat fungal, parasitic, and viral diseases. Chapter 12, on antifungal drugs, gives a detailed treatment of the new imidazole antibiotics (e.g., itraconazole) as well as the more traditional antifungal drugs. Chapters 13, 14, and 15, which deal with the antiparasitic drugs, review both parasite life cycles and the pathophysiology of various infections so that readers may understand the basis for therapy and the often complex interactions between the drugs, the parasites, and the host. In Chapter 16, on antiviral drugs, we first review viral replication and introduce readers to the parts of this process that are amenable to chemotherapeutic attack. This is followed by a discussion of the biology of interferon action, the results of clinical trials with interferons, and the human pharmacology and side effects of interferons. Then we discuss in detail the mechanism of action, pharmacology, and therapeutic efficacy of the antiviral drugs that are currently marketed in the United States. The number of new antiviral drugs has grown tremendously since the last edition of this book. We discuss ganciclovir, foscarnet, and several other new antivirals. Finally, we have added Chapter 17, a new chapter on the drugs used to treat the human immunodeficiency virus, including the nucleoside and non-nucleoside reverse transcriptase inhibitors as well as the protease inhibitors.

The University of Nebraska College of Medicine E.M.S.
Omaha
The University of Michigan W.B.P.
Ann Arbor
October 1999

Acknowledgments

The authors would like to thank Dr. Carl Gessert
for his careful reading of several chapters in this book.

Contents

PART I
PRINCIPLES OF ANTIMICROBIAL THERAPY

1. Determinants of Bacterial Response to Antimicrobial Agents   3
2. Drug Resistance   37

PART 2
DRUGS EMPLOYED IN THE TREATMENT OF BACTERIAL INFECTIONS

3. The Inhibitors of Cell Wall Synthesis, I   51
   Mechanism of Action of the Penicillins, Cephalosporins, Vancomycin, and Other Inhibitors of Cell Wall Synthesis
4. The Inhibitors of Cell Wall Synthesis, II   81
   Pharmacology and Adverse Effects of the Penicillins, Cephalosporins, Carbapenems, Monobactams, Vancomycin, and Bacitracin
5. Bactericidal Inhibitors of Protein Synthesis   127
   The Aminoglycosides
6. Bacteriostatic Inhibitors of Protein Synthesis   159
   Chloramphenicol, Macrolides, Clindamycin, Spectinomycin, Tetracyclines, and Streptogramins
7. The Antimetabolites   211
   The Sulfonamides and Trimethoprim (Trimethoprim-Sulfamethoxazole)
8. Antibiotics that Affect Membrane Permeability   234
   Polymyxin B, Colistin, and Gramicidin A
9. The Urinary Tract Antiseptics   242
   Nalidixic Acid and Cinoxacin; Nitrofurantoin; Methenamine; Fosfomycin
10. The Fluoroquinolones   257
11. Drugs that Act on Mycobacteria   280
    Isoniazid, Rifampin, Ethambutol, Streptomycin, and Pyrazinamide; The Second-Line Antituberculosis Drugs; Drugs Effective Against Leprosy; Drugs Effective Against the Mycobacterium avium Complex

PART 3
DRUGS EMPLOYED IN THE TREATMENT OF FUNGAL INFECTIONS

12. Antifungal Drugs   327
    The Polyene Antibiotics, Flucytosine, Azoles, Iodide, Griseofulvin, and Topical Agents

PART 4
DRUGS EMPLOYED IN THE TREATMENT OF PARASITIC DISEASE

13. Chemotherapy of Malaria   375
14. Chemotherapy of Protozoal Diseases   419
15. Chemotherapy of Helminthic Diseases   458

PART 5
DRUGS EMPLOYED IN THE TREATMENT OF VIRAL INFECTIONS

16. Chemotherapy of Viral Infections, I   491
        *Drugs Used to Treat Influenza Virus Infections, Herpesvirus Infections, and Drugs
        with Broad-Spectrum Antiviral Activity*

17. Chemotherapy of Viral Infections, II   550
        Antiretroviral Agents

     Index   587

Principles of Antimicrobial Therapy

Determinants of Bacterial Response to Antimicrobial Agents

Selective Toxicity

The formal definition of an antibiotic restricts the use of the term to chemicals that are produced by microorganisms and that have the capacity to inhibit the growth of, or to kill, bacteria and other microorganisms. This definition distinguishes between chemicals produced by microorganisms and antimicrobial compounds synthesized by chemists (e.g., sulfonamides, trimethoprim, isoniazid). The distinction is rather academic, and one finds that the word *antibiotic* is now often used to include both these groups of antimicrobial agents.

The central concept of antibiotic action is that of *selective toxicity*—that is, growth of the infecting organism is selectively inhibited, or the organism is killed, without damage to the cells of the host. The ideal antibiotic would have no deleterious effect on the patient but would be lethal to the organism. There is no ideal antibiotic. Perhaps penicillin G in the nonallergic patient comes as close to this goal as any antimicrobial drug.

To obtain selectivity of action the antibiotics exploit differences between the biochemistry of the infecting agent and that of the host. With the penicillins, for example, the basis for the selective effect is quite clear: they inhibit cell wall synthesis, a process that does not take place in mammalian cells, which lack a cell wall. This explains the selective action of the penicillins but not their relative lack of toxicity. Other inhibitors of cell wall synthesis, which include bacitracin, cycloserine, and vancomycin, also inhibit biochemical processes unique to bacterial cells, but when given systemically, such antibiotics act on the cells of the host in other ways, and this makes them quite toxic.

It is important that those who are beginning their study of antimicrobial agents do not confuse the concept of selective toxicity with that of therapeutic index, also called *therapeutic ratio*, which is the ratio of the toxic dose to the effective dose of a drug. In some cases, the selective toxicity will parallel the therapeutic index, as for the penicillins (see above). The polyene antibiotics (e.g., amphotericin B) have both a low degree of selective toxicity and a low therapeutic index. That is, they show little selectivity of action against fungi versus mammalian cells, and they are also quite toxic. With other antibiotics, there is little relationship between selective cellular toxicity and therapeutic index. Let us take the aminoglycosides as an example. These antibiotics are very selective with respect to killing bacterial versus host cells, but for some members of this class, unrelated effects on the patient's nervous system, kidneys, or inner ear (hearing, balance) result in a lower margin for therapeutic error than would be predicted on the basis of their selective action on cell viability. Major sections of this book will be devoted to explanations of the mechanisms of the selective action of antibiotics on microorganisms. Equally important sections will be devoted to explanations of the mechanisms by which these drugs cause the undesirable effects that contribute to the therapeutic index and thus impose limitations on their clinical use.

Antibiotic Effect—Cidal versus Static

In the chemotherapy of infectious disease, the goal is to assist the body in ridding itself of the infecting organism. In general, the human body is extraordinarily well equipped to fight bacterial invasion. The skin is very efficient at preventing entry of organisms, by virtue of both its physical properties and its ability to produce unsaturated fatty acids, which have antibacterial action. The mucous membranes and their secretions also efficiently prevent entry of microorganisms. And once invasion has taken place, the bacterium is confronted with a well-orchestrated set of responses, including antibody production, the complement system, inflammatory responses, cellular migration and phagocytosis, and intracellular killing mechanisms. The overall effect of the host defense is bacterial death, and the system is very effective. Most infections do not require therapy; they are taken care of by the body's defense mechanisms, and the individual may never be aware of them. For some infections, however, treatment with antibiotics may be required.

Antibiotics exert an effect in the patient that is either bactericidal or bacteriostatic. Those antibiotics that are generally *bacteriostatic* at concentrations that are achieved clinically (e.g., chloramphenicol, erythromycin, tetracyclines) inhibit bacterial cell replication but do not kill the organism. Other antibiotics (e.g., penicillins, cephalosporins, aminoglycosides) are usually *bactericidal*; they cause microbial cell death and lysis. A few compounds (e.g., sulfonamides) are either cidal or static according to the composition of the environment (blood, pus, urine, etc.) in which the infecting organisms are growing. These two effects can be demonstrated in vitro and are illustrated schematically in Figure 1–1.

Treatment with a bacteriostatic drug stops bacterial growth, thereby allowing the host defenses to catch up in their battle. Treat-

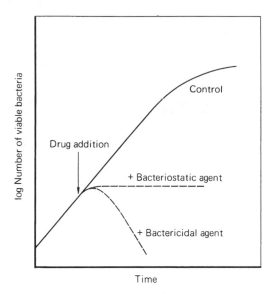

Figure 1–1. Bacteriostatic and bactericidal effects of antibiotics. A suspension of bacteria in the log phase of growth is divided into three parts. A bacteriostatic drug, such as chloramphenicol, is added to one culture and a bactericidal agent, such as penicillin, to another; the third is a control. At various times, samples are taken from each culture, diluted, and plated on agar with new growth medium. The number of colonies obtained is a measure of the number of viable cells per culture.

ment with a bactericidal agent superimposes the killing effect of the drug on the effect of the host defense. This is clearly somewhat oversimplied, since bactericidal drugs at low concentrations sometimes have a bacteriostatic effect, and bacteriostasis, if continued long enough, will be accompanied by a decrease in bacterial viability.

The distinction between the two types of antibiotics, cidal and static, is important in choosing a drug for therapy. In a patient with a severe infection, it is usually better (assuming that other considerations, such as organism sensitivity and the distribution properties, and the clinically undesirable effects of the drugs do not dictate otherwise) to choose a bactericidal, rather than a bacteriostatic, antibiotic. In some cases, the patient's natural ability to fight an infection may be lowered. This occurs, for example, in patients with disorders of the immune system, in patients with lymphoreticular diseases or diabetes mellitus, and in severely debilitated patients. Also, a growing number of patients are under treatment with drugs having immunosuppressive effects, and they often have virtually no ability to fight infection. In these cases, almost total reliance must be placed on a chemotherapeutic effect that is unaided by host defense mechanisms, and bactericidal antibiotics must be employed.

Determinants of Bacterial Response to Therapy

There are numerous reasons why a patient may not respond to therapy with antibiotics. One of the major factors is that the wrong antibiotic may have been prescribed since these drugs are extensively misused by physicians.[1-4] Most cases of antibiotic misuse are probably due to inappropriate choices based on considerations that do not fall within the purview of this book. These would include the administration of antibiotics to treat infections (particularly viral infections of the respiratory tract) against which they are inactive,[5] the use of antibiotics in conditions of noninfectious etiology because of misdiagnosis, and inappropriate prophylactic antibiotic therapy (a major problem in surgical services).[6,7] Antibiotics are commonly administered to hospitalized patients who show no evidence of infection; in fact, in some hospitals much of the antibiotic use may fall into this category.[8,9] It is also clear that there is considerable misuse of antibiotics by the patients themselves. Many outpatients fail to initiate or more often, fail to properly complete their prescribed course of therapy, and in some cases, patients treat themselves with antibiotics that were prescribed for a previous condition or obtained from relatives or friends.[10]

Host Determinants

Some of the factors a physician must consider when treating an infection with an antimicrobial drug include the sensitivity of the organism to the drug; the appropriate dosage, route of administration, and duration of therapy; and the special features of the patient that may alter the way a drug is handled by the body. These features, the *host determinants*, may result in an inadequate concentration of the active drug at the site of infection or they may render the patient more likely to suffer adverse drug effects.[11] The host determinants of particular importance in determining undesirable toxic and side effects will be discussed briefly in this chapter and in detail with each drug as it is presented in subsequent chapters. In this introduction, it is appropriate to mention a few host determinants that affect the response of the bacterium to the drug. Some examples have been given above. These include poor phagocytic activity, immunosuppression, serious disease of noninfectiuos etiology (diabetes mellitus, neoplasms), and physical debilitation, all of which compromise the ability of patients to call on or utilize their full complement of host defenses.

If a patient continues to demonstrate symptoms of infection despite appropriate antibiotic therapy, several host determinants must be considered. Is there an occult abscess responsible for the continuing problem? If such a focus of infection is located, it requires surgical drainage. Is there an obstruction (e.g., in the lungs or in the biliary or urinary tracts) creating conditions of stasis under which bacteria can multiply in poorly perfused pockets of infection? If so, surgical intervention may be necessary. Are there mechanical factors involved, such as a foreign body, or retained suture material that requires removal? Are continuous portals of bacterial entry being maintained unnecessarily or inappropriately (e.g., intravenous catheters left in for long periods of time, an unnecessary use of or inappropriate maintenance of a urinary catheter)? These are examples of host determinants that are subject to analysis and correction, but are often ignored by physicians who favor adding, or changing to, another antibiotic.

Some aspects of the host defense mechanisms are compromised when tissue necrosis and localized abscesses exist. For example, phagocytes function very poorly in such suppurative regions, and the local bactericidal response is diminished. The conditions of acidity, low oxygen tension, and lack of nutrients that impair phagocytic function in such areas can also affect bacterial growth. Since organisms that are not dividing are not killed by certain bactericidal drugs (e.g., penicillins, aminoglycosides), the bacterial response to the antibiotic may also be compromised. Abscess walls may be poorly vascularized; consequently, delivery of drug to the infection site is poor, and the local concentration of antibiotic may be inadequate. The antibacterial effect of some antibiotics (e.g., gentamicin) may be reduced in purulent infections because the antibiotic itself becomes extensively bound to components of pus.[12] Thus, in an abscess, both the host's response to the organism and the organism's response to the antibiotic may be compromised. Such closed infections require surgical drainage; reliance on chemotherapy alone is usually useless.

The Indigenous Microbial Flora—Superinfection

Another factor entering into the therapeutic response is difficult to classify as either a host or a bacterial determinant. While patients are being treated with an antibiotic, they can become infected with organisms other than those causing the original infection. This problem is more common when antibiotics having a broad spectrum of action or antibiotic combinations are employed. The organisms responsible for producing this secondary infection are usually normal residents of the host. The human body harbors a variety of microflora existing in ecologically balanced communities. The bowel is the largest and most obvious example of such a community. Other important areas normally colonized with bacteria include the oropharynx, skin, vagina, the genital and perineal areas, the external ear canals, and the conjuctivae. Usually resident bacteria in these areas are harmless and some perform important functions for the host, such as the synthesis of vitamin K by coliform organisms. The harmless resident bacteria also serve to control the growth of potentially pathogenic organisms.

The ecological balance of the microbial colonies is maintained by a variety of mechanisms referred to collectively as *microbial antagonism*. Two principal mechanisms of antagonism are competition for nutrients and the production of compounds that inhibit the growth of other organisms. Some enteric bacilli, for example, produce *colicins*, proteins that kill sensitive bacteria in very specific ways.[13] These colicins attach to specific receptors on the bacterial cell membrane where they may increase permeability to ions or inhibit active transport or oxidative phosphorylation. Some colicins act inside the cell to degrade DNA (e.g., Col E2) or to inhibit protein synthesis (e.g., Col E3, which cleaves a fragment from 16S ribosomal RNA). Resident bacteria can also alter the chemical environment so that it is unfavorable for the growth of less desirable organisms. For example, lactobacilli in the adult vagina help maintain an acidic pH (4.0 to 4.5), which is probably not optimal for the growth of a number of potential pathogens.

If the ecological balance of these microbial communities is disturbed, as it is when an antibiotic acts upon important resident bacteria, other microbes normally kept in check in the ecosystem can multiply and possibly cause complications. This phenomenon has been called *superinfection*.[14] The superinfecting organism may be a bacterium or a fungus and is either initially resistant to the antibiotic or has become resistant during therapy. The degree of discomfort and patient risk that can attend the complication of superinfection ranges from superficial irritation or mild diarrhea to severe oropharyngeal candidiasis or the potentially life-threatening condition of antibiotic-associated colitis (see Chapter 6). The risk of creating conditions that would lead to flora overgrowth and superinfection must be considered by the physician in the rational administration of antibiotics. It is important that physicians be aware of the general spectrum of action of an antibiotic, that they be attuned to the signs and symptoms signaling the presence of superinfection, and the they carefully consider the necessity for continuing the antibiotic treatment if superinfection ensues. The concept of superinfection will be discussed in more detail in Chapter 6 and throughout the text.

Identifying the Infecting Organism

In many patients with infections, the history, physical examination, and simple laboratory tests will indicate the probable diagnosis and etiologic agent. If, in addition, the susceptibility of the suspected pathogen is predictable, the choice of antimicrobial and ancillary therapy is relatively straightforward. In most patients, however, especially those who are critically ill because of infection or underlying diseases, only the general nature of the infection is known (i.e., pneumonia, cellulitis, or urinary tract infection), and the clinician must begin empiric therapy based on judgment of the probable etiologic agents and their characteristics. The organisms that are most likely to cause specific types of

acute infections are presented in Table 1–1. The organisms are listed roughly according to the frequency at which they are responsible for causing infection at each body site. A listing of probable etiologic agents such as this one is useful to the physician in providing a basis for empiric therapy that also must rely on the results of a few simple laboratory tests, especially the gram stain. For optimal therapy of patients who are infected by an unidentified organism, it is necessary to obtain cultures of exudates and body fluids in order to confirm or deny the presumptive diagnosis, to determine the actual etiologic agent, and especially to obtain information concerning the susceptibility of the probable responsible organism(s) to antimicrobials. This information, although not immediately available, is often useful later in modifying therapy (either by altering dosages or changing antimicrobial drugs) in the event that the patient has not responded, or has developed an adverse reaction, to the initial therapy.

Table 1–1. *Microorganisms most likely to cause acute infections at different body sites in noncompromised hosts.* These organisms are listed in the estimated order of frequency with which they cause infections at each site. Organisms not listed here may also be important occasional causes of these infections.

A. SKIN AND SUBCUTANEOUS TISSUES

Burns
1. *Staphylococcus aureus*
2. Group A β-hemolytic streptococcus (*S. pyogenes*)
3. *Pseudomonas aeruginosa*
4. *Enterobacteriaceae*

Skin Infections
1. *Staphylococcus aureus*
2. Group A β-hemolytic streptococcus (*S. pyogenes*)
3. Herpes simplex or zoster
4. Dermatophytes
5. Gram-negative bacilli
6. *Candida albicans*
7. *Trepnema pallidum*

Decubitus wound infections
1. *Staphylococcus aureus*
2. *Escherichia coli* (or other Enterobacteriaceae)
3. *Bacteroides*

4. Anaerobic streptococci
5. Group A β-hemolytic streptococcus (*S. pyogenes*)
6. *Clostridia*
7. *Pseudomonas aeruginosa*
8. *Enterococcus (Streptococcus faecalis)*

Traumatic and surgical wounds
1. *Staphylococcus aureus*
2. Group A β-hemolytic streptococcus (*S. pyogenes*)
3. Gram-negative bacilli
4. *Clostridia*
5. Anaerobic streptococci
6. *Enterococcus (Streptococcs faecalis)*

B. MOUTH (ORAL CAVITY)
1. Herpes virus, esp. type 1
2. *Candida albicans*
3. Vincent's fusospirochetes
4. Mixed anaerobic cocci
5. *Bacteroides*
6. *Treponema pallidum*

(continued)

Table 1–1. Continued

7. *Actinomyces*
8. *Capnocytophaga*

C. THROAT

1. Respiratory viruses
2. Group A β-hemolytic streptococcus (*S. pyogenes*)
3. *Neisseria gonorrhoeae*
4. *Corynebacterium diphtheriae*
5. *Candida albicans*
6. Vincent's fusospirochetes
7. *Neisseria meningitidis*
8. Groups C and G Streptococci
9. *Corynebacteria hemolyticum*
10. Epstein-Barr virus (infectious mononucleosis)

D. PARANASAL SINUSES

1. *Streptococcus pneumoniae*
2. Group A β-hemolytic streptococcus (*S. pyogenes*)
3. *Haemophilus influenzae*
4. *Klebsiella* (or other gram-negative bacilli)
5. *Staphylococcus aureus*
6. Anaerobic streptococci
7. Rhinovirus
8. *Mucor, Aspergillus* (esp. in diabetics)

E. EARS

Auditory Canal and Pinna

1. *Pseudomonas aeruginosa* (or other gram-negative bacilli)
2. *Staphylococcus aureus*
3. Group A β-hemolytic streptococcus (*S. pyogenes*)
4. *Streptococcus pneumoniae*
5. *Haemophilus influenzae* (children)
6. Fungi

Middle Ear (Otitis media)

1. *Streptococcs pneumoniae*
2. *Haemophilus influenzae* (children)
3. Group A β-hemolytic streptococcus (*S. pyogenes*)
4. *Staphylococcus aureus*
5. Anaerobic streptococci
6. *Bacteroides*
7. Other gram-negative bacilli (chronic)
8. *Mycoplasma pneumoniae*

F. EYES (CORNEA AND CONJUNCTIVA)

1. Herpes and other viruses
2. *Neisseria gonorrhoeae*
3. *Haemophilus influenzae* (children)
4. *Staphylococcus aureus*
5. *Pseudomonas aeruginosa*

6. *Moraxella*
7. *Haemophilus aegyptius* (Koch-Weeks bacillus)
8. *Streptococcus pneumoniae*
9. Other gram-negative bacilli
10. *Chlamydia*
11. Fungi

G. LARYNX, TRACHEA, AND BRONCHI

1. Respiratory viruses
2. *Streptococcus pneumoniae*
3. *Mycoplasma pneumoniae*
4. *Haemophilus influenzae*
5. *Chlamydia pneumoniae*
6. *Mycobacterium tuberculosis*
7. *Corynebacterium diphtheriae*
8. *Staphylococcus aureus*
9. Gram-negative bacilli
10. *Bordetella pertussis*
11. *Moraxella catarrhalis*

H. LUNGS

Pneumonia

1. *Streptococcus pneumoniae*
2. *Haemophilus influenzae*
3. *Mycoplasma pneumoniae*
4. *Chlamydia pneumoniae*
5. Respiratory viruses, esp. influenza, adenovirus
6. *Staphylococcus aureus*
7. *Klebsiella pneumoniae* (or other gram-negative bacilli)
8. Group A β-hemolytic streptococcus (*S. pyogenes*)
9. *Mycobacterium tuberculosis*
10. Cytomegalovirus
11. *Chlamydia psittaci*
12. *Bacteroides*, usually not *B. fragilis*
13. Anaerobic streptococci
14. *Pneumocystis carinii*
15. *Legionella pneumophila*
16. *Legionella micdadei*
17. *Nocardia*
18. Fungi
19. *Herpes simplex*
20. *Moraxella catarrhalis*

Abscess

1. Anaerobic streptococci
2. *Bacteroides* (up to 15% *B. fragilis*)
3. *Staphylococcus aureus*
4. *Klebsiella pneumoniae* (or other Enterobacteriaceae)
5. *Streptococcus pneumoniae* (type III)
6. Fungi

(continued)

8

Table 1–1. **Continued**

7. *Actinomyces, Nocardia*
8. *Pseudomonas aeruginosa*

I. ENDOCARDIUM (ENDOCARDITIS)

1. *Staphylococcus aureus*
2. Viridans group of *Streptococcus*
3. *Enterococcus (Streptococcus faecalis)*
4. *Staphylococcus epidermidis*
5. *Streptococcus bovis*
6. *Streptococcus pneumoniae*
7. Gram-negative bacilli
8. *Candida albicans* and other fungi
9. Group A β-hemolytic streptococcus
   (*S. pyogenes*)

J. PLEURA (EMPYEMA)

1. *Staphylococcus aureus*
2. *Streptococcus pneumoniae*
3. *Haemophilus influenzae*
4. *Mycobacterium tuberculosis*
5. Gram-negative bacilli
6. Anaerobic streptococci
7. *Bacteroides*
8. Group A β-hemolytic streptococcus
   (*S. pyogenes*)
9. *Actinomyces, Nocardia*
10. Fungi

K. BLOOD (SEPTICEMIA)

Newborn Infants

1. *Escherichia coli* (or other Enterobacteriaceae)
2. Group B streptococcus
3. *Staphylococcus aureus*
4. Group A β-hemolytic streptococcus
   (*S. pyogenes*)
5. *Enterococcus (Streptococcus faecalis)*
6. *Listeria monocytogenes*
7. *Streptococcus pneumoniae*

Children

1. *Streptococcus pneumoniae*
2. *Neisseria meningitidis*
3. *Haemophilus influenzae*
4. *Staphylococcus aureus*
5. Group A β-hemolytic streptococcus
   (*S. pyogenes*)
6. *Escherichia coli* (or other Enterobacteriaceae)

Adults

1. *Staphylococcus aureus*
2. *Streptococcus pneumoniae*
3. *Pseudomonas aeruginosa*
4. *Candida albicans*
5. *Neisseria meningitidis*

6. *Neisseria gonorrhoeae*
7. Group A β-hemolytic streptococcus
   (*S. pyogenes*)
8. *Enterococcus* spp.
9. *Escherichia coli* (or other Enterobacteriaceae)
10. *Bacteroides*, esp. *B. fragilis*

L. MENINGES (MENINGITIS)

1. Viral agens (enterovirus, mumps, herpes
   simplex, etc.)
2. *Neisseria meningitidis*
3. *Haemophilus influenzae* (esp. in children)
4. *Streptococcus pneumoniae*
5. Group B streptococcus (infants less than 2
   months old)
6. *Staphylococcus aureus* (after neurosurgery,
   brain abscess)
7. *Listeria moncytogenes*
8. Group A β-hemolytic streptococcus
   (*S. pyogenes*)
9. *Escherichia coli* (or other Enterobacteriaceae)
10. *Mycobacterium tuberculosis*
11. *Cryptococcus neoformans* and other
    fungi

M. BONES (OSTEOMYELITIS)

1. *Staphylococcus aureus*
2. Group A β-hemolytic streptococcus
   (*S. pyogenes*)
3. *Salmonella* (or other Enterobacteriaceae)
4. *Mycobacterium tuberculosis*
5. *Psuedomonas aeruginosa*

N. JOINTS (SEPTIC ARTHRITIS)

1. *Staphylococcus aureus*
2. Group A β-hemolytic streptococcus
   (*S. pyogenes*)
3. *Streptococcus pneumoniae*
4. *Neisseria gonorrhoeae*
5. Gram-negative bacilli
6. *Neisseria meningitidis*
7. *Haemophilus influenzae* (children)
8. *Mycobacterium tuberculosis*
9. *Sporothrix* and other fungi

O. GASTROINTESTINAL TRACT

1. Gastrointestinal viruses, esp. reoviruses, ro-
   taviruses
2. *Helicobacter pylori*
3. *Salmonella*
4. *Escherichia coli*
5. *Shigella*
6. *Clostridium difficile*
7. *Yersinia enterocolitica*

(continued)

Table 1–1.   Continued

8. *Vibrio cholerae*
9. *Vibrio parahaemolyticus*
10. *Staphylococcus aureus*
11. *Entamoeba histolytica*
12. *Giardia lamblia*
13. *Treponema pallidum* (anus)
14. *Neisseria gonorrhoeae* (anus)
15. *Stronglyoides stercoralis*
16. *Aeromonas*
17. *Campylobacter fetus*
18. *Bacillus cereus*
19. *Edwardsiella*

P. PERITONEUM (PERITONITIS)

1. Facultative gram-negative bacilli
2. Enterococcus *(Streptococcus faecalis)*
3. Anaerobic streptococci
4. *Bacteroides*, esp. *B. fragilis*
5. *Clostridium*
6. *Streptococcus pneumoniae*
7. Group B streptococcus
8. *Pseudomonas aeruginosa*
9. *Staphyloccus epidermidis*
10. *Candida albicans*
11. *Mycobacterium tuberculosis*

Q. URINARY TRACT

1. *Escherichia coli* (and other enteric gram-negative bacilli)
2. *Enterococcus* spp.
3. *Staphylococcus aureus* or *Staphylococcus saprophyticus*
4. *Candida albicans*
5. *Neisseria gonorrhoeae* (urethra)
6. *Chlamydia* (urethra)
7. *Treponema pallidum*
8. *Trichomonas vaginalis* (urethra)

R. FEMALE GENITAL TRACT

Vagina

1. *Trichomonas vaginalis*
2. *Candida albicans*
3. *Neisseria gonorrhoeae*
4. Group A β-hemolytic streptococcus (*S. pyogenes*)

5. *Gardnerella vaginalis*
6. *Treponema pallidum*
7. *Staphylococcus aureus*

Uterus

1. Anaerobic streptococci
2. *Bacteroides*, incl. *B. fragilis*
3. *Escherichia coli* (or other enteric gram-negative bacilli)
4. *Clostridium*
5. *Neisseria gonorrhoeae*
6. Herpes simplex, esp. type 2 (cervix)
7. Group A β-hemolytic streptococcus (*S. pyogenes*)
8. Groups B and C streptococcus
9. *Staphylococcus aureus*
10. *Enterococcus* spp.
11. *Treponema pallidum*

Fallopian Tubes

1. *Neisseria gonorrhoeae*
2. Facultative gram-negative bacilli (i.e., *Escherichia coli*)
3. Anaerobic streptococci
4. *Bacteroides*, incl. *B. fragilis*
5. *Chlamydia*

S. MALE GENITAL TRACT

Seminal Vesicles

1. Gram-negative bacilli
2. *Neisseria gonorrhoeae*

Epididymis

1. Gram-negative bacilli
2. *Neisseria gonorrhoeae*
3. *Chlamydia*
4. *Mycobacterium tuberculosis*

Prostate Gland

1. Gram-negative bacilli
2. *Neisseria gonorrhoeae*
3. *Mycobacterium tuberculosis*
4. *Cryptococcus neoformans*
5. *Histoplasma capulatum*
6. *Nocardia*

Gram Stain

The most important and the simplest and quickest test available to physicians treating infections empirically is a direct microscopic examination of a gram-stained smear of a fluid sample, such as sputum, urinary sediment, cerebrospinal fluid, or purulent drainage, from the site of the infection. Not only does this provide immediate clues as to the nature of the infection and its proper treatment but it can also aid in determining how the laboratory should process cultures and in the subsequent interpretation of culture results.

The usefulness of the gram stain in arriving at a presumptive diagnosis to guide empiric therapy is illustrated by the examination of sputum samples from a patient with pneumonia. If a gram stain of freshly expectorated sputum reveals many polymorphonuclear cells and a few epithelial cells, then it is probably a valid sample from the infected site in the lungs. If, in addition, the specimen reveals gram-positive lancet-shaped diplococci in large numbers adjacent to leukocytes, then the diagnosis is almost certainly pneumococcal pneumonia. If subsequent culture reports reveal organisms such as *Streptococcus viridans, Neisseria, Escherichia coli, Proteus,* or *Candida* that were not seen or were seen only in small numbers in the gram-stained smear, then in all likelihood these organisms are merely contaminants of normal mouth flora that overgrew the pneumococci that caused the infection. When gram-positive cocci located within granulocytes are seen on gram stains of sputum, then the clinician should be certain to treat adequately for *Staphylococcus aureus* as well as pneumococcal pneumonia, even though the detection of intracellular cocci does not prove the patient has a staphylococcal infection. If large gram-negative bacilli are seen near leukocytes in sputum from a patient who became ill at home (not in a hospital or nursing home), then *Klebsiella pneumoniae* should be suspected, and the therapeutic regimen should consist of one or preferably two antimicrobials that are probably active against this important respiratory pathogen, usually a cephalosporin and an aminoglycoside, or trimethoprim-sulfamethoxazole.

If sputum showing large gram-negative bacilli is obtained from a patient who developed pneumonia in the hospital, then antibiotic-resistant organisms such as *Enterobacter* or *Pseudomonas aeruginosa* should be suspected, as well as *Klebsiella.* If the patient is granulocytopenic and has pneumonia, *Pseudomonas, Enterobacter,* and *Klebsiella* should be suspected when the sputum shows gram-negative bacilli, even if few granulocytes are present. If a good specimen of sputum shows a mixture of many different types of organisms, then aspiration pneumonia or lung abscess due to organisms derived from infected gingivae should be suspected. This possibility becomes almost certain if the sputum is putrid or foul-smelling, the patient's dental hygiene is poor, there has been a recent episode of stupor or unconsciousness, and the patient's ability to clear tracheobronchial secretions is impaired. Gram-variable organisms with bizarre bulbous or elongated shapes are often seen in specimens from indolent infections, or from patients receiving partially effective therapy.

If the sputum shows few or no organisms on gram stain, then *Mycobacterium tuberculosis, Legionella pneumoniae, Pneumocytis carinii, Mycoplasma pneumoniae,* viral, rickettsial, or chlamydial pneumonia should be suspected, and appropriate diagnostic and therapeutic measures should be instituted. In this situation, *initial* treatment with erythromycin is particularly appropriate and should be given promptly, since results of the various cultures and serologic tests used to confirm these diagnoses often are delayed, and in many cases are not even readily available.

The importance of doing an acid-fast stain on sputum obtained from puzzling cases, especially when the gram stain has not been helpful, must be emphasized. Unfortunately, many younger physicians in developed countries are not accustomed to thinking of tuberculosis in patients with pneumonia.

Cultures

It is always important to indicate the most likely or suspected etiologic agents to laboratory personnel. There is no such thing as a "routine sputum culture for all pathogens." If nocardia, anaerobes, fungi, or mycobacteria are suspected, then special techniques may have to be used in order to isolate the organism. Since organisms may be present in small numbers (fewer than 5000/ml) in specimens obtained from infected sites in the lung, cultures should be processed in order to detect the presence of small numbers of highly pathogenic organisms (despite the possible presence of contaminants); in many cases it is also appropriate to determine their susceptibility to therapeutic agents. As another example, the numbers of cryptococci in cerebrospinal fluid from patients with meningitis may be in the range of one organism per 50 ml, and repeated specimens may have to be sent to the laboratory for culture, for India ink preparations, and to test for the presence of cryptococcal antigen in order to establish the diagnosis and justify the need for potentially toxic therapeutic regimens.

Other useful laboratory tests include dark-field examinations for the spirochetes of syphilis, stained blood smears to detect malaria parasites, Tzanck preparations from scrapings of lesions that suggest a viral etiology, and methylene blue stains of stools to detect leukocytes that suggest an inflammatory etiology of diarrheal illness.

In general, cultures should be obtained before beginning or changing antibiotic therapy. The techniques used should minimize contamination by the normal body flora or disinfectants, and should also prevent adverse transport conditions that can foster overgrowth of fastidious pathogens by hardy contaminants. Rapid transport of specimens to the laboratory and the use of protective transport media are highly desirable. Exposure of the specimen to antiseptics, oxygen or low temperatures, or the prior administration of antibiotics can prevent the detection of many pathogens. Direct aspiration from sites of infection is preferred for obtaining specimens, so long as this does not entail the risk of serious morbidity.

As mentioned, laboratory personnel should be given enough clinical information to enable them to predict the most likely pathogens so that appropriate culture methods are used. Cultures and serologic tests for viruses, mycoplasmas, and chlamydia are being employed more and more often now that specific treatment with effective chemotherapeutic agents is available. Rapid, sensitive, and specific diagnostic tests based on immunologic techniques that will detect spe-

cific antigens of the infecting organisms are also becoming available and promise to revolutionize diagnostic and therapeutic measures in the next few years.

Antimicrobial Susceptibility

Antimicrobial Susceptibility Tests

The most widely used method for testing the activity of antimicrobial drugs against aerobic and facultative anaerobic organisms is the *disk-diffusion test* (also called the *Kirby-Bauer test*)[15,16] in which antibiotic-impregnated paper disks are placed on agar plates inoculated with the bacterium. After 16 to 18 h, the plates are examined and the diameters of the clear zones around the disks indicating no bacterial growth are measured. The diameters of the zones for the individual drugs are translated into "susceptible," "intermediate," or "resistant" categories by referring to standardized values as shown in Table 1-2.[17] The diameters of the zones have been correlated with the minimum inhibitory concentrations (MICs) of the antibiotics obtained by serial dilution tests with standard bacterial inocula. Organisms are generally considered susceptible when the MIC is lower than the concentration of drug usually attainable in the serum (or urine if the urinary tract is the site of the infection).

The disk-diffusion test is standardized, reliable, and adequate for most pathogenic bacteria and infections. The diameter of the zone of inhibition for specific drug–organism combinations correlates well with quantitative susceptibility tests and with the likelihood of a successful therapeutic response if the antimicrobial is administered correctly. With some organisms, susceptibility is so predictable that susceptibility tests are not necessary. Unfortunately, this is becoming less and less common. With some organisms, a zone of inhibition is produced, but it is relatively small, and this is an indication that higher than ordinary dosages of the drug must be employed to treat a systemic infection successfully. Such organisms are considered to be moderately resistant (or only moderately susceptible), but may nonetheless respond to ordinary therapy if the uri-

Table 1–2. Zone diameter standards and approximate minimal inhibitory concentration (MIC) correlates for amikacin and gentamicin in the disk-diffusion (Kirby-Bauer) test. The antibiotic diffuses into the agar from the disk and the approximate concentration of the drug at the edge of the zone of no growth is the MIC. An organism is "susceptible" if it prevents growth at a concentration of drug that is readily achieved in serum. The last column in the table shows the peak serum levels of drug that are achieved in patients after normal dosage. See text for more detail.

	Content of antibiotic in disk (μg)	Zone diameter (mm)			Approximate MIC correlates (μg/ml)		Range of peak serum level after usual dosage (μg/ml)
		Resistant	Intermediate	Susceptible	Resistant	Susceptible	
Amikacin	30	$\leq$14	15–16	$\geq$17	$\geq$32	$\leq$16	15–30
Gentamicin	10	$\leq$12	13–14	$\geq$15	$\geq$8	$\leq$4	4–8

Source: The standard disk test data are from reference 17.

nary tract is the site of the infection and the antimicrobial is eliminated in its active form in the urine, where particularly high concentrations are achieved despite the fact that concentrations at other body sites are suboptimal. With some organisms, susceptibility tests are not well standardized and are unreliable, especially if the organisms are strict anaerobes or fastidious or grow slowly. The disk test is useless when a bactericidal drug is required, since the disk-diffusion test measures only bacteriostatic activity.

A more recently developed diffusion method is the *E test*. This test is becoming more and more popular. It enables the MIC of an antibiotic to be estimated directly. High standard concentrations of an antibiotic are taken and a series of twofold dilutions are made and distributed linearly along a special carrier strip. The strip is then applied to a suitably inoculated plate and, after an overnight incubation, the MIC is read where the inhibition ellipse intersects on the calibrated scale. This test appears to be especially useful to detect pneumococci with resistance to penicillins and/or certain cephalosporins and enterococci with resistance to aminoglycosides, ampicillin, or vancomycin.

Broth dilution susceptibility tests are used to determine the MIC and minimum bactericidal concentration (MBC) of antibiotics. In broth dilution procedures, the organism is incubated at 35°C for 16 to 20 h in the presence of serial dilutions of antibiotics in agar

or broth media.[19] This method is more labor-intensive and therefore more costly than the disk-diffusion test, but it yields a more accurate estimate of the MIC, which is the lowest concentration of antibiotic producing complete inhibition of visible growth. One may also use this test to obtain the MBC of the antibiotic by subculturing the tubes that show growth inhibition in a second medium that is antibiotic-free. The MBC is the lowest concentration of antibiotic that yields no growth or results in a 99.9% decline in the number of colonies counted in a standardized volume that is subcultured overnight in an antibiotic-free medium. The value of the MIC or MBC is that it can be compared to the concentration of drug that is assayed in plasma or in an appropriate body fluid (urine, cerebrospinal fluid, synovial fluid, etc.) obtained from the site of the infection, whereas the disk test result is reported as simply susceptible, resistant, or intermediate.

The disk-diffusion procedure may be used for routine susceptibility testing but MICs and MBCs determined by dilution tests are becoming routine, especially when there is a severe infection in hospitalized patients and more exact information is required. The quantitative broth dilution methods are especially useful for guiding therapy in severely ill or septic patients, in debilitated or compromised patients, in patients with bacterial endocarditis or meningitis, in patients who have failed to respond to a seemingly adequate antimicrobial regimen, and in patients for whom high and potentially toxic dosage regimens must be used to control the infection. The results of quantitative susceptibility tests must be considered in relation to the probable concentrations of antimicrobials achieved at various body sites. The interactions between antimicrobials must also be considered. *Streptococcus faecalis* (enterococcus) isolates, for example, are often reported resistant to gentamicin, but expert clinicians are aware that the seeming inactivity of the drug is caused by the inability of gentamicin to penetrate in adequate amounts to the interior of the enterococcus, where its ribosomal site of action is almost always highly susceptible to the bactericidal effects of the drug. Addition of other antibiotics such as penicillins or vancomycin that inhibit synthesis of the cell wall results in enhanced penetration of gentamicin through the bacterial cell wall. These drugs often produce a synergistic effect when combined with gentamicin, and a bactericidal effect is observed that is not detectable when either drug is used alone.

An estimation of the MBC is particularly useful in those severe infections, such as bacterial endocarditis or meningitis, where knowledge of the killing activity of the drug is considered to be an essential guide to therapy. In the case of bacterial endocarditis, some physicians use the serum bactericidal activity as a guide to treatment. In this test (the so-called Schlichter test), samples of serum from treated patients are incubated (in dilutions with broth or serum or both) with the infecting organism to determine the maximal dilutions that are bacteriostatic or bactericidal.[19] Serum samples may be obtained at times that coincide with the anticipated peak and trough levels of antimicrobial activity. In the treatment of bacterial endocarditis caused by gram-positive cocci, serum bactericidal titers of 1:8 are often considered necessary to ensure a successful outcome (although this clinical impression has not been confirmed by an appropriately designed clinical study).[15] Higher bactericidal activity appears necessary in many serious gram-negative bacteremic infections.

Some bacterial species have not developed appreciable resistance to the drug of choice and susceptibility testing is not necessary. The group A streptococci, for example, have remained sensitive to pencillin G, as have meningococci. Susceptibility testing is especially important with *Staphylococcus aureus* pneumococci and the gram-negative bacilli where resistance is widespread. In general, any bacterium that is isolated from a normally sterile body fluid (blood, cerebrospinal fluid, synovial fluid, etc.) in the presence of clinical signs of infection should be tested for antibiotic susceptibility. Organisms like *Staphylococcus epidermidis* and *Corynebacterium* species are often considered skin contaminants and are usually not tested. However, significant *S. epidermidis* infections are being recognized with increasing frequency in debilitated patients and in patients with implanted foreign bodies. Bacteria isolated from throat and stool cultures are tested only if they are appropriate potential pathogens for that site, and if resistance may be a problem.

Drugs of Choice for Empiric Therapy Prior to Availability of Susceptibility Tests

The most important consideration in choosing the appropriate antibiotic for therapy is the susceptibility of the organism. After identifying the organism directly in fluid specimens obtained from the patient or determining the most likely pathogen on the basis of clinical findings, therapy is initiated with one or more antibiotics to which the organism is likely to be susceptible. Particular antibiotics have been chosen as the best agents for treatment of certain infections on the basis of their high clinical efficacy and their low potential for producing toxicity. For each pathogen there is a drug or drug combination that is generally regarded as the therapy of first choice. If the organism isolated from the patient is known (or suspected) to be resistant to the drug of first choice or if the pharmacokinetic properties of the drug or a variety of host factors (see next section) indicate that another drug should be used, then therapy is initiated with alternative drugs. The drugs of first choice and appropriate alternative drugs for treating infections caused by various organisms are presented in Table 1–3. Similar recommendations for treatment of fungal infections are presented in Chapter 12.

The role of any drug in the treatment of infection is subject to constant revision. The recommendation for drug of choice may change quite suddenly because a more effective or less toxic drug is marketed, because a new and serious side effect of an older

Table 1–3. Recomended antimicrobial drugs for empiric therapy before susceptibility tests are available.

Organism	Disease	Drugs of choice	Alternative drugs
GRAM-POSITIVE COCCI			
Enterococcus	Endocarditis or other severe infection	Penicillin G or ampicillin + gentamcin or streptomycin	Vancomycin + gentamicin; teicoplanin (an investigational drug)
	Uncomplicated UTI	Ampicillin or amoxicillin	Nitrofurantoin; a fluoroquinolone[a]
Staphylococcus aureus or S. epidermidis			
Non-penicillinase-producing	Abscesses, bacteremia, endocarditis, pneumonia, osteomyelitis, cellulitis	Penicillin G or V	A cephalosporin; vancomycin; imipenem; clindamycin; a fluoroquinolone[a]
Penicillinase-producing		A penicillinase-resistant penicillin[b]	A cephalosporin; vancomycin; amoxicilin/clavulanic acid; ticarcillin/clavulanic acid; pipericillin/tazobactam; imipenem
Methicillin-resistant[c]		Vancomycin with or without gentamicin and/or rifampin	TMP-SMX; a fluoroquinolone; minocycline
Streptococcus pyogenes (groups A, C and G)	Pharyngitis, scarlet fever, otitis media, sinusitis, cellulitis, erysipelas, pneumonia, bacteremia, toxic shock–like syndrome	Penicillin G or V	Clindamycin;erythromycin; a cephalosporin; vancomycin
Group B streptococcus	Endocarditis, bacteremia, meningitis	Penicillin G or ampicillin	A cephalosporin; vancomycin; erythromycin
Streptococcus viridans group	Endocarditis, bacteremia	Penicillin G with or without gentamicin	A cephalosporin; vancomycin
Streptococcus bovis	Endocarditis, bacteremia	Penicillin G	A cephalosporin; vancomycin
Anaerobic *streptococci*	Endocarditis, bacteremia, brain and other abscesses, sinusitis	Penicillin G	A cephalosporin; vancomycin
Streptococcus pneumoniae (pneumococcus)	Pneumonia, arthritis, sinusitis	Penicillin G or V	A cephalosporin; erythromycin; vancomycin ± rifampin; TMP-SMX

(continued)

Table 1–3. *Continued*

Organism	Disease	Drugs of choice	Alternative drugs
GRAM-NEGATIVE COCCI			
Moraxella (Branhamella) catarrhalis	Otitis, sinusitis, pneumonia	TMP-SMX	A cephalosporin; erythromycin; clarithromycin; azithromycin; amoxicillin/clavulanic acid
Neisseria gonorrhoeae (gonococcus)	Gonorrhea	Ceftriazone or cefixime	Cefotaxime; a fluoroquinolone; spectinomicin; penicillin G
Neisseria meningitidis (meningococcus)	Meningitis	Penicillin G	Cefotaxime; ceftizoxime; ceftriaxone; chloramphenicol[d]; a sulfonamide[e]
GRAM-POSITIVE BACILLI			
Bacillus anthracis	Anthrax	Penicillin G	Erythromycin; a tetracycline
Bacillus cerus, B. subtilis		Vancomycin	Imipenem; clindamycin
Clostridium perfringens	Gas gangrene	Penicillin G	Imipenem; clindamycin; metronidazole; a tetracycline
Clostridium tetani	Tetanus	Antitoxin; penicillin G	A tetracycline
Clostridium difficile	AAPC	Metronidazole	Vancomycin
Corynebacterium diphtheriae	Diphtheria	Antitoxin; erythromycin	Penicillin G
Corynebacterim spp.	Endocarditis, infected foreign bodies, bacteremia	Vancomycin	Penicillin G ± gentamicin; erythromycin
Listeria monocytogenes	Meningitis, bacteremia	Ampicillin ± gentamicin	TMP-SMX
ENTERIC GRAM-NEGATIVE BACTERIA			
Bacteroides			
Oropharyngeal strains (not *Bacteroides fragilis* group)		Penicillin G or clindamycin	Cefoxitin; metronidazole; chloramphenicol; cefotetan
Gastrointestinal strains (*Bacteroides fragilis*)		Metronidazole	Clindamycin; imipenem; ticarcillin/clavulanic acid; piperacillin/tazobactam; cefoxitin; cefotetan; chloramphenicol
Campylobacter fetus	Dysentery	Imipenem	Gentamicin
Campylobacter jejuni	Dysentery	A fluoroquinolone or erythromycin	A tetracycline; gentamicin
Enterobacter		Imipenem[f]	Cefotaxime, ceftizoxime, ceftriaxone, or ceftazidime; gentamicin, tobramycin, or amikacin; TMP-SMX

(continued)

16

Table 1–3. Continued

Organism	Disease	Drugs of choice	Alternative drugs
Escherichia coli	UTI, other	Cefotaxime, ceftizoxime, ceftriaxone, or ceftazidime	Ampicillin + gentamicin, tobramycin or amikacin; ticarcillin, mezlocillin, or piperacillin; gentamicin, tobramycin, or amikacin; TMP-SMX; aztreonam; imipenem; a fluoroquinolone
Helicobacter pylorii	Peptic ulcer	Tetracycline HCL + metronidazole + bismuth subsalicylate	Tetracycline HCL + clarithromycin + bismuth subsalicylate; amoxicillin + metronidazole + bismuth subsalicylate
Klebsiella pneumoniae	UTI, pneumonia	Cefotaxime, ceftizoxime, ceftriaxone, or ceftazidime	Imipenem; gentamicin, tobramycin, or amikacin; carbenicillin, ticarcillin, mezlocillin, or piperacillin; amoxicillin/clavulanic acid
Proteus mirabilis	UTI, other	Ampicillin	A cephalosporin; gentamicin, tobramycin, or amikacin; ticarcillin, mezlocillin, or piperacillin; TMP-SMX
Proteus, indole-positive *(Providencia rettgeri, Morganella morganii,* and *Proteus vulgaris)*	UTI, other	Cefotaxime, ceftizoxime, ceftriaxone, or ceftazidime	Imipenem; gentamicin, tobramycin, or amikacin; amoxicilin/clavulanic acid; carbenicillin, ticarcillin, mezlocillin, or piperacillin;
Providencia stuartii		Cefotaxime, ceftizoxime, ceftriaxone, or ceftaxidime	Imipenem; ticarcillin/clavulanic acid; piperacillin/tazobactam; gentamicin, tobramycin, or amikacin
Salmonella typhi	Typhoid fever, bacteremia	A fluoroquinolone or ceftriaxone	Chloramphenicol; TMP-SMX; ampicillin or amoxicillin
Other *Salmonella*	Gastroenteritis, paratyphoid fever, bacteremia	A fluoroquinolone or ceftriaxone or cefotaxime	Chloramphenicol; TMP-SMX; ampicillin, amoxicillin, carbenicillin, ticarcillin, mezlocillin, or piperacillin,
Serratia marcescens	Various nosocomial and opportunistic infections	Cefotaxime[g] ceftizoxime, ceftriaxone or ceftazidime	Gentamicin or amikacin; imipenem; aztreonam; TMP-SMX
Shigella	Acute gastroenteritis	A fluoroquinolone	TMP-SMX; ampicillin; ceftriaxone

(continued)

Table 1–3.   *Continued*

Organism	Disease	Drugs of choice	Alternative drugs
OTHER GRAM-NEGATIVE BACILLI			
Acinetobacter	Various nosocomial infections	Imipenem	Amikacin, tobramyci, or gentamicin; doxycycyline; ticarcillin, mezlocillin, or piperacillin; TMP-SMX; a fluroroquinolone
Bordetella pertussis	Whooping cough	Erythromycin	TMP-SMX; ampicillin
Brucella	Brucellosis	A tetracycline + streptomycin or gentamicin	A tetracycline + rifampin; TMP-SMX ± gentamicin; chloramphenicol ± streptomycin
Calymmatobacterium granulomatis	Granuloma inguinale	A tetracycline	Streptomycin or gentamicin; TMP-SMX; erythromycin
Eikenella corrodens		Ampicillin	An erythromycin; a tetracycline; amoxicillin/clavulaic acid
Francisella tularensis	Tularemia	Streptomycin	Gentamicin; a tetracycline; chloramphenicol
Gardnerella vaginalis	Vaginosis	Oral metronidazole[h]	Topical clindamycin or metronidazole; oral clindamycin
Haemophilus ducreyi	Chancroid	Erythromycin or ceftriaxone or azithromycin	A fluoroquinolone
Haemophilus influenzae	Meningitis, epiglottitis, arthritis, and other serious infections	Cefotaxime or ceftriaxone	Cefuroxime (but not for meningitis); chloramphenicol
	Upper respiratory infections and bronchitis	TMP-SMX	Cefuroxime; amoxicillin/clavulanic acid; cefuroxime axetil, cefaclor, cefotaxime, or ceftizoxime
Legionella spp.	Legionaires' disease	Erythromycin ± rifampin	Clarithromycin; azithromycin; ciprofloxacin; TMP-SMX
Pasteurella multocida	Wound infection (animal bites), abscesses, bacteremia, meningitis	Penicillin G	A tetracycline; a cephalosporin; amoxicillin/clavulanic acid
Pseudomonas aeruginosa	UTI	A fluoroquinolone	Carbenicillin, ticarcillin, piperacillin, or mezlocillin; ceftazidime; aztreonam, imipenem, or meropenem; tobramycin, gentamicin, or amikacin

(continued)

Table 1–3. *Continued*

Organism	Disease	Drugs of choice	Alternative drugs
	Pneumonia, wound infections, bacteremia	Ticarcillin, mezlocillin, or piperacillin + tobramycin, gentamcin, or amikacin	Ceftazidime, imipenem, or aztreonam + tobramycin, gentamicin or amikacin; ciprofloxacin
Pseudomonas mallei	Glanders	Streptomycin + a tetracycline	Streptomycin + chloramphenicol
Pseudomonas pseudomallei	Melioidosis	Ceftazidime	Chloramphenicol + doxycycline + TMP-SMX; amoxicillin/clavulanic acid; imipenem
Spirillum minus	Rat bite fever	Penicillin G	A tetracycline; streptomycin
Streptobacillus moniliformis	Rat bite fever	Penicillin G	A tetracycline; streptomycin
Vibrio cholerae	Cholera[i]	A tetracycline	TMP-SMX; a fluoroquinolone
Yersinia pestis	Plague	Streptomycin	A tetracycline; chloramphenicol; gentamicin
ACID-FAST BACILLI			
Mycobacterium tuberculosis	Tuberculosis	Isoniazid + rifampin + pyrazinamide ± ethambutol or streptomycin	Ciprofloxacin or ofloxacin; cycloserine; capreomycin, kanamycin, or amikacin; ethionamide; clofazimine; paraaminosalicylic acid
Mycobacterium kansasii	Atypical tuberculosis	Isoniazid + rifampin ± ethambutol or streptomycin	Clarithromycin; ethionamide; cycloserine
Mycobacterium avium complex	Disseminated disease in AIDS	Clarithromycin or azithromycin + ethambutol, rifabutin, or ciprofloxacin	Rifampin; clofazimine; amikacin
Mycobacterium fortuitum complex		Amikacin + doxycycline	Cefoxitin; rifampin; a sulfonamide
Mycobacterium marinum		Minocycline	TMP-SMX; rifampin; clarithromycin
Mycobacterium leprae	Leprosy	Dapsone + rifampin ± clofazimine	Minocycline; ofloxacin; sparfloxacin; clarithromycin
ACTINOMYCETES			
Actinomyces israelii	Actinomycosis	Penicillin G	A tetracycline; erythromycin; clindamycin
Nocardia	Nocardiosis	TMP-SMX	Sulfisoxazole; amikacin; a tetracycline

(continued)

Table 1–3.   Continued

Organism	Disease	Drugs of choice	Alternative drugs
CHLAMYDIA			
Chlamydia psittaci	Psittacosis; ornithosis	A tetracycline	Chloramphenicol
Chlamydia trachomatis	Trachoma	Azithromycin	A tetracycline (topical + oral)
	Inclusion conjunctivitis or pneumonia	Erythromycin (oral or I.V.)	A sulfonamide
	Urethritis, cervicitis	Doxycycline or azithromycin	Erythromycin; ofloxacin; sulfisoxazole
	Lymphogranuloma venereum	A tetracycline	Erythromycin
MYCOPLASMA			
Mycoplasma pneumoniae	Pneumonia	Erythromycin or a tetracycline	Clarithromycin; azithromycin
Ureaplasma urealyticum	Urethritis	Erythromycin	A tetracycline; clarithromycin
RICKETTSIA			
	Rocky Mountain spotted fever, endemic typhus (murine), epidemic typhus (louse-borne), scrub typhus, trench fever, Q fever	A tetracycline	Chloramphenicol; a fluoroquinolone
SPIROCHETES			
Borrelia recurrentis	Relapsing fever	A tetracycline	Penicillin G
Borrelia burgdorferi	Lyme disease	Doxycycline or amoxicillin	Cefuroxime axetil; ceftriaxone; cefotaxime; penicillin G
Leptospira	Leptospirosis	Penicillin G	A tetracycline
Treponema pallidum	Syphilis	Penicillin G	A tetracycline; ceftriaxone
Treponema pertenue	Yaws	Penicillin G	A tetracycline,

AAPC, antibiotic-associated pseudomembranous colitis; TMP-SMX, trimethoprim-sulfamethoxazole; UTI, urinary tract infection.

[a] For most infections, ofloxacin or ciprofloxacin. For urinary tract infections, norfloxacin, lomefloxacin, or enoxacin can be used. Fluoroquinolones are not recommended for children or pregnant women. [b] For oral use against penicillinase-producing staphylococci, cloxacillin or dicloxacillin is preferred. For severe infections, a parenteral oxacillin or nafcillin should be used. [c] Many strains of coagulase-positive staphylococci and coagulase-negative staphylococci are resistant to penicillinase-resistant penicillins; these strains are also resistant to cephalosporins and imipenem. [d] Because of the possibility of serious adverse effects, chloramphenicol should only be used for severe infections when less hazardous drugs are ineffective. [e] Sulfonamide resistant strains are frequent in the United States. Sulfonamides should only be used when susceptibility is established by susceptibility tests. [f] In patients seriously ill with a gram-negative infection due to enteric gram-negative bacilli, most consultants would add gentamicin, tobramycin, or amikacin to regimens containing a cephalsoporin, penicillin, aztreonam, or imipenem. None of the aminoglycosides should be mixed in the same bottle with an antpseudomonal penicillin for I.V. administration. [g] In severely ill patients, most consultants would add gentamicin or amikacin to regimens containing a cephalosporin, imipenem, or aztreonam. [h] Metronidazole is effective for bacterial vaginosis even though it is not usually active against *Gardnerella* in vitro. [i] Antibiotic therapy is an adjunct to, and not a substitute for, prompt fluid and electrolyte replacement.

Drug recommendations are from *The Medical Letter on Drugs and Therapeutics,* with permission from The Medical Letter, Inc.

drug is discovered, or because an organism acquires resistance. The recommendations for treatment of *Haemophilus influenzae* meningitis, for example, have changed for all of these reasons. Because it readily passes into the cerebrospinal fluid and is effective against *H. influenzae*, chloramphenicol was, for many years, the drug of choice for treating *H. influenzae* meningitis. In the 1960s, ampicillin was introduced and shown to be equally effective against this infection.[20] By this time, it was recognized that chloramphenicol could produce aplastic anemia and the less toxic drug ampicillin became the drug of first choice. In 1974, ampicillin-resistant *H. influenzae* isolates were reported in the United States[21] and, subsequently, were encountered elsewhere. Ampicillin resistance was due to a β-lactamase that could be transferred to sensitive strains by conjugation. DNA hybridization studies showed considerable homology between the β-lactamase gene on the *H. influenzae* plasmid and the TEM β-lactamase gene, which is commonly found in other gram-negative bacteria. Thus, it seems that the TEM β-lactamase transposon (called TnA or transposon for ampicillin resistance) was transferred to *H. influenzae* from the existing reservoir of resistance in the enteric gram-negative bacilli.[22,23] Because of the emergence of ampicillin-resistant strains, it was recommended that initial therapy of serious infections (e.g., meningitis, epiglottitis) due to *H. influenzae* again include chloramphenicol.[24] *H. influenzae* isolates resistant to both chloramphenicol and ampicillin were subsequently reported.[25,26] As a result of this resistance and because chloramphenicol is only recommended for antimicrobial therapy when a safer drug is not effective, one of the β-lactamase–resistant third-generation cephalosporins, such as cefotaxime or ceftriaxone, is now the treatment of choice.[27,28]

These changes in the appropriate therapy of severe *H. influenzae* infection are presented here to demonstrate how important it is for the physician to have accurate and up-to-date guidelines for available therapy. In North America, one of the best ways for physicians to keep themselves informed of the relative efficacy of drugs in the treatment of specific infections is to read *The Medical Letter*. This biweekly review of therapeutics publishes a listing of the consensus recommendations of a number of experts in infectious disease therapy regarding the choice of antimicrobial drugs. The recommendations are updated continually as the therapeutic situation changes. We urge physicians to keep themselves informed by subscribing to *The Medical Letter* or *A Guide to Antimicrobial Therapy*.

Host Factors that Modify the Choice, Dose, or Route of Administration of Antimicrobial Drugs

A variety of host factors are important for determining the success of antimicrobial therapy. Some have been considered earlier in this chapter; others may modify the choice of an antimicrobial agent or influence the dosage or route of administration. At the end of an early and excellent review of these host determinants, Weinstein and Dalton[29] concluded the following: "Although information concerning the susceptibility of organisms to antibiotics and their potentially harmful effects are essential, the enthusiasm for the 'bug' and the 'drug' must never be permitted to outweigh careful consideration of the person who is to be treated. Studies of the factors that appear to influence the results of treatment with anti-infective compounds indicate very clearly that *the patient is a most important determinant* of their effects." The following discussion will mention some of these host factors in a general way; each of them is considered in greater detail in the chapters on the individual drugs.

Previous History of a Drug Reaction

A history of a previous drug reaction is a common reason for choosing an alternative to the drug of first choice. This is a particular problem with the penicillins because they are often drugs of first choice, there is a high incidence of allergy, and a large patient population has been exposed to these antibiotics.[30,31] The problem of hypersensitivity to the penicillins and cephalosporins is discussed in detail in Chapter 4. In general, when a patient offers a bona fide history of previous drug reaction, the physician initiates therapy with a suitable alternative agent in a different chemical class. Occasionally, it may be useful to skin test a patient with a history of drug reaction. This is done more often with the penicillins than with other classes of antibiotics. As many of the antibiotics are capable of causing severe reactions on rare occasion (e.g., chloramphenicol, aplastic anemia; sulfonamides, Stevens-Johnson syndrome; erythromycin estolate, hepatitis), the physician should ask about previous reactions to all drugs and not focus only on those with a high incidence of allergic reaction, such as the penicillins and sulfonamides.

Site of Infection

Although it has been shown in model systems that subinhibitory concentrations of antibiotics may work in cooperation with host defense mechanisms to produce a significant antibacterial effect,[32] in the treatment of serious, symptomatic infections it is desirable to have levels of free drug at the site of infection that are above the MIC for the organism. In many cases it is considered desirable to achieve levels that are at least three to five times the MIC to ensure optimal therapeutic response. If a drug does not adequately penetrate to the site of infection, then it must be administered directly into a fluid space or one must administer a drug with more favorable distribution properties. The penetration of aminoglycosides into the cerebrospinal fluid, for example, is simply insufficient to permit reliable treatment of meningitis by systemic administration and they must be administered intrathecally as well as parenterally in most cases.[33] In contrast, the sulfonamides and chloramphenicol penetrate well into cerebrospinal fluid and therapeutic levels are achieved even in the absence of meningeal inflammation. Although passage of penicillins into cerebrospinal fluid, synovial fluid, and ocular fluid is poor in the absence of inflammation, in the presence of inflammation of the menin-

ges, joint spaces, or the eye, adequate concentrations of drugs are achieved to treat meningitis, arthritis, and endophthalmitis.

If there is obstruction in the biliary or urinary tract, an antibiotic that might normally be present in bile or urine at levels that are higher than the MICs of many pathogens may not reach the site of infection at all. If there is biliary tract obstruction, for example, gentamicin does not penetrate into the bile in levels that are therapeutic.[34] Although nitrofurantoin is normally used only to treat infection in the urinary tract, the concentration of drug in the urine of uremic patients is not high enough to treat common urinary tract pathogens.[35]

Renal and Hepatic Function

Most antibiotics are excreted primarily by the kidneys, and their dosage may have to be modified if renal function is impaired (see Table 1–4.[36] It is particularly important to reduce dosage and to monitor serum drug levels when administering potentially toxic drugs like aminoglycosides, vancomycin, or flucytosine to patients with impaired renal function.[37] Methods of dosage reduction will be presented in the sections of this book concerned with the pharmacology of individual drugs. With patients who are receiving hemodialysis or peritoneal dialysis it may be necessary to administer a dose of antibiotic at the end of the procedure in order to replace drug and ensure appropriate antibacterial levels.

Tests of renal function, such as the creatinine clearance rate or the serum creatinine concentration, can often be used to predict the excretion rate of drugs in patients with compromised renal function and the results of such tests serve as a basis for making recommendations for dosage adjustment. The usual clinical tests of hepatic function do not accurately predict the ability of the damaged liver to excrete or metabolize antibiotics.[38] In some cases, recommendations for dosage reduction based on serum transaminase levels will be given in subsequent chapters. These guidelines are only very rough approximations, however, and serum drug levels or antibacterial activity must be used to

Table 1–4. Effect of impaired renal function on antibiotic dosage. Group I drugs are excreted or inactivated by nonrenal mechanisms, or modest elevations in their serum concentrations are usually well tolerated. Most group II drugs are eliminated by both renal and hepatic mechanisms and dosage redction is only required in severe renal failure. Group III drugs are potentially toxic and are eliminated exclusively by the renal route; they require marked dosage reduction and monitoring of serum concentrations. The risk of toxicity contraindicates administration of drugs in group IV to patients in renal failure. In the presence of combined hepatic and renal failure, marked dosage reduction may be required for many group I and II drugs.

GROUP I: NO OR MINOR REDUCTION OF DOSAGE	GROUP II: MODERATE REDUCTION OF DOSAGE	GROUP III: MARKED REDUCTION OF DOSAGE
Amoxicillin	Nalidixic acid	Pencillin G
Amphotericin B	Norfloxacin	Sparfloxacin
Ampicillin	Oxacillin	Sulfamethoxazole
Azithromycin	Piperacillin	Ticarcillin
Cefoperazone	Pyrazinamide	Trimethoprim
Ceftizoxime	Rifampin	Trimethoprim-Sulfamethoxazole
Ceftriaxone		
Chloroquine	**GROUP II: MODERATE REDUCTION OF DOSAGE**	**GROUP III: MARKED REDUCTION OF DOSAGE**
Ciprofloxacin	Azlocillin	Amikacin
Clarithromycin	Cefazolin	Carbenicillin
Clindamycin	Cefamandole	Ethambutol
Cloxacillin	Cefepime	Flucytosine
Dicloxacillin	Cefixime	Gentamicin
Doxycycline	Cefotaxime	Kanamycin
Enoxacin	Cefoxitin	Netilmicin
Erythromycin	Cefatzidime	Streptomycin
Ethambutol	Cefuroxime	Tobramycin
Ethionamide	Cephalexin	Vancomycin
Floxacin	Cephalothin	
Fluconazole	Cephapirin	**GROUP IV: CONTRA-INDICATED IN PATIENTS WITH RENAL FAILURE**
Isoniazid	Cephradine	Methenamine mandelate
Itraconazole	Imipenem	Nitrofurantoin
Ketoconzaole	Lincomycin	Tetracyclines (except for doxycycline)
Methicillin	Lomefloxacin	
Metronidazole	Loracarbef	
Mezlocillin	Meropenem	
Minocycline	Methicillin	
Nafcillin	Moxalactam	
	Ofloxacin	

Source: Modified from Hewitt and McHenry.[37]

guide therapy in patients with compromised hepatic function who are receiving potentially toxic drugs, such as chloramphenicol or clindamycin, that are excreted by the hepatic route.

Age

Several factors related to age have profound effects on the choice of an antibiotic and its dosage. The hepatic and renal physiology of the neonatal infant is different from that of the older child and the differences are re-sponsible for certain toxicities that are unique in this age-group.[39] Livers of newborn infants have low levels of glucuronyl transferase, an enzyme that is necessary to conjugate chloramphenicol to the glucuronide metabolite and detoxify the drug. Because of the deficiency in conjugating activity and a lower glomerular filtration rate in neonates, there is an inverse relationship between chloramphenicol half-life and an infant's age.[40] Before this difference was recognized, a number of infants died from cardiovascular collapse ("gray syndrome") as a result of the high levels of unconjugated chloramphenicol in the body. For this reason, chloramphenicol is administered at much lower doses to infants under 1 month of age. In contrast to chloramphenicol, a higher dosage of gentamicin is required in both infants and young children because the distribution volume occupies a greater percentage of the body weight than in older children and adults. Children under 5 years of age require almost twice as much gentamicin and some other aminoglycosides (in mg/kg body weight) than children older than 10 years or adults in order to achieve a similar peak concentration of drug.[41]

The sulfonamides bind to sites on plasma protein that are shared with bilirubin, and if sulfonamides are administered to neonates, this competition can result in high levels of free bilirubin, which can traverse the blood–brain barrier and become deposited in certain regions of the brain, causing a toxic encephalopathy called *kernicterus*.[42] For this reason, sulfonamides are contraindicated in the neonate. The tetracyclines are deposited in growing bone and enamel. This deposition is accompanied by a permanent discoloration of the teeth and tetracyclines should not be administered to pregnant women or to children less than 8 years of age.[43] For unknown reasons, some antibiotics (e.g., tetracyclines, nalidixic acid) occasionally produce reversible intracranial hypertension (pseudotumor cerebri) in infants and children. Age-related considerations such as these are based on physiological and developmental differences between infants, children, and adults. They are important host factors that determine differences in the way antibiotics are administered in pediatric and adult practice.[44]

There are a number of differences between elderly patients and younger adults which affect antibiotic use in the older population.[45] In some cases the older patient is more sensitive to toxic effects. This is the case with isoniazid, for example, where there is a definite relationship between the age of the patient and the development of overt drug-related hepatitis.[46] Because of the increased risk of hepatitis, routine preventive therapy with isoniazid is not employed in patients who have positive tuberculin tests and are over the age of 35 unless additional risk factors exist (see Chapter 11). Age-related increases in risk have also been demonstrated for nephrotoxicity with cephaloridine or colistin therapy and for ototoxicity with aminoglycoside therapy.[47–49]

The presence of degenerative diseases that are unique to elderly patients must be considered when choosing an antibiotic for therapy. Congestive heart failure, a common complication of coronary artery disease, occurs more often in elderly patients and it is not desirable to treat these patients with antibiotic regimens that deliver a large amount of sodium. Carbenicillin, for example, is provided as a disodium salt and in the treatment of serious infection as much as 3 g of sodium may be administered each day.[45] The salt load can be reduced somewhat by administering ticarcillin, which is more potent and can be given at lower dosage, or by administering mezlocillin or piperacillin, which have an even lower sodium content than ticarcillin. Patients with congestive heart failure are usually treated with digitalis and diuretic preparations, and therapy with high doses of penicillins or with amphotericin B can cause hypokalemic alkalosis, which may precipitate digitalis toxicity.

Pregnancy and Nursing

Pregnancy imposes an increased risk of adverse drug effects on both the mother and the fetus.[50] Since many of the antibiotics readily pass across the placenta, the fetus may experience toxicity. The example of tetracycline deposition in fetal bone and teeth has been mentioned above. In addition to the effect on the fetus, pregnant women, particularly women with renal disease, are especially vulnerable to developing tetracycline-induced hepatotoxicity.[51] The aminoglycosides are known to pass across the placenta and auditory toxicity has been reported in children born of mothers treated with streptomycin during pregnancy.[52] Because of a theoretical potential for teratogenicity, it is prudent not to administer some antimicrobial drugs to pregnant women (e.g., metronidazole, which is mutagenic, or griseofulvin, which can cause metaphase arrest in mammalian cells).

Most drugs ingested by the nursing mother are excreted to some extent in milk and in some cases they can be toxic to the infant.[53] Significant concentrations of sulfonamides may be present in breast milk and even small doses of an ingested sulfonamide may produce hyperbilirubinemia in premature nursing infants.[53] Hemolytic anemia has been reported in nursing infants with glucose-6-phosphate dehydrogenase deficiency after maternal ingestion of sulfonamides and nalidixic acid.[54,55] The physician should be aware of potential risk to the infant in treating the nursing mother and, if large amounts of an antibiotic must be administered, nursing should be temporarily interrupted.

Genetic Factors

Genetically determined deficiencies in enzyme activity can render certain patients more susceptible to the toxic effects of some antimicrobial drugs. The rate at which isoniazid is metabolized by N-acetylation in the liver is genetically regulated.[56] People who are slow acetylators of isoniazid experience a higher incidence of isoniazid—induced neuropathy[57] and hepatitis[58] than those who are rapid acetylators. Isoniazid is an inhibitor of diphenylhydantoin metabolism, and when both drugs are given, patients who are slow acetylators are more likely to develop symptoms of diphenylhydantoin toxicity.[59] Patients who have a genetically determined deficiency of glucose-6-phosphate dehydrogenase in their erythrocytes may experience hemolysis and methemoglobinemia when they are exposed to oxidant drugs. If possible, antimicrobial agents having a high oxidant activity (e.g., sulfonamides, sulfones, furazolidone, nitrofurantoin, nalidixic acid, primaquine) should be avoided in patients with a history of drug-induced hemolytic anemia and low glucose-6-phosphate dehydrogenase activity.[60] Sulfonamides also may cause hemolysis in patients with hemoglobinopathy of the hemoglobin Zurich or hemoglobin H variety.[61,62] The antifungal compound griseofulvin is prophyrogenic and,

although the effect on prophyrin metabolism is not usually of clinical consequence, in patients with porphyria, griseofulvin can precipitate acute attacks of the disease.[63]

Metabolic Abnormalities

The presence of metabolic abnormalities may modify the method of antibiotic administration or increase the risk of toxicity. If a patient has poor peripheral perfusion, antibiotics may not be absorbed rapidly from sites of intramuscular injection. Thus, patients who are in shock, for example, should receive intravenous therapy. Absorption of intramuscular antibiotics may also be impaired in some patients with severe diabetes.[29] When initiating therapy of severe infections with an aminoglycoside in diabetic patients, the drug should be administered intravenously.[45] It is important to remember that the amount of dextrose that is infused when antibiotics are administered intravenously may be sufficient to produce hyperglycemia and glucosuria in the diabetic patient. The sulfonamides are structural analogs of the sulfonylurea group of oral antidiabetic agents (e.g., tolbutamide and chlorpropamide) and they potentiate the hypoglycemic activity of these drugs in diabetic patients.[45] The presence of gastric achlorhydria (as with the concomitant use of cimetidine) may reduce the absorption of drugs like ketoconazole, which require an acid environment for dissolution and absorption. To obtain adequate absorption of ketoconazole in patients with pernicious anemia and in elderly patients with achlorhydria, it may be necessary to dissolve to dissolve the drug in 0.2N HC1 and administer it through a glass or plastic straw. Trimethoprim is an inhibitor of folate metabolism and patients with suboptimal folate nutrition (such as pregnant women, malnourished patients, and alcoholics) who are exposed to long-term therapy may develop megaloblastic anemia.[64]

Preexisting Dysfunction in Particular Organ Systems

Special care must be taken when choosing an antibiotic and monitoring for toxicity in patients who already have compromised organ function. Drugs that cause liver injury, for example, may be contraindicated or should be used only with special caution in patients with preexisting liver disease. Such drugs would include tetracyclines, nitrofurantoin, isoniazid, rifampin, pyrazinamide, and flucytosine. Potentially nephrotoxic drugs, such as aminoglycosides, tetracyclines, and amphotericin B, carry additional risk in the patient who already has decreased renal function. The physician must remember that the patient may be receiving nephrotoxic drugs to treat underlying conditions or as anesthetic agents, and in some cases (e.g., cisplatinum, methoxyflurane) the risk of renal damage with concomitant administration of a nephrotoxic antibiotic is clearly increased.[65,66] Prior or concomitant therapy with other ototoxic drugs (e.g., ethacrynic acid) increases the risk of ototoxicity occurring with aminoglycosides[67] (and perhaps with other ototoxic antibiotics like vancomycin).

When present at high concentration, the aminoglycosides, and possibly clindamycin, can produce neuromuscular blockade. Patients with myasthenia gravis and patients receiving ether anesthesia or a neuromuscular blocking agent during anesthesia are more likely to experience this complication.[68] Certain antibiotics that can stimulate the central nervous system, such as nalidixic acid and cycloserine, are contraindicated in patients with convulsive disorders. Ethambutol can produce optic neuritis and it is not advisable to administer the drug to a patient with limited vision. Nitrofurantoin produces pulmonary reactions and it should not be administered to a patient with already compromised pulmonary function. A unique host factor modifying antimicrobial therapy occurs with the administration of amphotericin B to patients who are also receiving leukocyte transfusions. Leukocyte recipients who receive amphotericin B are 10 times more likely to experience an acute pulmonary inflammatory reaction than leukocyte recipients who are not receiving the drug.[69] The pulmonary reaction can be fatal and the mechanism is not known. If an antibiotic that is toxic to an organ must be administered to a patient with preexisting dysfunction, then frequent plasma drug assays may be advisable and the patient's status should be frequently monitored by appropriate clinical assessment and laboratory tests.

Prophylactic Use of Antibiotics

From one-quarter to one-half of all antibiotic use in hospitals in the United States is for prevention of infection rather than for treatment of infection.[70,71] In many cases the benefit of prophylactic antibiotics to the patient has not been established by appropriately controlled clinical trials (for reviews see Jacoby et al.,[72] Goldman and Petersdorf,[73] Hirschmann and Inui[74]). Prophylactic use of antibiotics is most likely to be effective when the goal is to prevent infection by a single organism. The "shotgun" approach to preventing infection by any of a variety of organisms over a prolonged period is less likely to be successful, and the use of antibiotics in this manner accounts for a significant proportion of antibiotic misuse in nonsurgical practice.

There are a number of situations in which antibiotic prophylaxis is generally regarded as beneficial and is established medical practice. Antibiotics are sometimes administered in a prophylactic manner to patients with obstructive pulmonary disease or recurrent otitis media. Although the practice is widespread, it has not been unequivocally demonstrated to be beneficial or to retard progression of the pulmonary disease. It is clear that prophylactic antibiotics are not effective at preventing hospital-acquired pneumonia, infections due to indwelling catheters, or bacterial complications of viral respiratory infections. The largest area of controversy lies in the appropriate prophylactic use of antibiotics in the surgical setting.[74,75]

It is useful to group surgical procedures according to the frequency of postoperative infection.[73] Clean procedures are defined as nontraumatic uninfected operative wounds that do not involve entry into the bronchus, gastrointestinal tract, or urinary tract. In clean operations the infection rate is usually less than 5% and prophylactic antibiotics are not indicated unless there has been implantation of a foreign body (i.e., orthopedic prosthesis, prosthetic heart valve, or plastic vascular graft). *Clean-contaminated* operations are those in which the bronchus, the gastrointestinal tract, or the oropharyngeal cavity are entered without unusual contamination. In clean-contaminated operations the infection rate is generally less than 10%. In certain of these operations (e.g., vaginal or abdominal hysterectomy, high-risk cesarean section, elective colorectal surgery, head and neck surgery with entry of the orpharyngeal cavity, and elective high-risk gastric and biliary tract surgery) very short courses of prophylactic antibiotics begun just prior to surgery and continued for 24–48 hr probably reduce the postoperative infection rate and hospital charges without significant risk. *Contaminated* procedures include operations on open, fresh traumatic wounds, operations with a break in sterile technique, and incisions into areas of acute, nonpurulent inflammation. The anticipated infection rate is 20% in such cases and prophylactic antibiotics are often considered appropriate (e.g., open fractures). *Dirty* operations deal with perforated viscera or frankly infected wounds (e.g., abscesses, draining sinuses) and a postoperative infection rate of at least 30% may be anticipated. Dirty operations are already infected and require the administration of *therapeutic* antibiotic regimens. If gross contamination has occurred (as with penetrating wounds or perforated viscera) or if inflammatory disease is present (e.g., acute cholecystitis), the use of antibiotics should not be considered prophylactic—rather, it is therapeutic.

The efficacy of antibiotic prophylaxis in high-risk surgical patients has been shown to be efficacious and cost-beneficial. Several principles apply to prophylactic antibiotic use in surgery. The key to acceptable and effective antimicrobial prophylaxis in surgical patients is to begin an antibiotic that is effective against the most likely pathogens just a *short* time (30 mins) prior to the initial incision, so that effective concentrations of drug will be present in the tissues at the time of contamination or at most within an hour of contamination. If effective drug concentrations are maintained throughout most of the operation, then it is rarely necessary to continue antibiotics for more than 24 hr postoperatively, thus reducing expense and the likelihood of various adverse reactions to these antibiotics. This strategy of giving surgical prophylaxis is commonly referred to as *short-course perioperative prophylaxis*. It should be stressed that if there has been contamination of the tissues for more than 2 h prior to surgery and the administration of antimicrobials, then it is probably too late for prophylaxis, and the patient should be started on *treatment* with an appropriate antibiotic regimen, which is usually continued for 5 to 10 days.

Antibiotics are never a substitute for good surgical judgment and technique. Antibiotics will never sterilize skin or mucous membranes for more than a short time. They will reduce the number of organisms per gram of tissue or body fluid and thus may lower the likelihood of infection, but they will also alter the normal flora and select and encourage colonization with resistant organisms. *Prophylactic antibiotics are not needed when there is little or no contamination* in patients with normal host defenses. They are most effective when contamination is moderate and of brief duration. They are of little benefit when contamination is heavy and sustained. Therefore, the specific surgical procedure is the primary determinant of whether prophylaxis is needed and likely to be effective. Table 1–5 lists some recommendations for antimicrobial prophylaxis in surgical patients.

The two most common mistakes made in prophylaxis in the surgical setting are the use of antibiotics in clean operations where they are not justified and continuing administration of prophylactic antibiotics for several days after the operation. In a study of prophylactic antibiotic use in general hospitals in Pennsylvania, 70% to 90% of the courses of antimicrobial prophylaxis lasted more than 2 days after the operation, and the authors noted that once prophylaxis had been initiated, it tended to be continued for the remainder of the patient's hospitalization.[70] The problem with inappropriate antibiotic use could be lessened significantly if house

Table 1–5. *Antimicrobial prophylaxis in surgical patients.*

Type of operation and degree of contamination	Usual pathogens	Recommended prophylactic regimens[a]
I. CLEAN		
Cardiovasclar: prosthetic valve insertion, or arterial reconstruction involving a prosthesis or incision below the navel	*Staphylococcus aureus, S. epidermidis,* enteric gram-negative bacilli, Corynebacteria, fungi	Cefazolin 1.0 g IM or IV, or vancomycin 500 mg over 60 min IV just prior to induction of anesthesia and q6–8h for 24–48 h, or the duration of the procedure. Vancomycin is not for routine use. It should be used in infections with high likelihood of MRSA[b] or MRSE, or in patients with severe allergic reaction to β-lactams.
Orthopedic: total joint replacement, internal fixation of a proximal femoral fracture, or spinal fusion	*S. aureus, S. epidermidis*	Same as above
Immunocompromised hosts	*S. aureus,* streptococci, coliforms	Same as above
Long craniotomies	*S. aureus,* coliforms	Cefazolin 1.0 g IV at induction of anesthesia and q4–6h for duration of procedure
II. CLEAN-CONTAMINATED		
Head and neck surgery when the oral cavity or pharynx are incised	*S. aureus,* streptococci, oral anaerobes, coliform bacteria	Cefazolin 1.0–2.0 g IV and q6hr for 24 h, or penicillin G 1,000,000 U IV just prior to induction of anesthesia, or cefonicid 1.0 g IM or IV once per day
Gastroduodenal surgery, in high-risk patients only (bleeding, obstruction, carcinoma, achlorhydria)	Oral gram-positive cocci, facultative enteric gram-negative bacilli	Cefazolin or cefonicid as above
Biliary tract in high-risk patients only (elderly, acute cholecystitis, obstructed, stones)	As above, plus enterococci and clostridia	Cefazolin or cefonicid as above, or amplicillin with or without an aminoglycoside or ampicillin/sulbactam
Colorectal Surgery		
Elective	Enteric, gram-negative bacilli, *Bacteroides fragilis,* and other strict anaerobes, group D streptococci	Mechanical cleansing (2 days) plus oral erythromycin or metronidazole and neomycin, 1 g of each 1 P.M., 2 P.M., and 11 P.M. the day before operation. If high risk, add cefoxitin as below or other broad-spectrum agent.
Emergent or high-risk elective (after antibiotic bowel prep as above)	Same as above	Oral bowel prep followed by cefoxitin 2.0 g just prior to induction of anes-

(continued)

Table 1–5. Continued

Type of operation and degree of contamination	Usual pathogens	Recommended prophylactic regimens[a]
		thesia once or q6h × 2, or cefotaxime, 1 g IV just prior to surgery and (optional) 6 and 12 h later IV or IM, or doxycycline 100 mg IV just before anesthesia and 100 mg IV 12 and 24 h later.
Appendectomy	Facultative and obligate anaerobes	Cefoxitin 1.0 g IM or IV once, or clindamycin 600 mg IM or IV once, or doxycycline 200 mg IV once, at anesthesia induction
Vaginal or high-risk abdominal hysterectomy, or emergent Caesarian section	Enteric gram-negative bacilli, anaerobes, enterococci, group B streptococci. *B. fragilis* usually absent or present in low numbers	Cefazolin or cefoxitin 1.0 g IM or IV just before induction of anesthesia or after cord-clamping and q6h for 24 h. Alternatively, a single 1.0 g IM or IV dose of cefonicid
Abortion	Same as above	First trimester after pelvic inflammatory disease: penicillin G 1,000,000 units IV. Second trimester: cefazolin 1 g IM or IV
Neurosurgical, high-risk only (prolonged, or contaminated operative sites)	Staphylococci, gram-negative bacilli, streptococci	Cefotaxime 2 g IV just before induction of anesthesia and q6h for 24 h
III. CONTAMINATED AND DIRTY		
Ruptured viscus, severe appendicitis (gangrenous or perforated)	Enteric gram-negative bacilli, anaerobes (incl. *B. fragilis*), streptococci	Treatment IV with clindamycin or metronidazole plus an aminoglycoside or cefoxitin with or without an aminoglycoside begun as soon as possible and continued no more than 7 days postoperatively, even less with improvement.
Traumatic wounds	*S. aureus,* streptococci, *Clostridia*	Cefazolin (1 g q8h, IV)
Bites (animal and human)	*Eikenella,* staphylococci, and anaerobes, *Pasteurella multocida*	Penicillin G (1,000,000 units, q4h IV). Ampicillin/sulbactam IV or amoxicillin/clavulanate orally
Genitourinary surgery, i.e., prostatectomy	Coliforms	With pre- or postoperative bacteriuria, treat according to results of cultures and susceptibility tests

[a] Parenteral prophylactic antimicrobials for clean or clean-contaminated surgery can be given as a single dose just before induction of anesthesia. For prolonged operations, additional intraoperative doses can be given every 4–8 h for the duration of the procedure. If cephalosporins are used, a single daily dose of cefonicid is recommended instead of multiple doses of cefazolin. [b] MSRA, methicillin-resistant *S. aureus.*

Prepared by Eric Scholar with the assistance of Dr. Laurel Preheim, Department of Infectious Diseases and Dr. Jon Thompson, Department of Surgery, University of Nebraska College of Medicine.

officers would write orders to terminate prophylaxis at the end of or 24 h after the operation.

Therapy with Antibiotic Combinations

Synergism, Antagonism, and Indifference

In most cases, infections caused by a single defined organism are best treated with a single antibiotic. The use of multiple antibiotics simultaneously is usually not necessary: it exposes the patient to an increased risk of drug toxicity, it increases the cost of therapy, and it can sometimes be less effective than therapy with a single antibiotic. There are well-established clinical situations, however, when therapy with a combination of antibiotics (usually two) is clearly indicated. When an organism is exposed simultaneously to two antibiotics to which it is sensitive, the response to the combination will fall into one of three patterns: indifference, antagonism, or synergism.[76,77]

The three responses are diagrammed in Figure 1–2. In the *indifferent* (or additive) response, the drug combination is more effective than either antibiotic alone and the response represents roughly a summation of the two drug effects. This is probably the

most frequent outcome when two drugs are combined in therapy. Often, the added antibacterial effect of the second drug is not clinically significant.

The combination of two drugs may produce less of a response than one of the drugs alone. This is drug *antagonism*. Antagonism has been well demonstrated in vitro. It is more likely to occur when a bactericidal drug (e.g., a penicillin or an aminoglycoside) is combined with a primarily bacteriostatic drug (e.g., a tetracycline).[76,77] A common explanation of this observation is that many bactericidal agents have a killing effect only on cells that are growing or actively synthesizing protein and that bacteriostatic drugs prevent growth or protein synthesis and thereby counter the effect of a bactericidal drug. When there is drug antagonism, the effect of the combination is not likely to be less than the effect of the bacteriostatic agent alone.

There are only a few clear clinical examples of antagonism. In an early study of combined drug therapy, it was shown that the combination of penicillin and chlortetracycline was significantly less effective than penicillin alone against pneumococcal meningitis.[78] In another study, the mortality of children with acute bacterial meningitis (due

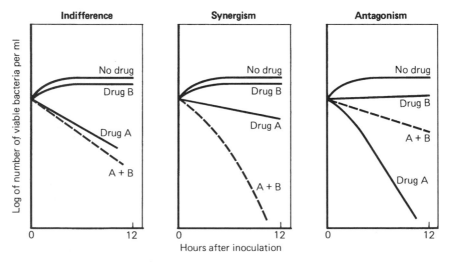

Figure 1–2. Patterns of response to therapy with two antibiotics. The response of bacteria suspended in growth medium to exposure to drug A or B alone is represented by the solid lines. The dashed lines represent the responses to simultaneous administration of the two drugs. (From Jawetz.[76])

to *Haemophilus influenzae, Streptococcus pneumoniae,* or *Neisseria meningitidis*) treated with ampicillin alone (3.9%) was found to be lower than that of a comparable group receiving a regimen of ampicillin and choloramphenicol supplmented with 2 days of streptomycin therapy (11.7%).[79] Antagonism between chloramphenicol (when present at its M.I.C) and ampicillin has also been shown with *H influenzae* growing in vitro.[80]

Fortunately, the undesirable interaction between antimicrobials that leads to antagonism is relatively rare. However, in treatment of infections in which a bactericidal action is essential or desirable (such as endocarditis, meningitis, or infection in granulocytopenic patients), it is best to avoid the use of drug combinations in which one member is only inhibitory, since the net result is likely to be only inhibitory. Many infections will often respond symptomatically to treatment with antagonistic regimens, but will be only suppressed and not cured; the result will be a relapse after the antibiotics are discontinued. However, when inhibition alone is adequate, the infection may be cured by antagonistic regimens. For example, in treatment of pneumonia or a wound infection in a patient with intact host defenses, the antagonism demonstrable in vitro may have no clinical significance. This distinction is justification for using combinations of bacteriostatic and bactericidal drugs to provide so-called empiric coverage for a large number of potential pathogens when the exact etiology of the infection is still unknown and a bactericidal effect is not essential.

A combination of antibiotics may have a greater effect than the sum of the two individual drug effects. This is called a *synergistic* response and it is seen in specific cases with mixtures of two bactericidal drugs. Synergism is obviously a therapeutically desirable response and it is one of the major clinical indications for the use of antibiotic combinations.

Clinical Indications for Combined Antimicrobial Therapy

SYNERGISM. Although there are methods that can distinguish between additive and synergistic responses to antibiotic combinations in vitro,[81] it is very difficult to clearly distinguish between the two responses in experimental infections in vivo.[82] If the response to an antibiotic combination in vivo is clearly superior to the effect of either agent alone, the response is often called *synergistic*. Synergism is usually defined as a fourfold or greater decrease in the minimal inhibitory or bactericidal concentrations of the individual antibiotics when they are present together. Lesser degrees of positive interaction are considered additive. There is a limited number of clinical situations involving infection by a single pathogen where it is well established that therapy with a combination of antimicrobial agents is superior to therapy with a single drug.[83]

The combination of an aminoglycoside with a drug that inhibits cell wall synthesis (a penicillin, a cephalosporin, vancomycin) may produce synergism. The best known example is the use of penicillin–aminoglycoside combinations in the treatment of enterococcal (*Streptococcus faecalis*) endocarditis (see Table 1–3).[83] Vancomycin also acts synergistically with an aminoglycoside against enterococci and is the recommended alternative in patients who are allergic to penicillins.[84] The combination of penicillin G and streptomycin is synergistic against *viridans* streptococci, but therapy with penicillin G alone is very effective and may be the preferred treatment for *S. viridans* endocarditis.[85] The combination of an antipseudomonal penicillin (carbenicillin, ticarcillin, mezlocillin, azlocillin, or piperacillin) with an aminoglycoside (gentamicin, tobramycin, or amikacin) is synergistic against many strains of *Pseudomonas aeruginosa* in vitro. In the treatment of moderate or severe *Pseudomonas* infection, an aminoglycoside is usually administered in addition to the penicillin. Synergism with cephalosporin–aminoglycoside combinations has been demonstrated against *Klebsiella pneumoniae* in vitro and it is possible that severe *K. pneumoniae* pulmonary infections respond better when synergistic therapy is employed.[83]

There is good evidence that the synergism that occurs with the combination of an aminoglycoside and an inhibitor of cell wall synthesis is due to increased entry of the aminoglycoside into the bacterium where it can interact with the ribosome and inhibit protein synthesis (see Chapter 5 for discussion of this mechanism). This general mechanism of synergy, where the effect of one drug permits increased entry of a second drug to its site of action inside the cell is also seen when the antifungal agent amphotericin B is combined with other drugs. Amphotericin B acts on fungal cell membranes and the combination of amphotericin B and flucytosine is synergistic against a few fungi growing in vitro,[86] especially cryptococci. Enhanced effects have been obtained with this drug combination against cryptococcal and candidal infections in mice (see Chapter 12),[87,88] and with cryptococci in humans.

A combination of drugs may result in synergism because one of the drugs inhibits the inactivation of the other. Clavulanic acid, for example, has little intrinsic antimicrobial activity, but it is an irreversible β-lactamase inhibitor and it is used in combined therapy with penicillins. Clavulanic acid acts synergistically with penicillins and some cephalosporins against a variety of β-lactamase-producing Enterobacteriaceae and *Staphylococcus aureus*.[89,90] A fixed-ratio combination of clavulanic acid and ampicillin is marketed under the trade name Augmentin.

If two drugs inhibit different steps in a critical metabolic pathway, synergism may result. Trimethoprim and sulfamethoxazole are combined in a single preparation for this purpose. Sulfonamides inhibit the synthesis of folic acid and trimethoprim inhibits the reduction of folate to tetrahydrofolate, which is the form of the cofactor that is utilized for one-carbon metabolism in the cell (see Chapter 8). The combination of these two drugs has been shown to be synergistic against a wide variety of bacteria.[91] Mecillinam is a unique β-lactam compound that is very effective against Enterobacteriaceae, in particular *Escherichia coli*.[92] Mecillinam interacts with one of the *E. coli* penicillin-binding proteins, a membrane-bound enzyme that is required for maintaining the "rod" shape of the organism. Synergy has been demonstrated in vitro when mecillinam is combined with penicillins or cephalosporins that interact preferentially with other penicillin-binding proteins, like the transpeptidases that are required for wall synthesis during elongation.[93] Synergy has also been observed in vivo against gram-negative bacillary infections in mice.[94]

PREVENTION OF RESISTANCE. The use of combinations of drugs having different mechanisms of action and different mechanisms of resistance should decrease emergence of resistant organisms during therapy. This principle has been effectively applied in the treatment of tuberculosis where initial intensive therapy of the disease is always carried out with two or three drugs. Combined drug treatment of tuberculosis results in markedly reduced selection of resistant mutants.[95]

DECREASED TOXICITY. Antibiotics have been used in combination to reduce toxicity. In clinical practice, the use of flucytosine in synergistic combination with amphotericin B permitted the use of a smaller dosage of amphotericin B for a shorter period of time in treating patients with cryptococcal meningitis.[96] Patients treated with the combination experienced less amphotericin B–induced nephrotoxicity. Sulfonamides have been combined in therapy to reduce crystalluria. The older sulfonamides are not very soluble in urine and they can crystallize out of solution in the kidney. The presence of one sulfonamide, however, does not affect the urine solubility of another. Thus, combinations of three sulfonamides were prepared in which each compound is present at a reduced dosage that is not likely to produce crystalluria, but the bacterium is exposed to the same aggregate antimicrobial activity.

MIXED INFECTIONS. A combination of antibiotics is used when an infection is caused by a mixture of organisms with different antibiotic susceptibilities.[97] Mixed infections occur commonly after perforation of a viscus, when there is pelvic infection, and in brain abscesses. Gram-positive and gram-negative aerobic and anaerobic bacterial species may be involved and therapy is initiated with a combination of antimicrobial agents.

In these situations, it is usual to administer an aminoglycoside such as gentamicin to cover facultative anaerobes of the coliform group, and another agent, such as clindamycin, cefoxitin, metronidazole, chloramphenicol, or ticarcillin, to provide coverage for obligate anaerobes, such as *Bacteroides fragilis*, peptostreptococci, and clostridia. Most of these drug regimens provide coverage for some staphylococci and most streptococci, but not enterococci. The latter organisms are usually ignored in polymicrobial or mixed infections unless they are present as the dominant organisms or are cultured from the blood. When it is necessary to provide coverage for enterococci in polymicrobial infections, high-dose intravenous penicillin or ampicillin is usually added to the treatment regimen. When reliable culture results become available, therapy should be changed to a more specific, less expensive and less toxic antimicrobial regimen.

INITIAL THERAPY OF SEVERE INFECTION. The most common clinical indication for combined antimicrobial therapy is the initiation of treatment of severe infection when the etiological agent is not known. Combination therapy is especially common in neutropenic patients. Patients with compromised host defense mechanisms may be infected with a wide variety of pathogens and early in the course of the infection they may not present clear-cut signs and symptoms of infection. Because infections progress rapidly in such patients, fever is treated empirically with an antibiotic combination and treatment is initiated immediately after obtaining appropriate cultures. In initial therapy of severe infection, an antibiotic combination is employed to obtain a broad spectrum of bactericidal action. In many cases an aminoglycoside is administered with either a penicillin having antipseudomonas activity (carbenicillin, ticarcillin, azlocillin, mezlocillin, or piperacillin) or a newer cephalosporin.[98,99] In patients with compromised renal function, a combination of an antipseudomonal penicillin and a cepahalosporin is often used to avoid the nephrotoxicity of the aminoglycosides; both antibiotics usually need to be given in high dosage. It is impor-

tant to emphasize that appropriate cultures must be obtained before therapy is started and that specific therapy should be employed when the infecting organism has been identified and its antibiotic susceptibility is established.

INFECTION AT SEQUESTERED SITES. It is sometimes necessary to administer a second antibiotic to provide good antibacterial activity at sequestered sites of infection when the primary drug does not reach effective concentrations there. An example of this is seen in the treatment of meningococcal meningitis, which is readily treated with penicillin G. However, the concomitant meningococcal carrier state is not eradicated by therapy with penicillin, because this antibiotic does not penetrate to the important colonization sites in the nasopharynx. Rifampin, minocycline, and sulfonamides, on the other hand, do get into tears, saliva, and mucous secretions that bathe the nasopharyngeal mucosa. They are usually effective at eradicating susceptible meningococci. Rifampin and minocycline, however, are not reliably effective by themselves in treatment of meningococcal meningitis. In this case, it is recommended that after treatment of meningitis is successful, a second drug be given to eradicate the carrier state.

REFERENCES

1. Kunin; C. M. Problems in antibiotic use. In *Principles and Practice of Infectious Diseases*, ed. by G. L. Mandell, R. G. Douglas, and J. E. Bennett. New York: Wiley, 1979, pp. 383–395.

2. Symposium (various authors). The impact of infections on medical care in the United States. Problems and priorities for future research. *Ann. Intern. Med.* 1978;89:737–866.

3. Buckwold, F. J., and A. R. Ronald. Antimicrobial misuse—effects and suggestions for control. *J. Antimicrob. Chemother.* 1979;5:129.

4. Simmons, H. E., and P. D. Stolley. This is medical progress? Trends and consequences of antibiotic use in the United States. *JAMA* 1974;227:1023.

5. Stolley, P. D. M. H. Becker, J. B. McEvilla, L. Lasagna, M. Gainor, and L. M. Sloan. Drug prescribing and use in an American community. *Ann. Intern. Med.* 1972;76:537.

6. Gardner, F. T., C. E. Jones, and H. C. Polk. Further definition of antibiotic use and abuse in the surgical setting. *Arch. Surg.* (1973);114:883.

7. Naqvi, S. H., L. M. Dunkle, K. J. Timmerman, R. M. Reichley, D. L. Stanley, and D. O'Connor. Antibiotic usage in a pediatric medical center. *JAMA* 1979; 242:1981.

8. Scheckler, W. E. and J. V. Bennett. Antibiotic usage in seven community hospitals. *JAMA* 1970;213:264.

9. Castle, M., C. M. Wilfert, T. R. Cate, and S. Osterhout. Antibiotic use at Duke University Medical Center. *JAMA* 1979;237:2819.

10. Chretien, J. H., M. Garvey, A. de Stwolinski, and J. G. Esswein. Abuse of antibiotics, a study of patients attending a university clinic. *Arch. Intern. Med.* 1975; 135:1063.

11. Weinstein, L., and A. C. Dalton. Host determinants of response to antimicrobial agents. *N. Engl. J. Med.* 1968;279:476–473;524–531;580–588.

12. Craig, W. A. and C. M. Kunin. Significance of serum protein and tissue binding of antimicrobial agents. *Annu. Rev. Med.* 1976;27:287.

13. Konisky J.; Colicins and other bacteriocins with established modes of action. *Annu. Rev. Microbiol.* 1982;36:125.

14. Weinstein, L., and D. M. Musher. Antibiotic-induced suprainfection. *J. Infect. Dis.* 1969;119:662.

15. Rosenblatt, J. E., Laboratory tests used to guide antimicrobial therapy. *Mayo Clin. Proc.* 1977;2:611.

16. Bauer, A. W., W. M. M. Kirby, J. C. Sherris, and M. Turck. Antibiotic susceptibility testing by a standardized single disk method. *Am. J. Clin. Pathol.* 1966; 45:493.

17. Barry, A. L., and C. Thornsberry. Susceptibility testing: diffusion test procedures. In *Manual of Clinical Microbiology*, 3rd ed., ed. by E. H. Lennette, A. Balows, W. J. Hausler, and J. P. Truant. Washington DC: American Society of Microbiology, 1980, pp. 463–474.

18. Acar, J. F. and F. W. Goldstein. Disk susceptibility test. In *Antibiotics in Laboratory Medicine*, 4th ed., ed. by V. Lorian. Baltimore: Williams and Wilkins, 1996, pp. 1–51.

19. Washington, J. A., and V. L. Sutter. Dilution susceptibility test: agar and macro-broth dilution procedures. In *Manual of Clinical Microbiology*, 3rd ed., ed. by E. H. Lennette, A. Balows, W. J. Hausler, and J. P. Truant. Washington DC: American Society of Microbiology, 1980, pp. 453–462.

20. Barrett, F. F., L. H. Taber, C. R. Morris, W. B. Stephenson, D. J. Clark, and M. D. Yow. A 12 year review of the antibiotic management of *Haemophilus influenzae* meningitis. *Pediatrics* 1972;81:370.

21. Thornsberry, C., and L. A. Kirven. Antimicrobial susceptibility of *Haemophilus influenzae*. *Antimicrob. Agents Chemother.* 1974;6:620.

22. DeGraaff, J. L. P. Elwell, and S. Falkow. Molecular nature of two β-lactamase-specifying plasmids isolated from *Haemophilus influenzae* type B. *J. Bacteriol.* 1976;126:439.

23. Murray, B. E., and R. C. Moellering. Patterns and mechanisms of antibiotic resistance. *Med. Clin. North Am.* 1978;62:899.

24. Committee on Infectious Diseases. Ampicillin-resistant strains of *Haemophilus influenzae* type B. *Pediatrics* 1975;55:145.

25. Kenny, J. F., C. D. Isburg, and R. H. Michaels. Meningitis due to *Haemophilus influenzae* type b resistant to both ampicillin and chloramphenicol. *Pediatrics* 1980;66:14.

26. Uchiyama, N., G. R. Greene, D. B. Kitts, and L. D. Thrupp. Meningitis due to *Haemophilus influenzae* type b resistant to ampicillin and chloramphenicol. *J. Pediat.* 1980;97:421.

27. Belohradsky, B. H., K. Bruch, D. Geiss, D. Kafetzis, W. Marget, and G. Peters. Intravenous cefotaxime in children with bacterial meningitis. *Lancet* 1980; 1:61.

28. Schaad, U. B., G. H. McCracken, N. Threlkeld, and M. L. Thomas. Clinical evaluation of a new broad-spectrum oxa-beta-lactam antibiotic, moxalactum, in neonates and infants. *J. Pediatr* 1981;98:129.

29. Weinstein, L., and A. C. Dalton. Host determinants of response to antimicrobial agents. *N. Engl. J. Med.* 1968;279:467–473;524–531;580–588.

30. Parker, C. W., Drug allergy. *N. Engl. J. Med.*, 1975;292: 511,732,957.

31. Dewdney, J. M. Immunology of the antibiotics. In *The Antigens*, Vol. 4, ed. by M. Sela. New York: Academic Press, 1977, pp. 73–245.

32. Ahlstedt, S., The antibacterial effects of low concentrations of antibiotics and host defense factors: a review. *J. Antimicrob. Chemother.* 1981;8(Suppl. C):59.

33. Barling, R. W. A., and J. B. Selkon. The penetration of antibiotics into cerebrospinal fluid and brain tissue. *Antimicrob. Chemother.* 1978;4:203.

34. Pitt, H. A., R. A. Roberts, and W. D. Johnson. Gentamicin levels in the human biliary tract. *J. Infect. Dis.* 1973;127:299.

35. Sachs, J., T. Geer, P. Noell, and C. M. Kunin. Effect of renal function on urinary recovery of orally administered nitrofurantoin. *N. Engl. J. Med.* 1968; 278:1032.

36. Bennett, W. M., R. S. Muther, R. A. Parker, P. Feig, G. Morrison, T. A. Golper, and I. Singer. Drug therapy in renal failure: dosing guidelines for adults. Part I: Antimicrobial agents, analgesics. *Ann. Intern. Med.* 1980;93:62.

37. Hewitt, W. L, and M. C. McHenry. Blood level determinations of antimicrobial drugs. Some clinical considerations. *Med. Clin. North Am.* 1978;62:1119.

38. Barrett, S. P. and P. J. Watt. Antibiotics and the liver. *J. Antimicrob. Chemother.* 1979;5:337.

39. McCraken, G. H., Pharmacological basis for antimicrobial therapy in newborn infants. *Am. J. Dis. Child* 1974;128:407.

40. Weiss, C. F., A. J. Glazko, and J. K. Weston. Chloramphenicol in the newborn infant: a physiologic explanation of its toxicity when given in excessive doses. *N. Engl. J. Med.* 1960;262:787.

41. Siber, G. R., P. Echevirria, A. L. Smith, J. W. Paisley, and D. H. Smith. Pharmacokinetics of gentamicin in children and adults. *J. Infect. Dis.* 1975;132: 637.

42. Anton, A. H. Increasing activity of sulfonamides with displacing agents: a review. *Ann. N.Y. Acad. Sci.* 1973;226:273.

43. Grossman, E. R., A. Walchek, and H. Freedman.

Tetracyclines and permanent teeth: the relation between dose and tooth color. *Pediatrics* 1971;47:567.

44. Eichenwald, H. F. and G. H. McCracken. Antimicrobial therapy in infants and children. *J. Pediatr.* 1978;93:337.

45. Moellering, R. C. Factors influencing the clinical use of antimicrobial agents in elderly patients. *Geriatrics* 1974;33:83.

46. A joint statement of the American Thoracic Society, American Lung Association, and The Center for Disease Control. Preventive therapy of tuberculosis infection. *Am. Rev. Respir. Dis.* 1974;110:371.

47. Ford, R. D., Cephaloridine, cephalothin and the kidney. *J. Antimicrob. Chemother.* 1975;1(Suppl.):119.

48. Koch-Weser, J., V. W. Sidel, E. B. Federman, P. Kanarek, D. C. Finer, and A. E. Eaton. Adverse effects of sodium colistimethate. *Ann. Intern Med.*, 1970;72:857.

49. Jackson, G. G., and G. Arcieri. Ototoxicity of gentamicin in man: survey and controlled analysis of clinical experience in the United States. *J. Infect. Dis.* 1971;124(Suppl.):130.

50. Moellering, R. C. Special consideration of the use of antimicrobial agents during pregnancy, post partum, and in the newborn. *Clin. Obstet. Gynecol.* 1979;22:373.

51. Schultz, J. C., J. S. Adamson, W. W. Workman, and T. D. Norman. Fatal liver disease after intravenous administration of tetracycline in high dosage. *N. Engl. J. Med.* 1963;269:999.

52. Conway, N. and B. D. Birt. Streptomycin in pregnancy: effect on the foetal ear. *BMJ* 1965;2:260.

53. Anderson, P. O. Drugs and breast feeding. *Drug Intel. Clin. Pharmacy* 1977;11:208.

54. Harley, J. D. and H. Robin. Jaundice of late onset. *Pediatrics* 1966;37:856.

55. Belton, E. M., and R. V. Jones. Hemolytic anemia due to nalidixic acid. *Lancet* 1965;2:691.

56. Weber, W. W. and D. W. Hein. Clinical pharmacokinetics of isoniazid. *Clin. Pharmacokinet.* 1979;4:401.

57. Devadatta, S., P. R. J. Gangadharam, R. H. Andrews, W. Fox, C. V. Ramakrishnan, J. B. Selkon, and S. Velu. Peripheral neuritis due to isoniazid. *Bull. World Health Organ.* 1960;23:587.

58. Musch, E., M. Eichelbaum, J. K. Wang, W. von Sassen, M. Castro-Parra, and A. J. Dengler. Die Häufigkeit hepatotoxisher Nebenwirkungen der Tuberkulostatischen Kombinationstherapie (INH, RMP, EMB) in Abhängigkeit vom Acetyliererphänotyp. *Klin. Wochenschr.* 1982;60:513.

59. Kutt, H., W. Winters, and F. H. McDowell. Depression of parahydroxylation of diphenylhydantoin by antituberculous chemotherapy. *Neurology* 1966;16:594.

60. Beutler, E. Drug-induced hemolytic anemia. *Pharmacol. Rev.* 1969;21:73.

61. Frick, P. G., W. H. Hitzig, and K. Betke. Hemoglobin Zürich. I. New hemoglobin anomaly associated with acute hemolytic episodes with inclusion bodies after sulfonamide therapy. *Blood* 1962;20:261.

62. Rigas, D. A., and R. D. Koler. Decreased erythrocyte survival in hemoglobin H disease as a result of abnormal properties of hemoglobin H: benefit of splenectomy. *Blood* 1961;18:1.

63. de Matteis, F. Disturbances of liver porphyrin metabolism caused by drugs. *Pharmacol. Rev.* 1967;19:523.

64. Chanarin, I., and J. M. England. Toxicity of trimethoprim-sulfamethoxazole in patients with megaloblastic haemopoiesis. *BMJ* 1972;1:651.

65. Mazze, R. I., and M. J. Cousins. Combined nephrotoxicity of gentamicin and methoxyfluorane anesthesia in man. *Br. J. Anesth.* 1973;45:394.

66. Dentino, M. E., F. C. Luft, M. H. Yum, and L. H. Einhorn. Long term effect of *cis*-diamminedichloride platinum on renal function and structure in man. *Cancer* 1978;41:1274.

67. West, B. A., R. E. Brummett, and D. L. Himes: Interaction of kanamycin and ethacrynic acid. *Arch. Otolaryngol.* 1973;998:32.

68. Pittinger, C., and R. Adamson. Antibiotic blockade of neuromuscular function. *Annu. Rev. Pharmacol.* 1972;12:169.

69. Wright, D. G., K. J. Robichaud, P. A. Pizzo, and A. B. Diesseroth. Lethal pulmonary reactions associated with the combined use of amphotericin B and leukocyte transfusions. *N. Engl. J. Med.* 1981;304:1185.

70. Shapiro, M., T. R. Townsend, B. Rosner, and E. H. Kass. Use of antimicrobial drugs in general hospitals. *N. Eng. J. Med.* 1979;301:351.

71. Kunin, C. M., T. Tupasi, and W. A. Craig. Use of antibiotics: a brief exposition of the problem and some tentative solutions. *Ann. Intern. Med.* 1979;79:555.

72. Jacoby, I., L. A. Mandell, and L. Weinstein. The chemoprophylaxis of infection. A brief review of recent studies. *Med. Clin. North Am.* 1978;62:1083.

73. Goldman, P. L., and R. G. Petersdorf. Prophylactic antibiotics: controversies give way to guidelines. *Drug Therapy* 1979;9:57.

74. Hirshman, J. V., and T. S. Inui. Antimicrobial prophylaxis: a critique of recent trials. *Rev. Infect. Dis.* 1980;2:1.

75. Chodak, G. W., and M. E. Plaut. Use of systemic antibiotics for prophylaxis in surgery. *Arch. Surg.* 1977;112:326.

76. Jawitz, E. The use of combinations of antimicrobial drugs. *Annu. Rev. Pharmacol.* 1968;8:151.

77. Rahal, J. J. Antibiotic combinations: the clinical relevance of synergy and antagonism. *Medicine* 1978;57:179.

78. Lepper, M. H., and H. F. Dowling. Treatment of pneumococcal meningitis with penicillin compared with penicillin plus aureomycin. *Arch. Intern. Med.* 1951;88:489.

79. Wehrle, P. F., A. W. Mathies, J. M. Leedom, and D. Ivler. Bacterial meningitis. *Ann. N.Y. Acad. Sci.* 1967;145:488.

80. Rocco, V., and G. Overturf. Chloramphenicol inhibition of the bactericidal effect of ampicillin against *Haemophilus influenzae*. *Antimicrob. Agents Chemother.* 1982;21:349.

81. Anhalt, J. P., L. D. Sabath, and A. L. Barry. Special tests: bactericidal activity, activity of antimicrobics in combination, and detection of β-lactamase produc-

tion. In *Manual of Clinical Microbiology*, 3rd ed., ed. by E. H. Lennette, A. Balows, W. J. Hausler, and J. P. Truant. Washington DC: American Society of Microbiology, 1980, pp. 463–474.

82. Ernst, J. D., and M. E. Sande. Antibiotic combinations in experimental infections in animals. *Rev. Infect. Dis.* 1982;4:302.

83. Eliopoulos, G. M., and R. C. Moellering. Antibiotic synergism and antimicrobial combinations in clinical infections. *Rev. Infect. Dis.* 1982;4:282.

84. Sande, M. A., and W. M. Scheld. Combination antibiotic therapy of bacterial endocarditis. *Ann. Intern. Med.* 1980;92:390.

85. Karchmer, A. W., R. C. Moellering, D. Maki, and M. N. Swartz: Single antibiotic therapy of streptococcal endocarditis. *JAMA* 1979;241:1801.

86. Medoff, G., and G. S. Kobayashi: Strategies in the treatment of systemic fungal infections. *N. Engl. J. Med.* 1980;302:145.

87. Block, E. R., and J. F. Bennett. The combined effect of 5-fluorocytosine and amphotericin B in the therapy of murine cryptococcosis. *Proc. Soc. Exp. Biol. Med.* 1973;142:476.

88. Titsworth, E., and E. Grumberg. Chemotherapeutic activity of 5-fluorocytosine and amphotericin B against *Candida albicans* in mice. *Antimicrob. Agents Chemother.* 1973;4:306.

89. Wise, R., J. M. Andrews, and K. A. Bedford. In vitro study of clavulinic acid in combination with penicillin, amoxycillin, and carbenicillin. *Antimicrob. Agents Chemother.* 1978;13:389.

90. Neu, H. C., and K. P. Fu. Clavulinic acid, a novel inhibitor of β-lactamases. *Antimicrob. Agents Chemother.* 1978;14:650.

91. Bach, M. C., M. Finland, O. Gold, and C. Wilcox. Susceptibility of recently isolated pathogenic bacteria to trimethoprim and sulfamethoxazole separately and combined. *J. Infect. Dis.* 1973;128(Suppl.):508.

92. Neu, H. C. Mecillinam: a novel penicillanic acid derivate with unusual activity against gram-negative bacteria. *Antimicrob. Agents Chemother.* 1976;9:793.

93. Neu, H. C. Synergy of mecillinam, a beta-lactam antibiotics. *Antimicrob. Agents Chemother.* 1976;10:535.

94. Grunberg, E., R. Cleeland, G. Beskid, and W. F. DeLorenzo. In vivo synergy between 6β-amidino penicillanic acid derivatives and other antibiotics. *Antimicrob. Agents Chemother.* 1976;9:589.

95. Cohn, M. L., G. Middlebrook, and W. F. Russell. Combined drug treatment of tuberculosis. I. Prevention of emergence of mutant populations of tubercle bacilli resistant to both streptomycin and isoniazid in vitro. *J. Clin. Invest.* 1959;38:1349.

96. Bennett, J. E., W. E. Dismukes, R. J. Duma, G. Medoff, M. A. Sande, H. Gallis, J. Leonard, B. T. Fields, M. Bradshaw, H. Haywood, Z. A. McGee, T. R. Cate, G. C. Cobbs, J. F. Warner, and D. W. Alling. A comparison of amphotericin B alone and combined with flucytosine in the treatment of cryptococcal meningitis. *N. Engl. J. Med.* 1979;301:126.

97. McGowan, K., and S. L. Gorbach. Combination antibiotics for mixed infections. In *Combination antibiotics Therapy in the Compromised Host*, ed. by J. Klastersky and M. J. Staquet. New York: Raven Press, 1982, pp. 167–190.

98. Wade, J. C., and S. C. Schimpff. Antibiotic therapy for febrile granulocytopenic patients. In *Combination Antibiotic Therapy in the Compromized Host*, ed. by J. Klastersky and M. J. Staquet. New York: Raven Press, 1982, pp. 125–146.

99. Klastersky, J. Treatment of severe infections in patients with cancer. The role of new acyl-penicillins *Arch. Intern. Med.* 1982;142:1984.

CHAPTER TWO

Drug Resistance

Drug resistance is one of the most important problems in present-day antimicrobial chemotherapy. Several diseases that for many years were sensitive to antibiotic therapy are suddenly no longer sensitive to the same drugs. This has created a major problem for treatment of these diseases. Classically, *Yersinia pestis*, the causative agent of plague, is uniformly susceptible to the antibiotics streptomycin, chloramphenicol, and tetracycline. Recently, however, high-level resistance to multiple antibiotics has been reported.[1] Tuberculosis, which was believed to be under control in the U.S., is once again a major problem in certain population groups, a result of the emergence of *Mycobacterium tuberculosis* strains resistant to multiple anti-TB drugs.[2] *Drug resistance* is a condition in which there is insensitivity or decreased sensitivity to drugs that ordinarily cause inhibition of cell growth or cell death. Resistance can be either natural or acquired. In *acquired resistance*, the populations are initially sensitive but undergo a change so that they become less sensitive or insensitive to the drug. Tables 2–1 and 2–2 summarize some of the more current and serious problems with drug resistance, both in terms of organisms and drugs.

Intrinsic Resistance

Intrinsic resistance refers to a microorganism's inherent insensitivity to a drug. If an organism lacks the receptor for the drug, it will not respond and is therefore inherently insensitive to the antibiotic action. The *poly-enes* (e.g., amphotericin B, nystatin) are antibiotics that kill fungi by altering the permeability of the cell membrane. These drugs bind tightly to sterols in the fungal cell membrane, and the presence of sterol is required for drug action. Since bacterial membranes do not contain sterols, they are insensitive to the antibiotic. Most bacteria do not respond to isoniazid, a drug used to treat tuberculosis. There is good evidence that isoniazid is effective against the mycobacteria because it inhibits the synthesis of mycolic acids, which are unique components of mycobacterial cell walls. Since other bacteria do not have the biochemical pathway containing the target for the drug action, they are inherently insensitive.

Bacteria often contain the drug receptor but do not respond because the concentration of antibiotic at the target side is inadequate. Although the organism is not insensitive, for all practical purposes it behaves as if it were with respect to the chemotherapeutic goal. The failure of fungi to respond to rifampin is an example of this type of intrinsic resistance. The site of action of rifampin is in the cell interior where inhibition of DNA-dependent RNA polymerase occurs. Although fungal polymerases are inhibited by the antibiotic, rifampin is not particularly effective against fungi because it does not readily pass through the fungal cell envelope to its site of action. This intrinsic resistance of the fungus can be altered by simultaneous exposure to a polyene antibiotic, such as amphotericin B. In the presence of a low concentration of amphotericin B, the entry of other drugs into the cell is in some way fa-

Table 2–1.   The most serious antibiotic-resistant bacteria.

Antibiotic	Organism	Disease
Aminoglycosides	*Mycobacteium* spp.	Tuberculosis
	Enterobacteriaceae	Bacteremia, pneumonia, and surgical wound infections
	Pseudomonas	Bacteremia, pneumonia, urinary tract infections
β-lactams (penicillins, cephalosporins, etc.)	Enterobacteriaceae	
	Neisseria gonorrhea	Gonorrhea
	Hemophilus influenzae	Pneumonia, sinusitis, epiglottitis, meningitis, ear infections
Vancomycin	*Staphylococcus aureus*	Bacteremia, pneumonia, surgical wound infections
	Enteroccocus	Catheter infections, blood poisoning
Clindamycin	*Bacteroides* spp.	Anaerobic infections, septicemia
Erythromycin	*Enterococcus* spp.	Meningitis, pneumonia
	Streptococcus pneumoniae	
Isoniazid, ethambutol, pyrazinamide, and rifampin	*Mycobacterium* spp.	Tuberculosis
Chloramphenicol, ampicillin, trimethoprim-sulfamethoxazole, tetracycline	*Shigella dysenteriae*	Severe diarrhea
Ciprofloxacin	*Pseudomonas aeruginosa, S. aureus*	

Source: Adapted from Davies.[3]

cilitated. Rifampin now enters the organism, sufficient concentrations of drug are achieved at the site of action, and the synthesis of fungal RNA is inhibited.

A major example of intrinsic resistance on the part of an organism that contains appropriate drug targets is provided by the gram-negative bacilli. The difference in the permeability barrier provided by the cell envelopes of gram-negative and gram-positive organisms is important in determining sensitivity patterns to the penicillins.[5] *Gram-positive bacteria* are encased in a cell membrane surrounded by a peptidoglycan wall. In these organisms, the penicillins have very easy access to their target sites, the

Table 2–2.   Some examples of current problems with antimicrobial drugs because of resistance, according to organism.

Mycobacterium spp.	Multidrug-resistant *Mycobacterium* tuberculosis; multidrug-resistant *M. avium* complex (MAC)
Gram-positive cocci	Methicillin-resistant *Staphylococcus aureus* and coagulase-negative staphylococci; multidrug-resistant *Enterococcus*
Gram-negative cocci	Penicillin-resistant meningococci; quinolone-resistant gonococci
Gram-negative bacilli	*Enterobacter* and Enterobacteriaceae with chromosomal β-lactamases; multidrug-resistant *Pseudomonas aeruginosa* with aminoglycoside modifying enzymes; Enterobacteriaceae with extended spectrum β-lactamases; multi-drug-resistant *Yersinia pestis* (plague)

Source: Modified from Moellering.[4]

penicillin-binding proteins, which are attached to the cytoplasmic membrane. The *gram-negative envelope* is much more complex (see Fig. 3–10)[6,7] and, in general, it is less permeable to the antibiotic. The gram-negative cell envelope has a second membrane external to the peptidoglygan wall, and a penicillin must pass through pores or channels that span the outer membrane and diffuse through the periplasmic space before reaching its site of action. Some penicillins (penicillin G and the other narrow-spectrum compounds) that are effective against gram-positive bacteria do not readily pass through the pores in the outer membrane of many gram-negative bacilli. The chemical modifications that yielded the broad-spectrum penicillins (e.g., ampicillin, carbenicillin) make it possible for these drugs to pass more easily through the pores in the outer layer of the envelope and thus be effective against many gram-negative infections.

Escape from the Antibiotic Effect

Sometimes bacteria are sensitive to an antibiotic and sufficient concentrations are achieved at the site of action, but the organism is able to escape the consequences of the drug effect. Sulfonamides prevent the normal production of purines, thymidine, methionine, and serine by blocking the synthesis of the folate cofactor. But if these compounds are present in the environment, the bacterium may be able to utilize them as precursors for further biochemical synthesis and escape the consequences of the drug blockade. In purulent infections, the pus may contain a considerable amount of these substances as a result of tissue necrosis and the efficacy of the sulfonamides is compromised.

Acquired Drug Resistance

Resistance is *acquired* when populations of microorganisms that are initially sensitive to a drug undergo a change so that they become less sensitive or insensitive.[8,9] A population of organisms can lose its sensitivity to an antibiotic while the patient is under treatment. In some cases, the loss of sensitivity may be slight, but often organisms become resistant to any clinically achievable concentration of drug. The relative abundance of resistant organisms in a microbial population increases as continuing antibiotic therapy preferentially eliminates drug-sensitive cells. This process of enrichment is called *selection*, and the continuing presence of the antibiotic is said to exert a selective pressure in favor of the resistant organisms.

Microorganisms become less sensitive to antibiotics through a variety of biochemical mechanisms (Table 2–3).[10,11] The major mechanisms of resistance determined for clinical microbial isolates will be discussed as each drug is presented in subsequent chapters. In addition to the clinically important mechanisms, some unique modes of resistance studied only in laboratory strains will be discussed. These examples will be presented either because the resistance mechanism has played an important role in defining the biochemical mechanism of the drug action or to point out some of the ingenious ways in which microorganisms can change in order to live in the presence of antibiotics.

Most antibiotic resistance in microorganisms fits one of several general mechanisms, which may be classified as follows:

1. *Decreased drug uptake or increased efflux of the drug*: The principal mechanism of tetracycline resistance in bacteria. In recent years active efflux systems have been responsible for resistance of mammalian cells to a variety of structurally unrelated antibiotics and toxic compounds. This mechanism is being recognized more frequently in a variety of bacteria.[12]
2. *Enzymatic inactivation of drug*: The principal mechanism of resistance to the penicillins, aminoglycosides, and chloramphenicol.
3. *Decreased conversion of a drug to the active growth inhibitory compound*: The antifungal drug flucytosine must be converted in the organism to fluorouracil, which is further metabolized to the active form of the drug. Fungi

become resistant to flucytosine by losing the activity of enzymes along the activation pathway.

4. *Increased concentration of a metabolite antagonizing the drug action*: This has been shown to occur rarely in bacteria resistant to sulfonamides (increased amounts of para-aminobenzoic acid).

5. *Altered amount of drug receptor*: Some organisms become resistant to trimethoprim by synthesizing large amounts of dihydrofolate reductase, the target of the drug action. The alteration may be in the direction of less receptor as well.

6. *Decreased affinity of receptor for the drug*: This mechanism has been defined in bacteria resistant to sulfonamides, trimethoprim, streptomycin, erythromycin, rifampin, and several other antibiotics.

Microbial populations, particularly large inocula, often contain a few resistant organisms before the initiation of therapy. In some cases, the initial population is comprised solely of drug-sensitive cells, but one or a few organisms subsequently become resistant and are selected out during therapy. Drug resistance is acquired in two ways: it may arise de novo by mutation or gene amplification, or it may be transferred to the infecting organism from other bacteria in the form of extrachromosomal pieces of DNA that contain the information for the resistance mechanism.

The chromosomal type of resistance that arises because of mutation may change antibiotic sensitivity greatly or moderately, depending upon the location, type, and biological consequence of the mutation. For example, a single point mutation in the part of a gene coding for the receptor site of a drug may have one of several effects. The receptor protein may be altered so that it will no longer be able to bind the drug, although it still can carry out its biological function (assuming that the protein is an enzyme) sufficiently well to permit survival of the microorganism. This would constitute an example of a large-step mutation to drug insensitivity and it occurs very rarely in the clinical setting (e.g., altered ribosomal protein conferring complete resistance to streptomycin;[13] altered binding proteins conferring high-level resistance to penicillin G in pneumococci[14]). Or the receptor protein may be altered so that it has less affinity for the drug. In this case, the antibiotic is still effective, but higher concentrations are required. Additional mutational events, each conferring a small degree of resistance by one of the general mechanisms outlined above, will lead eventually to the production of organisms that are resistant to the concentrations of antibiotic achievable in therapy. This is called the *multiple-step pattern of resistance* as opposed to the facultative large-step pattern. It has been well docu-

Table 2–3. *Mechanisms of resistance to antibacterial agents.*

Antibiotic	Major mechanisms of resistance
Penicillins and cephalosporins	Increased production of β-lactamase enzymes
Macrolides	Alterations in the bacterial ribosome
Quinolones	Alterations in DNA gyrase and decreased permeability because of an altered porin protein (OmpF)
Vancomycin	Modified cell wall precursors with decreased affinity for vancomycin
Aminoglycosides	Increased production of aminoglycoside modifying enzymes (acetylation, phosphorylation, or adenylation)
Chloramphenicol	Increased presence of a specific acetyl transferase that inactivates the drug
Tetracyclines	Decreased accumulation as a result of increased drug efflux resulting from acquisition of a plasmid encoding an efflux transporter

mented that the mutations that lead to resistance occur as random events in the bacterial population.[15,16] Thus, they occur whether or not the antibiotic is present and the drug only exerts a selection pressure.

Drug Resistance by Gene Transfer

Most of the antibiotic resistance that occurs clinically is due to the transfer of segments of DNA containing drug resistance genes from one bacterium to another. Transfer of the DNA may occur by transformation, transduction, or conjugation. In *transformation*, soluble pieces of DNA containing resistance genes are taken up from the environment by a drug-sensitive bacterium. This is probably not a common clinical mechanism by which resistance is transferred. In *transduction*, the genes for determining drug resistance are located in a plasmid and this extra-chromosomal DNA is transferred from one bacterium to another by a phage. This mechanism of transferring antibiotic resistance is of considerable clinical importance. The great majority of the penicillin-resistant staphylococci, for example, have acquired plasmids that contain genes for β-lactamases.[17] In *conjugation*, the drug resistance genes contained in a plasmid are passed from one cell to another through a direct contact formed by a sex pilus. Conjugation occurs primarily among the gram-negative bacilli and it is the principal mechanism by which resistance is transferred among the enterobacteria.[18] The plasmids that are transferred via conjugation usually contain genes determining resistance to multiple drugs. Thus, in the clinical setting, resistant organisms selected during therapy with a penicillin, for example, may also contain genes that code for enzymes that inactivate chloramphenicol or some of the aminoglycosides. The fact that resistance to multiple drugs can be transferred from one bacterium to another is of great epidemiologic importance. In order to understand the effect of antimicrobial drug use on the drug sensitivity of bacteria, both in the patient undergoing treatment and in the hospital environment in general, the physician must be familiar with the principles of resistance transfer.

R Factors and the Problem of Infectious, Multiple Drug Resistance

The First Observations

At the end of World War II, the sulfonamides were introduced into Japan for the treatment of bacillary dysentery. As a result, the incidence of the disease decreased by about 80% within 2 years.[19] After 1949, however, the incidence of dysentery rose above the level observed at the end of the war. This higher incidence was seen despite the extensive use of sulfonamides; most of the *Shigella* strains isolated from cases at that time were found to be resistant to the drug. After 1952, newer antibiotics, such as streptomycin, chloramphenicol, and the tetracyclines, were used to treat the sulfonamide-resistant shigellae. With the advent of these newer drugs, the number of dysentery patients fell somewhat, but within only 4 years it became clear that their therapeutic usefulness was also diminishing rapidly. After 1952, Japanese workers isolated one strain of *Shigella* from each dysentery epidemic and tested it for resistance to streptomycin, chloramphenicol, and the tetracyclines (see Table 2–4). By 1958, a number of the strains being recovered were simultaneously resistant to two or three of these antibiotics. Many of the strains listed in the table were resistant to sulfonamides as well.

In epidemiologic studies, *Shigella* strains isolated from some patients were completely sensitive, whereas serologically identical strains isolated from other patients in the same epidemic were resistant to a number of drugs. Stool cultures from a single patient were sometimes found to contain both sensitive and multiple drug–resistant strains of the same serological type. Finally, it was observed that the administration of chloramphenicol alone to patients infected with sensitive *Shigella* could result in the appearance of organisms that were resistant to many drugs. These findings were tied together when one of the Japanese investigators postulated that multiple drug resistance might

Table 2–4. Antibiotic resistance in Shigellae isolated from epidemics of bacillary dysentery in Japan. One strain of Shigella was isolated from each epidemic of bacillary dysentery occurring in Japan from 1953 to 1969 and tested for resistance to streptomycin (Sm), tetracycline (Tc), and chloramphenicol (Cm).

Year	Number of strains tested	Number of strains resistant to:						
		Sm	Tc	Cm	Sm, Cm	Sm, Tc	Cm, Tc	Sm, Cm, Tc
1953	4900	5	2	0	0	0	0	0
1956	4399	8	4	0	0	0	1	0
1958	6563	18	20	0	7	2	0	193
1960	3396	29	36	0	61	9	7	308

Source: Data from Watanabe.[19]

be transferred from multiple drug–resistant *E. coli* to shigellae in the patient's intestinal tract. It was demonstrated that multiple drug–resistant *E. coli* could be cultured in vitro with sensitive *Shigella* and that the multiple resistance could then be transferred to the shigellae without the simultaneous transfer of a number of genetic markers that are a part of the genome of *E. coli*.[20]

The Mechanism

Since the original observations of drug resistance transfer, we have come to know a great deal more about the mechanisms by which drug resistance determinants are maintained and transmitted from cell to cell.[18,21,22] The genes coding for drug resistance are located in circular pieces of extrachromosomal DNA called *R-determinants*. In Enterobacteriaceae, R-determinants can be transferred to other bacteria after they become linked to another extrachromosomal piece of DNA called a *resistance transfer factor* (RTF). The complete unit is called an *R factor* or *R plasmid* (Fig. 2–1). The RTF contains the information required for bacterial conjugation, permitting the transmission of drug resistance genes to the appropriate recipient bacteria. Both R-determinants and RTF can exist as separate closed circles of DNA or combined as a complete R factor. Each unit (R-determinant, RTF, or the combination of the two) is called a *plasmid*; it contains its own genes

for replication and it replicates autonomously, that is, its replication is not linked to that of the chromosomal DNA. Plasmids usually determine resistance to more than one antibiotic and are classified according to incompatibility groups. Plasmids of the same incompatibility group are similar (they possess, considerable DNA homology), but they cannot stably coexist with each other. They can, however, cohabitate with each member of any other incompatibility set, and a bacterial cell may contain multiple plasmids as long as they belong to different incompatibility groups.

Some resistance genes, such as the TEM β-lactamase gene of gram-negative bacteria (see detailed discussion of β-lactamases in Chapter 3), have been found in a wide variety of plasmids located in many different organisms. For a number of years, it was not understood how these drug resistance genes were disseminated so rapidly and widely. It is now clear that the dissemination is due to transposable genetic elements capable of integration into numerous nonhomologous sequences of DNA. The genes for the TEM β-lactamase, for example, can jump (transpose) from one plasmid to another, from a plasmid to the bacterial chromosome, and from a chromosome to a plasmid in a manner that does not require the recombination functions of the bacterium.[23,24] This ability to transpose drug resistance genes from one site to another depends on the presence of *insertion sequences* (IS), which are discrete

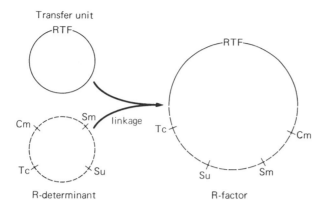

Figure 2–1. Diagram of the formation of an R factor that contains information for determining resistance to tetracycline (Tc), sulfonamide (Su), streptomycin (Sm), and chloramphenicol (Cm). Genetic determinants for antibiotic resistance (R determinants) can exist independently of the transfer factor or in combination with it. The transfer unit contains the genetic information that directs the transfer of the whole plasmid during bacterial conjugation.

DNA sequences that range in length from 800 to 1800 base pairs (bp).[25] A span of one or more genes with an insertion sequence at each end is called a *transposon* (Tn).

A well-studied transposon for tetracycline resistance is shown in the genetic map of plasmid R100 in Figure 2–2.[26] This R factor contains several IS elements and the transposon for tetracycline resistance, Tn10, which is composed of the determinants for tetracycline resistance bordered on each end by the insertion sequence IS10. Because the IS10 elements exist as inverted repeating sequences of DNA, they can join with each other, permitting the formation of loops containing the resistance gene which are then excised by endonucleases. As diagrammed in the bottom half of Figure 2–2, the excised Tn10 transposon then becomes integrated into another plasmid or into chromosomal DNA at certain favored "hot spots" for insertion.[25] The mechanisms by which transposable elements move from one genetic site to another are not yet completely defined, but the result is the transfer of the complete resistance gene from one locus to another. The existence of transposons combined with the selective pressure of widespread antibiotic use accounts for the rapid spread of resistance genes and the evolution of R factors containing multiple drug resistance determinants.

Nonconjugative drug resistance plasmids (r plasmids) are considerably smaller than conjugative plasmids (R factors or R plasmids) because they do not contain the genes for conjugal transfer. Such plasmids were first demonstrated in *Staphylococcus aureus* and have subsequently been isolated from a variety of gram-positive and gram-negative bacteria[21] These plasmids are transferred from one bacterium to another by transduction and their transfer is highly strain specific among the staphylococci. These plasmids encode mostly for resistance to a single antibiotic and, infrequently, for resistance to two antibiotics. Clinical isolates of *Staphylococcus aureus* may be resistant to multiple drugs because they contain several r plasmids, each of which exists in multiple copies in the cell.

In addition to plasmids and transposons, other gene transfer elements are important in the development of antibiotic resistance. Recently, for example, it has been recognized that conjugative transposons are now making a significant contribution to the spread of resistance genes, especially among the *Bacteroides* spp. and gram-positive bacteria.[27] Conjugative transposons are DNA segments ranging in size from 18 to over 150 kbp that are normally integrated into the bacterial genome.[28] To transfer, they first excise themselves to form a nonreplicating circular intermediate. The circular intermediate is then transferred by conjugation to a recipient, where it integrates into the recipient's genome. Conjugative transposons differ from conventional transposons in that they have a circular intermediate, transfer by conjugation, and do not create a target site duplication when they integrate. They were first discovered in gram-positive cocci and *Bacteroides* but are

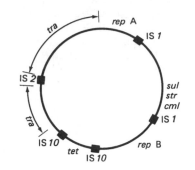

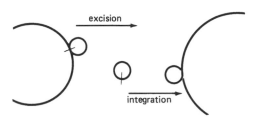

Figure 2–2. Genetic map of the resistance plasmid R100 and diagram of the transposition process. The determinants for tetracycline resistance *tet* are located in the 9.3 kilobase tetracycline resistance transposon, Tn10, which contains an IS10 insertion sequence at each end. The determinants governing conjugal transferability *tra* are split by another insertion sequence, IS2. *repA* and *repB* are genes governing replication of R plasmids and *sul, str,* and *cml* are resistance determinants for sulfanilamide, streptomycin, and chloramphenicol, respectively. The scheme at the bottom of the figure simply illustrates the excision and subsequent integration of the transposon into another plasmid or into bacterial chromosomal DNA. (Modified from Fig. 1 and 2 of Mitsuhashi.[26])

now found in a variety of genera including the enteric bacteria.[28,29] Conjugative transposons appear to be interactive with plasmids, resulting in a greater mobilization of these elements.[27] This is of great significance for bacterial resistance to antibiotics. Much of the literature on gene transfer elements has been concerned with the different elements acting in isolation. Yet conjugative transposons and other elements apparently can and often do work together. These interactions enhance their collective ability to

transfer resistance genes. Interactions between the elements may also be one explanation of why antibiotic resistance genes are so resistant to elimination.

The Clinical and Epidemiologic Problem

Many physicians outside the specialty of infectious disease do not fully appreciate the impact of plasmid-mediated resistance on antibiotic therapy. The most recognized example of the importance of plasmids in altering antibiotic use is probably the change that occurred in the sensitivity of *Staphylococcus aureus* to penicillin G during the first 20 years of penicillin therapy. Prior to the extensive use of penicillins, essentially all of the clinical isolates of *S. aureus* were sensitive to penicillin G.[30] In the late 1940s and '50s, however, the widespread use of penicillin was accompanied by a rapid increase in the resistance of *S. aureus* strains isolated in the hospital and a slower rise among community-acquired strains. By 1967, this difference had disappeared and the resistance rates reported for both hospital-acquired and community-acquired strains were in the range of 80% to 85%.[11] This increase in penicillin resistance was almost entirely due to the selection of *S. aureus* strains containing r plasmids encoding for β-lactamase. Conspicuous plasmid-mediated changes in drug sensitivity such as the emergence of penicillin resistance in *S. aureus*, ampicillin resistance in *Haemophilus influenzae* group B, or penicillin resistance in *Neisseria gonorrhoeae* are discussed broadly in the literature and are noticed by physicians in general, but the broader trends in resistance that lead up to these dramatic changes in antibiotic sensitivity are often not appreciated.

One fact that is not widely appreciated is that nonpathogenic coliform organisms serve as a reservoir of plasmid-mediated resistance that can be transmitted to pathogens. For example, the presence of carbenicillin resistance in *Pseudomonas aeruginosa* infecting patients in a burn unit has been shown to be due to determinants transmitted

Table 2–5.   Antibiotic resistance of coliform bacilli from sewers serving isolated premises. Coliform organisms were cultured from effluent of sewers serving restricted premises, such as hospitals or adjacent residential areas. The coliform bacilli were then tested for antibiotic sensitivity by the disk method.

Area	Premises	Number of samples	Percentage of coliform bacilli resistant to:		
			Streptomycin	Chloramphenicol	Tetracycline
A	General hospital	3	48.8	0.4	24.3
	Residential area	3	0.6	0.007	0.1
B	General hospital	3	34.7	0.7	32.0
BC	Residential area	3	6.5	0.02	1.3
C	Mental hospital	2	9.5	0.03	0.4

Source: From Linton et al.[32]

on R factors and derived from other bacteria resident in the alimentary tract.[31] The resulting clinical problem in the burn unit may be considered by the medical personnel to be an epidemic of a resistant bacterium, but from a microbiologist's point of view it is really an epidemic of the R factor. Treatment of a patient with an antibiotic to which R factor–mediated determinants exist is followed by the rapid conversion of the gut flora to the appropriate resistance pattern. (Sometimes as many as 90% of all strains isolated are resistant within a few days[31]). Since the resistance determinants are usually multiple, clinicians can enrich for coliform organisms resistant to penicillins and aminoglycosides, for example, while treating a patient with a tetracycline. When antibiotic treatment is ended, the percentage of resistant flora usually declines. This implies that R factors confer some growth disadvantage on the host bacteria.

The way antibiotic use can affect the resistance pattern of coliform bacteria can be appreciated from the data of Table 2–5.[32] In this study, researchers sampled the effluent of sewers draining hospitals and adjacent residential areas. Coliform bacteria were cultured and antibiotic sensitivity was determined on each strain. From the data, it is clear that there was high incidence of resistance in coliform organisms cultured from the sewers of general hospitals as compared to sewage draining from residential areas or a mental hospital. It was confirmed in the study that a much wider variety of antibiotics and many more courses of treatment were prescribed in the general hospital than in the large mental hospital.

In the above study, the coliform bacilli in the sewage from general hospitals had a much higher proportion of antibiotic resistance, more R factors, and a greater proportion of R factors carrying multiple resistance than sewage organisms from residential and other sources. Despite this enrichment in the effluent from general hospitals, it was calculated that 95% of the R factors in the total sewage output of this English city did not originate in hospitals. Thus, since the normal population appears to be the greatest source of R factors, one must ask what contributes to this drug resistance reservoir. The answer to the question is probably quite complex and it is certainly not yet defined.

One factor that may contribute to the maintenance of the pool of transmissible drug resistance plasmids is the selective pressure created by the widespread use of antibiotics in animal feeds. This practice has been the subject of wide discussion, both in the scientific community and in the popular press. The economic advantage of this practice has been clearly demonstrated. Although the basis for the effect is not well understood, the addition of certain antibiotics to animal feeds promotes growth.[33] The use of antibiotics as feed additives, even at very low concentrations, results in the emergence of resistance in a high percentage of the coliform bacteria.[34,35] There is clear evidence that the multiple drug resistance that has developed in animals emerges in the intestinal flora of farm personnel.[36-38] Tetracyclines are one of the major groups of antibiotics added to animal feed, and tetracycline resistance in both human and animal coliform bacteria has been studied in some detail. It has been shown that multiple drug–resistant *Salmonella* organisms derived from animals fed subtherapeutic amounts of chlortetracycline have caused serious illness in humans consuming processed meat that was sold in widely separated areas.[39] Thus, it is clear that animal-to-human transmission of antimicrobial-resistant enteric organisms occurs, but it is not clear to what extent the use of antibiotics as animal feed additives (this use accounts for about half of the antimicrobials produced yearly in the United States[40]) is responsible for the increased incidence of drug-resistant strains in humans. Some epidemiologic studies suggest that the main selective pressure for tetracycline resistance in the coliform organisms of humans who are not receiving the antibiotic lies in the use of the drug in human medicine rather than in its use as a growth supplement in livestock feed.[41]

Prevention of Resistance

The number of antibiotic-resistant strains of bacteria encountered in clinical settings is steadily increasing. However, there may be several steps that can be taken to prevent or decrease the incidence of resistance. Judicious use of antibiotics is one of the best measures. Physicians must be encouraged to restrict the prescribing of antibiotics for trivial complaints. In an ideal world, antibiotic sensitivity testing would be carried out before drugs are prescribed and the most appropriate agent or combination would be used, followed by more testing to ensure that the infection had been eliminated. Obviously, this is not practical and our best approach is to use more carefully those drugs for which there is the least evidence of resistance while concentrating efforts on developing new drugs to replace them.

There must also be a continuous effort to control the use of antibiotics in both humans and animals. The general public needs to be educated not to expect antibiotics to be used for everything and not to misuse them when they are prescribed. A recent report from the Hospital Infection Control Practices Advisory Committee on preventing the spread of vancomycin resistance stresses the need for professional and public educational programs, enhanced microbiological surveillance, enhanced surveillance among patients, effective implementation of infection control procedures as well as prudent use of antimicrobial agents for treatment and prophylaxis.[42] The use of antibiotics as animal food additives must also be limited. A comprehensive report by a National Academy of Science and Institute of Medicine panel on the risks and benefits of the use of antimicrobial agents in animal feed is an important effort dealing with this.[43]

Pharmaceutical and biotechnology firms are developing many potential new drugs intended to meet the challenge of resistant bacteria. Some of these new drugs work by unique mechanisms. For example, one drug company is investigating everninomicin, a drug that contains seven different sugars that are not involved in any class of medicine used in people.[44] Thus, no current form of drug resistance is likely to transfer to this antibiotic. Some companies are studying drugs that disable biochemical pumps that eject antibiotics as well as other drugs from resistant bacteria.[44]

Companies are also developing a variety of new vaccines to control bacterial infections.[44] Vaccines are now available against *Hemophilus influenzae* b as well as other infectious organisms, and new vaccines are being developed against the bacteria that commonly cause middle-ear infections in children.

Another strategy to prevent or decrease the incidence of resistance to antibacterial agents is combination chemotherapy. The probability of selecting cells that are resistant to therapy is decreased if two drugs with different mechanisms of action are administered together. The basis for this is the complete independence of mutational events leading to resistance. The probability is very small that a cell resistant to two drugs will arise. The first application of combination chemotherapy for suppression of drug resistance was in the treatment of tuberculosis. Combined therapy is now almost always used in this disease for this reason. Although it is an effective approach to prevent emergence of resistance in tuberculosis it is probably not effective for most bacterial infections in which resistance is due to transfer of multiple drug–resistant genes rather than mutation of chromosomal genes.

There must also be a continuing effort on the part of the pharmaceutical industry and scientists to better understand the mechanisms of drug resistance.[45] Agents targeted to block specific resistance mechanisms should be sought; examples are the β-lactamase inhibitors, such as clavulanic acid. Through the tools of molecular biology and computer modeling, more innovative ways of overcoming resistance will be discovered. For example, it may be possible to engineer genes capable of inactivating specific determinants of resistance.[46] Through the use of bioinformatics, the genetics of bacteria can be more easily studied and this in turn will help identify targets for attacking bacterial resistance. Furthermore, through the use of combinatorial chemistry, new drugs to use against bacterial resistance can be discovered much more quickly.

Regardless of what treatments are used, once people are infected with bacteria, everybody agrees that a crucial step in developing an effective offense against the bacteria must be the establishment of a strong surveillance system. This system should be able to identify resistance problems early, give clues as to why they are happening, and quickly provide critical information to public health officials worldwide. At present, there is no such system in place on a worldwide basis. There is one in the U.S. but the surveillance is uneven and has problems.[44]

REFERENCES

1. Galimand, M., A. Guiyoule, G. Gerband, B. Rasomanana, S. Chanteau, E. Carniel, and E. P. Courvalain. Multidrug resistance in *Yersinia pestis* mediated by a transferable plasmid. *N. Engl. J. Med.* 1997; 337:677.

2. Moore, M., I. M. Onorato, E. M. McCray, and K. G. Castro. Trends in drug-resistant tuberculosis in the United States, 1993–1996. *JAMA* 1997;278:833.

3. Davies, J. Bacteria on the rampage—the most serious antibiotic-resistant bacteria. *Nature* 1996;383: 219.

4. Moellering, R. Past, present and future of antimicrobial agents. *Am. J. Med.* 1995;99(Suppl. 6A): 6A.

5. Costerton, J. W., and K. J. Cheng. The role of the bacterial cell envelope in antibiotic resistance. *J. Antimicrob. Chemother.* 1975;1:363.

6. Nikaido, H., and T. Nakae. The outer membrane of gram-negative bacteria. *Adv. Microbiol. Physiol.* 1979;20:163.

7. DiRienzo, J. M., K. Nakamura, and M. Inouye. The outer membrane proteins of gram-negative bacteria: biosynthesis, assembly and functions. *Annu. Rev. Biochem.* 1978;47:481.

8. Bryan, L. E., ed. *Antimicrobial Drug Resistance.* Orlando, FL: Academic Press, 1984.

9. Mitsuhashi, S. ed. *Drug Resistance in Bacteria.* New York: Thiene-Stratton, 1982.

10. Davies, J., and D. I. Smith. Plasmid-determined resistance to antimicrobial agents. *Annu. Rev. Microbiol.* 1978;32:469.

11. Murray, B. E. and R. C. Moellering. Patterns and mechanisms of antibiotic resistance. *Med. Clin. North Am.* 1978;62:899.

12. Levy; S. B. Active efflux mechanisms for antimicrobial resistance. *Antimicrob. Agents Chemother.* 1992;36:695.

13. Shannon, K., and I. Phillips. Mechanisms of resistance to aminoglycosides in clinical isolates. *J. Antimicrob. Chemother.* 1982;9:91.

14. Williamson, R., S. Zighelboim, and A. Tomaz. Penicillin-binding proteins of penicillin-resistant and penicillin-tolerant *Streptococcus pneumoniae*. In *β-Lactam Antibiotics*, ed. by M. Salton and G. M. Shockman. New York: Academic Press, 1981, pp. 215–225.

15. Demerec, M. Origin of bacterial resistance to antibiotics. *J. Bacteriol.* 1948;56:43.

16. Goldstein, A., L. Aronow, and S. M. Kalman. Drug resistance. In *Principles of Drug Action.* New York: Wiley, 1974, pp. 517–567.

17. Lacey. R. W. Antibiotic resistance plasmids of *Staphylococcus aureus* and their clinical importance. *Bacteriol. Rev.* 1975;39:1.

18. Falkow, S. *Infectious Multiple Drug Resistance.* London: Pion Limited, 1975.

19. Watanabe, T. Infective heredity of multiple drug resistance in bacteria. *Bacteriol. Rev.* 1963;27:87.

20. Akiba, T., K. Koyama, Y. Ishiki, S. Kimura, and J. Fukushima. On the mechanism of the development of multiple-drug-resistant clones of Shigella. *Jpn. J. Microb.* 1960;4:219.

21. Mitsuhashi, S., ed. *R Factor Drug Resistance Plasmid.* Baltimore: University Park Press, 1977.

22. Mitsuhashi, S. Drug resistance plasmids. *Mol. Cell. Biochem.* 1979;26:135.

23. Cohen, S. N. Transposable genetic elements and plasmid evolution. *Nature* 1976;263:731.

24. Cohen, S. N., and D. J. Kopecko. Structural evolution of bacterial plasmids: role of translocating genetic elements and DNA sequence insertions. *Fed. Proc.* 1976;35:2031.

25. Kleckner, N. Transposable elements in prokaryotes. *Annu. Rev. Genet.* 1981;15:341.

26. Mitsuhashi, S. Translocatable drug resistance determinants. In *R Factor Drug Resistance Plasmid*, ed. by S. Mitsuhashi. Baltimore: University Park Press, 1977, pp. 73–87.

27. Salyers, A. A., and C. F. Amábile-Cuevas. Why are antibiotic resistance genes so resistant to elimination? *Antimicrob. Agents Chemother.* 1997;41:2321.

28. Salyers, A. A., N. B. Shoemaker, L. Y. Li, and A. M. Stevens. Conjugative transposons: an unusual and diverse set of integrated gene transfer elements. *Microbiol. Rev.* 1995;59:519.

29. Salyers, A. A., and N. B. Shoemaker. Resistance gene transfer in anaerobes: new insights, new problems. *Clin. Infect. Dis.* 1996;23(Suppl):536.

30. Finland, M. Changing patterns of susceptibility of common bacterial pathogens to antimicrobial agents. *Ann. Intern. Med.* 1972;76:1009.

31. Richmond M. H. R factors in man and his environment. In *Microbiology—1974*, ed. by D. Schlessinger. Washington, DC: American Society of Microbiology, 1975, pp. 27–35.

32. Linton, K. B., M. H. Richmond, R. Bevan, and W. A, Gillespie. Antibiotic resistance and R factors in coliform bacilli isolated from hospital and domestic sewage. *J. Med. Microbiol.* 1974;7:91.

33. Visek, W. J. The mode of growth promotion by antibiotics. *J. Anim. Sci.* 1978;46:1447.

34. Linton, K. B., P. A. Lee, and M. H. Richmond. Antibiotic resistance and transmissible R factors in the intestinal coliform flora of healthy adults and children in an urban and rural community. *J. Hygiene* 1972;70:99.

35. Pohl, P. Relationship between antibiotic feeding in animals and emergence of bacterial resistance in man. *J. Antimicrob. Chemother.* 1977;3(Suppl. C):67.

36. Fein, D., G. Burton, R. Tsutakawa, and D. Blenden. Matching of antibiotic resistance patterns of *Escherichia coli* of farm families and their animals. *J. Infect. Dis.* 1974;130:274.

37. Levy, S. B., G. B. FitzGerald, and A. B. Macone. Changes in intestinal flora of farm personnel after introduction of a tetracycline-supplemented feed on a farm. *N. Engl. J. Med.* 1976;295:583.

38. Marsik, F. J., J. T. Parisi, and J. C. Blenden. Transmissible drug resistance of *Escherichia coli* and *Salmonella* from humans, animals, and their rural environments. *J. Infect. Dis.* 1975;132:296.

39. Holmberg, S. D., M. T. Osterholm, K. A. Senger, and M. L. Cohen. Drug-resistant *Salmonella* from animals fed antimicrobials. *New Engl. J. Med.* 1984;311:617.

40. Holmberg, S. D., J. G. Wells, and M. L. Cohen. Animal-to-man transmission of antibiotic-resistant *Salmonella*: investigations of U.S. outbreaks, 1971–1983. *Science* 1984;225:833.

41. Richmond, M. H., and K. B. Linton. The use of tetracycline in the community and its possible relation to the excretion of tetracycline-resistant bacteria. *J. Antimicrob. Chemother.* 1980;6:33.

42. Food and Drug Administration. Anti-infective agent, biologics, and vaccines approved by the U.S. Food and Drug Administration's Center for Drug Evaluation and Research in 1993. *Antimicrob. Agents Chemother.* 1994;38:908.

43. Committee on Human Health Risk Assessment of Using Subtherapeutic Antibiotics in Animal Feed. Human health risks with the subtherapeutic use of a penicillin or tetracycline in animal feed. Washington, DC: National Academy Press, 1989.

44. Knudson, M. The hunt is on for new ways to overcome bacterial resistance. *Mitos. Tech. Rev.* 1998;100:22.

45. Gootz, T. D. Discovery and development of new antimicrobial agents. *Clin. Microb. Rev.* 1990;3:13.

46. Jacoby, G. A., and G. L. Archer. New mechanisms of bacterial resistance to antimicrobial agents. *N. Engl. J. Med.* 1991;324:601.

Drugs Employed in the Treatment of Bacterial Infections

CHAPTER THREE

The Inhibitors of Cell Wall Synthesis, I

Mechanism of Action of the Penicillins, Cephalosporins, Vancomycin, and Other Inhibitors of Cell Wall Synthesis

Discovery and Structure of the β-Lactam Antibiotics

The discovery of penicillin is a now classic story of serendipity in scientific investigation. In 1928, Fleming noted that bacteria growing in culture in the vicinity of a contaminating mold were lysed.[1] He followed up this observation by culturing the mold in broth and demonstrating that filtrates of the broth were bactericidal in vitro. Almost a decade later, a group at Oxford led by H. W. Florey isolated a crude preparation of the bactericidal agent from cultures of *Penicillium notatum*. These investigators subsequently demonstrated the usefulness of this antibiotic in the treatment of bacterial infections in humans. Although the basic unit of the penicillins has been synthesized, penicillin G, the most potent natural penicillin, is produced commercially by isolation from cultures of mold that have been genetically altered to produce a very high yield.

In many cases, a detailed knowledge of the structure of an antibiotic is not particularly critical for developing an understanding of the current state of knowledge regarding its mechanism of action. For the β-lactam antibiotics, however, a knowledge of the basic structure of the molecule is critical for understanding, at the molecular level, the basis of the mechanism of action, the development of bacterial cell resistance, and the mecha-

nisms underlying the allergic response. The basic penicillin structure is composed of a thiazolidine ring attached to a four-membered (β-lactam) ring and a side chain (R) attached in peptide linkage to the β-lactam ring. The four-membered ring is somewhat strained, and a number of important ring-opening reactions take place here. The cephalosporins and cephamycins have a similar basic structure with a β-lactam dihydrothiazine ring system.

Other β-lactams used clinically include the carbapenems and the monobactams, which are monocyclic β-lactams. The *carbapenems* have a carbon instead of a sulfur atom in the 1-position and an unsaturated bond between carbon atoms 2 and 3 in the five-membered ring.[2] At present, imipenem and meropenem are the only clinically available members of the carbapenems. In contrast to the bicyclic β-lactams, the *monobactams* are monocyclic β-lactam compounds. Aztreonam is the only clinically approved monobactam.

Mechanism of Action

Site of Action

The cell wall of a bacterium forms a rather rigid skeleton on the outer surface of the cell membrane. The bacterial cell membrane, in essence, encases a volume hypertonic to the environment of the organism. Although the

6-Aminopenicillanic acid

$$R-\overset{\overset{\displaystyle O}{\|}}{C}-NH-HC-HC\overset{S}{\diagdown}\overset{CH_3}{\underset{CH_3}{C}}$$

β-Lactam ring   Thiazolidine ring

Penicillins

7-Aminocephalosporanic acid

$$R_1-\overset{\overset{\displaystyle O}{\|}}{C}-NH-HC-HC\overset{S}{\diagdown}CH_2$$

COOH

R₂

Cephalosporins

Penam (penicillins)   Cepham (cephalosporins)

Carbapenem   Monobactam

β-Lactam core structures

longer viable, antibiotics that inhibit cell wall synthesis are usually bactericidal agents. The critical role of the autolysins in bringing about cell death after exposure to the penicillins and other drugs that inhibit cell wall synthesis will be expanded on later.

When the bacterium is growing in a medium isotonic to the cytoplasm, exposure to penicillin, rather than rupturing the bacterium, can lead to the production of organisms that have no cell wall.[3] Such bacteria, encased solely in their cell membrances, are called *protoplasts* or *spheroplasts*. The principal site of synthesis of the cell wall of many bacteria lies in a narrow growth zone that extends in a girdle around the organism. If *Escherichia coli,* for example, are exposed to penicillin, small protrusions of the cell

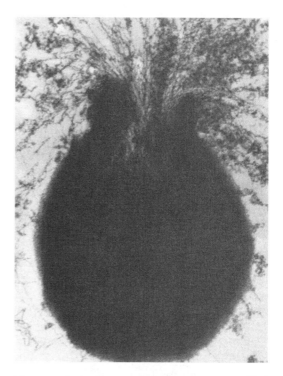

Figure 3–1. A staphylococcus, magnified 150,000 times, shown at the moment of exploding after exposure to a low concentration of an antibiotic that inhibits cell wall synthesis. At higher concentrations of drug, like those that are achieved in the clinical treatment of infection, the cell disintegrates in a more rapid and uniform manner. (Photograph kindly provided by Dr. Victor Lorian.)

cell membrane is critical to the maintenance of the osmotic gradient between the organism and its environment, it is not strong enough in itself to keep the hypertonic sac from rupturing by osmotic shock. Thus, the cell wall, which encases the cell membrane as a continuous, highly cross-linked molecule, prevents the cell membrane from rupturing. The drugs presented in this chapter all inhibit the synthesis of bacterial cell walls. Their killing effect results from continued activity of a group of bacterial surface enzymes, called *autolysins*, that cleave previously synthesized cell wall, creating weak points at which cell rupture eventually occurs (Fig. 3–1). Since the ruptured cell is no

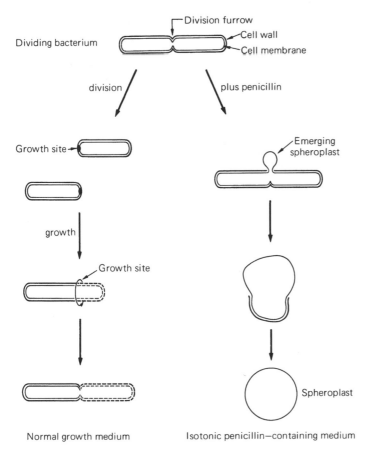

Figure 3–2. Normal cell growth and division compared to the formation of penicillin spheroplasts. Normal cell wall synthesis often takes place at a growth site that encircles the cell. In the presence of penicillin, cell wall synthesis is stopped, while nicking of the cell wall by autolytic enzymes (peptidoglycan hydrolases) continues, and the cell membrane protrudes out of the structurally defective cell wall.

membrane emerge at this division furrow.[4] One model of the sequence of events in bacterial cell growth and in the production of penicillin spheroplasts is presented schematically in Figure 3–2.

Early experiments by Park demonstrated that exposure of bacteria to penicillin resulted in the accumulation of cell wall precursors[5] and, in some bacteria like *Staphylococcus aureus*, penicillin caused a marked inhibition of radioactive precursor (lysine or phosphate) incorporation into the cell wall but not into bacterial protein or nucleic acid.[6] It was clear that the process of cell wall biosynthesis would have to be explained in order to understand its inhibition by antibiotics.

It is now known that cell wall synthesis is a complex process in which many enzymes involved in synthesis and lysis of the wall as well as maintenance of bacterial shape and other functions act in a coordinated manner during cell growth and division. Bacteria that are not growing and dividing are generally not killed by the antibiotics that inhibit these enzymes. Recently, it has been shown that the penicillins and cephalosporins can affect a variety of these enzymes, and although the result is usually lysis, nonlytic death and bacteriostasis may also occur.[7]

Inhibition of Cell Wall Synthesis

Synthesis of a bacterial cell wall can be divided into three stages according to where the reactions take place. The first series of reactions, resulting in the production of the basic cell building block (the UDP-acetylmuramyl-pentapeptide), takes place inside the cell. Cycloserine, a rather toxic antibiotic that is employed rarely in the treatment of mycobacterial infections, inhibits the terminal reactions in this sequence. In the second stage of cell wall synthesis, the precursor unit is carried from inside the cell membrane outside. During this process, a number of modifications occur in the chemical structure of the basic repeating unit of the cell wall, and the units are linked covalently to the preexisting cell wall. The antibiotics vancomycin and bacitracin act during this second stage. The third stage of the process takes place entirely outside the cell membrane and consists of a variety of reactions that cross-link and modify the wall components. The cross-linking enzymes (the transpeptidases) and some of the modifying enzymes are inhibited by penicillins and cephalosporins. Bacterial walls are complex structures and the composition of the peptidoglycan component is different in different types of bacteria. The pathway of peptidoglycan biosynthesis in *Staphylococcus aureus* will be presented to provide a specific framework for discussing the mechanism of antibiotic action.

STAGE I: PRECURSOR FORMATION. The sequence of reactions comprising the first stage of cell wall synthesis in *S. aureus* is presented in Figure 3–3. In the first reaction, UTP is

bound covalently to N-acetylglucosamine-1-P to form UDP-N-acetylglucosamine. Subsequent reactions add a three-carbon unit from phosphoenolpyruvate and three amino acids to form a UDP-acetylmuramyltripeptide. In the final reaction of this stage, a D-alanyl-D-alanine dipeptide is joined to the UDP-acetyl-muramyltripeptide to produce the UDP-acetylmuramyl-pentapeptide, which is then available to participate in the second stage of cell wall synthesis. Exposure of bacteria to the antibiotics that inhibit stages II and III of cell wall synthesis will result in an accumulation of the pentapeptide in the cell.

Exposure of organisms to cycloserine prevents the formation of the pentapeptide. D-cyloserine is a structural analog of D-alanine. The antibiotic inhibits alanine racemase,[8] D-alanyl-D-alanine synthetase,[9] and possibly also the ligase that connects the D-alanyl-D-alanine unit to the muramyl tripeptide.[10] It was originally thought that D-cycloserine was a competitive inhibitor of both the racemase and synthetase enzymes. Both enzymes were found to bind the antibiotic 100 times as strongly ($K_i = 5 \times 10^{-5}\ M$) as they bind the normal substrate ($K_m = 5 \times 10^{-3}\ M$). It is now clear, however, that D-cycloserine is a "suicide substrate" for the

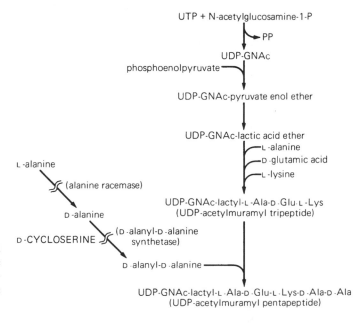

Figure 3–3. The first stage of cell wall synthesis in *S. aureus*. The reactions inhibited by D-cycloserine are indicated by the break marks.

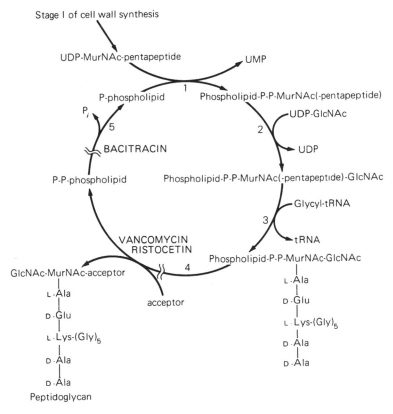

D-Cycloserine   D-Alanine
(zwitterion forms)

racemase. That is, the antibiotic occupies the substrate site on the racemase and forms a covalent complex with the enzyme, inactivating it in an irreversible manner.[11]

Fosfomycin is another antibiotic that inhibits cell wall synthesis at stage I. It was recently approved for use in the U.S. for treatment of urinary tract infections. Fosfomycin is an inhibitor of pyruvyl transferase, the enzyme that catalyzes the transfer of the enol pyruvate group to UDP-GlcNAc in the first stage of cell wall synthesis.[12]

STAGE II: FORMATION OF A LINEAR PEPTIDOGLYCAN. In the second stage of cell wall synthesis, the two uridine nucleotides UDP-acetylmuramyl pentapeptide and UDP-N-acetylglucosamine are linked together to form a linear polymer (Fig. 3–4). During this stage, the cell wall precursor units are attached to the cell membrane. In the first reaction, the sugar pentapeptide becomes attached by a pyrophosphate bridge to a phospholipid bound to the cell membrane. Then a second sugar derived from UDP-N-acetylglucosamine is added to form a disaccharide (-pentapeptide)-P-P-phospholipid. In *S. aureus,* this molecule is further modified by a series of reactions resulting in the addition of five glycines to the ε-amino group of lysine. In this unusual reaction sequence glycyl-tRNA serves as the amino acid donor molecule. The modified disaccharide is sub-

Figure 3–4. The second stage of cell wall synthesis in *S. aureus.* An ATP-requiring amidation of glutamic acid that occurs between reaction 2 and reaction 3 has been omitted. The sites of inhibition by bacitracin, vancomycin, and ristocetin are indicated by the break marks. (Modified from Strominger et al.[9])

sequently separated from the phospholipid and is covalently bonded to an acceptor molecule (i.e., preexisting portions of cell wall) to form a linear peptidoglycan polymer. In the terminal reaction of stage II, the phospholipid carrier molecule with two phosphate groups attached is dephosphorylated with the release of inorganic phosphate. The resulting phospholipid can again bind the end product of stage I synthesis, the UDP-N-acetylmuramyl pentapeptide, and continue on another cycle of the membrane-bound reactions.

During the course of the stage II reactions, the basic repeating units of the cell wall are put together to form a long polymer. All the events up to this point occur either inside the cell or at the cell membrane. The association of the wall precursor unit with the phospholipid is necessary for the transport of the unit from inside the cell and through the cell membrane to the outside. The precursor unit is apparently passing through the cell membrane as the stage II modifications are taking place at its inner surface. Two antibiotics that are employed clinically, vancomycin and bacitracin, inhibit the utilization of the lipid intermediates for the synthesis of the peptidoglycan. A third antibiotic, teicoplanin, which is an investigational drug in the U.S., is related structurally to vancomycin and has a similar mechanism of action.[12]

A major effect of vancomycin is to inhibit the reaction in which the finished unit is separated from the membrane-bound phospholipid and attached to the acceptor molecule (Reaction 4, Fig. 3–4). This reaction is directed by an enzyme called *peptidoglycan synthetase*. Vancomycin inhibits the formation of the peptidoglycan from the appropriate second-stage precursors at the same concentration at which it inhibits cell growth.[14] As seen in Table 3–1, exposure to penicillin will only inhibit the second-stage process at a concentration of antibiotic more than 6000 times that required to inhibit growth. In the presence of vancomycin, there is a normal synthesis of lipid intermediates, but they cannot be utilized for synthesis of the peptidoglycan.[15] Vancomycin can inhibit the reaction where the pentapeptide precursor unit is attached to the membrane carrier[16] (Reaction 1 in Fig. 3–4), but its primary effect appears to be inhibition of the utilization of lipid-linked intermediates for peptidoglycan synthesis.

The nature of vancomycin binding to bacterial components has been defined in some detail. Vancomycin-treated bacteria retain the drug tightly bound to cell wall precursor units.[17] The antibiotic binds with high affinity to both the UDP-acetylmuramyl-pentapeptide and to the membrane-bound intermediates.[18] It binds to the pentapeptide chain and there is a rather strict requirement for the presence of two alanines in the D configuration for tight binding of the drug to occur.[19] Vancomycin binds very tightly to short peptides that contain D-alanyl-D-alanine at the free carboxyl end.[20] The complex structure of vancomycin has now been determined by X-ray analysis[21] and the nature of the complex between vancomycin and acyl-D-alanyl-D-alanine has been determined by nuclear magnetic resonance (NMR) studies.[22–24]

It is postulated that the presence of vancomycin (molecular weight 1448) bound to

Table 3–1. Antibiotic sensitivity of cell growth and peptidoglycan synthetase in Staphylococcus aureus. *Antibiotics were introduced into cultures of growing cells, and cell growth and peptidoglycan synthetase activity were measured. The enzyme activity was assayed by incubating a particulate enzyme preparation from drug-treated cells with radioactive-labeled UDP-N-acetylmuramyl-pentapeptide and the appropriate substrates and then determining the amount of radioactivity incorporated into peptidoglycan. Ristocetin has a mechanism of action similar to that of vancomycin but is too toxic to be used clinically.*

| | Antibiotic concentration (μg/ml) required for 50% inhibition of: | |
Antibiotic	Growth	Peptidoglycan synthesis by particulate enzyme
Ristocetin	12	12
Vancomycin	6	6
Bacitracin	35	35
Penicillin	0.04	>250

Source: From Anderson et al.[14]

the peptide side chain of the membrane-linked precursor provides enough stearic hinderance to prevent it from occupying the substrate site on the synthetase enzyme. Thus, the membrane-linked cell wall precursor unit appears to be the most important receptor for the drug. In some cases, it has been found that a significant proportion of radiolabeled vancomycin bound by whole bacteria is associated with the cell wall itself.[25] This binding to cell wall could also produce effects that contribute to the antibacterial action.[26] The vancomycin story provides an elegant example of the development of knowledge regarding the mechanism of a drug action from the level of gross observation of the cell killing effect down to some understanding of the atomic perturbations that accompany the interaction of the drug with its receptor.

Bacitracin inhibits peptidoglycan synthesis by inhibiting the dephosphorylation of lipid pyrophosphate to lipid phosphate (Reaction 5, Fig. 3–4), a step essential to the regeneration of the lipid carrier.[27] In *S. aureus*, the lipid that attaches the precursor units to the cell membrane during the second stage of cell wall synthesis is a 55-carbon isoprenyl phosphate.[28] The dephosphorylation of the lipid pyrophosphate is carried out by a membrane-associated phosphatase.[29] Bacitracin forms a very tight complex with magnesium ion and the C_{55}-isoprenyl pyrophosphate,[30] and the formation of this complex is responsible for the inhibition of cell wall synthesis by the drug.[31]

STAGE III: CROSS-LINKING OF THE PEPTIDO-GLYCAN. The terminal reactions in cell wall synthesis take place outside the cell. At this stage, the glycopeptide polymers become cross-linked to each other by means of a transpeptidation reaction. The energy for the cross-linking reaction is derived from the peptide bond linking the two terminal D-alanine residues of each polypeptide side chain. As seen in Figure 3–5, transpeptidase enzymes direct the splitting of the terminal D-alanyl-D-alanine linkage and form a peptide bond between the terminal glycine of

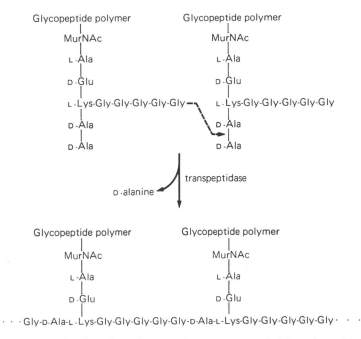

Figure 3–5. The third stage of cell wall synthesis in *S. aureus*: cross-linking of peptidoglycan polymers by the joining of the peptide side chains with the elimination of D-alanine. (Modified from Strominger et al.[9])

the pentaglycine side chain and the penulti-mate D-alanine of an adjacent peptidoglycan strand. Thus, each polypeptide side chain of each repeating unit becomes covalently linked to the side chains in two neighboring peptidoglycan strands.

The penicillins and the cephalosporins in-hibit this transpeptidation.[32] In the presence of penicillin, fibrous material, which can be seen by electron microscopy, accumulates at the growing point of the bacterium.[33] These fibers represent the accumulating petidogly-can strands, which cannot cross-link. In cer-tain organisms, exposure to penicillin under experimental conditions can be shown to ef-fect secretion of linear uncross-linked pepti-doglycan into the growth medium.[34] The in-hibition of transpeptidases by both penicillins and cephalosporins has been dem-onstrated in cell-free enzyme preparations that catalyze the cross-linking reaction.[35,36] The transpeptidases are membrane-bound enzymes, and in crude cell wall preparations from S. aureus that contain both cell membrane and peptidoglycan, inhibition of cross-linking by penicillin G occurs at the same drug concentrations that are effective in killing the organisms. This is consistent with the conclusion that inhibition of tran-speptidase activity is the important event that accounts for the penicillin effect in S. aureus.[36]

The mechanism of inhibition of tran-speptidase by penicillin has not been di-rectly demonstrated, but there is substan-tial evidence in support of the following model of Tipper and Strominger.[37] The structure of the penicillins is similar to that of the D-alanyl-D-alanine terminus of the polypeptide side chain of peptidogly-can.[37] Figure 3–6 shows this similarity in drawings of stereo models of the antibiotic and the dipeptide. The arrows point to the CO–N bond in the β-lactam ring of peni-cillin and the analogous peptide bond in D-alanyl-D-alanine. It is postulated that the penicillins and cephalosporins occupy the D-alanyl-D-alanine substrate site of the transpeptidase enzyme. In most cases the antibiotic then becomes covalently bound to the enzyme. This is supported by the observation that penicillin inhibition of transpeptidase is not reversed by washing the particulate enzyme preparation or by digestion with penicillinase.[35] According to this model, a penicillin would occupy the substrate site of transpeptidase, with the C–N bond of the β-lactam ring in the same orientation as the C–N peptide bond be-tween the two D-alanines. This is the pep-tide bond that is cleaved as part of the normal action of the enzyme. The highly reactive C–N bond of the β-lactam ring of the antibiotic opens in a similar manner, a

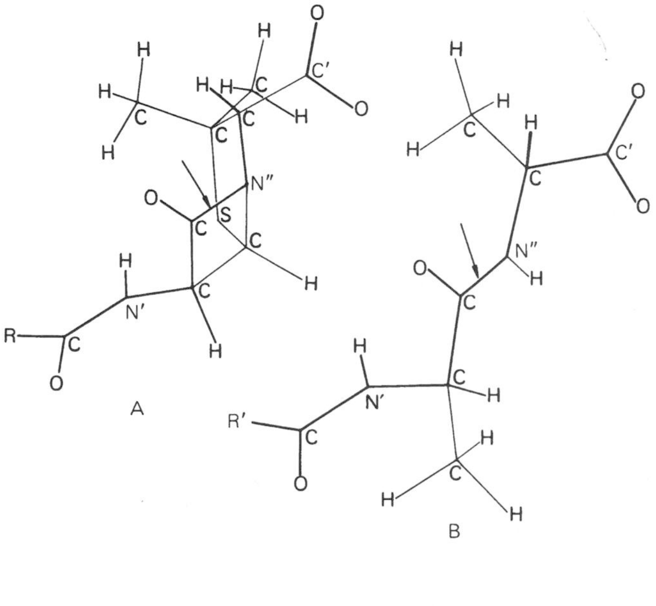

Figure 3–6. Stereomodels of pen-icillin (A) and of the D-alanyl-D-al-anine end of the peptidoglycan strand (B). The arrows indicate the CO-N bond in the β-lactam ring of penicillin and the CO-N bond in the D-alanyl-D-alanine at the end of the peptidoglycan strand. (From Strominger et al.[9])

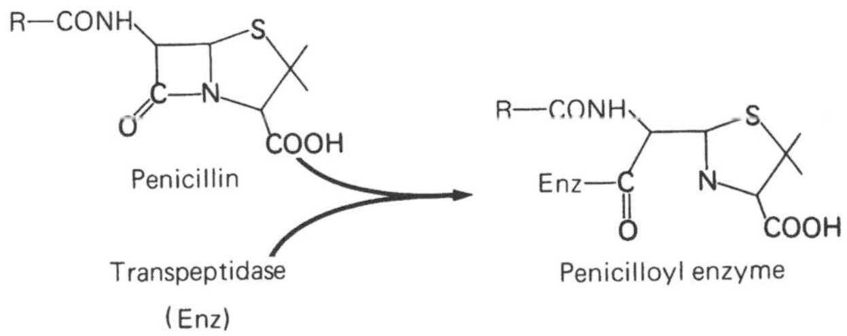

Figure 3–7. Proposed mechanism of transpeptidase inhibition by penicillin. Penicillin occupies the D-alanyl-D-alanine substrate site of transpeptidase, the reactive four-membered (β-lactam) ring is broken by cleavage at the CO-N bond, and the antibiotic becomes linked to the enzyme by a covalent bond. (From Tipper and Strominger.[37])

covalent bond with the transpeptidase is formed, and the enzyme is inactivated (Fig. 3–7). This substrate analog model is intellectually very attractive, and it is consistent with most experimental observations. The β-lactam antibiotic–transpeptidase complex can be regarded as an analog of the covalent transition state complex between the normal substrate and the enzyme. Penicillin degradation products are slowly released as a result of the action of the enzyme on the drug,[38] but the rate of release is very slow compared to the normal rate of enzyme activity and the enzyme remains inactivated for a long time.

Penicillin Binding Proteins

The *penicillin binding proteins* are the receptors for the β-lactam antibiotics. Although inhibition of transpeptidase is very important for the mechanism of action of the β-lactam antibiotics, additional targets for these drugs have been identified. They have collectively been called *penicillin binding proteins* (PBPs). All bacteria have several of these proteins with varying affinities for the different β-lactam drugs.[39]

The study of penicillin binding proteins in bacterial membranes has led to significant progress in understanding β-lactam antibiotic action. As these antibiotics bind to their receptors in a covalent manner, the drug–enzyme complexes can be easily identified in the following way. A radiolabeled penicillin or cephalosphorin is bound to bacterial cell envelopes that are prepared by sonication and differential centrifugation and the pro-

teins of the cell membrane are solubilized with a detergent. The different proteins are then separated by electrophoresis on polyacrylamide gels and those proteins with covalently bound radioactive antibiotic are detected by autoradiography. All bacteria that have been examined contain multiple penicillin binding proteins.[40] S. aureus has only four PBPs, but some gram-negative bacteria, like E. coli, have seven or more. Some of the PBPs are lethal targets for the action of β-lactam antibiotics (in general these are the high-molecular-weight PBPs) while others clearly are not.

The penicillin binding proteins of the inner membrane of E. coli K-12 are diagrammed in Figure 3–8.[41,42] PBP 1a and the proteins of the 1b group of E. coli are transpeptidases involved in peptidoglycan synthesis associated with cell elongation, and inhibition of these enzymes results in spheroplast formation and rapid lysis.[42,43] PBP 2 is involved in maintaining the "rod" shape of the bacterium, and selective inhibition of this enzyme causes the production of osmotically stable, ovoid, and round forms.[44] PBP 3 is required for septum formation at division[42] and selective inhibition causes the production of filamentous forms containing multiple rod-shaped units that cannot separate from each other. As with inhibition of the PBP 1 group, selective inhibition of PBP 2 is lethal, but lysis occurs very slowly and the mechanism of death is different from the rapid lytic death that follows PBP 1 inhibition. It has not yet been established that selective inhibition of PBP 3 is lethal.[40] Although PBPs 4, 5, and 6 account for almost 90% of the total binding

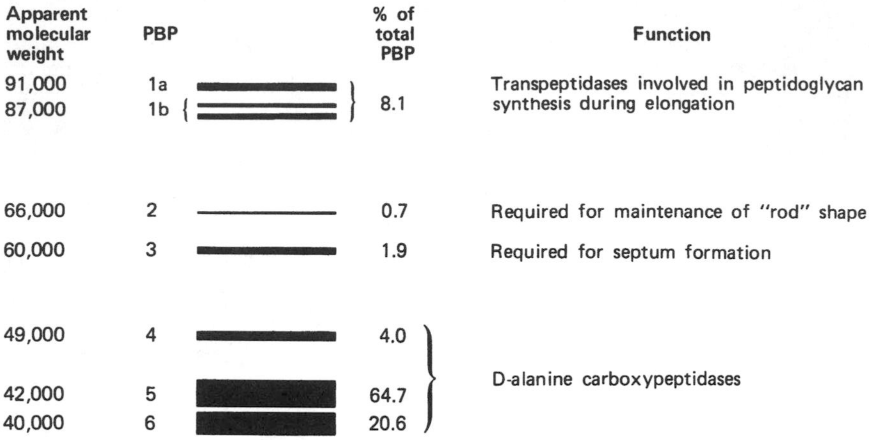

Apparent molecular weight	PBP		% of total PBP	Function
91,000	1a	▬▬▬▬	} 8.1	Transpeptidases involved in peptidoglycan synthesis during elongation
87,000	1b	{ ▬▬▬▬		
66,000	2	▬▬▬	0.7	Required for maintenance of "rod" shape
60,000	3	▬▬▬	1.9	Required for septum formation
49,000	4	▬▬▬	4.0 }	
42,000	5	▬▬▬▬	64.7 }	D-alanine carboxypeptidases
40,000	6	▬▬▬	20.6 }	

Figure 3–8. Penicillin binding proteins (PBPs) of *Escherichia coli* K-12. *E. coli* cell membranes were bound with benzyl[^{14}C]penicillin and the membrane proteins were solubilized with detergent and separated by sodium dodecyl sulfate polyacrylamide gel electrophoresis. The penicillin binding proteins were identified by autoradiography. The black bars indicate the relative location and amount of each labeled protein band on the autoradiogram. A high-molecular-weight band at 91,000 was originally thought to be a single protein but these were later resolved into bands la and lb. Subsequently, it has been found that lb is composed of two or perhaps three different components, giving a total of eight or nine PBPs in *E. Coli* K-12. (Compiled from data of Spratt.[42])

activity in *E. coli,* it is clear they are not lethal targets for β-lactam action.[45] These low-molecular-weight proteins are D-alanine carboxypeptidases that hydrolyze the peptide bond between terminal D-alanine residues of cell wall units.[46] When the terminal D-alanine is lost, the transpeptidation reaction cannot occur, and these enzymes are thought to play a role in limiting the extent of cross-linking in the peptidoglycan.

The β-lactam antibiotics vary with regard to their relative affinities for the critical binding proteins of *E. coli* K-12 (PBPs 1, 2, and 3).[47] In all cases the observed binding between the proteins and the antibiotic is covalent but this is preceded by a noncovalent interaction and the relative affinities of different antibiotics for the binding sites can be determined by competition experiments. For example, it can be observed that at low concentrations of drug, cephaloridine binds with very high affinity to PBP 1a and with much lower affinity to PBPs 2 and 3.[47] This binding preference is consistent with the observation that, even at low concentration, cephaloridine causes

rapid lysis of the bacterium (see Table 3–2). For a long time, it has been known that many penicillins and cephalosporins cause filament formation. Penicillin G binds preferentially to PBP 3 and causes filaments to form when it is present at low concentration. At higher concentrations, there is also binding to the proteins in group 1 and rapid lysis occurs. In contrast to other β-lactam antibiotics which can bind to PBPs 1, 2, and 3, mecillinam, an amidinopenicillin, binds only to PBP 2.[48] When gramnegative bacilli are exposed to mecillinam, the cells first become ovoid and later spherical.[49] This morphological change is followed by delayed lysis, in contrast to the rapid lysis that occurs with appropriate concentrations of the other β-lactam antibiotics. The pioneering work of Spratt led to this attractive and simple model which explains the different morphological effects of the different β-lactam antibiotics, and the concentration-dependent morphological effect of any one β-lactam antibiotic, on the basis of differential inhibition of distinct PBPs, each with a discrete function in the morphogenesis of *E. coli* K-12.[41]

Table 3–2.   Relationship between the relative affinities of β-lactam antibiotics for penicillin binding proteins and the effects of the antibiotics on Escherichia coli K-12. *Mecillinam binds only to protein 2.*

Relative affinities of binding proteins 1, 2, and 3 for a β-lactam antibiotic	Morphological effect produced at low or high concentration of antibiotic		β-lactam showing this behavior
	Low concentration	High concentration	
1 > 2 or 3	Lysis	Lysis	Cephaloridine
2 only	Ovoid cells	Ovoid cells	Mecillinam
3 > 1 > 2	Filaments	Lysis	Penicillin G

Source: From Spratt.[41]

Purification and Structure of Penicillin–Receptor Complexes

Several of the penicillin binding proteins have now been purified to apparent homogeneity. The method of purification employs affinity columns of Sepharose to which various β-lactam antibiotics are linked as ligands. When bacterial proteins are absorbed to the column, those proteins that interact with the β-lactam structure are retained as covalent Sepharose-penicilloyl-enzyme complexes and they can subsequently be eluted with neutral hydroxylamine.[50] Both the 1a and 1b proteins of *E. coli* K-12 have been purified in a form that is catalytically active and sensitive to inhibition by β-lactam antibiotics.[51] Each enzyme preparation was found to have both peptidoglycan synthetase (transglycosylase) and transpeptidase activity, suggesting that the same enzyme molecule may direct both the transfer of cell wall units from cell membrane to the peptidoglycan and the cross-linking of the resulting polymers. Only the transpeptidase activity was found to be sensitive to inhibition by the penicillins.[51]

Both high-molecular-weight PBPs (presumably transpeptidases) and the carboxypeptidases of *S. aureus* and *B. subtilis* have been shown to release covalently bound penicillin degradation products in catalyzed reaction.[38] The fact that the release of the drug products is catalyzed is consistent with the proposal that the penicillins are binding at the substrate site of the enzymes.

Because carboxypeptidases could be separated from cell membranes and obtained in good yield in catalytically active form much earlier than the high-molecular-weight binding proteins, their interaction with the penicillins has been studied in greater detail. Purified carboxypeptidase-[14C]penicillin complexes from *Bacillus subtilis* and *B. stearothermophilus* have been cleaved by digestion with protease and the fragment containing the covalently bound penicillin has been sequenced. In both cases the penicillin is bound as an ester to a serine located 36 amino acids from the NH$_2$-terminus of the protein.[52,53] The catalytically active end of the enzyme is located in the NH$_2$-terminal region[54] and the enzyme is connected to the bacterial membrane at the hydrophobic COOH-terminus.[55] The covalent intermediate formed between carboxypeptidase and a [14C]diacetyltripeptide substrate has also been sequenced and it was found that a labeled acyl group derived from the substrate is bound in the same manner to serine 36.[52,53] The demonstration that both the penicillin and the substrate are bound at exactly the same enzyme site in two bacilli fulfills an important prediction of the substrate analog model of penicillin action.

Autolytic Enzyme Activity and the Killing Effect

The antibiotics that inhibit cell wall synthesis are usually bactericidal when added to growing cultures of sensitive cells. Although we have described how these drugs inhibit various steps in cell wall biosynthesis, this does not explain how the drugs cause cell lysis and death. In most cases cell wall autolytic enzyme activity is required for lytic death to occur. The natural biological role of the autolysins (murein hydrolases) is subject to speculation. They may be required to make nicks in the cell wall that serve as points of attachment for new peptoglycan units.[56] or they may be necessary to separate two daughter cells from one another during division.[57] The growth of the cell wall may require both autolytic and synthetic activity. According to the "unbalanced growth" hypothesis, inhibition of biosynthesis by antibiotics in the presence of continued cell wall autolysis would produce weak points through which the cell membrane could extrude and eventually rupture would occur. It has become clear that the explanation of penicillin-mediated lysis may not be this simple. The relationship between autolytic enzyme activity and β-lactam antibiotic effects is complex and our understanding of the lytic process has not yet reached the level where simple, direct explanations of mechanisms can be offered. The goal of the next few paragraphs is to show how lytic enzymes activity affects the bacterium's response to the antibiotic, and the reader is referred to reviews of the literature for a discussion of the various hypotheses regarding the control of autolytic enzyme activity.[58,59]

One experimental approach demonstrating the requirement for autolytic enzyme activity in penicillin-induced lysis utilizes the observation that the autolytic activity of pneumococci is suppressed when cells are grown in the presence of ethanolamine rather than choline.[60] This is due to the inability of the autolytic enzyme of this organism to hydrolyze ethanolamine-containing cell walls. It was found that cycloserine and penicillin did not lyse the ethanolamine-containing cells.[61] When the cells were allowed to reincorporate choline into the cell wall, the normal lytic response to the antibiotics reappeared. The requirement for autolytic enzyme activity in penicillin-induced lysis was also supported by the observation

that an autolysin-defective mutant strain of pneumococcus did not lyse when treated with penicillin.[61] Subsequently, other laboratory strains of bacteria deficient in autolytic enzyme activity were shown not to undergo lysis after exposure to β-lactam antibiotics or other inhibitors of cell wall synthesis.[62,63]

"TOLERANCE" TO THE β-LACTAM ANTIBIOTICS. In the autolysin-deficient mutant bacteria, low concentrations of antibiotic stop cell growth, but the bacteria remain viable. Thus, the bactericidal antibiotic effect has been converted to a bacteriostatic effect (see Figure 3–9). These mutants are called "tol-

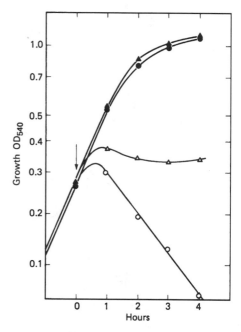

Figure 3–9. Effect of penicillin on the growth of a parent strain of *Bacillus subtilis* with normal autolytic enzyme activity and an autolysin-deficient mutant. Penicillin was added to cultures of *B. subtilis* in the middle log phase of growth and growth was assayed by turbidity at 540 nm. The arrow indicates the time of drug addition. ●, parent strain; ○, parent strain plus penicillin; ▲, autolysin-deficient mutant; △, mutant plus penicillin. The parent strain was lysed, whereas the growth of the mutant was halted without lysis. The same phenomenon was observed upon the addition of cycloserine, vancomycin, or bacitracin. (From Ayusawa et al.[63])

erant" organisms in that they are still suspectible to the growth-inhibiting effect of the antibiotic but they are tolerant with respect to the lytic action. Because these organisms are tolerant to the lytic action of cycloserine and vancomycin as well as the β-lactam antibiotics, they represent a unique mechanism of multiple drug resistance due to the modification of an enzymatic process that is unaffected by the drug but necessary for the drug effect (i.e., lysis).

The "tolerance" phenomenon is not limited to organisms selected under controlled laboratory conditions. Penicillin-tolerant strains of staphylococci[64,65] and streptococci[66,67] have been isolated from patients with persistant or relapsing infections. These tolerant organisms have the same minimum inhibitory concentrations (MICs) for β-lactam antibiotics as susceptible strains, but their minimum bactericidal concentrations (MBCs) are very high (see Table 3–3). Some tolerant organisms, like the laboratory strains of pneumococci, do not undergo lysis even after long exposure to high concentrations of antibiotic,[59] whereas others, such as the tolerant staphylococci obtained from patients with persistent infections,[65] slowly

Table 3–3. *Susceptibility of 60 strains of* Staphylococcus aureus *to oxacillin.* The minimum concentration of oxacillin required to inhibit growth (MIC) and the minimum concentration required to kill 99.9% of organisms (MBC) were determined for 60 randomly selected clinical isolates of *S. aureus.* The penicillin was bactericidal against 27 strains and only bacteriostatic against the other 33. It should be noted that the "tolerant" organisms will die very slowly if kept in the presence of a high concentration of oxacillin for many hours. The data represent the mean MIC and MBC for each group with the range of values shown in parenthesis.

Isolates	MIC (μg/ml)	MBC (μg/ml)
Sensitive group	0.30 (0.1–1.6)	2.2 (0.2–12.5)
"Tolerant" group	0.33 (0.1–0.8)	>100 (50->100)

Source: From Mayhall et al.,[65] Table 1.

become nonviable at very high antibiotic concentrations.

THE "TRIGGERING" HYPOTHESIS. The "unbalanced growth" hypothesis of penicillin-induced lysis is based on the assumption that continuous activity of cell wall degrading enzymes is essential for cell growth. This assumption is not consistent with the observation that many strains of pneumococci and some other organisms that are deficient in murein hydrolase activity grow with normal generation times (although some of these bacteria have a tendency to fail to separate).[59] The observation that much of the autolytic enzyme activity in pneumococci is apparently inhibited by teichoic acid components of the cell wall has led to an alternative hypothesis. It has been suggested that the inhibition of cell wall synthesis by *any* means "triggers" bacterial autolytic enzymes by in some way deinhibiting their activity.[68] Thus, according to this model, inhibition of cell wall synthesis by antibiotics leads to an increase in cell wall degrading activity.

Several observations support the "triggering" hypothesis.[58,59,68] Treatment of sensitive pneumococci with β-lactam antibiotics or other inhibitors of cell wall synthesis causes the escape of lipoteichoic acid (Forssman antigen) into the growth medium.[68] *Teichoic acids* are polymers of glycerol phosphate or ribitol phosphate found in the walls of most gram-positive bacteria where they are normally covalently linked to the peptidoglycan.[69] Lipoteichoic acid has been shown to inhibit purified *N*-acetylmuramyl-*L*-alanine amidase,[70] the major autolytic enzyme in pneumococci. Also, addition of purified lipoteichoic acid to the growth medium of wild-type pneumococci prevents penicillin-induced lysis of the cells.[71] The "autolysin triggering" hypothesis is a synthesis of several observations made in pneumococci, but because we are almost completely ignorant of the normal mechanisms by which autolytic enzyme activity is controlled, the hypothesis has not yet evolved into a clear and intellectually satisfying explanation of penicillin-induced lysis.

Since 1944, it has been recognized that inhibition of bacterial growth during exposure to penicillin protects the cells against both lysis and loss of viability.[72] The requirement that bacteria must be growing in order to be susceptible to lysis by penicillin has not been explained in a satisfactory manner. It is known that inhibition of protein synthesis in some bacteria arrests cell wall turnover catalyzed by autolysins,[58] and it is possible that the requirement for active growth and protein synthesis in penicillin-induced lysis is related in some way to the control of autolytic enzyme activity.

Penetration of β-Lactam Antibiotics through the Bacterial Cell Envelope: A Determinant of Their Spectrum of Action

Although some of the penicillins are relatively ineffective in inhibiting the growth of many gram-negative organisms, others (e.g., ampicillin and carbenicillin) are quite effective against certain gram-negative bacteria. These are the *broad-spectrum* penicillins. In this context "broad spectrum" is not equivalent to the term as it is applied to such truly broad-spectrum antibiotics as chloramphenicol or the tetracyclines. It merely refers to a broader spectrum of action than that of penicillin G and the penicillinase-resistant penicillins. In this restricted sense, the cephalosporins are also broad spectrum. The concept of broad versus narrow spectrum of action of the penicillins is of considerable clinical importance. The major reason for the broad-spectrum effect of certain penicillins is that they are better able to penetrate through the gram-negative cell envelope than the narrow-spectrum drugs.

The β-lactam antibiotics must first pass through the outer cell envelope in order to reach their cytoplasmic membrane-bound target enzymes. The outer envelope of gram-positive bacteria is composed of peptidoglycan with covalently linked teichoic acid and teichuronic acid polymers and of capsular proteins and carbohydrates located external to the peptidoglycan layer.[73] The gram-positive cell envelope does not present a significant barrier to the passage of small compounds like the β-lactams which can readily penetrate to their target enzymes.[74] The en-

velope of gram-negative bacteria is considerably more complex: a second membrane is covalently linked via lipoproteins bridges (Braun lipoproteins) to the peptidoglycan (see Fig. 3–10) and this outer membrane presents a physical barrier to the penetration of antibiotics. Although it was originally thought that all antibiotics might traverse the outer membrane by simple diffusion through the phospholipid bilayer, it has become clear that small hydrophilic drugs enter through pores in the outer membrane that are formed by proteins called porins (for reviews see refs. 75 and 76).

The role of the porins in the penetration of small hydrophilic compounds has been demonstrated by both genetic and reconstitution experiments. In mutant E. coli and S. typhimurium possessing a markedly reduced number of porins, the rate of penetration of β-lactam antibiotics is reduced by more than 90%.[76,77] The porin proteins from sensitive strains of these two gram-negative bacteria have been purified and reconstituted into membrane vesicles and lipid bilayers and shown to form transmembrane channels.[78,79] The gram-negative bacteria differ in the number and types of porins produced and in the size of their pores. The pores in E. coli and S. typhimurium permit the passage of hydrophilic molecules with molecular weights up to about 600 daltons,[78,80] whereas the porin system of P. aeruginosa permits the passage of molecules up to about 6,000 daltons.[81] Figure 3–10 is a diagram of the gram-negative cell envelope with the porins arranged in trimers as they are thought to exist in E. coli.[75,82]

The importance of the outer membrane in determining the spectrum of action of the penicillins is demonstrated by comparing the response of a permeability mutant of E. coli K-12 to that of its wild-type parent.[47] As in the clinical treatment of E. coli infection, the broad-spectrum drug amoxicillin is more active against the wild-type organism than the narrow-spectrum agent penicillin G. But the two penicillins have virtually the same ability to interact with the penicillin binding proteins of E. coli K-12.[47] The permeability properties of the outer membrane of the mutant bacterium are altered such that the pen-

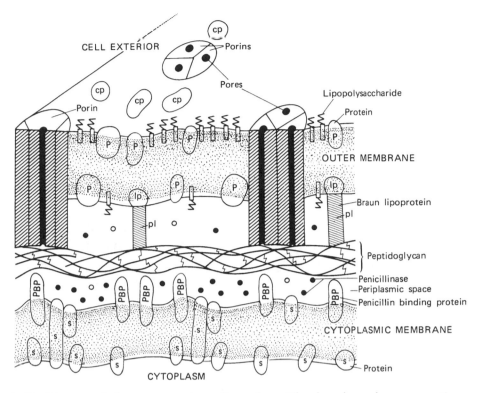

Figure 3–10. Diagram of the gram-negative cell envelope. The three-layered gram-negative envelope consists of two membranes separated by the periplasmic space containing the cross-linked peptidoglycan. Hydrophobic regions are stippled. Each membrane has protein as well as phospholipid and lipopolysaccharide components: s and p designate the protein components of these membranes. There are also extra-membrane proteins, some of which are capsular proteins (cp) and others are located in the periplasmic zone (O). β-Lactamase-producing gram-negative bacilli retain most of the enzyme (●) in the periplasmic space. The outer membrane is attached to the peptidoglycan by bridges of Braun lipoprotein; pl and lp refer to the protein and lipid portions of these bridging units. The penicillin binding proteins (PBP) are attached to the cytoplasmic membrane and extend into the periplasmic space. Antibiotics traverse the outer membrane by passing through pores formed by proteins called porins, which extend from outside the cell to the peptidoglycan. In *E. coli* and some other enterobacteria the porins are arranged as trimers with each monomeric unit contributing a channel. (Adapted from Costerton and Cheng,[73] Fig. 2; Nikaido and Nakae,[75] Fig. 11.)

icillins can readily enter the periplasmic space where the penicillin binding proteins are located. In the permeability mutant, penicillin G and amoxicillin are equally active and the drugs inhibit growth at the same concentration at which they interact with the critical binding proteins.[47]

The ease with which β-lactam antibiotics diffuse through the pores in the outer membrane varies according to their hydrophobicity and their charge.[76] It has been shown that the rate of penetration of β-

lactam antibiotics through the outer membrane of *E. coli* K-12 is more rapid with increasing hydrophilicity of the molecule.[76,83] Relatively hydrophobic, narrow-spectrum penicillins do not pass through the porin system as readily as the more hydrophilic broad-spectrum and extended-spectrum penicillins. In the *E. coli* system, the presence of positively charged groups, like the amino group on ampicillin or amoxicillin, also increases the penetration rate. In general, the cephalosporins in clinical use diffuse through the porin system more readily than the narrow-spectrum penicillins.[83,84]

The activity of a penicillin or a cephalosporin against gram-negative bacteria depends on three main properties: *(1)* its intrinsic ability to bind to the different target enzymes; *(2)* its ability to penetrate through the outer envelope; and *(3)* its sensitivity to inactivation by β-lactamase enzymes located in the periplasmic space between the inner and outer membranes. The third property is of particular importance in determining the enhanced effectiveness of the newer cephalosporins against certain gram-negative bacilli. The newer cephalosporins, such as cefoxitin, cefotaxime and cefepime are more effective clinically against some gram-negative bacilli because they are less sensitive than older cephalosporins, such as cephalothin and cephazolin, to digestion by β-lactamases produced by those organisms.

Resistance to the Penicillins and Cephalosporins

Mechanisms of Resistance

When the penicillins first came into wide use in the 1940s, relatively few infections due to penicillin-resistant gram-positive organisms were encountered. For example, no resistant strains were found in a study of 29 clinical isolates of *S. aureus* obtained in 1942.[85] During the late 1940s and the 1950s, however, an increasing proportion of *S. aureus* strains isolated from patients were found to be resistant to the penicillins. The growing incidence of resistance in *S. aureus* was accompanied by more frequent problems with penicillin resistance in other organisms as well.

Bacteria can become resistant to the action of penicillins in several ways. In the upper urinary tract, organisms can become refractory to the action of penicillins because L-forms (bacteria without cell walls) are created, and they can survive if the toxicity of the environment is high enough to prevent cell rupture.[86] This is an example of escape from the therapeutic effect of the drug but not true resistance. Resistance can result from changes in the penicillin binding proteins.[87] Altered binding proteins are responsible for the high-level resistance seen clinically with some organisms that are usually very sensitive to penicillins. Highly penicillin-resistant, non-β-lactamase–producing pneumococci isolated from patients,[88] have been shown to have several altered penicillin binding proteins.[89] Similarly, highly penicillin-resistant strains of *Neisseria gonorrhoeae* are being isolated from patients with increasing frequency. Most of these so-called intrinsically resistant strains also do not produce β-lactamase and several of them have been found to have markedly altered penicillin binding proteins.[90] Earlier in this chapter, we reviewed a mechanism of resistance called "tolerance," in which a deficiency of autolytic enzyme activity can cause resistance to the lytic effect of all of the antibiotics that inhibit cell wall synthesis. Staphylococci[64,65] and streptococci[66,67] isolated from patients with persistent infections have demonstrated a "tolerance" phenomenon (characterized by low MICs and unusually high MBCs for β-lactam antibiotics) that may be due to alterations in autolytic enzyme activity. Reduction in antibiotic penetration due to mutations affecting the porin system has accounted for β-lactam resistance in both laboratory and clinical strains of gram-negative bacilli.[76,77]

Resistance Due to Changes in Penicillin Binding Proteins

Resistance to β-lactams due to PBP modification occurs either through mutations in the chromosomal genes encoding the PBPs or through the acquisition of supplementary foreign genes encoding new PBPs.[91] This mechanism of resistance is important in gram-positive cocci such as *Staphylococcus aureus* but is seen to a much less degree in gram-negative bacteria.

Micorganisms can be intrinsically resistant to β-lactam antibiotics because of structural differences in the PBPs that are the targets of these drugs. Mecillinam, for example, is an amidinopenicillin that does not interact with appreciable affinity to most PBPs. It does, however, readily fit into the substrate site of an enzyme that is required for maintaining the shape of gram-negative enterobacteria. Consequently, although mecillinam has high activity against *E. coli* and other enterobacteria, it has very poor activity against gram-positive cocci.

Furthermore, acquired resistance to the β-lactams can occur as a result of mutations that alter the binding proteins. For example, resistance to cloxacillin has developed as a result of mutations in *Bacillus subtilis*. These mutants have a binding protein with altered affinity for cloxacillin but normal affinity for penicillin G.[87] Apparently the mutants have an altered configuration of the protein so that it no longer accepts the cloxacillin structure but does retain the ability to accept penicillin G. Other mutations in the binding proteins account for the highly penicillin-resistant strains of pneumococci and gonococci that have been isolated from patients.[73,90] The mutations that have occurred in these organisms arc vcry rarc cvents but the therapeutic and social consequences of infections caused by these resistant strains can be very serious.

Since the β-lactams inhibit many different PBPs in a single bacterium, the affinity for β-lactams must decrease for the organism to become resistant. Homologous recombination between PBP genes of different bacterial species can account for the altered PBPs with decreased affinity for β-lactam antibiotics. For example, four of the five high-molecular-weight PBPs of the most highly penicillin-resistant *Streptococcus pneumoniae* isolated clinically have decreased affinity for β-lactam antibiotics as a result of interspecies homologous recombination events.[92] On the other hand, bacteria isolated with a high level of resistance to some third-generation cephalosporins have been found to have alterations of only two of the five high-molecular-weight PBPs. Apparently, the other PBPs have an intrinsically low affinity for these compounds.

Resistance Due to Increased production of β-Lactamase Enzymes

The principal mechanism by which bacteria become resistant to the penicillins and ceph-alosporins is by producing enzymes that inactivate the drugs. Although β-lactam antibiotics can be inactivated in a number of ways, only the β-lactamases are important for the production of clinical resistance. The β-lactamases cleave the C–N bond on the β-lactam ring of the antibiotic (Fig. 3–11). As described earlier in the chapter, an intact β-lactam ring is an absolute requirement for interaction with the penicillin binding proteins, and cleavage of the ring destroys antibacterial activity. Bacteria can also produce amidohydrolases (penicillin acylases) that cleave the penicillins and cephalosporins between the β-lactam nucleus and the acyl substituent on the β-lactam ring, but this is not an important resistance mechanism.[93]

Origin of β-Lactamases and Resistance Transfer

Penicillinases clearly existed before the introduction of penicillin into therapy, but few strains of bacteria produced them. With the selection pressure caused by widespread antibiotic use, penicillinase-producing strains became more prevalent. It is interesting to speculate about what caused the β-lactamases to evolve in the first place. It is likely that the β-lactamases evolved from the penicillin binding proteins. Both the binding proteins and the β-lactamases have substrate sites that accommodate the β-lactam structure and cleave the C–N bond. If the binding proteins and the β-lactamases are evolutionally related, then one would expect that the amino acid sequences at the active sites of the enzymes would be similar. The NH_2-terminal regions of several β-lactamases and two D-alanine carboxypeptidases have been sequenced and considerable homology has been demonstrated.[52] In fact, in the region of the active site serine, the *Bacillus subtilis* carboxypeptidase is as homologous with the *E. coli* and *S. aureus* β-lactamses as several of the β-lactamases are with each other.[52] The sequence similarity supports the hypothesis that at least the penicillin-sensitive carboxypeptidases and penicillin-inactivating β-lactamases are related evolutionally. The β-lactamases must have played some needed role in the life of the bacterium before the

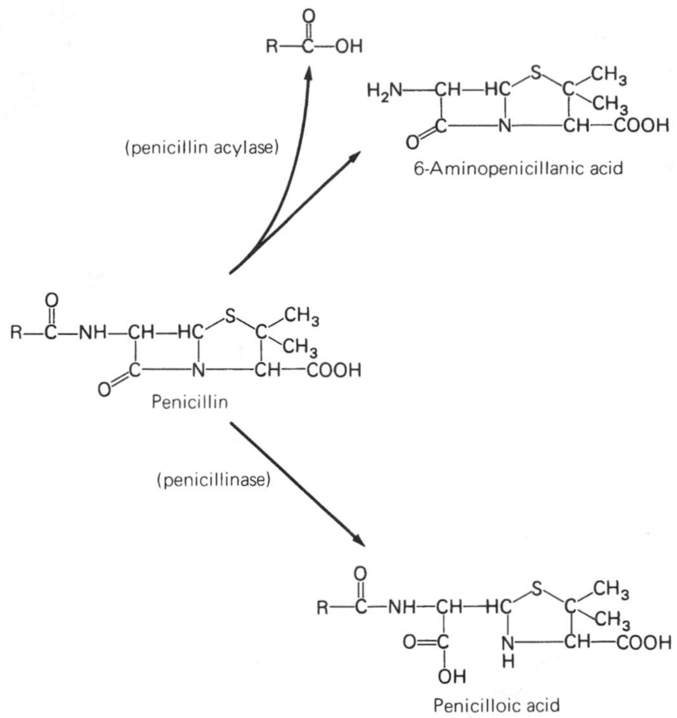

Figure 3–11. Enzymes that hydrolyze the β-lactam antibiotics. Bacteria produce two types of enzymes that hydrolyze the penicillins and cephalosporins. β-Lactamase (penicillinase) production is by far the most common form of resistance.

introduction of antibiotics. Those few strains of bacteria that acquired the ability to produce β-lactamases may have had some selective advantage if the enzymes acted as detoxifiers of penicillins and cephalosporins present in their natural environment.[94] This route of evolution is, of course, hypothetical, and alternative theories propose that the penicillinases evolved as peptidases that are required in the process of sporulation.[95] The hypothesis that the binding proteins and the β-lactamases are evolutionarily related is intriguing, since it provides a perspective for considering the enzymes that act in a specific manner on the β-lactam structure, both as drug receptors and as instruments of bacterial resistance.

The increase in *S. aureus* penicillin resistance that occurred as the clinical use of penicillin increased was not due just to selection of a few strains of mutant organisms that were capable of producing penicillinase before the introduction of the drug. The genetic information determining the production of resistance to the penicillins is carried in most cases in DNA that is located ex-

trachromosomally in plasmids. Both the genes determining penicillinase structure and the genes controlling its production can be carried in a single plasmid, and this information can be transferred from one organism to another by transduction in vivo.[96,97] Analysis of staphylococci isolated from hospital patients confirms the important role of plasmids in determining penicillinase production in the clinical environment.[98,99] In the enterobacteria, the genes determining penicillinase are also frequently located in plasmids. In this case the plasmids often contain determinants for resistance to other antibiotics and they can be transferred from one bacterium to another by conjugation (see discussion of multiple drug resistance in Chapter 2). The problem of penicillin resistance in *S. aureus* has been reviewed from an epidemiologic standpoint by Rolinson,[100] and a detailed review of the role of plasmids in antibiotic resistance in this organism has been published by Lacey.[101] It is not possible to extend this discussion here except to note that, because of extrachromosomal resistance transfer and the selective pressure of widespread antibiotic use, by 1960 many hospitals were reporting 60% to 80% of their *S. aureus* isolates resistant to penicillin. It was fortunate that methicillin, the first of the penicillinase-resistant penicillins, was introduced at about that time.

β-Lactamase Production

There are many different β-lactamases, and they can be distinguished on the basis of their substrate and inhibitor specificities, physical differences (pH optimum, isoelectric point), immunological differences, etc.[102] It is difficult to classify such a large variety of enzymes, but Table 3–4 presents a reasonable and complete scheme for classification of the β-lactamases.[103] The classification of these enzyme groups is based on their inhibition by clavulanic acid and EDTA. Additional subgroups are identified according to substrate hydrolysis profiles. Group 1 β-lactamases include the AmpC enzymes that are intrinsically resistant to β-lactamase inhibitors and are found in a variety of gram-negative bacteria. Group 2 β-lactamases include a variety of enzymes, which are all intrinsically susceptible to the β-lactamase inhibitors. Included in this group are the most prevalent plasmid-mediated, 2b β-lactamases found in *E. coli*

and *K. pneumoniae*, which are responsible for resistance to ampicillin and first-generation cephalosporins in these species.[104] Mutant forms of these enzymes are responsible for resistance to expanded-spectrum cephalosporins and aztreonam and for resistance to β-lactamase inhibitor/β-lactam drug combinations. Group 3 β-lactamases include the metallo-β-lactamases capable of hydrolyzing the carbapenems. Group 4 β-lactamases are those penicillinases not inhibited by clavulanic acid. Fortunately, they are not very common.

The β-lactamases vary considerably with respect to their ability to inactivate the penicillins and cephalosporins. Some of the enzymes primarily hydrolyze penicillins, some cephalosporins, and others hydrolyze a wide variety of β-lactam antibiotics. The β-lactamases produced by *S. aureus* are penicillinases, but the R factor–transmitted TEM enzyme which is widely distributed among gram-negative bacteria is an example of a β-lactamase that hydrolyzes a rather broad spectrum of substrates. Many bacteria produce a low level of β-lactamase that may be induced to higher levels by the presence of β-lactam antibiotics. This is particularly true in gram-positive organisms where most β-lactamases are inducible. Most of the older penicillins, including penicillinase-resistant

Table 3–4. *Classification of β-lactamases.*

Group	Characteristics	Representative enzymes
1	Cephalosporinases not inhibited by clavulanic acid	AmpC
2a	Penicillinases inhibited by clavulanic acid	PC1 *(S. aureus)*
2b	Broad-spectrum enzymes inhibited by clavulanic acid	TEM-1, TEM-2, SHV-1
2be	Extended broad-spectrum enzymes inhibited by clavulanic acid	TEM-3 to -28, SHV-2 to -6
2br	Broad-spectrum enzymes with reduced binding to clavulanic acid	TEM-30 to -36, TRC-1
2c	Carbenicillin-hydrolyzing enzymes inhibited by clavulanic acid	PSE-1, CARB-3
2d	Cloxacillin-hydrolyzing enzymes inhibited by clavulanic acid	OXA-1, PSE-2
2e	Cephalosporinases inhibited by clavulanic acid	*Proteus vulgaris*
2f	Carbapenem-hydrolyzing nonmetallo-β-lactamases	IMI-1, NMC-A, Sme-1
3	Carbapenem-hydrolyzing metallo-β-lactamases	L1
4	Penicillinases not inhibited by clavulanic acid	*Proteus cepacia*

Source: The β-lactamases of gram-negative bacteria are classified according to criteria by Pitout et al.[105]

penicillins, and cephalosporins can act as inducers. Some of the newer penicillins (e.g., piperacillin) and cephalosporins (e.g., moxalactam and cefoperazone) have very low inducer activity.[106]

Penicillinases are synthesized at the inner surface of the bacterial cell membrane and probably pass through the membrane to the external surface while they are being synthesized. In general, gram-positive bacteria produce large amounts of penicillinase, and most of it is released into the surrounding medium. This is called *exopenicillinase*. In contrast, gram-negative organisms usually produce β-lactamase in smaller amounts, and it remains largely in association with the surface structures external to the cytoplasmic membrane.[107]

The synthesis and processing of penicillinase by the gram-positive organism *Bacillus licheniformis* has been studied in some detail. This bacterium has a single structural gene for penicillinase.[108] It is typical of gram-positive bacteria to synthesize one β-lactamase but some naturally occurring strains of gram-negative bacteria produce more than one type of enzyme.[102] The enzyme of *B. licheniformis* exists in both hydrophilic and hydrophobic forms. The enzyme appears first in a hydrophobic form associated with the cell membrane or with small vesicles located at the cell membrane surface.[109] When the bacterium is exposed to inducers (e.g., a penicillin), there is a rapid increase in penicillinase production accompanied by the formation of numerous vesicles with high enzyme activity. The hydrophilic exopenicillinase is released from the cell by a proteolytic cleavage of the hydrophobic carboxy-terminal region of the membrane-bound enzyme.[110,111] The hydrophobic forms of β-lactamase should not be considered mere precursors of the free exoenzyme. Indeed, they play a very important role in protecting cells, particularly gram-negative bacteria, from the action of penicillins and cephalosporins.

There are significant differences in the way the β-lactamases protect gram-positive and gram-negative bacteria from β-lactam antibiotics.[93,112] In general, β-lactamase production in gram-positive organisms is inducible and large amounts of penicillinase are secreted into the surrounding medium. For example, when fully induced, clinical isolates of *S. aureus* can synthesize up to 1% of their dry weight as penicillinase.[112] The substrate affinities of β-lactamases produced by gram-positive bacteria are, in general, much higher than those of the enzymes synthesized by gram-negative bacteria. As the enzyme is diluted by diffusion into the medium, the ability to produce large amounts of enzyme with high substrate affinity would seem to be important for protecting the gram-positive organism against the antibiotic. Dilution of penicillinase into the surrounding medium accounts for the "inoculum effect" observed when the MIC values of penicillinase-producing staphylococci are being determined (see Table 3–5). At low cell concentrations, the level of penicillinase activity (after dilution) may not be sufficient to protect the organism from exposure to moderate amounts of penicillinase-sensitive penicillins, but at high cell concentrations an impressive drug-destroying activity exists and very large amounts of penicillin may be required to inhibit bacterial growth.[102] The penicillinase-sensitive penicillins may be par-

Table 3–5. *Effect of inoculum size on the resistance of a β-lactamase-producing strain of* Staphylococcus aureus *to penicillin G.*

	Minimum inhibitory concentration (µg/ml)			
Inoculum size (bacteria/ml)	10^1	10^3	10^5	10^7
S. aureus (nonpenicillinase-producing strain)	<0.5	<0.5	<0.5	<0.5
S. aureus (penicillinase-producing strain)	<0.5	<0.5	16	1250

Source: From Sykes and Mathew,[102] Table 8.

ticularly ineffective in treating infections, such as abscesses, where high concentrations of β-lactamase-producing organisms exist. Occasionally, infections have been noted to be clinically resistant to penicillin therapy even though the pathogen cultured from the infection site remained sensitive to antibiotic testing in vitro. Such apparent clinical resistance happens rarely with streptococcal infections in the respiratory tract.[113] The major pathogen is protected from the drug because the exopenicillinase produced by other organisms (eg., staphylocci) inactivates the antibiotic.

β-Lactamase-synthesizing gram-negative bacteria can attain a high level of penicillin resistance with the production of a relatively small amount of enzyme, much of which is retained in the periplasmic space between the cytoplasmic and outer membranes (see Fig. 3–10). As mentioned before, the gram-negative bacteria have a certain intrinsic resistance due to the barrier function of the outer membrane. The cell-bound β-lactamases of these organisms can provide a very effective level of activity in the periplasmic space. As shown in Figure 3–10, an antibiotic that traverses the pores in the outer membrane encounters the β-lactamase-containing environment of the periplasmic space before reaching its targets, the penicillin binding proteins. Thus, in gram-negative bacteria the effectiveness of a β-lactam antibiotic is a function of both its ability to diffuse through the porin system and its sensitivity to destruction by the periplasmic β-lactamase(s).

The interplay of permeability and enzymatic barriers in determining antibiotic sensitivity in gram-negative bacteria is illustrated by the potential response of E. coli producing the TEM-type of β-lactamase to exposure to ampicillin or cephaloridine.[112] The TEM β-lactamase can hydrolyze ampicillin and cephaloridine at similar rates,[114] yet cephaloridine has a much better ability to pass through the outer membrane of E. coli.[75,83] In organisms containing the TEM enzyme, clear resistance to ampicillin is often present, yet resistance to cephaloridine may be marginal.[112] In the case of cephaloridine, large amounts of drugs pass into the peri-

plasmic space and the β-lactamase activity may not be able to eliminate enough of the drug to prevent growth inhibition. Because ampicillin penetrates relatively poorly, the same amount of enzyme activity may be quite adequate to protect the cell. Although the penicillinase-resistant penicillins methicillin and cloxacillin are not inactivated by the TEM enzyme at all, E. coli are not susceptible to these drugs because they don't penetrate the outer membrane barrier.[112] It is clear that the interplay between the permeability barrier and β-lactamase activity in gram-negative bacteria is very important in determining the clinical efficacy of β-lactam antibiotics, and pharmaceutical manufacturers are devoting considerable effort to developing drugs that have both high permeability coefficients and improved β-lactamase resistance.

β-Lactamase-Resistant Penicillins and Cephalosporins

Methicillin, nafcillin, and the isoxazolyl penicillins (oxacillin, cloxacillin, and dicloxacillin) are semisynthetic penicillins that are resistant to cleavage by penicillinases. The affinity constants for methicillin and two penicillinase-sensitive penicillins for a staphylococcal penicillinase are shown in Table 3–6.[115] It is evident that methicillin has an affinity for the substrate site of the penicillinase some four orders of magnitude less than penicillin G, which is readily hydrolyzed. The penicillinase-resistant penicillins have proven to be very useful in treating penicillinase-producing staphylococcal infections. It is fortunate that even though these antibiotics have been used widely since the early 1960s, penicillinases capable of hydrolyzing the methicillin-oxacillin group have not been identified in clinical isolates of gram-positive bacteria.[116] Some gram-negative bacteria produce R plasmid-mediated β-lactamases that hydrolyze methicillin and some of the isoxazolyl penicillins more rapidly than penicillin G.[102]

The ability of a cephalosporin to act as a substrate for gram-negative β-lactamase is an important determinant of its spectrum of action. The cephalosporins that have been in

Table 3–6. *Affinity of penicillins for* Staphylococcus aureus *penicillinase.* The K_m was determined for each compound with free penicillinase in the broth from a culture of *S. aureus*.

Antibiotic	Effectiveness in treatment of penicillinase-producing staphylococci	$K_m(\mu M)$
Penicillin G	Ineffective	2.5
Phenoxymethyl penicillin	Ineffective	3.8
Methicillin	Effective	28,000

Source: From Novick.[115]

clinical use the longest, the so-called first-generation cephalosporins, are generally better substrates for gram-negative β-lactamases than newer second-generation cephalosporins, which are effective against a greater variety of gram-negative bacteria. The relative rates of hydrolysis of several first- and second-generation cephalosporins by several gram-negative β-lactamases are presented in Table 3–7.[117] The third-generation cephalosporins (e.g., cefotaxime, cefoperazone, ceftriaxone, ceftizoxime) are even more active against some β-lactamase-producing strains of gram-negative bacteria than the second-generation cephalosporins and cephamycins.

Table 3–7. *Relative rates of hydrolysis of first-and second-generation cephalosporins by some gram-negative β-lactamases.* Enzymes Ia and Id are cephalosporinases from *Enterobacter cloacae* and *Pseudomonas aeruginosa*; IIIa is the major broad-spectrum TEM enzyme found in a wide range of gram-negative species; IVc is a broad-spectrum β-lactamase from *Klebsiella aerogenes*. Rates are expressed relative to an arbitrary value of 100 for cephaloridine.

Antibiotic	Rate of hydrolysis			
	Ia	Id	IIIa	IVc
First generation				
Cephaloridine	100	100	100	100
Cephalothin	100	60	25	68
Cefazolin	45	110	15	75
Second generation				
Cefamandole	0.1	0	20	60
Cefoxitin	0	0.1	0	0
Cefuroxime	0	0	0.1	1.3

Source: From Richmond and Wotton,[117] Table 1.

The newest of the third-generation cephalosporins are inactivated by very few β-lactamases and have an even broader spectrum of action against gram-negative bacteria. They are, however, susceptible to hydrolysis by inducible, chromosomally encoded β-lactamases. Induction of β-lactamases by treatment of infections with second and third-generation cephalosporins and/or imipenem may result in resistance to all third-generation cephalosporins.

The newest class of cephalosporins introduced for clinical use is the fourth-generation compounds of which cefipime is the only available member at this time. These fourth-generation agents are dipolar ionic compounds in contrast to the anionic third-generation compounds. They also have a lower affinity for the β-lactamases of gram-negative organisms,[118] and are poor inducers of β-lactamases.[119] These drugs thus have a broad antimicrobial spectrum of activity.

β-Lactamase-Inactivating β-Lactam Drugs

An important advance in the development of β-lactam antibiotics has come with the introduction of drugs that inhibit β-lactamase enzymes. Several naturally occurring β-lactamase inhibitors have been isolated and others are being synthesized. Clavulanic

Clavulanic acid

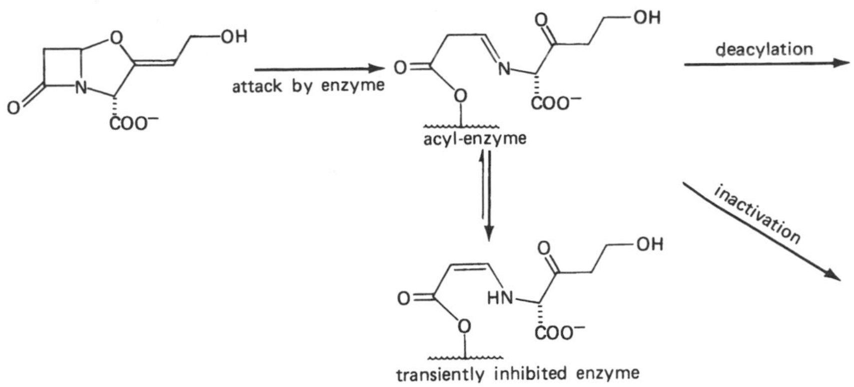

Figure 3–12. Formation of acyl-enzyme intermediate from clavulanic acid and β-lactamase and its conversion to the transiently inhibited form of the enzyme as proposed by Charnas and Knowles.[123]

acid, a β-lactam isolated from *Streptomyces clavuligerus*, was the first of these inhibitors.[120] This drug has only a weak antibacterial activity but it is a potent and progressive inhibitor of β-lactamases.[121] Detailed studies of the interaction of clavulanic acid with TEM β-lactamases show that the inhibition is complex. Clavulanic acid interacts with the enzyme in three ways: the clavulanic acid is destroyed catalytically and the enzyme is both transiently inhibited and irreversibly inactivated (Fig. 3–12).[122,123] As described previously for D-alanine carboxypeptidases, the reaction of β-lactamase with penicillins and cephalosporins normally proceeds via the formation of an acyl-enzyme intermediate.[124] Clavulanic acid is a substrate that can be both a mechanism-based inhibitor ("suicide substrate") and a

mechanism-based inactivator of β-lactamase. Clavulanic acid has been shown to act synergistically with penicillins and cephalosporins in vitro against clinical isolates of β-lactamase-producing strains of *S. aureus* and several gram-negative bacteria (see Table 3–8).[125,126] The combination of amoxicillin and clavulanic acid (trade name Augmentin) is marketed in Great Britain and the United States.

Tazobactam, the latest β-lactamase inhibitor to be developed, seems to be similar to clavulanic acid in activity and both it and the older inhibitor sulbactam are more potent than clavulanic acid. A relatively new combination agent is piperacillin-tazobactam, which has a broader spectrum of antibiotic activity than the amoxicillin-clavulanic acid combination.[127]

Table 3–8. *Activity of ampicillin alone and in the presence of sodium clavulanate against β-lactamase-producing strains of* Staphylococcus aureus, Proteus mirabilis, *and* Escherichia coli.

	Minimum inhibitory concentration (µg/ml)		
Antibiotic	*S. aureus*	*P. mirabilis*	*E. coli*
Sodium clavulanate alone	15	62–125	31
Ampicillin alone	500	>2000	>2000
Ampicillin in the presence of 5 µg/ml of Na clavulanate	0.02	8	4

Source: From Reading and Cole,[121] Table 3.

Methicillin-Resistant Staphylococci

Although staphylococci do not produce penicillinases that efficiently hydrolyze methicillin and other penicillinase-resistant penicillins, methicillin-resistant strains of *S. aureus* are a clinical problem. Strains of *S. aureus* resistant to methicillin at first were thought to be rare, but their prevalence has risen rapidly worldwide in recent years. The acquisition of this resistance in hospitals and nursing homes has caused severe administrative and clinical problems. The methicillin-resistant strains are usually resistant to many antibiotics.[128,129] Table 3–9 presents some data from a study of several cases of methicillin-resistant staphylococcal infections at the Boston City Hospital. In the strains tested there was resistance not only to the penicillinase-resistant penicillins but also to the other β-lactam antibiotics and to a number of antibiotics of widely differing structures and mechanisms of action. The methicillin-resistant staphylococci that have been reported in the literature, like those in this Boston study, have remained sensitive to vancomycin and this is the initial drug of choice for treating these infections.[130]

Methicillin resistance is clearly not due to a β-lactamase that hydrolyzes methicillin.[131] Although almost all the methicillin-resistant strains of staphylococci produce penicillin-ase, it has been shown that segregants that have lost the ability to produce penicillinase retain methicillin resistance.[132] Methicillin resistance is usually determined by a chromosomal gene,[133] it is transferred by transduction, and the recipient apparently must carry a penicillinase plasmid.[133, 134] Once established, the maintenance and expression of methicillin resistance is independent of either β-lactamase production or the presence of plasmid DNA.[135] The β-lactamase requirement for transduction of methicillin resistance has not been explained.

The mechanism of resistance is believed to be acquisition of supplementary penicillin binding proteins with a low affinity for methicillin and other β-lactams. Methicillin-resistant *S. aureus* (MRSA) strains were found to become resistant as a result of acquisition of an additional PBP (via a transposon) with a very low affinity for all β-lactams. The gene encoding this new PBP has also been found in certain coagulase-negative staphylococci and can account for methicillin resistance in these organisms.[92] The ability of a single PBP to take over the functions of the three normal high-molecular-weight PBPs of staphylococci was surprising, as multiple high-molecular-weight PBPs are thought to be required for the normal growth and morphogenesis of bacteria.[136] The PBP-mediated resistance in

Table 3–9. *Relative sensitivity of methicillin-sensitive and methicillin-resistant strains of* Staphylococcus aureus *to various antibiotics*. The minimum concentration of antibiotic required to prevent visible growth in cultures of *S. aureus* isolated from patients at the Boston City Hospital was determined. Results as concentration of drug at which growth was totally inhibited in 50% of the strains tested.

Antibiotic	Antibiotic concentration reqired for growth inhibition (μg/ml)		
	Methicillin-sensitive (291 strains)	Methicillin-resistant (22 strains)	Approximate-fold resistance
Methicillin	1.3	40	34
Cloxacillin	0.24	18	75
Cephalothin	0.24	20	83
Erythromycin	0.24	>100	>400
Tetracycline	1.6	70	44
Chloramphenicol	5	60	12
Vancomycin	2	1.4	0
Bacitracin	20	15	0

Source: Table constructed from data of Barrett et al.[128]

MRSA is analagous to bacterial resistance to the sulfonamides in which alternative target enzymes with low affinity are acquired.[137] The bacterial population is highly heterogeneous in its response to methicillin and only a small minority of cells may appear to be resistant in conventional media. The progeny of resistant colonies are also heterogeneous in their response to the drug. For these reasons standard susceptibility tests may not detect MRSA. The use of large inocula plus media supplemented with sodium chloride and/or incubation at 30°C is recommended.[138]

The MRSA are believed to be resistant to all β-lactam antibiotics, including imipenem, and to most antistaphylococcal antibiotics. Resistance has also been reported to occur to fluoroquinolones, such as ciprofloxacin. Vancomycin is the treatment of choice for MRSA, and some clinicians use a combination of vancomycin and rifampin, especially for life-threatening infections and those involving foreign bodies (e.g., prostheses). The two drugs appear to be synergistic against these organisms.

Resistance to Vancomycin

Resistance of enterococci to vancomycin has now become a major clinical problem. A major advantage of vancomycin therapy had been the virtual absence of resistant strains, but the recent emergence of vancomycin resistance in the clinic has been met with great apprehension. Both Van A resistance (resistance to both vancomycin and its close relative teicoplanin) and Van B and C resistance (resistance to vancomycin alone) have been extensively studied.[139] Van A resistance is inducible and is brought about by a cluster of genes that are on a transposable element and may be present on a transferable plasmid. Van B resistance is also inducible but is chromosomally mediated and generally not transferable.[140] The genes responsible for high-level vancomycin resistance in pathogenic enterococci have been cloned and sequenced.[141] Resistance involves the action of nine genes contained within the transposable element Tn 1536, which is carried on a plasmid.[142] Two of the genes are involved in pro-

moting mobilization of the transposable element from one DNA locus to another. The seven vancomycin-resistance genes are expressed only in the presence of the drug. Proteins produced by these genes result in resistance by a simple but clever mechanism: basically, the resistant cells have replaced the normal D-Ala-D-Ala peptidoglycan termini with D-Ala-D-lactate termini that are not recognized by vancomycin. One of the gene products is a reductase that produces the necessary lactate from the normal metabolites pyruvate and ketobutyrate. In vitro binding studies have shown that the affinity of vancomycin for N-acyl-D-Ala-D-lactate is 1000 times less than its affinity for N-acyl-D-Ala-D-Ala, paralleling the 1000-fold reduced sensitivity of vancomycin-resistant bacteria to the drug.[143] Thus, clinical resistance to vancomycin has emerged as a result of a simple switch of an ester bond for an amide bond.[141]

Vancomycin has been used with increasing frequency to treat severe staphylococcal infection because of both resistance and allergy to the β-lactams. This use has resulted in resistance to vancomycin in these bacteria as well. It has not yet been established whether a similar resistance gene has the potential for conferring vancomycin resistance on methicillin-resistant strains of *Staphylococcus aureus*. *S. aureus* resistance has been demonstrated in the laboratory and is associated with production of a 39 kilodalton cell wall protein that shows a low level of homology with a similar-sized molecule produced by enterococci exhibiting Van A resistance. Low-level resistance has been described in clinical isolates of coagulase-negative staphylococci. Such resistance has been attributed to alterations in cell wall structure, overproduction of the cell wall peptidoglycan, and binding to cell wall sites other than the primary target.[140] More research is needed to fully elucidate the mechanisms of resistance among the different phenotypes.

REFERENCES

1. Florey, H. W. *Antibiotics*, Vol. I, ed. by H. W. Florey et al. New York: Oxford University Press, 1949.

2. Norrby, S. R. Carbapenems. *Med. Clin. North Am.* 1995;79:745.

3. Lederberg, R. J. Bacterial protoplasts induced by penicillin. *Proc. Natl. Acad. Sci. U.S.A.* 1956;42:574.

4. Donachie, W. D., and K. J. Begg. Growth of the bacterial cell. *Nature* 1970;227:1220.

5. Park, J. T., and M. J. Johnson. Accumulation of labile phosphate in *Staphylococcus aureus* grown in the presence of penicillin. *J. Biol. Chem.* 1949;179:585.

6. Nathenson, S. G., and J. L. Strominger. Effects of penicillin on the biosynthesis of the cell walls of *Escherichia coli* and *Staphylococcus aureus. J. Pharmacol. Exp. Ther.* 1961;131:1.

7. Shockman, G. D., L. Daneo-Moore, T. D. McDowell, and W. Wong. Function and structure of the cell wall—its importance in the life and death of bacteria. In *β-Lactam Antibiotics*, ed. by M. Salton and G. M. Shockman. New York: Academic Press, 1981, pp. 31–65.

8. Roze, U., and J. L. Strominger. Alanine racemase from *Staphylococcus aureus*: conformation of its substrates and its inhibitor, D-cycloserine. *Mol. Pharmacol.* 1964;2:92.

9. Strominger, J. L., K. Izaki, M. Matsuhashi, and D. L. Tipper. Pepitdoglycan transpepidase and D-alanine carboxypeptidase: penicillin-sensitive enzymatic reactions. *Fed. Proc.* 1967;26:9.

10. Neuhaus, F. C., C. V. Carpenter, M. P. Lambert, and R. J. Wargel. D-cycloserine as a tool in studying the enzymes in the alanine branch of peptidoglycan synthesis. In *Molecular Mechanisms of Antibiotic Action on Protein Biosynthesis and Membranes*, ed. by E. Munoz, F. Ferrandiz, and D. Vasquez. Amsterdam: Elsevier, 1972, pp. 339–387.

11. Wang, E., and C. Walsh. Suicide substrates for the alanine racemase of *Escherichia coli* B. *Biochemistry* 1978;17:1313.

12. Kahan, F. M., J. S. Kahan, P. T. Cassidy, and H. Kropp. The mechanism of action of fosfomycin (phosphonomycin). *Ann. N.Y. Acad. Sci.* 1974;235:364.

13. Felmingham, D. Glycopeptides. In *Antibiotic and Chemotherapy*, 7th ed. by F. O'Grady, H. Lambert, R. G. Finch, and D. Greenwood. New York: Churchill Livingstone, 1997, pp. 363–368.

14. Anderson, J. S., M. Matsuhashi, M. A. Haskin, and J. L. Strominger. Lipid-phosphoacetylmuramyl-pentapeptide and lipid-phospho-disaccharide-pentapeptide: presumed membrane transport intermediates in cell wall synthesis. *Proc. Natl. Acad. Sci. U.S.A.* 1965;53:881.

15. Matsuhashi, M., C. P. Dietrich, and J. L. Strominger. Biosynthesis of the peptidoglycan of bacterial cell walls: the role of soluble ribonucleic acid and of lipid intermediates in glycine incorporation in *Staphylococcus aureus. J. Biol. Chem.* 1967;242:3191.

16. Perkins, H. R., and M. Nieto. The chemical basis for the action of the vancomycin group of antibiotics. *Ann. N.Y. Acad. Sci.* 1974;235:348.

17. Chatterjee, A. N., and H. R. Perkins. Compounds formed between nucleotides related to the biosynthesis of bacterial cell wall and vancomycin. *Biochem. Biophys. Res. Commun.* 1966;24:489.

18. Johnston, L. S., and F. C. Neuhaus. Initial membrane reaction in the biosynthesis of peptidogly-

can. Spin-labeled intermediates as receptors for vancomycin and ristocetin. *Biochemistry* 1975;14:2754.

19. Nieto, M., and H. R. Perkins. Modification of the acyl-D-alanine terminus affecting complex formation with vancomycin. *Biochem. J.* 1971;123:789.

20. Perkins, H. R. Specificity of combination between mucopeptide precursors and vancomycin or ristocetin. *Biochem. J.* 1969;111:195.

21. Sheldrick, G. M., P. G. Jones, O. Kennard, D. H. Williams, and G. Smith. Structure of vancomycin and its complex with acetyl-D-alanyl-D-alanine. *Nature* 1978;271:223.

22. Brown, J. P., J. Feeney, and A. S. V. Burgen. A nuclear magnetic resonance study of the interaction between vancomycin and acetyl-D-alanyl-D-alanine in aqueous solution. *Mol. Pharmacol.* 1975;11:119.

23. Brown, J. P., L. Terenius, J. Feeney, and A. S. V. Burgen. A structure-activity study by nuclear magnetic resonance of peptide interactions with vancomycin. *Mol. Pharmacol.* 1975;11:126.

24. Williams, D. H., and J. R. Kalman. Structural and mode of action studies on the antibiotic vancomycin. Evidence from 270-mHz proton magnetic resonance. *J. Am. Chem. Soc.* 1977;99:2768.

25. Perkins, H. R., and M. Nieto: The preparation of iodinated vancomycin and its distribution in bacteria treated with the antibiotic. *Biochem. J.* 1970;116:83.

26. Irving C. S., and A. Lapidot: Effects of binding and bactericidal action of vancomycin in *Bacillus licheniformis* cell wall organization as probed by ^{15}N nuclear magnetic resonance spectroscopy. *Antimicrob. Agents Chemother.* 1978;14:695.

27. Siewert, G., and J. L. Strominger. Bacitracin: an inhibitor of the dephosphorylation of lipid pyrophosphate, an intermediate in biosynthesis of the peptidoglycan of bacterial cell walls. *Proc. Natl. Acad. Sci. U.S.A.* 1967;57:767.

28. Higashi, Y., J. L. Strominger, and C. C. Sweeley. Biosynthesis of the peptidoglycan of bacterial cell walls: XXI. Isolation of free C_{55}-isoprenoid alcohol and of lipid intermediates in peptidoglycan synthesis from *Staphylococcus aureus. J. Biol. Chem.* 1970;245:3697.

29. Stone, K. J., and J. L. Strominger. Mechanism of action of bacitracin: complexation with metal ion and C_{55}-isoprenyl pyrophosphate. *Proc. Natl. Acad. Sci. U.S.A.* 1971;68:3223.

30. Storm, D. R., and J. L. Strominger. Complex formation between bacitracin peptides and isoprenyl pyrophosphates: the specificity of lipid-peptide interactions.*J. Biol. Chem.* 1973;248:3940.

31. Storm, D. R., and J. L. Strominger. Binding of bacitracin to cells and protoplasts of *Micrococcus lysodeikticus. J. Biol. Chem.* 1974;249:1823.

32. Tipper, D. J., and J. L. Strominger. Biosynthesis of the peptidoglycan of bacterial cell walls: inhibition of cross-linking by penicillins and cephalosporins. *J. Biol. Chem.* 1968;243:3169.

33. Fitz-James, P., and R. Hancock. The initial structural lesion of penicillin action in *Bacillus megaterium. J. Cell Biol.* 1965;26:657.

34. Mirelman, D., R. Bracha, and N. Sharon. Penicillin-induced secretion of a soluble, uncross-linked

peptidoglycan by *Micrococcus luteus* cells. *Biochemistry* 1974;13:5045.

35. Izaki, K., M. Matsuhashi, and J. L. Strominger. Biosynthesis of the peptidoglycan of bacterial cell walls: peptidoglycan transpeptidase and D-alanine carboxypeptidase; penicillin-sensitive enzymatic reaction in strains of *Escherichia coli*. *J. Biol. Chem.* 1968;243:3180.

36. Mirelman, D., and M. Sharon. Biosynthesis of peptidoglycan by a cell wall preparation of *Staphylococcus aureus* and its inhibition by penicillin. *Biochem. Biophys. Res. Commun.* 1972;46:1909.

37. Tipper, D. J., and J. L. Strominger. Mechanism of action of penicillins: a proposal based on their structural similarity to acyl-D-alanyl-D-alanine. *Proc. Natl. Acad. Sci. U.S.A.* 1965;54:1133.

38. Waxman, D. J., and J. L. Strominger. Cephalosporin-sensitive penicillin binding proteins of *Staphylococcus aureus* and *Bacillus subtilis* active in the conversion of [¹⁴C]penicillin G to [¹⁴C]phenylacetylglycine. *J. Biol. Chem.* 1979;254:12056.

39. Spratt, B. G. Biochemical and genetical approaches to the mechanism of action of penicillin. *Philos. Trans. R. Soc. Lond. (Biol.)* 1980;289:273.

40. Reynolds, P., and H. Chase. β-Lactam-binding proteins: identification as lethal targets and probes of β-lactam accessibility. In *β-Lactam Antibiotics*, ed. by M. Salton and G. M. Shockman. New York: Academic Press, 1981, pp. 153–168.

41. Spratt, B. G. Distinct penicillin binding proteins involved in the division, elongation, and shape of *Escherichia coli* K-12. *Proc. Natl. Acad. Sci. U.S.A.* 1975;72:2999.

42. Spratt, B. G. Properties of the penicillin-binding proteins of *Escherichia coli*. *Eur. J. Biochem.* 1977;72:341.

43. Tamaki, S., S. Nakajima, and M. Matsuhashi. Thermosensitive mutation in *Escherichia coli* simultaneously causing defects in penicillin-binding proteins 1B's and in enzyme activity for peptidoglycan synthesis in vitro. *Proc. Natl. Acad. Sci. U.S.A.* 1977;74:5472.

44. Spratt, B. G., and A. B. Pardee. Penicillin-binding proteins and cell shape in *E. coli*. *Nature* 1975;254:516.

45. Suzuki, H., Y. Nishimura, and Y. Hirota. On the process of cell division in *Escherichia coli*: a series of mutants of *E. coli* altered in the penicillin binding proteins. *Proc. Natl. Acad. Sci. U.S.A.* 1978;75:664.

46. Amanuma, H., and J. L. Strominger. Purification and properties of penicillin-binding proteins 5 and 6 from *Escherichia coli* membranes. *J. Biol. Chem.* 1980;255:11173.

47. Curtis, N. A. C., D. Orr, G. W. Ross, and M. Boulton. Affinities of penicillins and cephalosporins for the penicillin-binding proteins of *Escherichia coli* K-12 and their antibacterial activity. *Antimicrob. Agents Chemother.* 1979;16:533.

48. Spratt, B. G. Comparison of the binding properties of two 6β-amidinopenicillanic acid derivatives that differ in their physiological effects on *Escherichia coli*. *Antimicrob. Agents Chemother.* 1977;11:161.

49. Melchoir, N. H., J. Blom, L. Tybring, and A. Birch-Andersen. Light and electron microscopy of the early response of *Escherichia coli* to a 6β-amidinopenicillanic acid (FL 1060). *Acta Pathol. Microbiol. Scand. Sect. B.* 1973;81:393.

50. Blumberg, P. M., and J. L. Strominger. Isolation by affinity chromatography of the penicillin-binding components from membranes of *Bacillus subtilis*. *Proc. Natl. Acad. Sci. U.S.A.* 1972;69:3751.

51. Matsuhashi, M., F. Ishino, J. Nakagawa, K. Mitsui, S. Nakajima-Iijima, S. Tamaki, and T. Hashizume. Enzymatic activities of penicillin-binding proteins of *Escherichia coli* and their sensitivities to β-lactam antibiotics. In *β-Lactam Antibiotics*, ed. by M. Salton and G. M. Shockman. New York: Academic Press, 1981, pp. 169–184.

52. Waxman, D. J., and J. L. Strominger. Sequence of active site peptides from the penicillin-sensitive D-alanine carboxypeptidase of *Bacillus subtilis*. Mechanism of penicillin action and sequence homology to β-lactamases. *J. Biol. Chem.* 1980;255:3964.

53. Yocum, R. R., J. R. Rasmussen, and J. L. Strominger. The mechanism of action of penicillin. Penicillin acylates the active site of *Bacillus stearothermophilus* D-alanine carboxypeptidase. *J. Biol. Chem.* 1980;255:3977

54. Waxman, D. J., and J. L. Strominger. Limited proteolysis of the penicillin-sensitive D-alanine carboxypeptidase purified from *Bacillus subtilis* membranes. *J. Biol. Chem.* 1981;256:2059.

55. Waxman, D. J., and J. L. Strominger. Primary structure of the COOH-terminal mambranous segment of a penicillin-sensitive enzyme purified from two *Bacilli*. *J. Biol. Chem.* 1981;256:2067.

56. Shockman, G. D. Symposium on the fine structure and replication of bacteria and their parts. IV. Unbalanced cell-wall synthesis: autolysis and cell-wall thickening. *Bacteriol. Rev.* 1965;29:345.

57. Forsberg, C., and H. J. Rogers. Autolytic enzymes in growth of bacteria. *Nature* 1971;229:272.

58. Tomasz, A. The mechanism of the irreversible antimicrobial effects of penicillins. How the β-lactam antibiotics kill and lyse bacteria. *Annu. Rev. Microbiol.* 1979;33:113.

59. Tomasz, A. Penicillin tolerance and the control of murein hydrolases. In *β-Lactam Antibiotics*, ed. by M. Salton and G. M. Shockman. New York: Academic Press, 1981, pp. 31–65.

60. Tomasz, A. Biological consequences of the replacement of choline by ethanolamine in the cell wall of *Pneumococcus*: chain formation, loss of transformability, and loss of autolysis. *Proc. Natl. Acad. Sci. U.S.A.* 1968;59:86.

61. Tomasz, A., A. Albino, and E. Zanati. Multiple antibiotic resistance in a bacterium with suppressed autolytic system. *Nature* 1970;227:138.

62. Rogers, H. J., and C. W. Forsberg. Role of autolysins in the killing of bacteria by some bactericidal antibiotics. *J. Bacteriol.* 1971;108:1235.

63. Ayusawa, D., Y. Yoneda, K. Yamane, and B. Maruo. Pleiotropic, phenomena in autolytic enzyme(s) content, flagellation, and simultaneous hyperproduction of extracellular α-amylase and protease in a *Bacillus subtilis* mutant. *J. Bacteriol.* 1975;124:459.

64. Sabath, L. D., N. Wheeler, M. Laverdiere, D.

Blazevic, and B. J. Wilkinson. A new type of penicillin resistance of *Staphylococcus aureus*. *Lancet* 1977;1: 443.

65. Mayhall, C. G., G. Medoff, and J. J. Marr. Variation in the susceptibility of strains of *Staphylococcus aureus* to oxacillin, cephalothin, and gentamicin. *Antimicrob. Agents Chemother.* 1976;10:707.

66. Allen, J. L., and K. Sprunt. Discrepancy between minimum inhibitory and minimum bactericidal concentrations of penicillin for group A and group B β-hemolytic streptococci. *J. Pediatr.* 1978;93:69.

67. Savitch, C. B., A. L. Barry, and P. D. Hoeprich. Infective endocarditis caused by *Streptococcus bovis* resistant to the lethal effect of penicillin G. *Arch Intern. Med.* 1978;138:931.

68. Tomasz, A., and S. Waks. Mechanism of action of penicillin: triggering of the pneumococcal enzyme by inhibitors of cell wall synthesis. *Proc. Natl. Acad. Sci. U.S.A.* 1975;72:4162.

69. Baddiley, J. Overview of the chemistry and biochemistry of bacterial walls and unique prokaryotic polymers. In *β-Lactam Antibiotics*, ed. by M. Salton and G. M. Shockman. New York: Academic Press, 1981, pp. 13–30.

70. Holtje, J. V., and A. Tomasz. Purification of the pneumococcal N-acetylmuramyl-L-alanine amidase to biochemical homogeneity. *J. Biol. Chem.* 1976;251: 4199.

71. Holtie, J. V., and A. Tomasz. Biological effects of lipoteichoic acids. *J. Bacteriol.* 1975;124:1023.

72. Hobby, G. L., and M. H. Dawson. Effect of rate of growth of bacteria on action of penicillin. *Proc. Soc. Exp. Biol. Med.* 1944;56:181.

73. Costerton, J. W., and K.-J. Cheng. The role of the bacterial cell envelope in antibiotic resistance. *J. Antimicrob. Chemother.* 1975;1:363.

74. Sykes, R. B., and N. H. Georgopapadakou. Bacterial resistance to β-lactam antibiotics: an overview. In *β-Lactam Antibiotics*, ed. by M. Salton and G. M. Shockman. New York: Academic Press, 1981, pp. 199–214.

75. Nikaido, H., and T. Nakae. The outer membrane of gram-negative bacteria. *Adv. Microb. Physiol.* 1979;20:163.

76. Nikaido, H. Outer membrane permeability of bacteria: resistance and accesibility of targets. In *β-Lactam Antibiotics*, ed. by M. Salton and G. M. Shockman. New York: Academic Press, 1981, pp. 249–260.

77. Nikaido, H., S. A. Song, L. Shalteil, and M. Nurminen. Outer membrane of *Salmonella* XIV. Reduced transmembrane diffusion rates in porin-deficient mutants. *Biochem. Biophys. Res. Commun.* 1977;76: 324.

78. Nakae, T. Outer membrane of *Salmonella*. Isolation of protein complex that produces transmembrane channels. *J. Biol. Chem.* 1976;251:2176.

79. Schindler, H., and J. P. Rosenbusch. Matrix protein from *Escherichia coli* outer membranes forms voltage-controlled channels on lipid bilayers. *Proc. Natl. Acad. Sci. U.S.A.* 1978;75:3751.

80. Decad, G. M., and H. Nikaido. Outer membrane of gram-negative bacteria. XII. Molecular-sieving function of cell wall. *J. Bacteriol.* 1976;128:325.

81. Hancock, R. E. W. and H. Nikaido. Outer membranes of gram-negative bacteria. XIX. Isolation from *Pseudomonas aeruginosa* PA01 and use in reconstitution and definition of the permeability barrier. *J. Bacteriol.* 1978;136:381.

82. Steven, A. C., B. ten Heggler, R. Muller, J. Kistler, and J. P. Rosenbusch. Ultrastructure of a periodic protein layer in the outer membrane of *Escherichia coli*. *J. Cell Biol.* 1977;72:292.

83. Zimmerman, W., and A. Rosselet. Function of the outer membrane of *Escherichia coli* as a permeability barrier to β-lactam antibiotics. *Antimicrob. Agents Chemother.* 1977;12:368.

84. Richmond, M. H., D. C. Clark, and S. Wotton. Indirect method for assessing the penetration of beta-lactamase-nonsusceptible penicillins and cephalosporins in *Escherichia coli* strains. *Antimicrobi. Agents Chemother.* 1976;10:215.

85. Rammelkamp, C. H., and T. Moxon. Resistance of *Staphylococcus aureus* to the action of penicillin. *Proc. Soc. Exp. Biol. Med.* 1942;51:386.

86. Guze, L. B., and G. M. Kalmanson. Persistence of bacteria in "protoplast" form after apparent cure of pyelonephritis in rats. *Science* 1964;143:1340.

87. Buchanan, C. E., and J. L. Strominger. Altered penicillin-binding components in penicillin-resistant mutants of *Bacillus subtilis*. *Proc. Natl. Acad. Sci. U.S.A.* 1976;73:1816.

88. Jacobs, M. R., H. J. Koornhoff, R. M. Robbins-Browne, C. M. Stevenson, Z. A. Vermaak, I. Frieman, G. B. Miller, M. A. Witcomb, M. Isaacson, J. I. Ward, and R. Austrian. Emergence of multiply resistant pneumococci. *N. Engl. J. Med.* 1978;299:735.

89. Williamson, R., S. Zighelboim, and A. Tomasz. Penicillin-binding proteins of penicillin-resistant and penicillin-tolerant *Streptococcus pneumoniae*. In *β-Lactam Antibiotics*, ed. by M. Salton and G. M. Shockman. New York: Academic Press, 1981, pp. 215–225.

90. Dougherty, T. J., A. E. Koller, and A. Tomasz. Penicillin-binding proteins of penicillin-susceptible and intrinsically resistant *Neisseria gonorrhoeae*. *Antimicrob. Agents Chemother.* 1980;18:730.

91. Georgopapadakou, N. H. Penicillin-binding proteins and bacterial resistance to β-lactams. *Antimicrob. Agents Chemother.* 1993;37:2045.

92. Spratt, B. G. Resistance to antibiotics mediated by target alterations. *Science* 1994;264:388.

93. Richmond, M. H. Factors influencing the antibacterial action of the β-lactam antibiotics. *J. Antimicrob. Chemother.* 1978;4(Suppl. B):1.

94. Pollock, M. R. The function and evolution of penicillinase. *Proc. R. Soc. Lond. B* 1971;179:385.

95. Ozer, H. J., and A. K. Saz. Possible involements of β-lactamase in sporulation in *Bacillus cereus*. *J. Bacteriol.* 1970;102:65.

96. Novick, R. P. Analysis by transduction of mutants affecting penicillinase formation in *Staphylococcus aureus*. *J. Gen. Microbiol.* 1963;33:121.

97. Novick, R. P., and S. I. Morse. In vivo transmission of drug resistance factors between strains of *Staphylococcus aureus*. *J. Exp. Med.* 1967;125:45.

98. Dyke, K. G. H., M. T. Parker, and M. H. Rich-

mond. Penicillinase production and metal-ion resistance in *Staphylococcus aureus* isolated from hospital patients *J. Med. Microbiol.* 1970;3:125.

99. Lacey, R. W., and M. H. Richmond. The genetic basis of antibiotic resistance in *S. aureus*: the importance of gene transfer in the evolution of this organism in the hospital environment. *Ann. N.Y. Acad. Sci.* 1974; 236:395.

100. Rolinson, G. N. Bacterial resistance to penicillins and cephalosporins. *Proc. R. Soc. Lond. B* 1971; 179:403.

101. Lacey, R. W. Antibiotic resistance plasmids of *Staphylococcus aureus* and their clinical importance. *Bacteriol. Rev.* 1975;39:1.

102. Sykes, R. B., and M. Mathew. The β-lactamases of gram-negative bacteria and their role in resistance to β-lactam antibiotics. *J. Antimicrob. Chemother.* 1976; 2:115.

103. Bush, K., G. A. Jacoby, and A. A. Medeiras. A. functional classification scheme for β-lactamases and its correlation with molecular structure. *Antimicrob. Agents Chemother.* 1995;39:1211.

104. Sanders, C. C., and W. E. Sanders. β-lactam resistance in gram-negative bacteria: global trends and clinical impact. *Clin. Infect. Dis.* 1992;15:824.

105. Pitout, J. D. D., C. C. Sanders, and W. E. Sanders. Antimicrobial resistance with focus on β-lactam resistance in gram-negative bacilli. *Am. J. Med.* 1997; 103:51.

106. Mitsuhashi, S., and M. Inoue. New β-lactam antibiotics—antibacterial activities and inducibility of β-lactamase formation. In *β-lactam Antibiotics*, ed. by M. Salton and G. M. Shockman. New York: Academic Press, 1981, pp. 361–375.

107. Richmond, M. H., and N. A. C. Curtis. The interplay of β-lactamases and intrinsic factors in the resistance of gram-negative bacteria to penicillins and cephalosporins. *Ann. N.Y. Acad. Sci.* 1974;235:553.

108. Sherratt, D. J., and J. F. Collins. Analysis by transformation of the penicillinase system in *Bacillus licheniformis*. *J. Gen. Microbiol.* 1973;76:217.

109. Ghosh, B. K., J. O. Lampen, and C. C. Remsen. Periplasmic structure of frozen-etched and negatively stained cells of *Bacillus licheniformis* as correlated with penicillinase formation. *J. Bacteriol.* 1969;100:1002.

110. Simons, K., M. Sarvas, H. Garoff, and A. Helenius. Membrane-bound and secreted forms of penicillinase from *Bacillus licheniformis*. *J. Mol. Biol.* 1978; 126:673.

111. Izui, K., J. B. K. Nielsen, M. P. Caulfield, and J. O. Lampen. Large exopenicillinase, initial extracellular form detected in cultures of *Bacillus licheniformis*. *Biochemistry* 1980;19:1882.

112. Richmond, M. Beta-lactamases and bacterial resistance to beta-lactam antibiotics. In *β-Lactam Antibiotics*, ed. by M. Salton and G. M. Shockman. New York: Academic Press, 1981, pp. 261–273.

113. Weinstein, L., and A. C. Dalton. Host determinants of response to antimicrobial agents. *N. Engl. J. Med.* 1968;279:580.

114. Mathew, M. Plasmid-mediated β-lactamases of gram-negative bacteria: properties and distribution. *J. Antimicrob. Chemother.* 1979;5:349.

115. Novick, R. P. Staphylococcal penicillinase and the new penicillins. *Biochem. J.* 1962;83:229.

116. Dyke, K. G. H. Penicillinase production and intrinsic resistance to penicillins in methicillin-resistant cultures of *Staphylococcus aureus*. *J. Med. Microbiol.* 1969;2:261.

117. Richmond, M. H., and S. Wotton. Comparative study of seven cephalosporins: susceptibility to beta-lactamases and ability to penetrate the surface layers of *Escherichia coli*. *Antimicrob. Agents Chemother.* 1976; 10:219.

118. Goldfarb, J. New antimicrobial agents. *Pediatr. Clin. North Am.* 1995;42:717.

119. Sanders, C. C., and W. E. Sanders. Type I beta-lactamases of gram-negative bacteria: interactions with beta-lactam antibiotics. *J. Infect. Dis.* 1986;154:796.

120. Brown, A. G., D. Butterworth, M. Cole, G. Hanscomb, J. D. Hood, C. Reading, and G. N. Rolinson. Naturally occurring β-lactamase inhibitors with antibacterial activity. *J. Antibiot.* 1976;29:668.

121. Reading, C., and M. Cole. Clavulinic acid: a beta-lactamase-inhibiting beta lactam from *Streptomyces clavuligerus*. *Antimicrob. Agents Chemother.* 1977; 11:852.

122. Fisher, J., R. L. Charnas, and J. R. Knowles. Kinetic studies on the inactivation of *Escherichia coli* RTEM β-lactamase by clavulinic acid. *Biochemistry* 1978;17:2180.

123. Charnas, R. L., and J. R. Knowles. Inactivation of RTEM β-lactamase from *Escherichia coli* by clavulinic acid and 9-deoxyclavulinic acid. *Biochemistry* 1981;20:3214.

124. Fisher, J., J. G. Belasco, S. Khosla, and J. R. Knowles. β-Lactamase proceeds via an acyl-enzyme intermediate. Interaction of the *Escherichia coli* RTEM enzyme with cefoxitin. *Biochemistry* 1980;19:2895.

125. Wise, R., J. M. Andrews, and K. A. Bedford. In vitro study of clavulinic acid in combination with penicillin, amoxicillin, and carbenicillin. *Antimicrob. Agents Chemother.* 1978;13:389.

126. Neu H. C., and K. P. Fu. Clavulinic acid, a novel inhibitor of β-lactamases. *Antimicrob. Agents Chemother.* 1978;14:650.

127. Hishashitani, F., A. Hyodo, N. Ishida, M. Inune, and S. Mitsuhashi. Inhibition of beta-lactamases by tazobactam and in vitro antibacterial activity of tazobactam compared to piperacillin. *J. Antimicrob. Chemother.* 1990;25:507.

128. Barrett, F. F., R. F. McGehee, and M. Finland. Methicillin-resistant *Staphylococcus aureus* at Boston City Hospital. *N. Engl. Med.* 1968;279:441.

129. Plorde, J. J., and J. C. Sherris. Staphylococcal resistance to antibiotics: origin, measurement, and epidemiology. *Ann. N.Y. Acad. Sci.* 1974;236:413.

130. Peacock, J. E., F. J. Marsik, and R. P. Wenzel. Methicillin-resistant *Staphylococcus aureus*: introduction and spread within a hospital. *Ann. Intern Med.* 1980;93:526.

131. Dyke, K. G. H. Penicillinase production and intrinsic resistance to penicillins in methicillin-resistant cultures of *Staphylococcus aureus*. *J. Med. Microbiol.* 1969;2:261.

132. Seligman, S., Penicillinase-negative variants of

methicillin-resistant *Staphylococcus aureus*. *Nature* 1966;209:994.

133. Kayser, F. M., J. Wust, and P. Corrodi. Transduction and elimination of resistance determinants in methicillin-resistant *Staphylococcus aureus*. *Antimicrob. Agents Chemother.* 1972;2:217.

134. Cohen, S., and H. M. Sweeney. Transduction of methicillin-resistance in *Staphylococcus aureus* dependent on an unusual specificity of the recipient strain. *J. Bacteriol.* 1970;104:1158.

135. Stewart, G. C., and E. D. Rosenblum. Transduction of methicillin resistance in *Staphylococcus aureus*: recipient effectiveness and beta-lactamase production. *Antimicrob. Agents Chemother.* 1980;18:424.

136. Ghutsen, J. M. Serine β-lactamases and penicillin-binding proteins. *Annu. Rev. Microbiol.* 1991;45:37.

137. Then, R. L. Resistance to sulfonamides *Handbook of Experimental Pharmacology*, ed. by L. E. Byron, Springer-Verlag, Berlin, 1989, pp. 291–312.

138. Sutherland, R., β-lactams: penicillins. In *Antibiotics and Chemotherapy*, ed. by F. O'Grady, H. Lambert, R. Finch, and D. Greenwood. New York: Churchill-Livingstone, 1997, pp. 256–305.

139. Arthur, M., and P. Courvalain. Genetics and mechanisms of glycopeptide resistance in enterococci. *Antimicrob. Agents Chemother.* 1993;37:1563.

140. Woodford, N., A. P. Johnson, D. Morrison, and D. C. E. Speller. Current perspectives on glycopeptide resistance. *Clin. Microb. Revs.* 1995;8:585.

141. Walsh, C. T., Vancomycin resistance: decoding the molecular logic. *Science* 1993;261:308.

142. Leclerq, R., E. Derlot, J. Duval, and P. Courvalain. Plasmid-mediated resistance to vancomycin and teicoplanin in *Enterococcus faecium*. *N. Engl. J. Med.* 1988;319:157.

143. Bugg, T. D. H., G. D. Wright, S. Dutka-Malen, M. Arthur, P. Courvalain, and C. T. Walsh. Molecular basis for vancomycin resistance in *Enterococcus faecium* BM4147: biosynthesis of a depsipeptide peptidoglycan precursor by vancomycin resistance proteins Van H and Van A. *Biochemistry* 1991;30:10408.

CHAPTER FOUR

The Inhibitors of Cell Wall Synthesis, II

Pharmacology and Adverse Effects of the Penicillins, Cephalosporins, Carbapenems, Monobactams, Vancomycin, and Bacitracin

The Penicillins

Classification of the Penicillins

The penicillins can be classified according to their antibacterial spectrum of action as outlined in Table 4–1. Penicillin G (benzylpenicillin) has been in clinical use since the 1940s and is still the antibiotic of choice for treatment of a wide variety of infections (see tables on drugs of choice in Chapter 1 for a complete listing). Penicillin G is the antibiotic of choice for treatment of infections caused by most of the gram-positive cocci (the exceptions being *Streptococcus faecalis* and penicillinase-producing staphylococci), some gram-positive bacilli (e.g., *Bacillus anthracis*), a variety of anaerobic pathogens (gastrointestinal strains of *Bacteroides fragilis* are an exception), a few uncommon gram-negative bacilli (e.g., *Leptotrichia bucalis, Pasturella multocida, Streptobacillus moniliformis, Spirillum minus*), several spirochetes (*Treponema pallidum, Treponema pertenue, Leptospira*), and *Actinomyces israelii*. Although penicillin G is clinically useful in treatment of infections due to a variety of organisms, it is considered to have a narrow spectrum of action, as defined within the β-lactam antibiotic group. The penicillinase-resistant penicillins are also classified as narrow-spectrum and they are

used clinically only for treatment of penicillinase-producing strains of staphylococci. The aminopenicillins, such as ampicillin and amoxicillin, are effective against some gram-negative bacilli that do not respond to concentrations of penicillin G achieved in therapy. For this reason, they are referred to as broad spectrum penicillins. The aminopenicillins are not clinically effective against *Pseudomonas aeruginosa* but the penicillins of the carbenicillin group are effective against most strains of *P. aeruginosa* as well as *Enterobacter* and indole-positive *Proteus* and have been used for this purpose for many years. Extended-spectrum pencillins with increased activity against *P. aeruginosa* and *Bacteroides fragilis* have been available for several years.

Pharmacology of the Penicillins

Penicillin G (Fig. 4–1) is the prototype compound in the penicillin series, thus it is appropriate to begin a review of the penicillins with a summary of the pharmacology of this drug and its formulations. The pharmacology of the specialized penicillins is summarized in several tables and in discussions of each penicillin group in the next section of this chapter. An extensive discussion of the pharmacology of the individual penicillins in

Table 4–1. Classification of the penicillins.

Group	Characteristics	Generic name	Clinically useful antimicrobial spectrum
I	Narrow spectrum, penicillinase-sensitive penicillins	Penicillin G (benzylpenicillin) Penicillin V (phenoxymethyl-penicillin) Phenethicillin	*Streptococcus* species, *Neisseria* species, many anaerobes, spirochetes, others
II	Narrow spectrum, penicillinase-resistant penicillins	Methicillin Nafcillin Oxacillin Cloxacillin Dicloxacillin	*Staphylococcus aureus*
III	Broad spectrum, aminopenicillins	Ampicillin Amoxicillin Proampicillins Bacampicillin	*Haemophilus influenzae, Escherichia coli, Proteus mirabilis,* enterococci, *Neisseria gonorrhoeae*
IV	Broad spectrum, antipseudomonal penicillins	Carbenicillin Carbenicillin indanyl Ticarcillin Azlocillin	As for group III and *Pseudomonas aeruginosa, Enterobacter* species, indole-positive *Proteus*
V	Extended spectrum penicillins	Piperacillin Mezlocillin	As for group IV with increased activity against Enterobacteriaceae (esp. *Klebsiella*) and some anaerobes, including *Bacteroides fragilis.* Mezlocillin and piperacillin are very active against *Pseudomonas aeruginosa*

groups I–IV is presented in a review by Rolinson and Sutherland.[1]

ABSORPTION. Approximately one-third of an oral dose of penicillin G is absorbed from the gastrointestinal tract, primarily from the duodenum.[2] Maximum blood levels are reached in about 45 min. Penicillin G is unstable in acid,[3] and though one would assume from this that maximum absorption of penicillin G would be achieved if the drug were ingested when the gastric pH is highest, this is not the case. For maximum absorption, penicillin G should be taken either 1 h before or 2 to 3 h after a meal, as it has been clearly shown that the absorption is highest when the stomach is empty.[4] This, however, is the time when the pH is the lowest. Apparently the longer retention time of the drug in the food-containing stomach results in more extensive inactivation despite the higher pH. There is a great deal of variability in the amount of penicillin G that is absorbed with each oral administration in the same patient. This variability is probably due to different degrees of acid inactivation.

Penicillin V (phenoxymethyl penicillin) is a narrow-spectrum, penicillinase-sensitive penicillin that is more stable in acid than penicillin G; thus higher and more consistent blood levels are achieved with oral administration of this preparation.[5] Penicillin V has a spectrum of action similar to that of penicillin G, and because of the higher blood levels achieved, penicillin V is preferred for oral treatment of infections caused by nonpenicillinase-producing gram-positive cocci. Penicillin V is not recommended for treatment of gram-negative coccal infections, particularly gonorrhoea.

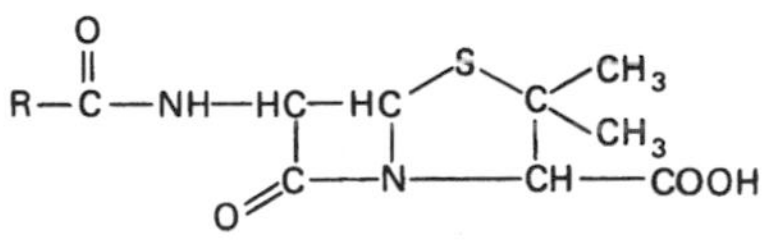

Penicillins

Name	**Side chain**	**Stability in acid**	**Routes of administration**	**Sensitivity to penicillinase**
Penicillin G	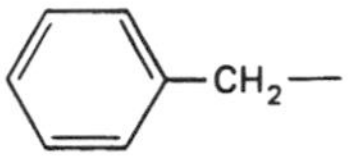	Poor	Oral, IM, IV	Sensitive
Phenoxymethyl penicillin (Pen V)	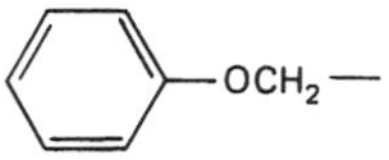	Good	Oral	Sensitive
Methicillin	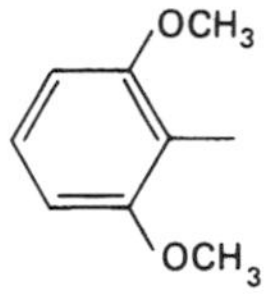	Poor (not given orally)	IM, IV	Resistant
Nafcillin	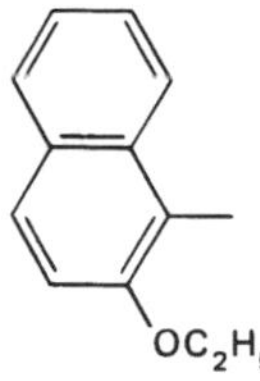	Poor	Oral*, IM, IV	Resistant
Oxacillin	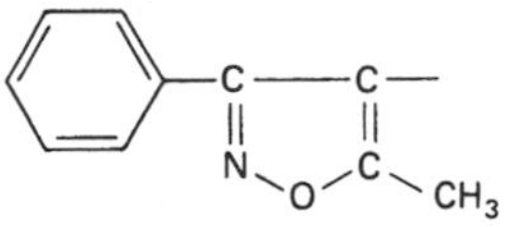	Good	Oral, IM, IV	Resistant
Cloxacillin	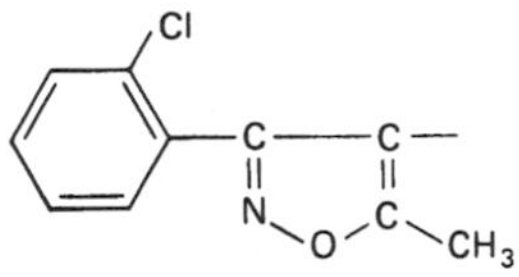	Good	Oral	Resistant
Dicloxacillin	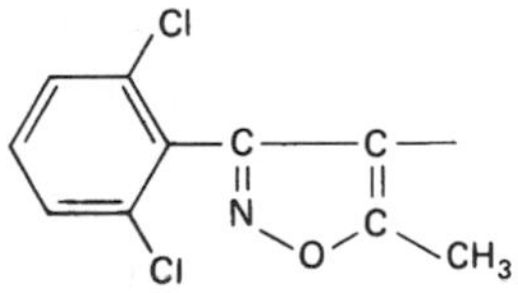	Good	Oral	Resistant

Figure 4–1. Structures and properties of the narrow spectrum penicillins. *An oral preparation of nafcillin is available but absorption is erratic and this route of administration is not recommended.

When penicillin G is administered intramuscularly, maximum blood levels are achieved in 15 min. In more severe infections, the antibiotic is administered parenterally at first, and oral penicillin is then utilized as the patient's condition permits. A schematic drawing of the relative blood levels and durations of action of penicillin G administered in various forms is presented in Figure 4–2. There are two parenteral prep-

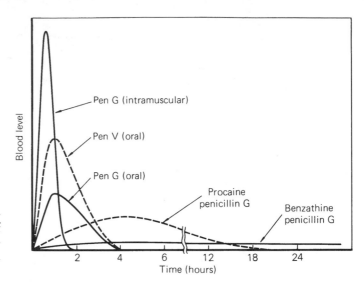

Figure 4–2. Schematic presentation of the blood concentration of various forms of penicillin G plotted as a function of time after oral or intramuscular administration.

arations of penicillin G that are very slowly absorbed from the site of intramuscular injection—procaine penicillin G and benzathine penicillin G. Procaine penicillin G yields peak blood levels in 2 to 4 h, and the blood concentration declines to negligible levels by 24 to 48 h. Benzathine penicillin G is absorbed from the injection site much more slowly, and very low serum levels of the antibiotic are detectable for 3 to 4 weeks after administration.[6,7] Since these two forms of the antibiotic result in low blood levels, they must be employed only in the treatment of organisms that are very sensitive to penicillin G. Obviously, benzathine penicillin G can be employed only with organisms that are exquisitely sensitive to the antibiotic, such as group A β-hemolytic streptococci and *Treponema pallidum*. Some physicians, in lieu of daily oral therapy, will treat selected patients with a single injection of benzathine penicillin G at monthly intervals as prophylaxis against rheumatic heart disease.

DISTRIBUTION AND EXCRETION. About 60% of the penicillin G in the serum is bound to plasma protein.[8] As shown in Table 4–2, the extent of protein binding ranges from about 20% for the aminopenicillins to 92% to 96% for the isoxazolyl group (oxacillin, cloxacillin, and dicloxacillin) of

penicillinase-resistant penicillins.[9] The free drug passes rapidly into interstitial fluid[10] and the peak concentration achieved in abscess fluid and fibrin clots is about 20% of the concentration of unbound penicillin in serum.[11]

The penicillins distribute widely throughout the body spaces. Passage into cerebrospinal, joint, and ocular fluids is poor in the absence of inflammation, however. In the presence of inflammation of the meninges, the joint spaces, or the eye, adequate concentrations of drug are achieved to treat meningitis,[12] arthritis,[13] and endophthalmitis caused by susceptible bacteria. The penicillins pass into the bile to varying extents and, in the absence of biliary obstruction, most (including those that are effective against gram-negative enteric organisms, like ampicillin or carbenicillin) achieve levels in the bile that are equal to or significantly greater than the serum levels. Unfortunately, in the presence of obstruction, significant concentrations are achieved only with nafcillin, which is a narrow-spectrum penicillin that is not effective against the common biliary tract pathogens.

Penicillin G is rapidly excreted by the kidney. In adults, most of an intramuscular dose of penicillin G (80% to 90%) is excreted by the kidney within an hour and a half. This rapid clearance is accomplished by

Table 4–2. Pharmacokinetic properties of the penicillins.

Penicillin	Major excretion routes	Half-life Normal (hours)	Half-life ESRD (hours)	Plasma protein binding (%)
Penicillin G	Renal (hepatic)	0.5	6–20	60
Methicillin	Renal (hepatic)	0.5	4	37
Nafcillin	Hepatic	0.5	1.2	90
Oxacillin	Renal (hepatic)	0.5	1	92
Cloxacillin	Hepatic (renal)	0.5	0.8	94
Dicloxacillin	Renal (hepatic)	0.5	1	96
Ampicillin	Renal (hepatic)	1.5	8–20	16–20
Amoxicillin	Renal	1	7	15–25
Carbenicillin	Renal (hepatic)	1.5	10–20	50
Ticarcillin	Renal	1–1.5	15	45

ESRD, end-stage renal disease.

Source: The values in the table have been taken from a review by Bennett et al.[9] (Table 1), to which the reader is referred for specific references on the pharmacokinetics of the individual drugs.

secretion in the proximal tubule[14] (about 80%) and by glomerular filtration (about 20%). After an intramuscular dose of a penicillin, 80% to 98% of the drug in the urine is present in the unaltered form.[15] Because these drugs are concentrated in the urine in their active forms, very high levels of antibacterial activity are attained. The half-life of penicillin G in older children and adults is about 30 min, but because of decreased tubular secretory capacity the half-life in infants during the first week of life is about 3.3 h and in infants 14 days of age and older it is about 1.4 h.[16] Metabolism of parenterally administered penicillins is minor; the chief metabolites are the corresponding penicilloic acids.[15]

Since penicillin G, the aminopenicillins, and the antipseudomonas penicillins are excreted predominantly by the renal route, their half-lives are significantly lengthened when renal function is markedly impaired (see Table 4–2) and their dosage should be modified to avoid the risk of neurotoxicity (see Table 4–3 for dosage modification). In contrast to penicillin G and the broad spectrum penicillins, nafcillin is eliminated almost solely by the hepatic route and no dosage adjustment is required with renal failure.[17,18] Oxacillin, cloxacillin, and dicloxacillin are efficiently eliminated by both renal and hepatic routes and, in the presence of renal failure and competent hepatic function, their half-lives are not significantly lengthened, so dosage reduction is not required.

The tubular secretion mechanism for penicillins is shared with a wide variety of organic acids. When penicillin was both scarce and expensive, it was often given with probenecid. Since probenecid is an organic acid that competes for the tubular transport of penicillins[19] (and possibly also for serum binding sites[12]), longer-lasting, higher levels of the drug result. However, probenecid is rarely used anymore because it can cause significant toxicity as a result of hypersensitivity reactions and gastrointestinal irritation. A similar active transport system for organic acids exists in the choroid plexus. In this case, organic acids such as 5-hydroxyindoleacetic acid, phenosulfonphthalein (PSP), and the penicillins are transported from the cerebrospinal fluid to the blood.[20] The cerebrospinal fluid levels of penicillins are increased in the presence of inflammation both because the rate of drug entry is increased and, perhaps more importantly, because the active efflux of drug from the cerebrospinal fluid is decreased.[21] It has been shown in animals that the administration of probenecid decreases the rate of efflux of penicillin from

Table 4–3. Adjustment of penicillin dosage in pateints with compromised renal function and after dialysis. The total daily dosage may be adjusted by maintaining the normal dosage interval and decreasing the dose per administration (the *dose reduction* method) or by keeping the dosage size normal and increasing the interval between administrations (the *interval extension* method). In the dose reduction method (D) the percentage of the usual dose that should be given at the normal dosage interval is presented. In the interval extension method (I) the interval in hours between doses of normal size is given.

Penicillin	Normal dose interval (hours)	Method of dosage adjustment	Creatinine clearance (ml/min)			Dialysis
			>50	10–50	<10	
Penicillin G	8	I	8	8	8–12	No (P)
		D	100	100	50	Yes (H)
Methicillin	4	I	4	4	8–12	No (H, P)
Nafcillin	6	I	Unch.	Unch.	Unch.	No (H)
Oxacillin	6	I	Unch.	Unch.	Unch.	No (H, P)
Cloxacillin	6	I	Unch.	Unch.	Unch.	No (H)
Dicloxacillin	6	I	Unch.	Unch.	Unch.	No (H)
Ampicillin	6	I	6	9	12–15	Yes (H)
						No (P)
Amoxicillin	8	I	8	12	16	Yes (H)
Carbenicillin	4	I	4	6–12	12–16	Yes (H)
		D	100	75	25–50	No (P)
Ticarcillin	4–6	I	4	8	12	Yes (H, P)
		D	100	50–75	50	

H, hemodialysis; P, peritoneal dialysis; Unch., unchanged. Yes, enough drug is removed to require supplementary dosage to insure adequate blood levels; No, a dosage supplement is not required with dialysis.

Source: The values in the table have been taken from a review by Bennet et al.[9] (Table 1), to which the reader is referred for specific references on the individual drugs.

the cerebrospinal fluid to the blood. In animals given penicillin intravenously, pretreatment with probenecid increases the concentration of penicillin in the cerebrospinal fluid as a result of the combined blockade of the active transport systems for penicillin in both the choroid plexus and the kidney.[22] An active transport system in the eye carries organic anions from the intraocular fluids to plasma,[23] and probenecid prolongs the intraocular half-life of penicillins.[24] The penicillins do not penetrate into prostatic fluid even when the prostate is inflamed. The prostate does not transport organic acids from prostatic fluid to plasma, and in this case the concentration of drug is very low because weak acids pass through the prostatic epithelium very poorly.[25]

TOXICITY AND SIDE EFFECTS OF THE PENICILLINS. Oral administration of penicillins may be accompanied by gastric distress or diarrhea, a problem that occurs more frequently in infants and young children than in adults. Superinfection of the gastrointestinal tract may occur during therapy with the broad spectrum penicillins and antibiotic associated (pseudomembranous) colitis occurs rarely. Penicillins produce several untoward effects that are the consequence of chemical irritation of the tissues. As with virtually any antibiotic administered intravenously, phlebitis can occur, and intramuscular injection may be especially painful when large amounts of penicillin are administered. Accidental injection of penicillin into the sciatic nerve is followed by pain and sensory and motor dysfunction that may last for weeks.[26] Intrathecal administration can cause meningeal irritation or encephalopathy[27] and the penicillins should not be administered by this route.

The penicillins have a very high therapeutic index and are among the least toxic of all drugs. Most of the undesirable effects rep resent hypersensitivity reactions. When large amounts of penicillin are administered, physicians should be aware that they are giving the patient large quantities of salt as well. This is particularly important in patients with compromised cardiac and renal function.

When penicillins are administered in very large doses by the intravenous route[28,29] or when high serum levels develop because of failure to adjust the dosage in patients with renal failure,[30] neurotoxic reactions may occur. The neurotoxicity is most frequently manifest as myoclonus or seizures but may present as agitated confusion and hallucination or lethargy and stupor that can progress to coma.[27,31] Although most reports have involved penicillin G, neurotoxicity has been reported with intravenous administration of large amounts of semisynthetic penicillins and cephalosporins as well.[27] Predisposing factors include impaired renal function, a daily dose of penicillin G exceeding 20 million units, patient age greater than 40 years, continuous intravenous infusion, and administration during cardiopulmonary bypass.[27] Considerable evidence supports the proposal that penicillin acts on synaptic transmission to reduce the inhibitory action of gamma aminobutyric acid (GABA).[32,33] In a direct study of the effect of penicillin on cultured mammalian spinal cord neurons, the drug was shown to selectively antagonize postsynaptic inhibition mediated by iontophoretically applied GABA.[34] In addition, it is possible that high concentrations of penicillin directly increase membrane excitability.[35]

Ampicillin, carbenicillin, and oxacillin have been reported to cause occasional anicteric hepatitis characterized by transient elevations in hepatic enzymes.[36,37] Although this usually occurs during high-dose therapy, it is possible that some cases reflect a hypersensitivity reaction. Penicillin G and several of the synthetic penicillins occasionally cause reversible granulocytopenia during high-dose therapy.[38,39] When large doses of penicillin are given for a prolonged period (typically, at least 10 million units daily for a week or more), hemolysis may occur. Al-though it is dose related, the hemolysis is due to a hypersensitivity, not a toxicity. Penicillin becomes bound to red cell membranes and antibodies of the IgG class react with the cell-bound drug.[40] Complement is not usually involved in this reaction and intravascular hemolysis rarely occurs. Cessation of penicillin therapy is followed by complete recovery.[40] Rarely, coagulation disorders have been observed after high-dose therapy with penicillin G and carbenicillin, especially in uremic patients. The bleeding diathesis apparently results from platelet dysfunction. At high concentrations, penicillin G and carbenicillin have been reported to interfere with the initial step in platelet activation by inhibiting the binding of activating agonists, such as ADP and epinephrine, to their receptors on the platelet membrane.[41]

The Semi-Synthetic Penicillins

The semi-synthetic penicillins were developed with the goals of obtaining resistance to β-lactamase digestion and an increased spectrum of antibacterial action. Many of the pharmacological properties of these drugs (including acid stability, routes of administration and elimination, serum half-lives, and degree of protein binding) are presented in Figures 4–2 and 4–3 and in Table 4–2. The reader is referred to a review of the literature for a detailed discussion of the pharmacology of each drug.[1]

THE PENICILLINASE-RESISTANT PENICILLINS. Structural modifications in the side chains of these penicillins (Fig. 4–1) provide enough steric hindrance to make them very poor substrates for most β-lactamases (see Chapter 3 for a complete discussion of the β-lactamases). The *penicillinase-resistant penicillins* have a narrow spectrum of action and they are used only for treatment of infections due to penicillinase-producing staphylococci. These penicillins are not as potent as penicillin G against nonpenicillinase-producing strains of staphylococci and they are not useful against gram-negative bacteria. The penicillinase-resistant penicillins are generally more resistant to staphylococcal β-lactamase than cephalosporins; the rank order of stability is methicillin > cloxacillin = dicloxacillin > oxacillin = cephalothin = cephradine = cephalexin > cefazolin.[42] The isoxazolyl penicillins and nafcillin have more intrinsic activity against staphylococci than methicillin; but methicillin has much less protein binding (see Table 4–2) and the activities of these drugs are roughly equivalent in the presence of serum.

The penicillinase-resistant penicillins available for parenteral use are methicillin, oxacillin, and nafcillin (Fig. 4–1). Methicillin has been in clinical use the longest, but it is no longer widely used. It is rapidly inactivated in acid and is thus given only parenterally. Methicillin has been associated with interstitial nephritis (described below under hypersensitivity reactions) more often than oxacillin or nafcillin. Oxacillin and nafcillin are both widely used for parenteral administration. Oxacillin given intravenously in high-dose therapy has been associated with hepatitis more often than the other penicillinase-resistant penicillins,[43,44] but, as it is less frequently associated with interstitial nephritis and produces less pain on intramuscular injection, many physicians consider it to be the preferred drug for parenteral use. Nafcillin is available in both oral and parenteral forms, but absorption from the gastrointestinal tract is poor and the oral route is not recommended. The apparent volume of distribution of nafcillin is larger than that of the other penicillinase-resistant penicillins and the blood levels achieved after intramuscular injection are lower than those achieved with oxacillin.[45] Intravenous nafcillin frequently causes reversible bone marrow suppression.

Of the penicillinase-resistant penicillins available for oral use in the United States, cloxacillin and dicloxacillin are the best absorbed.[46] Dicloxacillin is more completely absorbed and yields serum levels that are twice as high as those from cloxacillin but, after correction for protein binding, the levels of free drug in the serum are comparable.[1]

THE AMINOPENICILLINS: AMPICILLIN, AMOXICILLIN, AND CONGENERS As discussed in Chapter 3, the *aminopenicillins* have a broader spectrum of action than penicillin G and the penicillinase-resistant penicillins because they have a better ability to penetrate through the pores in the outer membrane of gram-negative bacteria. The increased spectrum of action is achieved by the addition of an amino group to the side chain of penicillin G (Fig. 4–3). The aminopenicillins are readily inactivated by both the gram-positive and gram-negative β-lactamases, and thus are ineffective for the treatment of most staphylococcal infections.

Ampicillin was the first aminopenicillin introduced into clinical use. However, in recent years, its use has been superceded in oral therapy by amoxicillin, which is more reliably absorbed from the stomach. The antibacterial spectra of the aminopenicillins are comparable, with few exceptions (for a review see Nathwani and Wood).[47]

The gram-positive antibacterial spectrum of these drugs is similar to that of penicillin G, but these compounds are more active against enterococci and *Listeria monocytogenes*. The aminopenicillins are susceptible to β-lactamases and thus most staphylococci are resistant to them. Most meningococci and pneumococci remain sensitive but pneumococcal strains that are highly resistant to penicillin G are also resistant to the aminopenicillins.

Most strains of *Hemophilus influenzae* are susceptible, but resistant β-lactamase-producing strains are prevalent in many areas. In contrast to penicillin G, the aminopenicillins are active against several aerobic gram-negative enteric bacilli, such as *E. coli*, *Proteus mirabilis*, *Salmonella*, and *Shigella*. However, in some areas, resistant strains are prevalent. Other Enterobacteriaceae, such as *Klebsiella*, *Enterobacter*, *Serratia*, indole-positive *Proteus*, and *Providencia*, are resistant, as is *Pseudomonas aeruginosa*.

There are very specific indications for the use of aminopenicillins (see tables listing drugs of choice in Chapter 1), yet these drugs are frequently inappropriately employed by physicians. The most common indiscretion is the use of ampicillin for treatment of gram-positive infections for which the narrower-spectrum agent penicillin G is the drug of choice.

Ampicillin is available for both oral and

Name	Side chain	Stability in acid	Routes of administration	Sensitivity to penicillinase
Ampicillin	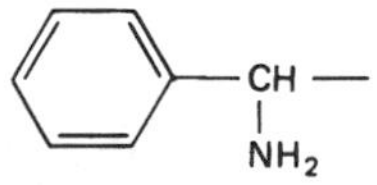	Good	Oral, IM, IV	Sensitive
Amoxicillin	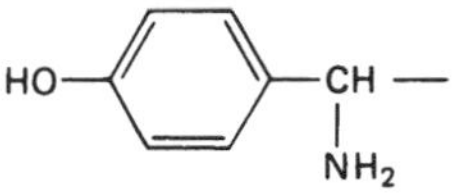	Very good	Oral	Sensitive
Carbenicillin	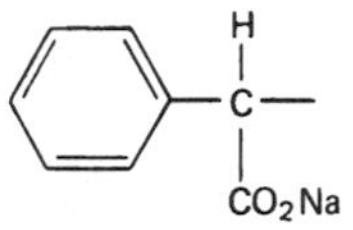	Poor (not given orally)	IM, IV	Sensitive
Carbenicillin indanyl sodium	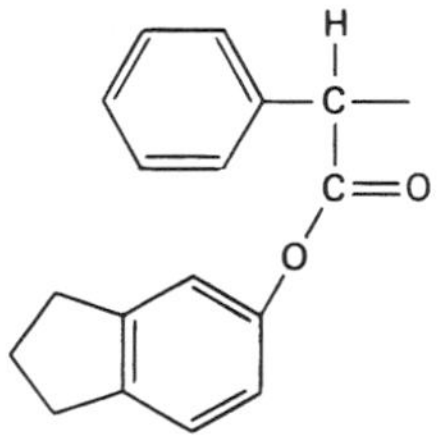	Good	Oral	Sensitive
Ticarcillin	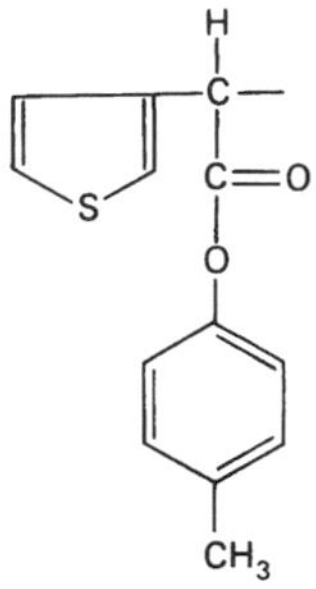	Poor (not given orally)	IM, IV	Sensitive
Azlocillin	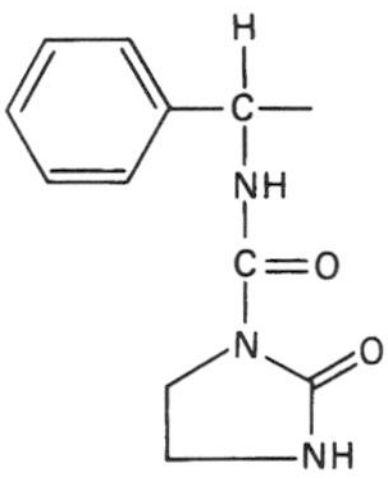	Poor (not given orally)	IM, IV	Sensitive

Figure 4–3. Structures and properties of the broad spectrum aminopenicillins and antipseudomonal penicillins.

parenteral administration. It is a bit more stable in acid and the half-life is somewhat longer than that of penicillin G, but the drug is distributed and excreted in a similar manner.[48] Amoxicillin differs from ampicillin in that it has a hydroxyl group at the *para* position of the benzene ring (see Fig. 4–3) that renders it very stable in acid. Amoxicillin is more readily absorbed from the gastrointestinal tract and yields blood levels of free drug that are two and a half times those obtained with ampicillin.[49,50] Unlike ampicillin, the absorption of amoxicillin is not significantly affected by food. The in vitro antibacterial activity of amoxicillin is the same as that of ampicillin.[49,51] Because of its better absorption and a lower incidence of diarrhea, amoxicillin is preferred over ampicillin in oral therapy. One exception is in the treatment of bacillary dysentery (shigellosis) where amoxicillin is less effective.[52]

The reason for the greater effectiveness of ampicillin in the treatment of shigellosis is not entirely clear. It may be that, since less ampicillin is absorbed, there is more drug left in the intestinal lumen to kill the bacteria. On the other hand, there is evidence that the serum concentration of antibiotic, not the intraluminal intestinal concentration, is the critical determinant of effectiveness against this infection.[53] In the absence of human serum, the two antibiotics have a nearly equivalent effect in vitro against *Shigella*. The difference in clinical efficacy seems to be determined by the presence of serum,[52] although the two drugs bind to serum protein to the same degree (see Table 3–2).[54]

Several proampicillins have been developed, but only one, bacampicillin,[55] is currently marketed in the United States.[56] Others include hetacillin,[56,57] cyclacillin,[1,58] pivampicillin, talampicillin, and epicillin. All of these are orally administered prodrugs that are rapidly hydrolyzed to ampicillin after absorption from the gastrointestinal tract, and they all yield peak serum levels of ampicillin that are twice as high as that achieved with oral administration of ampicillin itself but that are no higher than peak serum levels achieved with amoxicillin. The proampicillins and amoxicillin cause diarrhea less often (rate about 3%) than oral ampicillin (8%–10%)[59] It is possible that there is less diarrhea because more complete drug absorption leaves less drug in the intestine that can alter the flora. The proampicillin drugs do not seem to offer any advantage over amoxicillin in oral aminopenicillin therapy and they are usually more expensive.

THE ANTIPSEUDOMONAL PENICILLINS. *Pseudomonas aeruginosa* is one of the major pathogens responsible for nosocomial infections. Bacteremia caused by this organism

carries a high mortality rate even after the use of antipseudomonal agents. Carbenicillin was the first semisynthetic penicillin with good antipseudomonal activity. Over the years, increasing resistance to this agent has been observed and numerous agents with better activity have been introduced.[60] The *antipseudomonal* penicillins are now categorized into two groups: the *carboxypenicillins*, which include indanyl carbenicillin (an oral form of carbenicillin) and ticarcillin, and the *ureidopenicillins*, which include mezlocillin and piperacillin. Antipseudomonal penicillins retain most of the antibacterial activity of the natural penicillins and the aminopenicillins, but with added activity against gram-negative bacilli. Like the earlier penicillins these drugs are susceptible to many β-lactamases. Carbenicillin[61] and ticarcillin[62] are semisynthetic β-lactamase-sensitive penicillins that are active against *Pseudomonas aeruginosa* and indole-positive *Proteus* strains. These so-called antipseudomonal penicillins are as effective as ampicillin against nonpenicillinase-producing strains of gram-negative bacteria, such as *Haemophilus influenzae*, *Proteus mirabilis*, *Salmonella*, and *Shigella*, but they should be used clinically only to treat infections caused by organisms that are not susceptible to the aminopenicillins. In practical clinical application, this means that carbenicillin and ticarcillin are used primarily to treat infection with *Pseudomonas aeruginosa* and indole-positive *Proteus*. Other bacteria against which they are occasionally employed include *Enterobacter*, *Providentia stuarti*, *Serratia*, and *Acinetobacter*. At high concentration, carbenicillin, ticarcillin, piperacillin, and mezlocillin are active against many strains of *Bacteroides fragilis*.

Carbenicillin and ticarcillin are very acid-labile and are given only parenterally. Carbenicillin itself has been superceded for the most part by ticarcillin, although the orally available ester, indanyl carbenicillin, is still used. The pharmacology and spectrum of action of the two drugs are similar[63] and their principal difference is the fact that ticarcillin is about twice as active in vitro against *Pseudomonas aeruginosa* as carbenicillin.[64] This is important, because rather large amounts of carbenicillin (500 mg/kg/day) are required for the treatment of *Pseudomonas* infection and the use of carbenicillin has been associated with toxicity. Carbenicillin is provided as the disodium salt and large amounts of salt may be administered during therapy. Carbenicillin is excreted by the renal route and hypokalemia can occur because of obligatory excretion of cation with the drug. At high drug concentrations, carbenicillin[41] and ticarcillin[65] both interfere with platelet function and bleeding may occur because of abnormal platelet aggregation. As ticarcillin can be administered in lower dosage (300 mg/kg/day) than carbenicillin for treatment of *Pseudomonas* infection, the risk of these side effects is decreased. These drugs are excreted by the renal route and their half-lives are markedly prolonged in the presence of renal failure (Table 4–2). Thus, it is very important to modify the dosage when renal function is compromised (Table 4–3).

In the treatment of moderate or severe *Pseudomonas* infection, an aminoglycoside of the antipseudomonas group (gentamicin, tobramycin, or amikacin) is often adminis-

tered in addition to carbenicillin or ticarcillin. Such a combination is synergistic against many strains of *Pseudomonas*.[66,67] The basis for the synergism observed with combinations of β-lactam antibiotics and aminoglycosides is discussed in Chapter 5.

Indanyl carbenicillin is an acid-stable ester of carbenicillin that is well absorbed from the gastrointestinal tract.[68] This drug is useful only in the treatment of urinary tract infections, as blood levels are not adequate for treatment of infection elsewhere in the body.

THE EXTENDED SPECTRUM UREIDOPENICILLINS. The *ureidopenicillins* (mezlocillin and piperacillin) are semisynthetic derivatives of ampicillin with somewhat better activity against *Pseudomonas aeruginosa* than the carboxypenicillins. *Mezlocillin* (Fig. 4–4) is an acylureidopenicillin that is more active in vitro than carbenicillin or ticarcillin against enteric gram-negative bacilli, such as *Escherichia coli*, *Klebsiella* (only about 50% strains are sensitive), *Enterobacter*, *Citerobacter*, *Acinetobacter*, *Serratia*, and *Bacteroides fragilis*.[72] Its activity against *Pseudomonas aeruginosa* is comparable to that of ticarcillin.[73] Mezlocillin is acid-labile and

Structure	Name	Stability in acid	Routes of administration	Sensitivity to penicillinase	Half-life (hours)
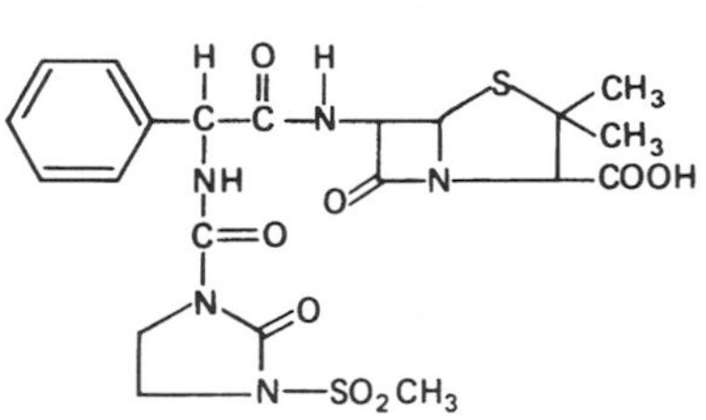	Mezlocillin	Poor (not given orally)	IM, IV	Sensitive	0.8–1.3
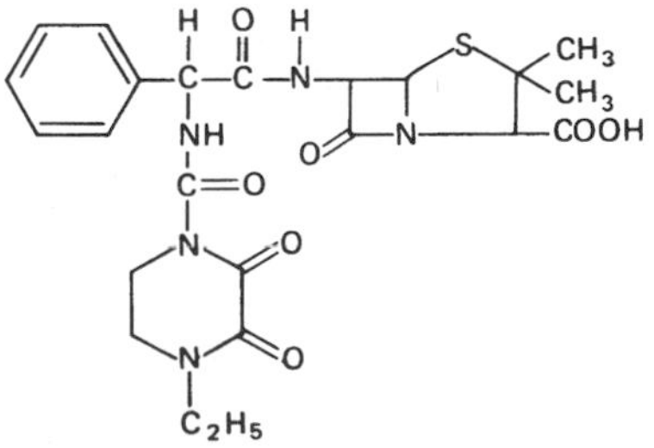	Piperacillin	Poor (not given orally)	IM, IV	Sensitive	0.6–1.0

Figure 4–4. Structures and properties of the ureidopenicillins. (Prepared from data in refs. 69–71.)

must be given parenterally. It is eliminated by both the renal and hepatic routes and, in the presence of competent hepatic function, the half-life is not markedly prolonged unless there is severe renal impairment.[70,74] When small doses are employed for treatment of very sensitive organisms, dosage adjustment may not be required, but in higher dose therapy the dosage should be reduced to one-half normal when the glomerular filtration rate (GFR) is between 10 and 30 ml/min and to one-third normal when the GFR is less than 10 ml/min.[75] The sodium content of mezlocillin is only about one-third that of ticarcillin or carbenicillin, a distinct advantage in patients with compromised cardiac function. The clinical experience with mezlocillin is reviewed in reference.[76]

Piperacillin is a piperazine derivative of ampicillin with increased activity against enterobacteria and the highest activity of any of the penicillins against *Pseudomonas aeruginosa*.[77,78] Both mezlocillin and piperacillin have been shown to be synergistic with aminoglycosides against gram-negative bacteria. Piperacillin is given parenterally and is excreted predominantly by the renal route. In the presence of normal renal function the half-life is in the range of 0.6 to 1 h but it increases to 4 or 5 h in patients with end-stage renal insufficiency.[79]

The ureidopenicillins also have several advantages over carboxypenicillins toxicologically. The sodium content is only about one-third that of ticarcillin or carbenicillin, a distinct advantage in patients with compromised cardiac function. They also produce hypokalemia less frequently, have reduced platelet dysfunction, and require minimal dosage adjustment in patients with renal failure.[60]

Penicillin Allergy

Hypersensitivity Reactions to β-Lactam Antibiotics

Hypersensitivity reactions are the most common type of adverse reaction associated with the use of the penicillins and the penicillins are probably the most common cause of drug allergy. Estimates of the incidence of allergic reaction to the penicillins range from 1% to 5% of patients treated.[80] The reactions encompass virtually every sort of allergic manifestation. Their onset may be immediate, accelerated (occurring 1 to 72 h after administration), or delayed for several days or even weeks (Table 4–4). Allergic responses to any of the penicillins can occur, and reactions are less frequent in children than in adults. Manifestations of allergy may be seen after any route of drug administration, but anaphylaxis (and perhaps other

Table 4–4. *Allergic reactions to penicillins.*

IMMEDIATE ALLERGIC REACTIONS	LATE ALLERGIC REACTIONS
(occur 2–30 min after penicillin)	(more than 72 h)
Urticaria	Morbilliform eruptions (occasionally occur as early as 18 h after initiation of penicillin)
Flushing	Urticarial eruptions
Diffuse pruritis	Erythematous eruptions
Hypotension or shock	Recurrent urticaria and arthralgia
Laryngeal edema	Local inflammatory reactions
Wheezing	
ACCELERATED URTICARIAL REACTIONS	**SOME RELATIVELY UNUSUAL LATE REACTIONS**
(1–72 h)	
Urticaria or pruritis	Immunohemolytic anemia
Wheezing or laryngeal edema	Drug fever
Local inflammatory reactions	Acute renal insufficiency
	Thrombocytopenia

Source: Modified from Levine et al,[80] Table 1.

types of allergic reaction) is less common with the oral than with the parenteral route.[81] The incidence of anaphylactic reaction appears to be higher in people with a history of atopy (e.g., asthma, hay fever, and other allergic diseases).[82]

Because of the high incidence of allergy to the penicillins and the large patient population exposed to these antibiotics, the mechanisms underlying the allergic reaction have been studied in greater detail than those for any other antibiotic. Indeed, most of our understanding of allergic responses to drugs in general has evolved from the study of penicillin hypersensitivity. The purpose of this section is to provide the reader with an overview of the mechanisms involved in the development of allergy to the β-lactam antibiotics, the methods of detecting penicillin allergy, and the principles and risks of treatment of the allergic patient. The reader is referred to two of the many reviews in the area for a more detailed discussion.[83,84]

IMMUNOCHEMISTRY. Before small molecules (such as most drugs) can elicit an immune response, they must become associated in an irreversible manner with large molecules in the host tissues. Antibodies to the complete antigen, the hapten-protein conjugate, then form. The hapten may be the unaltered drug, a metabolite, or a chemical degradation product. In the case of the penicillins, it is clear that penicillin itself is not the major form of the molecule that functions as a hapten. Rather, penicillin G can undergo a ring cleavage in solution to form small amounts of several degradation products.[85] One of the products resulting from the nonenzymatic cleavage of the thiazolidine ring is D-benzlypenicillenic acid. This is a very reactive isomer of penicillin, which can react irreversibly with sulfhydryl groups or amino residues in tissue proteins to form hapten-protein conjugates. The proposed mechanism is presented in Figure 4–5. Of primary importance is the chemically favored reaction of D-benzylpenicillenic acid with the ε-amino group of lysine residues on proteins[86] to form D-benzylpenicilloyl derivatives of tissue proteins, which then function

as complete penicillin antigens.

The results of one experiment supporting the proposal that the D-benzylpenicilloyl-ε-aminolysyl units are the primary antigenic determinants are presented in Figure 4–6. Serum from rabbits, which were exposed to penicillin G, contained an anti-penicillin antibody that precipitated when the serum was incubated with antigen—human gamma globulin containing a number of D-benzylpenicilloyl groups. These antigen–antibody precipitation reactions were carried out in the presence of increasing amounts of penicillin or penicilloylamide compounds to determine what concentration of penicillin G or penicillin derivative effectively competed for the antigen sites on the rabbit anti-penicillin serum antibodies. The more effective a compound was in associating with the antibody (thus preventing precipitation by the gamma globulin antigen) the more closely it would resemble the complete penicillin antigen that elicited antibody production. As seen in Figure 4–6, D-benzylpenicilloyl-ε-amino caproate, an analog of the ε-aminolysyl derivative, was effective in blocking the precipitation at one-hundredth the concentration at which penicillin G or D-benzylpenicilloc acid were effective. Similar experiments using serum from patients with penicillin allergy have shown that the majority of the antibodies formed are specific for the penicilloyllysyl group.[87] There is some evidence suggesting that penicillin itself can react with amino groups on proteins and form complete antigens without having to first proceed through the penicillenic acid intermediate.[88]

Penicillenic acid is not the only degradation product of penicillin that is capable of eliciting an antibody response. Others induce the production of antibodies that are different from the penicilloyl type—they are called *minor determinants*. Both the major and minor determinants elicit antibodies of several immunoglobulin classes. But at the risk of oversimplifying, it can be said that IgG is more often specific for the penicilloyl group and IgE reacts with a wider range of penicillin determinants, both major and minor. The IgE antibodies are responsible for

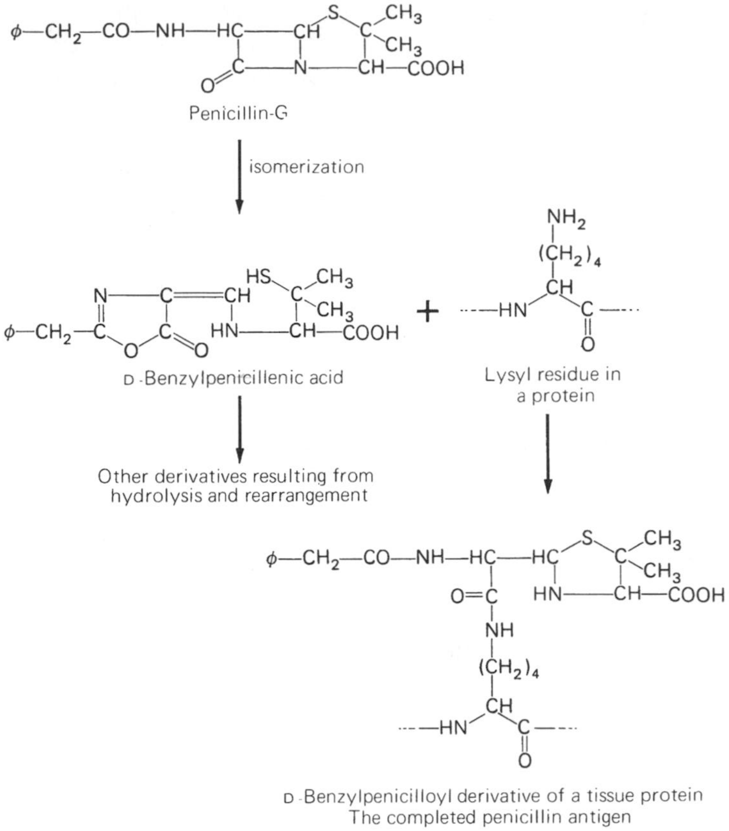

Figure 4–5. Proposed chemical pathway for the formation of the penicillin antigen. A very small percentage of penicillin G is isomerized at physiological pH to D-benzylpenicillenic acid, which then reacts with the ε-amino group of lysyl residues in proteins to form the complete penicillin antigen. (From Levine.[85])

the production of the wheal and flare reactions observed in skin testing and for such important immediate reactions as anaphylaxis.[89] In contrast, the serum sickness syndrome is an example of an allergic reaction mediated by antibodies of the IgG class (and possibly also by IgM).

Apparently allergic responses to commercial penicillin preparations are not always due to complete antigen formed between penicillin derivatives and tissue protein. Some preparations of penicillin have been found to contain a high-molecular-weight material responsible for producing allergic reactions.[90,91] In some cases, these high-molecular-weight antigens are penicilloyl-protein conjugates formed during the biosynthetic process used in production. In other cases high-molecular-weight penicillin polymers are formed that may themselves be immunogenic.[84] The extent to which the high-molecular-weight forms contribute to the immunogenicity of various penicillins is not clear, especially with the more purified preparations now available. In two studies it was shown that the incidence of reaction was lower when allergic patients were given skin tests using fresh preparations of penicillin from which the high-molecular-weight contaminants had been removed.[90-93]

Although the chemical structures of penicillins and cephalosporins are similar in several respects, there are distinct differences in their pathways of chemical degradation. In contrast to the penicilloyl group, which is the most common determinant of penicillin

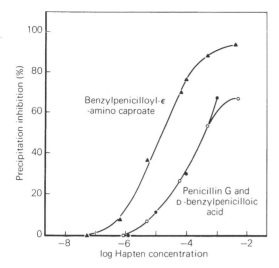

Figure 4–6. Inhibition of antibody precipitation by haptens related to penicillin. Rabbit anti-penicillin G serum was incubated with D-benzylpenicilloyl human gamma globulin in the presence of various concentrations of D-benzylpenicilloyl-ε-aminocaproate (▲-▲), D-benzylpenicilloic acid (●-●), or penicillin G (○-○). The amount of precipitate in each incubation was then assayed. (Data from Levine and Ovary.[87])

allergy, there is no conclusive evidence for the formation of an equivalent stable cephalosporyl group that is introduced into proteins.[84] Various degrees of cross-reactivity of antibodies to penicillins and cephalosporins have been demonstrated, both with test systems that detect IgG and IgM antibodies and with those that are specific for IgE antibodies.[94,95] The precise extent of cross-allergenicity between the penicillins and cephalosporins remains an unsettled issue,[96] and the determinants for cephalosporin allergy have not been defined as well as those for the penicillins.[84] In general, the cephalosporins are less immunogenic than the penicillins, and immunological specificity is more dependent on the nature of the side chain in the case of the cephalosporins.[84] Thus, cephalosporins with side chains similar to benzyl penicillin may be expected to cross-react more frequently than some of the newer cephalosporins, such as cefotaxime and cefuroxime, which have a very different side-chain structure and less cross-reactivity with human IgE antibodies induced by benzylpenicillin.[97]

SKIN TESTING FOR HYPERSENSITIVITY. A classic method of testing for drug allergy is to inject a small amount of the drug intradermally; if erythema develops, the patient is sensitive. This method of testing with penicillin is unsatisfactory for two reasons: *(1)* intradermal injection of penicillin can precipitate a full-blown anaphylactic response in the patient; and *(2)* the results are not completely reliable. One factor that apprently contributes to the production of false negatives is the phenomenon described by the curves in Figure 4–6. A small amount of the penicillin in the test injection is altered and forms the hapten-protein conjugate, but this complete antigen is prevented from reacting with the small amount of antibody in the area of injection because of competition for antibody sites by the relatively large amount of unaltered penicillin. A more reliable test substance than penicillin itself has been developed from the antigenic determinant we have just discussed; it is a penicilloyl derivative of lysine. Penicilloyl-polylysine is a multivalent antigen of approximately 20 lysine residues and 12 to 15 penicilloyl groups per unit. It is not immunogenic, its diffusion from the site of injection is slow because of its molecular size, and systemic response is rare. A small amount of the clear penicilloyl-polylysine solution is administered intradermally, and after 20 min the injected area is examined for evidence of a wheal-and-erythema response. The reaction is graded negative, 2+, or 4+, depending on the magnitude of the response.

The results of this test are more reliable, and the test is certainly less dangerous than the use of the drug itself as the test substance. A positive test reaction, however, is by no means an absolute indication that patients will have an allergic reaction if they are subsequently treated with penicillin.

Testing with benzylpenicilloyl-polylysine (PPL) is helpful, but the physician cannot rely on this test alone for predicting a patient's reaction to subsequent penicillin therapy. Patients who have a negative skin test with PPL may have developed an allergic response to minor determinants that do not react to the penicilloyl group. The use of the word "minor" to describe these determinants is unfortunate, since the clinical consequences of treating these patients with a penicillin can be major. People who are sensitive to minor determinants are more likely to experience an immediate anaphylactic reaction upon therapeutic administration of the drug. Thus it is critical to identify the patient's response to testing with the minor determinants as well as to PPL. There is no preparation of minor determinants available commercially, but pharmacies in the larger hospitals can prepare an appropriate test mixture. The minor determinant mixture (MDM) usually contains crystalline benzylpenicillin, 20 mM; sodium benzyl-penicilloate, 10 mM; and sodium-α-benzylpenicilloyl-amine, 10 mM.

The use of the two test procedures can be of great help to the physician.[98] It has been shown that the procedure can be applied by house officers in a ward setting in a useful and safe manner.[99,100] When MDM is not available, aqueous penicillin G can be used as a substitute.[101] PPL testing can be initiated with an intradermal injection. If this is negative, one may proceed to MDM (or penicillin G) scratch testing and then intradermal injection. No one should be tested for a drug sensitivity without trained personnel, syringes, epinephrine, and appropriate airway support immediately available.

It would be advantageous to have a method of testing for drug allergies that did not expose patients to the risk of injecting the antigen. Such methods have been developed,[84] but they are not yet rapid and definitive enough to be of clinical use.

TREATMENT OF THE PATIENT WITH PENICIL-LIN HYPERSENSITIVITY. When a patient with a history of penicillin allergy presents with an infection for which penicillin therapy is indicated, the physician may choose to treat with another antibiotic or test for penicillin hypersensitivity and proceed according to those results. In most cases, another antibiotic is chosen. In choosing an alternative to penicillin, there are several facts one should keep in mind.

Patients who are allergic to one penicillin must be assumed to be allergic to all penicillins. There are cases in which patients have been shown to be allergic to one penicillin and not to others,[98,102] but they are largely of academic interest. Clinically, physicians should never assume that they can substitute one penicillin for another in the treatment of allergic patients. One minimizes the risk of an allergic reaction by choosing an antibiotic that is not a member of the β-lactam group. Except in rare instances, a non-β-lactam antibiotic should be given if the patient has a history of anaphylaxis or other immediate-type penicillin hypersensitivity reaction. Because the choice of a non-β-lactam antibiotic may be associated with a higher risk of toxicity or less efficacy, it is often reasonable to use cephalosporins to treat appropriate infections in patients with a history of a less severe type of allergic reaction to penicillin. It should be remembered, however, that the cephalosporins are allergenic and some cross-reactivity with the penicillins exists, as determined both by serum tests[103,104] and by skin testing.[105]

The data in Table 4–5 give some indication of the frequency of reactions to several of the cephalosporins in patients presenting with a history of penicillin allergy.[95] Of 15,708 patients in these clinical trials, 701 (4.5%) had a history of allergy to penicillin and 57 (8.1%) of these had an allergic reaction to administration of cephalosporins. Of the 15,007 patients who did not have a history of penicillin allergy, 285 (1.9%) had an allergic reaction to cephalosporins. Thus, a patient with a history of penicillin allergy appears to be about four times as likely to have an allergic reaction to a cephalosporin as a patient without a history of penicillin allergy.[95] The physician should be aware that there have been several reports of anaphylaxis following administration of a cephalosporin to patients who were allergic to the penicillins.[106] When giving a cephalosporin to a patient with a history of penicillin allergy, appropriate precautions for treating an immediate reaction should be taken.

In the case of serious infection (e.g., an

Table 4–5. *Allergic reactions to cephalosporins in patients with and without a history of penicillin allergy.*

Cephalosporin, history of penicillin allergy (no. of patients)	No. with allergic reactions (%)
Cephaloridine	
No (3471)	86 (2.6)
Yes (109)	14 (13.0)
Cephalothin	
No (1045)	21 (2.0)
Yes (138)	8 (5.8)
Cephalexin	
No (7819)	87 (1.1)
Yes (291)	19 (6.5)
Cefazolin	
No (1369)	8 (0.6)
Yes (74)	3 (4.0)
Cefamandole	
No (1303)	83 (6.4)
Yes (89)	13 (14.6)
Total	
No (15,007)	285 (1.9)
Yes (701)	57 (8.1)

Source: From Petz,[95] Table 1.

endocarditis) for which a penicillin is clearly the drug of choice, one should skin test with both PPL and MDM. If the skin testing is negative, therapy with a penicillin may be initiated. If one or both of the skin tests are positive, treatment with another carefully chosen, potent antimicrobial is probably warranted.[107] In certain cases, in which the benefit of penicillin therapy outweighs the risk of immediate allergic reaction (for example, with an enterococcal endocarditis), treatment with a penicillin is begun with graduated doses of antibiotic according to a prudent desensitization schedule.[83,108] This is a dangerous procedure that should be carried out only in a hospital with maximum support and trained personnel available. Desensitization should be attempted only in life-threatening situations in which there is no equally effective alternative antibiotic. Desensitization may permit therapy with the penicillins to proceed, but often it simply does not work. If desensitization is success-

ful, the response of the patient to skin testing may change from positive to negative during therapy.[108,109] This may be due to depletion of the skin-sensitive IgE by the antigen and to the blocking action of increased IgG.

One possible method for controlling the allergic response may be to utilize stable univalent haptens to block the association of the multivalent antigens with the antibody. For example, *in vitro* studies such as the one presented in Figure 4–6 have shown that a stable, synthetic penicilloyl hapten (benzylpenicilloylformyllysine) is very efficient at blocking anti-penicilloyl antibodies.[110] This observation has been extended by administering the synthetic penicilloyl hapten to several patients who had allergic reactions and who required further penicillin therapy.[111] Most of the patients were able to continue or resume penicillin treatment without allergic symptoms under cover of the hapten. There is probably only a very small subgroup of the population in which this specific competing monovalent hapten would be effective, and the potential for the use of the technique is very limited. But it is a magnificent demonstration of the translation of basic molecular principles into therapy.

Several precautions can minimize the complications of penicillin allergy:

1. Always ask the patient about previous allergic reactions.
2. If the patient is given penicillin by injection, the patient should remain in the clinic or office 30 min after receiving the drug.
3. If the patient is to be given procaine or benzathine penicillin, some physicians prefer to give a small amount of penicillin G first and then inject the long-lasting preparation 30 min later. This is prudent, since it decreases the chance of having to treat a patient for a reaction when a lot of antigen is already in the body in a slow-release form.
4. Always have a syringe containing epinephrine (1:1000) on hand.
5. When using an alernative antibiotic, never substitute another penicillin.
6. Skin testing with PPL and MDM (or penicillin G) can be very helpful, par-

ticularly in identifying those patients who have a high risk of developing an immediate reaction.

7. Do not give a cephalosporin to a patient with a history of an immediate-type reaction to penicillins.

8. Cephalosporins are often appropriate alternatives in patients with a history of a less severe type of penicillin reaction. The best data suggest that there is about an 8% chance that these patients will have some type of allergic reaction to the cephalosporin, and approrpiate precautions should be taken in the event that anaphylaxis or another immediate-type reaction occurs.

AMPICILLIN RASHES. The incidence of skin rashes is about twice as high with ampicillin as with the other penicillins. In one study of 422 patients treated with ampicillin, for example, rashes occurred in 9.5%.[112] Most rashes associated with ampicillin are pruritic, maculopapular eruptions; a few are urticarial.[113] Although the variation is great, the time of onset of the maculopapular rashes associated with ampicillin is later (median 7 days) than penicillin rashes in general. The incidence of ampicillin rashes seems to be higher in children than in adults. The maculopapular rash might not have an allergic basis. The results of both skin testing and in vitro studies indicate that the rash is not mediated by IgE, and readministration of ampicillin to patients who have had the maculopapular type of rash produced no reaction.[113,114] The urticarial rashes seen with ampicillin clearly have an allergic basis, but the cause of the more common maculopapular rash is unknown.[84]

The incidence of rashes in patients with infectious mononucleosis who are also treated with ampicillin is extremely high (about 90%).[115,116] Again, the ampicillin rash is a pruritic, maculopapular eruption having a later onset and perhaps a somewhat different distribution than the similar rash that normally appears in 10% to 15% of patients with mononucleosis.[117] An antibody-like activity has been shown to be present in both the IgG and IgM fractions of serum from patients with infectious mononucleosis.[118]

INTERSTITIAL NEPHRITIS. Numerous specific reactions to the penicillins have been studied in detail, and the reader is referred to the review by Parker for an *entré* into the literature.[83] One rare complication of penicillin use that is particularly important to keep in mind if a patient's renal function begins to decline during therapy is interstitial nephritis. The clinical picture of the syndrome is characterized by fever, rash, and eosinophilia, with hematuria and proteinuria.[119] When penicillin therapy is stopped, there is usually recovery. The syndrome is more common with methicillin, but it can also be seen with penicillin G and ampicillin.[120,121] Both tubular damage and an interstitial accumulation of mononuclear cells and eosinophils are seen in specimens obtained by renal biopsy.[122] There are no glomerular abnormalities nor is there evidence of arteritis. The nephritis usually develops after high doses of methicillin or penicillin G, but this is clearly an allergic condition, not a toxicity. Methicillin haptenic groups have been demonstrated at the tubular basement membrane, and at least two patients have been shown to have antitubular basement membrane antibodies.[123,124] This finding suggests that penicillin may bind to the tubular basement membrane to form an antigen that can elicit the production of antitubular basement membrane antibodies. These antibodies are thought to be capable of reacting with the normal tubular basement membrane to produce the pathological changes of interstitial nephritis. As a result of the nephritis produced by methicillin, its use has declined and therapy with nafcillin is preferred.

The Cephalosporins

Classification of the Cephalosporins

The cephalosporins are among the most commonly prescribed antibiotics and their use continues to increase with the introduction of new members of this group. Because of the increasing incidence of hospital-acquired infections, the increase in antibiotic-resistant bacterial strains, and an increasing number of patients with depressed resistance to infection, physicians have considered the broad-spectrum bactericidal action, the relative β-lactamase resistance, and the comparatively low toxicity of the cephalosporins to be very attractive determinants in their choice of antibiotics. Modification of the basic cephalosporin structure has resulted in a very diverse group of drugs having unique antibacterial, pharmacokinetic, and pharmacological properties.

The explosive growth of the cephalosporins in recent years has led to the need for a satisfactory way of classifying these drugs. They may be classified in several ways according to their structures, pharmacological properties, sensitivity to β-lactamases, etc.[125] But, as with the penicillins, the meaningful basis of their classification from the standpoint of therapeutics is according to their spectrum of antibacterial action (see Table 4–6).

Thus, the cephalosporins are traditionally divided into first-generation, second-generation, third-generation, and the recently available fourth-generation compounds. The first cephalosporins that were made available, the so-called *first-generation cephalosporins*, do not have as broad a spectrum of action against gram-negative bacteria as the newer cephalosporins, but they have the greatest activity against gram-positive organisms. Most staphylococci (methicillin-resistant strains of *S. aureus* are an exception) and streptococci (enterococci and penicillin-resistant pneumococci are exceptions) are sensitive to these cephalosporins. The β-lactamases produced by *S. aureus* are primarily penicillinases and penicillinase-producing staphylococci are therefore susceptible to the cephalosporins, with cephalothin being the most resistant to hydrolysis by the staphylococcal enzymes.[126] Most strains of *Escherichia coli, Klebsiella pneumoniae*, and *Proteus mirabilis* acquired in the community are susceptible to the first-generation cephalosporins, but some hospital-acquired, R factor–containing (multiple drug–resistant) strains are resistant.

Most anaerobic species are susceptible in vitro, except for *Bacteroides fragilis*.[126] The first-generation cephalosporins have similar spectra of action and they differ primarily in their pharmacokinetic properties. Cephalothin has been in clinical use longer than the other first-generation cephalosporins and is considered the prototype compound in this class.

The *second-generation cephalosporins* have expanded activity against gram-negative organisms. As described in Chapter 3, the increased spectrum of action is due to increased affinity for penicillin binding proteins, increased penetration through the outer envelope of gram-negative bacteria, and increased resistance to hydrolysis by gram-negative β-lactamases. Thus, these drugs are active against many cephalothin-resistant *Escherichia coli, Klebsiella*, and *Proteus mirabilis* strains. Cefamandole is active against many strains of *Haemophilus influenzae, Enterobacter*, and indole-positive *Proteus* species and cefoxitin is particularly active against *Bacteroides fragilis*.

The third-generation compounds have substitutions in basic ring structure, which increases their affinity to penicillin binding proteins, thereby enhancing activity against gram-negative bacteria. There are currently five parenterally administered third-generation cephalosporins (ceftizoxime, cefotaxime, ceftriaxone, ceftazidime, and cefoperazone) and three oral drugs (cefpodoxime proxetil, cefixime, and ceftibuten). Third-generation compounds have an expanded spectrum of activity against gram-negative bacilli, and most Enterobacteriaceae are highly susceptible to these drugs, including some strains that are resistant to second-generation cephalosporins and aminoglycosides. Ceftazidime and cefoperazone are the two drugs in this class that have activity against *Pseudomonas aeruginosa*. *Neisseria* spp. and *Hemophilus influenzae* are susceptible to all third-generation members. Cefotaxime, cefoperazone, and ceftizoxime have the greatest activity against staphylococci and all of the third-generation cephalosporins except ceftazidime are active against methicillin-susceptible *Staphylococcus aureus*.

Table 4–6. Classification of the cephalosporins.

Class	Generic name	Clinically useful antimicrobial spectrum
FIRST-GENERATION		
Parenteral	Cephalothin Cefazolin Cephapirin Cephradine	Gram-positive: *Staphylococcus aureus* (except for methicillin-resistant strains), *Staphyococcus epidermidis, Streptococcus* species (except enterococci) Gram-negative: most strains of *Escherichia coli, Klebsiella pneumoniae,* and *Proteus mirabilis* Anaerobes: most anaerobes are susceptible in vitro except *Bacteroides fragilis*
Oral	Cephalexin Cefadroxil Cephradine	
SECOND-GENERATION		
Parenteral	Cefamandole Cefoxitin Cefuroxime Cefotetan Ceforanide Cefonicid	Less effective than first-generation cephalosporins against gram-positive organisms, but expanded activity against gram-negative organisms including cephalothin-resistant *Escherichia coli, Klebsiella,* and *Proteus mirabilis.* Cefamandole is particularly active against *Haemophilus influenzae, Enterobacter,* and indole-positive *Proteus* species. Cefoxitin and cefotetan have enhanced activity against *Bacteroides fragilis* and *Serratia marcescens.*
Oral	Cefaclor Cefuroxime axetil Loracarbef	
THIRD-GENERATION		
Parenteral	Cefotaxime Cefoperazone Ceftizoxime Ceftriaxone Ceftazidime	Increased activity against the gram-negative organisms cited above, *Providencia stuartii, Pseudominas aeruginosa,* and *Bacteroides fragilis.* Cefotaxime and ceftriaxone have especially high activity against β-lactamase-producing strains of *Haemophilus influenzae* and *Neisseria gonorrhoeae.*
Oral	Cefpodoxime proxetil Cefixime Ceftibuten	
FOURTH-GENERATION		
Parenteral	Cefepime	Comparable to the third-generation compounds but with more resistance to β-lactamases

The fourth-generation cephalosporins are the latest group of cephalosporins to be marketed. Of this group the only currently approved drug is cefepime, but others are under development. Chemical modifications to the basic cephem ring at position 7 enhance the stability of these cephalosporins against β-lactamases, which is the main characteristic of this generation of cephalosporins. Cefepime also has a positively charged quaternized *N*-methyl-pyrrolidine substitution at the 3 position of the cephem nucleus, making it a zwitterion. As a result, cefepime has an enhanced ability to penetrate the porins in the outer membrane of gram-negative bacteria.

Pharmacology of the Cephalosporins

The core structure of the cephalosporins is shown in Figure 4–7. The various cephalosporins differ in their chemical modifications at R_1 and R_2. In general, the pharmacology is similar to that described for the penicillins.

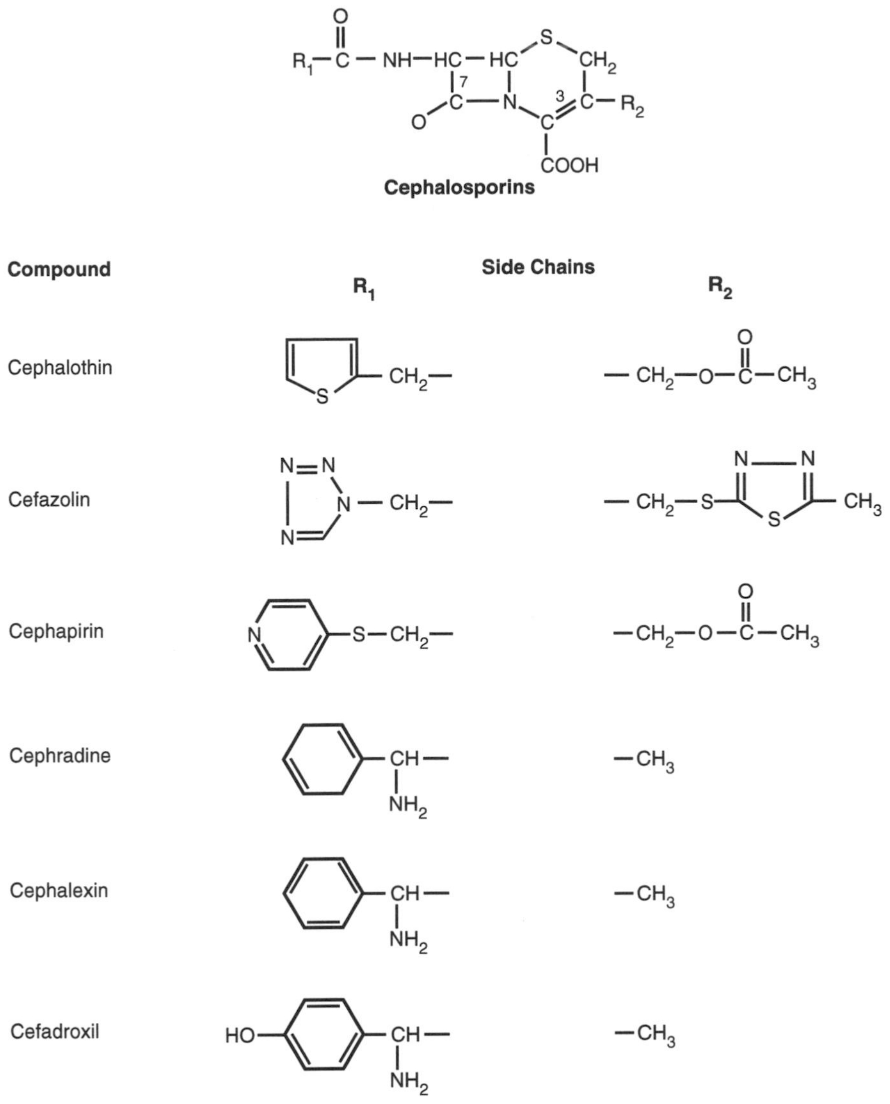

Cephalosporins

Compound	Side Chains	
	R₁	R₂

Figure 4–7. Structures of the first-generation cephalosporins.

As with the penicillins, the cephalosporins vary considerably with respect to their absorption, protein binding, and the relative extent of renal versus extrarenal routes of excretion. The pharmacokinetic properties of several selected first-, second-, and third-generation cephalosporins are presented in Tables 4–7 and 4–8.

ABSORPTION, METABOLISM, AND EXCRETION. There are now several cephalosporins that are absorbed well enough from the gastro-

intestinal tract to permit oral administration. These include some from each generation except the fourth. Cephalexin, cephradine, and cefaclor are rapidly absorbed, producing peak serum levels in 1 to 5 hs.[143] Absorption is slower when there is food in the stomach. Cephradine is the only cephalosporin available in the United States that is administered both orally and parenterally.

Those cephalosporins with an acetyl group at the 3 position (R_2 in Fig. 4–7) are deacetylated by liver esterases to form deriv-

Table 4–7. Pharmacokinetic properties of selected cephalosporins. The values in the table have been compiled from the indicated references.

Cephalosporin	Route of administration	Major route of excretion	Half-life Normal (hours)	Half-life ESRD (hours)	Plasma protein binding	Reference
FIRST GENERATION						
Cephalothin	IM, IV	Renal (hepatic)	0.5–0.9	3–18	65–79	9, 125, 126
Cefazolin	IM, IV	Renal	1.4–2.2	18–36	74–86	9, 126
Cephapirin	IM, IV	Renal (hepatic)	0.6	2.4	44–50	9, 125, 126
Cephradine	IM, IV Oral	Renal	0.6–0.9	8–15	6–20	9, 126
Cephalexin	Oral	Renal	0.6–0.9	5–30	10–15	9, 126, 127
SECOND GENERATION						
Cefamandole	IM, IV	Renal	1–1.5	10	67–80	9, 126, 128, 129
Cefoxitin	IM, IV	Renal	0.8	13–22	50–73	126, 128, 130
Cefaclor	Oral	Renal	0.5–1.0	2.3	22–25	126, 127
Loracarbef	Oral	Renal	1–1.2	32	25	131
Cefuroxime axetil	Oral	Renal	1.1–1.5	16.8	33	132
THIRD GENERATION						
Cefotaxime	IM, IV	Renal (hepatic)	0.9–1.4	11–14	35–45	125, 133, 134
Cefoperazone	IM, IV	Hepatic	1.6–2.1	2.2	89–91	135
Ceftriaxone	IM, IV	Renal	5.5–11	14.4–17	>95	136
Cefixime	Oral	Renal	3–4	10.5–12.5	60	137, 138
FOURTH GENERATION						
Cefepime	IM, IV	Renal	2.3	14	16–19	139

ESRD, end-stage renal disease; IM, intramuscular; IV, intravenous.

atives that are less active than the parent compounds.[144] Both the unaltered drug and the deacetylated metabolite are eliminated in the urine. Most of the cephalosporins are excreted in their unchanged form by active transport in the kidney and concomitant administration of probenecid increases their peak serum levels and half-lives. In the presence of impaired renal function, the half-lives of most of the cephalosporins are increased[145] (Table 4–7) and dosage reduction is recommended to avoid neurotoxicity (see Table 4–8 for dosage modification). Cephapirin and cefoperazone are more efficiently eliminated by the hepatic route than the other cephalosporins, and in patients with end-stage renal disease their half-lives are increased to only 2.2 to 2.4 h. Fourth-generation compounds like cefepime are excreted almost entirely in the urine unchanged. Dosage adjustments must be made when there is kidney failure.

DISTRIBUTION. The cephalosporins penetrate well into most fluid spaces. Penetration into fibrin clots and inflammatory peritoneal exudate is inversely related to the degree of serum protein binding, thus reflecting the free serum drug concentration.[11,146] Therapeutic concentrations of cephalosporins are achieved in pleural, pericardial, and peritoneal fluids and they are transferred through the placenta.[144,147] Several of the cephalosporins (e.g., cefazolin, cefamandole, and cefo-

Table 4–8.   Adjustment of dosage of selected cephalosporins in patients with compromised renal function and after dialysis. The total daily dosage may be adjusted by maintaining the normal dosage interval and decreasing the dose per administration (the "dose reduction" method) or by keeping the dosage size normal and increasing the interval between administration (the "interval extension" method). In the dose reduction method (D) the percentage of the normal dose that should be given at the normal dosage interval is presented. In the interval extension method (I) the interval in hours between doses of normal size is given.

Cephalosporin	Normal dose interval (hours)	Method of dosage adjustment	Creatinine clearance (ml/min)			Dialysis	Reference
			>50	1–50	<10		
FIRST GENERATION							
Cephalothin	4–6	I	6	6	8–12	Yes (H, P)	9
Cefazolin	8	I	8	12	24–48	Yes (H)	9
		D	100	50	25	No (P)	
Cephapirin	6	I	6	6	12	Yes (H)	9
Cephradine	6	D	100	50	25	Yes (H, P)	9
Cephalexin	6	I	6	6	6–12	Yes (H, P)	9
SECOND GENERATION							
Cefamandole	4–6	D	100	50–75	50	No (H, P)	9
		I	6	6–9	9		
Cefoxitin	6–8	I	8	12–24	24–48	Yes (H)	130
Cefaclor	6–8		Unch.	Unch.	Unch.	Yes (H)	127, 140
Cefuroxime	8	I	8	12	24	Yes (H), Poor (P)	132
THIRD GENERATION							
Cefotaxime	6–8	I	6	8–12	18–24	Yes (H)	133, 141
Cefoperazone	8–12		Unch.	Unch.	Unch.	?	135
Ceftriaxone	24	I	24	24	24	No (H, P)	136
Cefixime	12–24	I	12–24	24	24	No (H, P)	137, 138
FOURTH GENERATION							
Cefepime	12	D	100	25–50	6–2	Yes (H, P)	142

H, hemodialysis; P, peritoneal dialysis; Unch., unchanged. Yes, enough drug is removed to require supplementary dosage to insure adequate blood levels; No, a dosage supplement is not required with dialysis.

taxime) have been shown to achieve appropriate therapeutic concentrations in synovial fluid and bone.[144,148–151]

A number of the cephalosporins (e.g., cefazolin, cefamandole, cefoxitin, cefotaxime, and cefoperazone) are excreted into the unobstructed biliary tract in concentrations that are effective against gram-negative, enteric bacteria commonly encountered as biliary tract pathogens.[126,152,153] With the exception of cefoperazone, therapeutic levels of cephalosporins are not achieved in the presence of biliary tract obstruction.[126,151] Ce-

foperazone is eliminated predominantly (75%) by the hepatic route, and even with biliary obstruction, high concentrations of drug are achieved in bile. Although penetration into the eye is poor (for example, the concentration of cefazolin in the aqueous humor is about 10% of the serum concentration),[11,144] the cephalosporins can sometimes be administered systematically for the treatment of eye infections.

Even when there is meningeal inflammation, the first-and second-generation cephalosporins do not pass well into cerebrospinal fluid.[126,151] Higher cerebrospinal fluid levels are achieved with cefamandole and cefoxitin than with the other first- and second-generation compounds available in the United States, but a number of meningitis treatment failures have been reported,[154–156] and these drugs should not be relied upon for the treatment of bacterial meningitis.[126] In contrast to the older drugs, the cephalosporins of the third generation are very useful in the treatment of meningitis caused by enteric gram-negative bacilli. After large doses of drug are administered intravenously to patients with meningitis, ceftriaxone, cefotaxime, and ceftizoxime usually yield cerebrospinal fluid concentrations that are bactericidal for most susceptible gram-negative bacilli,[157–159] and these compounds are quite useful for the treatment of meningitis.

Fourth-generation cephalosporins have also good penetration into the CNS, but experience with treating gram-negative meningitis with these drugs is limited. In neonatal rats cefepime given parenterally was found to be as active as cefotaxime against *S. aureus* meningitis.[160]

Adverse Effects of the Cephalosporins

Compared to most of the antibiotics, the cephalosporins cause few significant side effects. Local reactions at the site of administration are the most frequent. Intramuscular administration may be painful and intravenous administration may cause thrombophlebitis.[161] As with the penicillins, intrathecal administration is hazardous and may cause convulsions.[162]

Hypersensitivity reactions are the most important systemic side effects; this subject has been discussed in detail in the preceding section of this chapter. It should be repeated here that some cross-reactivity exists between the penicillins and cephalosporins (Table 4–5), and although cephalosporins may be given to patients with a history of a mild reaction to penicillin, *cephalosporins should not be given to patients with a history of a severe reaction of the immediate type.* About 3% of patients receiving cephalosporins have positive Coomb's tests and

several cases of hemolytic anemia have been reported.[95]

The cephalosporins occasionally cause mild transient elevations of liver enzymes. If inordinately high serum levels are built up (as can occur when the dosage has not been modified in the presence of renal insufficiency), the cephalosporins can be neurotoxic[27] as described earlier for the penicillins. Repeated administration of large doses of cephalothin and cephaparin by rapid intravenous infusion over a prolonged period has been reported to cause an illness with symptoms like those of serum sickness.[163] The basis for this reaction is not known.

The cephalosporins can apparently cause two types of nephropathy.[164] At doses greater than 4 g daily, cephaloridine occasionally causes a renal tubular necrosis[165] that occurs rarely with other cephalosporins. Experiments in a rabbit model suggest that the necrosis occurs rather uniquely with cephaloridine because unusually high concentrations of the drug build up in the cells of the proximal tubule.[166] The second type of nephropathy is very rare and it appears to be similar to the allergic interstitial nephritis caused by methicillin.[164] Underlying renal disease or concomitant administration of other potentially nephrotoxic drugs may be predisposing factors in the development of toxic tubular necrosis.[164,165] There is evidence from carefully controlled prospective trials in humans that administration of cephalothin with an aminoglycoside is more nephrotoxic than administration of a penicillin with an aminoglycoside.[167,168] Gastrointesinal disturbances, primarily diarrhea, can result from cephalosporin administration and may be more frequent with ceftriaxone and cefoperazone[169]

Hematologic abnormalities can also occur after cephalosporin administration. These are usually reversible and include eosinophilia, thrombocytopenia, thrombocytosis, leukopenia, and a positive Coombs's reaction.[170] Cephalosporins with the methylthiotetrazole (MTT) side chain (e.g., cefoperazone) can interfere with vitamin K metabolism and have a greater potential for causing hypoprothrombinemia.[171] However, cephalosporins with this structure have not been associated with clinical bleeding. Administration of vitamin K rapidly reverses antibiotic-related hypothrombinemia in patients with nosocomial pneumonia treated with ceftazidime or cefoperazone. All cephalosporins may interfere with vitamin K–dependent clotting factors, but clinical bleeding relates to severity of illness, not the MTT side chain.[172] Cephalosporins having the MTT side chain may also cause a disulfiram-like reaction in patients who ingest alcohol.[173]

The Cephalosporin Preparations

THE FIRST-GENERATION DRUGS. The first-generation cephalosporins (see Fig. 4–7 for structures) have similar antibacterial activities in vitro, permitting routine sensitivity testing for all of these drugs with a single antibiotic disk containing cephalothin.[174] Cephalothin has been in clinical use longer than the other cephalosporins. It has the greatest resistance to hydrolysis by the staphylococcal β-lactamases and it is often considered to be the cephalosporin of choice when a cephalosporin is appropriate for treating severe staphylococcal infection. Intramuscular administration of cephalothin is often painful and intravenous administration frequently causes phlebitis. Cephalothin has a short half-life, and when treating severe infections intravenously, it is administered every 4 h.

Cefazolin[175,176] was introduced nearly a decade after cephalothin and it has pharmacological advantages that make it the first-generation cephalosporin that is preferred in most instances for parenteral administration. In contrast to cephalothin and cephaprin, which are metabolized to the less active desacetyl form, cefazolin remains unchanged. The longer serum half-life of cefazolin permits less frequent administration and lower dosage.[177] Although the protein binding is slightly higher than that of cephalothin, the serum concentration of free antibiotic achieved with cefazolin is 1.5 to 2 times that achieved with an equivalent dose of cephalothin.[178] Although cefazolin has a slower rate of renal clearance than the other cephalosporins, high urine concentrations are nevertheless achieved.[178] Cefazolin is well tolerated. It is less painful than cephalothin when given by intramuscular injection[179] and it produces less phlebitis when given intravenously.[161]

The other first-generation cephalosporins available for parenteral administration in the United States are cephaparin,[180] and cephradine.[180] Cephaparin is similar to cephalothin in its pharmacokinetic properties and toxic potential and it offers no particular advantages.[180] Cephradine is given both orally and parenterally, and when given intramuscularly, peak levels may be lower than those achieved after oral administration.[126] Another compound, cephaloridine,[165] causes less pain than cephalothin on intramuscular injection, but it is the most nephrotoxic cephalosporin and for that reason there is no indication for its use (cephaloridine is no longer marketed in the United States).

In addition to cephradine, two other first-generation drugs are available for oral use. Cephalexin[181] is acid stable and 80% to 100% of a dose is absorbed from the gastrointestinal tract.[144] Although cephradine and cephalexin are close chemical congeners and have nearly identical pharmacological properties[144] and indications for use, cephalexin has been in use longer and is preferred by many physicians. Cefadroxil is a long-acting, orally administered cephalosporin with a spectrum of action in vitro similar to cephalexin and cephradine.[182] The half-life in normal subjects is 1.2 to 1.6 h[183] and antibacterial levels of drug persist in the serum for 12 h. Because of the sustained levels in serum and urine, cefadroxil is administered only twice a day and for uncomplicated infections of the skin or lower urinary tract it may be given only once a day. In spite of its slow renal excretion, examination of cefadroxil kinetics in patients with renal insufficiency suggests that little accumulation occurs until the creatinine clearance is less than 25 ml/min.[184] Compared to other appropriate therapy, administration of cefadroxil can be expensive.[185]

THE SECOND-GENERATION DRUGS. The second-generation cephalosporins (Fig. 4–8) have a broader spectrum of gram-negative

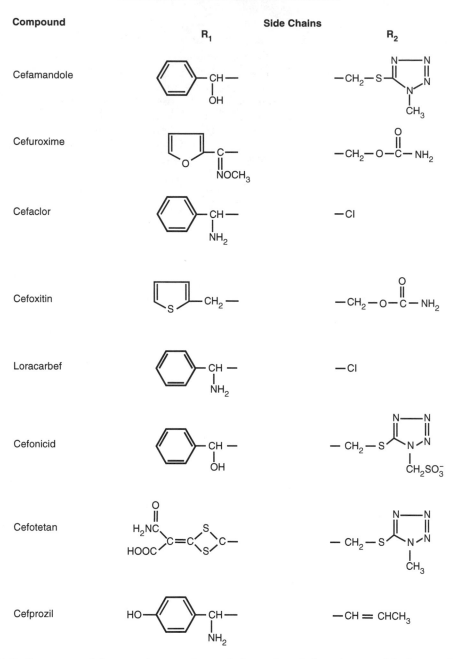

Figure 4–8. Structures of the second-generation cephalosporins. Cefuroxime axetil is the acetyloxyethyl ester of cefuroxime.

antimicrobial action than the first-generation drugs. This increased activity is due to a combination of increased affinity for the penicillin binding proteins, increased ability to penetrate through the outer bacterial membrane, and decreased sensitivity to gram-negative β-lactamases (see Table 3–7). Some of the second-generation drugs, such as cefoxitin, are more effective against gram-negative bacteria because they have an especially high resistance to hydrolysis by β-lactamases, whereas the enhanced spectrum of others, such as cefamandole, appears to be primarily due to particularly effective interaction with the penicillin binding proteins.[186] Thus the enhanced spectrum of these drugs depends on different combinations of properties and, unlike the first-generation cephalosporins, the second- and third-generation drugs vary in their spectra of action. The second- and third-generation cephalosporins are generally less active against gram-positive bacteria than the first-generation drugs.

Cefamandole[187] and cefoxitin[188] are the first parenterally administered second-generation drugs that were marketed in the United States. Both are active against some cephalothin-resistant strains of *Escherichia coli, Klebsiella,* and *Proteus mirabilis. Providentia* and *Serratia* strains are often susceptible. Cefamandole (but not cefoxitin) is active against some *Enterobacter* strains and it inhibits both ampicillin-sensitive and ampicillin-resistant strains of *Haemophilus influenzae.* Cefamandole should not be used to treat meningitis, as failure of therapy has been reported for some patients with *H. influenzae* meningitis.[155] Cefamandole has a half-life of 1 to 1.5 h in both adults[132] and newborn infants,[189] and it is usually administered every 4 to 6 h for severe infection.

Cefoxitin has a methoxy residue at position 7 in the β-lactam ring; thus, it is a cephamycin rather than a cephalosporin (see Fig. 4–8). Cefoxitin is the most active of the first- and second-generation drugs against *Bacteroides fragilis* and other anerobes.[188] Its pharmacology is similar to that of cephalothin. Intramuscular injection is painful and it is best to give the drug intravenously.[126] Cefuroxime is a parenteral cephalosporin with increased β-lactamase stability and increased activity in vitro against gram-negative bacteria.[190] Cefuroxime has a half-life of 1.6 to 2.2 h when renal function is normal and 14 to 28 h when the creatinine clearance is less than 10 ml/min.[191]

Cefaclor[192] is an orally administered cephalosporin that is more active against *Haemophilus influenzae,* including some β-lactamase-producing strains, than the first-generation drugs. Cefaclor is well absorbed, even when there is food in the stomach. The drug is hydrolyzed in human serum (decay half-life in serum at 37°C in vitro is 2.3 h)[193] and, apparently for this reason, it does not accumulate even in the presence of markedly depressed renal function.[130,192] Cefaclor is useful primarily for treating otitis media and respiratory tract infections.

Loracarbef is a second-generation cephalosporin but is also a carbacephem. It is the first available member of this new drug class. Structurally it is closely related to the cephalosporins, differing from cefaclor by a sulfur atom. Clinically, it is grouped with the second-generation cephalosporins. Loracarbef is orally administered, is more stable against some β-lactamases than other second-generation drugs, and has a half-life of about 1 h. It inhibits the growth of a variety of pathogens frequently isolated in respiratory, urinary, and skin and soft tissue infections such as *Streptococcus pneumoniae, Staphylococcus aureus, E. coli*, and *Haemophilus influenzae*. It is quite effective in the treatment of a variety of lower respiratory tract infections as well as infections of the skin and urinary tract.[131]

Cefuroxime axetil is the 1-acetoxyethyl ester of cefuroxime. Thirty to fifty percent of an oral dose is absorbed, and the drug is then rapidly hydrolyzed to the active parent compound cefuroxime. It has a half-life of about 2 h. Cefuroxime axetil has a broad spectrum of activity including methicillin-sensitive staphylococci and many common respiratory pathogens. It is an effective and convenient treatment for a wide range of infections and may be very useful for empirical treatment of community-acquired infections.[132]

Cefotetan is a cephamycin, and, like cefoxitin, it has good activity against *Bacteroides fragilis*. It is also effective against several other species of *Bacteroides* and is more active than cefoxitin against aerobic gram-negative organisms. It is usually given by intramuscular injection.

Cefprozil is a relatively new oral second generation cephalosporin. It can replace cefaclor as a standard oral second-generation agent. It is available as a palatable liquid and can be used to treat respiratory tract infections, otitis media and sinusitis.

THE THIRD-GENERATION CEPHALOSPORINS. The third-generation cephalosporins[194] represent an important therapeutic advance in the treatment of serious infection by gram-negative bacteria. As a group, they differ from the other cephalosporins on the basis of their particularly low MICs for most susceptible gram-negative organisms and their ability to penetrate into the cerebrospinal fluid when the meninges are inflamed. Cephalosporins of this generation are much less uniform than the first- and second-generation drugs in their in vitro activity. For example, although some maintain activity against gram-positive organisms, such as group A streptococcus, others have no activity. Cefotaxime[195] was the first of these extended-spectrum cephalosporins to be introduced in the United States. Most enteric gram-negative bacilli, including *Escherichia coli, Klebsiella, Proteus mirabilis*, indole-positive *Proteus, Citrobacter, Providencia*, and *Serratia marcescens*, are susceptible to the third-generation cephalosporins in vitro.[196,197] Even multiple drug–resistant strains may be sensitive to these drugs. *Neisseria* species and *Hemophilus influenzae* are susceptible to all third-generation agents and clinical experience in the treatment of severe infections by these organisms has been quite good. In fact, ceftriaxone is currently the drug of choice for most gonorrheal infections. Activity against staphylococci and streptococci is less with the third-generation compounds than with the first- and second-generation compounds. Cefotaxime, cefoperazone, and ceftizoxime have the greatest activity against staphylococci while methicillin-susceptible *Staphylococcus aureus* is susceptible to all third-generation drugs except ceftazidime.[198,199] Third-generation cephalosporins are active against *Streptococcus pyogenes* and most isolates of *S. Pneumoniae*, although penicillin-resistant pneumococcus is resistant to all of the third-generation compounds. Also resistant to the third-generation drugs are enterococci and *Listeria monocytogenes*. Activity against anaerobic bacteria varies with the different drugs and organisms, with cefotaxime and ceftizoxime being the most active against *Bacteroides fragilis*.[173,198] The only two third-generation cephalosporins with significant activity against *Pseudomonas aeruginosa* are ceftazidime and cefoperazone.[172] These two drugs are useful alternatives to the penicillins for treating *Pseudomonas* infection in patients with a history of penicillin hypersensitivity. If they are used to treat severe *Pseudomonas* infection outside the urinary tract, the third-generation cephalosporins should be used in conjunction with an aminoglycoside.

It is possible that the third-generation cephalosporins may have their greatest impact in the treatment of meningitis caused by gram-negative enteric bacteria (but not meningitis due to *Pseudomonas*, staphylococci, or pneumococci). Although all third-generation cephalosporins except cefoperazone are approved for therapy of gram-negative meningitis, cefotaxime, ceftriaxone, and ceftizoxime have been the most extensively used in this condition.[200,201] Like other β-lactam antibiotics, the third-generation cephalosporins do not pass into the cerebrospinal fluid in the absence of meningeal inflammation.[202] But it has been shown in both animal models[203,204] and in humans with meningitis[157–159] that they pass through the inflamed meninges to yield cerebrospinal fluid concentrations that exceed the minimum bactericidal concentrations for most Enterobacteriaceae and *Haemophilus influenzae*. Clinical experience in the treatment of gram-negative meningitis in infants and children has led to the third-generation cephalosporins being the drugs of choice.[157,158] Although all of the third-generation compounds have activity against anaerobes, ceftizoxime has the best activity and can be used to treat mixed aerobic/anerobic infections of the abdomen, female genital tract, and diabetic foot.[205]

The third-generation cephalosporins should be reserved for treatment of severe infections due to susceptible gram-negative bacilli. Although many gram-positive bacteria are also susceptible, these drugs are not as potent as cephalothin or cefazolin and they are not indicated for the treatment of any gram-positive infection. The third-generation cephalosporins should not be used on a frequent or routine basis because of selection of resistant organisms and because these drugs are very expensive.

Cefotaxime, ceftizoxime, ceftazidime, ceftriaxone, and cefoperazone (see Fig. 4–9 for structures) are all administered parenterally, as they are inactivated in the stomach and have limited absorption from the duodenum. The serum half-life for most third-generation drugs is 1–2 h, but ceftriaxone has a serum half-life of 5 to 10 h, so it can be given once a day.[206] Cefotaxime is metabolized to the desacetyl form and two other metabolites[207] and is excreted in the urine; about 60% is recovered as the parent compound.[208]

Cefotaxime is the only third-generation cephalosporin that is metabolized to a biologically active form. Desacetylcefotaxime has considerable antimicrobial activity, good penetration into extravascular tissue, and synergy with cefotaxime.[205,209] The serum half-life of cefotaxime in adults with normal renal function is in the range of 1 h, [130,208] but it is in the range of 3 to 4.5 h in newborn infants and higher values are observed in those with a low birth weight.[210] The drug distributes widely, with therapeutic levels reported in bile, bronchial secretions, ascitic fluid, cerebrospinal fluid, and the aqueous humor of the eye.[157,194,195,211]

All third-generation cephalosporins except cefoperazone are excreted mainly by the kidneys. Ceftriaxone has a dual mechanism of excretion with 40% of the drug being excreted in the bile. Cefoperazone is excreted predominantly by the liver. The serum half-life is 1.7 to 1.9 h in normal subjects and blood levels do not appear to be markedly elevated in patients with severe renal dysfunction.[135]

Cefixime, cefpodoxime and ceftibuten are third-generation cephalosporins that are available for oral administration. The first of these to come into clinical use was cefixime. It has a long half-life (about 3 h), which has allowed it to be given once a day. Cefixime has the best activity against gram-negative bacteria among the oral third-generation agents, but it is somewhat less active than the second-generation cephalosporins against *Streptococcus pneumoniae* and it has no activity against *Staphylococcus aureus*.[212] Cefixime is useful for treating pyelonephritis or other gram-negative infections caused by Enterobacteriaceae. It is also effective as a single oral dose for treating uncomplicated gonorrhea.[213]

Cefpodoxime proxetil is an oral third-generation agent very similar in activity to cefixime except that is more active against *S. aureus*. It is rapidly hydrolysed to its parent compound, cefuroxime. It has a half-life of about 2 h and is administered twice daily. It is associated with a low incidence of adverse effects and is an effective and convenient treatment for a wide range of infections.[132] The newest oral third-generation drug is ceftibuten. It can be given once or twice daily, is well tolerated, and is active against a wide spectrum of organisms.[214]

THE FOURTH-GENERATION CEPHALOSPORINS. In contrast to the anionic third-generation compounds, the fourth-generation cephalosporins are dipolar ionic compounds. These compounds diffuse more rapidly into gram-negative bacteria and they also have a lower affinity for β-lactamases located in the periplasmic space of gram-negative organisms. In vitro, they are poor inducers of β-lactamases, a property that is believed to correlate with a lower rate of development of clinical resistance among gram-negative bacteria. The fourth-generation drugs have a broad spectrum of antibacterial activity. Against the Enterobacteriaceae their activity surpasses that of the third-generation compounds. They have excellent activity against *Haemophilus influenzae*, *Neisseria gonorrea*, and *N. meningitidis*.[212] They are active against *Pseudomonas* and also have good activity against gram-positive bacteria. However, like the other cephalosporins, they are not active against enterococci nor against methicillin-resistant staphylococci.[215] Currently, the only approved fourth-generation drug is cefepime. The fourth-generation compounds should not be used for community-acquired infections but their broad spectrum of action should make them especially useful for the treatment of hospital-acquired infections, infections in

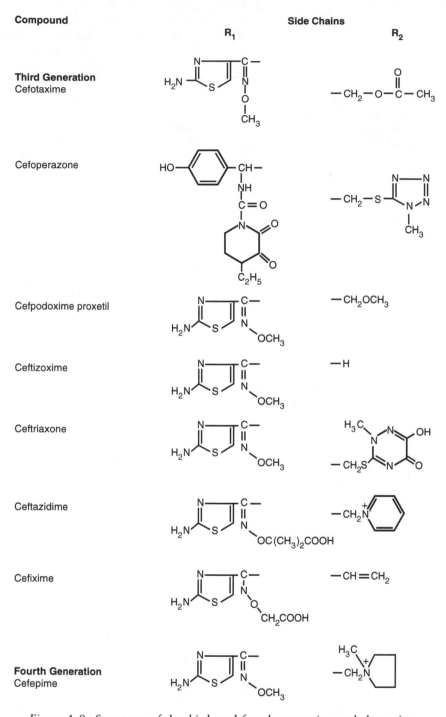

Compound	Side Chains	
	R_1	R_2

Third Generation
Cefotaxime

Cefoperazone

Cefpodoxime proxetil

Ceftizoxime

Ceftriaxone

Ceftazidime

Cefixime

Fourth Generation
Cefepime

Figure 4–9. Structures of the third- and fourth-generation cephalosporins.

110

immunocompromised hosts, and infections by highly resistant gram-negative bacteria. This will be a very important group of antibiotics if clinical experience supports their initial promise of less induction of resistance among hospital colonizing gram-negative organisms.

Carbapenems and Monobactams

Carbapenems

The *carbapenems* are β-lactam antibiotics that contain a carbon instead of a sulfur atom in the five-membered ring structure. The first carbapenem, thienamycin, was discovered as a natural product.[216] Because of its instability, it was synthetically modified to N-formimidoyl thienamycin, which was called *imipenem*. Several other carbapenems were subsequently synthesized, but the only one other than imipenem that is commercially available in the U.S. is meropenem. Like the penicillins and cephalosporins, the carbapenems are β-lactams and thus act by binding to penicillin binding proteins (PBPs). In gram-negative bacteria, carbapenems bind primarily to PBP1 and PBP2 rather than to PBP3, which is the main target of aminopenicillins.[217]

bacilli.[218] Methicillin-resistant strains of *Staphylococcus aureus* have varying susceptibility to carbapenems, as have pneumococci.[219] The carbapenems are highly resistant to hydrolysis by most β-lactamases.[220] They are potent inducers of chromosomal cephalosporinase, which hydrolyzes third-generation cephalosporins such as ceftazidime and ceftriaxone,[221] but they are not hydrolyzed by the enzyme.

All the carbapenems are water-soluble compounds that are not absorbed from the gastrointestinal tract after oral administration. Therefore, imipenem is given by intravenous infusion or by intramuscular administration and meropenem is given intramuscularly or by bolus or short-term infusion. Imipenem is hydrolyzed rapidly by a dipeptidase present in the brush border of the proximal renal tubule.[222] Consequently, it is administered as a preparation containing equal amounts of imipenem and cilastatin, an inhibitor of the dehydropeptidase. The dehydropeptidase enzyme catalyzing the reaction is dehydropeptidase-I,[222] which hydrolyzes and breaks the β-lactam bond in the carbapenem molecule, resulting in stable open lactam metabolites that are structurally similar to the penicilloyl moieties formed when the β-lactam bonds of penicillins are broken. When given as the combined preparation of imipenem and cilastatin, about 70% of the drug is excreted in the urine as active drug. Meropenem is unaffected by the dehydropeptidase and is not administered with cilastatin. About 30% of both imipenem and meropenem undergo nonrenal metabolism, and their dosages must be modified in the presence of renal failure.

Imipenem

Meropenem

Cilastatin

The carbapenems have a very broad antibacterial spectrum (see Table 4–9) and are active against most gram-negative and gram-positive aerobic and anaerobic cocci and

The carbapenems are well tolerated by adults and children. The incidence of hypersensitivity to the carbapenems is low, even though there is potential for cross-reactivity with other β-lactam antibiotics. Gastrointes-

Table 4–9. Antibacterial spectrum of carbapenems.

Susceptibility	Bacterial species
Generally highly susceptible (MIC_{90} <1 µg/ml)	*Acinetobacter* spp. *Bacteroids* *Citrobacter* spp. *Enterobacter* spp. *Escherichia coli* *Fusobacterium* spp. *Haemophilus influenzae* *Listeria monocytogenes* *Moraxella catarrhalis* *Morganella morganii* *Neisseria gonorrhoeae* *Neisseria meningitidis* *Proteus* spp. *Providencia* spp. *Salmonella* spp. *Staphylococcus aureus* (methicillin-sensitive) *Streptococcus pneumoniae* (penicillin MIC <1 µg/ml) *Streptococcus* spp. *Yersinia enteroclitica*
Varying susceptibility (MIC_{90} >1–<8 µg/ml)	*Pseudomonas aeruginosa* *Serratia* spp. *Staphylococcus aureus* (methicillin-resistant) *Staphylococcus* spp. (methicillin-resistant) *Streptococcus pneumoniae* (penicillin MIC <1 µg/ml)
Generally resistant (MIC_{90} >8 µg/ml)	*Corynebacterium jeikeium* *Enterococcus faecium* *Pseudomonas cepacia* *Xanthomonas maltophilia*

MIC_{90}, minimum concentration inibiting bacterial growth by 90%.
Source: Modified from Norrby.[217]

tinal reactions in the form of nausea and vomiting are the most common reactions associated with the use of these drugs. Even though minimal amounts of the carbapenems reach the intestine, diarrhea is rare, and the risk of pseudomembranous colitis seems low. Neurotoxicity associated with imipenem has limited the usefulness of this drug. Seizures can occur with high levels of the drug, particularly when there is renal failure or underlying central nervous system (CNS) injury.[223] This CNS toxicity has made the treatment of meningitis with imipenem less successful. Studies with meropenem indicate that seizures are not a major problem.

Imipenem, and probably meropenem, provide effective monotherapy for septicemia, neutropenic fever, and intraabdominal, lower respiratory tract, genitourinary, gynecological, skin and soft tissue, and bone and joint infections. For these indications, imipenem and meropenem have the same efficacy as broad-spectrum cephalosporins and are at least equivalent to standard combination drug regimens.[218] The carbapenems are useful for a variety of infections caused by mixed aerobes and anaerobes, as well as for infections caused by multiple drug–resistant nosocomial organisms. Meropenem is useful for treating bacterial meningitis. In general, the carbapenems are most useful for treating hospital-acquired resistant infections rather than community-acquired infections. Experience with meropenem is considerably less than with imipenem and further clinical experience is necessary to define its place in therapy.

Monobactams

The *monobactams* are monocyclic lactams. They are synthetic compounds, although they have been found in nature in various soil bacteria. Aztreonam is the only marketed monobactam; others are currently under investigation. Aztreonam is of clinical importance because of its unique spectrum of bactericidal action. Aztreonam has a sulfonic acid group on the nitrogen at the 1-position of the aminomonobactamic nucleus that causes it to bind preferentially to PBP-3 of gram-negative bacteria.[224] Because of its poor affinity for the PBPs in gram-positive and ananerobic organisms, its spectrum of activity is limited to aerobic, gram-negative bacteria. It is resistant to chromosomal and plasmid β-lactamases produced by gram-negative species.

Aztreonam

The antimicrobial activity (see Table 4–10) of aztreonam more closely resembles that of the aminoglycosides than that of other β-lactam compounds. Whereas gram-positive bacteria and anaerobic organisms are resistant to the drug, it has excellent activity against *Pseudomonas aeruginosa* and Enterobacteriaceae. It is also highly active against *Haemophilus influenzae* and gonococci, at least in vitro, whereas *Chlamydia* spp. and *Legionella* spp. are resistant.[225]

Absorption of aztreonam from the gut is poor because intestinal flora convert it into an inactive ring form, and the drug is administered parenterally. Rapid and complete absorption occurs following intramuscular

Table 4–10. Antibacterial spectrum of aztreonam.

Susceptibility	Organism
Generally high susceptible (MIC$_{90}$ <1 µg/ml)	E. coli Klebsiella pneumoniae Proteus mirabilis Proteus vulgaris Morganella morganii Haemophilus influenzae Salmonella spp. Yersinia Neisseria gonorrhoeae
Varying susceptibility (MIC$_{90}$ >1–<8 µg/ml)	Enterobacter cloacae Citrobacter freundii Pseudomonas aeruginosa Serratia marcescens
Generally resistant (MIC$_{90}$ >8 µg/ml)	Staphylococcus aureus Streptococcus pyogenes Streptococcus pneumoniae Streptococcus faecalis Bacteroides fragilis Enterobacter aerogenes

MIC$_{90}$, minimum inhibitory concentration at or below the value for 90% of isolates.

Source: Adapted from Johnson and Cunha.[225]

injection, with peak serum concentrations occurring within about 60 min. It can also be administered intravenously. The primary route of elimination is renal, by both glomerular filtration and tubular secretion; dosage adjustment is necessary in patients with renal impairment. Aztreonam is excreted as unchanged drug, with 58% to 74% of a dose excreted unchanged and 1%–7% as open-ring metabolites.[226] Aztreonam penetrates into the CNS, and in patients with uninflamed meninges, a 3 g dose of the drug produced concentrations of 0.5 µg/ml and 1 µg/ml in the cerebrospinal fluid at 1 and 4 h, respectively. Mean cerebrospinal fluid drug levels increased to 2 µg/ml and 3.2 µg/ml, respectively, when the meninges were inflamed.[227] Aztreonam is 45% to 60% bound to serum proteins in patients with normal serum albumin.[228]

Aztreonam has been used successfully in

the treatment of a variety of infections, such as bacteremias, urinary tract, pelvic, intraabdominal, and respiratory tract infections. It is often administered in combination with other drugs, and is a useful alternative to the aminoglycosides because of its lack of ototoxicity and nephrotoxicity. Aztreonam can also be used as a substitute for penicillins or cephalosporins, as it is not cross-allergenic to those compounds.

Aztreonam has a relatively low incidence of toxicity. The adverse effects are similar to those from other β-lactam antibiotics, the most common reactions being local, consisting of phlebitis or pain at the site of intramuscular injection. Some rash and gastrointestinal discomfort in the form of nausea, vomiting, and diarrhea have been reported. Because aztreonam contains the β-lactam ring structure, there is some concern about the possibility of cross-reactivity with the penicillins and the cephalosporins, but clinical studies have shown that fewer than 1% of β-lactam-allergic individuals had a possible hypersensitivity reaction to aztreonam. Nonetheless, it should be used with caution in persons with a history of immediate-type reactions to the other β-lactams. There have been no serious hematologic abnormalities associated with the use of this drug nor has there been any ototoxicity or nephrotoxicity.

β-Lactamase Inhibitor Combinations

Three β-lactamase inhibitors are available for clinical use in the United States. Their mechanism of action is discussed in Chapter 3. Tazobactam is the most active of the available inhibitors, with clavulanic acid being active against most β-lactamases and sulbactam against the least number of enzymes.[229] Combination drug preparations containing a penicillin and a β-lactamase inhibitor were developed to extend the therapeutic activity of the well-tolerated β-lactam antibiotics to β-lactamase-producing organisms.

The β-lactamase inhibitors are excreted mainly by the kidney, with half-lives of about 0.5 to 1 h. The elimination of all three inhibitors from the body is reduced in the elderly and in renal failure.[47] Clavulanic acid has been combined with amoxicillin as an oral preparation and with ticarcillin as a parenteral preparation. Sulbactam is similar in structure to clavulanic acid and, like clavulanic acid, it can be administered either orally or parenterally along with the penicillin. It is available combined with ampicillin as intravenous or intramuscular preparations. Tazobactam, a penicillanic acid sulfone, has been combined with piperacillin as a parenteral preparation.

Although the mechanism of action of all of these combinations is similar, they differ greatly in their antimicrobial spectrum as well as in their therapeutic uses. The antibacterial activity of the combinations is determined by both the antibacterial activity of the penicillin and the activity of the inhibitor against penicillinases. The inhibitor–penicillin combinations significantly extend the antibacterial spectrum of the penicillins alone. Amoxicillin–clavulanic acid, the only oral β-lactamase inhibitor combination currently available, is active in vitro against those organisms normally sensitive to amoxicilin, as well as to β-lactamase-producing strains of *Halmophilus influenzae, Bacteroides catarrhalis,* and *Staphylococcus aureus.*[229] The combinations ticarcillin–clavulanic acid and piperacillin-tazobactam generally show a significant increase in in vitro activity against methicillin-sensitive staphylococci, *H. influenzae, B. catarrhalis, E. coli, Acinetobacter,* and *Bacteroides fragilis.* However, the combination does not have increased activity against *Enterococcus* or *Pseudomonas.* Like the other inhibitors, tazobactam has good activity against many of the plasmid β-lactamases but poor activity against inducible, chromosomal β-lactamases (Table 4–11). In *Pseudomonas,* resistance is most likely due either to chromosomal β-lactamases or decreased permeability of piperacillin into the periplasmic space.[230] The combination drugs are beneficial in a variety of clinical situations; they are most useful for skin, soft tissue, and lower respiratory tract infections, as well as intraabdominal and gynecologic infections caused by susceptible pathogens.

Like the penicillin components themselves,

Table 4–11.   Relative in vitro activity of β-lactamase inhibitor combinations.

Class of organism	Amoxicillin/ clavulanic acid	Ampicillin/ sulbactam	Ticarcillin/ clavulanic acid	Piperacillin/ tazobactam
Gram-positive bacteria	+	+	+/++	++
Gram-negative bacteria	−	+	+/++	++
Pseudomonas	−	−	+	++
Anaerobic bacteria	−	+	+++	++

−, poor; +, some; ++, good; +++, very good.

Source: Adapted from Sensovic and Smith.[229]

the β-lactamase inhibitor combinations are relatively safe drugs. Skin rashes are seen in about 4% of patients,[229] and diarrhea and gastrointestinal upset are the most common adverse effects.

Vancomycin, Teicoplanin, and Bacitracin

Vancomycin

Vancomycin is a complex tricyclic glycopeptide of molecular weight 1448.[231] Although the molecule contains a disaccharide moiety, the carbohydrate components are not necessary for antibiotic activity. Vancomycin binds very tightly to the acyl-D-alanyl-D-alanine terminus of the cell wall precursor unit and this binding eventually leads to cell lysis as described in Chapter 3. The use, pharmacology, and toxicity of vancomycin has been the subject of several comprehensive reviews.[232–234]

SPECTRUM OF ACTION AND THERAPEUTIC USE. Vancomycin is active against most species of gram-positive cocci and bacilli, such as *Staphylococcus aureus* (including methicillin-resistant strains), *Staphylococcus epidermidis* (including multiple drug–resistant strains), *Streptococcus pneumoniae*, viridans group *Streptococcus*, enterococcus, *Streptococcus bovis*, *Clostridium* species, diphtheroids, *Listeria monocytogenes*, *Actinomyces* species, and *Lactobacillus* species.[235] *Neisseria gonorrhoeae* strains are usually susceptible, but gram-negative bacilli and mycobacteria are resistant. In recent years, there have been many reports of en-

terococci and staphylococci isolates that are resistant to vancomycin.[236–238]

Vancomycin was introduced, in 1956, for treatment of penicillinase-producing staphylococcal infections, but when the penicillinase-resistant penicillins became available, it was relegated to the role of alternative therapy. In later years, the use of this drug increased as more purified preparations became available and treatment extended to infections due to methicillin-resistant pathogens. Vancomycin is administered intravenously to treat serious infections due to staphylococci in patients who are intolerant to the penicillins or when the infection is caused by methicillin-resistant strains.[239] It is used as an alternative to β-lactam antibiotics in treating endocarditis caused by staphylococci and streptococci.[240,241] Vancomycin acts synergistically with aminoglycosides against both enterococcal (*Streptococcus faecalis*) and nonenterococcal (*Streptococcus bovis* and viridans group) streptococci.[242,243] As vancomycin is often not bactericidal for *Streptococcus faecalis*, it is usually combined with gentamicin for treating enterococcal endocarditis. Endocarditis due to *S. viridans* or *S. bovis* can be treated with vancomycin alone if the minimum bactericidal concentration for the isolate is low enough (not more than 10 μg/ml;[234] otherwise it should be combined with an aminoglycoside. Other serious infections due to resistant organisms that respond to vancomycin are *Corynebacterium* endocarditis and *Flavobacterium meningosepticum* meningitis.[234] Vancomycin may be administered orally to treat antibiotic-associated enterocolitis due to *Clostridium difficile*[244] and staphylococcal enterocolitis.[234]

Vancomycin has been considered an important drug for the treatment of enterococcal and staphylococcal infections, especially when there is resistance to several other drugs. Thus, the recent emergence of clinical resistance to vancomycin and, in some instances, other glycopeptides in nosocomial enterococcal infections has resulted in infections that are resistant to all clinically available antibiotics. The mechanism of this plasmid encoded vancomycin resistance is described in Chapter 3.

PHARMACOLOGY. Vancomycin is very poorly absorbed from the gastrointestinal tract. The oral route is used for treating enterocolitis and resulting stool concentrations of bactericidal activity are far above those required to inhibit *Clostridium difficile* and *Staphylococcus aureus* in vitro.[234] For other infections the drug is administered by slow intravenous infusion two or four times daily.

Vancomycin distributes widely in tissues[245] and penetrates into pleural, pericardial, synovial, and ascitic fluids in concentrations that are therapeutic for most sensitive organisms.[246] The drug does not concentrate in the bile. Vancomycin does not pass into the cerebrospinal fluid unless the meninges are inflamed. When meningitis is present, therapeutic levels of drug are often achieved in the cerebrospinal fluid; however, the concentration may not be adequate and concomitant intrathecal administration should be considered if response to parenteral therapy is poor.[247–249] Although only limited data are available, it seems that penetration of the drug into the cerebrospinal fluid is better in young children with meningitis than in adults.[246]

Vancomycin is 55% bound to serum protein and is excreted into the urine by glomerular filtration as the unchanged drug.[250] The elimination half-life in adults has been found to range from 5 to 11 h.[250] The half-life in children varies inversely with age; it is 6 to 10 h in newborns, 4 h in older infants, and 2 to 3 h in children.[249] The half-life is longer in adults because the apparent volume of distribution is somewhat higher and the plasma clearance rate is slower than in children.[249] As vancomycin is potentially toxic and is eliminated by the kidneys, it is very important that the dosage be modified in patients with renal failure. A convenient nomogram for modification of dosage according to creatinine clearance rate has been published.[251] Vancomycin serum levels should be assayed to confirm that drug concentrations are in the therapeutic range. In anephric patients the half-life of vancomycin is 7.5 days, and after giving a loading dose (1 g), the drug (500 mg) is administered only once every 7 or 8 days.[252] Little or no drug is removed with hemodialysis, [248,251] but as vancomycin passes across the peritoneum, the dosage may have to be increased during peritoneal dialysis.[253] Because of poor absorption from the gastrointestinal tract, vancomycin may be safely administered to functionally anephric patients for treatment of enterocolitis.[254]

ADVERSE EFFECTS. Rapid intravenous administration of vancomycin may cause a variety of alarming symptoms, including erythematous or urticarial reactions, flushing, tachycardia, and hypotension.[250,255] The extreme flushing that can occur has been called *red-neck* or *red-man syndrome*,[256] and it is thought to result from histamine release from cutaneous mast cells.[257] The incidence is related to both the dose and rapidity of infusion, affecting 80% of patients receiving a 1 g dose over 60 min.[258] Longer infusion times of up to 2 h may minimize the occurrence and the severity of symptoms.[250,257] Administration of the antihistaminic drug methapyrilene has been found to prevent hypotension caused by rapid administration of vancomycin to dogs,[259] suggesting that the syndrome in humans may be due to a vancomycin-induced release of histamine; However, there is evidence that other mediators may also be involved.[260] Phlebitis occurs occasionally and is reduced by dilution of the drug. Oral administration of vancomycin may cause vomiting, but the problem is often reduced by administering the drug through a nasogastric tube that has been passed beyond the pylorus.

Vancomycin is potentially ototoxic. Hearing loss is rarely seen when serum levels are kept below 30 μg/ml.[232] Patients receiving parenteral vancomycin, particularly those with compromised renal function, should have periodic audiography or frequent clinical assessment of hearing. Hearing loss is first observed in the high frequency range and is sometimes reversible after cessation of therapy.[241] Although a high incidence of nephrotoxicity, phlebitis, and fever was reported in early studies, these reactions were probably caused by impurities in the early vancomycin preparations, which have been eliminated with current manufacturing procedures.[241] Thus, although vancomycin was formerly considered to be very nephrotoxic, nephrotoxicity has not been clearly established in humans.[261] Vancomycin should nevertheless be used cautiously in patients with prior renal disease and renal function should be monitored before and during therapy. Concomitant administration of vancomycin and aminoglycosides significantly increases nephrotoxicity in rats[259] and special caution should be exerted in patients receiving both drugs, both with respect to nephrotoxicity and ototoxicity. Reversible neutropenia has been reported rarely with vancomycin therapy.[262] With appropriate administration, dosage adjustment, and assay of serum drug levels, vancomycin can be employed in a safe and reliable manner.

Teicoplanin

Teicoplanin is another glycopeptide antibiotic that is a complex of several molecules of similar antibiotic activity. Teicoplanin is structurally related to vancomycin but has certain advantages in terms of pharmacokinetics and toxicity. The five components of teicoplanin differ from each other by the acylaliphatic sidechain substitution present on one of the sugars, but they all have the same aglycone backbone.[263] Teicoplanin has a mechanism of action identical to that of vancomycin. It also has a spectrum of activity similar to that of vancomycin, with a few notable differences. For example, teicoplanin is more active than vancomycin against all streptococci and enterocci,[264,265] but it is less active against S. hemolyticus. Teichoplanin is very poorly absorbed from the gastrointestinal tract and, in contrast to vancomycin, it is safely administered intramuscularly or by rapid intravenous injection. It has a very long half-life, ranging from 33 to 190 h or longer, thus allowing once-daily maintenance dosing. Over 90% of the drug is bound to plasma protein, and almost all of teicoplanin is excreted via the kidney by glomerular filtration. Like vancomycin, the half-life of teichoplanin is substantially altered in renal failure and dosage adjustment is necessary.[265]

Unlike vancomycin, teicoplanin does not cause significant histamine release and the redman or redneck syndrome is seldom seen. The incidence of allergic cross-reactivity between vancomycin and teicoplanin is still somewhat controversial; several cases of cross-reactivity have been reported.[266] Given its long half-life, it is probably unwise to administer teicoplanin to any patient with a history of significant hypersensitivity reaction to vancomycin.[264] Nephrotoxicity and ototoxicity are uncommon to rare and are not dose related. Other toxicities are also uncommon; these include reaction at the site of injection, fever, altered liver function, and thrombocytopenia. Teicoplanin is an alternative to vancomycin in almost all clinical situations where vancomycin would be used, and it appears to be effective in vancomycin-resistant enterococcal infections. It is not yet approved for use in the U.S. but has undergone numerous trials in Europe.

Bacitracin

Bacitracin is a polypeptide antibiotic of molecular weight 1411 isolated from a strain of Bacillus subtilis.[267] Bacitracin inhibits cell wall synthesis by preventing the dephosphorylation of the lipid that attaches the cell wall precursor units to the cell membrane, an event that eventually leads to cell lysis as discussed in Chapter 3. When given systemically, bacitracin is very nephrotoxic,[267] and it is no longer administered parenterally. Bacitracin is not absorbed to an appreciable extent from the gastrointestinal tract. After oral administration, it has been reported to be effective in treatment of antibiotic-associated enterocolitis due to *Clostridium difficile*,[268] although some isolates are resistant and metronidazole or vancomycin is preferred,[244] and in treatment of vancomycin-resistant *Enterococcus faecium* infection.[269,270]

Bacitracin is particularly active against gram-positive cocci and bacilli. The unusual sensitivity of group A streptococci to very low concentrations of bacitracin has led to the use of the bacitracin-impregnated disk for identification of Lancefield group A streptococci in clinical isolates.[271] As bacitracin is very effective in vitro against staphylococci and group A streptococci, the most common pathogens in acute skin infections, it is included in a number of formulations that are used topically to treat superficial infections of the skin and eye. Topical bacitracin is not effective in treating impetigo and deeper skin infections,[272] and the value of any topical antibiotics in the treatment of minor superficial skin infections has not been clearly established. When given topically, bacitracin can cause local hypersensitivity reactions, but this is uncommon.[273]

The topical preparations often contain other antimicrobials like neomycin and polymyxin. Some preparations also contain corticosteroids. The rationale behind the inclusion of a corticosteroid with the antibiotics is subject to some dispute.[274] The shotgun use of both the steroid and the antibiotics permits treatment of dermatitis of both infectious and noninfectious etiology without having to make a definitive diagnosis. When one must deal with large numbers of patients this is convenient. Those who use the combined preparations draw support from the argument that the steroid reduces local discomfort and itching, thus decreasing irritation of the involved area by scratching. One can also argue, however, that the inclusion of the corticosteroid would seem to be frankly counter-productive in the case of superficial infection, since it suppresses both the local reaction and the healing process. When the dermatitis is not due to infection, antibiotics are clearly being used when they are not needed and the patient is exposed to the risk of developing hypersensitivity to one of the antibiotic components. There is good reason to question the role of these antibiotic-corticosteroid combinations in therapy. They are certainly overused and their efficacy against mild superficial infections is not well documented.

REFERENCES

1. Rolinson, G. N., and R. Sutherland. Semisynthetic penicillins. *Adv. Pharmacol. Chemother.* 1973; 11:152.
2. Rammelkamp, C. H., and C. S. Keefer. The absorption, excretion, and distribution of penicillin. *J. Clin. Invest.* 1943;22:425.
3. Rammelkamp, C. H., and J. D. Helm. Studies on the absorption of penicillin from the stomach. *Proc. Soc. Exp. Biol. Med.* 1943;54:324.
4. McDermott, W., P. A. Bunn, M. Benoit, R. DuBois, and M. E. Reynolds. The absorption, excretion and destruction of orally administered penicillin. *J. Clin. Invest.* 1946;25:190.
5. McCarthy, C. G., and M. Finland. Absorption and excretion of four penicillins. Penicillin G, penicillin V, phenethicillin and phenylmercaptomethyl penicillin. *N. Engl. J. Med.* 1960;263:315.
6. Wright, W. W., H. Welch, J. Wilner, and E. F. Roberts. Body fluid concentrations of penicillin following intramuscular injection of single doses of benzathine penicillin G and/or procaine penicillin G. *Antibiot. Med. Clin. Ther.* 1959;6:232.
7. Kaplan, J. M., and G. H. McCracken. Clinical pharmacology of benzathine penicillin G in neonates with regard to its recommended use in congenital syphilis. *J. Pediat.* 1973;82:1069.
8. Rolinson, G. N., and R. Sutherland. The binding of antibiotics to serum proteins. *Br. J. Pharmacol.* 1965; 25:638.
9. Bennett, W. M., L. Singer, T. Golper, P. Feig, and C. J. Coggins. Guidelines for drug therapy in renal failure. *Ann. Intern. Med.* 1977;86:754.
10. Barza, M., and L. Weinstein. Penetration of antibiotics into fibrin loci in vivo. I. Comparison of penetration of ampicillin into fibrin clots, abscesses, and "interstitial fluid". *J. Infect. Dis.* 1974;129:59.
11. Barza, M. T. Samuelson, and L. Weinstein. Penetration of antibiotics into fibrin loci in vivo. II. Comparison of nine antibiotics: effect of dose and degree of protein binding. *J. Infect. Dis.* 1974;129:66.
12. Fishman, R. A. Blood-brain and CSF barriers to penicillin and related organic acids. *Arch. Neurol.* 1966; 15:113.
13. Parker, R. H., and F. R. Schmid. Antibacterial activity of synovial fluid during therapy of septic arthritis. *Arthritis Rheum.* 1971;14:96.
14. Bergeron, M. G., F. J. Gennari, M. Barza, L. Weinstein, and S. Cortell. Renal tubular transport of penicillin G and carbenicillin in the rat. *J. Infect. Dis.* 1975;132:374.
15. Cole, M., M. D. Kenig, and V. A. Hewitt. Me-

tabolism of penicillins to penicilloic acids and 6-aminopenicillanic acid in man and its significance in assessing penicillin absorption. *Antimicrob. Agents Chemother.* 1973;3:463.

16. McCracken, G. H., C. Ginsberg, D. F. Chrane, M. L. Thomas, and J. L. Horton. Clinical pharmacology of penicillin in newborn infants. *J. Pediatr.* 1973; 82:692.

17. Rudnick, M., G. Morrison, B. Walker, and I. Singer. Renal failure, hemodialysis and nafcillin kinetics. *Clin. Pharmacol. Ther.* 1976;20:413.

18. Diaz, C. R., J. G. Kane, R. H. Parker, and F. R. Pelsor. Pharmacokinetics of nafcillin in patients with renal failure. *Antimicrob. Agents Chemother.* 1977;12: 98.

19. Barza, M., J. Brusch, M. G. Bergeron, O. Kemmotsu, and L. Weinstein. Extraction of antibiotics from the circulation by liver and kidney: effect of probenecid. *J. Infect. Dis.* 1975;131(Suppl.):S86.

20. Dixon, R. L., E. S. Owens, and D. P. Rall. Evidence of active transport of benzyl-^{14}C-penicillin from the cerebrospinal fluid to blood. *J. Pharm. Sci.* 1969; 58:1106.

21. Spector, R., and A. V. Lorenzo. Inhibition of penicillin transport from the cerebrospinal fluid after intracisternal innoculation of bacteria. *J. Clin. Invest.* 1974;54:316.

22. Spector, R., and A. V. Lorenzo. The effects of salicylate and probenecid on the cerebrospinal fluid transport of penicillin, aminosalicylic acid and iodide. *J. Pharmacol. Exp. Ther.* 1974;188:55.

23. Forbes, M., and B. Becker. The transport of organic anions by rabbit eye. II. In vitro transport of iodopyracet (diodrast). *Am. J. Ophthalmol.* 1960;50:867.

24. Barza, M., and J. Baum. Penetration of ocular compartments by penicillins: analysis of factors affecting intraocular concentration and half life. *Surv. Ophthalmol.* 1973;18:71.

25. Winningham, D. G., N. J. Nemoy, and T. A. Stamey. Diffusion of antibiotics from the plasma into prostatic fluid. *Nature* 1968;219:139.

26. Weinstein, L., and A. J. Weinstein. The pathophysiology and pathoanatomy of reactions to antimicrobial agents. *Adv. Intern. Med.* 1974;19:109.

27. Fossieck, B., and R. H. Parker. Neurotoxicity during intravenous infusion of penicillin. A review. *J. Clin. Pharmacol.* 1974;14:504.

28. Smith, H., P. I. Lerner, and L. Weinstein. Neurotoxicity and massive intravenous therapy with penicillin. *Arch. Intern. Med* 1967;120:47.

29. Seamans, K. B., A. R. C. Dobell, and J. D. Wyant. Penicillin-induced seizures during cardiopulmonary bypass. A clinical and electroencephalographic study. *N. Engl. J. Med.* 1968;278:861.

30. Bryan, C. S., and W. J. Stone. "Comparably massive" penicillin G therapy in renal failure. *Ann. Intern. Med* 1975;82:189.

31. Raichle, M., S. Louis, H. Kutt, and F. McDowell. Neurotoxicity of intravenous penicillin G and its analogs in cats. *Trans. Am. Neurol. Assoc.* 1968;93:266.

32. Curtis, D. R., C. J. A. Game, G. A. R. Johnston, R. M. McCulloch, and R. M. Maclachlan. Convulsive action of penicillin. *Brain Res.* 1972;43:242.

33. Davidoff, R. A. Penicillin and inhibition in the cat spinal cord. *Brain Res.* 1972;45:638.

34. Macdonald, R. L., and J. L. Barker. Specific antagonism of GABA-mediated postsynaptic inhibition in cultured mammalian spinal cord neurons: a common mode of convulsant action. *Neurology (Minneapolis)* 1978;28:325.

35. Kao, L. I., and W. E. Crill. Penicillin-induced segmented myoclonus. II. Membrane properties of cat spinal motoneurons. *Arch. Neurol.* 1972;26:162.

36. Dismukes, W. E. Oxacillin-induced hepatic dysfunction. *JAMA* 1973;226:861.

37. Wilson, F. M., J. Belamaric, C. B. Lauter, and A. M. Lerner. Anicteric carbenicillin hepatitis. Eight episodes in four patients. *JAMA* 1975;232:818.

38. Reyes, M. P., M. Palutke, and A. M. Lerner. Granulocytopenia associated with carbenicillin. *Am. J. Med.* 1973;54:413.

39. Homayouni, H., P. A. Gross, U. Setia, and T. J. Lynch. Leukopenia due to penicillin and cephalosporin homologues. *Arch. Intern. Med.* 1979;139:827.

40. Garraty, G., and L. D. Petz. Drug-induced immune hemolytic anemia. *Am. J. Med.* 1975;58:398.

41. Shattil, S. J., J. S. Bennett, M. McDonough, and J. Turnbull. Carbenicillin and penicillin G inhibit platelet function in vitro by impairing the interaction of agonists with the platelet surface. *J. Clin. Invest.* 1980;65: 329.

42. Basker, M. J., R. A. Edmundson, and R. Sutherland. Comparative stabilities of penicillins and cephalosporins to staphylococcal β-lactamase and activities against *Staphylococcus aureus. J. Antimicrob. Chemother.* 1980;6:333.

43. Onorato, I. M., and J. L. Axelrod. Hepatitis from intravenous high-dose oxacillin therapy: findings in an adult inpatient population. *Ann. Intern. Med.* 1978;89:497.

44. Pollack, A. A., S. A. Berger, M. S. Simberkoff and J. J. Rahal. Hepatitis associated with high dose oxacillin therapy. *Arch. Intern. Med.* 1978;138:915.

45. Kind, A. C., T. E. Tupasi, H. C. Standiford and W. M. Kirby. Mechanisms responsible for plasma levels of nafcillin lower than those of oxacillin. *Arch. Intern. Med.* 1970;125:685.

46. Marcy, S. M., and J. O. Klein. The isoxazolyl penicillins: oxacillin, cloxacillin and dicloxacillin. *Med. Clin. North Am.* 1970;54:1127.

47. Nathwani, D., and M. J. Wood. Penicillins. A current review of their clinical pharmacology and therapeutic use. *Drugs* 1993;45:866.

48. Neu, H. C. Amoxicillin. *Ann. Intern. Med.* 1979;90:356.

49. Neu, H. C. Antimicrobial activity and human pharmacology of amoxicillin. *J. Infect. Dis.* 1974; 129(Suppl.):S123.

50. Kirby, W. M., R. C. Gordon, and C. Regamey. The pharmacology of orally administered amoxicillin and ampicillin. *J. Infect. Dis* 1974;129(Suppl.):S154.

51. Finland, M., J. E. McGowan, C. Garner, and C. Wilcox. Amoxicillin: in vitro susceptibility of "blood culture strains" of gram-negative bacilli and comparisons with penicillin G, ampicillin, and carbenicillin. *J. Infect. Dis.* 1974;129(Suppl.):S132.

52. Nelson, J. D., and K. C. Haltalin. Amoxacillin less effective than ampicillin against *Shigella* in vitro and in vivo: relationship of efficacy to activity in serum. *J. Infect. Dis.* 1974;129(Suppl.):S222.

53. Haltalin, K. C., J. D. Nelson, L. V. Hinton, H. T. Kusmiesz, and M. Sladoje. Comparison of orally absorbable and nonabsorbable antibiotics in shigellosis. *J. Pediat.* 1968;72:708.

54. Neu, H. C., and E. B. Winshell. In vitro antimicrobial activity of 6-[D(−)-α-amino-β-hydroxyphenyl-acetamide]-penicillanic acid, a new semisynthetic penicillin. *Antimicrob. Agents Chemother.* 1971;11:407.

55. Symposium (various authors). Pulse dosing of antimicrobial drugs with special reference to bacampicillin. *Rev. Infect. Dis.* 1981;3:110–177.

56. Tuano, S. B., L. D. Johnson, J. L. Brodie, and W. M. M. Kirby. Comparative blood levels of hetacillin, ampicillin and penicillin G. *N. Engl. J. Med.* 1966; 275:635.

57. Sutherland, R. and O. P. W. Robinson. Laboratory and pharmacological studies in man with hetacillin and ampicillin. *BMJ* 1967;2:804.

58. Gold, J. A., C. P. Hegarty, M. W. Deitch, and B. R. Walker. Double-blind clinical trials of oral cyclacillin and ampicillin. *Antimicrob. Agents Chemother.* 1979;15:55.

59. Reves, D. S., and D. W. Bullock. The aminopenicillins: development and comparative properties. *Infection* 1979;7(Suppl. 5):S425.

60. Tan, J. S., and T. M. File. Antipseudomonal penicillins. *Med. Clin. North Am.* 1995;79:679.

61. Symposium (various authors). Symposium on carbenicillin: a clinical profile. *J. Infect. Dis.* 1970; 122(Suppl.):S1–S116.

62. Parry, M. F., and H. C. Neu. Ticarcillin for treatment of serious infections with gram-negative bacteria. *J. Infect. Dis.* 1976;134:476.

63. Libke, R. D., J. T. Clarke, E. D. Ralph, R. P. Luthy, and W. M. M. Kirby. Ticarcillin vs. carbenicillin: clinical pharmacokinetics. *Clin. Pharmacol. Ther.* 1975; 17:441.

64. Eickhoff, T. C., and J. M. Ehret. Comparative activity in vitro of ticarcillin, BL-P1654 and carbenicillin. *Antimicrob. Agents Chemother.* 1976;10:241.

65. Brown, C. H., E. A. Natelson, M. W. Bradshaw, C. P. Alfrey, and T. W. Williams. Study of the effects of ticarcillin on blood coagulation and platelet function. *Antimicrob. Agents Chemother.* 1975;7:652.

66. Smith, C. B., J. N. Wilfert, P. E. Dans, T. A. Kurrus, and M. Finland. In vitro activity of carbenicillin and results of treatment of infections due to *Pseudomonas* with carbenicillin singly and in combination with gentamicin. *J. Infect. Dis.* 1970; 122(Suppl.):S14.

67. Andreole, V. T. Synergy of carbenicillin and gentamicin in experimental infection with *Pseudomonas J. Infect. Dis.* 1971;124(Suppl):S46.

68. Symposium (various authors). Symposium on oral indanyl carbenicillin in the treatment of urinary tract infection. *J. Infect. Dis.* 1973;127(Suppl.):S93–S164.

69. Pancoast, S. J., and H. C. Neu. Kinetics of mezlocillin and carbenicillin. *Clin. Pharmacol. Ther.* 1978; 24:108.

70. Frimodt-Moller, N., S. Maigaard, R. Toothaker, R. W. Bundtzen, M. V. Brodey, W. A. Craig, P. G. Welling, and P. O. Madsen. Mezlocillin pharmacokinetics after single intravenous doses to patients with varying degrees of renal function. *Antimicrob. Agents Chemother.* 1980;17:599.

71. Tjandramaga, T. B., A. Mullie, R. Verbesselt, P. J. De Schapper, and L. Verbist. Piperacillin: human pharmacokinetics after intravenous and intramuscular administration. *Antimicrob. Agents Chemother.* 1978; 14:829.

72. Fu, K. P., and H. C. Neu. Azlocillin and mezlocillin: new ureido penicillins. *Antimicrob. Agents Chemother.* 1978;13:930.

73. Bodey, G. P., and T. Pan. Mezlocillin: in vitro studies of a new broad-spectrum penicillin. *Antimicrob. Agents Chemother.* 1977;11:74.

74. Kampf, D., R. Schurig, K. Weihermüller, and D. Förster. Effects of impaired renal function, hemodialysis and peritoneal dialysis on the pharmacokinetics of mezlocillin. *Antimicrob. Agents Chemother.* 1980;18:81.

75. Aronoff, G. R., Mezlocillin elimination in patients with impaired renal function. *J. Antimicrob. Chemother.* 1982;9(Suppl. A):77.

76. Symposium (various authors). Mezlocilin. *J. Antimicrob. Chemother.* 1982;9(Suppl. A):1–295.

77. Fu, K. P., and H. C. Neu. Piperacillin, a new penicillin active against many bacteria resistant to other penicillins. *Antimicrob. Agents Chemother.* 1978;13: 358.

78. Reeves, D. S., H. A. Holt, M. J. Bywater, and J. L. Bidwell. Comparative activity in vitro of piperacillin. *J. Antimicrob. Chemother.* 1982;9(Suppl.B):59.

79. De Schepper, P. J., T. B. Tjandramaga, A. Mullie, R. Verbesselt, A. van Hecken, R. Verberckmoes, and L. Verbist. Comparative pharmacokinetics of piperacillin in normals and in patients with renal failure. *J. Antimicrob. Chemother.* 1982;9(Suppl. B):49.

80. Levine, B. B., A. P. Redmond, H. E. Voss, and D. M. Zolov. Prediction of penicillin allergy by immunological tests. *Ann. N.Y. Acad. Sci.* 1967;145:298.

81. R. P Spark. Fetal anaphylaxis due to oral penicillin. *Clin. Pathol.* 1971;56:407.

82. Austen, K. F. Systemic anaphylaxis in the human being. *N. Engl. J. Med.* 1974;291:661.

83. Parker, C. W. Drug allergy. *N. Engl. J. Med.* 1975;292:511,732,957.

84. Dewdney, J. M. Immunology of the antibiotics. In *The Antigens*, Vol. 4, ed. by M. Sela. New York: Academic Press, 1977, pp. 73–245.

85. Levine, B. B. Studies on the mechanism of the formation of the penicillin antigen; delayed allergic cross-reactions among penicillin G and its degradation products. *J. Exp. Med.* 1960;112:1131.

86. Corran, P. H., and S. G. Waley. The reaction of penicillin with proteins. *Biochem. J.* 1975;149:357.

87. Levine, B. B., and Z. Ovary. Studies on the mechanism of the formation of the penicillin antigen. *J. Exp. Med.* 1961;114:875.

88. Parker, C. W. Mechanisms of penicillin allergy. *Pathobiol. Ann.* 1972;2:405.

89. Ishizaka, K., and T. Ishizaka. Human reaginic antibodies and immunoglobulin E. *J. Allergy* 1968;42:330.

90. Batchelor, F. R., J. M. Dewdney, J. G. Feinberg, and R. D. Weston. A penicilloylated protein impurity as a source of allergy to benzylpenicillin and 6-aminopenicillanic acid. *Lancet* 1967;1:1175.

91. Stewart, G. T. Allergenic residues in penicillins. *Lancet* 1967;1:1177.

92. Knudsen, E. T., O. P. W. Robinson, E. A. P. Croydon, and E. C. Tees. Cutaneous sensitivity to purified benzylpenicillin. *Lancet* 1967;1:1184.

93. Stewart, G. T. Allergy to pencillin and related antibiotics: antigenic and immunochemical mechanism. *Annu. Rev. Pharmacol.* 1973;13:309.

94. Levine, B. B. Antigenicity and cross-reactivity of penicillins and cephalosporins. *J. Infect. Dis.* 1973; 128(Suppl):S364.

95. Petz, L. D. Immunologic cross-reactivity between penicillins and cephalosporins: a review *J. Infect. Dis.* 1978;137(Suppl.):S74.

96. Delafuente, J. C., R. S. Panush, and J. R. Caldwell. Penicillin and cephalosporin immunogenicity in man. *Anal. Allergy* 1979;43:337.

97. de Weck, A. L., and C. H. Schneider. Allergic and immunological aspects of therapy with cefotaxime and other cephalosporins. *J. Antimicrob. Chemother.* 1980;6(Suppl. A):161.

98. Warrington, R. J., F. E. R. Simons, H. W. Ho, and B. A. Gorski. Diagnosis of penicillin allergy by skin testing: the Manitoba experience. *Can. Med. Assoc. J.* 1978;118:787.

99. Adkinson, N. F., W. L. Thomson, W. C. Maddrey, and L. M. Lichtenstein. Routine use of penicillin skin testing on an inpatient service. *New Engl. J. Med.* 1971;285:22.

100. Fellner, M. J., A. I. Weidman, M. V. Klaus, and R. L. Baer. The usefulness of immediate skin tests to haptens derived from penicillin. *Arch. Dermatol.* 1971; 103:371.

101. Green, G. R., A. H. Rosenblum, and L. C. Sweet. Evaluation of penicillin hypersensitivity: value of clinical history and skin testing with penicilloyl-polylysine and penicillin G. *J. Allergy Clin. Immunol.* 1977;60:339.

102. Van Dellen, R. G., W. E. Walsh, G. A. Peters, and G. J. Gleich. Differing patterns of wheal and flare skin reactivity in patients allergic to the penicillins. *J. Allergy* 1971;47:230.

103. Spath, P., G. Garratty, and L. Petz. Studies on the immune response to penicillin and cephalothin in humans: II. Immunohematologic reactions to cephalothin administration. *J. Immunol.* 1971;107:860.

104. Hamilton-Miller, J. M. T. and E. P. Abraham. Specificities of haemagglutinating antibodies evoked by members of the cephalosporin C family and benzylpenicillin. *Biochem. J.* 1971;123:183.

105. Perkins, R. L., and S. Saslaw. Experiences with cephalothin. *Ann. Intern. Med.* 1966;64:13.

106. Scholand, J. F., J. I. Tennenbaum, and G. J. Cerilli. Anaphylaxis to cephalothin in a patient allergic to penicillin. *JAMA* 1968;206:130.

107. Westenfelder, G. O., and P. Y. Paterson. Life-threatening infection: choice of alternate drugs when penicillin cannot be given. *JAMA* 1969;210:845.

108. Fellner, M. J., E. Van Hecke, M. Rozan, and R. L. Baer. Mechanisms of clinical desensitization in urticarial hypersensitivity to penicillin. *J. Allergy* 1970;45:55.

109. Gillman, S. A., J. L. Korotzer, and Z. H. Haddad. Penicillin desensitization. *Clin. Allergy* 1972;2:63.

110. deWeck, A. L., and C. H. Schneider: Specific inhibition of allergic reactions to penicillin in man by a monovalent hapten. I Experimental immunological and toxicologic studies. *Int. Arch. Allergy* 1972;42:782.

111. deWeck, A. L., and J. P. Girard. Specific inhibition of allergic reactions to penicillin in man by a monovalent hapten. II Clinical studies. *Int. Arch. Allergy* 1972;42:798.

112. Shapiro, S., D. Slone, and V. Siskind. Drug rash with ampicillin and other penicillins. *Lancet* 1969;2:969.

113. Bierman, C. W., W. E. Pierson, S. J. Zeitz, L. S. Hoffman, and P. P. VanArsdel. Reactions associated with ampicillin therapy. *JAMA* 1972;220:1098.

114. Haddad, Z. H., and J. L. Korotzer. In vitro studies on the mechanism of penicillin and ampicillin drug reactions. *Int. Arch. Allergy* 1971;41:72.

115. Patel, B. M. Skin rash with infectious mononucleosis and ampicillin. *Pediatrics* 1967;40:910.

116. Pullen, H., N. Wright, and J. M. Murdoch. Hypersensitivity reactions to antibacterial drugs in infectious mononucleosis. *Lancet* 1967;2:1176.

117. Weary, P. E., J. W. Cole, and L. H. Hickam. Eruptions from ampicillin in patients with infectious mononucleosis. *Arch. Dermatol* 1970;101:86.

118. McKenzie, H., D. Parratt, and R. G. White. IgM and IgG antibody levels to ampicillin in patients with infectious mononucleosis. *Clin. Exp. Immunol.* 1976; 26:214.

119. Galpin, J. E., J. H. Shinaberger, T. M. Stanley, and multiple authors. Acute interstitial nephritis due to methicillin. *Am. J. Med.* 1978;65:756.

120. Brauninger, G. E., and J. S. Remington. Nephropathy associated with methicillin therapy. *JAMA* 1968; 203:103.

121. Gilbert, D. N., R. Gourly, A. d'Agostino, S. H. Goodnight, and H. Worthen. Interstitial nephritis due to methicillin, penicillin and ampicillin. *Ann. Allergy* 1970;28:378.

122. Baldwin, D. S., B. B. Levine, R. T. McCluskey, and G. R. Gallo. Renal failure and interstitial nephritis due to penicillin and methicillin. *N. Eng. J. Med.* 1968; 279:1245.

123. Border, W. A., D. H. Lehman, J. D. Egan, H. J. Sass, J. E. Glode, and C. B. Wilson. Antitubular basement-membrane antibodies in methicillin-associated interstitial nephritis. *New Engl. J. Med.* 1974;291:381.

124. Bergstein, J., and N. Litman: Interstitial nephritis with anti-tubular-basement-membrane antibody. *N. Engl. J. Med.* 1975;292:875.

125. O'Callaghan, C. H. Description and classification of the newer cephalosporins and their relationships with the established compounds. *J. Antimicrob. Chemother.* 1979;5:635.

126. Murray, B. E., and R. C. Moellering. Cephalosporins. *Annu. Rev. Med.* 1981;32:559.

127. Spyker, D. A., B. L. Thomas, M. A. Sande, and W. K. Bolton. Pharmacokinetics of cefaclor and cephalexin: dosage nomograms for impaired renal function. *Antimicrob. Agents Chemother.* 1978;14:172.

128. Neu, H. C. Comparison of the pharmacokinetics of cefamandole and other cephalosporin compounds. *J. Infect. Dis.* 1978;137(Suppl.):S80.

129. Brogard, J. M., J. Kopferschmitt, M. O. Spach, O. Grudet, and J. Lavillaureix. Cefamandole pharmacokinetics and dosage adjustments in relation to renal function. *J. Clin. Pharmacol.* 1979;7:366.

130. Filastre, J. P., A. Leroy, M. Godin, G. Oksenhendler, and G. Humbert. Pharmoacokinetics of cefoxitin sodium in normal subjects in in uremic patients. *J. Antimicrob, Chemother.* 1978;4(Suppl. B):79.

131. Brogden, R. N., and D. McTavish. Loracarbef: a review. *Drugs* 1993; *45*:717.

132. Perry, C. M., and R. N. Brogden. Cefuroxime axetil: a review of its antibacterial activity, pharmacokinetic properties and therapeutic efficacy. *Drugs* 1996; 52:125.

133. Filastre, J. P., A. Leroy, G. Humbert, and M. Godin. Pharmacokinetics of cefotaxime in subjects with normal and impaired renal function. *J. Antimicrob. Chemother.* 1980;6(Suppl. A):103.

134. Esmieu, F., J. Guibert, H. C. Rosenkilde, I. Ho, and A. Le Go. Pharmacokinetics of cefotaxime in normal human volunteers. *J. Antimicrob. Chemother.* 1980;6(Suppl. A):83.

135. Symposium (various authors). Proceedings of the first international symposium on cefoperazone sodium. *Clin. Ther.* 1980;3(Special Issue):1–208.

136. Yuk, J. H., C. H. Nightingale, and R. Quintiliani. Clinical pharmacokinetics of ceftriaxone. *Clin. Pharmacokinet.* 1989;17:223.

137. Cove-Smith, R. Antibiotics in renal failure. *In Antibiotic and Chemotherapy*, ed. by F. O'Grady, H. P. Lamberty, R. G. Finch, and D. Greenwood, New York: Churchill Livingsone, 1997, pp. 70–90.

138. Guay, D. R. P., R. C. Meatherall, G. K. Harding, and G. R. Brown. Pharmacokinetics of cefixime (CL284,635; FK027) in healthy subjects and patients with renal insufficiency. *Antimicrob. Agents Chemother.* 1986;30:485.

139. Cunha, B. A., and M. V. Gill. Cefepime. *Med. Clin. North Am.* 1995;79:727.

140. Spyker, D. A., L. L. Gober, W. M. Scheld, M. A. Sande and W. K. Bolton. Pharmacokinetics of cefaclor in renal failure: effects of multiple doses and hemodialysis. *Antimicrob. Agents Chemother.* 1982; 21:278.

141. Glöckner, W. M., U. Höffler, J. Kindler, G. Peters, and H. G. Sieberth. Elimination kinetics of cefotaxime in patients with renal insufficiency requiring dialysis. *J. Antimicrob. Chemother.* 1980;6(Suppl. A): 219.

142. Okamoto, M. P., R. K. Nakahiro, A. Chin, and A. Bedikian. Cefepime clinical pharmacokinetics. *Clin. Pharmacokinet.* 1993;25:88.

143. Welling, P. G., S. Dean, A. Selen, M. J. Kendall, and R. Wise. The pharmacokinetics of the oral cephalosporins cefaclor, cephradine and cephalexin. *Int. J. Clin. Pharmacol. Biopharm.* 1979;17:397.

144. Brogard, J. M., F. Comte, and M. Pinget. Pharmacokinetics of cephalosporin antibiotics. *Antibiot. Chemother.* 1978;25:123.

145. Andreole, V. T. Pharmacokinetics of cephalosporins in patients with normal or reduced renal function. *J. Infect. Dis* 1978;137(Suppl.):S88.

146. Guerrero, I. C., and R. R. MacGregor. Comparative penetration of various cephalosporins into inflammatory exudate. *Antimicrob. Agents Chemother.* 1979; 15:712.

147. Nightingale, C. H., J. J. Klimek, and R. Quintiliani. Effect of protein binding on the penetration of non-metabolized cephalosporins into atrial appendage and pericardial fluids in open heart surgical patients. *Antimicrob. Agents Chemother.* 1980;17:595.

148. Reller, L. B., W. W. Kartney, H. N. Beaty, K. K. Holmes, and M. Turk. Evaluation of cefazolin, a new cephalosporin antibiotic. *Antimicrob. Agents Chemother.* 1973;3:488.

149. Leigh, D. A., J. Marriner, D. Nisbet, H. D. W. Powell, J. C. T. Church, and K. Wise. Bone concentrations of cefuroxime and cefamandole in the femoral head in 96 patients undergoing total hip replacement surgery. *J. Antimicrob. Chemother.* 1982;9:303.

150. Kosmidis, J., C. Stathakis, K. Mantopoulos, T. Pouriezi, B. Papathanassiou, and G. K. Daikos. Clinical pharmacology of cefotaxime including penetration into bile, sputum, bone, and cerebrospinal fluid. *J. Antimicrob. Chemother.* 1980;6(Suppl. A):147.

151. Quintiliani, R., M. French, and C. H. Nightingale. The first and second generation cephalosporins. *Med. Clin. North Am.* 1982;66:183.

152. Soussy, C. J., L. P. Deforges, J. Le Van Thoi, W. Feghali, and J. R. Duval. Cefotaxime concentration in the bile and wall of the gallbladder. *J. Antimicrob. Chemother.* 1980;6(Suppl. A):125.

153. Martinez, O. V., J. U. Levi, A. Livingstone, T. L. Malinin, R. Zeppa, D. Hutson, and N. Einhorn. Biliary excretion of moxalactam. *Antimicrob. Agents Chemother.* 1981;20:231.

154. Fisher, L. S., A. W. Chow, T. T. Yoshikawa, and L. B. Guze. Cephalothin and cephaloridine therapy for bacterial meningitis. An evaluation. *Ann. Intern. Med.* 1975;82:689.

155. Steinberg, E. A., G. D. Overturf, J. Wilkins, L. J. Baraff, J. M. Streng, and J. M. Leedom. Failure of cefamandole in treatment of meningitis due to *Haemophilus influenzae* type *b. J. Infect. Dis.* 1978; 137(Suppl.):S180.

156. Feldman, W. E., S. Moffitt, and N. S. Manning. Penetration of cefoxitin into cerebrospinal fluid of infants and children with bacterial meningitis. *Antimicrob. Agents Chemother.* 1982;21:468.

157. Belohradsky, B. H., K. Bruch, D. Geiss, D. Kafetzis, W. Marget, and G. Peters. Intravenous cefotaxime in children with bacterial meningitis. *Lancet* 1980; 1:61.

158. Schaad, U. B., G. H. McCracken, N. Threlkeld, and M. L. Thomas. Clinical evaluation of a new broad-spectrum oxa-beta-lactam antibiotic, moxalactam, in neonates and infants. *J. Pediatr.* 1981;98:129.

159. Kaplan, S. L., E. O. Mason, H. Garcia, S. J. Kvernland, E. M. Loiselle, D. C. Anderson, A. A. Mintz, and R. D. Feigen. Pharmacokinetics and cerebrospinal fluid penetration of moxalactam in children with bacterial meningitis. *J. Pediatr.* 1981;98:152.

160. Tauber, M. G., C. J. Hackbarth, K. G. Scott, M. G. Rusnak, and M. A. Sande. New cephalosporins cefotaxime, cefpimizole, BMT28142, and HR810 in experimental pneumococcal meningitis in rabbits. *Antimicrob. Agents Chemother.* 1985;27:340.

161. Shemonsky, N. K., J. Carrizosa, D. Kaye, and M. E. Levison. Double-blind comparison of phlebitis produced by cefazolin versus cephalothin. *Antimicrob. Agents Chemother.* 1975;7:481.

162. Yoshioka, H., H. Nambu, M. Fujiita, and H. Uehara. Convulsion following intrathecal cephaloridine. *Infection* 1975;3:123.

163. Sanders, W. E., J. E. Johnson, and J. G. Taggart. Adverse reactions to cephalothin and cephapirin: uniform occurrence on prolonged intravenous administration of high doses. *N. Engl. J. Med.* 1974;290:424.

164. Barza, M. The nephrotoxicity of cephalosporins: an overview. *J. Infect. Dis.* 1978;137(Suppl.):S60.

165. Mandell, G. L. Cephaloridine. *Ann. Intern. Med.* 1973;79:561.

166. Tune, B. M. Relationship between the transport and toxicity of cephalosporins in the kidney. *J. Infect. Dis.* 1975;132:189.

167. Klastersky, J., C. Hansgens, and L. Debusscher. Empiric therapy for cancer patients: comparative study of ticarcillin-tobramycin, ticarcillin-cephalothin, and cephalothin-tobramycin. *Antimicrob. Agents Chemother.* 1975;7:640.

168. Wade, J. C., C. R. Smith, B. G. Petty, J. J. Lipsky, G. Contrad, J. Ellner, and P. S. Lietman-Cephalothin plus an aminoglycoside is more nephrotoxic than methicillin plus an aminoglycoside. *Lancet* 1978;2:604.

169. Meyers, B. R. Comparative toxicity of the third-generation cephalosporins. *Am. J. Med.* 1985;79(Suppl. 2A):96.

170. Bang, N. U., and R. B. Kasmmer. Hematologic complications associated with β-lactam antibiotics. *Rev. Infect. Dis.* 1983;(Suppl. 2):S380.

171. Sattler, F. R., M. R. Weitkamp, and J. O. Ballard. Potential for bleeding with β-lactam antibiotics. *Ann. Intern. Med.* 1986;105:924.

172. Cunha, B. A. Third-generation cephalosporins: a review. *Clin. Ther.* 1992;14:616.

173. Klein, N. C., and B. A. Cunha. Third-generation cephalosporins. *Med. Clin. North Am.* 1995;79:705.

174. Washington, J. A. The in vitro spectrum of the cephalosporins. *Mayo Clin. Proc.* 1976;51:237.

175. Symposium (various authors). Clinical symposium on cefazolin. *J. Infect. Dis.* 1973;128(Suppl.):S307-S424.

176. Quintiliani, R., and C. H. Nightingale. Cefazolin. *Ann. Intern. Med.* 1978;89:650.

177. Kirby, W. M. M., and C. Regamey. Pharmacokinetics of cefazolin compared with four other cephalosporins. *J. Infect. Dis.* 1973;128(Suppl.):S341.

178. Craig, W. A., P. G. Welling, J. C. Jackson, and C. M. Kunin. Pharmacology of cefazolin and other cephalosporins in patients with renal insufficiency. *J. Infect. Dis.* 1973;128(Suppl.):S347.

179. Gold, J. A., J. J. McKee, and D. S. Ziv. Experience with cefazolin: an overall summary of pharmacologic and clinical trials in man. *J. Infect. Dis.* 1973;128(Suppl.):S415.

180. Murray, B. E., and R. C. Moellering. The cephalosporin and cephamycin antibiotics: a status report. *Clin. Ther.* 1979;2:155.

181. Symposium (various authors). Cephalexin and cephaloridine. *J. Antimicrob. Chemother.* 1975;1(Suppl.):1–139.

182. Buck, R. E., and K. E. Price. Cefadroxil, a new broad-spectrum cephalosporin. *Antimicrob. Agents Chemother.* 1977;11:324.

183. La Rosa, F., S. Ripa, M. Prenna, A. Ghezzi, and M. Pfeffer. Pharmacokinetics of cefadroxil after oral administration in humans. *Antimicrob. Agents Chemother.* 1982;21:320.

184. Cutler, R. E., A. D. Blair, and M. R. Kelley. Cefadroxil kinetics in patients with renal insufficiency. *Clin. Pharmacol. Ther.* 1979;25:514.

185. Two new oral cephalosporins. *Med. Lett.* 1979;21:85.

186. Richmond, M. H., and S. Wotton. Comparative study of seven cephalosporins: susceptibility to β-lactamases and ability to penetrate the surface layers of *Escherichia coli. Antimicrob. Agents Chemother.* 1976;10:219.

187. Symposium (various authors). Symposium on cefamandole. *J. Infect. Dis.* 1978;137(Suppl.)S1-S194.

188. Symposium (various authors). Cefoxitin: Microbiology, pharmacology and clinical use. *J. Antimicrob. Chemother.* 1978;4(Suppl. B):1–256.

189. Agbayani, M. M., A. J. Khan, P. Kemawikasit, W. Rosenfeld, D. Salazar, K. Kuman, L. Glass, and H. E. Evans. Pharmacokinetics and safety of cefamandole in newborn infants. *Antimicrob. Agents Chemother.* 1979;15:674.

190. O'Callaghan, C. H., R. B. Sykes, A. Griffiths, and J. E. Thornton. Cefuroxime, a new cephalosporin antibiotic: activity in vitro. *Antimicrob. Agents Chemother.* 1976;9:511.

191. van Dalen, R., T. B. Vree, J. C. M. Hafkenscheid, and J. S. F. Gimbrere. Determination of plasma and renal clearance of cefuroxime and its pharmacokinetics in renal insufficiency. *J. Antimicrob. Chemother.* 1979;5:281.

192. Symposium (various authors). Clinical advances in oral antibiotic therapy. *Postgrad. Med. J.* 1979;55(Suppl. 4):1–101.

193. Gillett, A. P., J. M. Andrews, and R. Wise. Comparative in vitro microbiological activity and stability of cefaclor. *Postgrad. Med. J.* 1979;55(Suppl. 4):9.

194. Cunha, B. A., and A. M. Ristuccia: Third generation cephalosporins. *Med Clin. North Am.* 1982;66:283.

195. Symposium (various authors). Cefotaxime: a new cephalosporin antibiotic. *J. Antimicrob. Chemother.* 1980;6(Suppl. A):1–303.

196. King, A., C. Warren, K. Shannon, and I. Philips. The in vitro antibacterial activity of cefotaxime com-

pared with that of cefuroxime and cefoxitin. *J. Antimicrob. Chemother.* 1980;6:479.

197. Jorgensen, J. H., S. A. Crawford, and G. A. Alexander. In vitro activities of moxalactam and cefotaxime against aerobic gram-negative bacilli. *Antimicrob. Agents Chemother.* 1980;17:937.

198. Thornsberry, C. Review of in vitro activity of third-generation cephalosporins and other new β-lactam antibiotics against clinically important bacteria. *Am. J. Med.* 1985;79:14.

199. Bryan, J., H. Rocha, H. Silva, A. Taveres, M. A. Sande, and W. M. Scheld. Comparison of ceftriaxone and ampicillin plus chloramphenicol for the therapy of acute bacterial meningitis. *Antimicrob. Agents. Chemother.* 1985;28:361.

200. Neu, H. C. Cephalosporins in the treatment of meningitis. *Drugs* 1987;34:135.

201. Overturf, G. D., D. C. Cable, D. N. Forthal, and C. Shikuma. Treatment of bacterial meningitis with ceftizoxime. *Antimicrob. Agents Chemother.* 1984; 25:258.

202. Karimi, A., K. Seeger, D. Stolke, and H. Knothe. Cefotaxime concentration in cerebrospinal fluid. *J. Antimicrob. Chemother.* 1980;6(Suppl. A):119.

203. Perfect, J. R., and D. T. Durack. Pharmacokinetics of cefoperazone, moxalactam, cefotaxime, trimethoprim and sulfamethoxazole in experimental meningitis. *J. Antimicrob. Chemother.* 1981;8:49.

204. Schaad, U. B., G. H. McCracken, C. A. Loock, and M. L. Thomas. Pharmacokinetics and bacteriologic efficacy of moxalactam, cefotaxime, cefoperazone, and rocephin in experimental bacterial meningitis. *J. Infect. Dis.* 1981;143:156.

205. Piro, J. T. D., and J. R. May. Use of cephalosporins with enhanced anti-anaerobic activity for treatment and prevention of anaerobic and mixed infections. *Clin. Pharmacokinet.* 1988;7:285.

206. Bergan, T. Pharmacokinetic properties of the cephalosporins. *Drugs* 1987;34(Suppl. 2):89.

207. Reeves, D. S., L. O. White, H. A. Holt, D. Bahari, M. J. Bywater, and R. P. Bax. Human metabolism of cefotaxime. *J. Antimicrob. Chemother.* 1980; 6(Suppl. A):93.

208. Neu, H. C., P. Aswapokee, K. P. Fu., I. Ho, and C. Matthijssen. Cefotaxime kinetics after intravenous and intramuscular injection of single and multiple doses. *Clin. Pharmacol. Ther.* 1980;27:677.

209. Jones, R. N. A review of cephalosporin metabolism: a lesson to be learned for future chemotherapy. *Diagn. Microbiol. Infect. Dis.* 1989;12:25.

210. McCracken, G. H., N. E. Threlkeld, and M. L. Thomas. Pharmacokinetics of cefotaxime in newborn infants. *Antimicrob. Agents Chemother.* 1982;21:683.

211. Busse, H., K. Seeger, and P. Wreesmann: Concentrations of cefotaxime in the anterior chamber of the eye in rabbits and humans. *J. Antimicrob. Chemother.* 1980;6(Suppl. A):143.

212. Goldfarb, J. New antimicrobial agents. *Pediatr. Clin. North Am.* 1995;42:717.

213. Handsfield, H. H., W. M. McCormack, E. W. Hook, J. M. Douglas, J. M. Covino, M. S. Verdon, C. A. Reichart, J. M. Ehret, and the Gonorrhea Study Group. A comparison of single-dose cefixime with cef-

triaxone for treatment of uncomplicated gonorrhea. *N. Engl. J. Med.* 1991;325:1337.

214. Wiseman, L. R., and J. A. Balfour. Cefibuten: a review of its antibacterial activity, pharmacokinetic properties and clinical efficacy. *Drugs* 1994;47:784.

215. Sanders, C. C. Cefepime: the next generation. *Clin. Infect. Dis.* 1993;17:369.

216. Kahan, J. S., F. M. Kahan, R. Goegelman, S. A. Currie, M. Jackson, E. O. Stapley, T. W. Miller, A. K. Miller, D. Herdlin, S. Mochales, S. Hernandez, H. B. Woodruff, and J. Birnbaum. Thienamycin, a new beta-lactam antibiotic. I. Discovery, taxonomy, isolation, and physical properties. *J. Antibiot.* 1979;32:1.

217. Norrby, S. R. Carbapenems. *Med. Clin. North Am.* 1995;79:745.

218. Balfour, J. A., H. M. Bryson, and R. N. Brogden. Imipenem/cilastatin: an update of its antibacterial activity, pharmacokinetics and therapeutic efficacy in the treatment of serious infections. *Drugs* 1996;51:99.

219. Kayser, F. H., G. Morenzoni, A. Strässle, and K. Hadorn. Activity of meropenem against gram-positive bacteria. *J. Antimicrob. Chemother.* 1989;24(Suppl. 2A):101.

220. Sanders, C. C., W. E. Sanders, K. S. Thomson, and J. P. Iaconis. Meropenem: activity against gram-negative bacteria and interactions with β-lactamases. *J. Antimicrob. Chemother.* 1989;24(Suppl. A):187.

221. Livermore, D. M. Mechanisms of resistance of β-lactam antibiotics. *Scand. J. Infect. Dis.* 1991; 78(Suppl.):7.

222. Kropp, H., J. G. Sundelof, R. Hajdu, and F. M. Kahan. Metabolism of thienamycin and related carbapenem antibiotics by the renal dipeptidase: dehydropeptidase-I. *Antimicrob. Agents. Chemother.* 1982;22:62.

223. Wang, C., G. B. Calandra, M. A. Aziz and K. R. Brown. Efficacy and safety of imipenem/cilastatin: a review of worldwide clinical experience. *Rev. Infect. Dis.* 1985;7(Suppl. 3):528.

224. Neu, H. C. Aztreonam: The first monobactam. *Med. Clin. North Am.* 1988;72:555.

225. Johnson, D. H., and B. A. Cunha. Aztreonam. *Med. Clin. North Am.* 1995;79:733.

226. Swabb, E. A., S. M. Singhvi, M. A. Leitz, M. Frantz, and A. A. Sugerman. Metabolism and pharmacokinetics of aztreonam in healthy subjects. *Antimicrob. Agents Chemother.* 1983;24:394.

227. Stutman, H. R., M. I. Marks, and E. A. Swabb. Single-dose pharmacokinetics of aztreonam in pediatric patients. *Antimicrob. Agents Chemother.* 1984;26:196.

228. Swabb, E. A. Review of the clinical pharmacology of the monobactam antibiotic aztreonam. *Am. J. Med.* 1985;78(Suppl. 2A):11.

229. Sensakovic, J. W., and L. G. Smith. Beta-lactamase inhibitor combinations. *Med. Clin. North Am.* 1995;79:695.

230. Mandell, G. L., and W. A. Petri. Penicillins, cephalosporins, and other β-lactam antibiotics. In The Pharmacological Basis of Therapeutics, ed. by J. Hardman, L. Limbird, P. Molinoff, R. Ruddon, and A. Gilman. New York: McGraw-Hill, 1995, pp. 1073–1081.

231. Sheldrick, G. M., P. G. Jones, O. Kennard, D. H. Williams, and G. A. Smith. Structure of vanco-

mycin and its complex with acetyl-D-alanyl-D-alanine. *Nature* 1978;271:223.

232. Geraci, J. E. Vancomycin. *Mayo Clinic Proc.* 1977;52:631.

233. Cook, F. V., and W. E. Farrar. Vancomycin revisited. *Ann. Intern. Med.* 1978;88:813.

234. Fekety, R. Vancomycin. *Med. Clin. North Am.* 1982;66:175.

235. Watanakunakorn, C. The antibacterial action of vancomycin. *Rev. Infect. Dis.* 1981;3(Suppl.):S210.

236. Hagman, H. M., and L. J. Strausbaugh. Vancomycin-resistant enterococci. *Postgrad. Med.* 1996;99:60.

237. Garrett, D. O., E. Jochimsen, and K. Murfitt. The impending apocalypse: the emergence of vancomycin resistance in *Staphylococcus* spp. [Abstract S1]. *Infect. Control. Hosp. Epidemiol.* 1997;18:P32.

238. Noskin, G. A. Vancomycin-resistant enterococci: clinical, microbiologic, and epidemiologic features. *J. Lab. Clin. Med.* 1997;130:14.

239. Kirby, W. M. M. Vancomycin therapy in severe staphylococcal infections. *Rev. Infect. Dis.* 1981;3(Suppl.):S236.

240. Geraci, J. E., and W. R. Wilson. Vancomycin therapy for infective endocarditis. *Rev. Infect. Dis.* 1981;3(Suppl.):S250.

241. Hook, E. W., and W. D. Johnson. Vancomycin therapy of bacterial endocarditis. *Am. J. Med.* 1978;65:411.

242. Watanakunakorn, C., and C. Bakie. Synergism of vancomycin-gentamicin and vancomycin-streptomycin against enterococci. *Antimicrob. Agents Chemother.* 1973;4:120.

243. Watanakunakorn, C. and C. Glotzbecker. Synergism with aminoglycosides of penicillin, ampicillin and vancomycin against non-enterococcal group-D streptococci and viridans streptococci. *J. Med. Microbiol.* 1977;10:133.

244. Fekety, R., J. Silva, J. Armstrong, M. Allo, R. Browne, J. Ebright, R. Lusk, G. Rifkin, and R. Toshniwal. Treatment of antibiotic-associated enterocolitis with vancomycin. *Rev. Infect. Dis.* 1981;3(Suppl.):S273.

245. Torres, J. R., C. V. Sanders, and A. C. Lewis. Vancomycin concentration in human tissues—preliminary report. *J. Antimicrob. Chemother.* 1979;5:475.

246. Moellering, R. C., D. J. Krogstad, and D. J. Greenblatt. Pharmacokinetics of vancomycin in normal subjects and in patients with reduced renal function. *Rev. Infect. Dis.* 1981;3(Suppl.):S230.

247. Gump, D. W. Vancomycin for treatment of bacterial meningitis. *Rev. Infect. Dis.* 1981;3(Suppl.):S289.

248. Schaad, U. B., J. D. Nelson, and G. McCracken. Pharmacology and efficacy of vancomycin for staphylococcal infections in children. *Rev. Infect. Dis.* 1981;3(Suppl.):S282.

249. Schaad, U. B., G. H. McCracken, and J. D. Nelson. Clinical pharmacology and efficacy of vancomycin in children. *J. Pediatr.* 1980;96:119.

250. Drogstad, D. J., R. C. Moellering, and D. J. Greenblatt. Single dose kinetics of intravenous vancomycin. *J. Clin. Pharmacol.* 1980;20:197.

251. Moellering, R. C., D. J. Krogstad, and D. J. Greenblatt. Vancomycin therapy in patients with impaired renal function: a nomogram for dosage. *Ann. Intern. Med.* 1981;94:343.

252. Cunha, B. A., R. Quintiliani, J. M. Deglin, M. W. Izard, and C. H. Nightingale. Pharmacokinetics of vancomycin in anuria. *Rev. Infect. Dis.* 1981; 3(Suppl.):S269.

253. Nielsen, H. E., I. Sorensen, and H. E. Hansen: Peritoneal transport of vancomycin during peritoneal dialysis. *Nephron* 1979;24:274.

254. Bryan, C. S., and W. L. White. Safety of oral vancomycin in functionally anephric patients. *Antimicrob. Agents Chemother.* 1978;14:634.

255. Newfield, P., and M. F. Roizen. Hazards of rapid administration of vancomycin. *Ann. Intern. Med.* 1979;91:581.

256. Davis, R. L., A. L. Smith, and J. R. Koup. The "red-man's syndrome" and "slow infusion of vancomycin." *Ann. Intern. Med.* 1986;104:285.

257. Wallace, M. R., J. R. Mascola, and E. C. Oldfield. The red-man syndrome: incidence, aetiology, and prophylaxis. *J. Infect. Dis.* 1991;164:1180.

258. Polk, R. E. Anaphylactoid reactions to glycopeptide antibiotics. *J. Antimicrob. Chemother.* 1991; 27(Suppl. B):17.

259. Wold, J. S., and S. A. Turnipseed. Toxicology of vancomycin in laboratory animals. *Rev. Infect. Dis.* 1981;2(Suppl.):S224.

260. O'Sullivan, T. L., M. J. Ruffing, K. C. Lano, L. H. Warbasse, and M. J. Rybak. Prospective evaluation of red-man syndrome in patients receiving vancomycin. *J. Infect. Dis.* 1993;168:773.

261. Appel, G. B., and H. C. Neu. The nephrotoxicity of antimicrobial agents (second of three parts). *N. Engl. J. Med.* 1977;296:722.

262. Borland, C. D. R., and W. E. Farrar. Reversible neutropenia from vancomycin. *JAMA* 1979; 242:2392.

263. Felmingham, D. Glycopeptides. In *Antibiotic and Chemotherapy*, ed. by F. O'Grady, H. P. Lamberty, R. G. Finch, and D. Greenwood. New York: Churchill Livingstone, 1997, pp. 363–370.

264. Shea, K. W., and B. A. Cunha. Teicoplanin. *Med. Clin. North Am.* 1995;79:833.

265. Brogden, R. N., and D. H. Peters. Teicoplanin: a reappraisal of its antimicrobial activity, pharmacokinetic properties and therapeutic efficacy. *Drugs* 1994; 47:823.

266. Davenport, A. Allergic cross-reactivity to teicoplanin and vancomycin. *Nephron* 1993;63:482.

267. Meleney, F. L., and B. A. Johnson. Bacitracin. *Am. J. Med.* 1949;7:794.

268. Chang, T., S. L. Gorbach, J. G. Bartlett, and R. Saginur. Bacitracin treatment of antibiotic-associated colitis and diarrhea caused by *Clostridium difficile* toxin. Gastroenterology 1980;78:1584.

269. Rupp, M. E., and M. Lewis. In vitro activity of bacitracin and bismuth subsalicylate against vancomycin-resistant *Enterococcus faecium*. *Proc. Infect. Dis. Soc. Am.* 1996;118.

270. O'Donovan, C. A., P. Fan-Havard, T. T. Tecson-Tumang, S. M. Smith, and R. H. K. Eng. En-

teric eradication of vancomycin-resistant *Enterococcus faecium* with oral bacitracin. *Diagn. Microbiol. Infect. Dis.* 1994;18:105.

271. Coleman, D. J., D. McGhie, and G. M. Tebbutt. Further studies on the reliability of the bacitracin inhibition test for the presumptive identification of Lancefield group A streptococci. *J. Clin. Path.* 1977; 30:421.

272. Dillon, H. C. The treatment of streptococcal skin infections. *J. Pediatr.* 1970;76:676.

273. Björkner, B., and H. Möller. Bacitracin: a cutaneous allergen and histamine liberator. *Acta Dermatovener.* 1973;53:487.

274. Marples, R. R., A. Rebora, and A. M. Kligman. Topical steroid antibiotic combinations. *Arch. Dermatol.* 1973;108:237.

Bactericidal Inhibitors of Protein Synthesis
The Aminoglycosides

The *aminoglycoside* group of antibiotics includes a large number of structurally related polycationic compounds containing two or more amino sugars connected by glycosidic linkage to a hexose core (see Fig. 5–1). The different aminoglycosides are distinguished by their amino sugars. Eight aminoglycosides are currently marketed in the United States. Streptomycin, neomycin, kanamycin, tobramycin, and paromomycin are derived from different species of *Streptomyces*; gentamicin and netilmicin are derived from *Micromonosporum* species; amikacin is produced through chemical modification of kanamycin. These drugs all inhibit protein synthesis, they are all bactericidal, and they have similar pharmacokinetic properties. Although the aminoglycosides are important drugs for treatment of gram-negative infections, their use is limited by serious toxicity. All members of this group have similar types of toxicity, particularly ototoxicity and nephrotoxicity. The earlier aminoglycosides, streptomycin, neomycin, and kanamycin, are very toxic and in systemic antibacterial therapy they have largely been replaced by the newer drugs, gentamicin, tobramycin, amikacin, and netilmicin. Paromomycin is unique among the aminoglycosides in that it is used only to treat two parasitic diseases, cestodiasis (tapeworm infection) and intestinal amebiasis.

Mechanism of Action

The aminoglycosides are known to be rapidly bactericidal and this killing effect depends on the concentration of drug. The higher the concentration of aminoglycoside, the greater the killing.[1,2] Aminoglycosides also have a residual bactericidal activity that is present after the serum concentration has fallen below the minimum inhibitory concentration (MIC). This effect probably explains the efficacy of once-daily dosing with aminoglycosides.

Aminoglycosides diffuse through aqueous channels formed by porin proteins in the outer membrane of gram-negative bacteria. Electron transport is necessary for further transport of the aminoglycosides across the cytoplasmic or inner membrane. This phase of transport is termed *energy-dependent phase I*. It is rate limiting and can be blocked by certain divalent ions, hyperosmolarity, pH reduction, and anaerobiasis. After transport across the cytoplasmic membrane, the aminoglycosides bind to polysomes and inhibit protein synthesis.

Bacteria exposed to aminoglycosides undergo a wide variety of metabolic changes, including changes in cell permeability and transport,[3] inhibition of protein synthesis,[4] and misreading of the genetic code.[5] When it was observed that certain highly

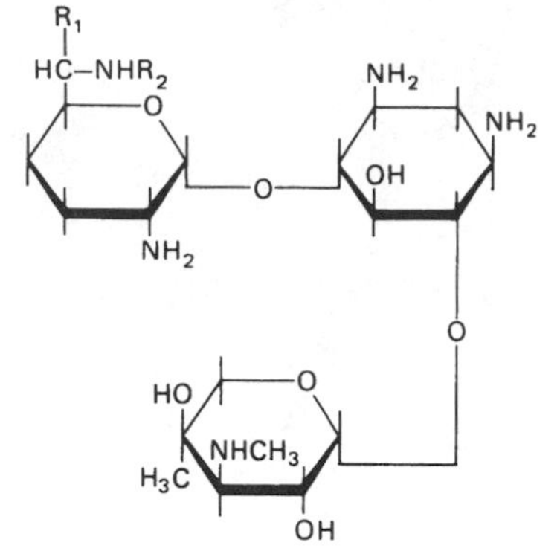

Gentamicin

Gentamicin C_1 : R_1 =CH_3; R_2 =CH_3
Gentamicin C_2 : R_1 =CH_3; R_2 =H
Gentamicin C_{1a} : R_1 =H ; R_2 =H

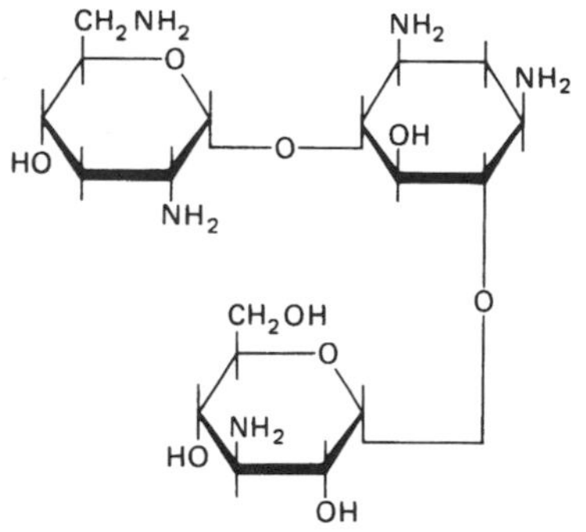

Tobramycin

Figure 5–1. Structures of gentamicin and tobramycin. The preparation of gentamicin that is used clinically is a mixture of equal amounts of gentamicin C_1, C_2, and C_{1a}. The three forms of gentamicin have equivalent antimicrobial activities and pharmacokinetic properties.

streptomycin-resistant mutant bacteria were no longer killed because they contained an altered ribosomal protein necessary for streptomycin binding, it was proposed that inhibition of protein synthesis leads to cell killing. It is not yet understood, however, why total inhibition of protein synthesis by streptomycin kills cells, whereas total blockade by some other antibiotics (erythromycin, tetracyclines, etc.) is bacteriostatic. Thus, although inhibition of protein synthesis is clearly important, the mechanism of cell killing has never been adequately explained. The following discussion will focus on the

effects of streptomycin on protein synthesis. Much of the early work on the mechanism of action of the aminoglycosides has been done with streptomycin. The reader should be aware in advance that all of the observations made with streptomycin cannot be extrapolated to other aminoglycosides, because there are clear differences in the way the various aminoglycosides interact with the protein synthetic machinery at the molecular level.

Protein Synthesis in Bacteria

It is appropriate to review our current understanding of protein synthesis in bacteria [6,7] before discussing inhibition of the process by drugs. Bacteria and eukaryotic systems have ribosomes of different structures. Ribosomes in prokaryotes are referred to as *70S ribosomes*, a measure of their sedimentation rate in a centrifuge and hence their size. A 70S ribosome consists of two subunits, 50S and 30S, each of which is made up of RNA and protein. Eukaryotic ribosomes are similar in structure although they are somewhat larger (80S) and contain mostly larger RNAs. These fundamental structural differences account for some of the selective toxicity shown by antibiotics toward bacterial systems. The synthesis of proteins, which, for the purpose of this discussion, equals the process of messenger RNA (mRNA) translation, can be conveniently divided into three stages: initiation, elongation, and termination. In each of these stages a different set of protein factors is utilized by the ribosome. These factors cycle on and off the ribosome and allow the ribosome to interact with them sequentially at a single site.

In the original model of ribosome function the ribosome was believed to interact with transfer RNA (tRNA) at two sites designated *A* (aminoacyl) and *P* (peptidyl). Recently, it became clear that three sites are involved with the third site referred to as the *E* (exit) site. This site is believed to be transiently occupied by tRNA before its exit from the ribosome.[8,9]

The first stage of protein synthesis involves the formation of an initiation

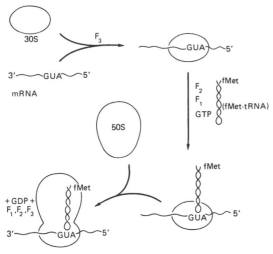

Figure 5–2. Steps in the formation of the 70S initiation complex in bacteria. F_1, F_2, and F_3 represent the initiation factors. The process of initiation is described in detail in the text. Note that protein synthesis will proceed in the 5' to the 3' direction along the mRNA and the initiation codon is oriented as (5')AUG(3').

complex (Fig. 5–2). In bacteria the first or N-terminal amino acid for all proteins is formylmethionine. Formylmethionine and its appropriate tRNA are first united under the direction of an aminoacyl-tRNA-synthetase to form aminoacyl-tRNA. The mRNA becomes attached to the 30S subunit, a process that requires the participation of a soluble protein called an *initiation factor* (F_3). The formylmethionine-charged tRNA then combines with the mRNA-30S-ribosomal complex. The anticodon triplet portion of the tRNA is juxtaposed to the initiation codon in the mRNA [which is (5')AUG(3')]. This requires the participation of two additional initiation factors (F_1 and F_2) and guanosine triphosphate (GTP). In the next step, the 50S ribosomal subunit becomes bound to the mRNA-30S-tRNA-amino acid complex, the bound GTP is hydrolyzed, and the initiation factors are released. The initiation complex is now complete.

At the conclusion of initiation the ribosome is ready to translate the reading frame

associated with the initiation codon. This is the elongation step (Fig. 5–3). Translation is accomplished by the sequential repetition of three reactions with each amino acid. Two of them require nonribosomal proteins known as *elongation factors*. GTP is also required. The first two tRNAs are now oriented appropriately with their anticodon ends opposite their respective code triplets on the mRNA and their attached amino acids adjacent to each other on the surface of the 50S portion of the ribosome. The two amino acids then become linked by a peptide bond. This step is called *peptidyl transfer* and is accomplished by an enzyme complex called *peptidyltransferase*. This is an integral part of the 50S subunit. Although there may be some ribosomal proteins that are a part of this enzymatic complex, the ribosomal RNA itself is believed to play a major role, functioning as a ribozyme.[9,10] The carboxyl group of formylmethionine is linked to the amino group of the second amino acid, and the dipeptide is now attached to the second tRNA, which is occupying the A site. After the formation of the peptide bond, a complicated translocation takes place. The tRNA for formylmethionine is released from the P site, the tRNA with the attached dipeptide moves from the A to the P site, and the 30S subunit moves one codon along the mRNA. The A site is now unoccupied and ready to receive the next aminoacyl-tRNA directed by the next code triplet on the mRNA. The process of elongation continues with the addition of single amino acid units until a termination sequence containing code triplets UAA, UGA, or UAG in the mRNA signals that the protein chain is complete. After the formation of the peptide bond, the final step in elongation occurs, or *termination*. This is catalyzed by an elongation factor (EF-G) that cycles on and off the ribosome and hydrolyzes GTP in the process. This last step in translation involves the cleavage of the ester bond that joins the peptide chain to the tRNA corresponding to its C-terminal amino acid.

When one of these nonsense (terminator) codons appears in the A site, no aminoacyl-tRNA is bound. Instead, the ribosome binds a protein, called a *termination release factor*,

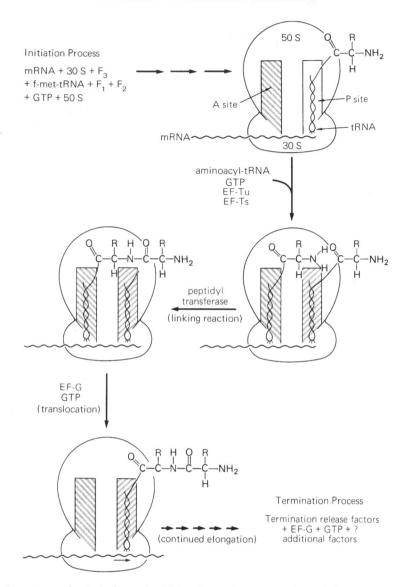

Figure 5–3. Protein synthesis in bacteria. This schematic presentation of this process is described in detail in the text. The shapes representing the tRNA and the ribosome are, of course, highly schematic and are not intended to represent their actual form. F_1, F_2, and F_3, refer to the three initiation factors and EF-Tu, EF-Ts, and EF-G represent the three elongation factors. As described in the text, these factors and the termination release factors are soluble proteins required for the processes of protein synthesis.

which recognizes the terminator codon. When the release factor recognizes the termination codon in the A site this results in an alteration of the peptidyl transferase center on the large, or 50S, ribosomal subunit so that it can accept water as the attacking nucleoplile rather than requiring the normal substrate, aa-tRNA. In other words, the termination reaction serves to convert the peptidyl transferase into an esterase. The ribosomes are apparently released as 70S units, which then become dissociated into 30S and 50S subunits in a process that requires the participation of a ribosome dissociation factor.[11] This factor is apparently the same as initiation factor 3. The 30S and 50S subunits then return to the cycle of events at initiation.

The Streptomycin Binding Site

Early studies of streptomycin inhibition of protein synthesis in cell-free preparations established that the drug altered the function of ribosomes and not other components of the system.[12,13] Streptomycin interacts specifically with the 30S subunit of the ribosome. This site of interaction was first indicated by experiments that utilized ribosomes from streptomycin-sensitive and streptomycin-resistant cells to support poly U–directed protein synthesis.[14] The 70S ribosome can be dissociated into its 50S and 30S subunits by lowering the Mg^{2+} concentration; raising the Mg^{2+} concentration permits reassociation. Accordingly, cell extracts of E. coli were made in buffer of low Mg^{2+} concentration and centrifuged on a sucrose gradient to separate the heavier 50S subunits from the 30S particles. Crossover experiments were then carried out by raising the Mg^{2+} concentration to produce hybrid 70S ribosomes with one subunit from sensitive cells and one from resistant cells. These reassociated ribosomes were then incubated with poly U and streptomycin in an appropriate system for protein synthesis. The results of the experiment, summarized in Table 5–1, demonstrate that substantial inhibition of protein synthesis is achieved only when the 30S subunit is derived from sensitive cells.

This type of experiment has been carried further by Nomura and co-workers; they separated purified 30S ribosomes into 16S RNA and 21 different proteins, which could be fractionated by phosphocellulose column chromatography.[15] These proteins and the 16S RNA were then reassociated into 30S ribosomal subunits that support protein synthesis. Protein-synthesizing experiments utilizing such reconstituted ribosomes prepared with 30S ribosomal protein purified from streptomycin-sensitive and streptomycin-resistant cells demonstrate that a single protein designated S12 in accordance with its migration on polyacrylamide gel electro-

Table 5–1. *The effect of streptomycin on the incorporation of phenylalanine in a system utilizing hybrid ribosomes from sensitive and resistant cells.* Ribosomes reconstituted from 30S and 50S subunits purified from streptomycin-sensitive and streptomycin-resistant E. coli were added to a phenylalanine incorporation system directed by poly U. Incubations were carried out with or without streptomycin ($5 \times 10^{-5}M$), and the amount of radioactivity incorporated into the acid-insoluble form was assayed. The results are presented as the average percent inhibition of incorporation by streptomycin for four experiments.

Constitution of hybrid ribosomes		Inhibition of phenylalanine incorporation by streptomycin (%)
30S	50S	
Sensitive	Sensitive	62
Sensitive	Resistant	60
Resistant	Resistant	6
Resistant	Sensitive	15

Source: Data from Davies.[14]

phoresis) determines the streptomycin sensitivity of the reconstituted particles (Table 5–2).[16]

Clearly the S12 protein is necessary not only for streptomycin sensitivity but also for streptomycin binding. This has been demonstrated by incubating reconstituted 30S particles with radioactive dihydrostreptomycin and then separating the bound 30S-streptomycin complex from the free drug by filtration.[17] The results presented in Table 5–3 show that there is significant binding of dihydrostreptomycin to ribosomes only when the S12 protein in the reconstituted ribosome is derived from sensitive cells. In dialysis experiments, S12 alone (that is, not in combination with RNA as a reconstituted 30S particle) does not bind the drug, whereas complete 30S particles under the same conditions bind well. Therefore some structure involving both S12 and other components of the 30S subunit of the ribosome is essential to the formation of the complete functioning receptor site for the drug.

The S12 protein is the product of the *str A* gene. Analysis of S12 proteins purified

Table 5–2.   Poly U–directed phenylalanine incorporation activity of reconstituted 30S ribosomal particles and their sensitivity to streptomycin. RNA prepared from 30S ribosomes and 30S ribosomal protein purified by phosphocellulose chromatogrphy from streptomycin-sensitive and streptomycin-resistant *E. coli* were reconstituted into 30S subunits. Two protein fractions were prepared: the protein S12, which was essentially pure, and the protein mixture containing all the other 30S subunit proteins except S12. Particles were reconstituted in the combinations indicated and assayed for their activity in poly U–directed phenylalanine incorporation with or without streptomycin $(5 \times 10^{-5}\text{M})$. Values are in counts per minute of phenylalanine incorporated per incubation.

Origin of proteins used for reconstituted 30S subunits		Incorporation activity (cpm)		Inhibition by streptomycin (%)
All proteins but S12	S12	−Sm	+Sm	
S	S	6354	4153	35
S	R	6209	5755	7
S	—	2926	3116	0
R	R	4214	4031	4
R	S	4236	2771	35

R, resistant; S, sensitive; Sm, streptomycin.
Source: Data from Ozaki et al.[16]

from several highly streptomycin-resistant (*str A*) mutants of *E. coli* demonstrated that resistance results from a single amino acid replacement at one of two positions in the molecule.[17] The bacterial ribosome is composed of many macromolecules that interact with each other in a complex manner[18] and it is difficult to envision how a single amino acid change in only one of these proteins has such a profound effect on the streptomycin-binding site. Several observations suggest that many proteins (and perhaps also the 16S ribosomal RNA[19]) contribute to this binding site.[20] For example, mutational alterations in three different 30S proteins (S4, S5, S12) have clearly been shown to affect streptomycin action.[20] Also, streptomycin analogs used as site-specific affinity labels have been found to attach to proteins S4, S7, and S14, indicating that all of these proteins are in, or close to, the binding site.[21,22]

Binding of streptomycin induces conformational changes in the ribosome that can be detected by various analytical techniques,[23–25] and the kinetics of the interaction between radiolabeled dihydrostreptomycin and native 70S ribosomes and ribosomal subunits purified from *E. coli* has been studied in

some detail.[26] At low drug concentrations, 70S ribosomes bind one molecule of streptomycin per ribosome in a tight but reversible manner $(K_D \sim 10^{-7}\text{M at } 25°\text{C})$.[26]. There is essentially no binding to 70S ribosomes or their subunits from streptomycin-resistant strains. The binding of streptomycin to purified 30S subunits is an order of magnitude weaker than that to 70S ribosomes. Thus, although binding to the 50S subunit alone is insignificant at low drug concentration, the presence of the 50S subunit in the 70S complex affects the confirmation of the high-affinity binding site. It is interesting to note that when a photoaffinity analog of streptomycin was irradiated in the presence of either 30S or 50S subparticles alone, the analog bound chiefly to the 30S particle, but when it was reacted with 70S ribosomes, the covalent label was equally distributed between the two subunits.[22] These observations suggest that the streptomycin binding site may lie near the interface of the ribosomal subunits. It is important to know that binding to the high-affinity site is reversible and the bound dihydrostreptomycin is readily exchanged by streptomycin but not by other aminoglycosides.[26]

Table 5–3. Binding of dihydrostreptomycin to reconstituted 30S ribosomal particles. 30S particles reconstituted from 16S RNA and purified 30S subunit protein from streptomycin-sensitive or streptomycin-resistant *E. coli* were incubated at 30°C with radioactive dihydrostreptomycin (3.4 μg/ml). After 20 min, the bound drug-30S complex was separated from the free drug by filtration on cellulose acetate. The radioactive drug remaining on the filter was assayed in a scintillation counter; values are in counts per minute of dihydrostreptomycin bound per 1.5 OD_{260} units of 30S particles.

Origin of proteins used for reconstituted 30S subunits: All proteins but S12	S12	Dihydrostreptomycin bound (cpm)
S	S	1198
S	R	65
S	—	83
R	R	31
R	S	691
Control 30S (S)		943
Control 30S (R)		35

R, resistant; S, sensitive.

Source: Data from Ozaki et al.[16]

At concentrations of streptomycin greater than $10^{-5}M$, there is weak binding ($K^D > 10^{-4}M$) to multiple sites on both the 30S and 50S portions of the ribosome.[26] It is not yet clear whether these weak interactions are entirely nonspecific or whether they contribute to streptomycin effects on protein synthesis. The question is important because streptomycin has different effects at high and low drug concentrations. At sublethal concentrations of streptomycin (e.g., 2 μg/ml), protein synthesis continues but there is an increase in the frequency of errors made during translation, whereas at high drug concentrations (>20 μg/ml) there is complete inhibition of protein synthesis and rapid cell death.[27]

Streptomycin-Induced Misreading of the Genetic Code

The effect of streptomycin on decreasing the fidelity of messenger translation can be seen in vitro as an increased incorporation of the "wrong" amino acid in protein synthesis directed by synthetic mRNA.[28] The effect can also be seen in vivo as "phenotypic suppression": that is, the drug masks the phenotypic expression of certain mutations.

Under routine assay conditions, poly U directs the incorporation of phenylalanine (codes UUU and UUC) much more readily than leucine, isoleucine, or serine, all of which have codons that differ from a phenylalanine codon by only one base. In the presence of streptomycin, neomycin, or gentamicin, however, the incorporation of isoleucine relative to phenylalanine increases several-fold.[28] This misreading effect of streptomycin has also been examined in a poly U–directed protein-synthesizing system utilizing ribosomes with reconstituted 30S particles, and the presence of protein S12 from sensitive cells was found to be a prerequisite for extensive streptomycin-induced incorporation of "wrong" amino acids (isoleucine, serine, and tyrosine). Streptomycin-induced misreading has been demonstrated with natural messengers as well as synthetic mRNAs.[29] The misreading appears to be due to stabilization of the aminoacyl-tRNA binding to the A site on the ribosome.[30] The stabilization is sufficient to overcome a single mismatch in the codon–anticodon interaction, thus bypassing the proofreading mechanism.

The distortion of codon recognition in intact, growing bacteria should result in the frequent insertion of "wrong" amino acids and a consequent alteration in (or loss of) activity of proteins. It is possible that abnormal proteins produced as a result of aminoglycoside action are inserted into the cell membrane and lead to altered permeability and a further stimulation of aminoglycoside transport.[31] This phase of transport, termed energy-dependent phase II, is not well understood, although it is believed to be linked with disruption of the cytoplasmic membrane. This action is consistent with the leakage of small ions followed by larger molecules and eventually by proteins from the bacterial cell prior to aminoglycoside-induced death. This action may partially explain the bactericidal effect of the aminoglycosides.[32,33]

Inhibition of Protein Synthesis by Streptomycin

When growing, sensitive bacteria are exposed to appropriate concentrations of streptomycin that are high enough to be bactericidal, protein synthesis is rapidly inhibited.[34] Two lines of evidence suggest that the major effect of streptomycin is to block protein synthesis at some step during or shortly after initiation. In one series of experiments in *Escherichia coli*, Luzzatto and colleagues[35] found that lethal concentrations of streptomycin cause the accumulation of 70S ribosomes that are incapable of protein synthesis. They called the 70S units that accumulated "streptomycin monosomes" and found that these units consist of a complex of 30S and 50S particles, mRNA, tRNA, and streptomycin. In their model, which is diagrammed in Figure 5–4, Luzzatto et al.[35] propose that the streptomycin-containing 70S units are abnormal initiation complexes that cannot elongate; therefore they accumulate irreversibly in the cell. This is what one would expect if the effect of streptomycin were to "freeze" protein synthesis at the initiation complex stage.

Davis and co-workers[36–39] developed a somewhat different model. They also found that the drug blocks initiation, but they did not find that the process is "frozen" in the 70S monosome state described by Luzzatto et al.[35] Rather, they found that initiation complexes and aberrant polyinitiation com-

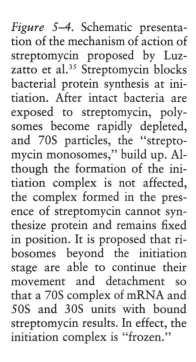

Figure 5–4. Schematic presentation of the mechanism of action of streptomycin proposed by Luzzatto et al.[35] Streptomycin blocks bacterial protein synthesis at initiation. After intact bacteria are exposed to streptomycin, polysomes become rapidly depleted, and 70S particles, the "streptomycin monosomes," build up. Although the formation of the initiation complex is not affected, the complex formed in the presence of streptomycin cannot synthesize protein and remains fixed in position. It is proposed that ribosomes beyond the initiation stage are able to continue their movement and detachment so that a 70S complex of mRNA and 50S and 30S units with bound streptomycin results. In effect, the initiation complex is "frozen."

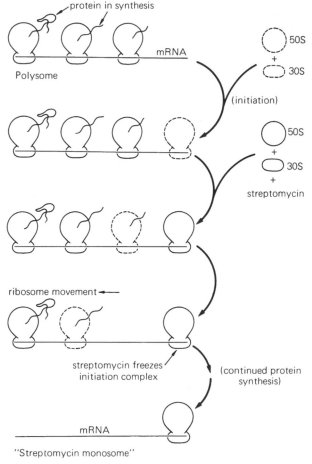

plexes are formed in a dynamic manner. Elongation of these complexes is prevented by streptomycin, but the 70S ribosome is gradually released from the RNA and the ribosomal subunits are returned to the ribosome pool.[38,39]

Differences between the Mechanisms of Action of Streptomycin and the Other Aminoglycosides

Although the other aminoglycosides used clinically bind to ribosomes and cause both misreading and inhibition of protein synthesis, they do not do so by occupying precisely the same binding site as streptomycin. Several observations point out large differences in the binding sites. Streptomycin-resistant (str A) mutants with altered S12 proteins and no streptomycin binding are usually sensitive to other aminoglycosides, such as gentamicin, neomycin, and kanamycin.[40] As mentioned above, other aminoglycosides do not compete for the binding of the streptomycin class compounds to 30S ribosomal subunits.[26] Other aminoglycosides can be shown to bind to 50S units as well as 30S units. At low concentrations of drug, 70S ribosomes from E. coli bind two molecules of kanamycin and each subunit possesses a tight binding site.[41] Similarly, an N-acetyl derivative of tobramycin was found to bind to both ribosomal subunits, and kanamycin and neomycin compete for the binding whereas streptomycin does not.[42] Gentamicin-resistant strains of E. coli have been found to have an altered protein (L6) in the 50S rather than in the 30S subunit.[43]

Differences have been observed in the misreading induced by aminoglycosides in different structural classes. As the concentration of neomycin, kanamycin, or gentamicin is raised from 10^{-6} to 10^{-4}M, there is a several-fold increase in the amount of misreading of synthetic RNA messengers.[44] In contrast, misreading by streptomycin remains constant over the concentration range. This and other experiments showing multiphasic effects of gentamicin over a wide range of drug concentrations[45,46] are consis-

tent with the interpretation that many aminoglycosides may interact with several ribosomal binding sites of different affinities.

On the basis of observations made with streptomycin, the aminoglycosides have been considered to be a group of antibiotics that cause misreading and inhibit protein synthesis by interacting with the 30S ribosomal subunit. It is clear, however, that at this stage of our understanding, the other aminoglycosides that are used clinically should be considered to intereact with both ribosomal subunits and perhaps at multiple binding sites that are different from the binding site that has been studied with the S12 protein mutants.

Resistance to the Aminoglycosides

Three mechanisms of aminoglycoside resistance have been identified in clinical isolates: (1) ribosomal resistance, (2) resistance due to decreased drug uptake, and (3) resistance caused by aminoglycoside modifying enzymes. This third mechanism is the most important explanation for the acquired microbial resistance that is encountered clinically.

Ribosomal resistance refers to resistance arising from mutations in genes coding for ribosomal proteins. The best known of these occur at the str A locus and confer a high degree of resistance to streptomycin. Ribosomal resistance to streptomycin occurs occasionally but ribosomal resistance to other aminoglycosides has not been found in clinical isolates.[47] This type of resistance is less relevant clincally for most bacterial infections, but in mycobacteria, ribosomal resistance may be the only kind of resistance. Diminished drug uptake due to altered components of the membrane transport system is responsible for a low level of aminoglycoside resistance that has been identified with increasing frequency in strains of Pseudomonas aeruginosa isolated from nosocomial infections.[48,49] Most aminoglycoside resistance in clinical isolates results from the production of enzymes that modify these antibiotics.[50,51]

In order to be susceptible to an aminoglycoside, the bacterium must take up the drug by an active process. Aminoglycosides are cationic, hydrophilic compounds that do not readily pass across membranes by simple passive diffusion. Bacterial uptake of aminoglycosides appears to occur in three phases.[52,53] Initially, there is energy-independent binding of the drug to cation binding sites (phospholipid phosphates) on the cell membrane. The binding is followed by an energy-dependent phase in which the aminoglycoside traverses the cell membrane by a mechanism that is linked to components used in the terminal electron transport phase of energy metabolism.[54] In this case the strongly cationic aminoglycoside appears to bind solely on the basis of charge to anionic transporters and to be driven across the cytoplasmic membrane by the membrane potential which is negative on the interior.[54] Several divalent cations, such as Mg^{2+} and Ca^{2+}, antagonize cell killing by aminoglycosides. This antagonism is due to inhibition of both ionic binding to the cell surface and energized uptake.[49] This phase of transport (termed *energy-dependent phase 1*) is associated with a low rate of drug accumulation that is rate limiting for susceptibility. A faster rate of aminoglycoside uptake (termed *energy-dependent phase II*) starts after aminoglycosides have bound to membrane-associated ribosomes and the mechanism of this uptake has not been defined.

Anaerobic bacteria are naturally resistant to these drugs because the transport of aminoglycosides across the cytoplasmic membrane is an oxygen-dependent, active process. These organisms thus lack the ability to take up these drugs. Similarly, facultative bacteria generally are much more resistant when they are grown under anerobic conditions.[55]

Aminoglycoside-modifying enzymes could cause resistance by blocking drug uptake or by inactivating the drug so that it can no longer affect ribosome function. Since it has been demonstrated that only a small fraction (less than 1%) of the total available, active aminoglycoside in the growth medium is detoxified, it has been argued that drug modification in some way blocks drug entry into the cell.[56] In certain instances it has been shown, however, that modified aminoglycosides do not inhibit protein synthesis by ribosomes under cell-free conditions.[57] Resistant bacteria with modifying enzymes can still take up aminoglycosides via energy-dependent phase I and it is perhaps best to think of this form of resistance as a competition between drug uptake and drug inactivation by modification.[58] The drug modifying enzymes are associated with the bacterial cell membrane and it is probably at the internal membrane surface, where the ATP and coenzyme A cofactors are readily available, that the aminoglycosides are inactivated. When the rate of drug modification exceeds the rate of uptake by energy-dependent phase I, most or all of the drug that is accumulated is inactivated and the bacterium is resistant.

The aminoglycoside-modifying enzymes are the subject of a large body of literature that has been reviewed in detail.[47,50,51] Three classes of enzymes are known: O-phosphotransferases, O-nucleotidyltransferases (adenylyltransferases), and N-acetyltransferases. More than 20 distinct enzymes have been identified. The genes for the aminoglycoside modifying enzymes are carried on plasmids, they are conjugally transmitted by R factors in gram-negative bacteria, and it is becoming more common to find clinical isolates with several plasmids conferring different modifying enzymes. Each antibiotic can be modified by more than one enzyme and each enzyme can modify more than one antibiotic; therefore, the resistance profiles are complex. A modification that inactivates one aminoglycoside may not markedly affect the antibacterial activity of another.[59] Elaboration of these enzymes also explains some of the cross-resistance or lack thereof that occurs among the different aminoglycosides in some bacteria. Different enzymes are responsible for inactivation of gentamicin and streptomycin and thus a small proportion of gentamicin-resistant strains of enterococci will be susceptible to streptomycin. On the other hand, resistance to gentamicin indicates resistance to tobramycin, amikacin, kanamycin, and netilmicin because the inactivating enzyme modifies all of these aminoglycosides.[60]

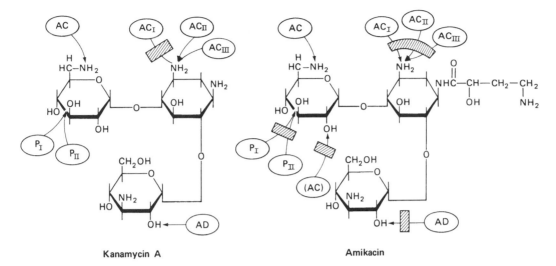

Figure 5–5. Sites of modification of kanamycin and amikacin by several aminoglycoside modifying enzymes. The arrows point to sites modified by *N*-acetyltransferases (AC), *O*-phosphotransferases (P) and an *O*-adenylyltransferase (AD). The hatched bars indicate that the enzyme is not able to modify the site. Kanamycin is shown to be attacked by six different enzymes but the modification of the kanamycin structure that yielded amikacin rendered the molecule able to be attacked by only one of those six. (From Moellering.)[61]

The characterization of the aminoglycoside-modifying enzymes has led to the design and synthesis of aminoglycosides that are not substrates for the enzymes and are therefore effective inhibitors of resistant strains. The most successful of these compounds introduced into clinical use is amikacin, a semisynthetic derivative of kanamycin. The structures of kanamycin A and amikacin and their sites of attack by several modifying enzymes are presented in Figure 5–5.[61] Kanamycin A, which is the major component of the commercial product, is a substrate for several aminoglycoside-modifying enzymes.[58] As a consequence, resistance to kanamycin is widespread and its clinical usefulness has greatly declined. In contrast, amikacin is a substrate for six modifying enzymes and three of these are produced only by staphylococci.[51] The relative insensitivity of amikacin to enzymatic modification is reflected in the relatively low incidence of amikacin resistance in clinical isolates.[62] Indeed, it has been found that the degree of effectiveness of the aminoglycosides is directly related to their degree of resistance to the modifying enzymes.[63]

Antibacterial Activity of the Aminoglycosides

The aminoglycosides are potent gram-negative antimicrobial drugs. Kanamycin, gentamicin, tobramycin, amikacin and netilmicin are used most commonly to treat infection by aerobic gram-negative bacilli. Kanamycin, like streptomicin, has a more limited spectrum compared to the other aminoglycosides. The activity of these drugs against enterococcus and selected gram-negative bacilli is presented in Table 5–4.[64] It should be noted that the in vitro activity of aminoglycosides is strongly dependent on the cation content and pH of the growth medium because these factors modify the ability of bacteria to actively take up the drugs.[49] Thus, MIC values like those presented in Table 5–4 vary among different laboratories. The aminoglycosides are not very active against gram-positive bacteria, except for most strains of staphylococci which are quite sensitive to gentamicin and tobramycin in vitro.[66] Enterococci and *Streptococcus viridans* are not usually susceptible to aminoglycosides alone, but streptomycin and

Table 5–4. Susceptibility of enterococci and selected aerobic gram-negative bacteria to the aminoglycosides expressed as the concentration that will inhibit growth in culture by 90% (MIC$_{90}$).

Organism	Kanamycin	Gentamicin	Tobramycin	Amikacin	Netilmicin
	\multicolumn{5}{c}{MIC$_{90}$ (μg/ml)}				
Enterobacter	3	64	0.5	2	0.5
Escherichia coli	16	1	0.5	2	0.25
Klebsiella pneumoniae	32	≥16	1	1	0.25
Proteus vulgaris	1	2	1	4	1
Providencia	128	16	4	2	16
Serratia marcescens	128	8	32	16	32
Pseudomonas aeruginosa	—	16	6	32	≥32
Acinetobacter	—	2	—	32	≥32
Enterococcus	—	16	32	≥64	32
Salmonella spp.	1	1	0.5	2	—

Source: Data from Wiedemann and Grimm.[65]

gentamicin are used to treat severe infections in combination with a penicillin because the combination is synergistic at concentrations of aminoglycoside that are achieved clinically. Some strains of enterococci have acquired high-level resistance to streptomycin, gentamicin, and tobramycin but not to amikacin. Anaerobic bacteria are not susceptible to aminoglycosides because active uptake of these drugs by the bacterium requires respiration (electron transport).[49]

The aminoglycosides are often used in combination with a β-lactam antibiotic because such combinations have been shown to be synergistic in vitro. There are several well-established examples. The combination of an antipseudomonas penicillin (e.g., carbenicillin, ticarcillin, azlocillin, mezlocillin, or piperacillin) with gentamicin, tobramycin, or amikacin is synergistic against many strains of *Pseudomonas aeruginosa.*[67–69] Aminoglycosides are synergistic with cephalosporins against some strains of *Klebsiella,*[70] and the combination of a penicillin and an aminoglycoside is synergistic against many strains of enterococci[71,72] and *Streptococcus viridans.*[73]

It has been shown that all the antibiotics that inhibit bacterial cell wall synthesis (cycloserine, bacitracin, vancomycin, and the β-lactam antibiotics) are synergistic with aminoglycosides against sensitive strains of enterococci in culture.[72] A mechanism for

the synergism is suggested by the experiment presented in Figure 5–6. When suspensions of enterococci are incubated with radioactive streptomycin, very little antibiotic becomes associated with the bacteria. But when the growing bacteria are exposed to penicillin as well as to radioactive streptomycin, increasing amounts of radioactivity are recovered with the organism. This suggests that inhibition of cell wall synthesis in some way permits the entry of the aminoglycoside into the cell. Thus, the role of the β-lactam antibiotic in the synergistic pair is to permit the aminoglycoside to have a greater effect. It is not at all clear how interference with cell wall synthesis would cause increased uptake of aminoglycosides.

The combination of chloramphenicol with an aminoglycoside may result in drug antagonism. This has been shown both in vitro[75,76] and in vivo,[77] and the reason for the antagonism has not been established. It has been suggested that chloramphenicol, by retarding the breakdown of polysomes,[78] tends to slow the return of ribosomal subunits into the free pool where they can be occupied by the aminoglycosides.

The individual aminoglycosides have variable activity against the aerobic gram-negative bacilli. Tobramycin and gentamicin show similar activity against most gram-negative bacilli although tobramycin usually is more active against *Pseudomonas aerugi-*

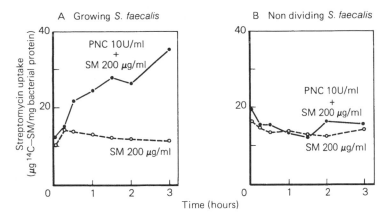

Figure 5–6. Effect of penicillin on the uptake of radioactive streptomycin by *Streptococcus faecalis*—a possible mechanism for synergism. Carbon 14-labeled streptomycin ([14C]-SM) was added to suspensions of *S. faecalis* in the presence or absence of 10 U/ml of penicillin (PNC). At various times, aliquots of the bacterial suspensions were filtered and the amount of radioactivity remaining on the filter with the bacteria was assayed. Graph A shows the effect of penicillin on streptomycin uptake in growing cultures and Graph B the effect in suspensions of nondividing bacteria. One explanation of the data is that penicillin, in inhibiting cell wall synthesis in the growing bacterium, lowers a permeability barrier to streptomycin passage through the cell wall to the cell membrane. Another possibility is that inhibition of wall synthesis and autolytic activity in some way increase the active transport of streptomycin across the cell membrane. Since higher intracellular streptomycin levels are obtained in the presence of penicillin, the combination of the two drugs is synergistic. (From Moellering and Weinberg.[74])

nosa and some *Proteus* species. Most gram-negative bacilli that are resistant to gentamicin are also resistant to tobramycin, although about 50% of *Pseudomonas* spp. resistant to gentamicin remain sensitive to tobramycin. In some hospitals there has been an increase in resistance to gentamicin and tobramycin over the past 20 years. The relative frequency of these changes in resistance patterns has varied dramatically.[79] Fortunately, amikacin and netilmicin have retained their activity in the treatment of most of these nosocomial infections and are particularly valuable agents for that reason.[80]

Pharmacology of the Aminoglycoside Antibiotics

The aminoglycosides have similar pharmacokinetic properties. This section will review the general pharmacology of these drugs. The reader who wishes more detailed information is referred to several reviews of the literature[81–83] and symposia concerned with the individual drugs.[84–87] A summary of the pharmacokinetic properties of the major aminoglycosides is presented in Table 5–5.

Absorption

Aminoglycosides are highly polar compounds that pass across membranes very poorly and only about 1% of an orally administered dose is absorbed from the gastrointestinal tract[88] even when there is intestinal inflammation or ulceration.[89] Aminoglycosides (principally neomycin and kanamycin) are administered orally to kill the bowel flora before intestinal surgery. Since there is essentially no absorption, this constitutes local administration of the drug. In this case, the aminoglycoside is often combined with another antibiotic that is effective against anaerobic bacteria.[90,91]

The aminoglycosides are routinely administered by intramuscular injection. They are absorbed well from intramuscular injection sites, and peak blood levels (see Table 5–5) are achieved in about 1 h. Gentamicin, tobramycin, amikacin, and netilmicin may be

Table 5–5. Pharmacokinetic characteristics of aminoglycosides.

Aminoglycoside	Routes of administration	Adult daily dose (mg/kg/day)	Normal dosage inteval (hours)	Range of peak serum level (µg/ml)	Half-life		Plasma protein binding (%)
					Normal (hours)	Anuric (hours)	
Streptomycin	IM	15–25	12	25–30[a]	2.5	50–110	35
Kanamycin	IM, IV	15	12	15–30	2–2.5	60–96	0
Gentamicin	IM, IV	3–5	8	4–8	2	48–72	0
Tobramycin	IM, IV	3–5	8	4–8	2	56–60	0
Amikacin	IM, IV	15	8 or 12	15–30	2–2.5	56–150	4
Netilmicin	IM, IV	2–6.5	12	4–12	2–2.5	NA[b]	0

[a] In adults, 1 g of streptomycin administered by intramusclar injection yields a peak plasma concentration of 25–30 µg/ml. [b] NA, not available.

Source: The values in the table were taken from a review by Leroy et al.[81] and from manufacturers' data.

administered intravenously for the treatment of severe infection. When given intravenously, the aminoglycosides should be administered slowly by continuous infusion over a 30- to 60-min period to avoid the risk of producing neuromuscular blockade. When a penicillin and an aminoglycoside are used together in therapy, it is important not to mix the two drugs in the same intravenous solution, because the penicillins in high concentration chemically inactivate the aminoglycosides.[92,93]

Aminoglycosides are present in many antibiotic formulations used in topical therapy and wound irrigation. Absorption through intact skin is minimal but there may be significant absorption if aminoglycosides are applied to burned areas or open wounds. The use of neomycin in wound-irrigating solutions, for example, may result in a substantial serum concentration of antibiotic[94] and ototoxicity and nephrotoxicity have been reported.[95]

Distribution

The literature on the pharmacokinetics of the aminoglycosides is extensive and sometimes conflicting. A detailed review of the field is provided by Pechere and Dugal.[96] The aminoglycosides are poorly distributed to most cells because of their polar nature. They also are excluded for the most part from the central nervous system and the eye because of their polar properties. The volume of distribution of aminoglycosides is calculated to be about 25% of the lean body weight when a two-compartment pharmacokinetic model is used for the analysis.[96] Thus, the volume of distribution is equal to the extracellular fluid volume. There is little or no binding of aminoglycosides to serum proteins.[97] The aminoglycosides accumulate to high levels in the kidney where tissue concentrations of amikacin and gentamicin have been reported to vary from 16 to 89 times the plasma concentration.[98] The binding of the drug in the kidney probably accounts for the fact that detectable concentrations of aminoglycosides persist in the urine for several weeks.[96]

The aminoglycosides penetrate into the interstitial fluid to levels that approximate those found in serum.[99] In the absence of obstruction, the concentration of gentamicin achieved in the bile is 25% to 50% of that in the serum,[100,101] but if there is biliary obstruction or severe hepatic damage, there may be no penetration into the biliary tract.[101] Concentrations of aminoglycosides in sputum or bronchial secretions have been reported to range from 25% to 67% of those in serum[102] and the concentration of tobramycin or gentamicin may achieve the MIC for many sensitive gram-negative bacilli.[103,104] The concentration of aminoglycosides achieved in pleural, pericardial, and ascitic fluids is approximately 50% that of serum.[83,100] There is good penetration into synovial fluid where drug levels are 50% to

Table 5–6. Relative diffusion of gram-negative antimicrobial agents from blood into cerebrospinal fluid. In general, the cephalosporins penetrate into the cerebrospinal fluid with meningeal inflammation better than the aminoglycosides but not as well as the penicillins. Results in treating meningitis with the first- and second-generation cephalosporins have been poor and they are not used to treat infection of the central nervous system.

Excellent with or without inflammation	Good only with inflammation	Minimal or not good with inflammation
Sulfonamides	Penicillins	Tetracycline
Chloramphenicol	Third-generation cephalosporins	Aminoglycosides
Metronidazole		First- and second-generation cephalosporins

100% of those in serum.[105] Penetration of aminoglycosides into the eye is very poor and subconjunctival injection is required to achieve intravitreal concentrations of drug that are in the therapeutic range.[106]

Penetration of aminoglycosides into the cerebrospinal fluid is very poor in the absence of inflammation, and although penetration is somewhat greater with inflammation,[107] the concentrations achieved are usually inadequate for treating meningitis in adults[108,109] (see Table 5–6 for comparative penetration of gram-negative antimicrobial agents into the cerebrospinal fluid). To achieve therapeutic levels, the drug must be administered directly into the cerebrospinal fluid. Injection of aminoglycosides into the lumbar subarachnoid space produces a high local concentration of drug, but the concentration achieved in ventricular fluid is very low.[109] It has been shown that the clinical outcome in infants with gram-negative meningitis is not improved with lumbar injection over systemic therapy alone.[110] Thus, to achieve high intraventricular levels, the aminoglycosides must be given by direct intraventricular administration.[108] Thus we are very fortunate that potent anitmicrobials, such as the third-generation cephalosporins, have been introduced to permit treatment of gram-negative meningitis with systemic administration.

Aminoglycosides pass across the placenta and the concentration of gentamicin in human fetal serum has been found to range from 20% to 40% of the maternal serum concentration.[111] Auditory toxicity has been reported in children born of mothers treated with streptomycin during pregnancy.[112]

Recent studies have compared tissue levels of the aminoglycosides after administration once a day or three-times a day. Daily administration promotes higher than proportional concentrations in bronchial secretions, facial sinuses, and pulmonary parenchyma. However, daily dosing decreases renal accumulation of gentamicin and tobramycin.[113,114]

Excretion

The aminoglycosides are not metabolized and they are excreted in their active forms by glomerular filtration.[96] Some tubular reabsorption occurs. In the patient with normal renal function, aminoglycoside half-lives are in the range of 2 to 3 h, but in the anuric individual the half-lives range from 50 to 100 h or more (Table 5–5). The aminoglycosides are all potentially nephrotoxic and ototoxic and their dosage must be modified when renal function is impaired. Because these drugs are not metabolized and are eliminated by glomerular filtration, it would seem at first glance that it would be rather simple to determine the glomerular filtration rate by assaying creatinine clearance and then adjusting the dose accordingly. The elimination rates of all of the aminoglycosides have been shown to be linearly related to the creatinine clearance rate.[115] The relationship between the elimination rate constant of gentamicin and the rate of creatinine clearance is shown in Figure 5–7 which also

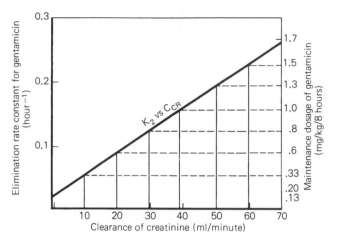

Figure 5–7. Relationship between the elimination rate constant for gentamicin and the rate of creatinine clearance. The elimination rate constant (K₂) for gentamicin was calculated from the values for the plasma half-life of the drug in 20 patients with differing degrees of renal failure. The elimination rate constant (left ordinate) when plotted against the creatinine clearance (C_CR) values determined in the same patients yields a straight line up to a creatinine clearance of 70 ml/minute. The figure also contains a nomogram for estimating the maintenance dosage of gentamicin (in mg/kg) that must be administered every 8 hours to sustain a safe antibacterial serum concentration between 3 and 8 µg/ml. The solid and dashed lines in the grid provide easier reading of the maintenance dosage at each ten units of creatinine clearance. As discussed in the text, it is always best to monitor aminoglycoside serum levels in patients with compromised renal function and to adjust the dose accordingly. (From Chan et al.)[116]

contains a nomogram for determining the maintenance dosage of gentamicin to be administered with various degrees of renal failure.[116] A number of nomograms and equations for dosage adjustment based on either the creatinine clearance rate or serum creatinine concentration have been published for the various aminoglycosides.[116-119] Clinical experience has shown, however, that these methods do not accurately predict aminoglycoside serum concentrations.[120] A wide variation in aminoglycoside elimination rates and distribution volumes exists among patients, and the same dosage of drug (in mg/kg body weight) can produce markedly different serum levels in different patients.

Factors that Influence Serum Drug Concentration

Several factors influence serum concentration of aminoglycosides and contribute to the wide interpatient variability. There are clear age-related differences in both distribution volumes and elimination rates of aminoglycosides. Neonates have distribution

volumes that may average 60% of body weight compared with 25% in adults.[96] Because of decreased glomerular filtration rates, the elimination half-life is 5–6 h during the first few days of life versus 2 h for adults.[96,121,122] To achieve similar peak serum concentrations, children under 5 years of age require almost twice as much gentamicin as children over 10 years or adults.[123] The age-related differences are diminished when doses are calculated on the basis of body surface area rather than body weight.[123]

The patient's pathophysiology may determine variations in serum levels achieved with aminoglycosides. Since fat contains less extracellular fluid than other tissues, the relative volume of distribution in obese patients is smaller than in those with normal body weight.[124] In obese subjects the serum aminoglycoside concentration is predicted best when dosage is calculated on the basis of ideal body weight plus a normalizing factor of 40% of the adipose mass.[124] Any factor that alters the extracellular fluid volume can have a marked effect on serum aminoglycoside concentration. In patients with marked edema or fluid collection (e.g., patients with ascites, congestive heart failure, etc.), serum levels will be lower than anticipated because of increased distribution volume.[125] In contrast, dehydration will lead to unusually high serum levels. The presence of fever or anemia are both associated with changes in serum aminoglycoside concentration. In volunteers subjected to drug-induced (etiocholanolone) fever, the average serum concentration of gentamicin was reduced by 40% compared to control individuals who were injected with the pyrogen but did not develop fever.[126] Fever is associated with a short gentamicin half-life[123] that apparently reflects an increased renal blood flow and a consequent increase in glomerular filtration rate. A significant inverse relation between hematocrit and peak serum level of gentamicin[100] and gentamicin half-life[120] has been reported in adults. Patients with major burns have increased glomerular filtration rates and shorter aminoglycoside half-lives.[127] Patients with cystic fibrosis appear to tolerate rather large doses of aminoglycosides.[103,128] Cystic fibrosis patients have a higher aminoglycoside clearance rate[129] and they tend to have hypervolemia with an increase in red blood cell mass and plasma volume,[130] both of which would tend to lower the effective free concentration of drug.

In a large study of 1640 patients with gram-negative infections receiving gentamicin, the daily dose necessary to obtain therapeutic serum concentrations ranged from 0.5 to 25.8 mg/kg in patients who had a normal serum creatinine.[131] This is perhaps an extreme example of interpatient variability, but it allows one to appreciate why it has been difficult to devise simple ways to predict appropriate aminoglycoside dosage and why monitoring of serum antibiotic concentrations is necessary for the proper administration of these drugs.

Serum Assay of Aminoglycosides, Dosing Strategies, and Dosage Adjustment

Several types of assays are available for monitoring aminoglycoside concentration in serum.[132] Bioassay techniques are inexpensive and easily done, but the methods are time consuming and results are delayed.[133] A quality control study of bioassays performed in Great Britain has raised questions about the reproducibility and accuracy of these assays performed in different laboratories.[134] Enzymatic radiochemical assays that measure the transfer of a radiolabeled adenyl or acetate moiety to aminoglycosides offer the advantage of specificity and rapidity, but scintillation counting facilities are required. It is somewhat ironic that the enzymes used for these assays are aminoglycoside-modifying enzymes produced by drug-resistant bacteria. Several types of immunoassays are now available, and they are the most sensitive and specific of the assay methods.[132]

Blood for assay of peak aminoglycoside concentration should be drawn 45–60 min after an intramuscular injection or within 15 min of the completion of an intravenous infusion.[135] Blood for trough levels should be drawn during the hour prior to injection of the next dose. It is often difficult to obtain the samples at appropriate times in the hospital situation, but it is necessary to do so if the values are to be meaningful. Peak serum levels for gentamicin and tobramycin should be over 4 μ/ml and below 10 μ/ml. This provides a peak level that is high enough to kill most susceptible bacteria but low enough to be safe. Peak concentrations of 4 μ/ml are adequate for obtaining synergism with penicillins. The peak concentration for amikacin should be 15 to 30 μ/ml. Several investigators have found that elevated trough levels, in particular, are associated with higher risk of toxicity. Patients with trough levels of gentamicin or tobramycin greater than 2 μ/ml or of amikacin greater than 10 μ/ml were found to have an increased risk of nephrotoxicity and ototoxicity.[136–138] It is possible that elevated trough levels are more indicative than elevated peak levels of an increased area under the serum concentration time curve (AUC), which is the major risk factor for toxicity.[125]

Some patients clearly need to have their serum levels monitored at greater frequency than others. Patients whose renal function changes quickly and unpredictably require frequent serum drug assays. Patients with serious infections (due to sensitive organisms) who are failing to respond should have careful serum assay to guide possible dosage adjustment. Special care should be taken to monitor serum drug concentrations frequently in patients who are at special risk of ototoxicity or nephrotoxicity (e.g., those with compromised hearing and those receiving other ototoxic or nephrotoxic drugs). When therapy is being initiated, it is important to assure that appropriate peak levels of drug are being achieved, but in the presence of stable renal function, it may be necessary to assay only once or twice a week thereafter. It is not necessary to monitor serum levels in patients with urinary tract infections. Aminoglycosides are concentrated in their active forms in the urine, and high levels of antibacterial activity result, especially if the urine is made slightly alkaline. It has been shown that it is the concentration of antibiotic in the urine, not that in the serum, that correlates with clinical success in the treatment of urinary tract infections. Because aminoglycosides are concentrated in the urine, lower doses are administered for treating infections of the urinary tract than infections elsewhere in the body.[100]

When initiating treatment, it is important to administer a loading dose of the drug so that therapeutic serum concentrations will be achieved rapidly. For most adult patients, an appropriate loading dose for gentamicin and tobramycin is 2 mg/kg (lean body weight) and for amikacin it is 10 mg/kg. In the patient with normal renal function this would be followed with a dose of 1.5 mg of gentamicin or tobramycin per kg every 8 h. A maintenance dosage for amikacin of 5 mg/kg every 8 h or 7.5 mg/kg every 12 h is generally recommended.[135] In the case of the patient with compromised renal function, the first dose after the loading dose is often calculated from a nomogram for dosage adjustment based on the serum creatinine concentration or the creatinine clearance rate [references containing nomograms for dosage adjustment of aminoglycosides are: kanamycin (118), gentamicin (116), tobramycin (117), and amikacin (119)]. Subsequent doses are adjusted on the basis of serum drug assay.

Another method of determining mainte-nance dosage is based on the serum assay of drug levels obtained immediately and at intervals after delivering the intial dose by infusion.[131] The data obtained provide an estimate of the elimination rate constant, the half-life, and the volume of distribution of the drug in each patient. The clearance of the aminoglycoside can then be determined from the product of the elimination rate constant and the distribution volume. Thus, the dosage is calculated on the basis of how the individual patient distributes and excretes the drug. This method requires facilities for rapid assay and considerable technical expertise, and it is expensive; but it can be done in the type of referral hospital setting where many of the more difficult patient management problems are encountered.[131] This method has received wide application in many clinical settings because it is the best and most accurate method of individualizing dosage regimens for aminoglycosides.

The aminoglycosides are removed from the body by both hemodialysis and peritoneal dialysis. The half-life of aminoglycosides during hemodialysis is in the range of 5 to 10 h.[96] Since approximately half the drug is removed during the dialysis period, a dose equivalent to one half the loading dose is usually administered at the end of dialysis to maintain the plasma concentration. Patients receiving hemodialysis must have their serum drug levels assayed frequently. Aminoglycoside half-life during peritoneal dialysis varies widely.[96] For replacement, 1 mg of gentamicin or tobramycin or 3 to 4 mg of kanamycin or amikacin is generally administered for every 2 liters of dialysate removed.[139] Although inactivation of aminoglycosides by penicillins in vivo is negligible in the presence of normal renal function, in patients with severe renal impairment in whom the half-life of aminoglycosides is greatly prolonged, simultaneous administration of carbenicillin or ticarcillin may reduce the half-life by 50%[140]

It is clear that the concentration of the drug must be assayed in the serum for rational therapy with aminoglycosides. Obviously, for serum assays to be valuable, the blood sample must be drawn at the correct time so that the results can be used to make appropriate decisions in patient care. In reality, this is often not done. In reviewing 212 serum gentamicin assays at a university-associated hospital, for example, investigators found that 110 samples (52%) were improperly drawn and the results of 85 samples (40%) were ignored.[141] Only 26 of the 62 samples (42%) that were correctly drawn and not ignored were appropriately acted on. The investigators felt that, at most, 42 of the 212 samples (20%) were appropriately used in making patient care decisions.

A recent trend in the use of aminoglycosides has been once-daily aminoglycoside administration instead of the conventional, more frequent administration of these drugs.[142] There are now at least 29 studies in humans comparing these two types of dosing.[143] None of these studies has shown an advantage for the conventional dosing schedule whereas seven studies have shown an advantage for once-daily dosing. Several pharmacodynamic features of the aminoglycosides favor the administration of larger doses given less frequently than in conventional therapy. There are convincing data that support this rationale. Aminoglycosides display concentration-dependent bacterial killing both in vitro and in vivo.[1,144,145] The use of a 24 h dose interval is largely based on convenience as the optimum dose and dose interval are yet to be determined. Many researchers now recommend once-daily aminoglycoside therapy in selected patient groups:[142] This once-a-day dosing may have the advantage of better efficacy, easier administration, and, perhaps best of all, less toxicity.

Toxicity of the Aminoglycosides

The aminoglycosides have a low therapeutic index compared with other systemic antibiotics. This makes the administration of these compounds difficult. The incidence of allergic reaction to systemically administered aminoglycosides is very low. The aminoglycosides are all toxic to the kidney and the inner ear and can produce neuromuscular blockade. Other toxicities occur rarely, and

they include neutropenia, agranulocytosis, and aplastic anemia. Transient elevations of hepatic enzymes occur occasionally. Unlike several other antibiotics, parenteral aminoglycosides are usually not associated with pseudomembranous colitis, probably because they do not affect the common anaerobic flora.

Neuromuscular Blockade

At very high concentrations, the aminoglycosides can produce a nondepolarizing type of neuromuscular blockade. This was first observed when neomycin was found to produce respiratory arrest after intraperitoneal administration. Neuromuscular blockade can occur after intravenous or intramuscular administration of aminoglycosides in patients who are receiving ether anesthesia or a neuromuscular blocking agent during anesthesia.[146] Patients with myasthenia gravis[147] and possibly patients with Parkinson's disease[148] are predisposed to neuromuscular blockade and constitute high-risk groups. Because physicians are aware of the risk and take appropriate precautions, aminoglycoside-induced neuromuscular blockade now occurs only rarely.

The aminoglycosides reduce the amount of acetylcholine released from motor nerve terminals.[149] The paralysis produced by aminoglycosides is completely reversed by calcium.[146]

Since calcium is required for the release of acetylcholine from the prejunctional membrane, it is postulated that the aminoglycosides (which are polycations) bind to the required calcium-binding sites on the presynaptic membrane to produce paralysis. Consistent with this hypothesis, neomycin has been shown to prevent the reuptake of calcium or its rebinding to superficial sites on the cell membrane in vascular smooth muscle preparations.[150] In addition to the prejunctional inhibition of acetylcholine release, aminoglycosides also decrease the sensitivity of the postjunctional endplate to the depolarizing action of acetycholine.[147] Some confusion exists in the literature regarding the relative importance of the two effects in producing the neuromuscular blockade. Apparently, this is because prejunctional inhibition is predominant in fast-twitch muscle preparations and postjunctional inhibition is predominant in slow-twitch preparations.[151] Since the prejunctional inhibition and the neuromuscular blockade are both reversed by calcium, the prejunctional effect is probably the most important component in aminoglycoside-induced blockade in humans.[152]

The neuromuscular reaction is potentially fatal, since respiratory paralysis may occur. The condition is treated by administering calcium gluconate and an anticholinesterase drug, such as neostigmine.

Ototoxicity

The aminoglycosides are ototoxic. Both the hearing and balance functions of the inner ear can be affected. The aminoglycosides differ with respect to the type of toxicity that occurs most often.[153] Streptomycin primarily affects the vestibular system, whereas neomycin, kanamycin, and amikacin are primarily toxic to the cochlea. Gentamicin and tobramycin show both vestibular and cochlear toxicity, with vestibular toxicity occurring more frequently. In a series of 11,000 hospitalized patients monitored for all types of drug reactions, aminoglycosides were associated with a higher frequency of drug-induced deafness than any other group of drugs.[154] In a review of the clinical literature up to 1976, investigators found that the relative incidence of ototoxicity (vestibular plus cochlear) among the commonly used aminoglycosides was kanamycin > amikacin > gentamicin = tobramicin.[155] Although it appears that netilmicin is less ototoxic than the other aminoglycosides, the incidence of ototoxicity is not negligible. In one trial it occurred in 10% of patients.[156] Predisposing factors include preexisting renal impairment, prior or concomitant therapy with other ototoxic drugs, and therapy for longer than 10 days.[155] If loss of hearing or balance is not extensive, termination of the drug therapy will usually result in complete return to normal function. After extensive damage, however, a permanent decrease in hearing acuity or even complete deafness can occur. The el-

derly also seem more susceptible to ototoxicity.

Patients treated with aminoglycosides should be carefully monitored for signs of ototoxicity. It is not enough to casually test for loss of hearing acuity by observing if the patient responds to questions asked in a low tone of voice. The first hearing loss that takes place is in the high-tone range, and there can be considerable loss of function before there is any noticeable change in the range of normal conversational speech. Therefore, a patient can suffer significant loss of ability to appreciate music, for example, if the drug is stopped only when the hearing decrement is readily apparent by voice testing. For this reason, patients receiving aminoglycosides should have their hearing acuity monitored by audiometry.[157] Vestibular function may be evaluated by quantitative caloric stimulation.[157] Patients should be advised to alert the physician if they experience tinnitus, a sensation of fullness in the ears, oscillopsia, ataxia, or vertigo. Although ototoxicity does not generally appear earlier than 5 days after initiation of therapy, changes in cochlear potential in response to a sound stimulus (detected by electrocochleography) may be transiently reduced in some patients after a single injection of aminoglycoside.[158]

Ototoxicity is the most frequent toxic effect that limits therapy with the aminoglycosides. Great caution must thus be taken to ensure appropriate reduction of the drug dosage and monitoring of serum levels in patients with compromised renal function. If possible, the aminoglycosides should not be used with other drugs that are ototoxic. Ethacrynic acid and furosamide are both potentially ototoxic and the risk of ototoxicity is increased in patients receiving either of these drugs and an aminoglycoside.[159–161]

The aminoglycosides readily penetrate into inner ear fluid and their half-lives in perilymph (10–12 h) are much longer than their serum half-lives (about 2 h).[162] Thus, tissues in contact with the perilymphatic and endolymphatic fluids are exposed to high concentrations of drug for long periods of time. It is clear that the primary toxic effect is on the peripheral sensory portions of the inner ear and not on the eighth nerve itself.[163,164] The primary pathophysiological lesion, both in patients who develop symptoms of ototoxicity[157,165] and in model animal systems,[166,167] is destruction of hair cells in the organ of Corti. At low doses, hair cells in the basal turn of the cochlea are affected first, with destruction progressing toward the apex as the aminoglycoside dosage is increased.[166,167] This progression is consistent with clinical experience, since the basal region responds to high-frequency sounds and the apex to low-frequency sounds.

The biochemical mechanism of the toxic effect has not been firmly established, but recent evidence strongly suggests that it is due to free radicals generated by an aminoglycoside-iron chelate. It seems clear that the ototoxicity is not caused by inhibition of protein synthesis.[168] Kanamycin has been shown to cause a marked decrease in the activity of several enzymes involved in carbohydrate metabolism and energy utilization in the organ of Corti,[169,170] but these are probably secondary effects. Aminoglycosides do not readily pass across cell membranes and it seems likely that at least the rapid and reversible toxicity results from an interaction of the drug with superficial membrane structures. At this stage in our understanding of the toxic effect, a model based on the interaction of aminoglycosides with acidic groups on membrane phospholipids deserves special attention. It has been known for many years that phosphatidylinositol is selectively active in binding calcium, and Corrado and colleagues[171] originally suggested that aminoglycosides block calcium flux through artificial membranes by binding to calcium binding sites on phosphatidylinositol. The likely binding sites for the calcium ion or for the strongly cationic aminoglycoside are the negatively charged phosphate groups on the phospholipid.

Several observations suggest that there may be a causal relationship between binding of aminoglycosides to polyphosphoinositides and ototoxicity.[172] It has been shown, for example, that perfusion of guinea pig cochlea with artificial perilymph containing a high concentration of neomycin causes a rapid reduction in its ability to generate an acoustic current (ac) potential in response to a sound stimulus.[173] If radioactive phosphate is also added to the artificial perilymph, neomycin decreases the incorporation of the phosphate into phosphatidylinositol diphosphate in the cochlear membrane.[168,174] If guinea pigs are subcutaneously injected with large doses of neomycin for 3 weeks, and the cochlea are then perfused for a short time with radioactive phosphate, the effect of the systemically administered drug can be studied by rapidly fixing the tissue to prevent biochemical degradation and removing individual components by microdissection. It has thus been shown that neomycin decreases incorporation of phosphate into phosphatidylinositol diphosphate but not into other phospholipids in both the organ of Corti and the stria vascularis.[174] This location of the drug effect on phosphatidylinositol metabolism agrees with the localization of early changes viewed by histological means.[164] Neomycin and the other aminoglycosides have also been shown to competitively inhibit the binding of radioactive calcium ion to homogenates of these tissues[174] and to phosphoinositides in artificial membranes.[175] Binding of aminoglycosides to phosphatidylinositol has been demonstrated directly.[176,177] In fact, a neomycin-containing affinity column has been used to isolate ^{32}P-labeled phophadidylinositol phosphate and diphosphate from inner ear tissues and kidney.[177]

The irreversible toxicity appears to result from progressive free-radical damage to the hair cells of the inner ear. This hypothesis derives from the demonstration that aminoglycosides by themselves are not toxic to isolated hair cells[178] but require activation to be cytotoxic.[179] The activator is iron. It has been shown, for example, that gentamicin acts as an iron chelator and, as with other metal chelates, the iron-gentamicin complex is a potent catalyst of free-radical formation.[180] The strong binding of aminoglycosides to phosphoinositides would facilitate the generation of free radicals at the cell membrane, leading to progressive hair cell destruction.[181]

The importance of this model mechanism is that it suggests a means of preventing the toxicity by preventing formation of the iron-aminoglycoside complex. Thus, coadministration of the iron chelators desferioxamine and dihydroxybenzoic acid were shown to protect guinea pigs from gentamicin ototoxicity.[182] Importantly, neither the serum level nor the antibacterial activity of gentamicin was affected by coadministration of the iron chelator. The effectiveness of this treatment extends to other aminoglycosides and to both vestibular and cochlear damage,[181,182] raising the possibility that coadministration of an iron chelator may become a standard component of aminoglycoside treatment.

Studies of a pharmacogenetic trait where there is a familial susceptibility to aminoglycoside antibiotic–induced deafness (AAID) have provided another mechanism for permanent deafness.[183] The predisposition to deafness is maternally transmitted; thus, AAID is a mitochondrial inheritance. In those families where the mitochondrial genome was sequenced, a single adenine-to-guanine substitution was found in the 12S rRNA.[184] The mutation is located in a highly conserved region of the 12S RNA in which the aminoglycosides are known to bind.[185] As a result of the 12S rRNA mutation, there is likely to be increased misreading of the genetic code and production of faulty mitochondrial proteins. Examination of the oxidative phosphorylation enzyme activity in lymphoblastoid cell lines from one AAID pedigree revealed normal activity for enzyme complexes I and IV but increased activity for complexes III and V in deaf individuals compared to unaffected siblings.[186] It is likely that a similar mitochondrial insult occurs in the cochlear cells of genetically normal people treated with aminoglycosides but at much lower incidence and severity than those with AAID.

Nephrotoxicity

The aminoglycosides cause a nephrotoxicity that usually presents as an acute tubular necrosis manifest by proteinuria, cylinduria, and inability to concentrate the urine.[139] This is followed by a reduction in glomerular filtration rate with a rise in serum creatinine and blood urea nitrogen. This toxicity apparently is a result of accumulation and retention of aminoglycoside in the proximal tubular cells. The renal damage is usually reversible on cessation of therapy. Neomycin is the most nephrotoxic aminoglycoside and streptomycin is the least nephrotoxic. The relative toxicity of the different aminoglycosides correlates with their concentration in the renal cortex in experimental animals, but clinical studies have not consistently agreed with this finding. Several controlled studies of gentamicin and tobramycin usage have given different estimates of their relative toxicities.[187–190] Although the relative nephrotoxic potential of the other aminoglycosides is difficult to assess, tobramycin appears to be about half as nephrotoxic as gentamicin or amikacin.[191,192] Nephrotoxicity is more common in elderly patients, those with pre-existing renal disease, and those receiving other nephrotoxic drugs, such as methoxyfluorane,[193] amphotericin B,[194] cephalothin,[195] or cisplatinum.[196] Those patients taking the drug for extended periods of time, and those exhibiting hypotension, volume depletion or high peak or trough serum concentrations are also at increased risk for nephrotoxicity.[142] Although preexisting renal impairment and old age have been identified as risk factors, the association is believed to result from inappropriate dosing in the presence of diminished renal function.[197,198]

Bennet et al.[199] have reviewed the pathophysiology of the nephrotoxicity in detail. As discussed previously, aminoglycosides are excreted by glomerular filtration and there is a small amount of tubular reabsorption. Reabsorption occurs in the proximal tubule[200] and the drugs accumulate to high levels in renal tissue.[198,201] Autoradiographic studies show that aminoglycosides are transported into proximal tubule cells by pinocytosis and the resulting phagocytic vacuoles fuse with lysosomes.[202,203] After aminoglycosides are taken up, prominent myeloid bodies appear in the lysosomes of proximal tubular cells.[204,205]

This pathway of events may very well be determined by the same interaction of aminoglycosides with polyphosphoinositides that was discussed in the previous section. High levels of polyphosphoinositides are found in kidney tissue.[206] It has been shown that neomycin binds to polyphosphoinositides[177] and inhibits their dephosphorylation in rat kidney[207] in the same way as discussed above for synaptosomes and tissues of the inner ear. Radiolabeled gentamicin has been shown to bind to a saturable number of sites ($K_D = 0.2$ mM) on the brush-border membranes of proximal tubular cells[208] and the uptake of gentamicin by renal cortical slices is inhibited by the other aminoglycosides.[200] Thus, the aminoglycosides bind first to a limited number of binding sites on the luminal surface of the proximal tubule cell and the binding occurs in the same concentration range as binding to purified phosphatidylinositol diphosphate.[175]

After binding to the luminal surface of the proximal tubule cell and internalization and fusion with lysosomes, the aminoglycosides may interfere with phospholipid metabolism. This is suggested by studies in cultured rat embryo fibroblasts which have been shown to accumulate aminoglycosides selectively within lysosomes[209] where they remain sequestered because of ion trapping.[210] Like renal tubular cells, fibroblasts exposed to gentamicin develop prominent myeloid bodies and chemical analysis of the lysosomes shows an increase in all of the major phospholipids,[211] including two polar lipids that may represent phosphatidylinositol phosphate and diphosphate. Interaction with phospholipids may impair the generation of membrane-derived autocoids and intracellular second messengers such as prostaglandins, inositol phosphates, and diacylglycerol. Changes in prostaglandin metabolism might explain the relationship between tubular damage and reduction in glomerular filtration rate.[212] Calcium has been shown to inhibit the uptake and binding of aminoglycosides to the renal brush-border luminal membrane in vitro and supplemental dietary calcium decreases nephrotoxicity in experimental systems.[213] As discussed above in regard to ototoxicity, iron chelators have been shown to reduce renal injury in rats,[214] suggesting that catalysis of free-radical formation by iron-aminoglycoside complexes may play an important role in nephrotoxicity.

Table 5–7. Precautions and contraindications of the aminoglycosides.

Aminoglycosides and various penicillins chemically interact in a 1:1 molar ratio, usually resulting in loss of aminoglycoside activity. Thus, simultaneous administration should be avoided.

The ototoxicity produced by ethacrynic acid can be additive with the aminoglycosides.

Additive or synergistic nephrotoxicity may occur when aminoglycosides are given with other nephrotoxic drugs such as vancomycin or amphotericin B.

The neuromuscular blockade produced by skeletal muscle relaxants can be potentiated by the aminoglycosides.

Table 5–7 describes the precautions and contraindications associated with the use of the aminoglycosides.

Properties and Therapeutic Uses of the Individual Aminoglycosides

Gentamicin, tobramycin, amikacin and netilmicin are the most important aminoglycosides for treatment of serious infection due to aerobic gram-negative bacilli. These drugs are active against most Enterobacteriaceae and *Pseudomonas aeruginosa* strains (see Table 5–4). These four drugs are often used interchangeably for the treatment of most of these infections. Because of their potent bactericidal action on gram-negative bacteria, one of these drugs is often used in combination with a β-lactam antibiotic when there is need for broad-spectrum bactericidal chemotherapy, as in treating serious infection due to suspected gram-negative pathogens and in treating bacteremia in the immunocompromised host.[215,216]

Gentamicin

Gentamicin has been in clinical use longer than the other broad-spectrum, antipseudomonal aminoglycosides.[84,85,217] Gentamicin is often used to treat serious infections due to gram-negative bacilli, particularly those due to *Pseudomonas aeruginosa, Enterobacter, Escherichia coli, Klebsiella*, indole-positive *Proteus* strains, and *Serratia*. It is used in combination with an appropriate β-lactam antibiotic for treatment of deep-seated and severe infections due to *Pseudomonas aeruginosa* because the combination is synergistic against many strains.[67-69] Gentamicin is synergistic with a penicillin[72] or vancomycin[218] against enterococci and with a penicillin against viridans group streptococci.[73] Gentamicin is active against most strains of *Staphylococcus aureus* but it is not used for this purpose clinically. Resistance to gentamicin is more common among hospital isolates and methicillin-resistant *S. aureus* strains than resistance to amikacin. Most gentamicin-resistant Enterobacteriaceae are cross-resistant to tobramycin but are susceptible to amikacin.[62] Many gentamicin-resistant strains of *Pseudomonas aeruginosa* are susceptible to both tobramycin and amikacin.[62] Gentamicin is more nephrotoxic than tobramycin, but roughly equivalent in ototoxic potential.

Tobramycin

Tobramycin is pharmacologically similar to gentamicin (cf. Table 5–5).[86] The spectrum of antibacterial activity is also similar, except that tobramycin is much less active against enterococci[219] and *Serratia* and it is two to four times more active against *Pseudomonas aeruginosa*.[220,221] Some strains of *P. aeruginosa* that are resistant to gentamicin retain sensitivity to tobramycin.[62] Indications for the use of tobramycin are essentially identical to those for gentamicin. In contrast to several of the aminoglycosides, tobramycin is not active against mycobacteria.[222] Tobramicin is less nephrotoxic than gentamicin[191,192] and roughly equivalent to gentamicin in its ototoxic potential.[155]

Amikacin

Amikacin[87] is produced by chemical modification of the kanamycin structure (see Figure 5–5). The chemical change makes the drug resistant to most of the aminoglycoside-modifying enzymes. As a consequence, there is a low incidence of ami-

kacin resistance among clinical isolates,[62] and amikacin has the broadest spectrum of activity of the aminoglycosides against gram-negative bacilli. Gram-negative bacteria that become resistant to amikacin are usually resistant to gentamicin and tobramycin.[62,63] The pharmacokinetics of amikacin are like those of its parent drug kanamycin and it is less active by weight than gentamicin or tobramycin.[87] Thus, like kanamycin, it is administered in higher dosage than gentamicin and tobramycin and peak serum levels are higher (see Table 5–5). Amikacin is reported to be more nephrotoxic than tobramycin[191] and it may be more ototoxic than either gentamicin or tobramycin,[155] although some studies show no difference.[223]

Amikacin is clearly a very useful addition to the drugs that are used to treat gram-negative infections in hospitalized patients. The use of this drug should be limited to the treatment of severe infection by *Pseudomonas aeruginosa* strains and enteric bacilli that are suspected of being resistant to gentamicin and tobramycin. Restriction of amikacin use is advocated to minimize the emergence of resistant strains of bacteria.

Netilmicin

Netilmicin is the newest of the aminoglycosides to be marketed. Netilmicin[217,224] is a semisynthetic aminoglycoside that is resistant to many of the aminoglycoside-modifying enzymes that inactivate gentamicin. The pharmacokinetics and the spectrum of activity of netilmicin are similar to those of gentamicin, and it is active against some gentamicin-resistant isolates of *Escherichia coli, Klebsiella*, and *Enterobacter*. It is less active than gentamicin against *Pseudomonas aeruginosa*.[224] Netilmicin has been found to be less ototoxic than other aminoglycosides in animal models[225] and it appears to be less ototoxic and nephrotoxic than gentamicin in clinical trials.[224]

Kanamycin

Kanamycin is active against enteric bacilli like *Klebsiella, Enterobacter, Escherichia coli*, and *Proteus*. It is not active against

Pseudomonas aeruginosa or *Serratia*. Because resistance is common and because it is somewhat more toxic than gentamicin or tobramycin, the use of kanamycin has declined markedly since the 1960s. Kanamycin is administered orally to kill the bowel flora prior to intestinal surgery.

Neomycin

Neomycin is very nephrotoxic and is no longer administered parenterally. Like kanamycin, neomycin is administered orally to kill the bowel flora prior to intestinal surgery, but this constitutes a local use because there is no absorption from the gastrointestinal tract. The primary use of neomycin is in the topical treatment of superficial infections of the skin and eye. Neomycin is present in a large number of topical formulations, many of which also contain bacitracin or polymixin B. The use of these preparations (of which there are at least 100 different forms) has been criticized because their value in the treatment of skin infections has not been clearly established and because neomycin produces contact allergic reactions. In several studies, neomycin has been found to be the most frequent cause of drug-induced contact sensitivity in humans.[226] Neomycin is often present in wound-irrigating solutions and enough drug can be absorbed from the wound area to produce both ototoxicity and nephrotoxicity.[95]

Streptomycin

The role of streptomycin in therapy has declined considerably since the advent of the newer aminoglycosides, the broad-spectrum penicillins, and the cephalosporins. It is still employed in combination with a penicillin to treat bacterial endocarditis due to *S. viridans* and enterococcus. Many physicians now employ gentamicin and ampicillin or penicillin G for the latter condition, however. Streptomycin is still used in the treatment of tuberculosis (see discussion of tuberculosis therapy in Chapter 11). Either alone or in combination with another antibiotic, streptomycin is still useful in the treatment of several rather uncommon infections including plague (*Yersinia pestis*), tularemia (*Franci-*

sella tularensis), glanders (*Pseudomonas mallei*), and severe cases of brucellosis (*Brucella abortus*).

Paromomycin

Paromomycin is a broad-spectrum aminoglycoside that is used only for treating intestinal amebiasis[227] and tapeworm infections. Paromomycin is given orally and it is not absorbed from the gastrointestinal tract. Thus, it is effective against organisms in the intestine and is not effective in treating amebic abscess in the liver.

REFERENCES

1. Kapusnik, J. E., C. J. Hackbarth, H. F. Chambers, T. Carpenter, and M. A. Sande. Single, large, daily doses versus intermittent dosing of tobramycin for treating experimental pseudomonas pneumonia. *J. Infect. Dis.* 1988;158:7.

2. Blaser, J. Efficacy of once and thrice daily dosing of aminoglycosides in in vitro models of infection. *J. Antimicrob. Chemother.* 1991;21(Suppl. C):21.

3. Hancock, R. E. W. Aminoglycoside uptake and mode of action—with special reference to streptomycin and gentamicin. II. Effects of aminoglycosides on cells. *J. Antimicrob. Chemother.* 1981;8:429.

4. Pestka, S. Inhibitors of ribosome functions. *Annu. Rev. Microbiol.* 1971;25:487.

5. Gorini, L. Streptomycin and misreading of the genetic code. In *Ribosomes*, ed. by M. Nomura, A. Tissieres, and P. Lengyel. Cold Spring Harbor: Cold Spring Harbor Laboratories, 1974, pp. 791–803.

6. Haselkorn, R., and L. B. Rothman-Denes. Protein synthesis. *Annu. Rev. Biochem.* 1973;42:397.

7. Weissbach, H., and S. Pestka, eds. *Molecular Mechanisims of Protein Synthesis*. New York: Academic Press, 1977.

8. Zubat, G. *Biochemistry*, 3rd ed. Dubuque, IA: William C. Brown, 1993.

9. Matthews, C. K., and K. E. van Holde. *Biochemistry*, 2nd ed. Redwood City, CA: Benjamin/Cumings Publishing, 1996.

10. Noller, H. F. tRNA-rRNA interactions and peptidyl transferase. *FASEB J.* 1993;7:87.

11. Davis, B. D. Role of subunits in the ribosome cycle. *Nature* 1971;231:153.

12. Flaks, J. G., E. C. Cox, M. L. Witting, and J. R. White. Polypeptide synthesis with ribosomes from streptomycin-resistant and dependent E. coli *Biochem. Biophys. Res. Commun.* 1962;7:390.

13. Speyer, J. F., P. Lengyel, and C. Basilio. Ribisomal localization of streptomycin sensitivity. *Proc. Natl. Acad. Sci. U.S.A.* 1962;48:684.

14. Davies, J. E. Studies on the ribosomes of streptomycin-sensitive and resistant strains of *Escherichia coli. Proc. Natl. Acad. Sci. U.S.A.* 1964;51:659.

15. Traub, P., and M. Nomura. Structure and func-

tion of *Escherichia coli* ribosomes; VI. Mechanism of assembly of 30S ribosomes studied in vitro. *J. Mol. Biol.* 1969;40:391.

16. Ozaki, M., S. Mizuchima, and M. Nomura. Identification and functional characterization of the protein controlled by the streptomycin-resistant locus in *E. coli. Nature* 1969;222:333.

17. Funatsu, G., and H. G. Wittman. Ribosomal proteins. XXXIII. Location of amino-acid replacements in protein S12 isolated from *Escherichia coli* mutants resistant to streptomycin. *J. Mol. Biol.* 1972; 68:547.

18. Brimacombe, R., G. Stöffler, and H. G. Wittmann. Ribosome structure. *Annu. Rev. Biochem.* 1978; 47:217.

19. Biswas, D. K., and L. Gorini. The attachment site of streptomycin to the 30S ribosomal subunit. *Proc. Natl. Acad. Sci. U.S.A.* 1972;69:2141.

20. Stöffler, G., and G. W. Tischendorf. Antibiotic receptor-sites in *Escherichia coli* ribosomes. In *Drug Receptor Interactions in Antimicrobial Chemotherapy*, ed. by J. Drews and F. E. Hahn. New York: Springer-Verlag, 1975, pp. 117–143.

21. Pongs, O., and V. A. Erdman. Affinity labeling of *E. coli* ribosomes with a streptomycin-analogue. *FEBS Lett.* 1973;37:47.

22. Girshovich, A. S., E. S. Bochkareva, and Y. A. Ovchinnikov. Identification of components of the streptomycin-binding center of *E. coli* MRE 600 ribosomes by photo-affinity labelling. *Mol. Gen. Genet.* 1976;144:205.

23. Sherman, M. I. The role of ribosomal conformation in protein biosynthesis. Further studies with streptomycin. *Eur. J. Biochem.* 1972;25:291.

24. Brakier-Gingras, L., G. Boileau, S. Glorieux, and N. Brisson. Streptomycin-induced conformational changes in the 70S bacterial ribosome. *Biochim. Biophys. Acta* 1978;521:413.

25. Martinez, O., D. Vazquez, and J. Modolell. Streptomycin- and viomycin-induced conformational changes of ribosomes detected by iodination. *FEBS Lett.* 1978;87:21.

26. Chang, F. N., and J. G. Flaks. Binding of dihydrostreptomycin to *Escherichia coli* ribosomes: characteristics and equilibrium of the reaction. *Antimicrob. Agents Chemother.* 1972;2:294.

27. Davis, B. D., P.-C. Tai, and B. J. Wallace. Complex interactions of antibiotics with the ribosome. In *Ribosomes*, ed. by M. Nomura, A. Tissieres, and P. Lengyel. Cold Spring Harbor: Cold Spring Harbor Laboratory, 1974, pp. 771–789.

28. Davies, J., L. Gorini, and B. D. Davis. Misreading of RNA codewords induced by aminoglycoside antibiotics. *Mol. Pharmacol.* 1965;1:93.

29. Tai, P.-C., B. J. Wallace, and B. D. Davis. Streptomycin causes misreading of natural messenger by interacting with ribosomes after initiation. *Proc. Natl. Acad. Sci. U.S.A.* 1978;75:275.

30. Hornig, H., P. Wooley, and R. Lührmann. Decoding at the ribosomal A site: antibiotics, misreading and energy of aminoacyl-tRNA binding. *Biochimie* 1987;69:803.

31. Busse, H. J., C. Wöstmann, and E. Bakker. The

bactericidal action of streptomycin. *J. Gen. Microbiol.* 1992;138:551.

32. Bryan, L. E. General mechanisms of resistance to antibiotics. *J. Antimicrob. Chemother.* 1988; 22(Suppl. A):1.

33. McCormack, J. P., and P. J. Jewesson. A critical evaluation of the "therapeutic range" of aminoglycosides. *Clin. Infect. Dis.* 1992;14:320–339.

34. Dubin, D. T., R. Hancock, and B. D. Davis. The sequence of some effects of streptomycin in *Escherichia coli. Biochim. Biophys. Acta* 1963;74:476.

35. Luzzatto, L., D. Apirion, and D. Schlessinger: Polyribosome depletion and blockage of the ribosome cycle by streptomycin in *Escherichia coli. J. Mol. Biol.* 1969;42:315.

36. Wallace, B. J., P.-C. Tai, E. L. Herzog, and B. D. Davis. Partial inhibition of polysomal ribosomes of *Escherichia coli* by streptomycin. *Proc. Natl. Acad. Sci. U.S.A.* 1973;70:1234.

37. Tai, P.-C., B. J. Wallace, E. L. Herzog, and B. D. Davis. Properties of initiation-free polysomes of *Escherichia coli. Biochemistry* 1973;12:609.

38. Modolell, J., and B. D. Davis. Breakdown by streptomycin of initiation complexes formed on ribosomes of *Escherichia coli. Proc. Natl. Acad. Sci. U.S.A.* 1970;67:1148.

39. Wallace, B. J., and B. D. Davis. Cyclic blockade of initiation sites by streptomycin-damaged ribosomes in *Escherichia coli*: an explanation for dominance of sensitivity. *J. Mol. Biol.* 1973;75:377.

40. Davies, J. Bacterial resistance to aminoglycoside antibiotics. *J. Infec. Dis.* 1971;124 Suppl:S7.

41. Misumi, M., T. Nishimura, T. Komai, and N. Tanaka. Interaction of kanamycin and related antibiotics with the large subunit of ribosomes and the inhibition of translocation. *Biochem. Biophys. Res. Commun.* 1978;84:358.

42. LeGoffic, F., M.-L. Capmau, F. Tangy, and M. Baillarge. Mechanism of action of aminoglycoside antibiotics: binding studies of tobramycin and its 6'-N-acetyl derivative to the bacterial ribosome and its subunits. *Eur. J. Biochem.* 1979;102:73.

43. Kühlberger, R., W. Piepersberg, A. Petzet, P. Buckel, and A. Böck. Alteration of ribosomal protein L6 in gentamicin-resistant strains of *Escherichia coli.* Effects on fidelity of protein synthesis. *Biochemistry* 1979;18:187.

44. Davies, J., and B. D. Davis. Misreading of ribonucleic acid code words induced by aminoglycoside antibiotics: the effect of drug concentration. *J. Biol. Chem.* 1968;243:3312.

45. Tai, P.-C., and B. D. Davis. Triphasic concentration effects of gentamicin on activity and misreading in protein synthesis. *Biochemistry* 1979;18:193.

46. Zierhut, G., W. Piepersberg, and A. Böck. Comparative analysis of the effect of aminoglycosides on bacterial protein synthesis. *Eur. J. Biochem.* 1979;98:577.

47. Shannon, K., and I. Phillips. Mechanisms of resistance to aminoglycosides in clinical isolates. *J. Antimicrob. Chemother.* 1982;9:91.

48. Bryan, L. E., R. Haraphongse, and H. M. Van Den Elzen. Gentamicin resistance in clinical isolates of

Pseudomonas aeruginosa associated with diminished gentamicin accumulation and no detectable enzymatic modification. *J. Antibiot.* 1976;29:743.

49. Hancock, R. E. W. Aminoglycoside uptake and mode of action—with special reference to streptomycin and gentamicin. I. Antagonists and mutants. *J. Antimicrob. Chemother.* 1981;8:249.

50. Davies, J., and D. I. Smith. Plasmid-determined resistance to antimicrobial agents. *Annu. Rev. Microbiol.* 1978;32:469.

51. Reynolds, A. V., and J. T. Smith. Enzymes which modify aminoglycoside antibiotics. *Rec. Adv. Infect.* 1979, 1:165.

52. Bryan, L. E., and H. M. Van Den Elzen. Streptomycin accumulation in susceptible and resistant strains of *Escherichia coli* and *Pseudomonas aeruginosa*. *Antimicrob. Agents Chemother.* 1976;9:928.

53. Bryan, L. E., and H. M. Van Den Elzen. Effects of membrane-energy mutations and cations on streptomycin and gentamicin accumulation by bacteria: a model for entry of streptomycin and gentamicin in susceptible and resistant bacteria. *Antimicrob. Agents Chemother.* 1977;12:163.

54. Bryan, L. E., T. Nicas, B. W. Holloway, and C. Crowther. Aminoglycoside-resistant mutation of *Pseudomonas aeruginosa* defective in cythochrome c_{552} and nitrate reductase. *Antimicrob. Agents Chemother.* 1980;17:71.

55. Mates, S. M., L. Patel, H. R. Kaback, and M. H. Miller. Membrane potential in anaerobically growing *Staph. aureus* and its relationship to gentamicin uptake. *Antimicrob. Agents Chemother.* 1983;23:526.

56. Davies, J., P. Courvalin, and D. Berg. Thoughts on the origins of resistance plasmids. *J. Antibiot. Chemother.* 1977;3(Suppl. C):7.

57. Yamada, T. D., D. Tipper, and J. Davies. Enzymatic inactivation of streptomycin by R-factor-resistant *Escherichia coli*. *Nature* 1968;219:288.

58. Dickie, P., L. E. Bryan, and M. A. Pickard. Effect of enzymatic adenylylation on dihydrostreptomycin accumulation in *Escherichia coli* carrying an R-factor: model explaining aminoglycoside resistance by inactivating mechanisms. *Antimicrob. Agents Chemother.* 1978;14:569.

59. Benveniste, R., and J. Davies. Enzymatic acetylation of aminoglycoside antibiotics by *Escherichia coli* carrying an R factor. *Biochemistry* 1971;10:1787.

60. Murray, B. E., New aspects of antimicrobial resistance and the relating therapeutic dilemmas. *J. Infect. Dis.* 1991;163:1184.

61. Moellering, R. C. Microbiological considerations in the use of tobramycin and related aminoglycosidic aminocyclitol antibiotics. *Med. J. Aust.* 1977; 2(Special Suppl.):4.

62. Moellering, R. C., C. Wennersten, L. J. Kunz, and J. W. Poitras. Resistance to gentamicin, tobramycin and amikacin among clinical isolates of bacteria. *Am. J. Med.* 1977;62:873.

63. Price, K. E., M. D. DeFuria, and T. A. Pursiano. Amikacin, an aminoglycoside with marked activity against antibiotic-resistant clinical isolates. *J. Infect. Dis.* 1976;134(Suppl.):S249.

64. Finland, M., C. Garner, C. Wilcox, and L. D.

Sabath. Susceptibility of "enterobacteria" to aminoglycoside antibiotics: comparisons with tetracyclines, polymyxins, chloramphenicol, and spectinomycin. *J. Infect. Dis.* 1976;134(Suppl.):S57.

65. Wiedemann, B., and H. Grimm. Susceptibility to antibiotics: species incidence and trends. In *Antibiotics in "Laboratory Medicine,"* 4th ed., ed. by V. Lorian. Baltimore: Williams and Wilkins, 1996, pp. 900–1168.

66. Richards, F., C. McCall, and C. Cox. Gentamicin treatment of staphylococcal infections. *JAMA*, 1971;215:1297.

67. Andreole, V. T. Synergy of carbenicillin and gentamicin in experimental infection with *Pseudomonas*. *J. Infect. Dis.* 1971;124(Suppl.):S46.

68. Smith, C. B., J. N. Wilfert, P. E. Dans, T. A. Kurrus, and M. Finland. In vitro activity of carbenicillin and results of treatment of infections due to *Pseudomonas* with carbenicillin singly and in combination with gentamicin. *J. Infect. Dis.* 1970;122(Suppl.):S14.

69. Fu, K. P., and H. C. Neu. Piperacillin, a new penicillin active against many bacteria resistant to other penicillins. *Antimicrob. Agents Chemother.* 1978;13:358.

70. D'Alessandri, R. M., D. J. McNeely, and R. M. Kluge. Antibiotic synergy and antagonism against clinical isolates of *Klebsiella* species. *Antimicrob. Agents Chemother.* 1976;10:889.

71. Jawetz, E., and M. Sonne. Penicillin-streptomycin treatment of enterococcal endocarditis: a re-evaluation. *N. Engl. J. Med.* 1966;274:710.

72. Moellering, R. C., C. Wennersten, and A. N. Weinberg. Studies on antibiotic synergism against enterococci. I. Bacteriologic studies. *J. Lab. Clin. Med.* 1971;77:821.

73. Duperval, R., N. J. Bill, J. E. Geraci, and J. A. Washington. Bactericidal activity of penicillin or clindamycin with gentamicin or streptomycin against species of *Viridans streptococci*. *Antimicrob. Agents Chemother.* 1975;9:673.

74. Moellering, R. C., and A. N. Weinberg. Studies on antibiotic synergism against enterococci. II. Effect of various antibiotics on the uptake of ^{14}C-labeled streptomycin by enterococci. *J. Clin. Invest.* 1971;50:2580.

75. Plotz, P., and B. D. Davis: Absence of a chloramphenicol-insensitive phase of streptomycin action. *J. Bacteriol.* 1962;83:802.

76. Klastersky, J., and M. Husson. Bactericidal activity of the combinations of gentamicin with clindamycin or chloramphenicol against species of *Escherichia coli* and *Bacteroides fragilis*. *Antimicrob. Agents Chemother.* 1977;12:135.

77. Sande, M. A., and J. W. Overton. In vivo antagonism between gentamicin and chloramphenicol in neutropenic mice. *J. Infect. Dis.* 1973;128:247.

78. Dresden, M. H., and M. B. Hoagland. Polyribosomes of *Escherichia coli*: breakdown during glucose starvation. *J. Biol. Chem.* 1967;242:1065.

79. Cross, A. S., S. Opal, and D. J. Kopecko. Progressive increase in antibiotic resistance of gram-negative bacterial isolates. Walter Reed Hospital, 1976–1980: specific analysis of gentamicin, tobramycin, and amikacin resistance. *Arch. Intern. Med.* 1983;143:2075.

80. O'Grady, F., H. P. Lambert, R. G. Finch, and D.

Greenwood. *Antibiotics and Chemotherapy*, 7th ed. New York: Churchill Livingstone, 1997.

81. Leroy, A., G. Humbert, G. Oksenhendler, and J. P. Fillastre. Pharmacokinetics of aminoglycosides in subjects with normal and impaired renal function. *Antibiotics Chemother.* 1978;25:163.

82. Mower, G. E. Aminoglycoside pharmacology. *Rec. Adv. Infect.* 1979;1:121.

83. Ristuccia, A. M., and B. A. Cunha. The aminoglycosides. *Med. Clin. North Am.* 1982;66:303.

84. International Symposium on Gentamicin. A new aminoglycoside antibiotic. *J. Infect. Dis.* 1969;119:540.

85. Second International Symposium on Gentamicin. An Aminoglycoside Antibiotic. *J. Infect. Dis.* 1971; 124(Suppl):S1–S300.

86. Symposium (various authors). Tobramycin. *J. Infect. Dis.* 1976;134(Suppl.):S1–S234.

87. Symposium (various authors). Advances in aminoglycoside therapy: amikacin. *J. Infect. Dis.* 1976; 134(Suppl.):S235–S460.

88. Kunin, C. M., T. C. Chalmers, C. M. Leevy, S. C. Sebastyen, C. S. Lieber, and M. Finland. Absorption of orally administered neomycin and kanamycin. *N. Engl. J. Med.* 1960;262:380.

89. Breen, K. J., R. E. Bryant, J. D. Levinson, and S. Schenker. Neomycin absorption in man; studies of oral and enema administration and effect of intestinal ulceration. *Ann. Intern. Med.* 1972;76:211.

90. Feathers, R. S., A. A. M. Lewis, G. R. Sagor, I. D. Amirak, and P. Noone. Prophylactic systemic antibiotics in colorectal surgery. *Lancet* 1977;2:4.

91. Clarke, J. S., R. E. Condon, J. G. Bartlett, S. L. Gorbach, R. L. Nichols and S. Ochi. Preoperative oral antibiotics reduce septic complications of colon operations: results of prospective, randomized, double-blind clinical study. *Ann. Surg.* 1977;186:251.

92. Noone, P., and J. R. Pattison. Therapeutic implications of interaction of gentamicin and penicillins. *Lancet* 1971;2:575.

93. Hale, D. C., R. Jenkins, and J. A. Matsen: In vitro inactivation of aminoglycoside antibiotics by perperacillin and carbenicillin. *Am. J. Clin. Pathol.* 1980; 74:316.

94. Weinstein, A. J., M. C. McHenry and T. L. Gavan. Systemic absorption of neomycin irrigating solution. *JAMA* 1977;238:152.

95. Davia, J. E., A. W. Siemsen, and R. W. Anderson. Uremia, deafness, and paralysis due to irrigating antibiotic solutions. *Arch. Intern. Med.* 1970; 125:135.

96. Pechere, J.-C., and R. Dugal. Clinical pharmacokinetics of aminoglycoside antibiotics. *Clin Pharmacokinet.* 1979;4:170.

97. Gordon, R. C., C. Regamey, and W. M. M. Kirby. Serum protein binding of the aminoglycoside antibiotics. *Antimicrob. Agents Chemother.* 1972;2:214.

98. Edwards, C. Q., C. R. Smith, K. L. Baugham, J. F. Rogers, and P. S. Leitman. Concentrations of gentamicin and amikacin in human kidneys. *Antimicrob. Agents Chemother.* 1976;9:925.

99. Dan, M., H. Halkin, and E. Rubinstein. Interstitial fluid concentrations of aminoglycosides. *J. Antimicrob. Chemother.* 1981;7:551.

100. Riff, L. J., and G. G. Jackson. Pharmacology of gentamicin in man. *J. Infect. Dis.* 1971;124(Suppl):S98.

101. Pitt, H. A., R. A. Roberts, and W. D. Johnson: Gentamicin levels in the human biliary tract. *J. Infect. Dis.* 1973;127:299.

102. Pennington, J. E. Penetration of antibiotics into respiratory secretions. *Rev. Infect. Dis.* 1981;3:67.

103. McCrae, W. M., J. A. Raeburn, and E. J. Hanson. Tobramycin therapy of infections due to *Pseudomonas aeruginosa* in patients with cystic fibrosis: effect of dosage and concentration of antibiotic in sputum. *J. Infect. Dis.* 1976;134(Suppl):S191.

104. Wong, G. A., T. H. Pierce, E. Goldstein, and P. Hoeprich. Penetration of antimicrobial agents into bronchial secretions. *Am. J. Med.* 1975;59:219.

105. Dee, T. H., and F. Kozin. Gentamicin and tobramycin penetration into synovial fluid. *Antimicrob Agents Chemother.* 1977;12:548.

106. Barza, M. Factors affecting the intraocular penetration of antibiotics. *Scand. J. Infect. Dis.* 1978; 14(Suppl.):151.

107. Strausbaugh, L. J., C. D. Mandaleris, and M. A. Sande. Comparison of four aminoglycoside antibiotics in the therapy of experimental *E. coli* meningitis. *J. Lab. Clin. Med.* 1977;89:692.

108. Rahal, J. J., P. H. Hyams, M. S. Simberkoff, and E. Rubinstein. Combined intrathecal and intramuscular gentamicin for gram-negative meningitis: pharmacologic study of 21 patients. *N. Engl. J. Med.* 1974;290: 1394.

109. Kaiser, A. B., and Z. A. McGee. Aminoglycoside therapy of gram-negative bacillary meningitis. *N. Engl. J. Med.* 1975;293:1215.

110. McCracken, G. H., and S. G. Mize. A controlled study of intrathecal antibiotic therapy in gram-negative enteric meningitis of infancy. *J. Pediatr.* 1976;89:66.

111. Kauffman, R. E., J. A. Morris, and D. L. Azarnoff. Placental transfer and fetal urinary excretion of gentamicin during constant rate maternal infusion. *Pediatr. Res.* 1975;9:104.

112. Conway, N., and B. D. Birt. Streptomycin in pregnancy: effect on the foetal ear. *BMJ* 1965;2:260.

113. Lortholary, O., M. Tod, Y. Cohen, and O. Petitjean. *Med. Clin. North Am.* 1995;79:761.

114. Verpooten, G. A., R. A. Giuliano, R. A., and L. V. Verbist. Once-daily dosing decreases renal accumulation of gentamicin and netilmicin. *Clin. Pharmacol. Ther.* 1989;45:22.

115. Cutler, R. E., and B. M. Orme. Correlation of serum creatinine concentration and kanamycin half-life. *JAMA* 1969;209:539.

116. Chan, R. A., E. J. Benner, and P. D. Hoeprich. Gentamicin therapy in renal failure: a nomogram for dosage. *Ann. Intern. Med.* 1972;76:773.

117. Pechere, J.-C., and R. Dugal. Pharmacokinetics of intravenously administered tobramycin in normal volunteers and in renal-impaired and hemodialyzed patients. *J. Infect. Dis.* 1976;134(Suppl.):S118.

118. Mower, G. E., S. B. Lucas, and J. G. McGough. Nomogram for kanamycin dosage. *Lancet* 1972;2:45.

119. Sarubbi, F. A., and J. H. Hull. Amikacin serum concentrations: prediction of levels and dosage guidelines. *Ann. Intern. Med.* 1978;89:612.

120. Barza, M., R. B. Brown, D. Shen, M. Gibaldi, and L. Weinstein. Predictability of blood levels of gentamicin in man. *J. Infect. Dis.* 1975;132:165.

121. McCracken, G. H., N. R. West, and L. J. Horton. Urinary excretion of gentamicin in the neonatal period. *J. Infect. Dis.* 1971;123:257.

122. Driessen, O. M. J., N. Sorgedrager, M. F. Michel, K. F. Kerrebijn, and J. Hermans. Pharmacokinetic aspects of therapy with ampicillin and kanamycin in newborn infants. *Eur. J. Clin. Pharmacol.* 1978;13:449.

123. Siber, G. R., P. Echeverria, A. L. Smith, J. W. Paisley, and D. H. Smith. Pharmacokinetics of gentamicin in children and adults. *J. Infect. Dis.* 1975;132:637.

124. Schwartz, S. N., G. J. Pazin, J. A. Lyon, M. Ho, and A. W. Pasculle. A controlled investigation of the pharmacokinetics of gentamicin and tobramycin in obese subjects. *J. Infect. Dis.* 1978;138:499.

125. Barza, M., and M. Lauermann. Why monitor serum levels of gentamicin? *Clin. Pharmacokin.* 1978;3:202.

126. Pennington, J. E., D. C. Dale, H. Y. Reynolds, and J. D. MacLowry. Gentamicin sulfate pharmacokinetics: lower levels of gentamicin in blood during fever. *J. Infect Dis.* 1975;132:270.

127. Loirat, P., J. Rohan, A. Baillet, F. Beaufils, R. David, and A. Chapman. Increased glomerular filtration rate in patients with major burns and its effect on the pharmacokinetics of tobramycin. *N. Engl. J. Med.* 1978;299:915.

128. Martin, A. J., C. A. Smalley, R. H. George, D. E. Healing, and C. M. Anderson. Gentamicin and tobramycin compared in the treatment of mucoid pseudomonas lung infections in cystic fibrosis. *Arch. Dis. Child* 1980;55:604.

129. Finkelstein, E., and K. Hall. Aminoglycoside clearance in patients with cystic fibrosis. *J. Pediatr.* 1979;94:163.

130. Rosenthal, A., L. N. Button, and K. T. Shaw. Blood volume changes in patients with cystic fibrosis. *Pediatrics* 1977;59:588.

131. Zaske, D. E., R. J. Cipolle, J. C. Rotschafer, L. D. Solem, N. R. Mosier and R. G. Strate. Gentamicin pharmacokinetics in 1,640 patients: method for control of serum concentrations. *Antimicrob. Agents Chemother.* 1982;21:407.

132. Reeves, D. S. Therapeutic drug monitoring of aminoglycoside antibiotics. *Infection* 1980;8(Suppl. 3):S313.

133. Wenk, M. Concepts for aminoglycoside serum level monitoring. *J. Antimicrob. Chemother.* 1982;9:171.

134. Reeves, D. S., and M. J. Bywater. Quality control of serum gentamicin assays—experience of national surveys. *J. Antimicrob. Chemother.* 1975;1:103.

135. Hewitt, W. L., and M. C. McHenry. Blood level determinations of antimicrobial drugs: some clinical considerations. *Med. Clin. North Am.* 1978;62:1119.

136. Dahlgren, J. G., E. T. Anderson, and W. L. Hewitt. Gentamicin blood levels: a guide to nephrotoxicity. *Antimicrob. Agents Chemother.* 1975;8:58.

137. Nordstrom, L., G. Banck, S. Belfrage, I. Jublin, O. Tjernstrom, and N. G. Toremalen. Prospective study of the ototoxicity of gentamicin. *Acta Pathol. Microbiol. Scand. B* 1973;81(Suppl. 241):58.

138. Black, R. E., W. K. Lau, R. J. Weinstein, L. S. Young, and W. L. Hewitt. Ototoxicity of amikacin. *Antimicrob. Agents Chemother.* 1975;9:956.

139. Appel, G. B., and H. C. Neu. The nephrotoxicity of antimicrobial agents. *N. Engl. J. Med.* 1977;296:663, 772, 784.

140. Ervin, F. R., W. E. Bullock, and C. E. Nuttall. Inactivation of gentamicin by penicillins in patients with renal failure. *Antimicrob. Agents Chemother.* 1976;9:1004.

141. Anderson, A. C., G. R. Hodges, and W. C. Barnes. Determination of serum gentamicin sulfate levels: ordering patterns and use as a guide to therapy. *Arch. Intern. Med.* 1976;136:785.

142. Begg, E. J., and M. L. Barclay. Aminoglycosides—50 years on. *Br. J. Clin. Pharmacol.* 1995;39:597.

143. Barclay, M. L., E. J. Begg, and K. G. Hickling. What is the evidence for once daily aminoglycoside therapy? *Clin. Pharmacol.* 1994;27:32.

144. Vogelman, B. S., and W. A. Craig. Kinetics of antimicrobial activity. *J. Pediatr.* 1986;108:835.

145. Dudley, M. N., and S. H. Zimmer. Single daily dosing of amikacin in an in vitro model. *J. Antimicrob. Chemother.* 1991;27:15.

146. Pittinger, C. B., Y. Eryasa, and R. Adamson. Antibiotic-induced paralysis. *Anesth. Analg.* 1970;49:487.

147. Pittinger, C., and R. Adamson. Antibiotic blockade of neuromuscular function. *Annu. Rev. Pharmacol.* 1972;12:169.

148. Holtzman, J. L. Gentamicin and neuromuscular blockade. *Ann. Intern. Med.* 1976;84:55.

149. Vital Brazil, O., and J. Prado-Franceschi. The nature of neuromuscular block produced by neomycin and gentamicin. *Arch. Intern. Pharmacodyn.* 1969;179:78.

150. Goodman, F. R., G. B. Weiss, and H. R. Adams. Alterations by neomycin of ^{45}Ca movements and contractile responses in vascular smooth muscle. *J. Pharmacol. Exp. Ther.* 1974;188:472.

151. Adams, H. R., B. P. Mathew, R. H. Teske, and H. D. Mercer. Neuromuscular blocking effects of aminoglycoside antibiotics on fast- and slow-contracting muscles of the cat. *Anesth. Analog.* 1976;55:500.

152. Sanders, W. E., and C. C. Sanders. Toxicity of antimicrobial agents: mechanism of action on mammalian cells. *Annu. Rev. Pharmacol. Toxicol.* 1979;19:53.

153. Brown, R. D., and A. M. Feldman: Pharmacology of hearing and otoxicity. *Annu. Rev. Pharmacol. Toxicol.* 1978;18:233.

154. Boston Collaborative Drug Surveillance Program. Drug-induced deafness. *JAMA* 1973;224:515.

155. Neu, H. C., and C. L. Bendush. Ototoxicity of tobramycin: a clinical overview. *J. Infect. Dis.* 1976;134(Suppl.):S206.

156. Trestman, I., J. Parsons, J. Santoro, G. Goodhart, and D. Kaye. Pharmacology and efficacy of netilmicin. *Antimicrob. Agents Chemother.* 1978;13:832.

157. Lerner, S. A., and G. J. Matz. Aminoglycoside ototoxiticy. *Am. J. Otolaryngol.* 1980;1:169.

158. Harpur, E. S., and P. G. Davey. Toxic effects of aminoglycosides. *J. Antimicrob. Chemother.* 1981;7: 313.

159. Meriwether, W. D., R. J. Mangi, and A. S. Serpick. Deafness following standard intravenous dose of ethacrynic acid. *JAMA* 1971;216:795.

160. West, B. A., R. E. Brummett, and D. L. Himes. Interaction of kanamycin and ethacrynic acid. *Arch. Otolaryngol.* 1973;98:32.

161. Quick, C. A., and W. Hoppe. Permanent deafness associated with furosamide administration. *Ann. Otol. Rhinol. Laryngol.* 1975;84:94.

162. Federspil, P., W. Schätzle, and E. Tiesler. Pharmacokinetics and ototoxicity of gentamicin, tobramycin, and amikacin. *J. Infect. Dis.* 1976;134(Suppl.): S200.

163. Wersäll, J., B. Bjorkroth, A. Flock, and P.-G. Lundquist. Experiments on ototoxic effects of antibiotics. *Adv. Otol.* 1973;20:14.

164. Hawkins, J. E. Biochemical aspects of ototoxicity. In *Biochemical Mechanisms in Hearing and Deafness*, ed. by M. M. Paparella. Springfield: Charles C. Thomas, 1970. pp. 323–339.

165. Lowry, L. D., M. May, and P. Pastore. Acute histopathologic inner ear changes in deafness due to neomycin: a case report. *Ann. Otol. Rhinol. Laryngol.* 1973;82:876.

166. Brummett, R. E., K. E. Fox, T. W. Bendrick, and D. L. Himes. Ototoxity of tobramycin, gentamicin, amikacin and sisomycin in the guinea pig. *J. Antimicrob Chemother.* 1978;4(Suppl. A):73.

167. Brummett, R. E. Effects of antibiotic-diuretic interactions on the guinea pig model of ototoxicity. *Rev. Infect. Dis.* 1981;3(Suppl):S216.

168. Stockhorst, E. and J. Schacht. Radioactive labeling of phospholipids and proteins by cochlea perfusion in the guinea pig and the effect of neomycin. *Acta Otolaryngol.* 1977;83:401.

169. Kaku, Y., J. C. Farmer, and W. R. Hudson. Ototoxic drug effects on cochlear histochemistry. *Arch. Otolaryngol.* 1973;98:282

170. Tachibana, M., O. Mizukoshi, and K. Kuriyama. Inhibitory effects of kanamycin on glycolysis in cochlea and kidney—possible involvement in the formation of oto- and nephrotoxicities. *Biochem. Pharmacol.* 1976;25:2297.

171. Corrado, A. P., W. A. Prado, and I. Pimenta de Morais. Competitive antagonism between calcium and aminoglycoside antibiotics in skeletal and smooth muscles. In *Concepts of Membranes in Regulation and Exitation*, ed. by M. Rocha e Silva and G. Suarez-Kurtz. New York: Raven Press, 1975, pp. 201–215.

172. Schacht J. Interaction of neomycin with phosphoinositide metabolism in guinea pig inner ear and brain tissues. *Ann. Otol. Rhinol. Laryngol.* 1974;83: 613.

173. Nuttall, A. L., D. M. Marques, and M. Lawrence. Effects of perilymphatic perfusion with neomycin on the cochlear microphonic potential in the guinea pig. *Acta Otolaryngol.* 1977;83:393.

174. Orsulakova, A., E. Stockhorst, and J. Schacht. Effect of neomycin on phosphoinositide labeling and calcium binding in guinea pig inner ear tissues in vivo and in vitro. *J. Neurochem.* 1976;26: 285.

175. Lodhi, S., N. D. Weiner, and J. Schacht. Interactions of neomycin and calcium in synaptosomal membranes and polyphosphoinositide monolayers. *Biochim. Biophys. Acta* 1976;426:781.

176. Alexander, A. M., I. Gonda, E. S. Harpur, and J. B. Kayes. Interaction of aminoglycoside antibiotics with phospholipid liposomes studied by microelectrophoresis. *J. Antibiot.* 1979;32:505.

177. Schacht, J. Isolation of an aminoglycoside receptor from guinea pig inner ear tissues and kidney. *Arch. Otorhinolaryngol.* 1979;224:129.

178. Dulon, D., G. Zajic, J. M. Aran, and J. Schacht. Aminoglycoside antibiotics impair calcium entry but not viability and motility in isolated cochlear outer hair cells. *J. Neurosci. Res.* 1989;24:333.

179. Crann, S. A., and J. Schacht. Activation of aminoglycoside antibiotics to cytotoxins. *Audiol. Neurootol.* 1996;1:80.

180. Priuska, E. M., and J. Schacht. Formation of free radicals by gentamicin and iron and evidence for an iron/gentamicin complex. *Biochem. Pharmacol.* 1995;50:1749.

181. Sha, S.-H., and J. Schacht. Prevention of aminoglycoside-induced hearing loss. *Keio J. Med.* 1997;46:115.

182. Song, B.-S., D. J. Anderson, and J. Schacht. Protection from gentamicin ototoxicity by iron chelators in guinea pig in vivo. *J. Pharmacol. Exp. Ther.* 1997;282: 369.

183. Weber, W. W. *Pharmacogenetics.* New York: Oxford University Press, 1997, pp. 279–283.

184. Prezant, T. R., J. V. Agapian, M. C. Bohlman, X. Bu, S. Oztas, W.-Q. Qiu, K. S. Arnos, G. A. Cortopassi, L. Jaber, J. I. Rotter, M. Shohat, and N. Fischel-Ghodsian. Mitochondrial ribosomal RNA mutation associated with both antibiotic-induced and non-syndromic deafness. *Nat. Genet.* 1993;4:289.

185. Moazed, D., and H. F. Noller. Interaction of antibiotics with functional sites in 16S ribosomal RNA. *Nature* 1987;327:389.

186. Prezant, T. R., M. Shohat, L. Jaber, S. Pressman, and N. Fischel-Ghodsian. Biochemical characterization of a pedigree with mitochondrially inherited deafness. *Am. J. Med. Genet.* 1992;44:465.

187. Fong, I. W., R. S. Fenton and R. Bird. Comparative toxicity of gentamicin versus tobramycin: a randomized prospective study. *J. Antimicrob. Chemother.* 1981;7:81.

188. Aronoff, G. R., S. T. Pottratz, M. E. Brier, N. E. Walker, N. S. Fineberg, M. D. Glant, and F. C. Luft. Aminoglycoside accumulation kinetics in rat renal parenchyma. *Antimicrob. Agents Chemother.* 1983;23: 74.

189. Keys, T. F., S. B. Kurtz, J. D. Jones, and S. M. Muller. Renal toxicity during therapy with gentamicin or tobramycin. *Mayo Clin. Proc.* 1981;56:556.

190. Lietman, P. S., and C. R. Smith. Aminoglycoside

nephrotoxicity in humans. *J. Infect. Dis.* 1983;5(Suppl.) 2:5284.

191. Schentag, J. J., M. E. Plaut, F. B. Cerra, P. B, Wels, P. Walczak, and R. J. Buckley. Aminoglycoside nephrotoxicity in critically ill surgical patients. *J. Surg. Res.* 1979;26:270.

192. Smith, C. R., J. J. Lipsky, O. L. Laskin, D. B. Hellmann, E. D. Mellits, J. Longstreth, and P. S. Lietman. Double-blind comparison of the nephrotoxicity and auditory toxicity of gentamicin and tobramicin. *N. Eng. J. Med.* 1980;302:1106.

193. Mazze, R. I., and M. J. Cousins: Combined nephrotoxicity of gentamicin and methoxyflurane anesthesia in man. *Br. J. Anesth.* 1973;45:394.

194. Churchill, D. N., and J. Seely. Nephrotoxicity associated with combined gentamicin-amphotericin B therapy. *Nephron* 1977;19:176.

195. Wade, J. C., C. R. Smith, B. G. Petty, J. J. Lipsky, G. Conrad, J. Ellner, and P. S. Lietman. Cephalothin plus aminoglycoside is more nephrotoxic than methicillin plus an aminoglycoside. *Lancet* 1978;2:604.

196. Dentino, M. E., F. C. Luft, M. N. Yum, and L. H. Einhorn. Long term effect of cis-diamminedichloride platinum on renal function and structure in man. *Cancer* 1978;41:1274.

197. Appel, G. B. Aminoglycoside nephrotoxicity. *Am. J. Med.* 1990;88(Suppl. C):16S.

198. Kaloyanides, G. J. Aminoglycoside nephrotoxicity. In *Diseases of the Kidney.* 5th ed. by R. W. Schrier and G. W. Gottschalk, Boston: Little Brown, 1992, p. 1131.

199. Bennett, W. M., F. Luft, and G. A. Porter. Pathogenesis of renal failure due to aminoglycosides and contrast media used in roentgenography. *Am. J. Med.* 1980;69:767.

200. Pastoriza-Munoz, E., R. L. Bowman, and G. L. Kaloyanides. Renal tubular transport of gentamicin in the rat. *Kidney Int.* 1979;16:440.

201. Schentag, J. J., W. J., Jusko, J. W. Vance, T. J. Cumbo, E. Abrutyn, M. Delattre, and L. M. Gerbracht. Gentamicin disposition and tissue accumulation on multiple dosing. *J. Pharmacokin. Biopharm.* 1977;5:559.

202. Kuhar, M. J., L. L. Mark, and P. S. Lietman. Autoradiographic localization of ^{3}H-gentamicin in the proximal renal tubules of mice. *Antimicrob. Agents Chemother.* 1979;15:131.

203. Silverblatt, F. J., and C. Kuehn. Autoradiography of gentamicin uptake by the rat proximal tubule cell. *Kidney Int.* 1979;5:335

204. Kosek, J. C., R. I. Mazze, and M. J. Cousins. Nephrotoxicity of gentamicin. *Lab. Invest.* 1974;30:48.

205. Houghton, D. C., M. Hartnett, M. Campbell-Boswell, G. Porter, and W. Bennett. A light and electron microscopic analysis of gentamicin nephrotoxicity in rats. *Am. J. Pathol.* 1976;82:591.

206. Hauser, G., and J. Eichberg. Improved conditions for the preservation and extraction of polyphosphoinostides. *Biochim. Biophys. Acta* 1973;326:201.

207. Schibeci, A., and J. Schacht. Action of neomycin on the metabolism of polyphosphoinositides in the guinea pig kidney. *Biochem. Pharmacol.* 1977;26:1769.

208. Just, M., and E. Haberman. The renal handling of polybasic drugs. 2. In vitro studies with brush border and lysosomal preparations. *Nauyn-Schmiedeberg's Arch. Pharmacol.* 1977;300:67.

209. Tulkens, P., and A. Truet. The uptake and intracellular accumulation of aminoglycoside antibiotics in lysosomes of cultured rat fibroblasts. *Biochem. Pharmacol.* 1978;7:415.

210. de Duve, C., T. de Barsy, B. Poole, A. Truet, P. Tulkens, and F. Van Hoof. Lysosomotropic agents. *Biochem. Pharmacol.* 1974;23:2495.

211. Aubert-Tulkens, G., F. Van Hoof, and P. Tulkens. Gentamicin-induced lysosomal phospholipidosis in cultured rat fibroblasts. *Lab. Invest.* 1979;40:481.

212. Chambers, H. F. and M. A. Sande. The aminoglycosides. In *Goodman and Gilman's The Pharmacological Basics of Therapeutics*, 9th ed. ed. by. J. G. Hardman, L. E. Limbird, P.. B. Molinoff, R. W. Ruddon, and A. G. Gilman. New York: McGraw-Hill, 1996, p. 1103.

213. Quarum, M. L., D. C. Houghton, D. N. Gilbert, D. A. McCarron, and W. M. Bennett. Increasing dietary calcium moderates experimental gentamicin nephrotoxicity. *J. Lab. Clin. Med.* 1984;103:104.

214. Walker, P. D. and S. V. Shah. Evidence suggesting a role for hydroxyl radical in gentamicin-induced acute renal failure in rats. *J.Clin. Invest.* 1988;81:334.

215. Young, L. S., D. V. Meyer-Dudnik, J. Hindler, and W. J. Martin. Aminoglycosides in the treatment of bacteremic infections in the immunocompromised host. *J. Antimicrob. Chemother.* 1981;8(Suppl. A):121.

216. Levin, S. Antibiotics of choice in suspected serious sepsis. *J. Antimicrob. Chemother.* 1981;8(Suppl. A): 133.

217. Appel, G. B., and H. C. Neu. Gentamicin in 1978. *Ann. Int. Med.* 1978;89:528.

218. Roberts, R. B., and M. A. Sande. Antimicrobial therapy of experimental enterococcal endocarditis. *Antimicrob. Agents Chemother.* 1975;8:564.

219. Moellering, R. C., O. M. Korzeniowski, M. A. Sande, and C. B. Wennersten. Species-specific resistance to antimicrobial synergism among enterococci. *J. Infect. Dis.* 1979;40:203.

220. Levison, M. E., R. Knight, and D. Kaye. In vitro evaluation of tobramycin, a new aminoglycoside antibiotic. *Antimicrob. Agents Chemother.* 1972;1:381.

221. Laxer, R. M., E. Mackay, and M. I. Marks. Antimicrobial activity of tobramycin against gram-negative bacteria and the combination of ampicillin/tobramycin against. *E. coli. Chemotherapy.* 1975;21:90.

222. Gangadharam, P. R. J., E. R. Candler, and P. V. Ramakrishna. In vitro anti-mycobacterial activity of some new aminoglycoside antibiotics. *J. Antimicrob. Chemother.* 1977;3:285.

223. Smith, C. R., K. L. Baughman, C. Q. Edwards, J. F. Rogers, and P. S. Lietman. Controlled comparison of amikacin and gentamicin. *N. Engl. J. Med.* 1977; 296:350.

224. Jahre, J. A., K. P. Fu, and H. C. Neu: Clinical evaluation of netilmicin therapy in serious infections. *Am. J. Med.* 1979;66:67.

225. Arpini, A., L. Cornacchia, L. Albiero, F. Bramonte, and L. Parravicini. Auditory function in guinea pigs treated with netilmicin and other aminoglycoside antibiotics. *Arch. Otorhinolaryngol.* 1979;224: 137.

226. Dewdney, J. M. Immunology of the antibiotics. In *The Antigens*, Vol. 4, ed. by. M. Sela. New York: Academic Press, 1977, pp. 73–245.

227. Simon, M., H. B. Shookhoff, and H. Terner. Paromomycin in the treatment of intestinal amebiasis: a short course of therapy. *Am. J. Gastroenterol.* 1967;48: 504.

CHAPTER SIX

Bacteriostatic Inhibitors of Protein Synthesis

Chloramphenicol, Macrolides, Clindamycin, Spectinomycin, Tetracyclines and Streptogramins

Like the aminoglycosides, the antibiotics presented in this chapter were originally isolated from soil actinomycetes discovered in large programs that screened extracts of plants and fungi for antibacterial properties. All of the drugs alter bacterial growth by inhibiting protein synthesis. But in contrast to the aminoglycosides, their effect at clinically achieved drug concentrations is bacteriostatic against most sensitive organisms. There is no preferred order for classifying these drugs. They are presented here according to their locus of action on the bacterial ribosome. Some of these antibiotics, such as chloramphenicol and macrolides like erythromycin, act on the 50S ribosomal subunit, whereas spectinomycin and the tetracyclines act on the 30S subunit.

Chloramphenicol

Chloramphenicol was the first broad-spectrum antibiotic to be discovered. It was originally isolated from the soil actinomycete *Streptomyces venezuelae*. It has the sim-

ple structure shown below and is now produced by chemical synthesis rather than by fermentation. The aromatic ring system (I) and the acyl side chain (III) can be extensively substituted without loss of bacteriostatic potency, whereas very little substitution is permitted in the propanediol moiety (II).[1,2] Replacement of the nitro group by other chemical moieties renders the parent compound less active. However, these derivatives also have less hematopoietic toxicity.

Mechanism of Action

THE RECEPTOR. In 1954 Wisseman et al. demonstrated that exposure of bacteria to chloramphenicol stopped protein synthesis immediately with no immediate effect on the synthesis of nucleic acids (Fig. 6–1).[3] The ability of an organism's ribosomes to bind chloramphenicol is related to its sensitivity to growth inhibition by the drug,[4] and only 70S ribosomes have the ability to bind the drug (see Table 6–1). The binding is readily reversible, and if a chloramphenicol-treated culture is diluted with new growth medium, the culture will begin growing again.

It is clear that interaction of chloramphenicol with the ribosome is responsible for the inhibition of protein synthesis by the drug. This inhibition of protein synthesis is maximal when one molecule of chloramphenicol

Chloramphenicol

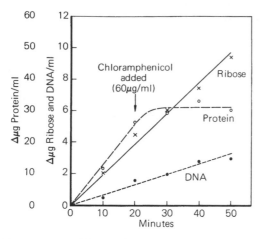

Figure 6–1. Chloramphenicol inhibition of protein synthesis in *Escherichia coli.* Chloramphenicol was added to *E. coli* in the logarithmic phase of growth, and portions of the culture were sampled at various time intervals and assayed for total cell protein and nucleic acid. The values represent the average of triplicate analyses expressed as increments in μg/ml over the initial concentration. (Reprinted from Wisseman et al.[3])

is bound per ribosome.[5] The results presented in Table 6–2 show that chloramphenicol inhibits protein synthesis in a cell-free system only when 70S ribosomes are present.[6] There is very little inhibition when protein synthesis is directed by a soluble fraction from *E. coli* and 80S ribosomes prepared from yeast. This is the basis for the selective toxicity of chloramphenicol. This selectivity is not complete, however. Although most protein synthesis in mammalian cells takes place on 80S ribosomes, the small amount of protein synthesis that takes place in mitochondria is inhibited by chloramphenicol.[7] It is hypothesized that mitochondria may have arisen from primitive infecting organisms that gradually became obligatory endosymbionts.[8] The mitochondria direct the synthesis of their own ribosomes, which behave in many ways like their bacterial 70S counterparts. As will be described later in this chapter, at least one of the major toxic effects of chloramphenicol may be explained on the basis of its inhibition of mitochondrial protein synthesis.

The affinity of 70S ribosomes for chlo-

ramphenicol is reasonably high ($K_D \sim 10^{-6}$M)[9] and nuclear magnetic resonance (NMR) studies indicate that the propanediol moiety (II) of the drug is most intimately associated with the ribosomal binding site.[10] The high-affinity binding site is located on the 50S subunit of the bacterial ribosome.[11] The 50S subunit can be separated into its protein and RNA components and then reconstituted. The reconstituted unit will bind chloramphenicol,[12] and reconstitution experiments with fractionated proteins show that protein L16 of the 50S subunit is required for chloramphenicol binding.[13] Protein L16 is preferentially labeled when ribosomes are exposed to monoiodochloramphenicol, a drug analog that acts as a site-specific affinity label.[14] These observations suggest that L16 is in the chloramphenicol binding site. Other proteins on the 50S subunit, including L2, L24, and L27, have been covalently bonded by other affinity labels[2] and have antigenic determinants that cluster in the region of peptidyl transferase.[15] The binding of chloramphenicol to ribosomes is inhibited by clindamycin and macrolide antibiotics, such as erythromycin.[16] But since the binding of erythromycin is not inhibited by chloramphenicol, it is clear that the binding sites are not identical.[17] Thus, it is likely that the receptor sites of erythromycin and chloramphenicol overlap or interact in some way. Clindamycin also has its receptor site in close proximity to, or shared with, the others. In addition to the high-affinity binding site on the 50S ribosomal subunit, there is a low-affinity chloramphenicol binding site ($K_D \sim 10^{-4}$M) on the 30S subunit,[18] but no relationship between this second binding site and chloramphenicol-mediated inhibition of protein synthesis has been established.

INHIBITION OF PROTEIN SYNTHESIS. In reviewing what we know of the mechanism of chloramphenicol action, it is useful to refer to the sequence of events in protein synthesis presented in Figure 5–3. It is clear that chloramphenicol does not preferentially inhibit the initiation of new protein chains or chain termination.[5] The binding of aminoacyl-tRNA[19] and the binding of mRNA[5] to the

Table 6–1. *Relationship between sensitivity to growth inhibition by chloramphenicol and the ability of isolated ribosomes to bind the radioactive-labeled drug.* Here ^{14}C-labeled chloramphenicol was added to ribosome suspensions prepared from various sources, and the amount of drug bound was assayed by centrifuging the samples and determining the radioactivity in the ribosomal pellet. The results are expressed as picograms of chloramphenicol bound per milligram of ribosomes.

Type of organism	Source of ribosomes	Response to chloramphenicol	Type of ribosome	In vitro binding to ribosomes
Bacterial	*Staphylococcus aureus*	Sensitive	70S	18
	Bacillus megaterium	Sensitive	70S	30
	Escherichia coli B	Sensitive	70S	29
Yeast	*Saccharomyces fragilis*	Resistant	80S	<1
Protozoan	*Strigomonas*	Resistant	80S	<1
Mammal	Rat liver	—	80S	<1

Source: Data compiled from Vazquez.[4]

30S ribosome subunit is not affected by the drug. In intact cells, the drug blocks the addition of new amino acids to the growing protein chains, which remain attached to the ribosomes.[5] Thus, chloramphenicol stabilizes polysomes. The results of a number of studies in cell-free protein-synthesizing systems support the conclusion that chloramphenicol inhibits peptide bond formation.[20,21]

The studies of chloramphenicol in cell-free protein synthesizing systems and the drug binding studies have led to a reasonable model for describing the mechanism of chloramphenicol action. If we visualize the orientation of the amino acid–charged tRNA on the ribosome, the tRNA is attached to the 30S portion in that region of the molecule containing the anticodon triplet. The region of the tRNA containing the attached amino acid must be correctly oriented on the surface of the 50S portion of the ribosome for peptide bond formation to take place. This can be inferred from the fact that the enzyme directing the synthesis of the peptide bond (peptidyl transferase) is a structurally integral part of the 50S ribosome subunit. In the presence of chloramphenicol the binding of tRNA at the codon recognition site is undisturbed, but the drug could inhibit peptide

Table 6–2. *Effect of chloramphenicol on* [^{14}C]*lysine incorporation with yeast and* Escherichia coli *supernatant and ribosomes.* Ribosomal and soluble (105,000 × *g* supernatant) fractions were prepared from *E. coli* and the yeast *S. fragilis.* The ribosomes and supernatant were incubated with [^{14}C]lysine and nonradioactive amino acids with or without chloramphenicol (2 μmoles/ml), and the amount of radioactivity incorporated into trichloroacetic acid-insoluble material was assayed. The results are expressed as counts per minute incorporated per incubation.

Supernatant	Ribosomes	Chloramphenicol	Amino acid incorporation		Average inhibition (%)
			Experiment 1	Experiment 2	
Escherichia coli	*Escherichia coli*	—	5625	3905	95
		+	196	239	
Escherichia coli	*Saccharomyces fragilis*	—	4804	10369	14
		+	4460	8236	

Source: From So and Davie.[6]

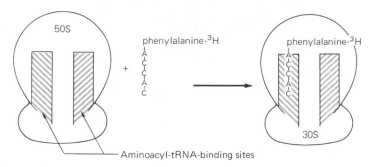

Figure 6–2. A schematic illustration of the binding of phenylalanyl-oligonucleotide to ribosomes. The binding of phenylalanyl-oligonucleotide to the ribosome is used here as a model of the specific binding of the amino acid–containing end of a complete aminoacyl-tRNA. The binding that does occur between the phenylalanyl-tRNA and the ribosome is inhibited by chloramphenicol but not by erythromycin. (Adapted from Pestka.[22])

bond formation by interfering with the binding of the amino acid–containing end of the tRNA to the 50S subunit.

This prediction has been tested directly: tRNA charged with tritium-labeled phenylalanine was digested with T₁ ribonuclease. After this limited digestion, a terminal aminoacyl tRNA "fragment" of [³H]phenylalanine-pentanucleotide was isolated. It was presumed that this radioactive amino acid–oligonucleotide represented the aminoacyl portion of an amino acid–charged tRNA. Several antibiotics were then tested for their effect on the ability of ribosomes to bind the radioactive phenylalanine-oligonucleotide (Fig. 6–2).[22] Chloramphenicol markedly inhibited the binding at concentrations that inhibited protein synthesis in in vivo systems. Subsequently, several other amino acid–oligonucleotides have been synthesized, and chloramphenicol inhibits the binding of all of them to bacterial ribosomes. Isomers of chloramphenicol that do not prevent bacterial growth do not prevent the binding of the amino acid–oligonucleotides.[9] There is evidence that this terminal fragment binding assay mimics the association between the aminoacyl terminal of the tRNA and the 50S ribosomal subunit.[23,24] These experiments, and others not discussed here, support the conclusion that chloramphenicol inhibits protein synthesis by binding in a reversible manner to a high-affinity binding site located at the peptidyl transfer-

ase center of the 50S ribosome subunit, preventing the attachment of the amino acid–containing end of the aminoacyl-tRNA to its binding region in the A site. This apparently prevents the appropriate association of peptidyl transferase with its amino acid substrate, and the peptide bond cannot be formed.[25]

Antimicrobial Activity of Chloramphenicol

Chloramphenicol has a broad spectrum of antibacterial activity. As shown in Table 6–3,[26] it is active against a wide variety of both gram-positive and gram-negative aerobic bacteria. Some of the Enterobacteriaceae, such as *Escherichia coli*, are very sensitive to chloramphenicol, whereas others, such as many strains of *Enterobacter, Serratia,* and *Klebsiella pneumoniae*, are relatively resistant.[27] Chloramphenicol is active in vitro against all types of anaerobes, including *Bacteroides fragilis*.[28] It is also active against most clinically important *Chlamydia* and *Mycoplasma*[29] as well as the majority of rickettsial organisms.[30,31] However, it is not active against *Pseudomonas aeruginosa* or fungi, yeasts, viruses, or protozoa.

Chloramphenicol has been generally regarded as strictly a bacteriostatic antibiotic, but this is not always the case. The action of chloramphenicol against *Haemophilus influenzae, Neisseria meningitidis,* and some strains of *Streptococcus pneumoniae* is bac-

Table 6–3.   Susceptibility of various bacteria to chloramphenicol.

	Very sensitive (MIC < 4.0 µg/ml)	Susceptible (MIC 4.0–12.5 µg/ml)	Relatively resistant (MIC 12.5–25.0 µg/ml)	Resistant (MIC > 25.0 µg/ml)
AEROBIC BACTERIA				
Gram-positive	Groups A and B streptocci Corynebacterium diphtheriae Bacillus anthracis	Staphylococcus aureus Streptococcus pneumoniae α-hemolytic streptococci	Group D streptococci	
Gram-negative	Neisseria meningitidis Neisseria gonorrhoeae Haemophilus influenzae Bordetella pertussis Burcella spp. Pasteurela multocida Shigella spp.	Escherichia coli Proteus mirabilis Salmonella spp. Vibrio cholerae Pseudomonas pseudomallei	Enterobacter spp. Serratia marcescens Klebsiella pneumoniae	Pseudomonas aeruginosa Indole-positive Proteus
ANAEROBIC BACTERIA				
Gram-positive	Peptococci and peptostreptococci Clostridium perfringens	Clostridium sp.		
Gram-negative	Veillonella spp. Fusobacterium fusiforme	Bacteroides fragilis		

MIC, minimum inhibitory concentration.
Source: Modified from Dajani and Kauffman.[26]

tericidal at concentrations of drug that are achieved clinically in cerebrospinal fluid.[32–34] It is not known why the drug kills these bacteria but has only a growth inhibitory effect against other bacteria. Chloramphenicol is effective in treating meningitis caused by these common meningeal pathogens, and the bactericidal action is probably a very important determinant of the drug's efficacy in the subarachnoid space where there is inefficient phagocytosis.[33]

RESISTANCE. The enteric bacteria generally become resistant to chloramphenicol by acquiring R factors that determine the production of chloramphenicol acetyltransferase.[35] The enzyme acetylates the drug at the 3-hydroxy position[36] in the propanediol moiety, a modification that renders it unable to bind to the high-affinity site on the 50S sub-

unit of the bacterial ribosome.[37] Three distinct types of acetyltransferases are determined by plasmids in gram-negative bacteria[38] and staphylococcal plasmids specify four closely related variants that are inducible.[39] The R factors in gram-negative bacteria carry determinants for multiple drug resistances and they can be passed from pathogens, such as *Salmonella typhi* or *Haemophilus influenzae*, to drug-sensitive strains of normal enteric bacteria, such as *Escherichia coli*.[40,41] It has also been shown that chloramphenicol resistance can be transferred from the induced-resistant *E. coli* to sensitive *Salmonella*.[40] This suggests that chloramphenicol resistance may be transmitted to enterobacteria in livestock in which the use of antibiotics in feed could enrich for the R factor–carrying organisms. The transfer of multiple drug resistance is particularly disturbing, because patients can become resistant to the major forms of therapy. This is seen, for example, with clinical isolates of *Haemophilus influenzae* that have acquired plasmids determining resistance to both chloramphenicol and ampicillin[42] and with strains of *Salmonella typhi* that have acquired resistance to chloramphenicol and trimethoprim-sulfamethoxazole.[43] Clinical resistance to chloramphenicol is becoming an increasing problem worldwide. This reflects the increased usage of this antibiotic, with over-the-counter sales compounding the problem in some places. In some countries this has led to increased resistance to chloramphenicol in *Salmonella typhi, Shigella, Enterobacter, Klebsiella, Neisseria menigitidis,* and *Haemophilus influenzae* as well as other organisms.[44–47]

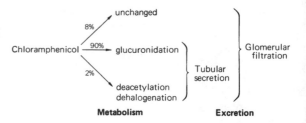

Pharmacology of Chloramphenicol

Chloramphenicol is well absorbed from the gastrointestinal tract, with peak serum levels attained in 1 to 2 h.[48] Because chloramphenicol is only slightly soluble in water, the water-soluble 3-monosuccinate ester is supplied for intravenous administration and the palmitate ester is used for preparing oral suspensions for pediatric use. The esters do not have antimicrobial activity and must be hydrolyzed in the body to release the active chloramphenicol base.[49] Because hydrolysis is not complete, the area under the plasma level curve after intravenous administration of the succinate ester to normal adults is about 70% of that obtained with an equivalent dose of chloramphenicol base administered by the oral route.[50] Chloramphenicol is available in ophthalmic solutions and ointments, and when applied topically to the eye, bacteriostatic concentrations of drug are achieved in the aqueous humor.[51,52] It is clear that chloramphenicol applied topically is absorbed into the bloodstream because aplastic anemia has been reported in patients treated with ophthalmic preparations.[53] Ophthalmologists should be aware of this potential hazard.

Chloramphenicol readily passes into the body fluid spaces including the pericardial, pleural, joint,[54] and cerebrospinal fluids. The level of drug achieved in cerebrospinal fluid is 40%–65% that of the plasma concentration,[55,56] and in brain tissue this lipophilic drug reaches a concentration level that is nine times that in the blood.[57] These distribution properties make chloramphenicol particularly useful in treating bacterial meningitis and brain abscess.

Chloramphenicol is metabolized in the liver by conjugation to the glucuronide.[58] Studies in both animal models[59] and humans[60] suggest that the rate of metabolism may be increased by concomitant administration of some other drugs, such as phenobarbital, leading to a significant decrease in the serum level of unaltered chloramphenicol. The glucuronide metabolite is neither toxic nor active against bacteria.[61] The glucuronide is excreted by the kidney, but the dosage of chloramphenicol does not have to be modified in the patient with compromised renal function.[62,63] Although higher levels of the drug build up in the patient who excretes it in reduced amounts, this accumulation is not of great consequence because it consists of nontoxic glucuronide. Since more than 90% of the drug is metabolized in the liver, compromised liver function would be expected to diminish drug metabolism and increase the serum concentration of the unaltered, toxic form. The incidence of bone marrow toxicity due to chloramphenicol is higher in patients who have extensive parenchymal damage in the liver.[61] Although some investigators have found significant correlations between serum bilirubin concentrations and chloramphenicol half-life,[58,64] other investigators have not found a clear relationship between the rate of chloramphenicol clearance and various indices of hepatic function.[65] Thus, liver function tests cannot be reliably used to determine dosage adjustment, and serum drug levels should be monitored frequently in patients with compromised hepatic function.

The average half-life of chloramphenicol in adults with normal liver function is 3 h (range 1 to 4.5 h).[62] In infants and children a wide interpatient variation in metabolism and excretion is responsible for a lack of correlation between the dose of chloramphenicol and the serum drug level.[49,55] Newborn infants are deficient in their ability to form glucuronide conjugates and have low glomerular filtration rates. Thus, there is an inverse relation between chloramphenicol half-life and age. High levels of the unaltered drug build up in the newborn if dosage is not adjusted appropriately (Figure 6–3)[66] and can result in the gray baby syndrome. Infants less than 1 month of age should receive a daily dosage of no more than 25 mg/kg of body weight, whereas 50 to 100 mg/kg/day is given to older infants and adults.

The rate of hydrolysis of chloramphenicol succinate to chloramphenicol varies among patients and is somewhat slower in infants less than 1 month of age.[49] About 50% of the chloramphenicol present in plasma is bound to albumin and the bound fraction may be lower in patients with liver disease or uremia.[67] Because of the wide variability in pharmacokinetics, serum drug concentrations should be carefully monitored in infants and children[49,55] as well as in older patients with significant hepatic disease. Several microbiological[68] and chemical[69] procedures are available for assaying the unaltered form of the drug. Most susceptible gram-negative bacteria are inhibited by the drug at a serum concentration of 5–15 µg/ml, and bone marrow depression occurs at concentrations greater than 25 µg/ml. Thus, for most infections, serum concentrations in the range of 10–20 µg/ml are desired. In those hospitals where sophisticated analytical services are available, physicians may find it useful to perform a serum drug assay several hours after the initial intravenous infusion to estimate the patient's chloramphenicol clearance rate; this can be used to calculate the daily dosage requirement.[70]

Clinically Undesirable Effects of Chloramphenicol

The most important adverse reactions to chloramphenicol are the gray syndrome, toxic bone marrow depression, and aplastic anemia. Hypersensitivity reactions in the form of skin rashes can occur, but these are rare.[29] Diarrhea, vomiting, and glossitis may develop with doses of 6 g/day given for more than 1 week.[29] Superinfection of the gastrointestinal tract may occur, and Herxheimer reactions have been observed during therapy for typhoid fever, syphilis, and brucellosis. Nervous system disorders, including digital paresthesias, peripheral neuritis, and acute encephalopathy, have been observed in younger patients with cystic fibrosis.[29] Occasionally, patients with cystic fibrosis experience an optic neuropathy characterized by reversible loss of visual acuity, central scotomas, and disturbances in red-green color discrimination.[71]

An interesting effect of chloramphenicol that has been examined in model animal systems is its ability to suppress the primary immune response at high doses.[72] The mechanism of this effect is not well understood, but it could involve an inhibition of the growth rate of the rapidly dividing, antigen-stimulated lymphocytes.[73] Chloramphenicol

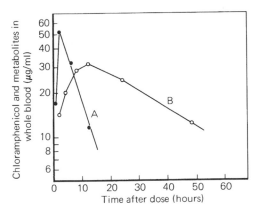

Figure 6–3. Mean whole-blood levels of free chloramphenicol and its metabolites in newborn infants and older children after oral administration of chloramphenicol palmitate in single doses of 50 mg/kg body weight. A, age 1 to 11 years (mean of 13 subjects); B, age 1 to 2 days (mean of five subjects). (From Weiss et al.[66])

inhibits the growth of leukemic lymphocytes at the same concentration at which it inhibits the growth mitochondrial protein synthesis.[74] It is tempting to speculate that the immunosuppressive effect, like the bone marrow toxicity, may be due to an inhibition of mitochondrial protein synthesis. Extensive depression of the immune system's ability to respond to an infection would be counterproductive. There is, however, no indication that chloramphenicol has a clinically significant immunosuppressive effect in the patient with infection.

GRAY SYNDROME. Chloramphenicol can produce a potentially fatal toxic reaction in newborn infants. The complex of symptoms is called the *gray syndrome*, which is characterized by abdominal distention, vomiting, progressive pallid cyanosis, irregular respiration, hypothermia, and finally, vasomotor collapse.[66] The syndrome is caused by high-level accumulation of the unaltered drug, which occurs because (1) newborn infants are unable to conjugate chloramphenicol to the glucuronide and (2) they excrete the drug more slowly since they have a lower glomerular filtration rate than older infants and children. The gray syndrome has been seen in newborns treated with doses of 100 mg/kg/day who have developed serum chloramphenicol concentrations in the range of 0.2–0.4 *mM*.[75] The syndrome has also been reported in older children (e.g., 25 months) who have high serum chloramphenicol levels.[76] These patients may conceivably have had a defect in glucuronidation, although there was no gross evidence of this. The syndrome may result from inhibition of mitochondrial oxidative phosphorylation. Chloramphenicol at these high concentrations interferes directly with electron transport in the NADH dehydrogenase portion of the mitochondrial respiratory chain.[75,77] In addition, at lower concentrations, the drug inhibits mitochondrial protein synthesis[78] and may alter oxidative phosphorylation secondarily by inhibiting the synthesis of components of the mitochondrial respiratory chain.[75] The gray syndrome usually reverses with termination of therapy at the onset of symptoms; however, infants with severe chloramphenicol intoxication have been treated by exchange transfusion[79] and charcoal-column hemoperfusion.[80] Because of gray syndrome toxicity, lower dosages (based on body weight) are given to infants less than 1 month old and special caution is advised. A similar condition has been reported in adults who were accidentally given excessive quantities of the drug.

EFFECTS OF CHLORAMPHENICOL ON THE HEMATOPOIETIC SYSTEM. Chloramphenicol affects the hematopoietic system in two ways: a toxic phenomenon manifested by bone marrow depression, and a likely idiosyncratic response manifested by aplastic anemia.

TOXIC BONE MARROW DEPRESSION. Chloramphenicol can cause a reversible, dose-related depression of bone marrow function, which presents as an anemia, sometimes with leukopenia or thrombocytopenia.[81] This effect can occur in anyone receiving high doses of drug. For example, in one well-controlled study, bone marrow depression developed in 2 of 20 patients given 2 g and in 18 of 21 receiving 6 g of the drug daily.[82] As a reference figure, approximately 4 g of the drug per day is administered routinely to adults in the treatment of typhoid fever.

There is considerable evidence that the toxic marrow depression is due to inhibition of mitochondrial protein synthesis.[83] Chloramphenicol readily penetrates mammalian mitochondria and binds to mitochondrial ribosomes. It inhibits protein synthesis in this organelle at concentrations of drug that exist in the serum during therapy.[84] Morphological changes have been demonstrated in the mitochondria of bone marrow cells taken from patients receiving chloramphenicol.[85] These changes, like the toxicity, are reversible. Chloramphenicol inhibits protein synthesis in human marrow cell mitochondria in vitro, and antibiotics that are not myelotoxic have no effect.[86] Chloramphenicol reversibly inhibits the growth of both human erythrocytic[87] and granulocytic[88,89] precursor cells in vitro.

APLASTIC ANEMIA. Another response of the hematopoietic cells to chloramphenicol is the development of aplastic anemia. Only after 3 years of extensive use did it become evident that chloramphenicol was able to completely depress bone marrow activity in some patients. In response to this 3-year delay the American Medical Association established the Registry on Blood Dyscrasias to collect data on such drug-associated reactions. Chloramphenicol has been implicated in more reports to the registry than any other single drug. This suppression of bone marrow activity differs from the toxic phenomenon just discussed (Table 6–4).[81] The response, characterized by pancytopenia with an aplastic marrow, can appear during treatment, but often it occurs long after treatment has ended; it is not dose related. The prognosis is very poor, with a high percentage of fatalities. Because the aplastic response does not occur frequently, it is difficult to arrive at a good estimation of its risk, although a value in the range of 1 in 24,000 to 1 in 40,000 courses of treatment is probably reasonable, given the available data.[90] Several patients who developed chronic bone marrow hypoplasia after chloramphenicol therapy subsequently developed acute myeloblastic leukemia.[91,92] Although the toxic bone marrow depression and the aplastic response are considered to be different entities, at least one patient has been reported to have features of both syndromes.[93]

The mechanism by which chloramphenicol causes bone marrow aplasia has not been defined. There is good reason to suggest that the aplasia represents an idiosyncratic drug response;[83] that is, it is a result of a genetically determined biochemical lesion. This would account for the rarity of the event and the fact that aplastic anemia has been observed on at least one occasion in identical twins given chloramphenicol.[94] One could postulate that the response stems from a rare biochemical abnormality in the undifferentiated stem cell compartment of the marrow, or that in individuals, altered routes of metabolism produce a toxic metabolite of chloramphenicol.

It has been proposed that the nitrobenzene moiety is the determining structural feature causing aplastic anemia.[83] Thiamphenicol, an analog of chloramphenicol in which the p-nitro group is replaced by a methylsulfonyl group, has been used extensively in Europe, but has apparently not been associated with the production of aplastic anemia.[95] Thiamphenicol produces reversible erythroid suppression and inhibits mitochondrial protein

Table 6–4. *Features of two types of blood dyscrasia resulting from treatment with chloramphenicol.* The hematopoietic system's two different responses to chloramphenicol, which were first characterized by Yunis and Bloomberg,[81] include the toxic effect (bone marrow depression) and the aplastic response.

Feature	Toxic effect	Aplastic response
Appearance of bone marrow smears	Normocellular	Hypoplastic or aplastic
Peripheral blood	Anemia (with or without leukopenia or thrombocytopenia)	Pancytopenia
Relation to dosage of drug given	Dose related	No dose relationship
Time of appearance	During therapy	Most often days to months after cessation of therapy
Most common presenting symptoms	Anemia	Purpura and/or hemorrhage
Prognosis	Recovery is usually complete on cessation of treatment	Fatal in many cases

Source: From Yunis and Bloomberg.[81]

synthesis with the same potency as chloramphenicol.[96] The reported lack of association of thaimphenicol with the aplastic response caused investigators to focus on the possible role of the *p*-nitro group of chloramphenicol in producing aplastic anemia. It has been suggested that in the predisposed host the *p*-nitro group is reduced, giving rise to highly reactive nitroso intermediates that lead to stem cell damage.[97] In support of this proposal, studies have shown that low concentrations of nitroso-chloramphenicol cause DNA strand breakage[98] and produce irreversible toxic effects on human bone marrow colony-forming cells.[97] The observations to date provide only indirect evidence for a role of the *p*-nitro group in the genesis of aplastic anemia. Nitroreduction by tissues of affected patients has not been demonstrated; it may be that nitroreduction is carried out by unique microflora in the gastrointestinal tract. A 1967 study noted that there were no reports of marrow aplasia occurring after parenteral administration, which suggests that gut flora could be responsible for producing metabolites that caused the syndrome.[99] On the basis of this report, physicians sometimes avoid the oral route, but it should be noted that several cases of aplastic anemia have been observed after parenteral administration[100,101] and there is no clear difference in risk based on the route of administration.

Drug Interactions

Chloramphenicol inhibits the hepatic microsomal drug-metabolizing system,[102] and it prolongs the half-life of drugs like dicumarol and phenytoin, which are metabolized by this system.[103] Severe toxcity and death have occurred when these effects have not been recognized. On the other hand, there are some drugs that will affect the metabolism of chloramphenicol. For example, chronic administration of phenobarbital or acute administration of rifampin shortens the half-life of chloramphenicol and may result in subtherapeutic concentrations of the drug. This probably results from induction of enzymes responsible for the metabolism of chloramphenicol.[104,105]

Therapeutic Indications for Chloramphenicol

When chloramphenicol came into clinical use, it was employed extensively in the treatment of a wide variety of infections. The clinical indications for its use became very restricted, however, when it became apparent that this drug could produce the fatal aplastic anemia. Nonetheless, chloramphenicol has been an important drug in the treatment of certain serious infections,[106,107] including typhoid fever and other types of salmonella infections. However, it is no longer the drug of choice, as other, safer drugs are also effective and the third-generation cephalosporins and quinolones are now preferred for treatment of this disease. In some regions of the world, for example, India and Southeast Asia,[46,108,109] a significant percentage of *Salmonella typhi* and other salmonella strains are now resistant to chloramphenicol.

Chloramphenicol has a bactericidal action against *Haemophilus influenzae* and until a few years ago chloramphenicol plus ampicillin was considered to be the regimen of choice for initial treatment of meningitis, epiglottitis, or arthritis due to this organism. Several cephalosporins (e.g., cefotaxime, ceftriaxone, and ceftizoxime) have replaced chloramphenicol as the treatment of choice for a variety of *H. influenzae* infections. Initially, chloramphenicol was commonly used for the treatment of *H. influenzae* meningitis, until 1965 when it became clear that the less toxic ampicillin was also effective. Ampicillin then supplanted chloramphenicol as the drug of choice. It has been difficult to determine which of these two antibiotics is the most efficacious drug for the treatment of *H. influenzae* meningitis.[110,111] In 1974, ampicillin-resistant strains of the bacterium began to appear[112] and because of the serious consequences of ineffective or delayed proper treatment of this condition, primary therapy for patients with confirmed or suspected infection due to *H.*

influenzae now included chloramphenicol. Thus, treatment was usually initiated with chloramphenicol alone or with chloramphenicol and ampicillin, and as soon as the ampicillin sensitivity of the organism was established, chloramphenicol therapy was stopped and treatment was continued with ampicillin. Under certain conditions, low concentrations of chloramphenicol may antagonize the bactericidal activity of ampicillin, but the effect of the combination is probably equivalent to treatment with chloramphenicol alone.[113] There have been many reports of *H. influenzae* isolates that are resistant to both chloramphenicol and ampicillin,[47,114,115] thus these drugs have been replaced by the third-generation cephalosporins in treating meningitis and other infections caused by *H. influenzae*.

Chloramphenicol is effective against many anaerobic bacteria,[28] the most common of which is *Bacteroides fragilis*. When a patient has a severe infection with *B. fragilis*, arising from a focus in the bowel or pelvis, chloramphenicol may be very useful in therapy.[116] Together with a penicillin it is often the preferred regimen for treatment of brain abscess.[106] However, many authorities now recommend penicillin plus metronidazole. Many of these infections result from anaerobic or mixed aerobic–anaerobic bacteria including *B. fragilis*. Chloramphenicol is very useful in the treatment of pneumococcal or meningococcal meningitis in penicillin-allergic patients. It is occasionally indicated for the treatment of rickettsial diseases, although the tetracyclines are usually preferred.[106] Chloramphenicol is the drug of choice for the treatment of rickettsial infections when patients are sensitized to the tetracyclines or when the tetracyclines can't be used for other reasons, as in patients with reduced renal function, pregnant women, or children less than 8 years of age.

The following guidelines should be employed in using chloramphenicol.

1. Chloramphenicol may be used for the treatment of anaerobic infections and in some cases typhoid fever (and invasive salmonellosis); brain abscess (in combination with a penicillin); and meningitis, epiglottitis, or arthritis due to *H. influenzae*. It should be employed only in severe (life-threatening) infections in which the drugs of choice cannot be used and chloramphenicol is clearly the superior alternative. It should never be used for prophylaxis or for the treatment of mild or uncharacterized infections.

2. Prolonged use and repeated exposure should be avoided.

3. It should not be used in a patient with a history of previous hematologic abnormalities induced by the drug, and should also be avoided in patients with a family history of chloramphenicol-induced blood dyscrasia.[117]

4. Leukocyte, reticulocyte, and platelet counts and hemoglobin determination should be performed at the outset of therapy. These studies should be repeated 1 week after the start of therapy and then approximately every 3 days if therapy is continued beyond 1 week.[117] Therapy should be discontinued if leukopenia occurs.

The Use of Chloramphenicol

A useful broad-spectrum antibiotic noted for its relative lack of adverse side effects, chloramphenicol was introduced to the American drug market in 1949 under a patent issued to Parke, Davis and Co. By 1950, however, it had become apparent that chloramphenicol produced aplastic anemia, a fatal side effect, in a few patients. A continuing argument regarding the proper use of this drug ensued. The drug firm and a number of physicians felt the risk of aplastic anemia was trivial compared with the therapeutic usefulness of the antibiotic. Expressing more caution about use of the drug were a steadily increasing number of authorities in the treatment of infectious disease, many hematologists, advisors in the Food and Drug Administration, and at least two congressional committees that held hearings on the drug (chaired by Senator

Estes Kefauver in 1960 and by Senator Gaylord Nelson in 1968). The controversy did not concern the right of the company to market the drug or the right of the physician to use it; rather, it concerned the way in which the drug company advertised its product and the uniformed way many physicians used the drug. Many critics felt that the company played down the problem of side effects in their advertisements to physicians. The story of the commercial side of the controversy has been reviewed in *Consumer Reports*.[118]

A great part of the problem with the use of this drug centered on the fact that many physicians lacked information about this drug. The indications given for therapy with chloramphenicol in those cases of chloramphenicol-associated blood dyscrasia reported to the Registry on Blood Dyscrasias from 1953 through 1964 demonstrate how ignorant many physicians were of the proper use of this antibiotic.[119] As seen in Figure 6–4, the second most common indication for therapy was the treatment of the common cold, a virus infection against which the drug is totally useless. In other cases, the drug was prescribed for minor infections where therapy with chloramphenicol is definitely not indicated. In a review of chloramphenicol use in office practice in Tennessee in 1974, it was found that the most common diagnosis for which chloramphenicol was prescribed was upper respiratory infection; the authors felt that most of the prescribing was

inappropriate.[120] After an informational letter was sent to the participating physicians, a second review in 1976 showed a reduction in chloramphenicol use.[121] In two studies of inpatient use of chloramphenicol during the 1970s, it was found that there were valid reasons for its use in 74% of cases reviewed in a university hospital[101] and in 78% of cases in a community hospital.[122] This suggests that physicians usually use the drug in an informed manner but that some misuse still occurs.

The use of chloramphenicol in some countries is much more lax than in the United States; in several countries, chloramphenicol is sold without a doctor's prescription.[123] In 1969, a correspondent wrote in the *New England Journal of Medicine* that chloramphenicol was being used by many people in South America as "...a daily self-medication for all ills and aches...."[124] In some places, appropriate warnings regarding the side effects and toxicities of chloramphenicol are not included in the drug package,[123] even in cases when it was manufactured in countries like Great Britain and the United States where there are strict laws regarding the presentation of this information with chloramphenicol sold within the country.[125] Travelers to countries with lax laws or no laws protecting the consumer have died from aplastic anemia following ingestion of chloramphenicol contained in cough preparations and other formulations sold over the counter.[126]

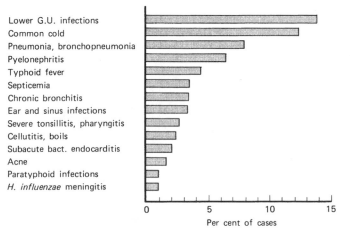

Figure 6–4. Some specific conditions for which chloramphenicol was given in instances of chloramphenicol-associated blood dyscrasia reported to the Registry on Blood Dyscrasias from 1953 through 1964. (From Best.[119])

Macrolide Antibiotics (Erythromycin, Clarithromycin, Azithromycin, and Dirithromycin)

Erythromycin is one of the macrolide antibiotics, which consist of a large lactone ring

Erythromycin

to which sugars are attached. Erythromycin, clarithromycin, azithromycin, and dirithromycin are the macrolides currently available for clinical use in the United States. Although erythromycin is still a very useful drug, the newer macrolides have a lower incidence of side effects than erythromycin. The newer macrolides produce less gastrointestinal irritability, are more stable in gastric acid, are better absorbed from the gut, have better tissue penetration, and possess longer half-lives, permitting once- or twice-daily administration.

Mechanism of Action

All the macrolides have a mechanism of action identical to that of erythromycin. Erythromycin binds in a specific manner to the 50S subunit of the bacterial ribosome.[127] It does not bind to mammalian 80S ribosomes, and this accounts in part for its selective toxicity.[128] Like chloramphenicol, erythromycin can inhibit protein synthesis on ribosomes from mammalian mitochondria.[129] Competition experiments indicate that the erythromycin binding site on the 50S ribosome subunit overlaps or interacts with the binding sites for chloramphenicol and the lincomycins. The binding of [14C]chloramphenicol to bacterial ribosomes is prevented by erythromycin and lincomycin,[17] but the binding of [14C]erythromycin is not inhibited by chloramphenicol[130] or lincomycin.[131] The binding of [14C]lincomycin is inhibited by erythromycin.[132]

Erythromycin binds in a reversible manner to a single high-affinity site ($K_D \sim 10^{-8}$M) on the bacterial ribosome.[133] Proteins L15 and L16 are absolutely required for erythromycin binding to the 50S subunit.[134] This was demonstrated by reconstitution experiments in which erythromycin binding capacity was restored to 50S ribosome subunit core particles. As described earlier in this chapter, protein L16 is also required for reconstituted 50S subunits to bind chloramphenicol.[13] Erythromycin prevents the binding of chloramphenicol to isolated 70S ribosomes but not to ribosomes in polysome form. If peptidyl-tRNA is removed from polyribosomes, however, chloramphenicol binding is inhibited by erythromycin.[135] This suggests that the erythromycin binding site is in the peptidyl-tRNA binding region (P site) on the 50S ribosome subunit. It is not completely clear whether erythromycin inhibits protein synthesis by inhibiting peptide bond formation[136] or by interfering with the subsequent translocation step (cf. Fig. 5–3). Several studies both in vivo and in vitro strongly suggest that erythromycin inhibits the translocation step.[137,138] The presence of erythromycin on the 50S subunit may inhibit translocation by preventing the proper association of the peptidyl-tRNA with its binding site after formation of the peptide bond.[139]

ERYTHROMYCIN RESISTANCE. Resistance to macrolides may stem from multiple mechanisms, some of them plasmid mediated and some due to chromosomal mutations. Laboratory strains of erythromycin-resistant *Escherichia coli* have been shown to have ribosomes that do not bind erythromycin. The resistance is due to a single amino acid replacement in the L4 protein of the 50S subunit.[140,141] Other erythromycin-resistant bacteria with altered 50S ribosomal protein have been identified, but they have not been well characterized.[142] The close relationship between the interactions of three structurally unrelated antibiotics with the 50S subunit has been demonstrated in experiments with ribosomal mutants of *E. coli*. One of the mutants with an altered L4 protein, for example, was also shown to bind chloramphenicol with decreased affinity.[143] A strain of *E. coli* that is absolutely dependent on the presence of erythromycin for growth has been selected.[144] Lincomycin and chloramphenicol also permitted growth of this mutant, although they were less effective than erythromycin. This again suggests a similarity in the interactions of the three antibiotics with the 50S subunit.

A unique form of inducible antibiotic resistance has been demonstrated in *Staphylococcus aureus*. Studies in the 1950s showed that some clinical isolates that were resistant to erythromycin were resistant to other macrolide antibiotics if they were grown in the presence of a very low concentration of erythromycin.[145,146] A subsequent study showed that exposure of the organisms to erythromycin at low concentration (about 10^{-8}M) results in resistance to high concentrations of erythromycin, the other macrolide antibiotics, and the lincosamides.[147] When the cells are initially exposed to high concentrations of erythromycin ($> 10^{-7}$M), their growth is inhibited and induction of the resistance is blocked because of inhibition of protein synthesis. The RNA portion of the 50S ribosomal subunits of organisms exposed to a low concentration of erythromycin contains a unique methylated component (a dimethyladenine).[148] Hybrid 50S ribosomal subunits have been assembled that utilize 23S RNA from drug-sensitive or induced-resistant *S. aureus* and other protein and RNA constituents derived from *Bacillus stearothermophilus*. The complete hybrid ribosomes support phenylalanine incorporation, and lincomycin inhibits the synthesis when the ribosomes contain 23S RNA from the drug-sensitive parent but not when they contain the methylated 23S RNA from the induced-resistant cells.[149] This strongly suggests that the alteration in the RNA is responsible for the drug resistance. These staphylococci apparently have acquired a plasmid that contains the gene for an inducible RNA methylase. In the presence of small amounts of erythromycin (concentrations too low to inhibit protein synthesis), the enzyme is induced, causing a change in the RNA so that upon subsequent exposure to the usual growth-inhibitory concentrations of lincosamides or erythromycin, the drugs are no longer effective. It is very interesting that of 10 streptomycetes tested for resistance to macrolide antibiotics and lincomycin, only *Streptomyces erythreus*, the organism used for production of erythromycin, was found to be resistant to both classes of antibiotics and to contain dimethyladenine in the 23S ribosomal RNA.[150] Thus, the organism that produces the antibiotic is protected from the drug effect in the same manner as resistant clinical isolates of *S. aureus*. Resistance to macrolides as a result of decreased permeability of the drugs through the cell envelope also occurs, in *Staphylococcus epidermidis*.[151]

Antimicrobial Activity and Therapeutic Indications

Erythromycin may be bacteriostatic or bactericidal, the nature of the response depending upon the bacterial species, the drug concentration, and the bacterial density.[152] Although erythromycin is used clinically to treat infections caused by both gram-positive and gram-negative bacteria, some gram-negative bacilli, notably the Enterobacteriaceae, are intrinsically resistant. Since cell-free protein-synthesizing systems from highly sensitive gram-positive bacteria and resistant enterobacteria are equally inhibited by erythromycin,[153] it is clear that the spectrum of drug action is not determined by intrinsic differences in ribosome sensitivity. It has been shown that enterobacteria (e.g., *Proteus mirabilis*) become sensitive to erythromycin when they are converted to stable L-forms that lack a cell envelope.[154] The concentration of erythromycin achieved in sensitive gram-positive organisms, such as *S. aureus*, is 100 times greater than that in intrinsically resistant enterobacteria, such as *E. coli*.[153] Thus the spectrum of antibacterial action of erythromycin appears to be largely determined by its ability to enter the organism. The drug is not actively transported into sensitive bacteria; rather, it enters by a passive process and is trapped by binding to the ribosomes.

The sensitivity of gram-negative bacilli to erythromycin increases markedly at alkaline pH.[152] As erythromycin is a weak base and becomes progressively less ionized as the pH of the growth medium is raised, it is likely that the unionized form of the drug passes most easily through the outer envelope of gram-negative bacteria.[155] This effect of pH on drug entry and bacterial sensitivity may be used to clinical advantage by alkalinizing the urine when erythromycin is used to treat urinary tract infections due to gram-negative bacilli.[156]

The activity of the macrolide antibiotics in vitro against selected bacteria is presented in Table 6–5.[157] Erythromycin is sometimes used as an alternative to penicillins in treating gram-positive infections in penicillin-allergic individuals (for reviews of clinical use see refs. 158–160). Erythromycin is, for example, an appropriate alternative to penicillin in the treatment of streptococcal infections and for prophylaxis of rheumatic fever in penicillin-allergic patients.[161] Pneumococcal infections generally respond well to erythromycin therapy. Occasional strains of both streptococci and pneumococci are resistant to erythromycin and may be resistant to clindamycin as well.[162,163] Erythromycin is useful for treating minor infections due to *Staphylococcus aureus* in penicillin-allergic individuals, but the drug is limited in use by the large number of strains that are resistant to it. Also, the need to use erythromycin has been reduced by the introduc-

Table 6–5. *Susceptibility of selected organisms to the macrolide antibiotics.*

Organism	Erythromycin (MIC$_{90}$)	Clarithromycin (MIC$_{90}$)	Azithromycin (MIC$_{90}$)
GRAM-POSITIVE AEROBES			
Methicillin-sensitive *Staphylococcus aureus*	>128	>128	>128
Methicillin-resistant *Staphylococcus aureus*	>128	>128	>128
Streptococcus pyogenes	0.03–4	0.012–2	0.12–4
Streptococcus pneumoniae	0.03–1	0.015–0.5	0.12–2
Enterococcus spp.	4	2	16
Listeria monocytogenes	0.5–2	0.12–2	2–4
GRAM-NEGATIVE AEROBES			
Moraxella catarrhalis	0.25–2	0.25–1	0.03–0.12
Neisseria gonorrhoeae	0.25–2	0.25–2	0.05–0.25
Legionella pneumophila	1–2	0.25	2
Haemophilus influenzae	4–32	2–16	0.5–4
ANAEROBES			
Bacteroides fragilis	4–32	2–8	2–6.25
Clostridium perfringens	1	0.5–2	0.25–0.78
OTHER PATHOGENS			
Chlamydia trachomatis	0.06–2	0.008–0.125	Data not available
Campylobacter spp.	1–4	1–8	0.5
Helicobacter pylori	0.25	0.03	0.25

MIC$_{90}$, minimum inhibitory concentration (μg/ml) at or below the given value for 90% of isolates.
Source: Data from Schlossberg.[157]

tion of the penicillinase-resistant penicillins, the cephalosporins, and the quinolones. Gram-positive bacilli are generally erythromycin sensitive. Erythromycin is the most active antibiotic against *Corynebacterium diphtheriae* and it is considered to be the drug of choice for eliminating the diphtheria carrier state.[164]

Among the gram-negative bacteria, *Bordetella pertussis* and *Legionella* are sensitive and an erythromycin is considered to be the drug of first choice for the treatment of whooping cough[165] and Legionnaire's disease.[166] Erythromycin is also an effective alternative to penicillin in the treatment of syphilis.[159] However, tetracyclines are the recommended alternative drugs in penicillin-allergic patients, and the U.S. Public Health Service recommends that pregnant patients with syphilis be hospitalized and desensitized to penicillin.[167] Erythromycin is active against some anaerobic bacteria[168] and it is used to eliminate *Clostridium tetani* from tetanus patients who are allergic to penicillin, but debridement, physiological support, and antitoxin are the main approaches to therapy. *Mycoplasma pneumoniae* is more sensitive to erythromycin than to tetracycline in vitro,[169] but the drugs produce equivalent clinical responses and both are considered to be drugs of first choice in the treatment of *Mycoplasma* infection. Many strains of *Chlamydia trachomatis* are sensitive to erythromycin,[158] which is administered topically for treating conjunctivitis[170] and systemically for treating pneumonia and urethritis. In most chlamydial infections a single dose of the related macrolide, azithromycin, is now preferred over erythromycin.[171] As more experience and knowledge is obtained, the other macrolides are gradually replacing erythromycin as the macrolide of choice.

Clarithromycin is two to four times more active against streptococci and staphylococci than erythromycin, but it has only modest activity against *Haemophilus influenzae* and *Neisseria gonorrhoeae*. Clarithromycin has the best activity among the macrolides against *Legionella* and *Chlamydia pneumoniae* and is superior to erythromycin against *Helicobacter* and most anaerobes. It

also has bactericidal activity against *Mycobacterium leprae*, including strains resistant to standard agents such as dapsone. Clarithromycin is superior to other macrolides for treating a variety of mycobacteria other than tuberculosis (MOTT).[157]

In contrast to clarithromycin, azithromycin is two to four times less active than erythromycin against streptococci and staphylococci, but it does inhibit most pathogenic streptococci, with the exception of enterococci. Azithromycin is more active than erythromycin or clarithromycin against *H. influenzae*. Its activity against MOTT is similar to that of clarithromycin. Azithromycin differs from the other macrolides in having good activity against certain aerobic gram-negative bacilli, such as salmonellae, shigellae, *Aeromonas*, *E. coli*, and *Yersinia*. It is superior to erythromycin for gram-negative organisms against which erythromycin has some activity, specifically *H. influenzae*, *Moraxella*, *Legionella*, *Neisseria*, and *Bordetella*. Azithromycin is superior to erythromycin for *Mycoplasma* and chlamydia as well as several anaerobes, including *Bacteroides*.[157,172]

Because of their good activity against *H. influenzae* and *Moraxella catarrhalis*, azithromycin and clarithromycin are the better choices than erythromycin for the treatment of community-acquired pneumonia. Both drugs are useful in treating infections by the *Mycobacterium avium* complex (MAC), disseminated forms of which are common in patients with advanced AIDS. The MAC is resistant to most antitubercular drugs, so the activity of clarithromycin and azithromycin against MAC is clinically very important, and both drugs are effective as prophylaxis against disseminated MAC in patients with AIDS.[173,174] Clarithromycin appears to be effective for both the treatment of and prophylaxis against MAC infections in patients with AIDS, while azithromycin is only effective for prophylaxis.[175] Both clarithromycin and azithromycin have good in vitro activity against *Helicobacter pylori*.[176] The antibacterial activity of dirithromycin is similar to that of erythromycin, and its role in treatment is still being determined.[177]

Pharmacology of Erythromycin

ABSORPTION AND BIOAVAILABILITY. Erythromycin base is inactivated by acid, its absorption is variable, and serum levels are higher if the drug is administered when the stomach is empty.[157] Azithromycin, clarithromycin, and dirithromycin are acid stable and better absorbed; thus their bioavailability is higher. Two approaches have been used to overcome the problem of acid lability and improve absorption of erythromycin. Several erythromycin preparations have an acid-resistant, enteric coating that protects the drug from degradation in the stomach. In other preparations, the chemical structure of the drug has been altered to decrease acid inactivation by forming a salt (the stearate), an ester (the ethyl succinate), or the estolate (the lauryl sulfate salt of the propionyl ester). The stearate salt dissociates in the intestine and the drug is absorbed as the base, whereas the ester derivatives are absorbed intact and partially hydrolyzed to the free base in the blood.[178] The esters do not have significant antibacterial activity until they have been hydrolyzed in the serum to erythromycin base.[179] The absorption of the ester derivatives is less affected by the presence of food in the stomach than that of the base, but even with the ester preparations the highest plasma levels are probably achieved when the drug is administered in the fasting state.[180]

The absorption of erythromycin base is erratic. The peak serum level achieved 4 h after oral administration of 500 mg of the free base ranges from 0.3 to 1.9 μg/ml.[158] The absorption of the stearate salt or the ethyl succinate ester is more consistent than that of the free base and the mean peak serum levels are the same as that achieved with the enteric-coated base. The estolate is absorbed from the gut as the propionate ester and there has been considerable controversy regarding the relative bioavailability of this preparation. Although more drug is absorbed from the gastrointestinal tract and serum levels of total drug are higher after ingestion of the estolate, only 20%–35% of the antibiotic in the blood is present in the active antibacterial form as the free base.[181]

It has been demonstrated that the plasma concentration of bioactive erythromycin is the same after administration of either enteric-coated base tablets or estolate capsules.[182]

Intravenous administration of the water-soluble lactobionate or glucoheptate salts produces serum levels that are consistently higher than those achieved with the oral preparations. Peak serum concentrations average about 10 μg/ml 1 h after infusion of 500 mg of the lactobionate.[183,184] Intramuscular injection of erythromycin is very painful and the drug should be administered intravenously to treat serious infections.

Clarithromycin is the best absorbed macrolide with a bioavailability of about 55%. It is acid stable and absorbed well with or without food (food increases its bioavailability). The opposite holds for azithromycin, which should be taken on an empty stomach, as food decreases its bioavailability.[157]

DISTRIBUTION, METABOLISM, AND EXCRETION. Only 5%–10% of an intravenous dose of erythromycin is excreted unchanged in the urine.[184] The drug is concentrated in the liver, and high concentrations of the unaltered, biologically active form are present in the bile.[185] It is not clear how extensively the drug is metabolized by humans. Studies in animals show that erythromycin is inactivated by N-demethylation in the liver,[186] and in the rat the drug induces its own transformation into a metabolite that forms a stable, inactive complex with the iron (II) of cytochrome P-450.[187] This type of inhibition may account for the potentiation of ergotamine and warfarin effects that have been reported in humans.[187] The half-life of erythromycin in the patient with normal renal and hepatic function is about 1.5 h,[183,184] and this increases to 4 to 6 h in anuric patients.[188] Because of the predominantly hepatic route of elimination, dosage reduction has not been recommended in renal failure,[188] but it should be noted that ototoxicity has been reported in a few elderly patients with renal insufficiency.[189] Erythromycin is not removed by peritoneal dialysis or hemodialysis.[188]

Clarithromycin is metabolized in the liver

by hydroxylation and *N*-demethylation. The 14-hydroxy metabolite is active, especially against *Haemophilus influenzae*. The metabolites are excreted by the kidney, with about 40% of a dose being recovered in the urine.[190] With azithromycin, most of the drug is eliminated in the gut or bile, with demethylation by the liver playing a minor role.[157] Most of the azithromycin in the body remains unmetabolized and any metabolites that do occur are not active. There is no need to alter dosage of azithromycin in either hepatic or renal failure.

The volume of distribution of erythromycin is greater than the extracellular fluid space but less than that of the total body water,[183,184] and the base is about 65% bound to plasma protein.[191] The concentration of drug achieved in ascitic and pleural fluid is about 50% of that found in the serum.[192] Erythromycin passes consistently into the prostatic fluid and semen, to a level that is approximately one-third of the blood level.[192] Erythromycin does not diffuse readily across the normal meninges, and although assayable concentrations of drug have been reported in the cerebrospinal fluid of patients with meningitis,[192] erythromycin cannot be reliably used to treat central nervous system infection. Erythromycin passes into middle-ear fluid in concentrations that are effective against group A β-hemolytic streptococci and pneumococci, but the drug concentration may not be sufficient to eradicate *Haemophilus influenzae*.[193] The drug passes across the placenta such that levels achieved in amniotic fluid and fetal tissues are 5%–10% of those in the maternal blood.[194] After oral administration of the base, erythromycin is present in the feces at concentrations (300–600 µg/ml)[192] that are an order of magnitude greater than those required to eliminate most anaerobic bacteria.[168] For this reason, erythromycin is often administered in addition to an oral aminoglycoside (aminoglycosides are not active against anaerobes) when antibiotics are given preoperatively to eliminate bowel flora before intestinal surgery.[195]

Clarithromycin is concentrated in tissues, and tissue-to-serum ratios are greater than those of erythromycin but less than those of azithromycin. The half-life of clarithromycin is longer than that of erythromycin but shorter than that of azithromycin. It penetrates tissue and cells, including alveolar macrophages, and polymorphonuclear leukocytes.[196] Protein binding of clarithromycin ranges from 40% to 70% and is concentration dependent.

Azithromycin is rapidly distributed into tissues but released slowly so that it has an extremely long half-life (>60 h).[157] High concentrations of azithromycin are achieved in phagocytes and macrophages.[197] The very high levels of azithromycin achieved in sputum, lung, tonsil, sinus, stomach, uterus, ovary, fallopian tube, cervix, and prostate can be 10 to 150 times the serum level. Effective tissue concentrations are achieved even when the serum level is below the minimum inhibitory concentration (MIC) of susceptible organisms. Thus azithromycin may be given over a relatively short course of treatment. Protein binding is relatively low at 51% and appears to be concentration dependent.[157]

Dirithromycin produces lower serum concentrations than the other macrolides but it is also concentrated in tissues. Dirithromycin has a long half-life (20 to 44 h), permitting once-daily administration.[177]

Adverse Effects of the Macrolides

As a group, the macrolides are relatively nontoxic antibiotics. The most common side effects with oral therapy are gastrointestinal disturbances in the form of epigastric pain, nausea, and mild diarrhea.[192] The gastrointestinal complaints are seen especially after high doses of erythromycin and are sometimes quite severe.[198,199] The mechanism underlying these effects is not clear, but erythromycin has been shown to be a motilin receptor agonist and thus stimulates gastrointestinal motility. The gastrointestinal symptoms appear to be dose related and occur more commonly in children and young adults.[198] In stomach acid erythromycin is converted to a cyclic hemiketal, which is the irritant that causes increased gastrointestinal motility. Clarithromycin and azithromycin do not cyclize and the incidence of gastric distress is much lower than with erythromycin. Intravenous administration of erythromycin frequently produces local pain during the infusion and rapid injection may cause faintness and dizziness.[184] Transient loss of hearing occurs rarely after intravenous administration,[189,200] and five cases of hypertrophic pyloric stenosis have been reported in infants receiving erythromycin estolate.[201] Hypersensitivity reactions are uncommon, but one in particular is of special interest. Erythromycin estolate can cause a cholestatic hepatitis characterized by fever, abdominal pain, eosinophilia, and elevated serum bilirubin and transaminase.[202] Other forms of erythromycin do not have this effect. The first reaction usually occurs 10 to 20 days after initiation of erythromycin estolate therapy, but in a patient who has had the reaction previously, it occurs within hours. The reaction is reversible upon withdrawal of the drug. Although this effect is often referred to as a *hepatotoxicity*, it has many of the characteristics of an allergic reaction. As yet, there has been no direct demonstration of an immunological mechanism in patients[203] and it has been suggested that the reaction may reflect an intrinsic toxicity to the liver coupled with a drug hypersensitivity.[204]

There are several observations that may shed light on the mechanism of the hepatitis. The liver normally concentrates erythromycin many-fold in the bile. Thus, the cells of this organ are exposed to very high concentrations of whichever erythromycin preparation is used. Erythromycin estolate is the lauryl sulfate salt of erythromycin propionate. Erythromycin propionate has been shown to rapidly reduce bile flow in the isolated, perfused rat liver, whereas erythromycin base has a minimal effect.[204] Erythromycin propionate is clearly toxic to liver cells in suspension in concentrations at which other forms of the drug have no effect.[205,206] The demonstration that erythromycin propionate is toxic in these in vitro systems, whereas other forms of erythromycin are not, is completely consistent with the clinical observation that cholestatic hepatitis occurs only with this compound. The argument supporting the hepatotoxicity of

erythromycin propionate is well substantiated. The rapid recurrence of symptoms when patients are rechallenged with the propionyl compound must be explained on an immunological basis. Thus, the interpretation that the cholestatic hepatitis is due to a summation of a hepatotoxic effect and a drug hypersensitivity seems a good one.

The proprietary name for erythromycin estolate is Ilosone. Because administration of the estolate does not yield higher serum levels of the bioactive form of the drug and since the estolate is uniquely associated with the production of cholestatic hepatitis, the Food and Drug Administration has raised the question of whether it should be withdrawn from the market in the United States. As of 1998, the estolate is still available. The estolate should not be administered to adults, in whom the incidence of hepatitis is much higher than in children.

Why isn't erythromycin base more toxic? Like chloramphenicol, erythromycin and lincomycin inhibit protein synthesis on mammalian mitochondrial ribosomes. As discussed earlier in this chapter, there is evidence that some toxic effects of chloramphenicol, such as reversible marrow suppression, result from an inhibition of mitochondrial protein synthesis in the cells of the patient. If that mechanism is valid, there must be a good reason why erythromycin and lincomycin do not produce similar toxic effects. Chloramphenicol inhibits protein synthesis in isolated intact mitochondria, but erythromycin and lincomycin do not.[84] When the mitochondrial membrane is ruptured, however, both these antibiotics produce a marked inhibition. Thus, the mitochondrial membrane acts as a permeability barrier to erythromycin and the lincomycins. This inability to penetrate into the mitochondria is probably an important factor in the selective toxicity of these agents. In addition, there is evidence that mammalian mitochondrial ribosomes are intrinsically less sensitive to lincomycin than bacterial ribosomes.[207] At very high concentrations (300 μg/ml), erythromycin inhibits the growth of cultured human cells (HeLa). It seems clear that this growth inhibition is due to an effect on mitochondrial function, since resistance to the drug effect is cytoplasmically inherited and, therefore, presumably encoded in the mitochondrial genome.[208]

The newer macrolides resemble erythromycin in toxicity but are even better tolerated. Clarithromycin, azithromycin, and dithromycin can produce occasional gastrointestinal toxicity but the incidences are less than with erythromycin. Cholestatic hepatitis has been reported with clarithromycin[209] as have nonspecific elevations in liver enzymes. Neither clarithromycin nor azithromycin has produced any of the reversible dose-related hearing loss seen with erythromycin. Patients with HIV infection may demonstrate more toxicity with clarithromycin, especially abdominal pain, nausea and vomiting, rash, and hematologic abnormalities.[157] No hematologic abnormalities have occurred in HIV negative patients.

Drug Interactions

Erythromycin and, to a lesser extent, clarithromycin are involved in several clinically significant drug interactions. The bulk of these reactions results from interference with cytochrome P-450-mediated metabolism of these drugs. Some of the macrolides inhibit the cytochrome P-450 3A enzyme,[210] which metabolizes cyclosporine, tacrolimus, theophylline, caffeine, carbamazepine, triazolam, rifabutin, and disopyramide, among others.[210] Drugs such as the antihistamines terfenadine or astemizole may produce *torsades de pointes* when given with erythromycin. The metabolism of clarithromycin has been reported to be affected by P-450 enzyme induction, with both rifampin and rifabutin inducing its metabolism.[210] Azithromycin does not interact with the hepatic cytochrome P-450 system and is not associated with the pharmacokinetic drug interactions seen with erythromycin. Dirithromycin does not appear to affect this system either.

In addition to effects on drug-metabolizing enzymes, other types of interactions can occur with the macrolides. When azithromycin is given with antacids, the resultant serum level is lowered, but the over-all absorption is the same. Clarithromycin interferes with zidovudine absorption in some patients, although the reverse effect is not seen. Azithromycin has no drug interactions with zidovudine. Erythromycin may cause increased serum levels of digoxin because it suppresses the gut flora that ordinarily metabolize digoxin.[157]

Clindamycin

Two lincosamide antibiotics are marketed in the United States, lincomycin and clindamycin. Lincomycin is produced by *Streptomyces lincolnensis*. Clindamycin, the 7-deoxy, 7-chloro derivative of lincomycin, is clinically the most important.

Clindamycin

Mechanism of Action

Lincomycin binds to the 50S ribosomal subunit.[132] As discussed in the preceding section on the mechanism of action of erythromycin, the lincomycin binding site appears to overlap the chloramphenicol and erythromycin receptor sites. In contrast to chloramphenicol, lincomycin and erythromycin do not interact with polysomes bearing nascent peptides but do bind to polysomes that are free of nascent peptides.[211] The mechanism of protein synthesis inhibition has not been worked out in detail. Some observations have suggested that the rate of chain initiation is affected,[212,213] but most of the observations made in cell-free systems support a mechanism based on inhibition of peptide bond synthesis.[214] The presence of lincomycin on the 50S ribosomal subunit apparently inhibits the peptidyl transferase reaction by interfering primarily with the binding of the aminoacyl-tRNA substrate to the A site.[214]

Antagonism between erythromycin and lincomycin has been reported, both for inhibition of bacterial growth and inhibition of cell-free protein synthesis.[214] The antagonism is due to the displacement of bound lincomycin by erythromycin, which has a tenfold higher affinity for the ribosome.

Antimicrobial Activity and Clinical Use

Clindamycin has an antibacterial spectrum that includes gram-positive cocci and anaerobes but not aerobic gram-negative organisms. Clindamycin is also active against certain protozoa. Lincomycin has the same spectrum of action as clindamycin, but it is less active both in vitro and in vivo,[215] and

it is used primarily in veterinary medicine. Clindamycin may be bacteriostatic or bactericidal; the response depends on the bacterial species and the growth conditions. It is active against many gram-positive cocci (see Table 6–6 for bacterial sensitivities[216]) and it was frequently used as an alternative to penicillins for treating infections due to *Staphylococcus aureus* and *Streptococcus pyogenes*. Because of the association of the drug with pseudomembranous colitis, the indications for its clinical use are now quite restricted. Clindamycin is largely used to treat anaerobic infections[217,218] and mixed intraabdominal and female genital tract infections (in combination with an aminoglycoside).[219-221] Clindamycin is considered to be the drug of choice for treating infection

Table 6–6. *Susceptibility of selected bacterial species to clindamycin.*

Organism	Range of minimum inhibitory concentration (μg/ml)
AEROBIC BACTERIA	
Gram-positive	
Staphylococcus aureus	0.05–1.5
Streptococcus pyogenes (group A)	0.025–0.05
Streptococcs pneumoniae	<0.002–0.05
Streptoccus, viridans group	0.005–0.05
Enterococcus	25–>100
Corynebacterium diphtheriae	0.2
Corynebacterium acnes	0.1–6.0
Gram-negative	
Escherichia coli	100
Neisseria gonorrhoeae	0.01–6.3
Neisseria meningitidis	6.3–25
Haemophilus influenzae	1.6–50
ANAEROBIC BACTERIA	
Gram-positive	
Peptococcus spp.	<0.01–6.2
Peptostreptococcus spp.	<0.1–1.6
Clostridium perfringens	0.025–0.1
Clostridium tetani	3.2
Gram-negative	
Bacteroides fragilis	<0.1–3.1
Bacteroides spp.	<0.1–1.6
Fusobacterium fusiforme	<0.1–1.6
Viellonella spp.	<0.1

Source: Data from Leigh.[216]

due to *Bacteroides fragilis* arising from a source in the abdomen or pelvis.[222,223] The drug is bactericidal against some strains of *B. fragilis* and bacteriostatic against others.[224] Clindamycin may be used as an alternative to penicillin G in treating infections due to other anaerobic bacteria, such as *Fusobacterium*, anaerobic streptococci, *Clostridium perfringens*, and oropharyngeal strains of *Bacteroides fragilis*. Clindamycin has also been used successfully in cases of osteomyelitis caused* by sensitive strains of *Staphylococcus aureus* and anaerobes. It has been of particular value for bone infections related to diabetic foot and decubitus ulcers in which a polymicrobial cause, including anaerobes, is common.[225] Clindamycin has been applied topically to treat acne vulgaris,[226,227] and it has been administered by the subconjunctival route to treat retinochoroiditis due to *Toxoplasma gondii*.[228]

Clindamycin (usually in combination with other agents) has good activity against certain protozoal pathogens, such as *Plasmodium* spp., *Pneumocytis carinii, Toxoplasma gondii,* and *Babesia* spp.[228,229,230] As a result, clindamycin has been used in combination with pyrimethamine for the acute treatment of encephalitis caused by *Toxoplasma gondii* in patients with AIDS.[230] In addition, clindamycin in combination with primaquine has been shown to be useful for the treatment of mild to moderate cases of *Pneumocystis carinii* pneumonia in AIDS patients.[231]

Bacteroides fragilis strains can become resistant to clindamycin, but the incidence of clinical resistance is low and has remained quite constant in most hospitals.[232] Staphylococci that have been induced by low concentrations of erythromycin to produce methylated 23S ribosomal RNA (see discussion of erythromycin resistance in the previous section) become resistant to high concentrations of both erythromycin and lincomycin.[147,233] At low concentration, clindamycin can also induce this type of ribosomal resistance in staphylococci[233] and *Corynebacterium diphtheriae*.[234] Some strains of staphylococci that are constitutively resistant to erythromycin remain sensitive to clindamycin, while others are cross-resistant.[147]

Methicillin-resistant strains of *Staphylococcus aureus* are resistant to clindamycin.

Pharmacology of Clindamycin

Clindamycin is absorbed from the gastrointestinal tract more readily than lincomycin and its absorption is not significantly affected by the presence of food in the stomach.[215] Because clindamycin yields higher serum levels and is more potent than lincomycin, it is the preferred drug, so the pharmacology of lincomycin will not be discussed here. Clindamycin is provided in two forms for oral administration, either as capsules of clindamycin hydrochloride or as the palmitate ester, which is used to prepare flavored suspensions for pediatric use. In adults, a peak serum level of 2.8 µg/ml is achieved 1 h after ingestion of 150 mg of clindamycin hydrochloride.[235] The palmitate is absorbed in the ester form and rapidly hydrolyzed to clindamycin, which is the biologically active form in the serum.[216] The phosphate ester of clindamycin is provided for intramuscular or intravenous administration. The phosphate ester is also rapidly hydrolyzed in the blood to bioactive clindamycin. After intramuscular administration of 300 mg of clindamycin phosphate to adults, peak serum levels of 4–5 µg/ml of clindamycin are achieved in 2 h.[236] After intravenous infusion of 300 mg clindamycin phosphate over 10 min in adults, peak serum levels of bioactive clindamycin are 5–6 µg/ml.[236]

Clindamycin is widely distributed in the tissues and body fluids,[216,237] with high levels being achieved in bone[238] and synovial, pleural, and peritoneal fluids.[237,239] Passage into the cerebrospinal fluid is very poor and the drug is not used to treat meningitis. Clindamycin is actively transported into polymorphonuclear leukocytes and macrophases where high concentrations are achieved.[240] Clindamycin readily passes across the placenta.[194] Sixty to ninety-five percent of the drug is bound to plasma protein.[188] The half-life of clindamycin in normal adults is 2 to 2.5 h.[216] Only 6% to 10% of a dose is eliminated in the urine in adults and about twice this amount in infants and children.[241] Extensive elimination occurs in the bile, where very high levels are achieved in the absence of biliary tract obstruction.[242] Two metabolites of clindamycin, the N-demethyl form and the sulfoxide, have been identified in human bile and urine.[236] Both of the metabolites are bioactive. Clindamycin undergoes enterohepatic circulation leading to a prolonged presence in stools, and changes in gut flora may last up to 2 weeks after the drug is discontinued.[243]

The half-life of clindamycin in anuric patients is extended to about 6 h,[294] but dosage adjustment is usually not necessary if hepatic function is normal.[188] The drug is not removed by hemodialysis or peritoneal dialysis.[188] In patients with moderate to severe hepatic dysfunction, the clindamycin half-life is prolonged and high serum concentrations result.[242,245] Recommendations for dosage reduction in the presence of hepatic failure have not been formulated. Serum clindamycin levels should be monitored in patients with severe renal and/or hepatic disease.

Adverse Effects of Clindamycin

The most common adverse effects of clindamycin are diarrhea and hypersensitivity reactions. Clindamycin may occasionally cause local irritation at intramuscular injection sites or local thrombophlebitis at sites of intravenous infusion. Hypotension and cardiovascular collapse have been reported after bolus injection, but this does not occur if the drug is infused over 10–60 min, as directed by the manufacturer. Clindamycin has neuromuscular blocking properties and caution should be employed with patients who are receiving neuromuscular blocking drugs.[246] Allergic reactions have been observed occasionally; they include morbilliform-like skin rashes, urticaria, and drug fever. Skin rashes may be more common in patients with human immunodeficiency virus (HIV) infection.[247] Rarely, instances of erythema multiforme (some resembling Stevens-Johnson syndrome) and anaphylactoid reactions have occurred.[216] Blood dyscrasias, including neutropenia, thrombocytopenia, and agranulocytosis, have been reported to occur rarely. Reversible rises in serum transaminases (SGOT and SGPT) occur frequently, but other evidence of hepatotoxicity is uncommon.[241,248] Clindamycin produces its most serious untoward effects in the gastrointestinal tract.

ANTIBIOTIC-ASSOCIATED (PSEUDOMEMBRANOUS) COLITIS. As with virtually any orally administered antibiotic,[249] clindamycin can cause a variety of untoward gastrointestinal effects, including nausea, vomiting, epigastric distress, and abdominal pain. Clindamycin commonly produces diarrhea. Reported incidence varies from 3.4% to 30%, with most of the estimates being in the range of 5%–10%.[250,251] Two forms of diarrhea occur. Mild to moderate diarrhea is most common, but it became clear in the 1970s that clindamycin could also produce a profuse, watery diarrhea and pseudomembranous colitis due to *Clostridium difficile*. The term *pseudomembranous colitis* was used because the intestinal lesions that are produced are covered by a pseudomembrane composed of polymorphonuclear leukocytes, fibrin, and necrotic cells. When the risk of pseudomembranous colitis was realized, the clinical indications for clindamycin use became quite restricted. Although it was the experience with clindamycin that led to detailed investigation of the etiology of pseudomembranous colitis, the condition can accompany the administration of a wide variety of antibiotics,[252] and it is now referred to as *antibiotic-associated colitis*. The clinical features and pathophysiology of this condition have been the subject of several symposia and reviews.[252–254]

The incidence of colitis with clindamycin therapy is not well defined; reported incidences range from 0.01% to 10%.[252] Although the symptoms usually begin within a week of initiating antibiotic therapy, they may occur up to 4–6 weeks after antibiotic therapy has stopped. Colitis is more common with oral administration of antibiotics, but occurs with parental therapy as well.[253] One case of colitis has been reported during topical therapy of acne,[255] but this should be a very rare event, as little drug is absorbed with topical use of a 1% solution.[256] Although the severity of the diarrhea is variable, most patients with biopsy-proven enterocolitis have 10–20 watery stools per day. Often there is blood and mucus in the stool. Abdominal tenderness is usually minimal, but some patients have diffuse cramping pain, abdominal rigidity, and toxic megacolon. Fever and hypoalbuminemia are seen in most patients, and peripheral leukocytosis is common.[253] If the condition is not recognized and appropriate therapy not initiated, the syndrome can be lethal.

The direct cause of the colitis is not the antibiotic, but a toxin or toxins produced by *Clostridium difficile*, a gram-positive anaerobic bacillus. Changes in normal flora related to antibiotic administration may promote overgrowth of *C. difficile* and elaboration of the toxin. Elderly patients, patients who are exposed to a nosocomial source of the organism, and patients whose normal resistance to colonization of the intestinal tract is impaired by disease or antibiotic therapy are at increased risk of having the pseudomembranous colitis. Some antibiotics are more likely than others to produce changes in the normal gastrointestinal flora. Certain properties of the antibiotic such as its spectrum of activity, its degree of intestinal absorption, and its enterohepatic recirculation may affect the indigenous flora.[257,258] Prolonged high intraluminal antibiotic levels promote selection of antibiotic-resistant strains and overgrowth of pathogens. Well-absorbed antibiotics that do not reach the colon are less likely to disrupt the microflora. The route of administration of the antibiotic may also affect the development of colitis. For example, the risk of colitis with clindamycin is about four times greater with oral than with intravenous therapy.[257]

The etiologic role of *C. difficile* was demonstrated in a hamster model. Hamsters were used for these studies because, after a single low dose of clindamycin, they develop a hemorrhagic enterocolitis with intestinal lesions that closely resemble those that occur with antibiotic-associated colitis in humans.[259,260] The cecal feces of antibiotic-treated hamsters contain an increased amount of *C. difficile*, and bacteria-free fecal filtrates from animals with antibiotic-induced colitis were shown to contain a cytotoxin that causes the colitis when introduced into the cecum of normal animals.[261,262] The effects of the hamster toxin were neutralized by antibodies raised against *Clostridium sordellii* toxin,[263] which is immunologically similar to that produced by *C. difficile*. Hamsters that were passively immunized with *C. sordellii* antitoxin survived lethal challenges of intracecally administered *C. difficile* toxin or a lethal challenge of antibiotic.[264] Thus, Koch's postulates were fulfilled, proving that clindamycin-induced colitis in the hamster model is caused by *C. difficile* toxin.

Observations made on clindamycin-induced colitis in humans have closely paralleled those in the hamster model. It was first shown that stools from clindamycin-treated patients with colitis contain a cytopathic toxin that is inactivated by clostridial antitoxins.[265,266] It was then shown that stool specimens from patients with clindamycin-induced colitis caused the syndrome when injected intracecally into hamsters.[267] The hamsters did not develop colitis if stool samples were first neutralized by clostridial antitoxin.[267] Subsequently, *C. difficile* was cultured from most patients with antibiotic-associated colitis.[252] The high incidence of *C. difficile* and toxin in patients with antibiotic-associated colitis is in contrast to an extremely low incidence in normal adults and in patients with other gastrointestinal diseases.[252] *C. difficile* is present, however, in a high percentage of stools obtained from infants, in whom this organism is usually benign.[252]

Antibiotic-associated colitis can be regarded as a superinfection of the bowel with *C. difficile*. Virtually all isolates of *C. difficile* are susceptible to vancomycin at levels less than 4 µg/ml.[268] The mean level of vancomycin in the stool of patients receiving 500 mg orally every 6 h is 3100 µg/g wet weight.[269] The antimicrobial drug of choice for antibiotic-associated colitis is either oral vancomycin at 125 mg four times a day, or oral metronidazole at 250 mg four times a day.[270,271] Treatment is usually continued for 7 to 10 days. Although oral vancomycin is expensive, it is still preferred for treatment of severe antibiotic-associated colitis. In some hospitals this use of vancomycin is discouraged in an effort to reduce selection of vancomycin-resistant bacteria. Metronidazole does have some disadvantages, in that it should not be used in pregnancy and it is so well absorbed in the small intestine that adequate levels of the drug may not reach the colon, particularly when intestinal motility is diminished. In addition, metronidazole-resistant strains of *C. difficile* have been reported. Patients who are severely ill require hospitalization and replacement of fluids and electrolytes.

Because of the risk of antibiotic-associated colitis, patients treated with clindamycin should be alerted to report significant diarrhea (more than five stools per day); if diarrhea occurs, the drug should be discontinued. In patients who develop colitis, diarrhea and clinical toxicity disappear within 3 to 5 days of starting therapy as does the toxin of *C. difficile* in fecal filtrates. The use of drugs that diminish intestinal mobility, such as atropine and opioids, should be avoided because they may worsen the condition.

Spectinomycin

Spectinomycin is an aminocyclitol antibiotic isolated from *Streptomyces spectabilis*. It produces a bacteriostatic effect at concentrations achieved clinically.

Spectinomycin

Spectinomycin interacts with the 30S ribosomal subunit and inhibits protein synthesis in a reversible manner.[272,273] Spectinomycin resistance can be conferred by amino acid replacements in protein S5 of the 30S ribosomal subunit[274,275] and these resistant ribosomes have lost the ability to bind the drug in a high-affinity manner.[276] The in vitro inhibition of protein synthesis by spectinomycin is strongly dependent on the composition of the synthetic RNA template, with inhibition becoming increasingly pronounced with increasing guanylic or cytidylic acid content.[273] The available evidence supports the hypothesis that the action of spectinomycin on the 30S ribosome subunit inhibits the translocation step in protein synthesis,[273,277] perhaps by interfering with the movement of mRNA with respect to the 30S ribosomal subunit.

Spectinomycin is active against a variety of gram-negative bacteria, but because resistance is rapidly acquired by most species, it is used clinically only for treatment of infection due to *Neisseria gonorrhoeae*. Resistance among enterobacteria is very common and is due to the acquisition of R factors that produce enzymes capable of inactivating the drug by adenylylation.[278,279] Resistance to spectinomycin in *N. gonorrhoeae* results from altered 30S ribosomal protein.[280] *N. gonorrhoeae* strains resistant to spectinomycin have now emerged in Southeast Asia, the United States, and the United Kingdom.[281]

The minimum inhibitory concentration (MIC) for the great majority of strains of *N. gonorrhoeae* is less than 15 μg/ml of spectinomycin.[282,283] The MICs for *Mycoplasma hominis* and *Ureaplasma urealyticum* range from 4 to 16 μg/ml.[284] Spectinomycin is not effective against *Chlamydia trachomatis*[285] or *Treponema pallidum* (syphilis).[286] Spectinomycin is now recommended for the treatment of uncomplicated gonococcal infection as an alternative regimen in patients who are intolerant or allergic to β-lactam antibiotics and quinolones. The recommended drugs of choice are ceftriaxone, cefixime, ciprofloxacin, or ofloxacin.[167] Two grams of spectinomycin hydrochloride in one intramuscular injection is the recommended dose. Spectinomycin is not useful for treating gonococcal pharyngitis[287] and it fails to abort incubating syphilis.[286]

Spectinomycin is not absorbed from the

gastrointestinal tract and is administered only by intramuscular injection. The average peak serum level achieved 1 h after injection of 2 g of spectinomycin hydrochloride is 74 μg/ml.[288] There is little or no binding to plasma protein and the half-life is about 2.5 h. Seventy-eight percent of the drug is excreted in the unmetabolized form in the urine within 8 h.[288] Concentrations of 1000 μg/ml may be achieved in urine.[289] Spectinomycin is well tolerated.[289,290] A single dose occasionally produces local pain at the injection site, dizziness, nausea, chills, fever, urticaria, and insomnia.

Tetracyclines

The tetracycline antibiotics are bacteriostatic agents with broad-spectrum antimicrobial activity. The tetracyclines were isolated from various species of *Streptomyces* recovered by large-scale screening of soil samples. The

Tetracycline

Tetracycline preparation	Substituents at position number 5	6	7
Chlortetracycline		—CH₃;—OH	—Cl
Oxytetracycline	—OH	—CH₃;—OH	
Demeclocycline		—OH	—Cl
Methacycline	—OH	=CH₂	
Doxycycline	—OH	—CH₃	
Minocycline			—N(CH₃)₂

first of these compounds, chlortetracycline (Aureomycin), was introduced in 1948. At present five tetracycline analogs are marketed in the United States. Tetracycline, oxytetracycline and demeclocycline are naturally derived compounds whereas doxycycline is derived semisynthetically from oxytetracycline and minocycline is prepared by chemical modification of tetracycline. Structurally, the tetracyclines are very closely related. All the tetracyclines contain a hydronaphthacene nucleus consisting of four fused rings. Differences among the various analogs

result from different substitutions on the basic structure. Their spectra of antimicrobial action are similar, although doxycycline and minocycline are active against some bacterial strains that may not respond to the other congeners.

Mechanism of Action

At the blood concentrations achieved in antibacterial therapy, the tetracyclines are bacteriostatic. At much higher concentrations, they are bactericidal. Various biochemical sites of action have been proposed for these drugs, based on reports of their inhibition of several bacterial enzyme systems, oxidative phosphorylation, glucose oxidation, and membrane transport.[291] One of the earliest studies demonstrated that protein synthesis is particularly sensitive to inhibition by the tetracyclines,[292] and it is now clear that inhibition of protein synthesis is responsible for the inhibition of growth by these drugs (for a review, see Kaji and Ryoji[293]).

The receptor for tetracyclines has not been defined as precisely as that for spectomycin or erythromycin. The tetracyclines bind to both ribosomes and mRNA. It is clearly the binding of the drug to the ribosome that inhibits protein synthesis.[294] This binding is largely reversible, and the bulk of the bound tetracycline is associated with the 30S ribosomal subunit.[295,296] A poly U–directed cell-free protein-synthesizing system from E. coli containing 30S ribosomal subunits from tetracycline-resistant cells is much less sensitive to inhibition by tetracycline than the same system containing 30S units from sensitive cells.[297] But it has not been demonstrated that the 30S particles from resistant cells do not bind the drug as well, as they do with streptomycin. A fluorescence study of the interaction of tetracycline with 70S ribosomes of E. coli identified a single, strong binding site that accounts for inhibition.[298] A photoaffinity study of tetracycline interaction with 70S ribosomes showed specific labeling of 30S subunit proteins S4 and S18, suggesting that they are either in or near the binding site.[299]

In bacteria, tetracycline inhibits protein synthesis by blocking the binding of

Table 6–7. The effect of tetracycline on the binding of phenylalanyl-tRNA to the 30S ribosomal subunit. Phenylalanyl-tRNA binding to ribosomes was measured by incubating ^{3}H-labeled phenylalanyl-tRNA with poly U and 30S subunits at 24°C for 20 min. After incubation, the samples were filtered and washed. The ribosome-bound radioactivity remained on the filter, while the unbound radioactive aminoacyl-tRNA passed through. The values in the table represent the total phenylalanyl-tRNA bound per 7 μg of 30S subunit.

	Binding of [^{3}H]phenylalanyl-tRNA	
Conditions of prebinding	Tetracycline added with 30S subunits	Tetracycline added 20 min after 30S subunits
Control	781	851
Tetracycline ($4.5 \times 10^{-4}M$)	226	674

Source: Data from Suzuka et al.[300]

aminoacyl-tRNA to the mRNA-ribosome complex. As shown in Table 6–7, when tetracycline and phenylalanyl-tRNA are added simultaneously to a system containing 30S subunits and poly U, binding of the radioactive phenylalanyl-tRNA to the 30S subunits is markedly inhibited.[300] When the phenylalanyl-tRNA is added to the system 20 min before the tetracycline, inhibition of binding is much less. Thus, once the aminoacyl-tRNA is bound to the 30S particles, tetracycline cannot dissociate it.

There are two binding sites for aminoacyl-tRNA on the mRNA-70S-ribosome complex (see Chapter 5). An aminoacyl-tRNA can bind to the first site, the A site, when the 30S subunit is present. It is only when the 50S subunit is bound to the 30S ribosome subunit that a second binding site (the P site) is generated. This second binding site normally binds the tRNA to which the growing polypeptide is attached. It has been shown that tetracycline inhibits the binding of lysyl-tRNA to the ribosome but has no effect on the binding of polylysyl-tRNA.[301] This indicates that the drug inhibits binding to the A site but not to the P site. A similar conclusion was reached by investigators who demonstrated that, although tetracycline inhibits virtually 100% of the protein synthesis, it can only inhibit 50%[302] of the binding of N-acetyl-phenylalanyl-tRNA. Protein synthesis is halted at the same concentration of

tetracycline that inhibits the binding of aminoacyl-tRNA to one-half of the tRNA binding sites on the ribosome.

The conclusion that tetracycline affects the binding to the acceptor site is supported by investigations using another antibiotic, puromycin, as an experimental tool. Puromycin is an analog of aminoacyl-tRNA.[303] It effects the separation of the growing peptide chain from the peptidyl-tRNA-messenger-ribosome complex, with the formation of peptidylpuromycin.[304] Puromycin does not prevent the binding of aminoacyl-tRNA to the A site nor does it effect the release of aminoacyl-tRNA from that site. It was reasoned that if tetracycline inhibits only the binding of aminoacyl-tRNA to the A site, then all of the aminoacyl-tRNA that remains bound in the presence of tetracycline should be occupying the peptidyl-tRNA (P) site and should be released by puromycin. Correspondingly, only one-half of the aminoacyl-tRNA bound in the absence of the drug should be sensitive to puromycin. In the experiment presented in Table 6–8 and Figure 6–5, only one-half of the aminoacyl-tRNA was bound in the presence of tetracycline, and all of this was released as phenylalanyl-puromycin.[305] In the absence of tetracycline, twice as much aminoacyl-tRNA was bound, and only one-half of it (presumably that portion occupying the P site) was released as phenylalanyl-puromycin.

Table 6–8.   *The release by puromycin of radioactive phenylalanyl-tRNA prebound to ribosomes: with and without tetracycline.* ^{14}C-labeled phenylalanyl-tRNA was bound to ribosomes with and without tetracycline. The phenylalanyl-tRNA was present in amounts sufficient to assure maximal binding. Puromycin was then added, incubation was continued for 1 h, and the amount of phenylalanyl-puromycin formed was extracted and assayed. Values represent the number of $\mu\mu$moles of phe-tRNA bound or phenylalanyl-puromycin released per incubation.

Conditions of prebinding	Phenylalanyl-tRNA prebound ribosomes ($\mu\mu$moles)	Phenylalanyl-puromycin synthesized and released ($\mu\mu$moles)	Prebound phenylalanine released by puromycin (%)
Control	14.1	6.74	47.7
Tetracycline ($6 \times 10^{-4}M$)	7.35	7.21	98.1

Source: From Sarkar and Thach.[305]

Figure 6–5. The release by puromycin of phenylalanyl-tRNA bound to ribosomes with and without tetracycline. A: In the normal process of mRNA translation, the tRNA with the attached peptide occupies the P site (I). When puromycin is added, an aminoacyl-tRNA can still bind in the A site; puromycin, however, becomes linked by a peptide bridge to the carboxy terminal of the growing peptide (II), and this complex is released as peptidyl-puromycin (III). B, C: The experiment as carried out with tetracycline by Sarkar and Thach.[305] When phenyalanyl-tRNA is bound to ribosomes in the presence of tetracyline (B), tetracycline blocks binding to the A site, but binding to the P site is permitted. When the bound complex is exposed to puromycin, all the phenylalanine is released as phenylalanyl-puromycin. In the absence of tetracycline (C), phenylalanyl-tRNA can bind to both the A and P sites; therefore, twice as much is bound. Since puromycin can release only the phenylalanine occupying the P site, one-half of the bound phenylalanine is released as phenylalanyl-puromycin. P, puromycin; T, tetracycline; phe, phenylalanine; aa, amino acid.

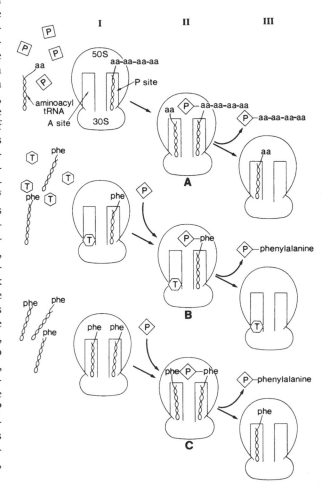

Basis for the Selective Toxicity of the Tetracyclines

When they are present in sufficient concentration, tetracyclines can inhibit protein synthesis in cell-free systems from mammalian cells.[306,307] As in bacteria, they appear to act by inhibiting the binding of aminoacyl-tRNA to the mRNA-ribosome complex.[307,308] The selective toxicity of these antibiotics cannot be explained solely in terms of different drug sensitivities of the ribosomes from the two sources. An important component of their selective toxicity resides in their differential entry into bacterial cells.

The tetracyclines are accumulated in both gram-positive and gram-negative bacteria in an energy-dependent manner.[309,310] Two types of uptake systems are involved in tetracycline accumulation.[311,312] There is an initial, rapid uptake that is driven by the protonmotive force and appears to reach an equilibrium with the tetracycline in the medium in about 5 min. A slow, second uptake system then becomes evident; it accumulates tetracycline over a period of hours and is energy dependent. Both uptake systems contribute to bacterial sensitivity to the drug. In gram-negative bacteria the tetracyclines must pass through the outer membrane to reach the uptake systems. The hydrophilic congeners, such as tetracycline, chlortetracycline, and oxytetracycline, pass preferentially through pores in the outer membrane, which in E. coli K-12 are formed from porin Ia.[313] Minocycline is much more lipophilic and appears to penetrate the outer membrane by diffusing through the lipid matrix.[314] Doxycycline may also be too hydrophobic to pass through the outer membrane pores.[314] The lipophilic properties of minocycline and doxycycline may account for their ability to inhibit some bacterial strains that are not susceptible to the more hydrophilic congeners.[315]

Mammalian cells (other than those involved in absorption and excretion of the drug) do not actively accumulate these antibiotics. When present at high concentration, however, tetracyclines can inhibit the growth of mammalian cells in culture,[316] and at concentrations achieved in therapy, tetracyclines inhibit both the migration and phagocytic function of human leukocytes.[317,318] Tetracyclines can extensively inhibit protein synthesis by mammalian cells in culture if their entry into the cell is facilitated by drugs, such as amphotericin B or polymyxin B, that alter membrane permeability.[319] Although some of the selective toxicity may be explained on the basis of differential entry into bacteria, differences in sensitivity at the ribosomal level must also be important. This is inferred from the fact that tetracyclines are used to treat infection due to rickettsiae and chlamydiae. These organisms grow intracellularly, and thus their protein synthesis must be more sensitive than the host cells' process of protein synthesis.

Antimicrobial Activity and Resistance

The tetracyclines have a very broad spectrum of antibacterial action that includes both gram-positive and gram-negative species.[320,321] The minimum inhibitory concentrations (MICs) of tetracycline and doxycycline for a variety of common aerobic bacteria are presented in Table 6–9.[322] In general, the newer, more lipophilic agents, doxycycline and minocycline, are more active against gram-positive organisms than the older tetracyclines.[320] For example, doxycycline, and minocycline are more active against Staphylococcus aureus and various streptococci than tetracycline. Many strains of gram-positive cocci are now resistant to tetracyclines, as indicated by the wide range of MICs in Table 6–9. Because resistance is common and because narrower-spectrum, less toxic, bactericidal antibiotics are available, the tetracyclines are generally not useful for treating infections due to gram-positive cocci. However, it is not widely appreciated that doxycycline and minocycline are very active against Streptococcus pneumoniae. Resistance of S. pneumoniae is minimal with these tetracyclines in contrast to the older ones. For this reason, doxycycline monotherapy remains useful in the treatment of community-acquired pneumonias whereas conventional tetracyclines should be avoided.[323] The tetracyclines are

Table 6–9.   *Activity of tetracycline and doxycycline against aerobic bacteria,* Mycoplasma, *and* Chlamydia.

| | Minimum inhibitory concentration (μg/ml) | | | |
| | Tetracycline | | Doxycycline | |
	Median	(Range)	Median	(Range)
GRAM-POSITIVE BACTERIA				
Staphylococcus aureus	3.1	(1.6–>100)	1.6	(0.39–>100)
Streptococcus pyogenes (group A)	0.78	(0.19–50)	0.39	(0.09–25)
Streptococcus pneumoniae	0.8	(0.2–100)	0.2	(0.1–12)
Streptococcus, viridans group	3.1	(0.9–100)	0.39	(0.09–50)
Enterococcus	>100	(6.3–>100)	50	(1.6–>100)
GRAM-NEGATIVE BACTERIA				
Escherichia coli	12.5	(3.1–500)	12.5	(1.6–500)
Enterobacter	25	(6.3–50)	25	(12.5–25)
Klebsiella	50	(6.3–500)	50	(6.3–300)
Serratia	200	(200)	50	(50)
Proteus mirabilis	>100	(50–>100)	>100	(50–>100)
Haemophilus influenzae	1.6	(0.8–3.1)	1.6	(0.8–3.1)
Shigella	100	(1.6–>500)	100	(1.6–500)
Pseudomonas aeruginosa	200	(50–300)	100	(25–300)
Neisseria gonorrhoeae	0.78	(0.39–6.3)	0.39	(0.09–3.1)
Neisseria meningitidis	0.8	(0.3–3.1)	1.6	(0.8–6)
MYCOPLASMA AND CHLAMYDIA				
Mycoplasma pneumoniae	1.6	(1.6–3.1)	1.6	(1.6)
T-mycoplasmas	0.4	(0.2–0.8)	0.1	(0.05–0.2)
Chlamydia	2.0	(0.5–4.0)	2.0	(0.5–4.0)

Source: Data from Neu[322] and Steigbigel et al.[320]

active against Neisseria, including both *N. gonorrhoeae* and *N. meningitidis*, although tetracycline-resistant *N. gonorrhoeae* strains are being identified with increasing frequency.

Among the common gram-negative bacilli, there is a wide range of activity against *Escherichia coli, Klebsiella,* and *Enterobacter;* however, many strains are resistant especially in the hospital environment. *Proteus mirabilis* and *Pseudomonas aeruginosa* strains are resistant; most strains of *Haemophilus influenzae* have remained susceptible. Many anaerobic bacteria are resistant to clinically achievable blood concentrations of tetracycline or doxycycline, but minocycline has somewhat greater activity, with 70% of strains being inhibited by 2.5 μg/ml, a concentration that is readily achievable in

the blood after therapeutic doses.[324] The tetracyclines are not generally recommended for treatment of anaerobic infections unless the in vitro sensitivity of the specific organism has been established.

Tetracyclines are active against several unusual gram-negative bacteria, including *Brucella* species, *Francisella tularensis, Pasturella multocida,* and *Yersinia pestis.* They are also active against spirochetes (including *Treponema pallidum, Treponema pertenue, Leptospira, Borrelia recurrentis,* and *Borrelia burgdorferi*), *Actinomyces,* some atypical mycobacteria (e.g., *Mycobacterium fortuitum* and *M. marinum*), *Mycoplasma, Chlamydia,* and rickettsia. Tetracyclines are not effective against fungi because they don't penetrate into the cell. However, if a low concentration of amphotericin B is present in vitro, entry of minocycline and doxycycline into the cell is facilitated, resulting in synergism against *Candida* strains.[325] The broad spectrum of action of the tetracyclines is reflected in their effectiveness against several protozoa, including *Entamoeba histolytica* and *Plasmodium falciparum*.[326]

RESISTANCE. Tetracycline resistance in clinical isolates is associated with a decreased ability to accumulate the antibiotic.[314] Most of the resistance in both gram-positive and gram-negative bacteria is determined by plasmids,[327] although clinical isolates of *N. gonorrhoeae* are resistant because of mutations in chromosomal genes.[328] In most bacteria with plasmid-determined resistance, the property is inducible; that is, the level of resistance increases in response to the presence of subinhibitory concentrations of the drug.[327] The mechanism of plasmid-mediated resistance has been studied in greatest detail in *E. coli*, where decreased accumulation of tetracycline has been shown to result both from decreased influx of the

antibiotic[329,330] and from the acquisition of an energy-dependent system that actively transports the antibiotic out of the cell.[330,331] This efflux system is inducible by tetracycline.[331] Although decreased accumulation of antibiotic may not account entirely for the 200-fold resistance that some plasmids confer, it is clearly a major component of the resistance mechanism. The emergence of resistance to tetracyclines has been a growing problem worldwide and of increasing concern. The addition of these drugs to animal feeds has been an important factor in the spread of the resistance.

Pharmacology of the Tetracyclines

The tetracyclines can be divided into three groups according to their duration of action. Their pharmacological properties are summarized in Table 6–10.

The short-acting tetracyclines, tetracycline, chlortetracycline, and oxytetracycline, were the first to be marketed. These were followed by demeclocycline and methacyc-

Table 6–10. Pharmacokinetic characteristics of the tetracyclines.

Tetracycline preparation	Usual oral dose in adults (mg)	Usual dosage interval (hours)	Oral dose obsorbed (%)	Primary route of elimination	Half-life Normal (hours)	Half-life Anuric (hours)	Plasma protein binding (%)
SHORT-ACTING							
Tetracycline hydro-chloride	500	6	77–80	Renal	8	c	55–64
Oxytetracycline	500	6	58	Renal	9	c	27–35
INTERMEDIATE-ACTING							
Demeclocycline	300	12	66	Renal (hepatic)	12–14	c	75–91
LONG-ACTING							
Doxycycline	100[a]	24	93	Hepatic (renal)	15–21	15–36	82–93
Minocycline	100[b]	12	98	Hepatic	12–13	17–30	76

[a] A loading dose of 200 mg (100 mg every 12 h) is administered on the first day and 100 mg is given every 24 h thereafter. [b] A loading dose of 200 mg is administered, then 100 mg every 12 h thereafter. [c] Prolonged half-lives and high serum levels occur in anuric patients. These tetracyclines should not be given to patients with compromised renal function.

Source: The values in the table are taken from Bennett et al.,[188] Fabre et al.,[332] Macdonald et al.,[333] Rosenblatt et al.,[334] and Kunin et al.[335]

line, both of which have longer half-lives that permit them to be administered twice daily, rather than every 6 h. Chlortetracycline is only available as an ophthalmic ointment in the United States; methacycline is no longer available. The newest tetracyclines, doxycycline and minocycline, are more lipophilic, are excreted by predominantly extrarenal mechanisms, and have longer half-lives. The general pharmacology of the tetracyclines will be presented here, and the reader is referred to several comprehensive reviews of the extensive literature for additional specific details concerning the human pharmacology of the individual drugs.[322,332,336]

ABSORPTION. The tetracyclines are absorbed from the stomach and upper intestinal tract. Absorption in the acid environment of the stomach is probably passive, but absorption in the intestine appears to be mediated by a transport mechanism.[337] The tetracyclines form stable chelates with a number of metal ions, such as calcium, magnesium, iron, and aluminum.[338] The formation of an insoluble complex with any of these compounds decreases absorption of the drug.[339] Therefore, tetracyclines should never be administered with milk, which contains calcium, or with antacids, such as Maalox, which contains magnesium and aluminum hydroxide, or Amphojel, which is an aluminum hydroxide gel. Ferrous sulfate administered with a tetracycline markedly reduces the absorption of the antibiotic,[340] so even small doses of iron should be avoided during tetracycline therapy. It has been suggested that increasing gastric pH impairs tetracycline absorption.[341] It is clear, however, that the absorption of tetracycline products with good bioavailability is not impaired in patients with achlorhydria who have a high gastric pH.[342] Concomitant administration of drugs that block acid production, such as cimetidine, or antacids that do not contain metal ions, such as sodium bicarbonate, does not appear to significantly affect tetracycline absorption.[343]

The different tetracyclines are absorbed to different extents from the gastrointestinal tract, ranging from oxytetracycline at 58% absorption to minocycline, which is com-

pletely absorbed. In contrast to the shorter-acting preparations, the absorption of doxycycline and minocycline is not affected by food.[334] Peak plasma levels of about 3 µg/ml are achieved after oral administration of 250 mg of tetracycline or oxytetracycline every 6 h and peak plasma levels of 4 to 5 µg/ml are achieved with 500 mg administered every 6 h. After intravenous administration of 500 mg of the short-acting tetracyclines, peak plasma levels are 6–10 µg/ml at the end of infusion and the levels decline to 2–4 µg/ml after 6 h.[335] Oral administration of the intermediate-acting and long-acting tetracyclines in the dosage and at the intervals indicated in Table 6–10 yields plasma levels that are maintained between a peak of 3–5 µg/ml and a trough of 1 µg/ml.[332,333] Because the absorption of doxycycline and minocycline is essentially complete, serum levels after oral or intravenous administration are the same.[333,344]

DISTRIBUTION. The tetracyclines distribute into a space that is larger than the body water.[335] With the exception of oxytetracycline, most of the drug in the serum is bound to protein (see Table 6–10).[345] Protein binding is highest with doxycycline, intermediate with minocycline, and lowest with oxytetracycline. The tetracyclines readily penetrate into most tissues; particularly high levels are achieved in the liver and kidney, and the levels in most other tissues are as high or higher than those in the serum.[332,333] Tissue penetration is directly related to the lipid solubility of the individual tetracyclines. Both doxycycline and minocycline are lipid soluble and thus these drugs have excellent tissue penetration. Minocycline is 10 times more soluble and doxycycline 5 times more soluble than tetracycline.[346] Bacteriostatic levels are achieved in pleural and synovial fluids,[332] in the aqueous humor,[347] and in abscess fluid.[332] Penetration into cerebrospinal fluid is poor and does not increase significantly in the presence of meningeal inflammation.[332] The levels achieved in the cerebrospinal fluid are insufficient to render these drugs useful in the treatment of meningeal infection. The tetracyclines readily pass across the human placenta and enter the fetal circulation and amniotic fluid.[348] The levels achieved in bile are several times larger than those in the serum and the concentration of minocycline in bile in the absence of obstruction is 38 times the serum concentration.[333] The lipophilic behavior of minocycline probably accounts for the observation that higher levels of this drug are achieved in brain tissue and in saliva and tears than with the other tetracyclines. The concentration of minocycline achieved in saliva and tears is equal to or greater than the average MIC for *Neisseria meningitidis*[349] and accounts for the unique effectiveness of minocycline in eradicating the meningococcal nasopharyngeal carrier state.[350]

In general, the association of the tetracyclines with tissues is rapidly reversible; however, these drugs can be permanently sequestered in newly forming bone and teeth.[351] The tetracyclines do not bind to bone that is already formed but are incorporated into calcifying tissue as a tetracycline-calcium orthophosphate complex. This drug deposition is not unique to the modern era of antibiotic therapy. Tetracycline that was apparently ingested in streptomycete-contaminated grain has been detected in the bones of mummified Nubians that lived 1400 years before the antibiotic era.[352] The deposition of tetracyclines in growing enamel of teeth and in growing nails is responsible for some cosmetically undesirable effects of these drugs.[353] Tetracyclines are also retained (probably as chelate complexes with calcium) in some tumor cells and in areas of infarcted myocardium where the presence of the drug can be detected by fluorescence techniques.[354–357]

ELIMINATION. The tetracyclines are eliminated by both renal and extrarenal mechanisms. All of the tetracyclines are excreted by the liver into the bile by an active transport mechanism.[358] Most of these drugs are reabsorbed during passage through the intestinal tract. The short-acting and intermediate-acting drugs are ultimately excreted in their active forms by glomerular filtration in the kidney. Because these drugs accumulate with impaired renal function, they should not be administered to patients with renal failure.[359] In contrast to the older drugs, doxycycline and minocycline are excreted to a much lesser extent by the kidney (only about 5% of minocycline is recovered in the urine during the first 24 h)[336] and their half-lives are not markedly prolonged in the presence of renal failure.[188,332,336] Doxycycline is eliminated primarily through the digestive tract, with up to 90% excreted in the feces as an inactive conjugate or as a chelate. Approximately 19% to 23% is excreted by glomerular filtration.[360] Because the half-life of doxycycline is the least affected by decreased renal function, it is the tetracycline of choice if tetracycline therapy is required in a patient with renal failure.[332,359] The tetracyclines are not removed by peritoneal dialysis or hemodialysis.[188]

The metabolism of the tetracyclines has not been well defined. Clearly, some metabolism of doxycycline occurs, because the half-life is reduced to approximately 7 h in patients who are receiving drugs like barbiturates or phenytoin, which induce the hepatic drug metabolizing system.[361,362] Only 30% of a dose of minocycline is accounted for by bioassay in urine and feces,[333] suggesting that the remaining drug may be inactivated by metabolism or chelation. As minocycline is very lipophilic, it is possible that some of the drug is stored in fat and slowly released.

Adverse Effects

IRRITATIVE EFFECTS. Although as a group, tetracyclines are considered to be relatively safe drugs, a number of adverse reactions can occur. The tetracyclines are irritative substances. When given intravenously, they cause thrombophlebitis. Intramuscular administration is painful and this route of administration is not recommended. Given orally, tetracyclines can cause epigastric burning, abdominal discomfort, nausea, and vomiting. If gastric distress is severe, symptoms can sometimes be controlled, at the risk of some impairment of absorption, by having the patient take tetracyclines immediately after meals. The irritative property of the tetracyclines can be appreciated from the fact that they have on rare occasion caused esophageal ulceration.[363] To avoid this complication, the tetracyclines should not be administered at bedtime and, if possible, they should not be given to patients with symptoms of esophageal reflux. Diarrhea caused by the direct irritative effects of the tetracyclines on the bowel mucosa is relatively common. Diarrhea occurs more often with the poorly absorbed tetracyclines and rarely with the well-absorbed tetracyclines, such as doxycycline. Diarrhea can also result from superinfection of the bowel.

SUPERINFECTION. Because they are broad-spectrum antibiotics, therapy with tetracyclines is associated with a higher incidence of superinfection than therapy with many other antibiotics, particularly in patients with diabetes and other conditions that reduce the natural host defense mechanisms. Superinfection of the bowel is due to the growth of drug-resistant bacteria or yeasts, and when severe diarrhea occurs, it must be viewed with concern. Occasionally, tetracycline therapy is associated with the production of enterocolitis due to *Clostridium difficile* or staphylococci. Antibiotic-associated colitis due to *C. difficile* is a potentially life-threatening condition that is reviewed in detail in an earlier section of this chapter. Staphylococcal enterocolitis is also a life-threatening condition that is characterized by severe diarrhea, fever, and leukocytosis. It can be differentiated from milder forms of diarrhea by the presence of large numbers of gram-positive cocci and leukocytes in profuse liquid stools that often contain blood. The condition occurs rarely and many cases of diarrhea that were labeled staphylococcal enterocolitis in the past may actually have represented antibiotic-associated colitis due to *C. difficile*. However, when either condition appears, tetracycline therapy must be stopped, vigorous fluid and electrolyte management begun, and oral treatment with vancomycin initiated immediately.

Superinfection with *Candida albicans* occurs in the oropharynx, vagina, and bowel; it can even occur as a systemic infection. Some tetracycline preparations used to contain both a tetracycline and nystatin, an antifungal agent included to suppress superinfection of the bowel with *Candida*. This does not constitute rational prophylactic use of an antibiotic. The use of these two drugs in a fixed-ratio combination has not been demonstrated to reduce the incidence of intestinal superinfection with *Candida*. As stated in a drug efficacy study conducted by the National Academy of Sciences, "it is preferable . . . to prescribe antifungal drugs when clinically indicated, rather than to use them indiscriminately as 'prophylaxis' against an uncommon clinical entity seen during therapy with tetracyclines and other antibiotics."[364] Upon careful review of the patient, the physician often will find that the tetracycline therapy can be simply discontinued when superinfection intervenes. When this is not possible, nystatin or another antifungal agent should be given in the appropriate form by the appropriate route. The use of the fixed-ratio drug combination represents a violation of several fundamental precepts of rational chemotherapy.

EFFECTS ON TEETH AND BONE. The unique property of the tetracyclines that causes them to be incorporated into growing teeth produces a cosmetically undesirable effect that is manifest as a yellow or brownish discoloration of the enamel. This effect is clearly related to the dose of the drug,[365] and if exposure is high, tooth deformity may result from faulty enamel formation.[366] Increasing exposure to tetracyclines produces a progressively darker yellow shade in the teeth, and if there is a deep yellow color it may be converted to brown, a process accelerated by exposure to light. The change in color is probably due to photooxidation products formed from tetracycline. The tetracyclines can cross the placenta, and their administration to a pregnant woman can discolor the deciduous teeth of the infant.[353] These drugs also appear in the milk of lactating patients. As would be expected, tetracycline taken by the mother during pregnancy does not affect the color of the child's permanent teeth.[367] The cosmetically undesirable discoloration occurs when the tetracycline is deposited in the crown of the anterior teeth. Crown formation in these teeth is complete by 6 years in girls and 7 years in boys.[365] Oxytetracycline binds calcium less readily than the other tetracyclines[368] and there is some suggestion that it is less likely to produce a noticeable discoloration.[365,366] In children under 8 years of age, the risk of discoloration of permanent teeth must be taken into account when the tetracyclines are being considered for therapy. Long-term therapy and repeat exposure should be avoided. The use of oxytetracycline (and possibly doxycycline) may further diminish the risk of dental staining. The period of greatest risk to the deciduous teeth is after the fourth month of gestation, thus tetracycline therapy should be avoided during pregnancy. Tetracyclines have been reported to depress long bone growth in premature infants.[369] Although it is often assumed that inhibition of skeletal growth is related to tetracycline deposition in bone, it may reflect an antianabolic action on osteoblasts. After short-term administration, the inhibition of bone growth is readily reversible.

HEPATIC AND RENAL TOXICITY. Tetracyclines cause a hepatotoxicity that presents clinically as lethargy and jaundice and that may progress to overwhelming liver failure.[370] The syndrome is characterized histologically by diffuse fatty infiltration of the liver.[371] The hepatotoxicity develops predominantly in patients who are receiving 2 g or more of the drug daily by parenteral administration.[372] Pregnant and postpartum women with renal disease are especially vulnerable to developing hepatotoxicity.[373]

The metabolic effects of tetracyclines can aggravate azotemia in patients with preexisting renal disease. If administered to patients with renal failure, most of the tetracyclines accumulate to toxic levels in the body and may produce progressive azotemia.[374] It has been postulated that the azotemia is secondary to inhibition of protein synthesis in the tissues with a consequent decrease in amino acid utilization leading to an increase in urea production.[375] In addition to an increasing blood urea nitrogen (BUN), acidosis and sodium and water loss may also occur. The glomerular filtration rate may be further reduced, sometimes irreversibly.[374] Elevated BUN values are more frequently seen with patients who are also receiving diuretics.[376] This is probably not the result of a drug interaction but represents the use of tetracyclines in a subpopulation with already compromised renal function. Since doxycycline does not accumulate to toxic levels in patients with renal failure, it does not increase urea production.[377] Clearly, tetracyclines other than doxycycline (and perhaps minocycline) should not be given to patients with renal failure. It has been noted that tetracycline therapy is sometimes associated with increased excretion of nitrogen and a negative nitrogen balance in surgical patients and in patients who are undernourished.[372] This effect could also be related to an inhibition of protein synthesis.

Several direct renal effects of the tetracyclines have been reported. The administration of demeclocycline has been associated with the production of a dose-dependent and reversible nephrogenic diabetes insipidus.[378] This side effect has been exploited with some success in treating the chronic syndrome of inappropriate antidiuretic hormone secretion with demeclocycline.[379] The ingestion of outdated tetracyclines has been associated with a reversible Fanconi syndrome, a proximal tubular defect leading to proteinuria, glycosuria, amino aciduria, and hypocalcemia.[380,381] Patients have symptoms of polyuria and polydipsia. The syndrome is reversible and it may be due to the presence of small amounts of anhydroepitetracycline, which can produce a similar syndrome in rats and dogs.[382] Tetracycline preparations that are now marketed do not contain citric acid as a preservative, a precaution that has prevented recurrences of the Fanconi syndrome.[383] Nevertheless, care should be taken that outdated preparations of tetracyclines are discarded.

EFFECTS ON SKIN. All the tetracyclines can cause a phototoxicity manifested by abnormal sunburn reactions or paresthesias (tingling sensations) in exposed parts.[384] These reactions are rapidly reversible. The mechanism of these reactions is not defined. As mentioned above, the tetracyclines fluoresce when exposed to light in the ultraviolet range. The sunburn reaction is also precipitated by that component of light falling in the ultraviolet spectrum (260 to 320 nm). Ultraviolet irradiation may promote the formation of photodecomposition products that are responsible for the sunburn effect, but other explanations are also possible. Demeclocycline and doxycycline cause these reactions more frequently than the other tetracyclines and the frequency is lowest with minocycline.[384,385] In addition to phototoxicity, porphyria-like changes consisting of fragility and blistering of the sun-exposed skin may occur with tetracycline therapy.[386] Several of the tetracyclines, including minocycline, have been reported to cause a photosensitivity reaction of the nails (photo-onycholysis).[387] Long-term and high-dose therapy with minocycline is rarely associated with the appearance of blue or blue-black regions of hyperpigmentation, predominantly affecting the skin of the lower extremities and atrophic scars.[388,389] The color is caused by the accumulation of electron-dense, iron-containing particles within the histiocytes of the dermis; the mechanism that causes the accumulation is unknown.[389]

MISCELLANEOUS EFFECTS. In addition to the major classes of clinically undesirable effects noted above, the tetracyclines rarely cause allergic reactions, central nervous system side effects, and effects on blood cells.[370] Anaphylaxis and anaphylactoid reactions have been reported but are rare. Other allergic reactions have occurred, including fixed-drug reactions involving the genitalia and other areas and contact dermatitis.[390] Fever and eosinophilia have been reported occasionally.

Tetracyclines rarely elevate intracranial pressure in infants[390] and in young women.[391] This benign intracranial hypertension (pseudotumor cerebri) may occur when the drug is administered at low dosage. In infants, it presents as bulging fontanelles, but there are no convulsions or focal signs of neural impairment. Young adults complain of headache, nausea, vomiting, and diplopia. The symptoms disappear soon after the drug is stopped, but papilledema may persist for several months in some patients.[391] The

pathogenesis of the syndrome has not been defined.[392]

Administration of minocycline may cause dizziness, vertigo, and ataxia, often with nausea and vomiting.[336] The syndrome is dose related and the symptoms start soon after the initiation of therapy; they subside when the drug is discontinued. Although the symptoms are exaggerated when the patient assumes erect posture, this is not due to orthostatic hypotension.[350] The incidence of the vestibular symptoms is higher in women, apparently because women, with their relatively smaller size, have a higher serum level of drug than men after standard dosage.[393] The symptoms are usually mild and estimates of their frequency vary tremendously.[370]

Leukocytosis, atypical lymphocytes, toxic granulation of granulocytes, thrombocytopenic purpura, and hemolytic anemia have rarely been associated with tetracycline use.[370] Tetracyclines have been reported to inhibit chemotaxis and phagocytosis by human leukocytes[317,318] and to decrease the bactericidal effect of human serum.[394] This interference with the host response may not be significant in the patient with normal immunological defense mechanisms, but it might contribute to failure of therapy in the patient with borderline function.

Drug Interactions

A number of drugs interact with the tetracyclines. The most prominent effects are on absorption and metabolism of the tetracyclines. As noted above, concomitant administration of ferrous sulfate or antacids containing calcium, magnesium, or aluminum may impair the oral absorption of tetracyclines, resulting in decreased serum levels. Antacids may enhance total body clearance and renal clearance of intravenously administered doxycycline.[395] It is recommended that tetracyclines should not be taken within 1 to 2 h of antacid administration.

Doxycycline may also be less effective in patients receiving long-term anticonvulsant therapy with phenytoin or carbamazepine because the half-life of doxycycline is shortened by 50%, owing to enhanced hepatic metabolism.[396] Barbiturates and long-term alcohol consumption also reduce the half-life of doxycycline for similar reasons.[397,398] Enhancement of the anticoagulant effect of warfarin and clinical bleeding has been noted during combination therapy with doxycycline. This interaction may involve the competition for plasma protein binding sites or the inhibition of warfarin hepatic metablism by doxycycline. Therefore, close monitoring of the prothrombin time is warranted in patients undergoing concomitant doxycycline and warfarin therapy.[399]

Therapeutic Use of the Tetracyclines

Tetracyclines are used to treat a variety of infections, including those involving the respiratory and urinary tracts. Because of the development of tetracycline resistance and the availability of less toxic antibiotics, the tetracyclines are rarely the drugs of first choice for common bacterial infections. The tetracyclines are indicated in the treatment of a wide variety of uncommon infections, both on a first-choice basis and as alternatives to less toxic agents (see refs. 400 and 401 for reviews of the clinical literature). The broad-spectrum antimicrobial action of the tetracyclines is reflected in their proven effectiveness in the treatment of diseases caused by *Rickettsia, Chlamydia, Mycoplasma, Spirochetes,* and protozoa, as well as the variety of gram-negative and anaerobic bacteria presented in Table 6–11.

In routine outpatient practice, tetracy-

Table 6–11. *Therapeutic indications for the use of tetracyclines.*

Tetracyclines—drugs of first choice	Tetracyclines—valuable alternatives to drugs of first choice
INFECTIONS DUE TO	INFECTIONS DUE TO
Bacteria	Bacteria
Brucellosis (with or without streptomycin)	Anthrax (penicillin G)
Granuloma inguinale	Tetanus (penicillin G)
Peptic ulcer *(Helicobacter pylori)* (with metronidazole and bismuth subsalicylate)	Tularemia (streptomycin)
Melioidosis	*Haemophilus influenzae,* respiratory infection (ampicillin or amoxicillin)
Cholera	Chancroid (trimethoprim-sulfamethoxazole
Spirochetes	Vincent's infection, *Leptotrichia buccalis* (penicillin G)
Relapsing fever *(Borrelia)*	Rat bite fever (penicillin G)
Lyme disease *(Borrelia burgdorferi)*	*Pasturella multocida* (penicillin G)
Chlamydia	Plague (streptomycin)
Psittacosis *(Chlamydia psittaci)*	Spirochetes
Urethritis, and lymphogranuloma venerum *(Chlamydia trachomatis)*	Syphilis (penicillin G)
Erlichia	Yaws (penicillin G)
Mycoplasma pneumonia (or erythromycin)	Leptospirosis (penicillin G)
Rickettsia	*Actinomyces israelii* (penicillin G)
Rocky Mountain spotted fever, Q fever, scrub typhus, typhus, rickettsial pox	Chlamydia
	Trachoma *(Chlamydia trachomatis)* (azithromycin)
SYNDROMES	Mycoplasma
	Ureaplasma urealyticum (an erythromycin)
Nongonococcal urethritis	Protozoa
Acne vulgaris (when systemic antibiotic is required)	Chloroquine-resistant *Plasmodium falciparum*
Chronic bronchitis, acute exacerbations	PROPHYLAXIS
Malabsorption syndromes	Meningococcal carrier state, minocycline only (rifampin)
	Traveler's diarrhea (doxycycline)

clines are commonly used in the management of acute anogenital, pharyngeal, and pelvic gonococcal infection where they are as effective as penicillin G, ampicillin, or spectinomycin regimens against sensitive strains.[287,402] Because of their activity against *Chlamydia trachomatis* and genital mycoplasmas, the tetracyclines are highly effective in the treatment of nongonococcal urethritis,[403,404] The tetracyclines are useful in the treatment of other venereal diseases. They are drugs of choice for lymphogranuloma venerum and granuloma inguinale; for treating syphilis they are used as alternatives to penicillin G.[400] Tetracyclines are frequently used in community practice to treat acute flare-ups of chronic bronchitis as they shorten the course of symptoms and prevent deterioration of the clinical status in patients with mild to moderate exacerbations.[400] Tetracyclines also reduce the morbidity associated with *Mycoplasma pneumoniae* pneumonitis,[405] and either a tetracycline or an erythromycin is considered to be the drug of choice for treating mycoplasma pneumonia.

The tetracyclines and chloramphenicol are effective and may be life saving in rickettsial infections of all types, including Rocky Mountain spotted fever and Q fever. Doxycycline is effective for treating the early phases of Lyme disease and preliminary data also indicate its efficacy against new and emerging pathogens, such as penicillin-resistant *Streptococcus pneumoniae* and vancomycin-resistant enterococci.[406] In peptic ulcer where *Helicobacter pylori* plays a major role, tetracycline is often used as part of a three-drug combination along with metronidazole and bismuth subsalicylate. Doxycycline is now relatively inexpensive and is the tetracycline of choice in many infections where a tetracycline is called for.[406]

The tetracyclines are often used prophylactically: a single daily dose of doxycycline is used to prevent traveler's diarrhea caused by enterotoxigenic *E. coli* and to prevent chloroquine-resistant malaria. Minocycline has been widely used for the chemoprophylaxis of meningococcal disease.[350] Its unique effectiveness in eradicating meningococci from carriers is apparently due to the fact that higher levels of minocycline are achieved in saliva compared to other tetracyclines.[349] Because minocycline is less effective than rifampin at eliminating the most pathogenic strains of meningococci from carriers and because it produces a vestibular toxicity, rifampin is now considered the drug of choice for meningococcal prophylaxis.

TETRACYCLINES IN TREATMENT OF ACNE. Tetracycline is given orally in low doses for the treatment of chronic severe acne vulgaris. Appropriate studies support the clinical effectiveness of long-term tetracycline therapy.[407,408] The use of a broad-spectrum antibiotic in long-term therapy for a relatively minor clinical indication like acne requires special comment. With the usual therapeutic dosage, this form of therapy would be accompanied by an inappropriate risk of adverse drug effects. Although therapy of acne may be initiated with normal dosage, the low amount of antibiotic required to maintain the beneficial response (usually 250 or 500 mg/day) has proven to be quite safe.[409] The only common complications are *Candida* vaginitis and minor gatrointestinal irritation. Rarely, the development of allergic reactions, gram-negative folliculitis,[410] or benign intracranial hypertension[392] have required cessation of therapy. Topical administration of tetracyclines is effective in the management of many patients with acne vulgaris.[256,411] Temporary yellow discoloration of the skin and skin fluorescence are unique side effects associated with this route of administration.

It is not completely clear why low-dose tetracycline therapy works in the treatment of acne, an inflammatory lesion of the pilosebaceous follicle.[227] Onset occurs when there is a marked increase in the activity of the sebaceous glands in response to androgenic hormones. The only bacteria regularly recoverable from acne lesions are *Propionobacterium acnes, Staphylococcus epidermidis*, and *Pityrosporum ovale*; all of these are normal, resident skin bacteria. The most important one is probably *P. acnes*, but several studies have failed to show any correlation between the number of bacteria present and the severity of acne.[227] Patients with severe acne may initially require 1 g/day of tetracycline and those with moderate acne, 250 or 500 mg/day. At the end of 2 to 3 months, the dosage for patients initially receiving 1 g/day is gradually reduced to 500 mg/day, depending on the progress of the disease. At 1 g/day tetracycline reduces the number of *P. acnes* in the skin,[412] but at a dosage of 500 mg/day the number of *P. acnes* does not decrease.[227] At the lower dosage, however, bacterial metabolism is altered such that there is decreased production of biologically active substances (e.g., free fatty acids) that mediate inflammation.[227,408] As other antibiotics, such as erythromycin, trimethoprim-sulfamethoxazole, and clindamycin (although the toxicity of this last drug makes oral use inappropriate in acne), are also effective, the therapeutic benefit must be due to an antibacterial effect.

In summary, the use of antibiotics in trivial acne is not justified, but most dermatologists would accept that long-term, low-dose oral tetracycline therapy is appropriate in chronic, severe acne.[407] The use of topically applied tetracycline (and other antibiotics) appears to be effective[256] and it eliminates the potential problems of *Candida* superinfection of the vagina and gastrointestinal upset. The primary mechanism of the beneficial effect at low drug dosage probably reflects an inhibition of bacterial metabolism, resulting in a decreased production of bioactive substances that mediate inflammation without any accompanying gross change in bacterial colony count.

Streptogramins

Streptogramins are a group of natural cyclic peptides produced by a number of species of bacteria. They represent a unique class of antibacterials in that each member of the class consists of at least two structurally unrelated molecules: group A streptogramins (macrolactones) and group B streptogramins (cyclic hexadepsipeptides). One of these streptogramins, quinupristin/dalfopristin, is

approved by the Food and Drug Administration.

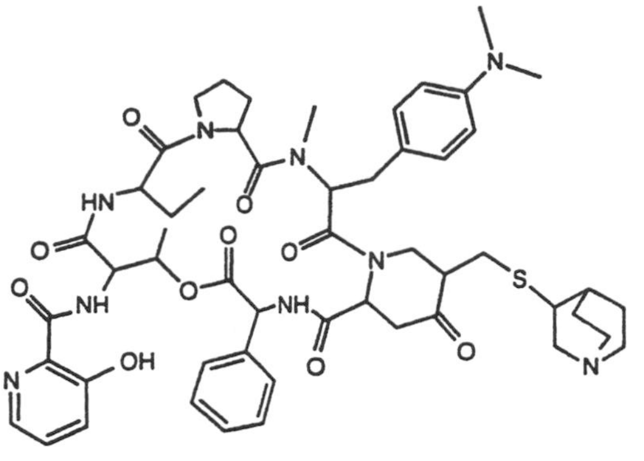

Quinupristin

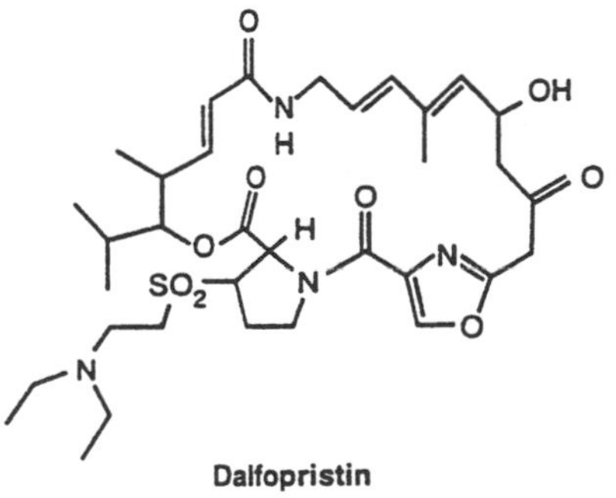

Dalfopristin

Both groups of streptogramins inhibit protein synthesis by acting on the peptidyltransferase domain of the 50S ribosomal subunit, and the streptogramins share many similarities in mechanism of action to the macrolides and lincosamide group of antibiotics.[413] Group A streptogramins inactivate the donor and acceptor sites of peptidyltransferase, thus interfering with the function of this enzyme and blocking two of the peptide chain elongation steps. Group B streptogramins interfere with the correct positioning of peptidyl-tRNA at the P site, thus they inhibiting peptide bond formation, interfering with the formation of long polypeptides, and causing premature detachment of incomplete peptide chains.[413,414] Group A and B streptogramins act synergistically against bacteria, apparently because type A streptogramins induce conformational changes in the peptidyl transferase center that increase ribosome affinity for type B streptogramins. Synergy also results from inhibition of both early and late stages of protein synthesis.[413,415] Because, of this synergism, the likelihood of resistance developing to the combination is reduced, and the antibacterial spectrum is extended beyond those of the individual agents. While the effect of each component alone is bacteriostatic, the effect of the combination is bactericidal. The mechanisms of acquired resistance to the streptogramins are similar to those of the macrolides and lincosamides, including modification of the drug target, drug inactivation, and active efflux.

Antibacterial Activity and Therapeutic Potential of Streptogramins

Quinopristin-dalfopristin is approved in the United States for use in patients with severe gram-positive infections who cannot tolerate or do not respond to the established clinically appropriate antibiotics.[416] Streptogramins in general have inhibitory activity against a wide range of aerobic and anaerobic gram-positive organisms and against a limited number of gram-negative bacteria. The streptogramins offer promise in the treatment of multi-resistant infections such as methicillin-resistant staphylococcal infections and enterococcal infections that are resistant to vancomycin. They may also be useful as therapy in patients with multidrug-resistant infections who are unable to tolerate vancomycin, including patients with skin and soft tissue infections, osteomyelitis, foreign body–associated infections, endocarditis, and sepsis due to gram-positive bacteria.[417]

Pharmacokinetics

Quinupristin-dalfopristin is the most studied of the streptogramins. With this drug the mean maximum blood concentration at the end of a 1-h infusion ranged from 9.97 µg/ml for a 1.4 mg/kg dose to 24.2 µg/ml for a 29.4 mg/kg dose. There was a linear correlation between dose and mean area under the concentration–time curve, and mean half-life ranged from 1.37 to 1.63 h.[418,419]

The drug undergoes extensive hepatic metabolism and appears to be rapidly converted to primary active metabolites that contribute to the total antibacterial activity.

Adverse Reactions

The most common local adverse reactions to quinupristin-dalfopristin include inflammation (42%), pain (40%), edema (17.3%), infusion site reaction (13.4%), and thrombophlebitis (2.4%). The most common systemic adverse reactions reported include nausea (4.6%), diarrhea (2.7%), vomiting (2.7%), rash (2.5%), headache (1.6%), pruritis (2.5%), and pain (1.46%).[418,420,421] No cases of ototoxicity, nephrotoxicity, or red man syndrome were reported in clinical trials.

REFERENCES

1. Hahn, F. E., and P. Gund. A structural model of the chloramphenicol receptor site. In *Drug Receptor Interactions in Antimicrobial Chemotherapy*, ed. by J. Drews and F. E. Hahn. New York: Springer-Verlag, 1975, pp. 245–266.

2. Pongs, O. Chloramphenicol. In *Antibiotics, V-1*, ed. by F. E. Hahn. New York: Springer-Verlag, 1979, pp. 26–42.

3. Wisseman, C. L., J. E. Smadel, F. E. Hahn, and H. E. Hopps. Mode of action of chloramphenicol. I. Action of chloramphenicol on assimilation of ammonia and on synthesis of proteins and nucleic acids in *Escherichia coli*. *J. Bacteriol.* 1954;67:662.

4. Vazquez, D. Uptake and binding of chloramphenicol by sensitive and resistant organisms. *Nature* 1964;203:257.

5. Das, H. K., A. Goldstein, and L. C. Kanner. Inhibition by chloramphenicol of the growth of nascent protein chains in *Escherichia coli*. *Mol. Pharmacol.* 1966;2:158.

6. So, A. G., and E. W. Davie. The incorporation of amino acids into protein in a cell-free system from yeast. *Biochemistry* 1963;2:132.

7. Perlman, S., and S. Penman. Protein-synthesizing structures associated with mitochondria. *Nature* 1970; 227:133.

8. Roodyn, D. B., and D. Wilkie. *The Biogenesis of Mitochondria*. London: Methuen, 1968. An extensive discussion of the possible evolutionary origin of mitochondria and a review of the effects of chloramphenicol on mitochondrial protein synthesis.

9. Lessard, J. L., and S. Pestka. Studies on the formation of transfer ribonucleic acid-ribosome complexes: chloramphenicol, aminoacyl-oligonucleotides, and *Escherichia coli* ribosomes. *J. Biol. Chem.* 1972; 247:6909.

10. Tritton; T. R. Ribosome-chloramphenicol interactions: a nuclear magnetic resonance study. *Arch. Biochem. Biophys.* 1979;197:10.

11. Vazquez, D. The binding of chloramphenicol by ribosomes from *Bacillus megaterium*. *Biochem. Biophys. Res. Commun.* 1964;15:464.

12. Nierhaus, K. H., and F. Dohme. Total reconstitution of functionally active 50S ribosomal subunits from *Escherichia coli*. *Proc. Natl. Acad. Sci. U.S.A.* 1974;71:4713.

13. Nierhaus, D., and K. H. Nierhaus. Identification of chloramphenicol-binding protein in *Escherichia coli* ribosomes by partial reconstitution. *Proc. Natl. Acad. Sci. U.S.A.* 1973;70:2224.

14. Pongs, O., R. Bald, and V. A. Erdman. Identification of chloramphenicol binding protein in *Escherichia coli* ribosomes by affinity labeling. *Proc. Natl. Acad. Sci. U.S.A.* 1973;70:2229.

15. Stöffler, G., and H. G. Wittmann. Primary structure and three dimensional arrangement of proteins within the *Escherichia coli* ribosome. In *Molecular Mechanisms of Protein Biosynthesis*, ed. by H. Weissbach and S. Pestka. New York: Academic Press, 1977, pp. 117–202.

16. Vazquez, D. Binding of chloramphenicol to ribosomes; the effect of a number of antibiotics. *Biochim. Biophys. Acta* 1966;114:277.

17. Oleinick, N. L., J. M. Wilhelm, and J. W. Corcoran. Nonidentity of the site of action of erythromycin A and chloramphenicol on *Bacillus subtilis* ribosomes. *Biochim. Biophys. Acta* 1968;155:290.

18. Grant, P. G., B. S. Cooperman, and W. A. Strycharz. On the mechanism of chloramphenicol-induced changes in the photoinduced affinity labeling of *Escherichia coli* ribosomes by puromycin. Evidence for puromycin and chloramphenicol sites on the 30S subunit. *Biochemistry* 1979;18:2154.

19. Cannon, M., R. Krug, and W. Gilbert. The binding of sRNA by *Escherichia coli* ribosomes. *J. Mol. Biol.* 1963;7:360.

20. S. Pestka. Inhibitors of ribosome functions. *Annu. Rev. Microbiol.* 1971;25:487.

21. Pestka, S. Studies on transfer ribonucleic acid-ribosome complexes: effect of antibiotics on peptidyl puromycin synthesis on polysomes from *Escherichia coli*. *J. Biol. Chem.* 1972;247:4669.

22. Pestka, S. Studies on the formation of transfer ribonucleic acid-ribosome complexes. XI. Antibiotic effects on phenylalanyloligonucleotide binding to ribosomes. *Proc. Natl. Acad. Sci. U.S.A.* 1969;64:709.

23. Pestka, S., T. Hishizawa, and J. L. Lessard. Studies on the formation of transfer ribonucleic acid-ribosome complexes: aminoacyl oligonucleotide binding to ribosomes: characteristics and requirements. *J. Biol. Chem.* 1970;245:6208.

24. Lessard, J. L., and S. Pestka. Studies on the formation of transfer ribonucleic acid-ribosome complexes: binding of aminoacyl-oligonucleotides to ribosomes. *J. Biol. Chem.* 1972;247:6901.

25. Vasquez, D., M. Barbacid, and R. Fernandez-Munoz. Antibiotic action on the ribosomal peptidyl transferase centre. In *Drug Receptor Interactions in Antimicrobial Chemotherapy*, ed. by J. Drews and F. E. Hahn. New York: Springer-Verlag, 1975, pp. 193–216.

26. Dajani, A. S., and R. E. Kauffman. The renaissance of chloramphenicol. *Pediatr. Clin. North Am.* 1981;28:195.

27. Finland, M., C. Garner, C. Wilcox, and L. D. Sabath. Susceptibility of "Enterobacteria" to aminoglycoside antibiotics: comparisons with tetracyclines, polymyxins, chloramphenicol and spectinomycin. *J. Infect. Dis.* 1976;134(Suppl.):S57.

28. Finegold, S. M. Therapy for infections due to anaerobic bacteria: an overview. *J. Infect. Dis.* 1977; 135(Suppl.):S25.

29. Cody Meissner, H., and A. L. Smith. The current status of chloramphenicol. *Pediatrics* 1979; 64:348.

30. Smadel, J. E., Chloramphenicol (chloromycetin) in the treatment of infectious diseases. *Am. J. Med.* 1949;7:671.

31. McClean, I. W., J. L. Schwab, A. B. Hillegas, and A. S. Schlingman. Susceptibility of microorganisms to chloramphenicol (chloromycetin). *J. Clin. Invest.* 1949;28:953.

32. Turk, D. C., A comparison of chloramphenicol and ampicillin as bactericidal agents for *Haemophilus influenzae* type B. *J. Med. Microbiol.* 1977;10:127.

33. Rahal, J. J., and M. S. Simberkoff. Bactericidal and bacteriostatic action of chloramphenicol against meningeal pathogens. *Antimicrob. Agents Chemother.* 1979;16:13.

34. O'Grady, F., N. J. Pearson, and C. Dennis. Thiamphenicol and chloramphenicol: an in vitro comparison with particular reference to bactericidal activity. *Chemotherapy* 1980;26:116.

35. Benveniste, R., and J. Davies. Mechanisms of antibiotic resistance in bacteria. *Annu. Rev. Biochem.* 1973;42:471.

36. Thibault, G., M. Guitard, and R. Daigneault. A study of the enzymatic inactivation of chloramphenicol by highly purified chloramphenicol acetyltransferase. *Biochim. Biophys. Acta* 1980;614:339.

37. Piffaretti, J.-C., and Y. Froment. Binding of chloramphenicol and its acetylated derivatives to *Escherichia coli* ribosomal subunits. *Chemotherapy* 1978; 24:24.

38. Gaffney, D., T. J. Foster, and W. V. Shaw. Chloramphenicol acetyltransferases determined by R plasmids from gram-negative bacteria. *J. Gen. Microbiol.* 1978;109:351.

39. Sands, L. C., and W. V. Shaw. Mechanism of chloramphenicol resistance in staphylococci: characterization and hybridization of variants of chloramphenicol transferase. *Antimicrob. Agents Chemother.* 1973; 3:299.

40. Lawrence, R. M., E. Goldstein, and P. Hoeprich. Typhoid fever caused by chloramphenicol-resistant organisms. *JAMA* 1973;224:861.

41. van Klingeren, B., J. D. A. van Embden, and M. Dessens-Kroon. Plasmid-mediated chloramphenicol resistance in *Haemophilus influenzae*. *Antimicrob. Agents Chemother.* 1977;11:383.

42. Roberts, M. C., C. D. Swenson, L. M. Owens, and A. L. Smith. Characterization of chloramphenicol-

resistant *Haemophilus influenzae*. *Antimicrob. Agents Chemother.* 1980;18:610.

43. Datta, N., H. Richards, and C. Datta. *Salmonella typhi* in vivo acquires resistance to both chloramphenicol and co-trimoxazole. *Lancet* 1981;1:1181.

44. Friedland, I. R., and K. P. Klugman. Failure of chloramphenicol therapy in penicillin-resistant pneumococcal meningitis. *Lancet* 1992;339:405.

45. Givner, L. B., J. S. Abramson, and B. Wasilauskas. Meningitis due to *Haemophilus influenza* type b resistant to ampicillin and chloramphenicol. *Rev. Infect. Dis.* 1989;11:329.

46. Mirza, S. H., N. J. Beeching, and C. A. Hauk. Multi-virus resistant typhoid; a global problem. *J. Med. Microbiol.* 1996;44:317.

47. Wallace, R. J., Jr., L. C. Steele, D. L. Brooks, G. D. Forrester, J. G. N. Garcia, J. I. Laman, R. W. Wilson, S. Shephard, and J. Mclarty. Ampicillin, tetracycline, and chloramphenicol resistant *Haemophilus influenza* in adults with chronic lung disease. *Am. Rev. Respir. Dis.* 1988;137:695.

48. Ley, H. L., J. E. Smadel, and T. T. Crocker. Administration of chloromycetin to normal human subjects. *Proc. Soc. Exp. Biol. Med.* 1948;68:9.

49. Kauffman, R. E., J. N. Miceli, L. Strebel, J. A. Buckley, A. K. Done, and A. S. Dajani. Pharmacokinetics of chloramphenicol and chloramphenicol succinate in infants and children. *J. Pediatr.* 1981;98:315.

50. Glazko, A. J., W. A. Dill, A. W. Kinkel, J. R. Goulet, W. J. Holloway, and R. A. Buchanan. Absorption and excretion of parenteral doses of chloramphenicol sodium succinate (CMS) in comparison with peroral doses of chloramphenicol. *Clin. Pharmacol. Ther.* 1977;21:104.

51. George, F. J., and C. Hanna. Ocular penetration of chloramphenicol. *Arch. Ophthalmol.* 1977;95:879.

52. Beasley, H., J. J. Boltralik, and H. A. Baldwin. Chloramphenicol in aqueous humor after topical application. *Arch. Ophthalmol.* 1975;93:184.

53. Abrams, S. M., T. J. Degnan, and V. Vinciguerra. Marrow aplasia following topical application of chloramphenicol eye ointment. *Arch. Intern. Med.* 1980;140:576.

54. Rapp, G. R., R. S. Griffith, and W. M. Hebble. The permeability of traumatically inflamed synovial membrane to commonly used antibiotics. *J. Bone Jt. Surg.* 1966;48-A:1534.

55. Friedman, C. A., F. C. Lovejoy, and A. L. Smith. Chloramphenicol disposition in infants and children. *J. Pediatr.* 1979;95:1071.

56. Rensimer, E. R., L. K. Pickering, C. D. Ericsson, and W. G. Kramer. Sequential CSF concentration of chloramphenicol after administration of oral chloramphenicol palmitate. *Lancet* 1981;1:165.

57. Kramer, P. W., R. S. Griffith, and R. L. Campbell. Antibiotic penetration of the brain. *J. Neurosurg.* 1969;31:295.

58. Azzolini, F., A. Gazzaniga, E. Lodola, and R. Natangelo. Elimination of chloramphenicol and thiamphenicol in subjects with cirrhosis of the liver. *Int. J. Clin. Pharmacol. Ther. Toxicol.* 1972;6:130.

59. Stramentinoli, G., A. Gazzaniga, and D. Della Bella. Increase of chloramphenicol glucuronidation in

rats treated with phenobarbital. *Biochem. Pharmacol.* 1974;23:1181.

60. Bloxham, R. A., G. M. Durbin, T. Johnson, and M. H. Winterborn. Chloramphenicol and phenobarbitone—a drug interaction. *Arch. Dis. Child.* 1979;54:76.

61. Suhrland, L. G., and A. S. Weisberger. Chloramphenicol toxicity in liver and renal disease. *Arch. Intern. Med.* 1963;112:747.

62. Kunin, C. M., A. J. Glazko, and M. Finland. Persistence of antibiotics in blood of patients with acute renal failure. II. Chloramphenicol and its metabolic products in the blood of patients with severe renal disease or hepatic cirrhosis. *J. Clin. Invest.* 1959;38:1498.

63. Lindberg, A. A., L. H. Nilsson, H. Bucht, and L. O. Kallings. Concentration of chloramphenicol in the urine and blood in relation to renal function. *BMJ* 1966;2:724.

64. Koup, J. R., A. H. Lau, B. Brodsky, and R. L. Slaughter. Chloramphenicol pharmacokinetics in hospitalized patients. *Antimicrob. Agents Chemother.* 1979;15:651.

65. Slaughter, R. L., J. A. Pieper, F. B. Cerra, B. Brodsky, and J. R. Koup. Chloramphenicol sodium succinate in critically ill patients. *Clin. Pharmacol. Ther.* 1980;28:69.

66. Weiss, C. F., A. J. Glazko, and J. K. Weston. Chloramphenicol in the newborn infant; a physiologic explanation of its toxicity when given in excessive doses. *N. Engl. J. Med.* 1960;262:787.

67. Grafnetterova, J., D. Grafnetter, O. Schuck, D. Tomkova, and J. Blaha. The effect of endogenous compounds, isolated from sera of uremic patients on chloramphenicol binding to proteins. *Biochem. Pharmacol.* 1979;28:2923.

68. DeLouvois, J., A. Mulhall, and R. Hurley. Comparison of methods available for assay of chloramphenicol in clinical specimens. *J. Clin. Pathol.* 1980;33:575.

69. Petersdorf, S. H., V. Raisys, and K. E. Opheim. Micro-scale method for liquid-chromatographic determination of chloramphenicol in serum. *Clin. Chem.* 1979;25:1300.

70. Koup, J. R., C. M. Sack, A. L. Smith, N. N. Neely, and M. Gibaldi. Rapid estimation of chloramphenicol clearance in infants and children. *Clin. Pharmacokinet.* 1981;6:83.

71. Godel, V., P. Nemet, and M. Lazar. Chloramphenicol optic neuropathy. *Arch. Ophthalmol.* 1980;98:1417.

72. Weisberger, A. S., and T. M. Daniel. Suppression of antibody synthesis by chloramphenicol analogs. *Proc. Soc. Exp. Biol. Med.* 1969;131:570.

73. Della Bella, D., D. Petrescu, G. Marca, and M. Veronese. Humoral antibody, plaque, and rosette formation in mice treated with chloramphenicol. *Chemotherapy* 1973;18:99.

74. Liberman, D. F., and J. L. Roti Roti. Effect of chloramphenicol on the growth and viability of exponentially growing mouse leukemic cells (L5178Y). *Exp. Cell Res.* 1973;77:346.

75. Hallman, M. Oxygen-uptake in neonatal rats: a developmental study with particular reference to the effects of chloramphenicol. *Pediatr. Res.* 1973;7:923.

76. Craft, A. W., J. T. Brocklebank, E. N. Hey, and

R. H. Jackson. The "grey toddler:" chloramphenicol toxicity. *Arch. Dis. Child.* 1974;49:235.

77. Freeman, K. B., and D. Halder: The inhibition of mammalian mitochondrial NADPH oxidation by chloramphenicol and its isomers and analogues. *Can. J. Biochem.* 1968;46:1003.

78. Abou-Khalil, S., W. H. Abou-Khalil, and A. A. Yunis. Differential effects of chloramphenicol and its nitrosoanalogue on protein synthesis and oxidative phosphorylation in rat liver mitochondria. *Biochem. Pharmacol.* 1980;29:2605.

79. Kessler, D. L., A. L. Smith, and D. E. Woodrum. Chloramphenicol toxicity in a neonate treated with exchange transfusion. *J. Pediatr.* 1980;96:140.

80. Mauer, S. M., B. M. Chavers, and C. M. Kjellstrand. Treatment of an infant with severe chloramphenicol intoxication using charcoal-column hemoperfusion. *J. Pediatr.* 1980;96:136.

81. Yunis, A. A., and G. R. Bloomberg. Chloramphenicol toxicity, clinical features and pathogenesis. *Prog. Hematol.* 1964;4:138.

82. Scott, J. L., S. M. Finegold, G. A. Belkin, and J. S. Lawrence. A controlled double-blind study of the hematologic toxicity of chloramphenicol. *New Engl. J. Med.* 1965;272:1137.

83. Yunis, A. A., Chloramphenicol-induced bone marrow suppression. *Semin. Hematol.* 1973;10:225.

84. Ibrahim, N. G., J. P. Burke, and D. Beattie. The sensitivity of rat liver and yeast mitochondrial ribosomes to inhibitors of protein synthesis. *J. Biol. Chem.* 1974;249:6806.

85. Yunis, A. A., U. S. Smith, and A. Restrepo. Reversible bone marrow suppression from chloramphenicol: a consequence of mitochondrial injury. *Arch. Intern. Med.* 1970;126:272.

86. Martelo, O. J., D. R. Manyan, U. S. Smith, and A. A. Yunis. Chloramphenicol and bone marrow mitochondria. *J. Lab. Clin. Med.* 1969;74:927.

87. Yunis, A. A., and J. W. Adamson. Differential in vitro sensitivity of marrow erythroid and granulocytic colony forming cells to chloramphenicol. *Am. J. Hematol.* 1977;2:355.

88. Ratzan, J., M. A. S. Moore, and A. A. Yunis. Effect of chloramphenicol and thiamphenicol on the in vitro colony-forming cell. *Blood* 1974;43:363.

89. Miller, A. M., M. A. Gross, and A. A. Yunis. Heterogeneity of human colony-forming cells (CFU$_c$) with respect to their sensitivity to chloramphenicol. *Exp. Hematol.* 1980;8:236.

90. Wallerstein, R. O., P. K. Condit, C. K. Kasper, J. W. Brown, and F. R. Morrison. Statewide study of chloramphenicol therapy and fatal aplastic anemia. *JAMA* 1969;208:2045.

91. Brauer, M. J., and W. Dameshek. Hypoplastic anemia and myeloblastic leukemia following chloramphenicol therapy. *N. Engl. J. Med.* 1967;277:1003.

92. Cohen, T., and W. P. Creger: Acute myeloid leukemia following seven years of aplastic anemia induced by chloramphenicol. *Am. J. Med.* 1967;43:762.

93. Daum, R. S., D. L. Cohen, and A. L. Smith. Fatal aplastic anemia following apparent "dose-related" chloramphenicol toxicity. *J. Pediatr.* 1979;94:403.

94. Nagao, T., and A. M. Mauer. Concordance for drug-induced aplastic anemia in identical twins. *N. Engl. J. Med.* 1969;281:7.

95. Keiser, C., and U. Buchegger. Hematological side effects of chloramphenicol and thiamphenicol. *Helv. Med. Acta* 1973;37:265.

96. Manyan, D. R., G. K. Arimura, and A. A. Yunis. Comparative metabolic effects of chloramphenicol analogues. *Mol. Pharmacol.* 1975;11:520.

97. Yunis, A. A., A. M. Miller, Z. Salem, M. D. Corbett, and G. K. Arimura. Nitroso-chloramphenicol: possible mediator in chloramphenicol-induced aplastic anemia. *J. Lab. Clin. Med.* 1980;96:36.

98. Skolimowski, I. M., D. A. Rowley, R. C. Knight, and D. I. Edwards. Reduced chloramphenicol-induced damage to DNA. *J. Antimicrob. Chemother.* 1981;7:593.

99. Holt, R. The bacterial degradation of chloramphenicol. *Lancet* 1967;1:1259.

100. Polin, H. B., and M. E. Plaut. Chloramphenicol. *N.Y. State J. Med.* 1977;77:378.

101. Fink, T. J., and D. W. Gump. Chloramphenicol: an inpatient study of use and abuse. *J. Infect. Dis.* 1978;138:690.

102. Adams, H. R., E. L. Isaacson, and B. S. Masters. Inhibition of hepatic microsomal enzymes by chloramphenicol. *J. Pharmacol. Exp. Ther.* 1977;203:388.

103. Rose, J. L., H. K. Choi, and J. J. Schentag. Intoxication caused by interaction of chloramphenicol and phenytoin. *JAMA* 1977;237:2630.

104. Powell, D. A., M. C. Nahata, D. C. Durrell, J. P. Glanzer, and M. D. Hilty. Interactions among chloramphenicol, phenytoin and phenobarbital in a pediatric patient. *J. Pediatr.* 1981;98:1001.

105. Prober, C. G. Effect of rifampin on chloramphenicol levels. *New Engl. J. Med.* 1985;312:788.

106. Kucers, A. Current position of chloramphenicol chemotherapy. *J. Antimicrob. Chemother.* 1980;6:1.

107. D. W. Gump. Chloramphenicol. A 1981 view. *Arch. Intern. Med.* 1981;141:573.

108. Miller, S. J., E. L. Hohmann, and D. A. Pegues. Salmonella (including *Salmonella typhi*). In *Principles and Practice of Infectious Diseases*, 4th ed., ed. by G. L. Mandell, J. E. Bennett, and R. Dolin. New York: Churchill Livingstone, 1995, pp. 2013–2032.

109. Sharma, K. B., M. B. Bhat, A. Pasricha, and S. Vaze. Multiple antibiotic resistance among salmonellae in India. *J. Antimicrob. Chemother.* 1979;5:15.

110. Shackelford, P. G., J. E. Bobinski, R. D. Feigin, and J. D. Cherry. Therapy of *Haemophilus influenzae* meningitis reconsidered. *N. Engl. J. Med.* 1972;287:634.

111. Barrett, F. F., L. H. Taber, C. R. Morris, W. B. Stephenson, D. J. Clark, and M. D. Yow. A 12 year review of the antibiotic management of *Haemophilus influenzae* meningitis. *Pediatrics* 1972;81:370.

112. Committee on Infectious Diseases. Ampicillin-resistant strains of *Haemophilus influenzae* type B. *Pediatrics* 1975;55:145.

113. Mackenzie, A. M. R. Combined action of chloramphenicol and ampicillin on *Haemophilus influenzae*. *J. Antimicrob. Chemother.* 1979;5:693.

114. Kenny, J. F., C. D. Isburg, and R. H. Michaels.

Meningitis due to *Haemophilus influenzae* type b resistant to both ampicillin and chloramphenicol. *Pediatrics* 1980;66:14.

115. Uchiyama, N., G. R. Greene, D. B. Kitts, and L. D. Thrupp. Meningitis due to *Haemophilus influenzae* type b resistant to ampicillin and chloramphenicol. *J. Pediatr.* 1980;97:421.

116. Harding, G. K. M., F. J. Buckwold, A. R. Ronald, T. J. Marrie, S. Brunton, J. C. Koss, M. J. Gurwith, and W. L. Albritton. Prospective, randomized comparative study of clindamycin, chloramphenicol, and ticarcillin, each in combination with gentamicin, in therapy for intraabdominal and female genital tract sepsis. *J. Infect. Dis.* 1980;142:384.

117. Oski, F. A. Hematologic consequences of chloramphenicol therapy. *J. Pediatr.* 1979;94:515.

118. *Consumer Reports*, October 1970, p. 616.

119. Best, W. R. Chloramphenicol-associated blood dyscrasias. *JAMA* 1967;201:99.

120. Ray, W. A., C. F. Federspiel, and W. Schaffner. Prescribing of chloramphenicol in ambulatory practice. An epidemiologic study among Tennessee medicaid recipients. *Ann. Intern. Med.* 1976;84:266.

121. Schaffner, W., W. A. Ray, and C. F. Federspiel. Surveillance of antibiotic prescribing in office practice. *Ann. Intern. Med.* 1978;89:796.

122. Feder, H. M., C. Osier, and E. G. Maderazo. An audit of chloramphenicol use in a large community hospital. *Arch. Intern. Med.* 1981;141:597.

123. Dunne, M., A. Herxheimer, M. Newman, and H. Ridley. Indications and warnings about chloramphenicol. *Lancet* 1973;2:781.

124. Aladiem, S. Chloramphenicol in South America. *N. Engl. J. Med.* 1969;281:1369.

125. Schreier, H. A., and L. Berger. On medical imperialism. [Letter]. *Lancet* 1974;1:1161.

126. Ryrie, D. R., J. Fletcher, M. J. S. Langman, and H. E. Daniels. Chloramphenicol over the counter [letter]. *Lancet* 1973;1:150.

127. Mao, J. C. H., and M. Putterman. The intermolecular complex of erythromycin and ribosome. *J. Mol. Biol.* 1969;44:347.

128. Mao, J. C. H., M. Putterman, and R. G. Wiegand. Biochemical basis for the selective toxicity of erythromycin. *Biochem. Pharmacol.* 1970;19:391.

129. Ibrahim, N. G., and D. S. Beattie. Protein synthesis on ribosomes isolated from rat liver mitochondria: Sensitivity to erythromycin. *FEBS Lett.* 1973;36:102.

130. Tanaka, K., H. Teraoka, T. Nagira, and M. Tamaki. [^{14}C] Erythromycin-ribosome complex formation and non-enzymatic binding of amino-acyl-transfer RNA to ribosome-messenger RNA complex. *Biochim. Biophys. Acta* 1966;123:435.

131. Teraoka, H., K. Tanaka, and M. Tamaki. The comparative study on the effects of chloramphenicol, erythromycin and lincomycin on polylysine synthesis in an *Escherichia coli* cell-free system. *Biochim. Biophys. Acta* 1969;174:776.

132. Chang, F. N., and B. Weisblum. The specificity of lincomycin binding to ribosomes. *Biochemistry* 1967; 6:836.

133. Pestka, S. Binding of ^{14}C-erythromycin to *Escherichia coli* ribosomes. *Antimicrob. Agents Chemother.* 1974;6:474.

134. Teraoka, H., and K. H. Nierhaus. Proteins from *Escherichia coli*. ribosomes involved in the binding of erythromycin. *J. Mol. Biol.* 1978;126:185.

135. Pestka, S. Antibiotics as probes of ribosome structure: binding of chloramphenicol and erythromycin to polyribosomes; effect of other antibiotics. *Antimicrob. Agents Chemother.* 1974;5:255.

136. Mao, J. C. H., and E. E. Robishaw. Erythromycin, a peptidyltransferase effector. *Biochemistry* 1972;11:4864.

137. Cundliffe, E., and K. McQuillen. Bacterial protein synthesis: the effects of antibiotics. *J. Mol. Biol.* 1967;30:137.

138. Tanaka, S., T. Otaka, and A. Kaji. Further studies on the mechanism of erythromycin action. *Biochim. Biophys. Acta* 1973;331:128.

139. Otaka, T., and A. Kaji. Release of (oligo) peptidyl-tRNA from ribosomes by erythromycin A. *Proc. Natl. Acad. Sci. U.S.A.* 1975;72:2649.

140. Otaka, E., H. Teraoka, M. Tamaki, K. Tanaka, and S. Osawa. Ribosomes from erythromycin-resistant mutants of *Escherichia coli* Q13 *J. Mol. Biol.* 1970;48:499.

141. Wittmann, H. G., G. Stöffler, D. Aprion, L. Rosen, K. Tanaka, M. Tamaki, R. Takata, S. Dekio, E. Otake, and S. Osawa. Biochemical and genetic studies on two different types of erythromycin resistant mutants of *Escherichia coli* with altered ribosomal proteins. *Mol. Gen. Genet.* 1973;127:175.

142. Stöffler, G., and G. W. Tischendorf. Antibiotic receptor-sites in *Escherichia coli* ribosomes. In *Drug Receptor Interactions in Antimicrobial Chemotherapy*, ed. by J. Drews and F. E. Hahn. New York: Springer-Verlag, 1975, pp. 117–143.

143. Tanaka, K., M. Tamaki, R. Takata, and S. Osawa. Low affinity for chloramphenicol of erythromycin resistant *Escherichia coli* ribosomes having an altered protein component. *Biochem. Biophys. Res. Commun.* 1972;46:1979.

144. Sparling, P. F., and E. Blackman. Mutation to erythromycin dependence in *Escherichia coli* K-12 *J. Bacteriol.* 1973;116:74.

145. Chabbert, Y. Antagonisme in vitro entre l'erythromycine et la spiramycine. *Ann. Inst. Pasteur* 1956;90:787.

146. Garrod, L. P. The erythromycin group of antibiotics. *BMJ* 1957;2:57.

147. B. Weisblum, C. Siddhikol, C. J. Lai, and V. Demohn. Erythromycin-inducible resistance in *Staphylococcus aureus*: requirements for induction. *J. Bacteriol.* 1971;106:835.

148. Lai, C. J., and B. Weisblum. Altered methylation of ribosomal RNA in an erythromycin-resistant strain of *Staphylococcus aureus*. *Proc. Natl. Acad. Sci. U.S.A.* 1971;68:856.

149. Lai, C. J., B. Weisblum, S. R. Fahnstock, and M. Nomura. Alteration of 23S ribosomal RNA and erythromycin-induced resistance to lincomycin and spiramycin in *Staphylococcus aureus*. *J. Mol. Biol.* 1973; 74:67.

150. Graham, M. Y., and B. Weisblum. 23S Riboso-

mal ribonucleic acid of macrolide-producing streptomycetes contains methylated adenine. *J. Bacteriol.* 1979;137:1464.

151. Lampson, B. C., W. von David and J. T. Parisi Novel mechanism for plasmid-mediated erythromycin resistance by PNE24 from *Staphylococcus epidermidis*. *Antimicrob. Agents Chemother.* 1986;30:653.

152. Haight, T. H., and M. Finland. The antibacterial action of erythromycin. *Proc. Soc. Exp. Biol. Med.* 1952;81:175.

153. Mao, J. C. H., and M. Putterman. Accumulation in gram-positive and gram-negative bacteria as a mechanism of resistance to erythromycin. *J. Bacteriol.* 1968;95:1111.

154. Taubeneck, U. Susceptibility of *Proteus mirabilis* and its stable L-forms to erythromycin and other macrolides. *Nature* 1962;196:195.

155. Sabath, L. D., D. A. Gerstein, P. B. Loder, and M. Finland. Excretion of erythromycin and its enhanced activity in urine against gram-negative bacilli with alkalinization. *J. Lab. Clin. Med.* 1968;72:916.

156. Zinner, S. H., J. I. Casey, L. D. Sabath, and M. Finland. Erythromycin and alkalinization of the urine in the treatment of urinary-tract infections due to gram-negative bacilli. *Lancet* 1971;1:1267.

157. Schlossberg, D. Azithromycin and clarithromycin. *Med. Clin. North Am.* 1995;79:803.

158. Nicholas, P. Erythromycin: clinical review. I. Clinical pharmacology. *N.Y. State J. Med.* 1977;77:2088.

159. Nicholas, P. Erythromycin: clinical review. II. Therapeutic uses. *N.Y. State J. Med.* 1977;77:2243.

160. McKendrick, M. W. Erythromycin revisited. *J. Antimicrob. Chemother.* 1979;5:493.

161. Shapera, R. M., K. A. Hable, and J. M. Matsen. Erythromycin therapy twice daily for streptococcal pharyngitis: controlled comparison with erythromycin or penicillin phenoxymethyl four times daily or penicillin G benzathine. *JAMA* 1973;226:531.

162. Dixon, J. M. S. Pneumococcus resistant to erythromycin and lincomycin. *Lancet* 1967;1:573.

163. Sanders, E., M. T. Foster, and D. Scott. Group A beta-hemolytic streptococci resistant to erythromycin and lincomycin. *N. Engl. J. Med.* 1968;278:538.

164. McCloskey, R. V., J. J. Eller, M. Green, C. U. Mauney, and S. E. M. Richards. The 1970 epidemic of diphtheria in San Antonio. *Ann. Intern. Med.* 1971;75:495.

165. Bass, J. W., E. L. Klenk, J. B. Klotheimer, C. C. Linnemann, and M. H. D. Smith. Antimicrobial treatment of pertussis. *J. Pediatr.* 1969;75:768.

166. International symposium on Legionnaire's disease. *Ann. Intern. Med.* 1979;90:489.

167. Centers for Disease Control. Sexually transmitted diseases treatment guidelines. *MMWR Morb. Mortal. Wkly. Rep.* 1993;42:14.

168. Harvey, K. J., H. Miles, A. Hurse, and M. Carson. In vitro activity of erythromycin against anaerobic microorganisms. *Med. J. Aust.* 1981;1:474.

169. Jao, R. L., and M. Finland. Susceptibility of *Mycoplasma pneumoniae* to 21 antibiotics in vitro. *Am. J. Med. Sci.* 1967;253:639.

170. Hammerschlag, M. R., J. W. Chandler, E. R. Alexander, M. English, W. Chiang, L. Koutsky, D. A. Eschenbach, and J. R. Smith. Erythromycin ointment for ocular prophylaxis of neonatal chlamydial infection. *JAMA* 1980;244:2291.

171. Charles, L., and J. Segreti. Choosing the right macrolide antibiotic. *Drugs* 1997;53:349.

172. Dunn, C. J., and L. B. Barradell. Azithromycin. A review of its pharmacological properties and use as 3-day therapy in respiratory tract infections. *Drugs* 1996;51:483.

173. Dautzenberg, B., C. C. Tuffot, S. Legris, M. C. Meyohas, H. C. Berlie, A. Mercat, S. Chevret, and J. Grosset. Activity of clarithromycin against *Mycobacterium avium* infection in patients with acquired immune deficiency syndrome. *Am. Rev. Respir. Dis.* 1993;144:564.

174. Shafran, S. D., J. Singer, D. P. Zarowny P. Phillips, I. Salit, S. Walmsley, I. Fong, J. Gill, A. Rachlis, R. Lalomde, M. Fanning, and C. Tsoukas. A comparison of two regimens for the treatment of Mycobacterial avium complex bacteremia or AIDs: rifabutin, ethambutol, and clarithromycin versus rifampin, ethambutol, clofazimine and ciprofloxacin. *New Engl. J. Med.* 1996;335:377.

175. Pierce, M., S. Crampton, D. Henry L. Heifets, A. LaMarca, M. Montecalvo, G. Wounser, H. Jabloworski, J. Jemsek M. Cynamon, B. Yangro, G. Notario, and J. C. Craft. A randomized trial of clarithromycin as prophylaxis against disseminated mycobacterium avium complex infection in patients with advanced acquired immunodeficiency syndrome. *N. Engl. J. Med.* 1996;335:385.

176. Hardy, D. J., C. W. Hanson, D. M. Hensey, J. Beyer, and P. B. Fernandes. Susceptibility of *Campylobacter pylori* to macrolides and fluoroquinolones. *J. Antimicrob. Chemother.* 1988;22:631.

177. Brogden, R. N., and D. H. Peters. Dirithromycin. A review of its antimicrobial activity, pharmacokinetic properties and therapeutic efficacy. *Drugs* 1994;48:599.

178. Bechtol, L. D., V. C. Stephens, C. T. Pugh, M. B. Perkal, and P. A. Coletta. Erythromycin esters—comparative in vivo hydrolysis and bioavailability. *Curr. Ther. Res.* 1976;20:610.

179. Tardrew, P. L., J. C. H. Mao, and D. Kenney. Antibactrial activity of 2'-esters of erythromycin. *Appl. Microbiol.* 1969;18:159.

180. Thompson, P. J., K. R. Burgess, and G. E. Marlin. Influence of food on absorption of erythromycin ethylsuccinate. *Antimicrob. Agents Chemother.* 1980;18:829.

181. Stephens, V. C., C. T. Pugh, N. E. Davis, M. M. Hochin, S. Ralston, M. C. Sparks, and L. Thomkins. A study of the propionyl erythromycin in blood by a new chromatographic method. *J. Antibiot.* 1969;22:51.

182. DiSanto, A. R., K. Y. Tserng, D. J. Chodos, K. A. DeSante, K. S. Albert, and J. G. Wagner. Comparative bioavailability evaluation of erythromycin base and its salts and esters. I. Erythromycin estolate capsules versus enteric-coated erythromycin base tablets. *J. Clin. Pharmacol.* 1980;20:437.

183. Houin, G., J. P. Tillement, F. Lhoste, M. Rapin, C. J. Soussy, and J. Douval. Erythromycin pharma-

cokinetics in man. *J. Int. Med. Res.* 1980;8(Suppl. 2):9.

184. Austin, K. L., L. E. Mather, C. R. Philpot, and P. J. McDonald. Intersubject and dose-related variability after intravenous administration of erythromycin. *Br. J. Clin. Pharmacol.* 1980;10:273.

185. Hammond, J. B., and R. S. Griffith. Factors affecting the absorption and biliary excretion of erythromycin and two of its derivatives in humans. *Clin. Pharmacol. Ther.* 1961;2:308.

186. Mao, J. C. H., and P. L. Tardrew. Demethylation of erythromycins by rabbit tissues in vitro. *Biochem. Pharamacol.* 1965;14:1049.

187. Danan, G., V. Descatoire, and D. Pessayre. Self-introduction by erythromycin of its own transformation into a metabolite forming an inactive complex with reduced cytochrome P-450. *J. Pharmacol. Exp. Ther.* 1981;218:509.

188. Bennett, W. M., R. S. Muther, R. A. Parker, P. Feig, G. Morrison, T. Golper, and I. Singer. Drug therapy in renal failure: dosing guidelines for adults. Part I: Antimicrobial agents, Analgesics. *Ann. Intern. Med.* 1980;93:62.

189. Mery, J. P., and A. Kanfer. Ototoxicity of erythromycin in patients with renal insufficiency. *N. Eng. J. Med.* 1979;301:944.

190. Fraschini, F., F. Scagliono, and G. DeMartini. Clarithromycin. *Clin. Pharmacokinet.* 1993;25:189.

191. Prandota, J., J. P. Tillement, P. d'Athis, H. Campos, and J. Barre. Binding of erythromycin base to human plasma proteins. *J. Int. Med. Res.* 1980;8(Suppl.)2:1.

192. Griffith, R. S., and H. R. Black. Erythromycin. *Med. Clin. N. Am.* 1970;54:1199.

193. Bass, J. W., R. W. Steele, R. A. Wiebe, and E. P. Dierdoff. Erythromycin concentrations in middle ear exudates. *Pediatrics* 1971;48:417.

194. Philipson, A., L. D. Sabath, and D. Charles. Transplacental passage of erythromycin and clindamycin. *N. Engl. J. Med.* 1973;288:1219.

195. Clarke, J. S., R. E. Condon, J. G. Bartlett, S. L. Gorbach, R. L. Nichols, and S. Ochi. Peroperative oral antibiotics reduce septic complications of colon operations: results of prospective, randomized, double-blind clinical study. *Ann. Surg.* 1977;186:251.

196. Rodvold, K. A., and S. C. Piscitelli. New oral macrolides and fluoroquinolone antibiotics: An overview of pharmacokinetics, interactions and safety. *Clin. Infect. Dis.* 1993;17(Suppl. 1):192.

197. McDonald, P. J., and H. Praul. Phagocyte uptake and transport of azithromycin. *Eur. J. Clin. Microbiol. Infect. Dis.* 1991;10:828.

198. Seifert, C. F., R. J. Swaney, and R. A. Bellagen-McCleery. Intravenous erythromycin lactobionate-induced severe nausea and vomiting. *DICP* 1989;23:40.

199. Bowler, W. A., C. Hosttettler, D. Samuelson, B. S. Lavin and E. C. Oldfield. Gastrointestinal side effects of intravenous erythromycin: incidence and reduction with prolonged infusion time and glycopyrrolate pretreatment. *Am. J. Med.* 1992;92:249.

200. Karmody, C. S., and L. Weinstein. Reversible sensorineural hearing loss with intravenous erythromycin lactobionate. *Ann. Otol. Rhinol. Laryngol.* 1977; 86:9.

201. Filippo, J. A. Infantile hypertrophic pyloric stenosis related to ingestion of erythromycin estolate: a report of five cases. *J. Pediatr. Surg.* 1976;11:177.

202. Braun, P. Hepatotoxicity of erythromycin. *J. Infect. Dis.* 1969;119:300.

203. Tolman, K. G., J. J. Sannella, and J. W. Freston. Chemical structure of erythromycin and hepatotoxicity. *Ann. Intern. Med.* 1974;81:58.

204. Kendler, J., S. Anuras, O. Laborda, and H. J. Zimmerman. Perfusion of the isolated rat liver with erythromycin estolate and other derivatives. *Proc. Soc. Exp. Biol. Med.* 1972;139:1272.

205. Dujovne, C. A., D. Shoeman, J. Biachine, and L. Lasagna. Experimental bases for the different hepatotoxicity of erythromycin preparations in man. *J. Lab. Clin. Med.* 1972;79:832.

206. Dujovne, C. A., and A. S. Salhab. Erythromycin estolate vs. erythromycin base, surface excess properties and surface scanning changes in isolated liver cell systems. *Pharmacology* 1980;20:285.

207. Denslow, N. D., and T. W. O'Brien. Antibiotic susceptibility of the peptidyl transferase locus of bovine mitochondrial ribosomes. *Eur. J. Biochem.* 1978;91: 441.

208. Doersen, C. J., and E. J. Stanbridge. Cytoplasmic inheritance of erythromycin resistance in human cells. *Proc. Natl. Acad. Sci. U.S.A.* 1979;76:45.

209. Yew, W. W., C. H. Chau, and J. Lee. Cholestatic hepatitis in a patient who received clarithromycin therapy for a *M. chelonae* lung infection. *Clin. Infect. Dis.* 1994;18:1025.

210. Langtry H. D., and R. N. Brogden. Clarithromycin. A review of its efficacy in the treatment of respiratory tract infections in immunocompetent patients. *Drugs* 1997;53:973.

211. Contreras, A. and D. Vasquez. Cooperative and antagonistic interactions of peptidyl-tRNA and antibiotics with bacterial ribosomes. *Eur. J. Biochem.* 1977; 74:539.

212. Cundliffe; E. Antibiotics and polyribosomes. II. Some effects of lincomycin, spiramycin, and streptogramin A in vivo. *Biochemistry* 1969;8:2063.

213. Reusser, F. Effect of lincomycin and clindamycin on peptide chain initiation. *Antimicrob. Agents Chemother.* 1975;7:32.

214. Change, F. N. Lincomycin. In *Antibiotics, V-1*, ed. by F. E. Hahn. New York: Springer-Verlag, 1979, pp. 127–134.

215. McGehee, R. F., C. B. Smith, C. Wilcox, and M. Finland. Comparative studies of antibacterial activity in vitro and absorption and excretion of lincomycin and clindamycin. *Am. J. Med. Sci.* 1968;256:279.

216. Leigh, D. A. Antibacterial activity and pharmacokinetics of clindamycin. *J. Antimicrob. Chemother.* 1981;7(Suppl. A):3.

217. Ball, A. P. Clindamycin in the 1980s. *J. Antimicrob. Chemother.* 1981;7(Suppl. A):81.

218. Klastersky, J., L. Coppens, and G. Mombelli. Anaerobic infection in cancer patients: comparative evaluation of clindamycin and cefoxitin. *Antimicrob. Agents Chemother.* 1979;16:366.

219. Harding, G. K. M., F. J. Buckwold, A. R. Ronald, T. J. Marrie, S. Brunton, J. C. Koss, M. J. Gurwith, and W. L. Albritton. Prospective, randomized compar-

ative study of clindamycin, chloramphenicol, and ticarcillin, each in combination with gentamicin, in therapy for intraabdominal and female genital tract sepsis. *J. Infect. Dis.* 1980;142:384.

220. Smith, J. A., A. G. Skidmore, A. D. Forward, A. M. Clarke, and E. Sutherland. Prospective, randomized, double-blind comparison of metronidazole and tobramycin with clindamycin and tobramycin in the treatment of intra-abdominal sepsis. *Ann. Surg.* 1980;192:213.

221. Louria, D. B. Clindamycin and other agents in the treatment of lung and pelvic infections. *J. Antimicrob. Chemother.* 1981;7(Suppl. A):37.

222. Symposium (various authors). The role of clindamycin in anaerobic bacterial infections. *J. Infect. Dis.* 1977;135(Suppl.):S1–S132.

223. Fass, R. J., J. F. Scholand, G. R. Hodges, and S. Saslaw. Clindamycin in the treatment of serious anaerobic infections. *Ann Intern. Med.* 1973;78:853.

224. Nastro, L. J., and S. M. Finegold. Bactericidal activity of five antimicrobial agents against *Bacteroides fragilis. J. Infect. Dis.* 1972;126:104.

225. Templeton, W. C., A. Wawrukiewicz, J. C. Nelo, M. Schiller, and M. Raff. Anaerobic osteomyelitis of long bones. *Rev. Infect. Dis.* 1983;5:692.

226. Stoughton, R. B., R. C. Cornell, R. W. Gange, and J. F. Walter. Double-blind comparison of topical 1 percent clindamycin phosphate (Cleocin T) and tetracyline 500 mg/day in the treatment of acne vulgaris. *Cutis* 1980;26:424.

227. Adams, S. J., E. M. Cooke, and W. J. Cunliffe. The use of oral and topical antibiotics in acne. *J. Antimicrob. Chemother.* 1981;7(Suppl. A):75.

228. Ferguson, J. G. Clindamycin therapy for toxoplasmosis. *Ann. Ophthalmol.* 1981;13:95.

229. Falagas, M. E., and S. L. Gorbach. Clindamycin and metronidazole. *Med. Clin. North Am.* 1995;79:845.

230. Dannemann, B., J. A. McCutchan, D. Israelski, D. Ontoniskis, D. Leport, B. Lutt, J. Nussbaum, N. Clumeck, P. Morlat, J. Chiu, J.-L. Vilde, M. Ovellana, D. Feigal, A. Bartok, P. Hesestine, J. Leedom, J. Rimington, and the California Collaborative Treatment Group. Treatment of toxoplasmic encephalitis in patients with AIDS. A randomized trial comparing pyrimethanine plus clindamycin to pyrmethamine plus sulfadiazine. *Ann. Intern. Med.* 1992;116:33.

231. Black, J. R., J. Feinberg, R. L. Murphy, R. J. Farr, D. Finkelstein, B. Akil, S. Safrin, J. T., Carey, J. Stansell, J. F. Plouffe, W. H. B. Shelton and F. R. Sattler. Clindamyacin and primaquine therapy for mild to moderate episodes of *Pneumocystis carinii* pneumonia in patients with AIDS. AIDS Clinical Trials Group 044. *Clin. Infect. Dis.* 1994;18:905.

232. Philips, I. Past and current use of clindamycin and lincomycin. *J. Antimicrob. Chemother.* 1981; 7(Suppl. A):11.

233. McGehee, R. F., F. F. Barrett, and M. Finland. Resistance of *Staphylococcus aureus* to lincomycin, clindamycin and erythromycin. *Antimicrob. Agents Chemother*—1968. 1969;392.

234. Coyle, M. B., B. H. Minshew, J. A. Bland, and P. C. Hsu. Erythromycin and clindamycin resistance in *Corynebacterium diphtheriae* from skin lesions. *Antimicrob. Agents Chemother.* 1979;16:525.

235. DeHaan, R. M., C. M. Metzler, and D. Schellenberg. Pharmacokinetic studies of clindamycin hydrochloride. *Int. J. Clin. Pharmacol.* 1972;6:105.

236. DeHann, R. M., C. M. Metzler, D. Schellenberg, and W. D. Vandenbosch. Pharmacokinetic studies of clindamycin phosphate. *J. Clin. Pharmacol.* 1973;13:190.

237. Panzer, J. D., D. C. Brown, W. L. Epstein, R. L. Lipson, H. W. Mahaffey, and W. H. Atkinson. Clindamycin levels in various body tissues and fluids. *J. Clin. Pharmacol.* 1972;12:259.

238. Baird, P., S. Hughes, M. Sullivan, and I. Wilmot. Penetration into bone and tissue of clindamycin phosphate. *Postgrad. Med. J.* 1978;54:65.

239. Rosen, A., R. S. Kanwar, G. Dempsey, and L. G. Brookes. Serum and peritoneal fluid concentrations of clindamycin and lincomycin in the mouse. *J. Pharmacol.* 1979;31:734.

240. Prokesch, R. C., and W. L. Hand. Antibiotic entry into human plymorphonuclear leukocytes. *Antimicrob. Agents Chemother.* 1982;23:373.

241. Kauffman, R. E., D. W. Shoeman, S. H. Wan, and D. L. Azarnoff. Absorption and excretion of clindamycin-2-phosphate in children after intramuscular injection. *Clin. Pharmacol. Ther.* 1972;13:704.

242. Williams, D. N., K. Crossley, C. Hoffman, and L. D. Sabath. Parenteral clindamycin phosphate: pharmacology with normal and abnormal liver function and effect on nasal staphylococci. *Antimicrob. Agents Chemother.* 1975;7:153.

243. Kager, L., L. Liljequist, A. S. Malmborg, and C. E. Nord. Effect of clindamycin prophylaxis on the colonic microflora in patients undergoing colorectal surgery. *Antimicrob. Agents Chemother.* 1981;20:736.

244. Joshi, A. M., and R. M. Stein. Altered serum clearance of intravenously administered clindamycin phosphate in patients with uremia. *J. Clin. Pharmacol.* 1974;14:140.

245. Eng, R. H. K., S. Gorski, A. Person, C. Mangura, and H. Chmel. Clindamycin elimination in patients with liver disease. *J. Antimicrob. Chemother.* 1981 8:277.

246. Pittinger, C., and R. Adamson. Antibiotic blockade of neuromuscular function. *Annu. Rev. Pharmacol.* 1972;12:169.

247. Kapusnik-Uner, J. E., M. A., Sande, and H. F. Chambers. Tetracyclines, chloramphenicol, erythromycin, and miscellaneous antibacterial agents. In *The Pharmacological Basis of Therapeutics*, 9th ed., ed. by J. G. Hardman, L. E. Limbird, P. B. Molinoff, and R. W. Ruddon. New York: McGraw-Hill, 1996, p. 1123.

248. Fass, R. J., and S. Saslaw. Clindamycin: clinical and laboratory evaluation of parenteral therapy. *Am. J. Med. Sci.* 1972;263:369.

249. Fekety, F. R. Gastrointestinal complications of antibiotic therapy. *JAMA* 1968;203:210.

250. Brause, B. D., J. A. Romankiewicz, V. Gotz, J. E. Franklin, and R. B. Roberts. Comparative study of diarrhea associated with clindamycin and ampicillin therapy. *Am. J. Gastroenterol.* 1980;73:244.

251. Leigh, D. A. K. Simmons, and S. Williams. Gastrointestinal side effects following clindamycin and lin-

comycin treatment—a follow up study. *J. Antimicrob. Chemother.* 1980;6:639.

252. Boriello, S. P., and H. E. Larson. Antibiotic and pseudomembranous colitis. *J. Antimicrob. Chemother.* 1981;7(Suppl. A): 53.

253. Silva, J., and R. Fekety. Clostridia and antimicrobial enterocolitis. *Annu. Rev. Med.* 1981;32:327.

254. Symposium (various authors). Antibiotic-associated colitis. *Microbiology* 1979;257–279.

255. Milstone, E. B., A. J. McDonald, and C. F. Scholhamer. Pseudomembranous colitis after topical application of clindamycin. *Arch. Dermatol.* 1981;117:154.

256. Stoughton, R. B. Topical antibiotics for acne vulgaris. *Arch. Dermatol.* 1979;115:486.

257. Hooker, K. D., and J. T. DiPiro. Effect of antimicrobial therapy on bowel flora. *Clin. Pharmacol.* 1988;7:878.

258. Kelly, C. P., C. Pothoulakis, and J. T. LaMont. *Clostridium difficile* colitis. *New Engl. J. Med.* 1994; 330:257.

259. Bartlett, J. G., A. B. Onderdonk, A. B. Cisneres, and D. L. Casper. Clindamycin-associated colitis due to toxin producing species of clostridium in hamsters. *J. Infect. Dis.* 1977;136:701.

260. Lusk, R. H., R. Fekety, J. Silva, R. A. Browne, D. H. Ringler, and G. D. Abrams. Clindamycin-induced enterocolitis in hamsters. *J. Infect. Dis.* 1978;137:464.

261. Rifkin, G. D., J. Silva, and R. Fekety. Gastrointestinal and systemic toxicity of fecal extracts from hamsters with clindamycin-induced colitis. *Gastroenterology* 1978;74:52.

262. Abrams, G. D., M. Allo, G. D. Rifkin, R. Fekety, and J. Silva. Mucosal damage mediated by clostridial toxin in experimental clindamycin-associated colitis. *Gut* 1980;21:493.

263. Rifkin, G. D., R. Fekety, and J. Silva. Neutralization by *Clostridium sordellii* antitoxin of toxins implicated in clindamycin-induced cecitis in the hamster. *Gastroenterology* 1978;75:422.

264. Allo, M., J. Silva, R. Fekety, G. D. Rifkin, and H. Waskin. Prevention of clindamycin-induced colitis in hamsters by *Clostridium sordellii* antitoxin. *Gastroenterology* 1979;76:351.

265. Larson, H. E., and A. B. Price. Pseudomembranous colitis: presence of a clostridial toxin. *Lancet* 1977; 2:1312.

266. Rifkin, G. D., F. R. Fekety, and J. Silva. Antibiotic-induced colitis; implication of a toxin neutralized by *Clostridium sordellii* antitoxin. *Lancet* 1977; 2:1103.

267. Bartlett, J. G., T. W. Chang, M. Gurwith, S. L. Gorbach, and A. B. Onderdonk. Antibiotic-associated pseudomembranous colitis due to toxin-producing clostridia. *N. Engl. J. Med.* 1978;298:531.

268. Dzink, J., and J. G. Bartlett. In vitro susceptibility of *Clostridium difficile* isolates from patients with antibiotic-associated diarrhea or colitis. *Antimicrob. Agents Chemother.* 1980;17:695.

269. Tedesco, F., R. Markham, M. Gurwith, D. Christie, and J. G. Bartlett. Oral vancomycin for antibiotic-associated pseudomembranous colitis. *Lancet* 1978;2:226.

270. Fekety, R. Antibiotic-associated colitis. In *Principles and Practice of Infectious Diseases*, 3 ed., ed. by G. L. Mandell, R. G. Douglas, and J. E. Bennet. New York: Churchill Livingstone, 1990, pp. 863–869.

271. Jacobs, N. F. Antibiotic-induced diarrhea and pseudomembranous colitis. *Postgrad. Med.* 1994;95: 111.

272. Davies, J., P. Anderson, and B. D. Davis. Inhibition of protein synthesis by spectinomycin. *Science* 1965;149:1096.

273. Anderson, P., J. Davies, and B. D. Davis. Effect of spectinomycin on polypeptide synthesis in extracts of *Escherichia coil. J. Mol. Biol.* 1967;29:203.

274. Bollen, A., J. Davies, M. Ozaki, and S. Mizushima. Ribosomal protein conferring sensitivity to the antibiotic spectinomycin in *Escherichia coli. Science* 1969;165:85.

275. DeWilde, M., and B. Wittman-Liebold. Localization of the amino acid exchange in protein S5 from *Escherichia coli* mutant resistant to spectinomycin. *Mol. Gen. Genet.* 1973;127:273.

276. Bollen, A., T. Helser, T. Yamada, and J. Davies. Altered ribosomes in antibiotic-resistant mutants of *E. coli. Cold Spring Harb. Symp. Quant. Biol.* 1969;34: 95.

277. Burns, D. J. W., and E. Cundliffe. Bacterial-protein synthesis. A novel system for studying antibiotic action in vivo. *Eur. J. Biochem.* 1973;37:570.

278. Smith, D. H., J. A. Janigian, N. Prescott, and P. W. Anderson. Resistance factor-mediated spectinomycin resistance. *Infect. Immun.* 1970;1:120.

279. Benveniste, R., T. Yamada, and J. Davies. Enzymatic adenylylation of streptomycin and spectinomycin by R-factor-resistant *Escherichia coli. Infect. Immun.* 1970;1:109.

280. Maness, M. J., G. C. Foster, and P. F. Sparling. Ribosomal resistance to streptomycin and spectinomycin in *Neisseria gonorrhoeae. J. Bacteriol.* 1974;120: 1293.

281. Phillips, I., and K. P. Shannon. Aminoglycosides and aminocyclitols. In *Antibiotics and Chemotherapy*, ed. by F. O'Grady, H. P. Lambert, R. G. Finch, and D. Greenwood. New York: Churchill Livingstone, 1997, pp. 164–201.

282. Duncan, W. C., W. R. Holder, D. P. Roberts, and J. M. Knox. Treatment of gonorrhea with spectinomycin hydrochloride: comparison with standard penicillin schedules. *Antimicrob. Agents Chemother.* 1972; 1:210.

283. Porter, I. A., and W. J. Wood. Spectinomycin: minimum inhibitory concentrations for *Neisseria gonorrhoeae. Br. J. Vener. Dis.* 1974;50:289.

284. Lee, Y., S. Alpert, P. E. Bailey, A. Duancic, and W. M. McCormack. In vitro and in vivo activity of spectinomycin against the genital mycoplasms. *J. Am. Vener. Dis. Assoc.* 1974;1:38.

285. Oriel J. D., G. L. Ridgway, S. Techamouroff, and J. Owen. Spectinomycin hydrochloride in the treatment of gonorrhoea: its effect on associated *Chlamydia trachomatis* infections. *Br. J. Vener. Dis.* 1977;53:226.

286. Petzoldt, D. Effect of spectinomycin on *T. pallidum* in incubating experimental syphilis. *Br. J. Vener. Dis.* 1975;51:305.

287. Karney, W. W., A. H. B. Pedersen, M. Nelson, H. Adams, R. J. Pfeifer, and K. K. Holmes. Spectinomycin versus tetracycline for the treatment of gonorrhea. *N. Engl. J. Med.* 1977;296:889.

288. Schroeter, A. L., G. H. Reynolds, K. K. Holmes, T. Pyke, and P. J. Wiesner. Spectinomycin in the treatment of gonorrhea. *J. Am. Vener. Dis. Assoc.* 1975;1:139.

289. Schoutens, E., M. Peromet, and E. Yourassowsky. Microbiological and clinical study of spectinomycin in urinary tract infections: reevaluation with hospital strains. *Curr. Ther. Res.* 1972;14:349.

290. Novak, E., J. E. Gray, and R. T. Pfeifer. Animal and human tolerance of high-dose intramuscular therapy with spectinomycin. *J. Infect. Dis.* 1974;130:50.

291. Laskin, A. I. Tetracyclines. In *Antibiotics,* Vol. 1, ed. by D. Gotlieb and P. D. Shaw. New York: Springer-Verlag, 1967, pp. 331–359.

292. Gale, E. F., and J. P. Folkes. The assimilation of amino acids by bacteria. Actions of antibiotics on nucleic acid and protein synthesis in *Staphylococcus aureus. Biochem. J.* 1953;53:493.

293. Kaji, A., and M. Ryoji. Tetracycline. In *Antibiotics V-1,* ed. by F. E. Hahn. New York: Springer-Verlag, 1979, pp. 304–328.

294. Day, L. E. Tetracycline inhibition of cell-free-protein synthesis. II. Effect of the binding of tetracycline to the components of the system. *J. Bacteriol.* 1966;92:197.

295. Connamacher, R. H., and H. G. Mandel. Binding of tetracycline to the 30S ribosomes and to polyuridylic acid. *Biochem. Biophys. Res. Commun.* 1965;20:98.

296. Maxwell, I. H. Studies of the binding of tetracycline to ribosomes in vitro. *Mol. Pharmacol.* 1968;4:25.

297. Craven, G. R., R. Gavin, and T. Fanning. The transfer RNA binding site of the 30S ribosome and the site of tetracycline inhibition. *Cold Spring Harb. Symp. Quant. Biol.* 1969;34:129.

298. Tritton, T. R. Ribosome-tetracycline interactions. *Biochemistry* 1977;16:4133.

299. Goldman, R. A., B. S. Cooperman, W. A. Strycharz, B. A. Williams, and T. R. Tritton. Photoincorporation of tetracycline into *Escherichia coli* ribosomes: identification of labeled proteins and functional consequences. *FEBS Lett.* 1980;118:113.

300. Suzuka, I., H. Kaji, and A. Kaji. Binding of specific sRNA to 30S ribosomal subunits: effect of 50S ribosomal subunits. *Proc Natl. Acad. Sci. U.S.A.* 1969;55:1483.

301. Gottseman, M. E. Reaction of ribosome-bound peptidyl transfer ribonucleic acid with aminoacyl transfer ribonucleic acid or puromycin. *J. Biol. Chem.* 1967;242:5564.

302. Suarez, G. and D. Nathans. Inhibition of aminoacyl-tRNA binding to ribosomes by tetracycline. *Biochem. Biophys. Res. Commun.* 1965;18:743.

303. Yarmolinsky, M., and G. de la Haba. Inhibition by puromycin of amino acid incorporation into protein. *Proc. Nat. Acad. Sci. U.S.A.* 1959;45:1721.

304. Smith, J. D., R. R. Traut, G. M. Blackburn, and R. E. Monroe. Action of puromycin in polyadenylic acid-directed polylysine synthesis. *J. Mol. Biol.* 1965;13:617.

305. Sarkar, S., and R. E. Thach. Inhibition of formyl-methionyl-transfer RNA binding to ribosomes by tetracycline. *Proc. Nat. Acad. Sci. U.S.A.* 1968;60:1479.

306. Franklin, T. J. The inhibition of incorporation of leucine into protein of cell-free systems from rat liver and *Escherichia coli* by chlortetracycline. *Biochem. J.* 1963;87:449.

307. Beard, H. S., S. A. Armentrout, and A. S. Weisberger. Inhibition of mammalian protein synthesis by antibiotics. *Pharmacol. Rev.* 1969;21:213.

308. Battaner, E., and D. Vazquez. Inhibitors of protein synthesis by ribosomes of the 80-S type. *Biochim. Biophys. Acta* 1971;254:316.

309. Franklin, T. J., and B. Higginson. Active accumulation of tetracycline by *Escherichia coli. Biochem. J.* 1970;116:287.

310. Dockter, M. E., and J. A. Magnuson. Characterization of the active transport of chlortetracycline in *Staphylococcus aureus* by a florescence technique. *J. Supramol. Structure* 1974;2:32.

311. McMurry, L., and S. B. Levy. Two transport systems for tetracycline in sensitive *Escherichia coli*: critical role for an initial rapid uptake system insensitive to energy inhibitors. *Antimicrob. Agents Chemother.* 1978;14:201.

312. Fayolle, F., G. Privitera, and M. Sebald. Tetracycline transport in *Bacteroides fragilis. Antimicrob. Agents Chemother.* 1980;18:502.

313. Chopra, I., and S. J. Eccles. Diffusion of tetracycline across the outer membrane of *Escherichia coli* K-12: involvement of protein I_a. *Biochem. Biophys. Res. Commun.* 1978;83:550.

314. Chopra, I., and T. G. B. Howe. Bacterial resistance to the tetracyclines. *Microbiol. Rev.* 1978;42:707.

315. Kuck, N. A., and M. Forbes. Uptake of minocycline and tetracycline by tetracycline-susceptible and -resistant bacteria. *Antimicrob. Agents Chemother.* 1973;3:662.

316. Li, L. H., S. L. Kuentzel, K. D. Shugars, and B. K. Bhuyan. Cytotoxicity of several marketed antibiotics on mammalian cells in culture. *J. Antibiot.* 1977;30:506.

317. Martin, R. R., G. A. Warr, R. B. Couch, H. Yeager, and V. Knight. Effects of tetracycline on leukotaxis, *J. Infect. Dis.* 1974;129:110.

318. Forsgren, A., D. Schmeling, and P. G. Quie. Effect of tetracycline on the phagocytic function of human leukocytes. *J. Infect. Dis.* 1974;130:412.

319. Medoff, G., C. N. Kwan, D. Schlessinger, and G. S. Kobayashi. Potentiation of rifampicin, rifampicin analogs, and tetracycline against animal cells by amphotericin B and polymyxin B. *Cancer Res.* 1973;33:1146.

320. Steigbigel, N. H., C. W. Reed, and M. Finland. Susceptibility of common pathogenic bacteria to seven tetracycline antibiotics in vitro. *Am. J. Med. Sci.* 1968;255:179.

321. Finland, M. Changing patterns of susceptibility of common bacterial pathogens to antimicrobial agents. *Ann. Intern. Med.* 1972;76:1009.

322. Neu, H. C. A symposium on the tetracyclines: a major appraisal. Introduction. *Bull. N.Y. Acad. Med.* 1978;54:141.

323. Klein, N. C., and B. A. Cunha. Tetracyclines. *Med. Clin. North Am.* 1995;79:789.

324. Chow, A. W., V. Patten, and L. B. Guze. Comparative susceptibility of anaerobic bacteria to minocycline, doxycycline, and tetracycline. *Antimicrob. Agents Chemother.* 1975;7:46.

325. Lew, M. A., K. M. Beckett, and M. J. Levin. Antifungal activity of four tetracycline analogues against *Candida albicans* in vitro: potentiation by amphotericin B. *J. Infect. Dis.* 1977;136:263.

326. Colwell, E. J., R. L. Hickman, R. Intrprasert, and C. Tirabutana. Minocycline and tetracycline treatment of acute falciparum malaria in Thailand. *Am. J. Trop. Med. Hyg.* 1972;21:144.

327. Chopra, I., T. G. B. Howe, A. H. Linton, K. B. Linton, M. H. Richmond, and D. C. E. Speller. The tetracyclines: prospects at the beginning of the 1980s. *J. Antimicrob. Chemother.* 1981;8:5.

328. Warner, P. F., L. J. Zubrzycki, and M. Chila. Polygenes and modifier genes for tetracycline and penicillin resistance in *Neisseria gonorrhoeae. J. Gen. Microbiol.* 1980;117:103.

329. Levy, S. B., and L. McMurry. Plasmid-determined tetracycline resistance involves new transport systems for tetracycline. *Nature* 1978;276:90.

330. Ball, P. R., S. W. Shales, and I. Chopra. Plasmid-mediated tetracycline resistance in *Escherichia coli* involves increased efflux of the antibiotic. *Biochem. Biophys. Res. Commun.* 1980;93:74.

331. McMurry, L., R. E. Petrucci, and S. B. Levy. Active efflux of tetracycline encoded by four genetically different tetracycline resistant determinants in *Escherichia coli. Proc. Natl. Acad. U.S.A.* 1980;77:3974.

332. Fabre, J., E. Milek, P. Kalafopoulos, and G. Mérier. La cinétique de tétracyclines chez l'homme. *Schweitz. Med. Wochenschr.* 1971;101:593–598;625–633.

333. Macdonald, H., R. G. Kelley, S. Allen, J. F. Noble, and L. A. Kanegis. Pharmacokinetic studies on minocycline in man. *Clin. Pharmacol. Ther.* 1973;14:852.

334. Rosenblatt, J. E., J. E. Barrett, J. L. Brodie, and W. M. M. Kirby. Comparison of in vitro activity and clinical pharmacology of doxycycline with other tetracyclines. *Antimicrob. Agents Chemother.* 1967;134.

335. Kunin, C. M., A. C. Dornbush, and M. Finland. Distribution and excretion of four tetracycline analogues in normal young men. *J. Clin. Invest.* 1959;38:1950.

336. Brogden, R. N., T. M. Speight, and G. S. Avery. Minocycline: a review of its antibacterial and pharmacokinetic properties and therapeutic use. *Drugs* 1975;9:251.

337. Banerjee, S., and K. Chakrabarti. The transport of tetracyclines across the mouse ileum in vitro: the effect of cations and other agents. *J. Pharm. Pharmacol.* 1976;28:133.

338. Albert, A., and C. W. Ross. Avidity of tetracyclines for the cations of metals. *Nature* 1956;177:433.

339. Kunin, C. M., and M. Finland. Clinical pharmacology of the tetracycline antibiotics. *Clin. Pharmacol. Ther.* 1961;2:51.

340. Neuvonen, P. J., G. Gothoni, R. Hackman, and K. Bjorksten. Interference of iron with the absorption of tetracyclines in man. *BMJ* 1970;4:532.

341. Barr, W. H., J. Adir, and L. Garrettson. Decrease of tetracycline absorption in man by sodium bicarbonate. *Clin. Pharmacol. Ther.* 1971;12:779.

342. Kramer, P. A., D. J. Chapron, J. Benson and S. A. Merick. Tetracycline absorption in elderly patients with achlorhydria. *Clin. Pharmacol. Ther.* 1978;23:467.

343. Garty, M., and A. Hurwitz. Effect of cimetidine and antacids on gastrointestinal absorption of tetracycline. *Clin. Pharmacol. Ther.* 1980;28:203.

344. Leibowitz, B. J., J. L. Hakes, M. M. Cahn, and E. J. Levy. Doxycycline blood levels in normal subjects after intravenous and oral administration. *Curr. Ther. Res.* 1972;14:820.

345. Bennett, J. V., J. S. Mickelwait, J. E. Barrett, J. L. Brodie, and W. M. M. Kirby. Comparative serum binding of four tetracyclines under simulated in vivo conditions. *Antimicrob. Agents Chemother.*—1965. 1966;180.

346. Cunha, B. A., and S. M. Garabedian-Ruffalo. Tetracyclines in urology: current concepts. *Urology* 1990;36:548.

347. Poirier, R. H., and A. C. Ellison. Ocular penetration of orally administered minocycline. *Ann. Ophthalmol.* 1979;11:1859.

348. LeBlanc, A. L., and J. E. Perry. Transfer of tetracycline across the human placenta. *Texas Rep. Biol. Med.* 1967;25:541.

349. Hoeprich, P. D., and D. M. Warshauer. Entry of four tetracyclines into saliva and tears. *Antimicrob. Agents Chemother.* 1974;5:330.

350. Devine, L. F., D. P. Johnson, C. R. Hagerman, W. E. Pierce, S. L. Rhode, and R. O. Peckinpaugh. The effect of minocycline on meningococcal carrier state in naval personnel. *Am. J. Epidemiol.* 1971;93:337.

351. Milch, R. A., D. P. Rall, and J. E. Tobie. Bone localization of the tetracyclines. *J. Natl. Cancer Inst.* 1957;19:87.

352. Bassett, E. J., M. S. Keith, G. J. Armelagos, D. L. Martin, and A. R. Villanueva. Tetracycline-labeled human bone from ancient Sudanese Nubia (A.D. 350). *Science* 1980;209:1532.

353. Douglas, A. C. The deposition of tetracycline in human nails and teeth. A complication of long-term treatment. *Br. J. Dis. Chest* 1963;57:44.

354. Rall, D. P., T. L. Loo, M. Lane, and M. G. Kelley. Appearance and persistence of fluorescent material in tumor tissue after tetracycline administration. *J. Natl. Cancer Inst.* 1957;19:79.

355. Klinger, J., and R. Katz. Tetracycline fluorescence in diagnosis of gastric carcinoma. Preliminary report. *Gastroenterology* 1961;41:29.

356. Dunn, R. J., and K. D. Devine. Tetracycline-induced fluorescence of laryngeal, pharyngeal, and oral cancer, *Laryngoscope* 1972;82:189.

357. Malek, P., J. Kolc, V. L. Zastava, F. V. Zak, and B. Peleska. Fluorescence of tetracycline analogues fixed in myocardial infarction. *Cardiologia* 1963;42:303.

358. Lanman, R. C., S. Muranishi, and L. S. Schankar. Hepatic uptake and biliary excretion of tetracycline in the rat. *Am. J. Physiol.* 1973;225:1240.

359. Whelton, A. Tetracyclines in renal insufficiency: resolution of a therapeutic dilemma. *Bull. N.Y. Acad. Med.* 1978;54:223.

360. Fabre, J., E. Milek, P. Kalfopoulos, and G. Mérier. Kinetics of tetracycline in man. II. Excretion, penetration in normal and inflammatory tissues, behavior in renal insufficiency and hemodialysis. *Schweiz. Med. Wochenschr.* 1971;101:625.

361. Penttila, O., P. J. Neuvonen, K. Aho, and R. Lehtovaara. Interaction between doxycycline and some antiepileptic drugs. *BMJ* 1974;1:470.

362. Neuvonen, P. J., and O. Penttila. Interaction between doxycycline and barbiturates. *BMJ* 1974;1:535.

363. Channer, K. S., and D. Hollanders. Severe tetracycline-induced oesophageal ulceration. *BMJ* 1981; 2:1359.

364. Editorial. *Candida* infections. *Med. Lett.* 1970; 12:29.

365. Grossman, E. R., A. Walchek, and H. Freedman. Tetracyclines and permanent teeth: the relation between dose and tooth color. *Pediatrics* 1971; 47:567.

366. Wallman, I. S., and H. B. Hilton. Teeth pigmented by tetracycline. *Lancet* 1962;1:827.

367. Anthony, J. R. Effect on deciduous and permanent teeth of tetracycline deposition in utero. *Postgrad. Med.* 1970;48:165.

368. Schach von Wittenau, M. Some pharmacokinetic aspects of doxycline metabolism in man. *Chemotherapy* 1968;13:41.

369. Cohlan, S. Q., G. Bevlander, and T. Tiamsic. Growth inhibition of prematures receiving tetracycline: clinical and laboratory investigation. *Am. J. Dis. Child.* 1963;105:453.

370. Siegel, D. Tetracyclines: new look at old antibiotic. I. Clinical pharmacology, mechanism of action, and untoward effects. *N.Y. State J. Med.* 1978; 78:950.

371. Loyd-Still, J. D., R. J. Grand, and G. F. Vawter. Tetracycline hepatotoxicity in the differential diagnosis of postoperative jaundice. *J. Pediatr.* 1974;84:366.

372. Lepper, M. H., C. K. Wolfe, H. J. Zimmerman, E. R. Caldwell, H. W. Spies, and H. F. Dowling. Effect of large doses of aureomycin on human liver. *Arch. Intern. Med.* 1951;88:271.

373. Schultz, J. C., J. S. Adamson, W. W. Workman, and T. D. Norman. Fatal liver disease after intravenous administration of tetracycline in high dosage. *N. Engl. J. Med.* 1963;269:999.

374. Philips, M. E., J. B. Eastwood, J. R. Curtis, P. E. Gower, and H. E. DeWardener. Tetracycline poisoning in renal failure. *BMJ* 1974;2:149.

375. Shils, M. E. Some metabolic aspects of the tetracyclines. *Clin. Pharmacol. Ther.* 1962;3:321.

376. Boston Collaborative Drug Surveillance Program. Tetracycline and drug-attributed rises in blood urea nitrogen. *JAMA* 1972;17:377.

377. Morgan T., and N. Ribush. The effect of oxytetracycline and doxcycline on protein metabolism. *Med. J. Austr.* 1972;1:55.

378. Singer, I., and D. Rotenberg. Demeclocycline-induced nephrogenic diabetes insipidus. In-vivo and in-vitro studies. *Ann. Intern. Med.* 1973;79:679.

379. Forrest, J. N., M. Cox, C. Hong, G. Morrison, M. Bia, and I. Singer. Superiority of demeclocycline over lithium in the treatment of inappropriate secretion of antidiuretic hormone. *N. Engl. J. Med.* 1978;298: 173.

380. F. Mavromatis. Tetracycline nephropathy. *JAMA* 1965;193:91.

381. Gross, J. M. Fanconi syndrome (adult type) developing secondary to the ingestion of outdated tetracycline. *Ann. Intern. Med.* 1963;58:523.

382. Benitz, K. F., and H. F. Diermeier. Renal toxicity of tetracycline degradation products. *Proc. Soc. Exp. Biol. Med.* 1964;115:930.

383. Appel, G. B., and H. C. Neu. The nephrotoxicity of antimicrobial agents (second of three parts). *N. Engl. J. Med.* 1977;296:722.

384. Frost, P., G. D. Weinstein, and E. C. Gomez. Phototoxic potential of minocycline and doxycycline. *Arch. Dermatol.* 1972;105:681.

385. Frost, P., G. D. Weinstein, and E. C. Gomez. Methacycline and demeclocycline in relation to sunlight. *JAMA* 1971;216:326.

386. Epstein, J. H., D. L. Tuffanelli, J. S. Seibert, and W. L. Epstein. Porphyria-like cutaneous changes induced by tetracycline hydrochloride photosensitization. *Arch. Dermatol.* 1976;112:661.

387. Kestel, J. L. Photo-onycholysis from minocycline. *Cutis* 1981;28:53.

388. McGrae, J. D., and A. S. Zelickson. Skin pigmentation secondary to minocycline therapy. *Arch. Dermatol.* 1980;116:1262.

389. Sato, S., G. F. Murphy, J. D. Bernhard, M. C. Mihm, and T. B. Fitzpatrick. Ultrastructural and X-ray microanalytical observations of minocycline-related hyperpigmentation of the skin. *J. Invest. Dermatol.* 1981; 77:271.

390. Opfer, K. The bulging fontanelle. *Lancet* 1963; 1:116.

391. Walters, B. N. J., and S. S. Gubbay. Tetracycline and benign intracranial hypertension: report of five cases. *BMJ* 1981;282:19.

392. Chadwick, D. Antibiotics and benign intracranial hypertension. *J. Antimicrob. Chemother.* 1982;9: 88.

393. Fanning, W. L., D. W. Gump, and R. A. Sofferman. Side effects of minocycline: a double-blind study. *Antimicrob. Agents Chemother.* 1977;11:712.

394. Forsgren, A., and H. Gnarpe: Tetracyclines and host-defense mechanisms. *Antimicrob. Agents Chemother.* 1973;3:711.

395. Nguyen, V. X., D. E. Nix, S. Gillikin, and J. J. Schentag. Effect of oral antacid administration on the pharmacokinetics of intravenous doxycycline. *Antimicrob. Agents Chemother.* 1989;33:434.

396. Neuvonen, P. J., O. Pentilla, R. Lehtovaara, and K. Aho. Effect of anti-epileptic drugs on the elimination of various tetracycline derivatives. *Eur. J. Clin. Pharmacol.* 1975;9:147.

397. Neuvonen, P. J., and O. Pentillä, Interaction between doxycycline and barbiturates. *BMJ* 1974;1:535.

398. Neuvonen, P. J., O. Pentillä, M. Roose, and J. Tirkkonen. Effect of long-term alcohol consumption on the half life of tetracycline and doxycycline in man. *Int. J. Clin. Pharmacol.* 1974;14:303.

399. Caraco, Y., and A. Rubinow. Enhanced anticoagulant effect of coumarin derivatives induced by doxycycline coadministration. *Ann. Pharmacother.* 1992; 26:1084.

400. Siegel, D. Tetracyclines: new look at old antibiotic. II. Clinical use. *N.Y. State J. Med.* 1978; 78:1115.

401. Symposium (various authors). Symposium on the tetracyclines: a major appraisal. *Bull. N.Y. Acad. Med.* 1978;54:141–249.

402. Kauffman, R. E., R. E. Johnson, H. W. Jaffe, C. Thornsberry, G. H. Reynolds, P. J. Wiesner, and the Cooperative Study Groups. National gonorrhea therapy monitoring study. Treatment results. *N. Engl. J. Med.* 1976;294:1.

403. Dunlop, E. M. C. Treatment of patients suffering from chlamydial infections. *J. Antimicrobial Chemother.* 1977;3:377.

404. Schachter, J. Chlamydial infections (second of three parts). *N. Engl. J. Med.* 1978;298:490.

405. Denny, F. W., W. A. Clyde, and W. P. Glezen. *Mycoplasma pneumoniae* disease: clinical spectrum, pathophysiology, epidemiology, and control. *J. Infect. Dis.* 1971;123:74.

406. Joshi, N., and D. Miller. Doxycycline revisited. *Arch. Intern. Med.* 1997;157:1421.

407. Ad Hoc Committee on the Use of Antibiotics in Dermatology. Systemic antibiotics for treatment of acne vulgaris. *Arch. Dermatol.* 1975;111:1630.

408. Cunliffe, W. J., R. A. Forster, N. D. Greenwood, C. Hetherington, K. T. Holland, R. L. Holmes, S. Khan, C. D. Roberts, M. Williams, and B. Williamson. Tetracycline and acne vulgaris: a clinical and laboratory investigation. *BMJ* 1973;4:332.

409. Delaney, T. J., B. J. Leppard, and D. M. MacDonald. Effects of long term treatment with tetracycline. *Acta Derm. Venerol.* (Stockh) 1974;54:487.

410. Leyden, J. J., R. R. Marples, O. H. Mills, and A. M. Kligman. Gram-negative folliculitis—a complication of antibiotic therapy in acne vulgaris. *Br. J. Dermatol.* 1973;88:533.

411. Melski, J. W., and K. A. Arndt. Topical therapy for acne. *N. Engl. J. Med.* 1980;302:503.

412. Marples, R. M., and A. M. Kligman. Ecological effects of oral antibiotics on the microflora of human skin. *Arch. Dermatol.* 1971;103:148.

413. Vannuffel, P., and C. Cocito. Mechanism of action of streptogramins and macrolides. *Drugs* 1996; 51(Suppl. 1):20.

414. Pechere, J.-C. Streptogramins. A unique class of antibiotics. *Drugs* 1996;51(Suppl. 1):13.

415. Cocito, C., M. DiGiambattista, E. Nysren, and P. Vannuffer. Inhibition of protein synthesis by streptogramins and related antibiotics. *J. Antimicrob. Chemother.* 1997;39(Suppl. A):7.

416. Griswold, M. W., B. M. Lomaestro, and L. L. Briceland. Quinupristin-dalfopristin (RP59500): an injectable streptogramin combination. *Am. J. Health Systems Pharm.* 1996;53:2045.

417. Rubinstein, E., and N. Keller. Future prospects and therapeutic potential of streptogramins. *Drugs* 1996;(Suppl. 1):38.

418. Etienne, S. D., G. Montay, A. LeLiboux, A. Frydman, and J. J. Garaud. A Phase I, double-blind, placebo-controlled trial of the tolerance and pharmacokinetic behavior of RP 59500. *J. Antimicrob. Chemother.* 1992;30(Suppl A):123.

419. Bernard, E., M. Bensoussen, F. Bensoussen, S. Etienne, I. Cazenave, E. Carsenti-Etesse, Y. LeRoux, G. Montay, and P. Dellamonica. Pharmacokinetics and suction blister fluid penetration of a semisynthetic injectable streptogramin RP59500 (RP57669/RP 54470). *Eur. J. Clin. Microbiol. Infect. Dis.* 1994;13:768.

420. Data on file. Rhone-Poulenc Rorer Pharmaceuticals, Inc., Collegeville, PA, 1998.

421. Bombart, F., M. B. Dorr, T. Bekele, S. Barriere, J. Rey, C. Vessereau, and G. H. Talbot. Overview of the safety and tolerability of quinupristin/dalfopristin (Synercid, RP59500) in the global development program. Proceedings: 8th European Congress on Clinical Microbiology and Infectious Diseases, 1997, p. 70.

CHAPTER SEVEN

The Antimetabolites

The Sulfonamides and Trimethoprim
(Trimethoprim-Sulfamethoxazole)

Sulfonamides

Discovery and Structure

The sufonamides were the first effective chemotherapeutic agents to be used systematically for the treatment of bacterial infections. Sulfonamide-containing compounds were synthesized early in this century by German chemists for use as dyes. Their therapeutic potential was not exploited until 1935, when Domagk demonstrated that one of these dyes, prontosil, was effective in treating mice infected with streptococci. Later it was found that prontosil is metabolized in the tissues to para-aminobenzenesulfonamide (sulfanilamide), the chemotherapeutically active part of the molecule. Subsequently, thousands of compounds were synthesized, and many were introduced for the treatment of infection.

The sulfonamides are structural analogs of para-aminobenzoic acid (PABA). The para-amino group is required for antibacterial activity and most of the clinically useful compounds have been prepared by adding various moieties to the amide group (N^1). It was originally proposed that the antibacterial activity would reflect the pK_a of the sulfonamide group, with the most active compounds being those with the pK_a of about 6.7.[1] There are, however, many exceptions to this prediction, although within a very homologous series of sulfonamides it is possible to show a linear relationship between the pK_a and the minimum inhibitory concentration (MIC).[2,3]

para-Aminobenzoic acid   Sulfonamides

Mechanism of Action

The sulfonamides usually produce a bacteriostatic effect. When they are added to a culture of bacteria, there is a delay period of several cell replications before there is inhibition of growth (Figure 7–1). These drugs arrest cell growth by inhibiting the synthesis of folic acid by the bacterium. During the delay period, before cell growth is arrested, the bacterium is exhausting its stores of folic acid.

Folic acid is required for growth by both bacterial and mammalian cells. Because animal cells are unable to synthesize folate, this compound must be supplied in the diet. Folic acid is taken into mammalian cells by an active transport mechanism. Since it does not enter most bacterial cells, bacteria must synthesize the compound intracellularly. This difference between the biochemistry of the bacterial and mammalian cell is the basis of the selective toxicity of the sulfonamides, para-aminosalicylic acid, and the sulfones.

A reduced form of folic acid functions as a coenzyme, which transports one-carbon

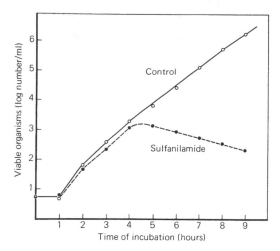

Figure 7–1. Early growth of hemolytic strepto-cocci in blood broth without (O-O) and with (●-●) 10^{-5} *M* sulfanilamide. (From Woods.[4])

units from one molecule to another. Such one-carbon transfer reactions are essential for the synthesis of thymidine, all the purines, and several amino acids. Thymidine is necessary for DNA synthesis, and the purines are necessary for all nucleic acid synthesis in the cell. When folate synthesis is inhibited, cell growth is arrested because of the cell's inability to synthesize these essential macromolecular precursors (see Fig. 7–5).

Folic acid consists of a pteridine unit, PABA, and glutamate. Some time ago it was postulated that the sulfonamides, being structural analogs of PABA, might compete for the incorporation of this subunit into the folate molecule. Also, the effect of sulfonamides in bacteria capable of taking up folic acid could be reversed in a noncompetitive manner by adding to the culture such products of the inhibited reaction sequence as

folic acid or leucovorin, a reduced and methylated form of folic acid. If the mechanism of growth inhibition by the sulfonamides is competition for PABA, then increasing the level of PABA in the culture medium should reverse the action of sulfonamide in a competitive manner. Figure 7–2 shows these effects in cultures of *Clostridium tetanomorphum.* Folic acid can enter these cells, and, in the presence of folic acid sufficient to maintain normal growth, the cell is not affected by any concentration of sulfonamide. In the presence of increasing concentrations of sulfanilamide, however, higher and higher concentrations of PABA are required to maintain growth.

The development of a cell-free system from bacteria that can form folate compounds from pteridines, PABA, and glutamic acid has permitted a more detailed analysis of the mechanism of sulfonamide action. Sulfonamides inhibit the incorporation of PABA into dihydropteroic acid in such a system, but inhibition is not solely competitive.[5] If sulfathiazole and PABA are added to the in vitro system simultaneously, then competition can be demonstrated. If the enzyme system is first preincubated with sulfathiazole, PABA cannot then completely reverse the inhibitory effect of the drug. The enzyme that directs the incorporation of PABA and the pteridine moiety into dihydropteroic acid (dihydropteroate synthetase) has been purified 50-fold from *Escherichia coli*[6] and sulfadiazine has been shown to inhibit the partially purified enzyme in a competitive manner when both PABA and the drug are added simultaneously.[7] If the enzyme is preincubated with a sulfonamide, the enzyme incorporates the drug into a product that is an adduct of the sulfonamide and the

pteridine moiety   PABA   glutamate

Folic acid

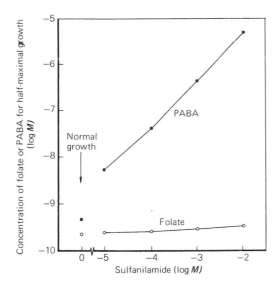

Figure 7–2. The requirement of *Clostridium tetanomorphum* for para-aminobenzoic acid (PABA) or folic acid for growth in the presence of varying concentrations of sulfanilamide. PABA (●-●); folic acid (○-○). (From Woods.[4])

pteridine moiety.[8] This preincubation depletes the system of pteridine, and when PABA is subsequently added, there is little remaining pteridine to permit folate synthesis. The formation of a drug-containing folate analog has also been demonstrated in growing bacterial cultures.[8] Thus, the sulfonamides have the potential to interfere with folate metabolism in two ways: the most important is competitive inhibition of PABA utilization in folate synthesis, but sulfonamide-containing analogs of folic acid are also formed and these could interfere with other aspects of folic acid metabolism.

The inhibition of cell growth by sulfonamides may be reversed by adding the end products of one-carbon transfer reactions (thymidine, purines, methionine, and serine) to the growth medium. This reversal is of some clinical significance; in purulent infections the pus may contain a considerable amount of these substances as a result of cell breakdown. This may substantially decrease the efficacy of the sulfonamides in the treatment of these infections.[9] Also, the presence of PABA in the culture medium in which organisms are grown in the laboratory can

lead to false conclusions regarding the drug sensitivity of clinical specimens. It is not uncommon to receive a report that a bacterium is resistant to sulfonamides when it is really quite sensitive to these drugs.

SULFONAMIDES AND "THYMINELESS DEATH." The sulfonamides are generally regarded as bacteriostatic drugs, but under special growth conditions, they can be bactericidal. When bacteria are grown in medium containing amino acids and a source of purines, but no thymine, exposure to sulfonamide is bactericidal.[10] The killing effect is overcome by the addition of thymine. When the same organism is grown in the absence of amino acids, purines, and thymine, the sulfonamides are bacteriostatic. This poorly understood killing phenomenon is called *thymineless death*, and it occurs when DNA synthesis is blocked (in this case because methylene tetrahydrofolate is required for the synthesis of thymidine monophosphate, which in turn is required for the synthesis of DNA) in the presence of continued protein synthesis. This is not merely of academic interest, since it has been shown that the sulfonamides can be bactericidal in human blood and urine as well as in synthetic media.[10,11] Thus, it is possible that these drugs are bactericidal in some body fluids containing little or no thymine. As mentioned earlier, sulfonamides are relatively ineffective in purulent wounds where liberation of thymine as a product of tissue breakdown may overcome any possible bactericidal effect. Obviously, if enough products of the blocked reactions are present, the drug will be ineffective.

PARA-AMINOSALICYLIC ACID AND THE SULFONES. Para-aminosalicylic acid (PAS) and the sulfones are also structural analogs of PABA. PAS is used to treat tuberculosis and the sulfones are used to treat leprosy. The pharmacology and toxicity of these drugs are discussed in Chapter 11. The antibacterial action of PAS and sulfones is antagonized by PABA;[12,13] PAS, like the sulfonamides, is joined to a pteroic acid moiety by the bacterial enzyme systems to produce PAS-containing folate analogs.[14] The sulfones, like the sulfonamides, have been shown to be competitive inhibitors of partially purified dihydropteroate synthetase from *Escherichia coli*[8] and from the malarial parasite *Plasmodium berghei.*[15]

COOH

OH

NH$_2$

para-Aminosalicylic acid

H$_2$N—⬡—S—⬡—NH$_2$

Diaminodiphenylsulfone
(dapsone)

There is a great deal of difference between the spectrum of antibacterial action of PAS and that of the sulfonamides. Para-aminosalicylic acid is an effective drug in *Mycobacterium tuberculosis*, but most organisms are not very sensitive to this compound. Sulfonamides are ineffective against *M. tuberculosis*, but they inhibit a number of organisms that are quite insensitive to PAS. There may be considerable variation in bacteria with regard to their relative permeability to these agents, but this cannot entirely explain the different sensitivities seen. Since both the sulfonamides and PAS inhibit growth by competing for PABA, it seems entirely possible that the enzyme responsible for incorporating PABA into the folate molecule may vary considerably from one type of bacterium to another. Thus, the PABA substrate site in *M. tuberculosis* may preferentially accept PAS over the sulfonamides. In other organisms, this same site may have another configuration, allowing good fit for PABA and the sulfonamides but not for PAS. This possibility is suggested by work carried out with mutant strains of pneumococci, which demonstrated varying degrees of resistance to the sulfonamides.[16] Cell-free extracts of the resistant cells, which incorporated PABA into folic acid, were found to

Table 7–1. *Relative effect of sulfanilamide and para-aminosalicylic acid (PAS) in inhibiting folic acid synthesis in cell-free extracts of pneumococci.* Cell-free extracts were prepared from two sulfanilamide-resistant strains of pneumococci and a wild type. The concentration of sulfanilamide or PAS required to reduce folic acid synthesis in each incubation to a fixed quantity was compared to that required for inhibition of the enzyme system from the wild type to the same level.

Strain	Sulfanilamide	PAS
Wild type	1	1
Fa	4	7.5
Fd	7	0.1

Source: Data from Wolf and Hotchkiss.[17]

require higher concentrations of sulfanilamide for inhibition of folate production than the wild type.[17] As shown in Table 7–1, the concentration of PAS required for inhibition of in vitro folate synthesis was higher in one resistant strain than in the wild type; but in the other resistant strain, the enzyme was 10 times more sensitive to PAS. Other experiments demonstrated that one of the altered enzymes (Fd) was heat sensitive and had an affinity for PABA that differed from that of the wild-type enzyme. A model system is available, therefore, which permits us to deduce that some of the great differences in sensitivity of different bacteria to growth inhibition by various members of three groups of drugs (the sulfonamides, PAS, and the sulfones) that act in a similar manner at the same receptor site may be explained by genetically determined variations in the structure of the receptor site.

Antimicrobial Activity and Clinical Use

The sulfonamides have a broad spectrum of antimicrobial action that includes gram-positive and gram-negative bacteria, *Actinomycetes, Chlamydiae,* and even some protozoa like *Toxoplasma* and *Plasmodia.* The use of sulfonamides as single drugs in the treatment of infection has diminished continually as less toxic, bactericidal antibiotics have been introduced and as the incidence of sulfonamide resistance has increased. Sulfonamides have been used for many years to treat acute urinary tract infection, which is the most common indication for their use. Resistance among community-acquired strains of *E. coli* and other urinary tract pathogens is no longer rare and sensitivity testing is recommended. The sulfonamides were formerly used to treat bacillary dysentery, but as discussed in Chapter 2, R factor–mediated resistance spread rapidly among the enteric pathogens. Similarly, *Neisseria meningitidis* strains are commonly resistant and active infection is treated with penicillin G or a third-generation cephalosporin. In some areas of the world, sulfonamides are used for prophylaxis of those in close contact with patients infected with proven sensitive strains of *N. meningitidis,* but rifampin is generally considered to be the agent of choice for prophylaxis. *Shigella* species are another group of bacteria for which resistance to the sulfonamides is now widespread.[18]

Nocardia asteroides is sensitive to the sulfonamides[19] and a sulfonamide or trimethoprim-sulfamethoxazole is the drug of choice for nocardiosis. The sulfonamides are useful alternatives to a tetracycline or an erythromycin in the treatment of trachoma and inclusion conjunctivitis. Toxoplasmosis is treated with pyrimethamine and a sulfonamide administered simultaneously. The sulfonamide yields an enhanced antibacterial effect with pyrimethamine, but should not be used alone. As discussed in Chapter 13, a sulfonamide plus pyrimethamine is useful in both treatment and suppression of malaria due to chloroquine-resistant strains of *Plasmodium falciparum.*

Several mechanisms of sulfonamide resistance have been demonstrated in both laboratory and clinical strains of bacteria. A few resistant strains of *Staphylococcus aureus* have been shown to produce increased amounts of PABA.[20] Some resistant bacteria synthesize an altered dihydropteroate synthetase with a decreased affinity for sulfonamides,[17,21] whereas others may produce increased amounts of the enzyme.[22] Resistance among the enteric bacteria is usually mediated by R factors. In some cases this resistance is due to transfer of determinants for the production of dihydropteroate synthetase with decreased affinity for the drug,[21] but the most common type of resistance appears to result from reduced drug uptake.[22,23] The biochemical mechanism for the reduced uptake is not known. There is complete cross-resistance among all the sulfonamides.

Sulfonamide Preparations

A large number of sulfonamide preparations have been marketed. The important drugs in each class of orally administered compounds are presented in Table 7–2, where the preparations have been classified according to their duration of action. Some references classify the sulfonamides by their speed of absorption and excretion. In the classification scheme in this chapter most of the short- and intermediate-acting sulfonamides are rapidly absorbed and excreted. The structures of selected sulfonamides are shown in Figure 7–3.

The *short-acting* sulfonamides are used mainly to treat urinary tract infections. Sulfisoxazole is rapidly absorbed and rapidly excreted in the urine, about 30% of the drug in the urine is in the inactive, acetylated form. Because high urine concentrations are achieved and its urine solubility is much higher than that of the older sulfonamides (see Table 7–3), sulfisoxazole replaced the older agents as the preferred drug for treating urinary tract infections. Sulfacytine is a newer sulfonamide that is slightly more potent and more soluble than sulfisoxazole.[24] The half-life of sulfacytine (4 h) is shorter than that of sulfisoxazole (5-6 h) and it is usually administered at one-fourth the dosage. Similar urine concentrations are achieved with the two drugs, but sulfisoxazole has the advantage of being the less expensive form of therapy. Sulfamethizole is also rapidly excreted, with about 80% of a dose recoverable in the urine within 8 h, largely (95%) as the unaltered drug. The plasma concentrations achieved with both sulfacytine and sulfamethizole are lower than those achieved with sulfisoxazole and

Table 7–2. *Selected orally administered sulfonamides classified according to their duration of action.* Sulfadoxine, sulfamethoxypyridazine, and sulfameter are not available in the United States.

Class	Preparation	Usual dosage interval (hours)	Serum half-life (hours)	Comment
Short-acting	Sulfisoxazole	4–5	5–6	Most soluble sulfona-mides
	Sulfacytine	6	4	
	Sulfadiazine	4–6	10	
	Sulfamethizole	6	6	
Intermediate-acting	Sulfamethoxazole	12	9–11	Given in combination with trimethoprim
Long-acting	Sulfamethoxypyridazine	Daily	40	High incidence of Stevens-Johnson syndrome, use not recommended
	Sulfameter	Daily	40	
Extra long-acting	Sulfadoxine	Weekly	100–120	Marketed in fixed-dose combination with pyrimethamine for prophylaxis of chloroquine-resistant *P. falciparum* malaria

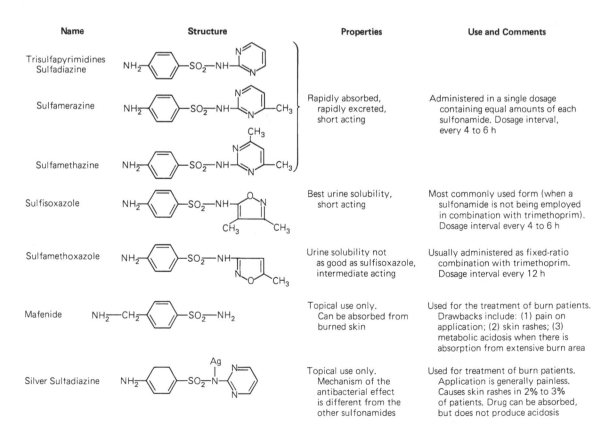

Figure 7–3. Structures and properties of selected sulfonamides.

the former drugs should be used only to treat infections in the urinary tract.

Sulfadiazine has a half-life of 10 h, but it is administered at intervals of 4–6 h and is classified as a short-acting sulfonamide. Sulfadiazine is less bound to serum protein than the other short-acting sulfonamides and the free form of the drug readily passes into the cerebrospinal fluid. Because sulfadiazine has a high intrinsic antibacterial potency (equivalent to sulfisoxazole) and high levels of drug are achieved in the cerebrospinal fluid, it is regarded as the best sulfonamide for treating meningitis. About 30% of the drug is recovered in the urine as the acetylated metabolite and it is less soluble in the urine than the other short-acting preparations. For this reason, special caution must be exercised to ensure good hydration and urine flow.

Sulfamethoxazole is an *intermediate-acting* sulfonamide with lower urine solubility than sulfisoxazole. Because the half-life of sulfamethoxazole (9–11 h) is similar to that of trimethoprim, it was the sulfonamide chosen for combined therapy with trimethoprim ($t^{1/2}$ 10–12 h). In the United States, sulfamethoxazole is available as a single drug preparation for treating both systemic and urinary tract infections, but its principal application is in fixed-dose combination therapy with trimethoprim. The pharmacokinetic properties of sulfamethoxazole are summarized in Table 7–8.

Sulfamethoxypyridazine and sulfameter (sulfamethoxydiazine) are slowly excreted sulfonamides with half-lives of about 40 h; the usual dosage interval is once daily. These *long-acting* drugs have been associated with a high incidence of Stevens-Johnson syndrome and they are no longer marketed in the United States. Sulfadoxine (sulfamethoxine) is a *very long-acting* sulfonamide (half-life 100–120 h) that is administered on a once-weekly basis as a fixed-dose combination with pyrimethamine for prophylaxis of *P. falciparum* malaria.

Several poorly absorbed sulfonamides (e.g., sulfaguanidine and sulfathalidine) were marketed for their local effects against intestinal bacteria. The only compound of this nature that is still of note is sulfasalazine, which is used for treatment of ulcerative colitis and regional enteritis.[25,26] The mechanism of the beneficial effect of this drug has not been completely defined, but it appears to be due to 5-aminosalicylic acid, which is released from the sulfapyridine moiety in the intestine.[27]

Several sulfonamides are available for topical use. Although topical sulfonamides are usually discouraged because of a lack of efficacy and a high risk of sensitization, sulfacetamide has certain benefits. Very high aqueous concentrations are nonirritating to the eye and are quite effective against many susceptible bacteria. Sulfacetamide penetrates into ocular fluids and tissues in high concentration and is not irritating like some of the sodium salts of the other sulfonamides. Hypersensitivity reactions following ophthalmic use of sulfacetamide are rare, but isolated reports of severe allergic reactions such as Stevens-Johnson syndrome[28] and systemic lupus erythematosis[29] have been published, thus ophthalmic solutions should not be administered to patients with known sulfonamide sensitivity.

Two topical preparations, mafenide and silver sulfadiazine, are used to prevent bacterial colonization of burns. The older preparation, mafenide,[30] produces pain at the site of application, and when it is applied to an extensive burn area, enough of the drug can be absorbed to cause metabolic acidosis.[31] The acidosis results from mafenide inhibition of carbonic anhydrase in the kidney, which reduces the body's ability to excrete acid. In contrast to mafenide, silver sulfadiazine may be applied less often and is generally painless. Significant quantities of the drug are absorbed, and serum levels of sulfadiazine can approach those obtained with systemic administration.[32] Therefore, toxic reactions similar to those with the other sulfonamides are possible with silver sulfadiazine, but this has not been a clinical problem. In contrast to mafenide, the use of silver sulfadiazine is not complicated by metabolic acidosis,[33] and silver sulfadiazine is generally considered to be the drug of choice for prevention of burn colonization.

The mechanism of action of silver sulfadiazine is not entirely clear. The antibacterial effect of this drug is not prevented by PABA,[34] which suggests that the principal effect is due to the silver. This is not surprising because many silver compounds (e.g., silver nitrate) have antiseptic properties. The silver dissociates from the sulfadiazine and becomes associated with the bacteria.[35,36] Although it has been suggested that silver at low concentration may be bactericidal as a result of an interaction with DNA,[35] the mechanism of the cell-killing effect is not known.[37,38] The spectrum of action of silver sulfadiazine is not restricted to bacteria. Several of the fungi that commonly infect the skin (dermatophytes) are sensitive to the drug.[39]

Pharmacology

ABSORPTION AND DISTRIBUTION. The sulfonamides are well absorbed from the gastrointestinal tract and are routinely given orally. Peak plasma levels are achieved in 2–3 h.

The sulfonamides bind to plasma protein to various extents;[40] the level of binding for the short-acting drugs ranges from a low of 35%–50% for sulfadiazine to 80%–95% for sulfisoxazole and many of the others.[41] The extent of protein binding decreases with severe renal failure.[42,43] These drugs readily pass into body fluids, including pleural, synovial, and ocular fluids. The sulfonamides are one of the few groups of antimicrobial agents that readily pass into the cerebrospinal fluid, even in the absence of inflammation. The cerebrospinal fluid levels achieved by the short-acting sulfonamides are 30%–80% of the level simultaneously present in the blood. Because of its relatively low binding to plasma protein and its longer half-life, which yields more sustained blood levels of free drug, the highest cerebrospinal fluid levels are most readily achieved with sulfadiazine. Sulfonamides readily pass through the placenta and into the fetal circulation.

METABOLISM AND EXCRETION. The sulfonamides are metabolized to various degrees—primarily by acetylation on the para-amino moiety, with some glucuronidation occurring also. The acetylated metabolites have no

antibacterial activity; however, they are still toxic and they are less soluble in the urine. Excretion of both the parent drug and the major acetylated metabolite is primarily renal, and the rate of excretion largely determines the duration of action. The sulfonamides are filtered and exhibit varying degrees of tubular reabsorption. In acid urine, the older sulfonamides are quite insoluble and will precipitate out in crystalline aggregates. These crystal deposits in the kidney and ureters can produce symptoms of urinary tract obstruction. This used to be a fairly frequent complication, but it is unusual with modern therapy. The problem of sulfonamide insolubility has been approached in three ways:

1. Ensuring good urine output by a high daily fluid intake minimizes the problem. The sulfonamides are more soluble in an alkaline urine (see Table 7–3), so bicarbonate or lactate can be administered if the urine pH is very low.
2. Sulfonamide analogs with higher urine solubility have been synthesized to overcome this problem. Sulfisoxazole and sulfacytine are such compounds.
3. Moderate doses of three different sulfonamides may be administered simultaneously. The presence of one sulfonamide does not decrease the solubility of another in the same aqueous solution. Thus, triple sulfonamides produce a higher total sulfonamide concentra-

Table 7–3. Solubility of sulfonamides in acid and alkaline urine.

Drug	Urine pH	Urine solubility at 37°C (mg/100 ml)
Sulfadiazine	5.5	18
	7.5	200
Sulfamerazine	5.5	35
	7.5	160
Sulfisoxazole	5.5	150
	7.5	14,500

Source: Data from Weinstein.[44]

tion than a single sulfonamide, without causing crystalluria. The triple sulfonamide combination, called *trisulfapyrimidines*, consists of sulfadiazine, sulfamerazine, and sulfamethazine (all short-acting drugs). Patients receiving trisulfapyrimidines for long periods of time should have the pH of their urine examined occasionally, and if it is unusually low, alkalinization may be advisable.

The soluble sulfonamides can be used in renal failure. The half-life of sulfisoxazole increases from 4–7 h to 6–12 h in end-stage renal disease and it is recommended that the dosage interval be increased from every 6 h to every 8–12 h when the glomerular filtration rate (GFR) is 10–50 ml/min and to every 18–24 h when the GFR is less than 10 ml/min.[45] Sulfisoxazole is removed by both peritoneal and hemodialysis.[45]

Adverse Effects

The sulfonamides can cause a variety of undesirable side effects,[46] with hypersensitivity reactions and effects on the hematopoietic system being particularly important. Oral administration is occasionally accompanied by nausea, vomiting, and diarrhea.

HYPERSENSITIVITY REACTIONS. Hypersensitivity reactions, particularly rashes, eosinophilia, and drug fever, occur in about 3% of patients receiving sulfisoxazole or sulfamethoxazole, the two oral preparations most commonly administered in the United States.[47] Because topical administration of the sulfonamides produced a high incidence of local hypersensitivity reactions and occasionally initiated systemic hypersensitivity, this route of administration has been largely discontinued. The exceptions are the use of ophthalmic preparations, the use of mafenide and silver sulfadiazine to reduce bacterial colonization of burns, and occasional use of vaginal preparations.

In addition to causing a variety of rashes, sulfonamides can cause a rare but severe form of erythema multiforme associated with widespread lesions of the skin and mu-

cous membranes that is called the *Stevens-Johnson syndrome*. This phenomenon can be caused by a wide variety of antigenic substances in addition to drugs. Systemic manifestations of fever, malaise, dehydration, and generalized toxemia may occur. The incidence of Stevens-Johnson syndrome was thought to be especially high with the long-acting sulfonamides,[48] which have been withdrawn from the market in the United States; but on rare occasions it can occur with the short-acting drugs in current use.[49] Although the reaction occurs rarely, it is important to identify it early and discontinue therapy, since it can be fatal. The sulfonamides, like the tetracyclines, occasionally cause photosensitivity reactions.[50]

The sulfonamides rarely produce a serum sickness-like syndrome, with delayed onset of fever, joint pain, urticaria, and sometimes bronchospasm. Drug fever occurring a few days to a week after the initiation of therapy is relatively common (1–2% of patients). The fever may be accompanied by headache, pruritis, and skin rash and it readily reverses on cessation of treatment. Sulfonamides rarely cause a vasculitis like that of periarteritis nodosa and several sulfonamides have been implicated in the production of a drug-induced lupus syndrome.[51] Sulfonamides very rarely cause hepatic necrosis, which also appears to have an allergic basis.[52] Immediate reactions of the anaphylactoid type occur rarely in previously sensitized individuals and a sulfonamide should not be administered to patients with a history of prior allergic reaction to these drugs.

TOXICITY TO THE HEMATOPOIETIC SYSTEM. The sulfonamides are among the large group of drugs that can cause hemolytic anemia in patients with a genetically determined deficiency of glucose-6-phosphate dehydrogenase activity in red blood cells. The mechanism of this effect is discussed in detail in Chapter 13. Acute hemolytic anemia may rarely occur in patients who do not have glucose-6-phosphate dehydrogenase deficiency. The sulfonamides rarely cause agranulocytosis, which is reversible on withdrawal of therapy. Thrombocytopenia has been reported, as has a very rare aplastic anemia.

TOXICITY TO THE URINARY TRACT. In the early days of sulfonamide therapy, renal damage due to deposition of drug crystals in the kidney occurred frequently. As mentioned earlier, this problem has been nearly eliminated with the use of the very soluble sulfonamides and care to ensure proper hydration and urine flow. In some cases, patients who have marked hypoproteinemia may be prone to develop crystalluria because there is a higher free component of drug available for filtration in the kidneys. Caution should be taken with these patients when drugs with moderate urine solubility, such as sulfamethoxazole, are administered.[53]

Precautions

The sulfonamide binding sites on plasma protein are also binding sites for bilirubin.[41] Thus, in the presence of sulfonamides, less bilirubin is bound and more of this compound circulates in the free form. In the newborn infant, free bilirubin can pass the blood-brain barrier and become deposited in the basal ganglia and subthalamic nuclei of the brain, causing a toxic encephalopathy called *kernicterus*. Therefore, sulfonamides should not be used for treating newborn infants, particularly those born prematurely. Since sulfonamides pass through the placenta and are excreted in the milk, they should not be administered during pregnancy approaching term or during nursing. Sulfonamides may displace certain drugs from plasma albumin and/or inhibit their biotransformation, thus potentiating their pharmacologic effects. Sulfonamides should thus be used cautiously when given along with coumarin anticoagulants, uricosuric agents, methotrexate, phenytoin, and thiopental since they have been reported to enhance the action of these drugs.

Three classes of drugs were developed by exploiting the side effects of the sulfonamides. Patients given sulfanilamide tended to develop metabolic acidosis with an alkaline urine. The finding that this was caused by the inhibition of carbonic anhydrase by sulfanilamide[54] led to the development of acetazolamide and other diuretics of the carbonic anhydrase-inhibitor class. The observation that sulfonamide treatment caused hypoglycemia in some patients led to the development of the sulfonylurea group of oral antidiabetic agents. Finally, the observation that rats treated with sulfaguanidine developed goiters led to the development of the thiouracil group of antithyroid drugs. The interesting story of these developments is related in detail by Goldstein et al.[55]

Trimethoprim (Trimethoprim-Sulfamethoxazole)

The development of trimethoprim is an example of rational drug design based on the results of basic research. During the process of characterizing the properties (pH optima, Michaelis constants) of folate reductases from various sources, it became clear that large differences existed between the bacterial and mammalian enzymes.[56,57] Trimethoprim was one of several compounds that were synthesized to maximize selective toxicity by exploiting these differences. The history of the development of trimethoprim, pyrimethamine, and the other diaminopyrimidines has been reviewed by Burchall.[58]

Mechanism of Action

Trimethoprim is a structural analog of the pteridine portion of dihydrofolic acid (Fig. 7–4). It is a competitive inhibitor of dihydrofolate reductase,[56] the enzyme that reduces dihydrofolate (FAH_2) to tetrahydrofolate (FAH_4) in the presence of NADPH. This reduction must take place before the molecule can be converted to the various one-carbon cofactors required for the synthesis of thymidine, purines, methionine, glycine, and formylmethionine (Fig. 7–5). Thus, when trimethoprim is added to a culture of bacteria growing in minimal medium, DNA, RNA, and protein synthesis are all affected.

In contrast to the sulfonamides, trimethoprim rapidly inhibits bacterial growth. Although the sulfonamides rapidly block synthesis of new folate, bacteria can continue to grow for several generations as their preex-

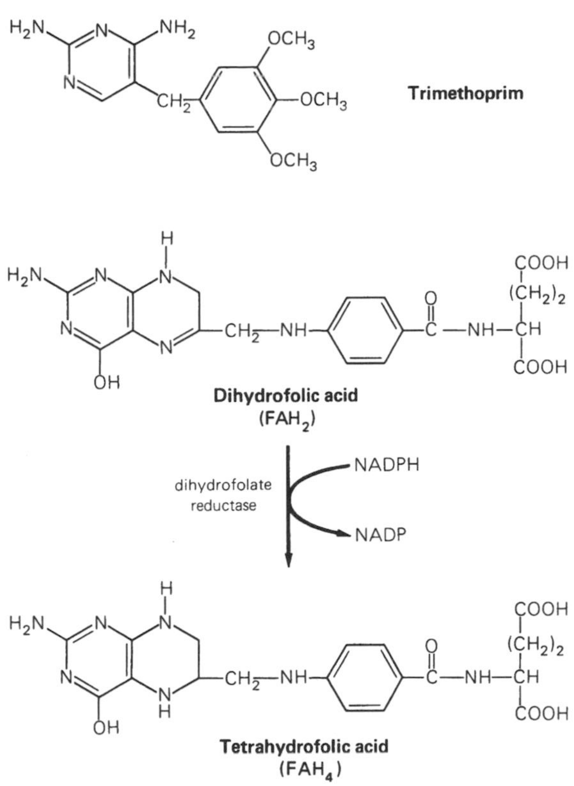

Figure 7-4. Trimethoprim and the reduction of dihydrofolate to tetrahydrofolate. Dihydrofolate must be reduced to tetrahydrofolate before the molecule can accept a one-carbon unit and act as a cofactor in subsequent reactions. This reaction is directed by dihydrofolate reductase and inhibited by trimethoprim. Trimethoprim is presented above to demonstrate its structural similarity to the pteridine portion of the normal substrate FAH_2.

isting folate pools decline (Fig. 7–1). In the presence of the trimethoprim block, FAH_4 is rapidly depleted and trapped in the unusable FAH_2 form.[59] Since the reutilization of FAH_2 is prevented, growth inhibition occurs very early. In most of the one-carbon transfer reactions, the one-carbon unit is simply transferred to a precursor to make a product, and FAH_4 is regenerated. But, when the one-carbon unit is transferred in the thymidylate synthetase reaction, dihydrofolic acid is formed. To keep the system running, the FAH_2 must be reduced to FAH_4 (Figure 7–6). Stoichiometric amounts of FAH_4 cofactor are required for the critical synthetase reaction, and in the absence of dihydrofolate reductase activity, the supplies of active folate cofactors are rapidly depleted.[60]

The composition of the growth medium determines whether the response to trimethoprim will be cidal or static. When cells are grown in medium that does not contain any of the products of one-carbon metabolism, trimethoprim is bacteriostatic. When thy-

mine is absent, but other products of one-carbon metabolism are supplied, trimethoprim is bactericidal. As is the case with sulfonamides, the addition of thymine reverses this effect.[61] Thus, the critical cellular lesion for the killing effect of the drug is inhibition of the thymidylate synthetase reaction.[62] In an appropriate low-thymine, amino acid–containing environment (e.g., human blood), bacteria exposed to trimethoprim will undergo thymineless death.[63]

In the presence of trimethoprim and the low-molecular-weight products of one-carbon metabolism, sustained exponential growth of *E. coli* can occur even when formylation of methionine-tRNA is undetectable.[64] In this case, one would expect cell growth to cease because formylmethionine-tRNA is utilized for the initiation of protein synthesis (see Figure 5–2). The continuation of reduced cell growth in the absence of folate-dependent formation of f-met-tRNA is consistent with observations suggesting that the methionine-initiation-tRNA without

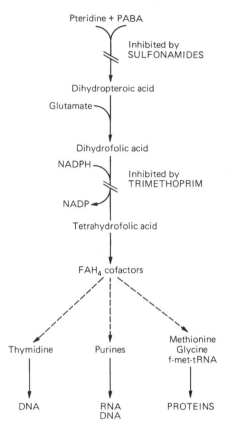

Figure 7–5. Schematic presentation of the sites of action of sulfonamides and trimethoprim in tetrahydrofolate (FAH₄) synthesis. The FAH₄ cofactors denote (dashed lines) one-carbon fragments required for the synthesis of protein and nucleic acid precursors.

the *N*-formyl group will permit some initiation of protein synthesis in intact bacteria.[65,66]

SELECTIVE TOXICITY. Trimethoprim is a much more potent inhibitor of bacterial than of mammalian folate reductases. This difference in intrinsic sensitivity of the enzyme targeted by the drug is the primary basis for the selective toxicity of trimethoprim. The inhibitory potency of trimethoprim against some bacterial and mammalian folate reductases is presented in Table 7–4. In this system, 20–60 thousand times as much drug is required to inhibit the human reductase as is required to inhibit the bacterial enzymes. The difference in sensitivity probably reflects changes in the structure of the enzyme that occurred during the evolution of the higher organisms.

Direct studies of the ternary complex formed between purified bacterial folate reductase, trimethoprim, and the NADPH coenzyme show that the presence of the inhibitor markedly affects the environment of the nicotinamide ring of the coenzyme[67] and decreases the rate constant of NADPH dissociation by more than 100-fold.[68] As has been observed in a number of other drug receptor systems, dihydrofolate reductase appears to assume an equilibrium between two conformational states in the absence of coenzyme or inhibitor. The interactions between the

Figure 7–6. Synthesis of thymidine monophosphate from deoxyuridine monophosphate. In this critical reaction, a methyl group is transferred from the tetrahydrofolate cofactor to dUMP forming TMP and dihydrofolate (FAH₂). Tetrahydrofolate (FAH₄) is then regenerated by reduction of FAH₂. This reaction is blocked by trimethoprim, bringing the cycle to a halt with the folate in the inactive dihydro-form.

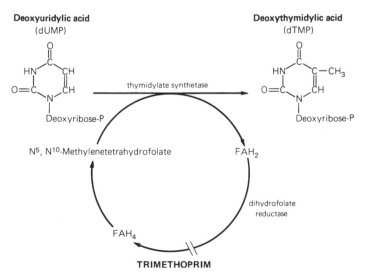

Table 7–4. Binding of trimethoprim to bacterial and mammalian dihydrofolate reductases. Folate reductase, purified from bacteria or from mammalian livers, was incubated with 50 μM dihydrofolate, NADPH, and varying concentrations of trimethoprim. Enzyme activity was recorded by the change in absorbance at 340 nm. The values in the table represent the concentrations of trimethoprim required for 50% inhibition of the enzyme activity. Thus, 60,000 times as much trimethoprim is required to inhibit the human enzyme as is required to inhibit that of *E. coli*.

Source of enzyme	Trimethoprim concentration required for 50% inhibition (nM)
BACTERIAL	
Escherichia coli	5
Staphylococcus aureus	15
Proteus vulgaris	5
MAMMALIAN	
Rat	260,000
Rabbit	370,000
Human	300,000

Source: Data from Burchall and Hitchings.[56]

enzyme, the coenzyme, and trimethoprim are complex, but it is clear that the binding of the drug and the coenzyme markedly alter the position of this conformational equilibrium.[69,70]

Synergism with Sulfonamides and Trimethoprim

The combination of trimethoprim (TMP) and a sulfonamide has been demonstrated to be synergistic in affecting cell growth. Although synergism has been shown with many sulfonamides,[71,72] the combined formulation used in therapy is that of trimethoprim-sulfamethoxazole (TMP-SMX). In sensitive bacteria, TMP is usually 20–100 times more active on a molar basis than the sulfonamide.[73] The concentrations of TMP, SMX, and TMP-SMX required for inhibition of growth of several bacteria are presented in Table 7–5. The increase in activity obtained with the combined formula-

tion is substantial. There is a wide variation in sensitivity to TMP or SMX, and the optimal ratio of the components in the mixture will also differ from one organism to another. Fortunately, potentiation occurs over a wide range of ratios, with the modal optimum being around 1 part trimethoprim to 20 parts sulfamethoxazole.[73] Synergy of the combined formulation of TMP-SMX has been demonstrated after oral administration to animals with different bacterial infections.[73,74]

The synergism between sulfonamides and trimethoprim has been attributed to the fact that the drugs inhibit different enzymes in the same biosynthetic pathway.[75] According to earlier studies, such a sequential blockade might often produce a synergistic effect.[76,77] There are several well-documented examples of potentiation resulting from the combination of two drugs that produce sequential blockade, and it has been clearly demonstrated that sequential reactions can be inhibited by drugs without the occurrence of a synergistic response.[78,79] The concept of sequential blockade does not take into account the type of enzyme inhibition produced by the drug, the presence of rate-limiting steps in a series of reactions, or the complex series of events that control the synthesis and degradation of enzymes in intact cells. The synergism between TMP and a sulfonamide can probably be best explained as follows[59]: Trimethoprim is a competitor for the substrate FAH_2 and its effect is reduced as FAH_2 accumulates, both as a result of the thymidylate synthetase reaction and new FAH_2 synthesis (Figs. 7–5 and 7–6). When new synthesis is inhibited by a sulfonamide, there is less substrate to compete with TMP, and the effectiveness of the drug is enhanced, a reasonable explanation for this type of drug synergism. One study suggests that synergism between TMP and SMX results from cooperative binding of both drugs to dihydrofolate reductase[80] but this is clearly not the case.[81]

As with the use of the individual drugs, the effect of TMP-SMX depends on the environment in which the bacteria are growing.[82] In minimal medium, the effect is bacteriostatic. In a low-thymine, amino acid–

Table 7–5. Effect of trimethoprim (TMP) and sulfamethoxazole (SMX) alone and in combination on several common pathogenic bacteria growing in vitro. The minimum inhibitory concentration (MIC) of TMP alone, SMX alone, or a mixture of one part TMP and 20 parts SMX was determined for several bacteria in culture.

| | MIC (µg/ml) | | | |
| | SMX | | TMP | |
Organism	Alone	Mixture	Alone	Mixture
Staphylococcus aureus	3	0.3	1	0.015
Streptococcus pneumoniae	30	2	2	0.1
Haemophilus influenzae	10	0.3	1	0.015
Shigella sonnei	10	1	0.3	0.05
Proteus vulgaris	30	3	3	0.15

Source: Data from Bushby.[73]

containing environment, the effect is bactericidal because of the production of thymineless death. The TMP-SMX formulation is bactericidal in human blood and urine, and its effect is overcome by the addition of thymine.[11] The addition of PABA to the medium will reduce the effect of the combination to that of TMP alone.[82]

In addition to synergism, TMP-SMX may have a somewhat broader spectrum of clinically useful action than TMP or SMX individually.[59] The use of two drugs concomitantly reduces the rate of emergence of resistance to therapy, and the combination is more often bactericidal than either drug used alone.[82]

Antimicrobial Activity and Clinical Use

Both TMP and SMX have a broad spectrum of antimicrobial action in vitro. The TMP-SMX combination is active against a wide range of both gram-positive and gram-negative bacteria (Table 7–6).[73,83,84] Most of the Enterobacteriaceae are susceptible to TMP-SMX; however, *Bacteroides* is an exception. TMP-SMX is also active against *Bordetella pertussis*, *Brucella*, *Vibrio cholerae*, and *Yersinia pestis*. *Pseudomonas aeruginosa* is not susceptible, but the combination is active against some other *Pseudomonas* species, such as *P. pseudomallei* and *P. cepacia*. *Neisseria meningitidis*

Table 7–6. Spectrum of in vitro antibacterial activity of trimethoprim-sulfamethoxazole.

Consistently susceptible	Frequently susceptible	Resistant
Streptococcus pneumoniae	*Staphylococcus aureus*	*Mycobacterium tuberculosis*
Escherichia coli	*Streptococcus pyogenes*	*Treponema pallidum*
Proteus mirabilis	Indole-positive *Proteus*	*Pseudomonas aeruginosa*
Salmonella typhi	*Serratia marcescens*	*Ureaplasma urealyticum*
Non-*typhi Salmonella*	*Klebsiella pneumoniae*	
Shigella species	Non-*aeruginosa Pseudomonas*	
Vibrio cholerae	*Brucella* species	
Haemophilus influenzae	*Bordetella pertussis*	
Yersinia pestis	*Neisseria gonorrhoeae*	
	Neisseria meningitidis	

Source: Modified from Wormser and Keusch.[84]

and *Neisseria gonorrhoeae* strains are usually susceptible. The TMP-SMX combination is inactive against *Mycoplasma, Mycobacterium tuberculosis,* and *Treponema pallidum,* but it is clinically effective against infections caused by *Nocardia,*[85] *Mycobacterium marinum,*[86] and some protozoa (*Pneumocystis carinii*[87] and *Plasmodium species*[88]).

The MICs of TMP alone, SMX alone, and TMP in a TMP-SMX mixture against selected gram-positive and gram-negative bacteria are presented in Table 7–7. The activities of trimethoprim and the TMP-SMX combination vary considerably with the growth medium that is used for the assay and the density of the bacterial inoculum.[83] Some bacterial growth media contain a low concentration of thymidine, which can reduce or eliminate the antibacterial activity. The data presented in Table 7–7 were obtained after 1000-fold dilution of the inoculum. When the same assays were performed using undiluted inocula, only 23% of *Hae-* *mophilus influenzae* and 15% of *Serratia marcescens* isolates were inhibited by TMP-SMX at a concentration of less than 1 μg TMP/ml. This contrasts with sensitivity in 100% and 90% of isolates in assays using the respective diluted inocula.[83]

The clinical experience with TMP-SMX in the treatment of various infections has been presented in several comprehensive reviews[84,89] and symposia.[90,91] The principal use of TMP-SMX is in the treatment of infections of the urinary and respiratory tracts. Most of the common urinary tract pathogens are susceptible (see Table 7–6) and TMP-SMX has proven to be effective in treating both chronic and recurrent urinary tract infections.[91] The TMP-SMX penetrates into the prostatic secretions[92] and is effective in the treatment of bacterial prostatitis.[89] The usual dose for treating urinary tract infection or prostatitis is two tablets (each tablet contains 400 mg SMX plus 80 mg TMP) every 12 h. A small dose of one-half tablet per day or one tablet on alternate nights

Table 7–7. *Susceptibility of selected bacteria to trimethoprim alone (TMP), sulfamethoxazole alone (SMX), and to trimethoprim in the mixture of 1 part TMP and 16 parts SMX. The minimum inhibitory concentrations (MICs) are determined by the serial dilution method in Mueller-Hinton agar at dilute inoculum. The MICs for TMP and SMX determined in different laboratories vary according to the growth medium, the innoculum size, and the method of assay. The righthand column shows the percentage of strains of each species inhibited by TMP-SMX at a concentration of less than 1 μg of TMP/ml.*

	Median MIC (μg/ml)			Strains inhibited by 1 μg TMP/ml in TMP-SMX combination (%)
	TMP	SMX	TMP in TMP-SMX	
Straphylococcus aureus	0.8	50	0.04	100
Enterococcus	0.1	>1000	0.04	100
Streptococcus pneumoniae	0.4	50	0.1	100
Streptococcus pyogenes	0.1	12.5	0.04	100
Escherichia coli	0.4	100	0.1	100
Enterobacter	0.8	50	0.1	100
Klebsiella pneumoniae	3.1	1000	0.2	91
Proteus species	3.1	100	0.2	90
Salmonella species	0.1	1000	0.04	100
Shigella species	0.4	>1000	0.04	100
Serratia marcescens	0.8	>1000	0.4	90
Providencia	1.6	100	0.4	63
Haemophilus influenzae	0.8	1000	0.4	100
Pseudomonas aeruginosa	1000	1000	6.3	0

Source: Data from Bach et al.[83]

given on a long-term basis is effective in suppressing recurrent urinary tract infections in females.[89]

Trimethoprim-sulfamethoxazole is effective in treating acute exacerbations of chronic bronchitis, but its role in chronic treatment has not been well established.[84] It is not indicated for the treatment of specific gram-positive infections. It is clearly inferior to penicillin in the treatment of streptococcal pharyngitis and is contraindicated in this infection.[84] Treatment with TMP-SMX is effective against acute otitis media, which is most often caused by *Haemophilus influenzea* and *Streptococcus pneumoniae*.[89] Ampicillin-resistant strains of *H. influenzae* have generally been found to be sensitive to TMP-SMX, and TMP-SMX is useful in treating acute sinusitis caused by susceptible strains of *H. influenzae* and *S. pneumoniae*.

The TMP-SMX combination is particularly useful in treating gastrointestinal infections. It is effective therapy for shigellosis, and is an alternative for the fluoroquinolones in this disease. However, resistance to the sulfonamide-trimethoprim combination has become increasingly common. Antibacterial agents shorten the duration of illness and decrease the relapse rate in this disease. Trimethoprim-sulfamethoxazole is an alternative treatment for typhoid fever as well as other systemic *Salmonella* infections. Third-generation cephalosporins, ampicillin, amoxicillin, chloramphenicol, and certain fluoroquinolones are also used to treat salmonelloses. Treatment with TMP-SMX reduces the duration and the severity of symptoms of travelers' diarrhea[93] and may be used prophylactically[94] to prevent this infection, which is usually caused by enterotoxigenic strains of *Escherichia coli*.

The TMP-SMX combination is effective in high-dose therapy (TMP, 20 mg/kg/day: SMX, 100 mg/kg/day) of *Pneumocystis carinii* pneumonia[87] in patients with acquired immunodeficiency syndrome (AIDS). Presently, it is the preferred treatment, having replaced pentamidine.[95] The incidence of side effects is high with both treatments. *Pneumocystis carinii* is an opportunistic infection that frequently occurs in immunocompromised patients, and is particularly common in patients with AIDS. In low-dose regimens TMP-SMX has proven to be effective for prophylaxis of infection by *Pneumocystis carinii* in patients with AIDS.[96] Adverse reactions are less frequent with these lower prophylactic doses. Trimethoprim-sulfamethoxazole is also effective in reducing gram-negative bacteremia in neutropenic patients and in otherwise immunocompromised hosts.[91] It has been used effectively to treat some uncommon infections, including brucellosis, plague (*Yersinia pestis*), nocardiosis,[85] melioidosis (*Pseudomonas pseudomallei*), and cutaneous infection due to *Mycoplasma marinum*.[84,89]

RESISTANCE. Since there are two drugs in the TMP-SMX formulation, there are several patterns of resistance to consider. An organism may remain sensitive to TMP and become resistant to sulfonamides. Such an organism may retain a synergistic response to the TMP-SMX combination.[97,98] With many TMP-sensitive, SMX-resistant organisms, however, synergy is not observed.[99,100] Synergy with TMP-SMX can also be seen with bacteria that are SMX-sensitive and moderately TMP-resistant.[97,98] *Neisseria* have relatively high MICs for TMP alone, for example, but still respond synergistically to the TMP-SMX combination.[101] With the exception of bacteria like *N. gonorrhoeae*, which are intrinsically more susceptible to the sulfonamide, susceptibility to TMP is usually more critical for the efficacy of the combination.[84]

Resistance to sulfonamides is widespread; the mechanisms have been discussed earlier in this chapter. Bacteria can become resistant to both SMX and TMP, and resistance to TMP-SMX therapy can develop during treatment.[100,102] Trimethoprim resistance may be due to cellular impermeability to the drug, to mutation to thymine dependence, to overproduction of dihydrofolate reductase, or to the production of TMP-resistant forms of dihydrofolate reductase.[101–104] The mechanism of greatest clinical importance is the production of dihydrofolate reductase with reduced affinity for TMP.[101] The production of TMP-resistant dihydrofolate reductase is mediated by either R factors or chromosomal genes.[100,102,105] The TMP-resistant reductases that have been characterized differ from all other dihydrofolate reductases in molecular weight, subunit structure, and kinetic properties.[104]

Emergence of resistance to TMP (alone or as a component of TMP-SMX) varies among countries, cities within countries, and individual hospitals. Results from several sequential studies generally suggest that TMP resistance, particularly high-level plasmid-mediated resistance, has been gradually increasing in developed countries, such as Finland, Great Britain, and the United States. Most of these surveys indicate that 3% to 20% of *E. coli* strains in developed countries are now resistant to this drug,[106–108] with concentrations of resistance in certain cities,[109] hospitals,[110] and even day care centers.[111,112] Resistance to TMP or TMP-SMX is also increasing in many developing countries.[113]

Pharmacology of Trimethoprim and Sulfamethoxazole

Trimethoprim is available in 100 mg tablets for use as a single agent for treatment of initial episodes of uncomplicated urinary tract infections.[114] The TMP-SMX combination (also called co-trimoxazole) is available as tablets and suspensions for oral administration and in sterile solution for intravenous infusion. Tablets are available in two sizes—a single-strength tablet containing 400 mg SMX and 80 mg TMP and a double-strength tablet containing 800 mg SMX and 160 mg TMP. The usual adult dosage is two single-strength tablets or one double-strength tablet taken every 12 h.

The pharmacokinetic properties of TMP and SMX are presented in Table 7–8 (see Patel and Welling[115] and Wilkinson and Reeves[116] for detailed reviews). Sulfamethoxazole was originally chosen for the formulation because its half-life is similar to that of trimethoprim. Other pharmacokinetic properties differ, however, and the differences markedly affect the ratio of the bioactive forms of each component in different tissues and body fluids. Both TMP and SMX are well absorbed from the gastrointestinal tract, with peak levels of SMX being achieved in 3–4 h and TMP in 2–3 h.[117] After a single oral administration of 800 mg SMX and 160 mg TMP, the peak plasma level of SMX is 30–60 µg/ml and that of TMP is 1.2–2 µg/ml.[115] The minimal steady-state levels of each drug achieved with oral administration of the TMP-SMX combination every 12 h are similar to the peak levels after the single administration.[115,118] Higher plasma levels of each component may be obtained by intravenous administration.[119] Forty-five percent of TMP and 66% of SMX in plasma is bound to protein.[115]

Because of its greater lipid solubility, TMP passes more readily across biological mem-

Table 7–8. *Pharmacokinetic properties of trimethoprim and sulfamethoxazole. Reported values for the half-life of sulfamethoxazole in renal failure vary widely.*

		Half-life				
	Apparent volume of distribution (liters)	Normal (hours)	Renal failure (hours)	Plasma protein binding (%)	Peak serum levels after usual adult dose (µg/ml)	Minimum serum levels with repeated doses every 12 h (µg/ml)	Percentage of drug in unmetabolized form in urine
Trimethoprim	100–120	10–12	15–30	45	1.2–2	1.3–2.8	80–90
Sulfamethoxazole	12–18	9–11	20–35	66	30–60	30–60	20–40

Source: The values presented here are from Craig and Kunin[42] for patients with a creatinine clearance less than 10 ml/min. The rest of the data were compiled from reviews by Patel and Welling[115] and Wilkinson and Reeves.[116]

Table 7–9. Concentration of trimethoprim (TMP) achieved in selected tissues and body fluids and approximate ratio of sulfamethoxazole (SMX) to TMP. The concentration of TMP is expressed relative to a simultaneous serum concentration of 1.

Tissue or body fluid	Concentration of TMP relative to plasma concentration	Approximate ratio of bioactive SMX to TMP
Saliva	1	0.5
Bronchial secretion	1–2	—
Lung tissue	1.5–3.5	—
Prostatic fluid	1–2	2.5–5
Prostatic tissue	2	2.5–4
Vaginal fluid	5	<0.04
Bile	0.2–0.8	2.5–10
Aqueous humor	0.1	40
Synovial fluid	1	20
Cerebrospinal fluid	0.3–0.4	10
Skin blister fluid	0.6–0.8	15

Source: Data were taken from Wilkinson and Reeves,[116] Hansen et al.,[120] Bruun et al.,[121] and Fries et al.[124]

branes and its apparent volume of distribution is greater than that of the body water. In contrast, SMX is confined to a volume that approximates the extracellular fluid space.[116] The differences in distribution volume determine the ratio chosen for the two components in the formulation. The ratio of SMX to TMP in the formulation is 5:1, but after the components have been absorbed and distributed throughout the body, the ratio of bioactive forms in the plasma is about 20:1,[117,118] which is the modal optimum ratio for production of synergy against bacteria. As shown in Table 7–9, the distribution properties of the components result in different SMX-to-TMP ratios in different tissues and body fluids. In most body fluids and secretions, the ratio of SMX to TMP is in the range of 2:1 to 5:1.[116] These low ratios are not optimal for synergy. Ratios of 20:1 and 40:1 are achieved in synovial fluid and aqueous humor.[116] The efficacy of the TMP-SMX combination in the treatment of respiratory and urinary tract infections correlates with the tissue distribution properties

of TMP. Therapeutic concentrations of TMP in excess of serum levels are achieved in lung tissue and bronchial secretions,[120] in prostate[92] and kidney[122] tissue, and in prostatic[92] and vaginal[123] fluids (Table 7–9). Cerebrospinal fluid levels of TMP are 30%–40% percent of serum levels.[124] Both TMP and SMX cross the human placenta.[115]

Both TMP and SMX are excreted predominantly in the urine, with 60% of a dose of TMP being excreted in the urine in 24 h. Ten to twenty percent of TMP is metabolized, primarily by oxidation and conjugation.[115] Metabolism of SMX occurs predominantly by N-acetylation and the biologically inactive metabolite accounts for 20% of the total drug in the serum and 60% to 80% of the drug in the urine.[115,118] The ratio of unaltered, bioactive SMX to TMP in the urine is generally low (ranging from 1:1 to 5:1[125,126]) and is dependent on the urine pH.[42] Because the ratio in the urine is low, it is unlikely that the effect of the combination in the treatment of urinary tract infections reflects synergism. High concentrations of TMP are achieved in urine, and even in uremic patients, the urine concentrations of both TMP and SMX are higher than the MICs for most susceptible urinary tract organisms.[42,115] The half-life of TMP is shorter in children (5.6 h in children less than 10 years of age) than in elderly patients (16 h).[119] There is a linear relationship between the serum creatinine and the TMP half-life,[119] and the rates of elimination of both drugs are decreased in uremic patients (see Table 7–8).[42,126] Patients with severe uremia (creatinine clearance less than 10 ml/min) should be given a full loading dose followed by half the loading dose once daily, and patients with moderate uremia (creatinine clearance between 10 and 30 ml/min) should receive half the loading dose twice daily.[42] Both TMP and SMX are removed by hemodialysis.[42] The serum protein binding of SMX, but not TMP, is reduced in uremic patients.[42,126]

Adverse Effects of Trimethoprim

The TMP-SMX combination is generally well tolerated. The most common adverse effects are gastrointestinal upset (mainly nausea and vomiting; diarrhea is rare), which occurs in about 4% of patients, and skin reactions, which occur in about 3%[127] Although serious reactions are rare, all of the types of adverse reactions that are associated with sulfonamides have been reported with the TMP-SMX combination, including Stevens-Johnson syndrome, toxic epidermal necrolysis (Lyell's syndrome), granulocytopenia, agranulocytosis, and aplastic anemia.[89,128] Patients with a history of hypersensitivity to sulfonamides should not receive TMP-SMX. Mild and transient jaundice has been seen occasionally.[89] Subjective experiences of headache, depression, and hallucinations, which are known to occur with sulfonamides, occur occasionally with TMP-SMX.[128]

Even though TMP has a good therapeutic index on the basis of its high affinity for bacterial folate reductases and low affinity for the human enzyme, folate deficiency can be produced in some patients. Megaloblastic anemia does not occur in patients in a normal dietary state receiving the usual oral therapy with TMP. People with suboptimal folate nutrition, such as pregnant women, malnourished patients, and alcoholics, who are exposed to long-term therapy may develop megaloblastic anemia, granulocytopenia, or thrombocytopenia.[129,130] The megaloblastosis can be reversed by administering folinic acid, which shunts around the TMP block in the cells of the marrow, but does not reduce the antibacterial effect because bacteria (enterococcus is an exception) cannot transport folinic acid.[131] Thrombocytopenia may occur more frequently with high-dose intravenous therapy.[119,130] At concentrations that are achieved in patients with renal failure (4.5–7µg/ml), TMP inhibits the growth of human bone marrow cells in culture (granulocytic colony forming units) and the inhibition is reversed by folinic acid.[132,133]

The TMP-SMX combination is rarely associated with the production of acute interstitial nephritis.[134] Crystalluria from the sulfonamide is a side effect that is avoided by adequate fluid intake. Deterioration of renal function has been reported after administration of TMP-SMX to patients with renal impairment.[135] However, the incidence of renal toxicity is very low.[127] The drug can cause an increase in serum creatinine that does not reflect nephrotoxicity. It interferes with creatinine secretion into the renal tubules[136] and causes an increase in serum creatinine without altering the glomerular filtration rate.[137]

Precautions and Drug Interactions of Trimethoprim-Sulfamethoxazole Therapy

Because of the sulfonamide component, TMP-SMX may potentiate the effects of warfarin, phenytoin, and oral hypoglycemic agents.[89] Patients receiving antimetabolites, such as 6-mercaptopurine or azothioprine,[132] and those receiving other antifolates, such as methotrexate or pyrimethamine, have an increased risk of bone marrow suppression when TMP is administered concomitantly. Care should be taken to perform blood counts and to monitor drug levels when patients with impaired renal function are treated with TMP-SMX. If possible, TMP-SMX should not be given to patients with serious hematologic disorders.[89] Although fetal abnormalities have not been reported, the manufacturers recommend that the drug not be used during pregnancy. For unknown reasons, patients with AIDS and AIDS-associated *Pneumocystis carinii* infection have a high incidence (45%–65%) of adverse reactions (rash, leukopenia) to TMP-SMX. The high incidence of reactions is not observed in patients with other immunosuppressive diseases.

REFERENCES

1. Bell, P. H., and R. O. Roblin. Studies in chemotherapy. VII. A theory of the relation of structure to activity of sulfanilamide type compounds. *J. Am. Chem. Soc.* 1942;64:2905.

2. Seydel, J. K. Sulfonamides, structure-activity relationship, and mode of action. *J. Pharm. Sci.* 1968;57:1455.

3. Seydel, J. K. Physicochemical factors in drug-receptor interactions demonstrated on the example of the sulfonamides. In *Drug Receptor Interactions in Antimicrobial Chemotherapy*, ed. by J. Drews and F. E. Hahn. New York: Springer-Verlag, 1975, pp. 25–43.

4. Woods, D. D. The biochemical mode of action of the sulfonamides. *J. Gen. Microbiol* 1962;29:687.

5. Brown, G. M. The biosynthesis of folic acid: inhibition by sulfonamides. *J. Biol. Chem.* 1962;237:536.

6. Richey, D. P., and G. M. Brown. The biosynthesis of folic acid: purification and properties of the enzymes required for the formation of dihydropteroic acid. *J. Biol. Chem.* 1969;244:1582.

7. McCullough, J. L., and T. H. Maren. Inhibition of dihydropteroate synthetase from *Escherichia coil* by sulfones and sulfonamides. *Antimicrob. Agents Chemother.* 1973;3:665.

8. Bock, L., G. H. Miller, K. J. Schaper, and J. K. Seydel. Sulfonamide structure-activity relationships in a cell-free system. 2. Proof for the formation of a sulfonamide-containing folate analog. *J. Med. Chem.* 1974;17:23.

9. Feingold, D. S. Antimicrobial chemotherapeutic agents; the nature of their action and selective toxicity. *N. Engl. J. Med.* 1963;269:957.

10. Then, R., and P. Angehrn. Sulfonamide-induced "Thymineless Death" in *Escherichia coli. J. Gen. Microbiol.* 1973;76:255.

11. Then, R., and P. Angehrn. Nature of the bactericidal action of sulfonamides and trimethoprim, alone and in combination. *J. Infect. Dis.* 1973; 128(Suppl.):S498.

12. Hurni, H. Uber die quantitativen Verhältnisse beim Antagonisms zwischen p-Aminosalicylsaure (PAS) und p-Aminobenzoesaure (PABA). *Schweiz. Z. Path. Bakt.* 1949;12:282.

13. Brownlee, G., A. F. Green, and M. Woodbine. Sulfetrone: a chemotherapeutic agent for tuberculosis. *Br. J. Pharmacol. Chemother.* 1948;3:15.

14. Wacker, A., H. Kolm, and M. Ebert. Uber den Stoffwecshel der p-Aminosalcysaure and Salicylsaure bei *Enterococcus. Z. Naturforsch.* 1958;13b:147.

15. McCullough, J. L., and T. H. Maren. Dihydropteroate synthetase from *Plasmodium berghei*: isolation, properties, and inhibition by dapsone and sulfadiazine. *Mol. Pharmacol.* 1974;10:140.

16. Hotchkiss, R. D. and A. H. Evans. Fine structure of a genetically modified enzyme as revealed by relative affinities for modified substrate. *Fed. Proc.* 1960;19:912.

17. Wolf, B., and R. D. Hotchkiss, Genetically modified folic acid synthesizing enzymes of *Pneumococcus. Biochemistry* 1963;2:145.

18. Mandell, G. L., and W. A. Petri. Sulfonamides, trimethoprim-sulfamethoxazole, quinolones, and agents for urinary tract infections. In *Goodman & Gilman's The Pharmacological Basis of Therapeutics*, 9th ed., ed. by J. G. Hardman, L. E. Limbird, P. Molinoff, and R. Ruddon. New York: McGraw-Hill, 1995, pp. 1057–1072.

19. Black, W. A., and D. A. McNellis. Susceptibility of Nocardia species to modern antimicrobial agents. *Antimicrob. Agents Chemother—1970.* 1971;34b.

20. Landy, M., N. W. Larkum, E. J. Oswald, and F. Streightoff. Increased synthesis of p-aminobenzoic acid associated with the development of sulfonamide resistance in *Staphylococcus aureus. Science* 1943; 97:265.

21. Skold, O. R-factor-mediated resistance to sulfonamides by a plasmid-borne, drug-resistant dihydro-pteroate synthetase. *Antimicrob. Agents Chemother.* 1976;9:49.

22. Brown, G. M. Methods for measuring inhibition by sulfonamides of the enzymatic synthesis of dihydropteroic acid. *Methods Med. Res.* 1964;10:233.

23. Benveniste, R. and J. Davies. Mechanism of antibiotic resistance in bacteria. *Annu. Rev. Biochem.* 1973;42:471.

24. Hughes, J., L. C. Roberts, and A. J. Coppridge. Sulfacytine: a new sulfonamide. Double-blind comparison with sulfisoxazole in acute uncomplicated urinary tract infections. *J. Urol.* 1975;114:912.

25. Anthonisen, P., F. Bavany, O. Folkenborg, A. Holtz, S. Jarnum, M. Kristensen, P. Riis, A. Walan, and H. Worning. The clinical effect of salazosulphapyridine (Salazopyrin') in Crohn's disease. *Scand. J. Gastroenterol.* 1974;9:549.

26. Summers, R. W., D. M. Switz, T. J. Sessions, J. M. Becktel, W. R. Best, F. Kern, and J. W. Singleton. National cooperative Crohn's disease study: results of drug treatment. *Gastroenterology* 1979;77:847.

27. Azad Khan, A. K., J. Piris, and S. C. Truelove. An experiment to determine the active therapeutic moiety of sulphasalzine. *Lancet* 1977;2:892.

28. Gottschalk, H. R. and O. J. Stone. Stevens-Johnson syndrome from ophthalmic sulfonamide. *Arch. Dermatol.* 1976;112:513.

29. Mackie, B. S., and L. E. Mackie. Systemic lupus erythematosus-dermatomyositis induced by sulfonamide eye drops. *Australas J. Dermatol.* 1979;20:49.

30. Boswick, J. A. Topical therapy of the burn wound with mafenide acetate. In *Contemporary Burn Management*, ed. by H. C. Polk and H. H. Stone. Boston: Little, Brown. 1971, pp. 193–202.

31. Harrison, H. N., H. W. Bales, and F. Jacoby. The absorption into burned skin of sulfamylon acetate from 5 per cent aqueous solution. *J. Trauma* 1972;12: 994.

32. Ballin, J. C. Evaluation of a new topical agent for burn therapy: silver sulfadiazine (Silvadene). *JAMA* 1974;230:1184.

33. Baxter, C. R. Topical use of 1.0% silver sulfadiazine. In *Contemporary Burn Management*, ed. by H. C. Polk and H. H. Stone. Boston: Little, Brown, 1971, pp. 217–225.

34. Fox, C. L., B. W. Rappole, and W. Stanford. Control of *Pseudomonas* infection in burns by silver sulfadiazine. *Surg. Gynecol. Obstet.* 1969;128:1021.

35. Modak, S. M., and C. L. Fox. Binding of silver sulfadiazine to the cellular components of *Pseudomonas aeruginosa. Biochem. Pharmacol.* 1973;22:2391.

36. Fox, C. L., and S. M. Modak. Mechanism of silver sulfadiazine action on burn wound infections. *Antimicrob. Agents Chemother.* 1974;5:582.

37. Rosenkranz, H. S., and H. S. Carr. Silver sulfadiazine: effect on the growth and metabolism of bacteria. *Antimicrob. Agents Chemother.* 1972;2:367.

38. Rosenkranz, H. S., and S. Rosenkranz. Silver sulfadiazine: interaction with isolated deoxyribonucleic acid. *Antimicrob. Agents Chemother.* 1972;2:373.

39. Speck, W. T., and H. S. Rosenkranz. Activity of silver sulfadiazine against dermatophytes. *Lancet* 1974; 2:895.

40. Hsu, P.-L., J. K. H. Ma, H. W. Jun, and L. A. Luzzi. Structure relationship for binding of sulfonamides and penicillins to bovine serum albumin by flurescence probe technique. *J. Pharma. Sci.* 1974;63:27.

41. Anton, A. H. Increasing activity of sulfonamides with displacing agents: A review. *Ann. N.Y. Acad. Sci.* 1973;226:273.

42. Craig, W. A., and C. M. Kunin. Trimethoprim-sulfamethoxazole: pharmacodynamic effects of urinary pH and impaired renal function. *Ann. Intern. Med.* 1973;78:491.

43. Levy, G., T. Baliah, and J. A. Procknal. Effect of renal transplantation on protein binding of drugs in serum of donor and recipient. *Clin. Pharmacol. Ther.* 1976;20:512.

44. Weinstein, L. Sulfonamides. In *The Pharmacological Basis of Therapeutics,* ed. L. S. Goodman and A. Gilman. New York: Macmillan, 1970, p. 1197.

45. Bennett, W. M., R. S. Muther, R. A. Parker, P. Feig, G. Morrison, T. A. Golper, and I. Singer. Drug therapy in renal failure: dosing guidelines for adults. *Ann. Intern. Med.* 1980;93:62.

46. Weinstein, L., M. A. Madoff, and C. M. Samet. The sulfonamides. *N. Eng. J. Med.* 1960;263: 793,842,900.

47. Koch-Weser, J., V. W. Sidel, M. Dexter, C. Parish, D. C. Finer, and P. Kanarek. Adverse reactions to sulfisoxazole, sulfamethoxazole, and nitrofurantoin: manifestations and specific reaction rates during 2,118 courses of therapy. *Arch. Intern. Med.* 1971;128:399.

48. Carroll, O. M., P. A. Bryan, and R. J. Robinson. Stevens-Johnson syndrome associated with long acting sulfonamides. *JAMA* 1966;195:179.

49. Bianchine, J. R., P. F. J. Macaraeg, L. Lasagna, D. L. Azarnoff, S. F. Brunk, E. F. Hvidberg, and J. A. Owen. Drugs as etiologic factors in the Stevens-Johnson syndrome. *Am. J. Med.* 1968;44:390.

50. Harber, L. C., and R. L. Baer. Pathogenic mechanisms of drug-induced photosensitivity. *J. Invest. Dermatol.* 1972;58:327.

51. Alarcon-Segovia, D. Drug-induced lupus syndromes. *Mayo Clin. Proc.* 1969;44:664.

52. Dujovne, C. A., C. H. Chan, and H. J. Zimmerman. Sulfonamide hepatic injury: review of the literature and report of a case due to sulfamethoxazole. *N. Engl. J. Med.* 1967;277:785.

53. Buchanan, N. Sulfamethoxazole, hypoalbuminaemia, crystalluria and renal failure. *BMJ* 1978;2:172.

54. Coleman, J. E. Chemical reactions of sulfonamides with carbonic anhydrase. *Annu. Rev. Pharmacol.* 1975;15:221.

55. Goldstein, A., L. Aronow, and S. M. Kalman. *Principles of Drug Action.* New York: Wiley, 1974, pp. 766–773.

56. Burchall, J. J., and G. H. Hitchings. Inhibitor binding analysis of dihydrofolate-reductases from various species. *Mol. Pharmacol.* 1965;1:126.

57. Burchall, J. J; Comparative biochemistry of dihydrofolate reductase. *Ann N.Y. Acad. Sci.* 1971;186: 143.

58. Burchall, J. J. The development of the diaminopyrimidines. *J. Antimicrob. Chemother.* 1979 5(Suppl. B):3

59. Hitchings, G. H. Mechanism of action of trimethoprim-sulfamethoxazole—I. *J. Infect. Dis.* 1973; 128(Suppl.):S433.

60. Dunlap, R. B., N. G. L. Harding, and F. M. Huennekens. Thymidylate synthetase and its relationship to dihydrofolate reductase. *Ann. N.Y. Acad. Sci.* 1971;186:153.

61. Koch, A. E., and J. J. Burchall. Reversal of the antimicrobial activity of trimethoprim by thymidine in commercially prepared media. *Appl. Microbiol.* 1971; 22:812.

62. Dale, B. A., and G. R. Greenberg. Effect of the folic acid analogue, trimethoprim, on growth, macromolecular synthesis, and incorporation of exogenous thymine in *Escherichia coli. J. Bacteriol.* 1972; 110:905.

63. Cohen, S. S. On the nature of thymineless death. *Ann. N.Y. Acad. Sci.* 1971;186:153.

64. Harvey, R. J. Growth and initiation of protein synthesis in *Escherichia coli* in the presence of trimethoprim. *J. Bacteriol* 1973;114:309.

65. Samuel, C. E., L. D'Ari and J. C. Rabinowitz. Evidence against the folate-mediated formylation of formyl-accepting methionyl transfer ribonucleic acid in *Streptococcus faecalis* R. *J. Biol. Chem.* 1970;245:5115.

66. Pine, M. J., B. Gordon, and S. S. Sarimo. Protein initiation without folate in *Streptococcus faecium. Biochim. Biophys. Acta* 1969;179:439.

67. Hyde, E. I., B. Birdsall, G. C. K. Roberts, J. Feeney, and A. S. V. Burgen. Proton magnetic resonance saturation transfer studies of coenzyme binding to *Lactobacillus caesei* dihydrofolate reductase. *Biochemistry* 1980;19:3738.

68. Birdsall, B., A. S. V. Burgen, and G. C. K. Roberts. Binding of coenzyme analogues to *Lactobacillus casei* dihydrofolate reductase: binary and ternary complexes. *Biochemistry* 1980;19:3723.

69. Cayley, P. J., S. M. J. Dunn, and R. W. King. Kinetics of substrate, coenzyme, and inhibitor binding to *Escherichia coli* dihydrofolate reductase. *Biochemistry* 1981;20:874.

70. Gronenborn, A., B. Birdsall, E. Hyde, G. Roberts, J. Feeney, and A. Burgen. ^{1}H and ^{31}P NMR characterization of two conformations of the trimethoprim-NADP$^+$-dihydrofolate reductase complex. *Mol. Pharmacol.* 1981;20:145.

71. Bushby, S. R. M., and G. H. Hitchings. Trimethoprim, a sulfonamide potentiator. *Br. J. Pharmacol. Chemother.* 1968;33:72.

72. Darrell, J. H., L. P. Garrod, and P. M. Waterworth. Trimethoprim:laboratory and clinical studies. *J. Clin. Pathol.* 1968;21:202.

73. Bushby, S. R. M. Trimethoprim-sulfamethoxazole: In vitro microbiological aspects. *J. Infect. Dis.* 1973;128(Suppl.):S442.

74. Grunberg, E. The effect of trimethoprim on the activity of sulfonamides and antibiotics in experimental infections. *J. Infect. Dis.* 1973;128(Suppl.):S478.

75. Hitchings, G. H., and J. J. Burchall. Inhibition of folate biosynthesis and function as a basis for chemotherapy. In *Advances in Enzymology,* Vol. 27, (ed. by F. F. Nord). New York: Wiley, 1965, pp. 417–468.

76. Potter, V. R. Sequential blocking of metabolic

pathways in vivo *Proc. Soc. Exp. Biol. Med. 1951;76: 41.*

77. Black, M. L. Sequential blockage as a theoretical basis for drug synergism. *J. Med. Chem.* 1963;6:145.

78. Rubin, R. J., A. Reynard, and R. E. Handschumacher. An analysis of the lack of drug synergism during sequential blockade of de novo pyrimidine biosynthesis. *Cancer Res.* 1964;24:1002.

79. Harvey, R. J. Synergism in the folate pathway. *Rev. Infect. Dis.* 1982;4:255.

80. Poe, M. Antibacterial synergism: a proposal for chemotherapeutic potentiation between trimethoprim and sulfamethoxazole. *Science* 1976;194:533.

81. Baccanari, D. P., and S. S. Joyner. Dihydrofolate reductase hysteresis and its effect on inhibitor binding analyses. *Biochemistry* 1981;20:1710.

82. Bushby, S. R. M. Combined antibacterial action in vitro of trimethoprim and sulfonamides: the in vitro nature of synergy. *Postgrad. Med. J.* 1969;45:10.

83. Bach, M. C., M. Finland, O. Gold, and C. Wilcox. Susceptibility of recently isolated pathogenic bacteria to trimethoprim and sulfamethoxazole separately and combined. *J. Infect. Dis.* 1973;128(Suppl.):S508.

84. Wormser, G. P., and G. T. Keusch. Trimethoprim-sulfamethoxazole in the United States. *Ann. Intern. Med.* 1979;91:420.

85. Wallace, R. J., E. J. Septimus, T. W. Williams, R. H. Conklin, T. K. Satterwhite, M. B. Bushby, and D. C. Hollowell. Use of trimethoprim-sulfamethoxazole for treatment of infections due to *Nocardia. Rev. Infect. Dis.* 1982;4:315.

86. Wallace, R. J., K. Wiss, M. B. Bushby, and D. C. Hollowell. In vitro activity of trimethoprim and sulfamethoxazole against the nontuberculous mycobacteria. *Rev. Infect. Dis.* 1982;4:326.

87. Lau, W. K., and L. S. Young. Trimethoprim-sulfamethoxazole treatment of *Pneumocystis carinii* pneumonia in adults. *N. Engl. J. Med.* 1976;295:716.

88. Hutchinson, D. B. A., and J. A. Farquhar. Trimethoprim-sulfamethoxazole in the treatment of malaria, toxoplasmosis, and pediculosis. *Rev. Infect. Dis.* 1982;4:419.

89. Salter, A. J. Trimethoprim-sulfamethoxazole: an assessment of more than 12 years of use. *Rev. Infect. Dis.* 1982;4:196.

90. Symposium (various authors). Trimethoprim-sulfamethoxazole. *J. Infect. Dis.* 1973;128(Suppl.):425–816.

91. Symposium (various authors). Trimethoprim-sulfamethoxazole revisited. *Rev. Infect. Dis.* 1982;4:185–618.

92. Dabhiolwala, N. F., A. Bye, and M. Claridge. A study of concentrations of trimethoprim-sulfamethoxazole in the human prostate gland. *Br. J. Urol.* 1976;48:77.

93. DuPont, H. L., R. R. Reves, E. Galindo, P. S. Sullivan, L. V. Wood, and J. G. Mendiola. Treatment of travelers' diarrhea with trimethoprim-sulfamethoxazole and trimethoprim alone. *N. Engl. J. Med.* 1982;307:841.

94. DuPont, H. L., E. Galindo, D. G. Evans, F. J. Cabada, P. Sullivan, and D. J. Evans. Prevention of travelers' diarrhea with trimethoprim-sulfamethoxazole and trimethoprim alone. *Gastroenterology* 1983;84:75.

95. Santamauro, J. T., and D. E. Storer. *Pneumocystis carinii* pneumonia. *Med. Clin. North Am.* 1997; 81:299.

96. Gallant, J. E., R. D. Moore, and R. E. Chaisson. Prophylaxis for opportunistic infections in patients with HIV infection. *Ann. Intern. Med.* 1994;120:932.

97. Amyes, S. G. B. Bactericidal activity of trimethoprim alone and in combination with sulfamethoxazole on susceptible and resistant *Escherichia coli* K-12. *Antimicrob. Agents Chemother.* 1982;21:288.

98. Acar, J. F., F. Goldstein, and Y. A. Chabbert. Synergistic activity of trimethoprim-sulfamethoxazole on gram-negative bacilli: observations in vitro and in vivo. *J. Infect. Dis.* 1973;128(Suppl.):S470.

99. Waterworth, P. M., Practical aspects of testing sensitivity to trimethoprim and sulfonamide. *Postgrad. Med. J.* 1969;45:21.

100. Hamilton-Miller, J. M. T. Mechanisms and distribution of bacterial resistance to diaminopyrimidines and sulfonamides. *J. Antimicrob. Chemother.* 1979; 5(Suppl. B):61.

101. Then, R. L. Mechanisms of resistance to trimethoprim, the sulfonamides, and trimethoprim-sulfamethoxazole. *Rev. Infect. Dis.* 1982;4:246.

102. Lacey, R. W., D. M. Bruten, W. A. Gillespie, and E. L. Lewis. Trimethoprim-resistant coliforms. *Lancet* 1972;1:409.

103. Centers for Disease Control: Drug-resistant *Streptococcus pneumoniae*—Kentucky and Tennessee. *MMWR Morb. Mortal. Wkly Rep.* 1994;43:23,31.

104. Burchall, J. J., L. P. Elwell, and M. E. Fling. Molecular mechanisms of resistance to trimethoprim. *Rev. Infect. Dis.* 1982;4:246.

105. Grey, D., J. M. T. Hamilton-Miller, and W. Brumfit. Incidence and mechanisms of resistance to trimethoprim in clinically isolated gram-negative bacteria. *Chemotherapy* 1979;25:147.

106. Huovinen, P. Trimethoprim resistance. *Antimicrob. Agents Chemother.* 1987;31:1451.

107. Towner, K. J., and R. C. B. Slack. Effect of changing selection pressures on trimethoprim resistance in Enterobacteriaceae. *Eur. J. Clin. Microbiol.* 1986;5: 502.

108. Mayer, K. H., M. Fling, J. Hopkins, and T. O'Brien. Trimethoprim resistance in multiple genera of Enterobacteriaceae at a U.S. hospital: spread of type II dihydrofolate reductase gene by single plasmid. *J. Infect. Dis.* 1985;151:783.

109. Goldstein, F. W., B. Papadopoulou, and J. Acar. Changing pattern of trimethoprim resistance in Paris, with review of worldwide experience. *Rev. Infect. Dis.* 1986;8:725.

110. Heikkilä, E., L. Sundstrom, and P. Huovinen. Trimethorprim resistance in *Escherichia coli* isolates from a geriatric unit. *Antimicrob. Agents Chemother.* 1990;34:2013.

111. Reves, R. R., B. Murray, L. Pickering, D. Prado, M. Maddock, and A. Bartlett III. Children with trimethoprim- and ampicillin-resistant fecal *Escherichia coli* in day care centers. *J. Infect. Dis.* 1987;156:758.

112. Reves, R. R., M. Fong, L. Pickering, A. Bartlett, M. Alvarez, and B. Murray. Risk factors for fecal col-

onization with trimethoprim-resistant and multiresistant *Escherichia coli* among children in day-care centers in Houston, Texas. *Antimicrob. Agents Chemother.* 1990;34:1429.

113. Murray, B. E., T. Alvarado, K.-H. Kim, M. Vorachit, P. Jayanetra, M. Levine, I. Prenzel, M. Fling, L. Elwell, G. McCracken, G. Madrigal, C. Odio, and L. Trabulsi. Increasing resistance to trimethoprim/sulfamethoxazole among isolates of *Escherichia coli* in developing countries. *J. Infect. Dis.* 1985;152:1107.

114. Neu, H. C. Trimethoprim alone for treatment of urinary tract infection. *Rev. Infect. Dis.* 1982; 4:366.

115. R. B. Patel and P. G. Welling. Clinical pharmacokinetics of co-trimoxazole (trimethoprim-sulfamethoxazole). *Clin. Pharmacokinet.* 1980;5:405.

116. Wilkinson, P. J., and D. S. Reeves. Tissue penetration of trimethoprim and sulfonamides. *J. Antimicrob. Chemother.* 1979;5(Suppl. B):159.

117. Kaplan, S. A., R. E. Weinfeld, C. W. Abruzzo, K. McFaden, M. L. Jack, and L. Weissman. Pharmacokinetic profile of trimethoprim-sulfamethoxazole in man. *J. Infect. Dis.* 1973;128(Suppl.):S547.

118. Kremers, P., J. Duvivier, and C. Heusghem. Pharmacokinetic studies of co-trimoxazole in man after single and repeated doses. *J. Clin. Pharmacol.* 1974;14:112.

119. Siber, G. R., C. C. Gorham, J. F. Ericson, and A. L. Smith. Pharmacokinetics of intravenous trimethoprim-sulfamethoxazole in children and adults with normal and impaired renal function. *Rev. Infect. Dis.* 1982;4:566.

120. Hansen, I., M. L. Nielsen and S. Bertelsen. Trimethoprim in human saliva, bronchial secretion and lung tissue. *Acta Pharmacol. Toxicol.* 1973;32:337.

121. Bruun, J. N., N. Ostby, J. E. Bredesen, P. Kierulf, and P. K. M. Lunde. Sulfonamide and trimethoprim concentrations in human serum and skin blister fluid. *Antimicrob. Agents Chemother.* 1981;19:82.

122. Trottier, S., M. G. Bergeron, and C. Lessard. Intrarenal distribution of trimethoprim and sulfamethazole. *Antimicrob. Agents Chemother.* 1980;17:383.

123. Stamey, T. A., and M. Condy. The diffusion and concentration of trimethoprim in human vaginal fluid. *J. Infect. Dis.* 1975;131:261.

124. Fries, V. N., U. Keuth, and J. S. Braun. Untersuchungen zur Liquorgängigkeit von Trimethoprim im Kindesalter. *Fortschr. Med.* 1975;93:1178.

125. Schwartz, D. E., and J. Rieder. Pharmacokinetics of sulfamethoxazole and trimethoprim in man and their distribution in the rat. *Chemotherapy* 1970;15:337.

126. Welling, P. G., W. A. Craig, G. L. Amidon, and C. M. Kunin. Pharmacokinetics of trimethoprim and sulfamethoxazole in normal subjects and in patients with renal failure. *J. Infect. Dis.* 1973;128(Suppl.): S556.

127. Jick, H. Adverse reactions to trimethoprim-sulfamethoxazole in hospitalized patients. *Rev. Infect. Dis.* 1982;4:426.

128. Frisch, J. M. Clinical experience with adverse reactions to trimethoprim-sulfamethoxazole. *J. Infect. Dis.* 1973;128(Suppl.):S607.

129. Chanarin, I., and J. M. England. Toxicity of trimethoprim-sulfamethioxazole in patients with megaloblastic haemopoiesis. *BMJ* 1972;1:651.

130. Kobrinsky, N. L., and N. K. Ramsay. Acute megaloblastic anemia induced by high-dose trimethoprim-sulfamethoxazole. *Ann. Intern. Med.* 1981;94:780.

131. Jewkes, R. F., M. S. Edwards, and J. B. Grant. Haematological changes in a patient on long-term treatment with a trimethoprim-sulfonamide combination. *Post-grad. Med. J.* 1970;46:723.

132. Bradley, P. P., G. D. Warden, J. G. Maxwell, and G. Rothstein. Neutropenia and thrombocytopenia in renal allograft recipients treated with trimethoprim-sulfamethoxazole. *Ann. Intern. Med.* 1980;93:560.

133. Golde, D. W., N. Bensch, and S. G. Quan. Trimethoprim and sulfamethoxazole inhibition of haematopoiesis in vitro. *Br. J. Haematol.* 1978;40:363.

134. Richmond, J. M., J. A. Whitworth, K. F. Fairley, and P. Kincaid-Smith. Co-trimoxazole nephrotoxicity. *Lancet* 1979;1:493.

135. Kalowski, S., R. S. Nanra, T. H. Mathew, and P. Kinkaid-Smith. Deterioration in renal function in association with co-trimoxazole therapy. *Lancet* 1973;1:394.

136. Berglund, F., J. Killander, and R. Pompeius. Effect of trimethoprim-sulfamethoxazole on the renal excretion of creatinine in man. *J. Urol.* 1975;114:802.

137. Kainer, G., and A. R. Rosenberg. Effect of co-trimoxazole on the glomerular filtration rate of healthy adults. *Chemotherapy* 1981;27:229.

CHAPTER EIGHT

Antibiotics that Affect Membrane Permeability

Polymyxin B, Colistin, and Gramicidin A

This chapter will deal with the antibiotics that kill bacteria by virtue of their effect on the permeability of the cell membrane. Some antibiotics, for example, bacitracin and vancomycin, have a locus of action at the membrane, but their principal effect is to specifically inhibit bacterial call wall synthesis. The antibiotics to be considered here interact specifically with membranes, and this interaction alters the function of the cell membrane in a manner incompatible with the survival of the bacterium. There are two groups of membrane antibiotics employed in the therapy of bacterial infection: the *polymixins*, which are used for the treatment of certain infections by gram-negative bacteria, and the *gramicidins*, which are included in some topical antibiotic preparations. Some of the most interesting antibiotics acting on the cell membrane belong to the polyene group. These drugs do not affect bacteria; they are used only in the treatment of fungal infections, and they will be discussed in Chapter 12.

The Polymyxins

Of the polymyxin group of antibacterial agents, polymyxin B and colistin (polymyxin E) are the least toxic and the only polymyxins used clinically. They contain both hydrophilic and hydrophobic portions and behave

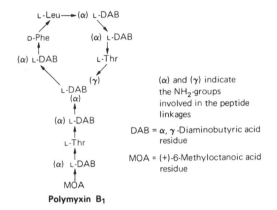

Polymyxin B₁

(α) and (γ) indicate the NH₂-groups involved in the peptide linkages

DAB = α, γ-Diaminobutyric acid residue

MOA = (+)-6-Methyloctanoic acid residue

as cationic surface-active compounds at physiological pH. The antibacterial activity of the polymyxins decreases in the presence of anionic compounds, such as soaps and phospholipids.[1]

Mechanism of Action

CELL KILLING IS DUE TO AN EFFECT ON CELL PERMEABILITY. The mechanism of action of the polymyxins has been reviewed by Storm et al.[2] The polymyxins are bactericidal for a broad range of gram-negative bacteria, but they have very little effect on gram-positive bacteria. A 1953 study showed that polymyxins cause leakage of small molecules, such as phosphate and nucleosides, from sensitive bacteria. The extent of the leakage, as measured by the amount of small molecular size material appearing in the growth medium, is proportional to the killing effect of the drug.[3] Changes in cellular permeability as a result of exposure to polymyxin have also been demonstrated with a dye compound. The dye N-toly-α-napthylamine-8-sulfonic acid fluoresces under ultraviolet light when it is bound to protein. *Pseudomonas* cells exposed to the dye did not fluoresce; but when a polymyxin was added to the cell suspension, the permeability characteristics of the cell exterior were altered, the dye was permitted to penetrate the cell membrane, and fluorescence resulted from the association of the dye with cellular protein.[4] This evidence of a change in the permeability of bacterial cells in the presence of polymyxins is supported by a number of other studies.[2] Alterations in membrane permeability are one of the earliest changes caused by the polymyxins, and their effects on other cellular functions, such as respiration and ATP levels, are thought to be entirely secondary to membrane damage.[2]

It is likely that the polymyxins are not active against gram-positive bacteria because the thick cell wall prevents access to the cell membrane. This proposal is consistent with the observation that protoplasts prepared from a gram-positive bacterium, *Bacillus subtilis,* are sensitive to the drug, whereas the intact bacterium is not.[5] To effect a change in the membrane permeability of gram-negative bacteria, a polymyxin must either first disrupt the permeability of the outer membrane or pass through the outer membrane and interact with the cytoplasmic membrane. At low concentrations, polymyxin B causes changes in the morphology of the outer membrane[6] and causes the selective release of proteins that are located in the periplasmic space between the inner and outer membranes.[2] This suggests that at least the initial effect is on the outer membrane. Experiments with polymyxin B bound covalently to agarose beads have shown that the drug does not have to enter the cell to inhibit bacterial growth.[5]

THE SITE OF ACTION—THE CELL MEMBRANE. The polymyxins have been shown to bind to the cell envelope. In 1955, Newton demonstrated that when *Pseudomonas aeruginosa* or *Bacillus megaterium* were exposed to a fluorescent DANSyl-derivative of polymyxin, the drug accumulated in the periphery of the cell.[7] Protoplasts obtained from such cells also fluoresced, and after disruption, the drug was recovered in the fraction containing the cell envelope. Early studies also showed that preparations of cell membrane from organisms resistant to the polymyxins bind much less drug than those from sensitive cells.[8,9]

Several investigators have used model membrane systems to try to further determine the requirements for polymyxin binding. Liposomes prepared by sonicating phospholipids in the presence of glucose form a simple system in which polymyxin effects can be assayed by monitoring the release of glucose after drug addition. Polymyxin B rapidly causes release of trapped glucose and the drug shows a preference for lysosomes prepared with negatively charged phospholipids.[10,11] The naturally resistant organism *Acholeplasma laidlawii* B can be made sensitive to polymyxin by fusing it with vesicles containing acidic phospholipids, such as cardiolipin or phosphatidylglycerol. The phospholipids diffuse into the membrane and the fusion product binds 12 times as much polymyxin B as the normal organism and is 10- to 30-fold more susceptible to the drug.[12] Polymyxin B binds to negatively charged phospholipid monolayers,[13] and from physical observations made on such phospholipid-drug complexes, it has been determined that the drug penetrates into the monolayer.[14–16] The studies in model membrane systems have led to the proposal that the fatty acid tail of the polymyxin penetrates into the hydrophobic regions of the phospholipid and the polypeptide ring binds electrostatically to the exposed phosphate groups. The binding of polymyxin B to negatively charged lipid bilayer membranes and the effects of the drug on bacterial permeability and growth are antagonized by calcium.[2,17]

Although studies in model membrane systems, such as liposomes and monolayers, have provided considerable information that may be directly applicable to polymyxin effects on spheroplasts and L forms which lack an outer envelope, these systems are not close analogs of the immediate target of polymyxin action in intact gram-negative bacteria. That target is the outer surface of the gram-negative outer membrane, which is composed largely of lipopolysaccharide rather than phospholipid (see Fig. 3–10). The importance of the outer membrane in determining the polymyxin sensitivity of gram-negative bacteria is underlined by studies with polymyxin-resistant organisms. The natural polymyxin resistance of some gram-negative bacteria is a function of cell structures located outside the cytoplasmic membrane. For example, the sensitivity of *Proteus mirabilis* to polymyxin B is increased 400-fold by converting it to the spheroplast or L form.[18] These forms are as susceptible to polymyxin B as normally susceptible gram-negative bacteria, and upon reconversion to the bacillary form, they become resistant again.[18] Polymyxin-resistant mutants of normally sensitive gram-negative bacilli have been shown to have defective outer membranes[19,20] that bind less drug[21] and contain much less lipopolysaccharide.[20,21] Polymyxins bind to a high-affinity binding site on lipopolysaccharides that is also a binding site for calcium and magnesium ions.[22]

At the current stage in our understanding of polymyxin action, the divalent cation binding site on the lipopolysaccharide component of the gram-negative outer membrane is thought to be the primary site of electrostatic interaction with amino groups in the cyclic peptide portion of the drug. The fatty acid tail of the polymyxin penetrates into the hydrophobic region of the outer membrane, disrupting the membrane packing and increasing its permeability to polar molecules. The studies with agarose-bound polymyxin B suggest that this interaction at the outer membrane is sufficient to cause inhibition of cellular respiration and death.[5] With the free drug, however, it is possible that subsequent interaction of the drug with the cytoplasmic membrane contributes to the bactericidal effect.

Antimicrobial Activity and Clinical Use

Polymyxin B and colistin have the same spectra of antibacterial action and show complete cross-resistance.[23,24] The spectrum of clinical action of the polymyxins is limited to gram-negative bacilli. Gram-positive bacteria and obligate anaerobes are resistant. Ninety nine percent of *Pseudomonas aeruginosa* strains are inhibited in vitro by 4 μg of colistin per ml.[25] *Escherichia coli, Klebsiella pneumoniae, Enterobacter, Salmonella, Shigella, Vibrios, Haemophilus, Pasturella,* and *Bordetella* isolates are usually susceptible. *Proteus, Providencia, Serratia,* and *Neisseria* isolates are usually resistant. Polymyxin have been shown to be synergistic with trimethoprim and sulfamethoxazole against several multiple drug–resistant, gram-negative bacilli (e.g., *Serratia, Pseudomonas cepacia,* and *P. maltophilia*).[26–28] Synergism has also been demonstrated with rifampin against multiresistant *Serratia.*[29] The mechanism of the synergism is probably the same as that observed with polymyxin B and tetracyclines against fungi at concentrations where each drug alone has no effect.[30] The polymyxin B increases the permeability of the yeast cell membrane to tetracycline, which then inhibits protein synthesis and causes cell death.[30]

Because of severe toxicity, Polymxin and colistin are rarely administered by systemic routes but they are available in several topical preparations. Polymyxin B is administered topically in otic and ophthalmic solutions to treat external otitis and corneal ulcers which are frequently caused by *Pseudomonas aeruginosa.* Polymyxin B is present in a wide variety of topical preparations that are used in outpatient practice to treat superficial infections of the skin. These topical preparations usually contain another antibiotic, such as neomycin or bacitracin, and sometimes a corticosteroid is also included. These topical antibiotic formulations are discussed briefly at the end of Chapter 4.

Pharmacology

Polymyxin B sulfate is available for parenteral and topical administration. Colistin sulfate is available for topical use, and sodium colistimethate (the methane sulfonate) is the form of colistin used for parenteral injection. The antibacterial activity of colistimethate depends on hydrolysis to colistin in vivo.[31] Administration of 150 mg of sodium colistimethate to an adult by intramuscular injection yields peak serum levels of 2–5 µg/ml of colistin (assayed as antibacterial activity) in 4 h.[32] Intravenous infusion of 2.5 mg of polymyxin B yields a peak serum concentration of approximately 5 µg/ml. Neither polymyxin B nor colistin is absorbed from the gastrointestinal tract. Colistin sulfate was formerly available as an oral preparation for infants and children for treatment of gastroenteritis due to enteropathogenic *E. coli*. After oral administration, the drug remains in the intestinal lumen and is not present in the tissues of the bowel wall. Polymyxins are poorly absorbed from the skin, even when it is partially denuded by burns. The drugs are absorbed from serous cavities like the peritoneum, and toxicity (apnea) can occur if infection sites are irrigated with solutions containing polymyxin.

The pharmacokinetics of polymyxins are complex. Both polymyxin B and colistin have a large volume of distribution because they are extensively bound to membrane phospholipids in the tissues.[33,34] Colistimethate is not extensively bound. The calcium in human serum decreases the antibacterial activity of polymyxins in vitro,[35] thus, these drugs may be less active in the patient than is suggested by in vitro sensitivity testing. The polymyxins do not pass into body fluid spaces, such as ocular, pleural, or peritoneal fluids, and they do not enter the cerebrospinal fluid, even when there is inflammation of the meninges. Thus, when they are employed for the treatment of gram-negative meningitis, they must be given intrathecally.[36] Polymyxins do cross the human placenta.[37]

The polymyxins are excreted into the urine by glomerular filtration. Polymyxin B is excreted slowly. The drug persists in the body because of extensive tissue binding,[38] but after a delay of several hours, it appears in the urine where concentrations of 20–100 µg/ml are achieved.[23] Sodium colistimethate is relatively poorly bound to tissue and is more rapidly excreted in the urine (serum half-life, 4.5 h).[24] After intramuscular injection of 150 mg of sodium colistimethate, urine levels of about 100 µg/ml of the bioactive form, colistin, are achieved in 4 h, and 12 h after administration, the urine level of colistin is in the range of 35 µg/ml.[32] The half-lives of polymyxin B and colistin increase markedly in renal failure (colistimethate half-life in end-stage renal disease is 10–20 h),[39] and the dosage of both drugs must be reduced according to guidelines that alter either the dosage interval[23] or the dosage amount.[40] Polymyxins are slowly removed by peritoneal dialysis but not by hemodialysis.[39]

Adverse Effects

Polymyxins are most often administered topically and topical sensitization occurs only rarely. Many topical formulations with polymyxin B also contain neomycin, however, and contact allergic reactions to the neomycin component are relatively common. Intramuscular injection of polymyxin B commonly produces pain at the injection site; this may be reduced by mixing the drug with a local anesthetic.[41] Injection of colistimethate is less painful.[24] Intrathecal administration may be accompanied by headache and other signs of meningeal irritation.

Given the rather nonspecific interaction between polymyxins and membranes that was discussed earlier in this chapter, it is not surprising that the polymyxins are toxic antibiotics. It is clear that high concentrations of polymyxin B (50 µg/ml) do alter the permeability of mammalian cells in culture and permit the entry of other antibiotics, such as tetracyclines.[42] The extensive tissue binding of polymyxins is largely accounted for by binding to membrane phospholipid. Both the neurotoxicity and the nephrotoxicity of polymyxins may reflect their effects on mammalian cell membranes. Occasional patients receiving parenteral polymyxins develop flushing and other subjective side effects of histamine release.[43] These drugs have been shown to induce histamine release in experimental animal models and from mast cells in vitro.[44] The in vitro degranulation of mast cells occurs in the absence of components of the immune system, which suggests that the drug interacts directly with the mast cells, and it is likely that direct membrane effects are involved.[43,44]

Polymyxins cause two types of neurotoxicity. About 7% of patients experience circumoral or "stocking-glove" paresthesias, sometimes accompanied by dizziness, vertigo, ataxia, slurred speech, drowsiness, or confusion.[45,46] These effects are dose related and disappear when the drug is discontinued. A second type of neurotoxicity is a noncompetitive neuromuscular blockade that causes a reversible respiratory paralysis.[47] The blockade usually occurs at high serum concentrations of drug and patients with impaired renal function clearly constitute a high-risk group.[47] The neuromuscular blocking effect is additive with that produced by aminoglycosides.[48] Polymyxins produce both pre- and postjunctional inhibition, with the postjunctional effect predominating.[49] In contrast to the neuromuscular blockade produced by the aminoglycosides, the block produced by polymyxins is only partially and unreliably reversed by calcium.[49,50] From electrophysiological studies, it is apparent that polymyxins cause a persistant blockade of acetylcholine-activated endplate channels.[51,52] An endplate channel block accounts for the noncompetitive nature of the effect and the inability of neostigmine to reverse it.[47,50]

The most common side effect of the polymyxins is a dose-related nephrotoxicity.[53] Signs of nephrotoxicity have been detected in approximately 20% of patients receiving normal therapeutic doses of colistimethate.[46] The nephrotoxicity is characterized by proteinuria, cylinduria, and the presence of cellular elements in the urine.[53] At doses of 3 mg/kg/day, nitrogen retention and decreased glomerular filtration rate occur in patients with previously normal renal function.[53] Acute tubular necrosis is reported to occur at a frequency of 1%–2%.[46] Renal damage is generally reversible with cessation of therapy. Elderly patients, those with impaired renal function, and those receiving other nephrotoxic drugs have a higher risk of developing nephrotoxicity when treated with polymyxin. Renal function should be carefully monitored in patients receiving polymyxin B and colistimethate; dosages should be reduced in the presence of renal failure; and these drugs should be used only when less toxic drugs are not available. Studies of renal function in dogs indicate that colistimethate is less nephrotoxic than polymyxin B;[54,55] although when antibacterial potency is taken into account, the difference in toxicity may be minimal. The mechanism of nephrotoxicity is not clearly defined. It is known that polymyxins are bound by the kidneys, mostly to membranes,[33,34] and the drugs can be extracted in their active bactericidal form from the renal phospholipid.[56] It is reasonable to postulate that the nephrotoxicity results from the interaction of the unaltered drug with the renal tubular cell membrane.[21]

Gramicidin A

There are several antibiotics that have been shown to cause rather specific changes in the cation permeability of membranes and lipid

$$HCO{-}L{-}Val{-}Gly{-}L{-}Ala{-}D{-}Leu{-}L{-}Ala{-}$$
$$L{-}Trp{-}D{-}Leu{-}L{-}Trp{-}D{-}Val{-}L{-}Val{-}D{-}Val{-}$$
$$D{-}Leu{-}L{-}Trp{-}D{-}Leu{-}L{-}Trp{-}NH_2CH_2{-}CH_2{-}OH$$

Gramicidin A

bilayers. These agents are generally too toxic to be clinically useful, but one of them, gramicidin A, is present in some topical antibiotic preparations. Gramicidin A was originally isolated from a mixture of antibiotics produced by *Bacillus brevis*. Gramicidin A is an open-chain polypeptide, with 15 amino acid residues in which D- and L-forms alternate in the sequence (this can be seen in the structure presented above), since glycine is ambivalent.

Gramicidin A is only used topically. It is provided in formulations that contain other antibiotics such as neomycin or polymyxin B. Gramicidin A is primarily active against gram-positive bacteria. It kills bacteria by acting as an ionophore and altering the cation permeability of the bacterial membrane.[57] The term *ionophore* refers to the ability of certain antibiotics to carry ions across such lipid barriers as cell membranes and artificial lipid bilayers. The study of these molecules has been very helpful in developing our understanding of membrane transport processes at the molecular level.

The lipid components of biological membranes are oriented in a more-or-less ordered way, such that their polar groups face the membrane surface and the nonpolar hydrocarbon chains form the membrane interior. The nonpolar components of the membrane form an extremely efficient barrier to the passage of such small ions as sodium or potassium. There are two principal mechanisms by which ionophores facilitate the passage of small ions across this barrier. Some ionophores, for example, valinomycin and monactin, form a three-dimensional cage around the cation (Fig. 8–1). The exterior of the antibiotic cage is quite hydrophobic and the ion–antibiotic complex is thus lipid sol-

uble. The antibiotic binds a cation at one membrane interface by forming ion-dipole interactions that replace the water of hydration normally surrounding the ion. The antibiotic with the cation bound in its center is then able to diffuse to the opposite membrane surface where the cation is released (Figure 8–1). These antibiotics are called *carrier type ionophores*. They can be very efficient, one molecule facilitating the passage of thousands of ions per second.[58]

Another group of ionophores is called the *channel-formers*, and gramicidin A belongs to this group.[59] Here, the antibiotic forms a tube that passes from one surface of the membrane to the other (Fig. 8–1). The ions enter the tube at one membrane interface and diffuse through the interior of the channel to the other side. Although the structure of gramicidin A has been presented above in linear form it is clear that it can assume three-dimensional conformations consistent with the formation of such an ion-conducting channel. It has been established that the channel is composed of a gramicidin A dimer and two conformations have been

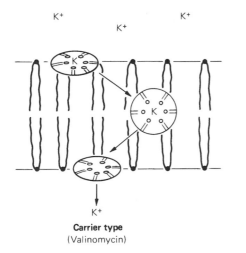

Carrier type
(Valinomycin)

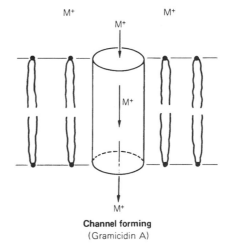

Channel forming
(Gramicidin A)

Figure 8–1. Schematic models of the mechanisms by which the carrier and the channel-forming type of ionophore antibiotics facilitate the passage of cations across biological and artificial membranes. The solid circles oriented at the membrane surface represent the polar head groups of the phospholipids, and the wavy lines denote the hydrophobic fatty acid chains. Valinomycin (an antibiotic not used clinically) is used as an example of the carrier type. In general, the carrier ionophores are much more specific with regard to the ions with which they interact, valinomycin being quite selective for potassium (K^+). The channel-formers are less selective, and in the case of gramicidin A, a variety of monovalent metal cations (M^+) are able to diffuse through the pore formed in the center of the antibiotic channel.

proposed for the channel structure.[60] One structure is a double-helical dimer in which two chains of gramicidin A are coiled around a common axis[61] and a second structure is a helical dimer that is formed by head-to-head association of two gramicidin A monomers.[62] The channel formed by the antibiotic permits the passage of univalent cations but completely excludes anions and polyvalent cations.[63,64] The gramicidin A channels are not static; they are constantly forming and disappearing. Cell death apparently results from changes in cellular cation content, principally the loss of potassium ion.[57]

REFERENCES

1. Bliss, E. A., C. A. Chandler, and E. B. Schoenbach. In vitro studies of polymyxin. *Ann. N.Y. Acad. Sci.* 1949;51:944.

2. Storm, D. R., K. S. Rosenthal, and P. E. Swanson. Polymyxin and related antibiotics. *Annu. Rev. Biochem.* 1977;46:723.

3. Newton, B. A. The release of soluble constituents from washed cells of *Pseudomonas aeruginosa* by the action of polymyxin. *J. Gen. Microbiol.* 1953;9:54.

4. Newton, B. A. Site of action of polymyxin on *Pseudomonas aeruginosa*; antagonism by cations. *J. Gen. Microbiol.* 1954;10:491.

5. LaPorte, D. C., K. S. Rosenthal, and D. R. Storm. Inhibition of *Escherichia coli* growth and respiration by polymyxin B covalently attached to agarose beads. *Biochemistry* 1977;16:1642.

6. Schindler, P. R. G., and M. Teuber. Action of polymyxin B on bacterial membranes: morphological changes in the cytoplasm and in the outer membrane of *Salmonella typhimurium* and *Escherichia coli* B. *Antimicrob. Agents Chemother.* 1975;8:95.

7. Newton, B. A. A fluorescent derivative of polymyxin; its preparation and use in studying the site of action of the antibiotic. *J. Gen. Microbiol.* 1955;12:226.

8. Few, A. V., and J. H. Schulman. The absorption of polymyxin E by bacteria and bacterial cell walls and its bactericidal action. *J. Gen. Microbiol.* 1953;9:454.

9. Newton, B. A. The properties and mode of action of the polymyxins. *Bacteriol. Rev.* 1956;20:14.

10. Imai, M., K. Inoue, and S. Nojima. Effect of polymyxin B on liposomal membranes derived from *Escherichia coli* lipids. *Biochim. Biophys. Acta* 1975;375:130.

11. HsuChen, C.-C., and D. S. Feingold. The mechanism of polymyxin B action and selectivity toward biologic membranes. *Biochemistry* 1973;12:2105.

12. Teuber, M., and J. Bader. Action of polymyxin B on bacterial membranes: phosphatidylglycerol- and cardiolipin-induced susceptibility to polymyxin B in *Acholeplasma laidlawii* B. *Antimicrob. Agents Chemother.* 1976;9:26.

13. Teuber, M., and I. R. Miller. Selective binding of polymyxin B to negatively charged lipid monolayers. *Biochim. Biophys. Acta* 1977;467:280.

14. Pache, W., D. Chapman, and R. Hillaby. Interaction of antibiotics with membranes: polymyxin B and gramicidin S. *Biochim. Biophys. Acta* 1972;255:358.

15. Sixl, F., and H.-J. Galla. Cooperative lipid-protein interaction: effect of pH and ionic strength on polymyxin binding to phosphatidic acid membranes. *Biochim. Biophys. Acta* 1979;557:320.

16. Galla, H.-J., and J. R. Trudell. Pressure-induced changes in the molecular organization of a lipid-peptide complex. *Biochim. Biophys. Acta* 1980;602:522.

17. Six, F., and H. J. Galla. Polymyxin interaction with negatively charged lipid bilayer membranes and the competitive effect of Ca^{2+}. *Biochim. Biophys. Acta* 1981;643:626.

18. Teuber, M. Susceptibility to polymyxin B of penicillin G-induced *Proteus mirabilis* L forms and spheroplasts. *J. Bacteriol.* 1969;98:347.

19. Vaara, M., and T. Vaara. Outer membrane permeability barrier disruption by polymyxin in polymyxin-susceptible and -resistant *Salmonella typhimurium. Antimicrob. Agents. Chemother.* 1981;19:578.

20. Gilleland, H. E., and R. D. Lyle. Chemical alterations in cell envelopes of polymyxin resistant *Pseudomonas aeruginosa* isolates. *J. Bacteriol.* 1979;138:839.

21. Vaara, M., T. Vaara, and M. Sarvas. Decreased binding of polymyxin-resistant mutants of *Salmonella typhimurium. J. Bacteriol.* 1979;139:664.

22. Schindler, M., and M. J. Osborn. Interaction of divalent cations and polymyxin B with lipopolysaccharide. *Biochemistry* 1979;18:4425.

23. Hoeprich, P. D. The polymyxins. *Med. Clin. North Am.* 1970;54:1257.

24. Goodwin, N. J. Colistin and sodium colistimethate. *Med. Clin. North Am.* 1970;54:1267.

25. Duncan, I. B. R. Susceptibility of 1,500 isolates of *Pseudomonas aeruginosa* to gentamicin, carbenicillin, colistin, and polymyxin B. *Antimicrob. Agents Chemother.* 1974;5:9.

26. Nord, E. E., T. Waldstrom, and B. Wretlind. Synergistic effect of combinations of sulfamethoxazole, trimethoprim, and colistin against *Pseudomonas maltophilia* and *Pseudomonas cepacia. Antimicrob. Agents Chemother.* 1974;6:521.

27. Rosenblatt, J. E., and P. R. Stewart. Combined activity of sulfamethoxazole, trimethoprim, and polymyxin B against gram-negative bacilli. *Antimicrob. Agents Chemother.* 1974;6:84.

28. Thomas, F. E., J. M. Leonard, and R. H. Alford. Sulfamethoxazole-trimethoprim-polymyxin therapy of serious multiply drug-resistant *Serratia* infections. *Antimicrob. Agents Chemother.* 1976;9:201.

29. Ostenson, R. C., B. T. Fields, and C. M. Nolan. Polymyxin B and rifampin: new regimen for multiresistant *Serratia marcescens* infections. *Antimicrob. Agents Chemother.* 1977;12:655.

30. Schwartz, S. N., G. Medoff, G. S. Kobayashi, C. N. Kwan, and D. Schlessinger. Antifungal properties of polymyxin B and its potentiation of tetracycline as

an antifungal agent. *Antimicrob. Agents Chemother.* 1972;2:36.

31. Barnett, M., S. R. M. Bushby, and S. Wilkinson. Sodium sulfomethyl derivatives of polymyxins. *Br. J. Pharmacol.* 1964;23:552.

32. Sande, M. A., and D. Kaye. Evaluation of methods for determining antibacterial activity of serum and urine after colistimethate injection. *Clin. Pharmacol. Ther.* 1970;11:873.

33. Craig, W. A., and C. M. Kunin. Dynamics of binding and release of the polymyxin antibiotics by tissues. *J. Pharmacol. Exp. Ther.* 1973;184:757.

34. Kunin, C. M. Binding of antibiotics to tissue homogenates. *J. Infect. Dis.* 1970;121:55.

35. Davis, S. D., A. Iannetta, and R. J. Wedgewood. Activity of colistin against *Pseudomonas aeruginosa*: inhibition by calcium. *J. Infect. Dis.* 1971;124:610.

36. Wise, B. L., J. L. Mathis, and E. Jawetz. Infections of the central nervous system due to *Pseudomonas aeruginosa*. *J. Neurosurg.* 1969;31:432.

37. MacAulay, M. A., and D. Charles. Placental transmission of colistimethate. *Clin. Pharmacol. Ther.* 1967;8:578.

38. Kunin, C. M., and A. Bugg. Binding of polymyxin antibiotics to tissues: the major determinant of distribution and persistence in the body. *J. Infect. Dis.* 1971; 124:394.

39. Goodwin, N. J., and E. A. Friedman. The effects of renal impairment, peritoneal dialysis, and hemodialysis on serum sodium colistimethate levels. *Ann. Intern. Med.* 1968;68:984.

40. Bennett, W. M., R. S. Muther, R. A. Parker, P. Feig, G. Morrison, T. A. Golper, and I. Singer. Drug therapy in renal failure: dosing guidelines for adults. *Ann. Intern. Med.* 1980;93:62.

41. Fekety, R. Polymyxins. In *Principles and Practice of Infectious Diseases*, ed by G. L. Mandell, R. G. Douglas, and J. E. Bennett. New York: Wiley, 1979, pp. 300–304.

42. Medoff, G., C. N. Kwan, D. Schlessinger, and G. S. Kobayashi. Potentiation of rifampicin, rifampin analogs, and tetracycline against animal cells by amphotericin B and polymyxin B. *Cancer Res.* 1973;33: 1146.

43. Sanders, W. E., and C. C. Sanders. Toxicity of antibacterial agents: mechanism of action on mammalian cells. *Ann. Rev. Pharmacol. Toxicol.* 1979; 19:53.

44. Tizard, I. R., and W. L. Holmes. Degranulation of sensitized rat peritoneal mast cells in response to antigen, compound 48/80 and polymyxin B. A scanning electron microscope study. *Int. Arch. Allergy Appl. Immunol.* 1974;46:867.

45. Fekety, F. R., P. S. Norman, and L. E. Cluff. The treatment of gram-negative bacillary infections with colistin: the toxicity and efficacy of large doses in forty-eight patients. *Ann. Intern. Med.* 1962;57:214.

46. Koch-Weser, J., V. W. Sidel, E. B. Federman, P. Kanarek, D. C. Finer, and E. A. Eaton. Adverse effects of sodium colistimethate: manifestations and specific reaction rates during 317 courses of therapy. *Ann. Intern. Med.* 1970;72:857.

47. Lindesmith, L. A., R. D. Baines, D. B. Bigelow,

and T. L. Petty. Reversible respiratory paralysis associated with polymyxin therapy. *Ann. Intern. Med.* 1968; 68:318.

48. Lee, C., and A. J. C. deSilva. Interaction of neuromuscular blocking effects of neomycin and polymyxin B. *Anesthesiology* 1979;50:218.

49. Singh, Y. N., I. G. Marshall, and A. L. Harvey. Depression of transmitter release and postjunctional sensitivity during neuromuscular block produced by antibiotics. *Br. J. Anesth.* 1979;51:1027.

50. Singh, Y. N., A. L. Harvey, and I. G. Marshall. Antibiotic-induced paralysis of the mouse phrenic nerve-hemidiaphragm preparation, and reversibility by calcium and by neostigmine. *Anesthesiology* 1978;50: 418.

51. Durant, N. N., and J. J. Lambert. The action of polymyxin B at the frog neuromuscular junction. *Br. J. Pharmacol.* 1981;72:41.

52. Fiekers, J. F. Neuromuscular block produced by polymyxin B: interaction with end-plate channels. *Eur. J. Pharmacol.* 1981;70:77.

53. Appel, G. B., and H. C. Neu. The nephrotoxicity of antimicrobial agents (second of three parts). *N. Engl. J. Med.* 1977;296:722.

54. Vinnicombe, J., and T. A. Stamey. The relative nephrotoxicities of polymyxin B sulfate, sodium sulfomethyl-polymyxin B, sodium sulfomethyl-colistin (colymycin), and neomycin sulfate. *Invest. Urol.* 1969; 6:505.

55. Pedersen, M. F., J. F. Pedersen, and P. O. Madsen. A clinical and experimental comparative study of sodium colistimethate and polymyxin B sulfate. *Invest. Urol.* 1971;9:234.

56. Kunin, C. M., and A. Bugg. Recovery of tissue bound polymyxin B and colistimethate. *Proc. Soc. Exp. Biol. Med.* 1971;137:786.

57. Harold, F. M., and J. R. Baarda. Gramicidin, valinomycin and cation permeability of *Streptococcus faecalis*. *J. Bacteriol.* 1967;94:53.

58. Bakker, E. P. Ionophore antibiotics. In *Antibiotics V-1*, ed. by F. E. Hahn. New York: Springer-Verlag, 1979, pp. 67–97.

59. Ovchinnikov, Y. A. Physico-chemical basis of ion transport through biological membranes: ionophores and ion channels. *Eur. J. Biochem.* 1979;94:321.

60. Urry, D. W. Molecular perspectives of monovalent cation selective transmembrane channels. *Int. Rev. Neurobiol.* 1979;21:311.

61. Veatch, W. R., E. T. Fosel, and E. R. Blout. The conformation of gramicidin A. *Biochemistry* 1974;13: 5249.

62. Urry, D. W., M. C. Goodall, J. D. Glickson, and D. F. Mayers. The gramicidin A transmembrane channel: characteristics of head-to-head dimerized helices. *Proc. Natl. Acad. Sci. U.S.A.* 1971;68:1907.

63. Bamberg, E., H.-J. Apell, H. Alpes, E. Gross, J. L. Morell, J. F. Harbaugh, K. Janko, and P. Läuger. Ion channels formed by chemical analogs of gramicidin A. *Fed. Proc.* 1978;37:2633.

64. Hladky, S. B., and D. A. Haydon. Ion transfer across lipid membranes in the presence of gramicidin A. I. Studies of the unit conductance channel. *Biochim. Biophys. Acta* 1972;274:204.

CHAPTER NINE

The Urinary Tract Antiseptics

Nalidixic Acid and Cinoxacin; Nitrofurantoin; Methenamine; Fosfomycin

Several of the drugs that have already been discussed are used in the treatment of urinary tract infections. The sulfonamides, ampicillin, the fluoroquinolomes, and the tetracyclines are the principal drugs employed in treating acute, uncomplicated infections of the urinary tract. Trimethoprim-sulfamethoxazole (TMP-SMX) is often used to treat chronic or recurrent infection. Others, such as the aminoglycosides, cephalosporins, and carbenicillin, are used much less often for restricted indications. There are several drugs that are concentrated in the urine and employed only in treating patients with infection of the urinary tract. These drugs are called *urinary tract antiseptics*, and the group includes nalidixic acid, cinoxacin, nitrofurantoin, methenamine, and fosfomycin.

Nalidixic Acid and Cinoxacin

Nalidixic acid and cinoxacin are structurally analogous, synthetic antimicrobial drugs that have the same mechanism of action but differ somewhat with respect to intrinsic potency and pharmacokinetic properties. The effects of nalidixic acid on bacterial growth and nucleic acid synthesis have been reviewed by Pedrini[1] and effects on DNA topoisomerases have been reviewed by Cozzarelli[2] and by Gellert.[3]

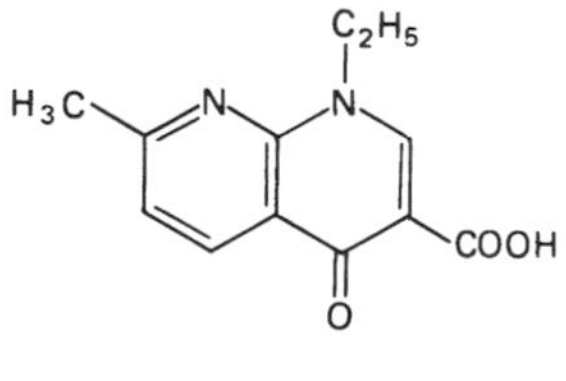

Nalidixic acid

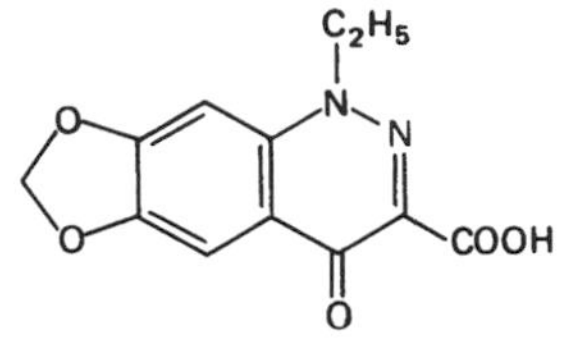

Cinoxacin

Mechanism of Action

Nalidixic acid and cinoxacin, although urinary tract antiseptics, are quinolones; their mechanism of action is thoroughly discussed in Chapter 10 along with the other fluoroquinolones. All members of this class inhibit DNA replication in susceptible bacteria by inhibiting the enzyme DNA gyrase.

Antimicrobial Activity and Resistance

Nalidixic acid is more active against gram-negative bacteria than gram-positive bacteria.[4] The great majority of strains of *Escherichia coli, Klebsiella, Enterobacter,* and *Proteus (mirabilis, morganii, vulgaris)* are

242

susceptible to 20 µg/ml of nalidixic acid.[5,6] Other gram-negative aerobic bacilli that are usually susceptible include *Providencia*, *Pasturella multocida*, *Salmonella* spp., and *Shigella* spp.[7] *Pseudomonas aeruginosa* isolates are invariably resistant, as are anaerobic bacteria, and in general, gram-positive, aerobic cocci are resistant.[7] Nalidixic acid and cinoxacin have the same antibacterial potency.[8]

At bactericidal concentrations, nalidixic acid and its analogs inhibit DNA replication, but protein and RNA synthesis continue. Continued RNA and protein synthesis are necessary for DNA degradation, which correlates with lethality.[9] When the drug is present at very high concentration, inhibition of RNA and protein synthesis occurs and less killing and more bacteriostasis is observed.[10] The peak concentrations of nalidixic acid that are achieved in the urine with usual dosage are often higher than the most lethal concentration for urinary pathogens.[10]

In the United States, nalidixic acid[7] and cinoxacin[11,12] are used principally to treat patients with recurrent uncomplicated urinary tract infections caused by susceptible gram-negative bacilli. Resistance to all of these agents may arise during therapy,[13,14] and the reported incidences of resistance vary widely. Several variables influence the frequency at which resistance is observed, including the drug dosage, the duration of treatment, the site of infection, and the rate of reinfection by resistant organisms in the reservoir of perineal and fecal flora. Administration of the drug at less than full dosage may result in low urinary drug concentrations that favor the selection of resistant bacteria.[15] The influence of infection site and duration of therapy is suggested by a study showing that after administration of nalidixic acid in full dosage (1 g four times a day) to women with bacteriuria, the incidence of resistance was 3% after 3 days of therapy in patients with bladder infections and 16% after 14 days of therapy in patients with renal infections.[16] It should be noted that the rate at which nalidixic acid resistance develops in the fecal and periurethral flora is less than that reported for sulfonamides, tetracyclines, ampicillin, and cephal-

exin.[15,16] This probably reflects the fact that nalidixic acid resistance in Enterobacteriaceae is not carried on R factors and multiply resistant organisms may retain sensitivity to nalidixic acid.[15]

Mutation at the *nalA* locus results in resistance to high concentrations of nalidixic acid (>40 µg/ml). These resistant bacteria have an altered DNA gyrase A subunit and are cross-resistant to cinoxacin.[1] A second class of nalidixic acid–resistant bacteria (growth at 4 µg/ml but no growth at 10 µg/ml) are transport mutants.[17] Resistance to the nalidixic acid class of drugs develops rapidly by a stepwise process when sensitive bacteria are grown in low concentrations of drug.[18,19] This resistance probably reflects the selection of bacteria that are deficient in drug uptake.

Pharmacology

The pharmacokinetic characteristics of the nalidixic acid class of drugs are presented in Table 9–1.[20–22] Nalidixic acid is almost completely (96%) absorbed from the gastrointestinal tract.[23] It is rapidly metabolized by the liver to the biologically active compound 7-hydroxynalidixic acid and to glucuronide conjugated products, which are inactive.[22,23] One-third of the biologically active drug in the plasma is present as the hydroxylated metabolite, which is 63% bound to plasma protein, and the rest is the parent compound, which is 80%–93% bound.[20,24] Peak plasma levels (see Table 9–1) are achieved in 2 h. Although the peak levels in plasma are lower if these drugs are ingested with food, the urine drug concentrations are not significantly altered.[21] In animal studies it was shown that nalidixic acid does not associate with tissues, the kidney being the only organ found to have a higher level of drug than plasma.[23] Nalidixic acid does not distribute into prostatic fluid.[25] This is important, since chronic bacterial prostatitis is a very common cause of recurrent urinary tract infections in male patients. Thus, even in the presence of effective clearance of bacteria from the urinary tract in response to the drug, the organism can become reinstated because of seeding of the urine from foci of

Table 9–1. Pharmacokinetic characteristics of the nalidixic acid group of urinary tract antiseptics.

Drug	Usual adult dosage	Usual dosage interval (hours)	Peak plasma concentration of bioactive forms after usual dosage (μg/ml)	Plasma protein binding (%)	Peak concentration of total drug in urine 2–4 h after usual dosage (μg/ml)	Amount of drug in urine as unaltered drug or bioactive metabolite (%)	Amount of drug in urine as unaltered drug or bioactive metabolite (μg/ml)
Nalidixic acid	1 g	6	25–40	80–93	1200–1800	13–20	250–350
Cinoxacin	500 mg	12	10–20	63–73	400–600	50–60	200–300
	250 mg	6					

Source: Data from Mannisto,[20] Black et al.,[21] and Ferry et al.[22]

infection in the prostate, which is not exposed to the antibacterial action.

Nalidixic acid and its metabolites are excreted almost completely via the kidney. Over 80% of the drug in the urine is present as inactive glucuronide conjugates. About 25% of the unconjugated drug in the urine is present as 7-carboxynalidixic acid, which is biologically inactive.[22] This metabolite has not been detected in the plasma and is probably formed in the kidney.[22] Most of the rest of the unconjugated drug is present as the biologically active hydroxylated metabolite (which is more potent than nalidixic acid itself).[20,24] The therapeutic effect of this drug in the treatment of urinary tract infection is primarily due to the action of that metabolite, hydroxynalidixic acid. Half-lives of 1.5–6 h have been reported for nalidixic acid in patients with normal renal function.[20,22,23]

Because nalidixic acid is efficiently conjugated to the inactive glucuronide by the liver, bioactive forms of nalidixic acid do not accumulate in the serum of patients with renal failure.[26,27] The serum levels of the biologically inactive (but possibly toxic) monoglucuronides increase when the drug is given without dosage reduction to patients with renal failure.[28] Although increased toxicity has not been observed in patients with renal failure, nalidixic acid probably should not be used when the glomerular filtration rate is less than 10 ml/min.[29] The dialysis properties of nalidixic acid have not been well defined.[7] Adequate bactericidal activity is achieved in the urine of patients with moderate to severe renal failure.[26,27]

The pharmacology of cinoxacin is similar to that of nalidixic acid. Cinoxacin differs from nalidixic acid, however, in that it is less bound to serum protein and undergoes much less inactivation by conjugation.[21] As a result, similar levels of bactericidal activity may be achieved in the urine with cinoxacin when it is administered at one-fourth the daily dosage of nalidixic acid. Because plasma levels achieved with these drugs are low and because distribution across membranes is poor, they have been used in the United States only for treating urinary tract infections. In some countries, however, nalidixic acid has been administered parenterally for treating gram-negative infections outside the urinary tract.

Adverse Effects

Therapy with nalidixic acid and its analogs has been associated with a substantial incidence of adverse reactions.[14,30] Nausea is the most frequent adverse effect.[14] Other gastrointestinal effects include diarrhea, vomiting, and abdominal pain. A variety of skin reactions has been reported, including urticaria, pruritis, and erythematous and maculopapular rashes.[31] In addition to nonspecific rashes, nalidixic acid and its analogs produce a photosensitivity response most commonly manifested as a sunburn-like reaction and less often as a bullous eruption that tends to occur on the hands, feet, and legs.[32,33] The bullae usually resolve without scarring within 2 weeks of discontinuing therapy, but minor abnormal reactions to sunlight may persist for as long as several months after therapy is stopped.[32] Patients receiving nalidixic acid or its analogs should be cautioned to avoid excessive exposure to direct sunlight.

Nalidixic acid occasionally produces central nervous system side effects. Dizziness and headache are the most common complaints; weakness, drowsiness, restlessness, insomnia, and mild disorientation may also occur.[31] Rarely, severe reactions, such as convulsions[34] and toxic psychosis, have been reported. These drugs should not be given to patients with convulsive disorders or symptoms of cerebrovascular insufficiency. In infants and children, nalidixic acid has occasionally produced intracranial hypertension (pseudotumor cerebri) with papiledema, bulging fontanelles, headache, and vomiting.[35,36] The syndrome is reversible, although papiledema may persist for several months.[35] For this reason, nalidixic acid and its analogs should not be administered to infants and, if possible, their use should be avoided in young children. The mechanism for the benign intracranial hypertension has not been defined.[37] A variety of visual disturbances have been reported to occur occasionally during therapy with these drugs; they include blurring of vision, diplopia, difficulty of accommodation, photophobia, and changes in color perception.[7] The visual abnormalities all reverse upon cessation of therapy.

Nalidixic acid has rarely been associated with a variety of other side effects, including cholestatic jaundice, blood dyscrasias, hemolytic anemia (sometimes associated with glucose-6-phosphate dehydrogenase deficiency), and metabolic acidosis (see ref. 7 for review). It has been found that cinoxacin causes lameness, soreness, and swelling of weight-bearing joints in juvenile dogs.[38] Nalidixic acid also causes arthropathy in immature animals. This has not been reported in humans, but it is another reason to avoid the use of these drugs in pregnant

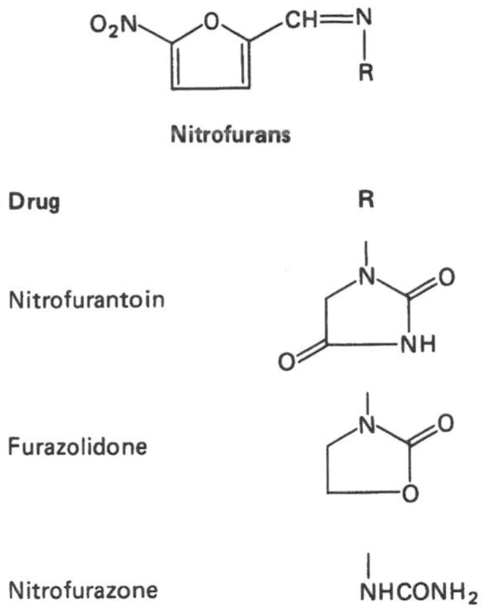

Figure 9–1. Structures of selected nitrofurans.

women and in children. The glucuronic acid liberated from the glucuronide conjugates of these agents in the urine can cause a false-positive reaction for glucose with certain test procedures. It has been suggested that cinoxacin causes fewer adverse reactions than nalidixic acid,[39] but the data are still too limited to establish a clear difference.

Nitrofurantoin

Several nitrofuran derivatives are being used clinically (see Fig. 9–1). Nitrofurazone, which is available in topical formulations, has a broad antibacterial effect against common skin pathogens. Furazolidone is a nitrofuran compound, which is marketed in oral preparations for treating intestinal infections caused by such organisms as *Salmonella, Shigella, Vibrio cholerae,* and *Giardia lamblia.*[40] Nitrofurantoin is available for use as a urinary tract antiseptic. The nitrofurans have been reviewed by Chamberlain[41] and by McCalla.[42]

Mechanism of Action

The nitrofurans inhibit a wide variety of enzyme systems in bacteria,[43,44] but their ability to cause DNA damage appears to be the primary event that leads to cell death. The use of mutant strains of *Escherichia coli* that are either resistant or supersensitive to nitrofurans has proved to be instrumental in developing a concept of their mechanism of action. The study of drug effects in nitrofurazone-resistant mutants first established that reduction of nitrofurans produces compounds that are more toxic than the nitrofurans themselves. Asnis and coworkers[45,46] selected mutants that were 10-fold resistant to nitrofurazone and showed that the resistant *E. coli* lacked a NADPH-dependent enzyme (nitrofuran reductase I) that reduces nitrofurazone and other nitrofuran derivatives, including nitrofurantoin. *E. coli* contain a second nitro reductase system (nitrofuran reductase II) that requires NADH, is inhibited by oxygen, and is therefore active only under anaerobic growth conditions. When the resistant strains lacking the oxygen-insensitive reductase I activity were incubated under anaerobic conditions, nitrofuran sensitivity was restored.[45,46] It has subsequently been demonstrated that lethality, mutation rate, and amount of DNA breakage are all markedly increased when these resistant *E. coli* are grown under anaerobic conditions in the presence of nitrofurazone.[47] These observations provide considerable evidence that reductive activation of nitrofurans is important for both DNA breakage and the bactericidal effect.

Reduction of nitrofurans by reductase I leads to end products with no antibacterial activity, but highly reactive, short-lived intermediates are formed during the course of the reduction.[48] These intermediates are thought to be responsible for DNA strand breakage, either through direct reaction with the DNA or through their ability to generate oxygen free-radicals. Additional evidence showing that DNA damage is a primary event leading to bacterial cell killing comes from studies comparing the sensitivity of wild-type *E. coli* to that of mutants that are defective in DNA repair. Both *E. coli* mutants that lack the ability to carry out post replication repair (*recA* mutants) and mutants that lack the "excision repair" system (*uvr* mutants) are more sensitive to nitrofurantoin than the nonmutant parent strains.[49,50] As the sensitivity of the cell varies inversely with its capacity to repair drug-induced DNA damage, it is reasonable to propose that DNA damage is the major factor behind the cytotoxic effect.[50]

The basis for the selective toxicity of nitrofurantoin probably rests on both its pharmacokinetic properties and selective activation in bacterial cells. Nitrofurantoin is rapidly excreted and the levels of drug in the plasma and tissues are low in comparison with that achieved in the urine. Mammalian tissues, such as liver and lung, can activate nitrofurantoin by reduction but bacteria reduce the drug much more rapidly.[42] It has been estimated, for example, that the specific activity of "nitrofurantoin reductase" in crude homogenates of mouse liver is at least 200 times lower than that of *E. coli*.[42]

Antimicrobial Activity and Clinical Use

Nitrofurantoin is active in vitro against a wide spectrum of gram-positive and gram-negative bacteria. As shown in Table 9–2, nitofurantoin is very active against staphylococci, streptococci, *Neisseria*, and *Bacteroides*.[51] The great majority (96%) of *Escherichia coli* strains are sensitive to 32 μg/ml or less of nitrofurantoin, whereas a minority (36%) of *Klebsiella* and *Enterobacter* species are sensitive at this level of drug.[52] *Proteus* are variably resistant and *Pseudo-*

Table 9–2. Susceptibility of selected organisms to nitrofrantoin.

Organism	MIC (μg/ml)
Staphylococcus aureus	6–12
Streptococcus pyogenes	3–12
Streptococcus faecalis	12–25
Neisseria gonorrhoeae	0.3–0.7
Bacteroides spp.	1.6–7
Escherichia coli	6–>200
Klebsiella-Enterobacter spp.	25–>200
Proteus spp.	32–>200
Pseudomonas aeruginosa	>200

MIC, minimum inhibitory concentration.

Source: Table modified from Chamberlain.[41]

monas aeruginosa is essentially always resistant.[52]

With standard oral therapy, nitrofurantoin does not yield sufficient serum or tissue levels of antimicrobial activity to permit its use in treating infection outside the urinary tract. It is employed for treatment of acute urinary tract infections by sensitive bacteria in patients who may not tolerate therapy with penicillins, sulfonamides, or tetracyclines. Because of the low tissue levels, nitrofurantoin should not be used to treat urinary tract infections with associated renal cortical or perinephric abscess. Its use for the initial treatment of acute infections has declined over the years because of the rather high frequency of gastrointestinal side effects associated with administration at the recommended doses (50–100 mg every 6 h for adults). But it has been shown that nitrofurantoin given in smaller amounts (50 to 100 mg/day) on a daily basis over a period of many months will reduce the frequency of recurrent urinary tract infections in females.[53–55] Continuous prophylaxis has also been reported to be beneficial in selected male patients with chronic or recurrent urinary tract infections.[56] Organisms isolated from the urine of women with recurrent infections generally remain sensitive to nitrofurantoin even after many courses of therapy, because nitrofurantoin does not appear in measurable amounts in the stool and resistance to nitrofurantoin is not transferable;[41] consequently, the sensitivity of intestinal flora is not altered.[57] Since reinfection from the bowel flora is the most common cause of recurrence of uncomplicated urinary tract infections in females, the fact that these organisms remain sensitive to nitrofurantoin is an advantage in both continuous prophylaxis and repeated courses of therapy.

Pharmacokinetics

Nitrofurantoin is provided in tablets and suspensions for oral administration and in sterile solution for intravenous administration. The drug is essentially completely absorbed (94%) from the gastrointestinal tract and the extent of absorption is not decreased when it is taken with food.[58] The oral preparation is provided in microcrystalline and macrocrystalline form. The macrocrystalline form was prepared in order to slow the rate of absorption from the gastrointestinal tract and decrease the amount of nausea and vomiting that patients experience with this drug. Several reports indicate that the incidence of gastrointestinal reactions may be lower with the macrocrystalline preparation.[59,60] Although the macrocrystalline form is absorbed more slowly, the percentage of drug recovered in the urine in 24 h (38%) is nearly the same as with the microcrystalline form (43%),[61] and the two preparations are therapeutically equivalent.[59,60]

Only very low levels of nitrofurantoin (less than 1 μg/ml) are achieved in the plasma after a normal therapeutic dosage of 50 or 100 mg,[61,62] and there is no accumulation of drug in the tissues or in body fluids other than urine and bile.[63] Nitrofurantoin is excreted by both glomerular filtration and tubular secretion and there is significant reabsorption when the urine is acid.[64] Although the urine concentration of nitrofurantoin can be increased by alkalinization, the antibacterial activity is decreased.[65] Thus, efforts to increase pH are nonproductive.[65] Nitrofurantoin is also excreted into the bile, but there is extensive reabsorption from the intestine[66] and the principal route of excretion of the active drug is via the kidney. In patients with normal renal function, the serum half-life is short (0.6–1.2 h)[58,62,67] because of both rapid excretion in the kidney and rapid enzymatic degradation of the drug in the tissues.[43,44] Nitrofurantoin has been shown by autoradiographic techniques to be present in the interstitial fluid of the renal medulla[68] and bacteriological methods have shown that it achieves a several-fold higher concentration in the lymphatics draining the medulla than in the plasma.[69] With normal renal function, the peak urine concentration of nitrofurantoin after oral administration of a 100 mg tablet ranges between 50 and 250 μg/ml.[58,70] The recovery of drug from the urine is linearly related to the rate of creatinine clearance, and the drug concentration in the urine of uremic patients is not high enough to treat common urinary tract pathogens.[70] Nitrofurantoin is contraindicated in patients with imparied renal function (creatinine clearance less than 40 ml/min),[70] both because inadequate urine concentrations are achieved and the risk of developing neuropathy may be increased.[71]

Adverse Effects

The most common undesirable effects associated with nitrofurantoin therapy are nausea and vomiting.[55,72] The frequency increases with the daily dosage per unit body weight.[72] Nausea and vomiting appear to result from an action of the drug on the central nervous system rather than on the gastrointestinal tract.[72] This proposal is consistent with the observation that symptoms of local gastric irritation, such as heartburn, abdominal pain, or gastrointestinal bleeding, are rare and the observation that nausea and vomiting occur after intravenous injection of nitrofurantoin.[72] In some patients, nausea and vomiting may be controlled by lowering the dosage or slowing the rate of absorption by ingesting the drug with food or administering the macrocrystalline form.[59,60]

Table 9–3 compares the incidence of untoward effects of nitrofurantoin therapy to those of two sulfonamides commonly employed in the treatment of urinary tract infections. The overall incidence of reaction severe enough to require discontinuation of nitrofurantoin therapy (9.2% in this study) is significantly higher than that observed with the sulfonamides; also, most nitrofurantoin reactions are toxic in nature, whereas

reactions to the sulfonamides are predominantly of the allergic type.[72] The allergic reactions to nitrofurantoin include a variety of rashes, urticaria, pruritis, angioneurotic edema, eosinophilia, and drug fever. Nitrofurantoin is rarely associated with the production of anaphylaxis, a "lupus-like" syndrome, vasculitis, arthralgia, and the precipitation of acute asthmatic attacks in asthmatic patients.

A few cases of hematologic reaction have been reported, including granulocytopenia, leukopenia, and megaloblastic anemia.[41,72] These reactions have been reversible on discontinuation of therapy. Acute hemolytic anemia can occur in patients with inherited glucose-6-phosphate dehydrogenase deficiency and in infants with immature enzyme systems involved in glutathione synthesis. For this reason, the drug is contraindicated in pregnant patients at term and in infants under 1 month of age. The hemolysis probably results from damage to erythrocyte membranes, which is caused by lipid peroxidation. Nitrofurantoin metabolites produce active oxygen species and have been shown to deplete glutathione content in human lymphocytes.[73] In the red cell, glutathione peroxidase appears to be the major mechanism of defense against oxidative membrane damage that leads to hemolysis[74] (see discussion of glucose-6-phosphate dehydrogenase deficiency in Chapter 13). Thus, the patient who has a reduced capacity to synthesize glutathione may experience hemolytic anemia during nitrofurantoin therapy.[73]

Table 9–3. *Incidence of adverse reactions to nitrofurantoin and two soluble sulfonamides commonly used to treat urinary infections.* Adverse reactions were monitored during 2118 courses of therapy with sulfisoxazole, sulfamethoxazole, or nitrofurantoin in a prospective study.

Drug	Number of courses of therapy	Total reactions		Toxic reactions		Allergic reactions	
		Number	Reaction rate (%)	Number	Reaction rate (%)	Number	Reaction rate (%)
Sulfisoxazole	1002	30	3.1	3	0.3	28	2.8
Sulfamethoxazole	359	12	3.3	1	0.3	11	3.0
Nitrofurantoin	757	70	9.2	39	5.1	31	4.1

Source: Data from Koch-Weser et al.[72]

Nitrofurantoin causes two types of pulmonary reactions.[75-77] The acute reaction is characterized by fever, cough, and dyspnea starting an average of 9 days after the initiation of treatment.[78] The chest X-ray generally shows infiltration, especially in the base of the lungs, and pleural effusion often occurs. Eosinophilia is present in 60%–80% of cases.[77,78] Patients with this acute reaction recover within 2–3 weeks after stopping the drug. Several features of the acute reaction strongly suggest that it is immunologically mediated,[76,77] particularly the fact that the entire syndrome recurs after rechallenge with the drug.[79] There is some evidence implicating cell-mediated immunity as a mechanism for this type of nitrofurantoin sensitivity.[80]

The second type of pulmonary reaction is rare, and it occurs almost solely in patients who are on continuous long-term therapy.[77] In this chronic reaction, the onset of symptoms is insidious, and consists primarily of exertional dyspnea and cough.[76] The pathological features are those of interstitial fibrosis with or without interstitial pneumonitis. Most patients with the chronic type of pulmonary reaction improve when therapy is stopped, but in two-thirds of these patients there is some residual radiological evidence of fibrotic changes.[78] There is good experimental support for the proposal that the chronic pulmonary reaction is a toxic effect due to the production of active species of oxygen that cause the tissue damage. Addition of nitrofurantoin to aerobic incubation mixtures containing rat lung microsomes and NADPH causes the production of superoxide anion and other active oxygen species as a result of redox cycling of the drug as shown in Figure 9–2.[81] Subcutaneous administration of nitrofurantoin to rats causes severe pulmonary damage and the acute lethality of nitrofurantoin in this animal model is promoted if the animals are fed a diet deficient in vitamin E (α-tochopherol), which acts as a free-radical scavenger, and if the animals are exposed to an oxygen-enriched atmosphere.[82] These results, coupled with the demonstration of redox cycling of the drug with the generation of reactive oxygen, suggest that the syndrome may result from peroxidative destruction of pulmonary membrane lipid by reactive oxygen derivatives as shown in the model presented in Figure 9–2. The high oxygen tension of lung tissue presumably could promote high rates of redox cycling of the drug and account for manifestation of the toxicity in this organ.

Nitrofurantoin has rarely been associated with both acute and chronic types of liver injury. Both hepatocellular and cholestatic forms of acute, reversible injury have been reported.[83] In many cases, the acute injury appears to have an allergic basis.[83] A few patients receiving long-term therapy have developed chronic, active hepatitis.[84,85] Although there have been a couple of deaths, patients with hepatitis generally improve when the drug is withdrawn. Some features of the chronic hepatitis suggest that it also has an immunologic basis; for example, most these patients have antinuclear antibodies.[84,85] About 40% of patients with the chronic pulmonary reaction to nitrofurantoin have elevated transaminase activities, indicating some degree of liver injury.[77,78] Direct toxic effects may also play a role in the genesis of the chronic, active hepatitis. It has been shown, for example, that liver microsomal enzymes reduce nitrofurantoin, and under aerobic conditions, autooxidation of the drug is accompanied by the generation of active oxygen species that could produce hepatic damage.[86] In addition to chronic, active hepatitis, there are isolated reports of nitrofurantoin-induced granulomatous hepatitis.[87] Clearly, patients on prolonged nitrofurantoin therapy should have their liver function monitored periodically.

Nitrofurantoin occasionally causes headaches, dizziness, nystagmus, drowsiness, and peripheral neuropathy. The latter is typically an ascending sensorimotor peripheral neuropathy and the mechanism is unknown.[88] Impaired renal function probably increases the risk of developing neuropathy,[71] but it may occur in patients with normal renal function receiving normal dosage, and therapy should be terminated if signs of peripheral neuritis occur. Several of the nitrofuran derivatives have been shown to arrest spermatogenesis in animals.[43] At high local concentrations, nitrofurantoin immobilizes hu-

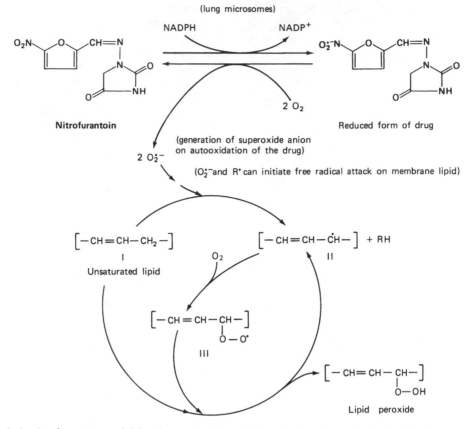

Figure 9–2. A schematic model for the mechanism of chronic nitrofurantoin-induced pulmonary injury via lipid peroxidation. After nitrofurantoin undergoes a one-electron reduction that is catalyzed by a NADPH-dependent microsomal reductase in lung tissue, the drug is regenerated autocatalytically with the production of superoxide anion ($O_2^{\cdot-}$). The $O_2^{\cdot-}$ and reactive species derived from it (R·), such as peroxy radicals and hydroxyl radicals, can remove hydrogen from unsaturated fatty acid (I) to yield the fatty acid free radical (II), which reacts with oxygen to produce a fatty acid peroxy radical (III). In some cases a cycle may be set up in which III can abstract a proton from another molecule of I to yield an unsaturated fatty acid hydroperoxide and another molecule of II, which can continue the autocatalytic chain reaction of lipid peroxidation. Continued lipid peroxidation destroys membranes, impairing the function of cell organelles (e.g., mitochondria) and producing the degenerative changes that lead eventually to pulmonary fibrosis. Based on observations by Sasame and Boyd[81] and Boyd et al.[82])

man sperm, and it has been suggested that irrigation of the vas deferens with the drug during male sterilization may eliminate the postoperative interval before the viable sperm count drops to zero.[89] Nitrofurantoin and nitrofurazone have also been shown to have radiosensitizing properties in hypoxic cells,[90] and nitrofurazone (but not nitrofurantoin) has been shown to produce double-stranded DNA breaks in mammalian cells under anaerobic conditions.[91] A number of the nitrofuran compounds are both mutagenic and carcinogenic. Nitrofurantoin is

weakly mutagenic,[42] but it has not been shown to be carcinogenic.[50,92] However, nitrofurantoin, like the carcinogenic nitrofurans, is metabolized by mammalian cells to a product that reacts covalently with cellular macromolecules.[93]

Methenamine

Methenamine has been used as a urinary tract antiseptic for many years; most of the details of its pharmacology and action were

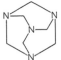

Methenamine

worked out in 1913.[94] Methenamine itself is not bactericidal, but it is hydrolyzed at acid pH to ammonia and formaldehyde, which is the active bactericidal agent. Formaldehyde

$$N_4(CH_2)_6 + 6H_2O + 4H^+ \rightarrow 4NH_4^+ + 6HCHO$$

is probably bactericidal by virtue of its ability to denature protein. If bacteria are exposed to formaldehyde and then washed and suspended in formaldehyde-free medium, there is a delay before the remaining viable organisms begin growing again.[95] This bacteriostatic effect may be useful in therapy, since the organisms that remain in the bladder after voiding may function as a less effective inoculum in the fresh urine that is subsequently produced. Exposure to at least 25 µg of formaldehyde per ml of urine for at least 2 h is required for a good bacteriostatic effect against gram-negative bacteria.[95]

Methenamine is well absorbed from the gastrointestinal tract;[96] the usual dosage is 1 g given orally four times a day. Some drug is lost because of hydrolysis in the stomach, so enteric-coated preparations have been made available with the intention of reducing this loss. Methenamine distributes widely in the body spaces. But since almost no formaldehyde is generated at physiological pH, there is no antibacterial activity in blood, tissues, or body fluids. The elimination half-life is about 4 h.[97] The concentration of formaldehyde achieved in the urine will vary according to the urine pH, the concentration of methenamine, and the time of retention of urine in the bladder.[95,98] Since formaldehyde is formed only in an acid environment, it is important that the urine be at pH 5.6 or lower. Normally an acidifying agent, such as ascorbic acid, has been administered with methenamine. But this practice has been questioned because the customary doses of ascorbic acid fail to influence the urinary pH and there is no documentation that its administration en-

hances the therapeutic activity of the methenamine compounds.[96]

Methenamine may also be obtained as the mandelic or hippuric acid salt. These formulations were prepared in order to provide the drug with its own acidifying agent. Although they are popular preparations, there is no evidence that these organic acids affect the urine pH at all when they are administered in the amount provided in the formulations. Mandelic and hippuric acids have some antibacterial effect of their own. Their antibacterial action is due to the undissociated form of the acid, which is only present in significant amounts at acid pH, but the concentration of these acids likely to be obtained after therapeutic doses is insufficient to produce an antibacterial effect alone.[99] At the recommended dosage (which is the same as the dosage for the pure base), the mandelic and hippuric acid salts contain less methenamine. Thus, the salts are probably not superior to administering methenamine itself, and they may provide less antibacterial activity.

Methenamine is used only for prophylactic or suppressive therapy. It has been shown to be useful in the management of recurrent urinary tract infection in females,[55,96] although it does not appear to be as effective as trimethoprim-sulfamethoxazole (TMP-SMX) administered once daily.[100] Methenamine has also been reported to be useful in prophylactic therapy of males with chronic bacteriuria.[56] Methenamine does not prevent infection in patients with indwelling catheters or in those undergoing intermittent catheterization.[101] The drug cannot be used to treat infections of the upper urinary tract because there is inadequate time for the generation of sufficient amounts of formaldehyde during the passage of urine through the kidney. Thus, methenamine is employed to sterilize the lower urinary tract between acute episodes of infection that are better treated with other drugs. Methenamine is generally not useful against such urea-splitting organisms as *Proteus*. These bacteria produce urease, an enzyme that breaks down urea into ammonia, thus raising the pH of the urine. In the presence of these organisms, it may be difficult or impossible to acidify the urine to the point at which sufficient formaldehyde is generated from methenamine. Acetohydroxamic acid, a urease inhibitor, has been shown to be synergistic with methenamine against *Proteus* in some culture systems in vitro.[102] Such a combined approach could prove useful in therapy if a nontoxic urease inhibitor were available.

Methenamine is usually well tolerated, with gastric distress and allergic reactions occurring occasionally.[96] Some patients complain of symptoms of bladder irritation (dysuria, frequency, hematuria, urgency). The mandelic acid salt should not be given to patients in renal failure, since it can cause crystalluria if urine flow is inadequate.[96] Methenamine should not be given to patients with hepatic insufficiency because ammonia is produced in the acid environment of the stomach and urine. Methenamine and sulfonamides should not be given concomitantly because formaldehyde forms an insoluble product with some of the sulfonamides.[103]

Fosfomycin

Fosfomycin is a broad-spectrum antibiotic that has been used parenterally in Europe for many years and it is approved by the Food and Drug Administration for single-dose treatment of uncomplicated urinary tract infections in women.

Fosfomycin

Fosfomycin, a *cis*- 1,2-epoxypropylphosphonic acid, is an organic phosphonate. It was originally isolated as a fermentation product from certain *Streptomyces* species but is now produced synthetically. It is available in the United States as the soluble sodium salt of fosfomycin trometamol.

Antimicrobial Activity and Mechanism of Action

Fosfomycin is moderately active against a wide range of pathogens, but its activity in vitro is reduced at an alkaline pH and by the presence of glucose, phosphates, or sodium chloride in the culture medium. Consequently, different sensitivity data may be obtained, depending on the medium used. It is in general more active against gram-negative bacilli than gram-positive cocci, although most strains of *Staphylococcus aureus* (including methicillin-resistant strains) are susceptible and *Pseudomonas aeruginosa* is usually resistant.[104] Fosfomycin is moderately active against *E. coli* and many other common pathogens of uncomplicated urinary tract infections. It is also active against most strains of enterococci, including some strains resistant to other antibiotics.

Fosfomycin and related organic phosphonates interfere with synthesis of the bacterial cell wall by inhibiting the enzyme phosphoenolpyruvate transferase, which catalyzes the first step in peptidoglycan synthesis.[105] Fosfomycin enters the bacterial cell via an active transport system for hexose phosphates. In many gram-negative bacteria (e.g., *E. coli*), this pathway is induced by glucose 6-phosphate, thus potentiating the activity of fosfomycin in vitro. As with other drugs that interfere with cell wall synthesis, synergy has been demonstrated against some organisms when fosfomycin is administered with an aminoglycoside.[105] Resistance to fosfomycin emerges rapidly if given in multiple doses, but cross-resistance to other important antibiotics does not occur and it is active against many strains resistant to other antibiotics.[106,107]

Pharmacokinetics

Fosfomycin can be administered both parenterally (disodium salt) and orally (calcium and trimethamine salts). The trometamol (trimethamine) salt is very well absorbed after oral administration and peak serum concentrations of drug are achieved in less than 2 h.[108] The sodium salt is only administered parenterally, as it causes gastric irritation. Fosfomycin is widely distributed throughout body fluids and tissues. Levels in the cerebrospinal fluid are about 10% of serum levels; increased drug levels are achieved when there is meningeal inflammation.[109] Fosfomycin is excreted as the unchanged drug by glomerular filtration into the urine where high concentrations accumulate (in excess of 200 mg/liter for 24 to 48 h) after a single dose.[104] The serum half-life is 4 h after an oral dose.[108]

Clinical Uses and Adverse Effects

Fosfomycin has been used in Europe to treat respiratory, gastrointestinal, and urinary tract infections. The trometamol salt has been particularly effective for the single-dose treatment of urinary tract infections in women. Single-dose or very short therapy for the treatment of urinary tract infections has several potential advantages, including less alteration of the bowel flora from which resistant strains may emerge and cause reinfection, fewer adverse effects, better compliance, and decreased cost.[106] In three randomized trials, a single dose of fosfomycin was compared to multiple doses of nitrofurantoin, norfloxacin, or cephalexin in treatment of women with uncomplicated urinary tract infections. Treatment with fosfomycin eradicated bacteriuria in over 90% of the women, a rate similar to those with norfloxacin and nitrofurantoin and superior to that of cephalexin.[110–112]

Fosfomycin is generally well tolerated. Adverse reactions have been observed in about 10%–17% of patients, with gastrointestinal disorders, principally diarrhea, being most common. Vaginitis occurrs in a smaller number of patients, and reversible elevations in serum transaminase may occur.

REFERENCES

1. Pedrini, A. M. Nalidixic acid. In *Antibiotics V-1*, ed. by F. E. Hahn. New York: Springer-Verlag, 1979, pp. 154–175.

2. Cozzarelli, N. R. DNA gyrase and the supercoiling of DNA. *Science* 1980;207:953.

3. Gellert, M. DNA topoisomerases. *Annu. Rev. Biochem.* 1981;50:879.

4. Deitz, W. H., J. H. Bailey, and E. J. Froelich. In vitro antibacterial properties of nalidixic acid, a new drug active against gram-negative organisms. *Antimicrob. Agents Chemother*—1963 1964;583.

5. Brumfitt, W., and R. Pursell. Observations on bacterial sensitivities to nalidixic acid and critical comments on the 6-centre survey. *Postgrad. Med. J.* 1971;47(Suppl.):16.

6. Stamey, T. A. Observations on the clinical use of nalidixic acid. *Postgrad. Med. J.* 1971;47(Suppl.):21.

7. Gleckman, R., S. Alvarez, D. W. Joubert, and S. J. Mathews. Drug therapy reviews: nalidixic acid. *Am. J. Hosp. Pharm.* 1979;36:1071.

8. Wick, W. E., D. A. Preston, W. A. White, and R. S. Gordee. Compound 64716, a new synthetic antibacterial agent. *Antimicrob. Agents Chemother.* 1973;4:415.

9. Bauernfeind, A. Mode of action of of nalidixic acid. *Antibiot. Chemother.* 1971;17:122.

10. Stevens, P. J. E. Bactericidal effect against *Escherichia coli* of nalidixic acid and four structurally related compounds. *J. Antimicrob. Chemother.* 1980;6:535.

11. Bucy, J. G. A clinical comparison of cinoxacin and nalidixic acid in the treatment of urinary tract infection. *J. Urol.* 1981;125:822.

12. Schaeffer, A. J., S. Flynn, and J. Jones. Comparison of cinoxacin and trimethoprim-sulfamethoxazole in the treatment of urinary tract infections. *J. Urol.* 1981;125:825.

13. Ronald, A. R., M. Turck, and R. G. Petersdorf. A critical evaluation of nalidixic acid in urinary-tract infections. *N. Engl. J. Med.* 1966;275:1081.

14. Atlas, E., H. Clark, F. Silverblatt, and M. Turck. Nalidixic acid and oxolinic acid in the treatment of chronic bacteriuria. *Ann. Intern. Med.* 1969;70:713.

15. Stamey, T. A. Resistance to nalidixic acid: a misconception due to underdosage. *JAMA* 1976;236:1857.

16. Preiksaitis, J. K., L. Thompson, G. K. M. Harding, T. J. Marrie, S. Hoban, and A. R. Ronald. A comparison of the efficacy of nalidixic acid and cephalexin in bacteriuric women and their effect on fecal and periurethral carriage of Enterobacteriaceae. *J. Infect. Dis.* 1981;146:603.

17. Bourguignon, G. T., M. Levitt, and R. Sternglanz. Studies on the mechanism of action of nalidixic acid. *Antimicrob. Agents Chemother.* 1973;4:479.

18. Giamarellou, H., and G. G. Jackson. Antibacterial activity of cinoxacin in vitro. *Antimicrob. Agents Chemother* 1975;7:668.

19. Lumish, R. M., and C. W. Norden. Cinoxacin: in vitro antibacterial studies of a new synthetic organic acid. *Antimicrob. Agents Chemother.* 1975;7:159.

20. Mannisto, P. T. Pharmacokinetics of nalidixic acid and oxolinic acid in healthy women. *Clin. Pharmacol. Ther.* 1976;19:37.

21. Black, H. R., K. S. Israel, R. L. Wolan, G. L. Brier, B. O. Obermeyer, E. A. Ziege, and J. D. Wolny. Pharmacology of cinoxacin in humans. *Antimicrob. Agents Chemother.* 1979;15:165.

22. Ferry, N., G. Cuisinaud, N. Pozet, P. Y. Zech, and J. Sassard. Nalidixic acid kinetics after single and repeated oral doses. *Clin. Pharmacol. Ther.* 1981;29:695.

23. McChesney, E. W., E. J. Froelich, G. Y. Lesher, A. V. R. Crain, and D. Rosi. Absorption, excretion and metabolism of a new antibacterial agent, nalidixic acid. *Toxicol. Appl. Pharmacol.* 1964;6:292.

24. Portmann, G. A., E. W. McChesney, H. Stander, and W. E. Moore. Pharmacokinetic model for nalidixic acid in man. II. Parameters for absorption, metabolism and elimination. *J. Pharm. Sci.* 1966;55:72.

25. Stamey, T. A., E. M. Meares, and D. G. Winningham. Chronic bacterial prostatitis and the diffusion of drugs into prostatic fluid. *J. Urol.* 1970;103:187.

26. Stamey, T. A., N. J. Nemoy, and M. Higgins. The clinical use of nalidixic acid: a review and some observations. *Invest. Urol.* 1969;6:582.

27. Mohring, K., and P. O. Madsen. Treatment of urinary tract infections with oxolinic acid in patients with normal and impaired renal function. *Del. Med. J.* 1971;43:376.

28. Adam, W. R., and J. K. Dawborn. Plasma levels and urinary excretion of nalidixic acid in patients with renal failure. *Aust. N.Z. J. Med.* 1971;1:126.

29. Bennett, W. M., R. S. Muther, R. A. Parker, P. Feig, G. Morrison, T. A. Golper, and I. Singer. Drug therapy in renal failure: dosing guidelines for adults. *Ann. Intern. Med.* 1980;93:62.

30. Ghatikar, K. N. A multicentric trial of a new synthetic antibacterial in urinary tract infections. *Curr. Ther. Res.* 1974;16:130.

31. Australian Drug Evaluation Committee. Adverse effects of drugs commonly used in the treatment of urinary tract infection. *Med. J. Aust.* 1972;1:435.

32. Ramsay, C. A., and E. Obreshkova. Photosensitivity from nalidixic acid. *Br. J. Dermatol.* 1974;91:523.

33. Brauner, G. J. Bullous photoreaction to nalidixic acid. *Am. J. Med.* 1975;58:576.

34. Fraser, A. G., and A. D. B. Harrower. Convulsions and hyperglycemia associated with nalidixic acid. *BMJ* 1977;2:1518.

35. Cohen, D. N. Intacranial hypertension and papilledema associated with nalidixic acid therapy. *Am. J. Ophthalmol.* 1973;76:680.

36. Rao, K. G. Pseudotumor cerebri associated with nalidixic acid. *Urology* 1974;4:204.

37. Chadwick, D. Antibiotics and benign intracranial hypertension. *J. Antimicrob. Chemother.* 1982;9:88.

38. Howard, L. C., D. C. VanSickle, K. Deshmukh, W. J. Griffing, and N. V. Owen. Cinoxacin induced arthropathy in juvenile beagle dogs. *Toxicol. Appl. Pharmacol.* 1979;48:A145.

39. Drylie, D. M. Cinoxacin and nalidixic acid in treatment of urinary tract infections. *Urology* 1981;17:500.

40. Craft, J. C., T. Murphy, and J. D. Nelson. Furizolidone and quinacrine. Comparative study of therapy for giardiasis in children. *Am. J. Dis. Child.* 1981;135:164.

41. Chamberlain, R. E. Chemotherapeutic properties of prominent nitrofurans. *J. Antimicrob. Chemother.* 1976;2:325.

42. McCalla, D. R. Nitrofurans. In *Antibiotics V-1*, ed. by F. E. Hahn. New York: Springer-Verlag, 1979, pp. 176–213.

43. Paul, H. E., and M. F. Paul. The nitrofurans—chemotherapeutic properties (first of two parts). In *Experimental Chemotherapy*, Vol. 2, ed. by R. J. Schnitzer

and F. Hawking. New York: Academic Press, 1964, pp. 307–370.

44. Paul, H. E., and M. F. Paul. The nitrofurans—chemotherapeutic properties (second of two parts). In *Experimental Chemotherapy*, Vol. 4, ed. by R. J. Schnitzer and F. Hawking. New York: Academic Press, 1966, pp. 521–536.

45. Asnis, R. E., F. B. Cohen, and J. S. Gots. Studies on bacterial resistance to furacin. *Antibiot. Chemother.* 1952;2:213.

46. Asnis, R. E. The reduction of furacin by cell-free extracts of furacin-resistant and parent susceptible strains of *Escherichia coli*. *Arch. Biochem. Biophys.* 1957;66:208.

47. McCalla, D. R., P. Olive, Y. Tu and M. L. Fan. Nitrofurazone-reducing enzymes in *E. coli* and their role in drug activation in vivo. *Can. J. Microbiol.* 1975;21:1484.

48. McCalla, D. R., A. Reuvers, and C. Kaiser. Mode of action of nitrofurazone. *J. Bacteriol.* 1970;104:1126.

49. Jenkins, S. T., and P. M. Bennett. Effect of mutations in deoxyribonucleic acid repair pathways on the sensitivity of *Escherichia coli* K-12 strains to nitrofurantoin. *J. Bacteriol.* 1976;125:1214.

50. McCalla; D. R. Biological effects of nitrofurans. *J. Antimicrob. Chemother.* 1977;3:517.

51. Ralph, E. D. The bactericidal activity of nitrofurantoin and metronidazole against anaerobic bacteria. *J. Antimicrob. Chemother.* 1978;4:177.

52. Turck, M., A. R. Ronald, and R. G. Petersdorf. Susceptibility of Enterobacteriaceae to nitrofurantoin correlated with eradication of bacteriuria. *Antimicrob. Agents Chemother—1966.* 1967;446.

53. Stamey, T. A., M. Condy, and G. Mihara. Prophylactic efficacy of nitrofurantoin macrocrystals and trimethoprim-sulfamethoxazole in urinary infections. *N. Engl. J. Med.* 1977;296:780.

54. Lohr, J. A., D. H. Numley, S. S. Howards, and R. F. Ford. Prevention of recurrent urinary tract infections in girls. *Pediatrics* 1977;59:562.

55. Brumfitt, W., J. Cooper, and J. M. T. Hamilton-Miller. Prevention of recurrent urinary tract infections in women: a comparative trial between nitrofurantoin and methenamine hippurate. *J. Urol.* 1981;126:71.

56. Freeman, R. B., W. M. Smith, J. A. Richardson, P. J. Hennelly, R. J. Thurm, C. Urner, J. A. Vaillancourt, R. J. Griep, and L. Bromer. Long-term therapy for chronic bacteriuria in men: U.S. Public Health Service cooperative study. *Ann. Intern. Med.* 1975;83:133.

57. Winberg, J., T. Bergstrom, K. Lincoln, and G. Lidin-Janson. Treatment trials in urinary tract infection (UTI) with special reference to the effect of antimicrobials on the fecal and periurethral flora. *Clin. Nephrol.* 1973;1:142.

58. Hoener, B., and S. E. Patterson. Nitrofurantoin disposition. *Clin. Pharmacol. Ther.* 1981;29:808.

59. Kalowski, S., N. Radford, and P. Kincaid-Smith. Crystalline and macrocrystalline nitrofurantoin in the treatment of urinary-tract infection. *N. Engl. J. Med.* 1974;290:385.

60. Hailey, F. J., and H. W. Glascock. Gastrointestinal tolerance to a new macrocrystalline form of nitro-

furantoin: a collaborative study. *Curr. Ther. Res.* 1967; 9:600.

61. Conklin, J. D., and F. J. Hailey. Urinary drug excretion in man during oral dosage of different nitrofurantoin formulations. *Clin. Pharmacol. Ther.* 1969; 10:534.

62. Maier-Lenz, H., L. Ringwelski, and A. Windorfer. Comparative pharmacokinetics and relative bioavailability for different preparations of nitrofurantoin. *Arzneim-Forsch.* 1979;29:1898.

63. Conklin, J. D. Biopharmaceutics of nitrofurantoin. *Pharmacology* 1972;8:178.

64. Schirmeister, J., F. Stephani, H. Willmann, and W. Hallauer. Renal handling of nitrofurantoin in man. *Antimicrobial Agents and Chemotherapy—1965.* 1966; 223.

65. Brumfitt, W., and A. Percival. Laboratory control of antibiotic therapy in urinary tract infection. *Ann. N.Y. Acad. Sci.* 1967;145:329.

66. Conklin, J. D., R. J. Sobers, and D. L. Wagner. Further studies on nitrofurantoin excretion in dog hepatic bile. *Br. J. Pharmacol.* 1973;48:273.

67. Liedtke, R. K., S. Ebel, B. Missler, W. Haase, and I. Stein. Single dose pharmacokinetics of macrocrystalline nitrofurantoin formulations. *Arzneim.-Forsch.* 1980;30:833.

68. Currie, G. A., P. J. Little, and S. J. McDonald. The localization of cephaloridine and nitrofurantoin in the kidney. *Nephron* 1966;3:282.

69. Katz, Y. J., A. T. K. Cockett, and R. S. Moore. Renal lymph and antibacterial levels in the treatment of pyelonephritis. *Life Sci.* 1964;3:1249.

70. Sachs, J., T. Geer, P. Noell, and C. M. Kunin. Effect of renal function on urinary recovery of orally administered nitrofurantoin. *N. Engl. J. Med.* 1968; 278:1032.

71. Felts, J. H., D. M. Hayes, J. A. Gergen, and J. F. Toole. Neural, hematologic and bacteriologic effects of nitrofurantoin in renal insufficiency. *Am. J. Med.* 1971; 51:331.

72. Koch-Weser, J., V. W. Sidel, M. Dexter, C. Parish, D. C. Finer, and P. Kanarek. Adverse reactions to sulfisoxazole, sulfamethoxazole, and nitrofurantoin. *Arch. Intern. Med.* 1971;128:399.

73. Spielberg, S. P., and G. B. Gordon. Nitrofurantoin cytotoxicity: in vitro assessment of risk based on glutathione metabolism. *J. Clin. Invest.* 1981;67:37.

74. Cohen, G., and P. Hochstein. Glutathione peroxidase: the primary agent for elimination of hydrogen peroxide in erythrocytes. *Biochemistry* 1963; 2:1420.

75. Hailey, F. J., H. W. Glascock, and W. F. Hewitt. Pleuropneumonic reactions to nitrofurantoin. *N. Engl. J. Med.* 1969;281:1087.

76. Holmberg, L., G. Boman, L. E. Bottinger, B. Eriksson, R. Spross, and A. Wessling. Adverse reactions to nitrofurantoin. Analysis of 921 reports. *Am. J. Med.* 1980;69:733.

77. Holmberg, L., and G. Boman. Pulmonary reactions to nitrofurantoin, *Eur. J. Respir. Dis.* 1981;62: 180.

78. Sovijarvi, A. R. A., M. Lemola, B. Stenius, and J. Idanpaan-Keikkila. Nitrofurantoin-induced acute,

subacute and chronic pulmonary reactions. *Scand. J. Respir. Dis.* 1977;58:41.

79. Nicklaus, T. M., and A. B. Snyder. Nitrofurantoin pulmonary reaction: a unique syndrome. *Arch. Intern. Med.* 1968;121:151.

80. Pearsall, H. R., J. Ewalt, M. S. Tsoi, S. Sumida, D. Bachus, R. H. Winterbauer, D. R. Webb, and H. Jones. Nitrofurantoin lung sensitivity: report of a case with prolonged nitrofurantoin lymphocyte sensitivity and interaction of nitrofurantoin-stimulated lymphocytes with alveolar cells. *J. Lab. Clin. Med.* 1974;83: 728.

81. Sasame, H. A., and M. R. Boyd. Superoxide and hydrogen peroxide production and NADPH oxidation stimulated by nitrofurantoin in lung microsomes: possible implications for toxicity. *Life Sci.* 1979;24: 1091.

82. Boyd, M. R., G. L. Catignani, H. A. Sasame, J. R. Mitchell, and A. W. Stiko. Acute pulmonary injury in rats by nitrofurantoin and modification by vitamin E, dietary fat, and oxygen. *Am. Rev. Respir. Dis.* 1979; 120:93.

83. Goldstein, L. I., K. G. Ishak, and W. Burns. Hepatic injury associated with nitrofurantoin therapy. *Am. J. Digest. Dis.* 1974;19:987.

84. Sharp, J. R., K. G. Ishak, and H. J. Zimmerman. Chronic active hepatitis and severe hepatic necrosis associated with nitrofurantoin. *Ann. Intern. Med.* 1980; 92:14.

85. Black, M., L. Rabin, and N. Schatz. Nitrofurantoin-induced chronic active hepatitis. *Ann. Intern. Med.* 1980;92:62.

86. Jonen, H. G., Reductive and oxidative metabolism of nitrofurantoin in rat liver. *Naunyn-Schmied. Arch. Pharmacol.* 1980;315:167.

87. Sippel, P. J., and W. A. Agger. Nitrofurantoin-induced granulomatous hepatitis. *Urology* 1981;18: 177.

88. Toole, J. F., and M. L. Parrish. Nitrofurantoin polyneuropathy. *Neurology* 1973;23:554.

89. Albert, P. S., D. J. Mininberg, and J. E. Davis. Nitrofurans: sperm-immmobilizing agents. Their tissue toxicity and clinical application. *Urology* 1974;4:307.

90. Chapman, J. D., A. P. Reuvers, J. Borsa, A. Petkau, and D. R. McCalla. Nitrofurans as radiosensitizers of hypoxic mammalian cells. *Cancer Res.* 1972;32: 2616.

91. Olive, P. L., and D. R. McCalla. Damage to mammalian cell DNA by nitrofurans. *Cancer Res.* 1975;35:781.

92. Morris, J. E., J. M. Price, J. J. Lalich, and R. J. Stein. The carcinogenic activity of some 5-nitrofuran derivatives in the rat. *Cancer Res.* 1969;29:2145.

93. Boyd, M. R., A. W. Stiko and H. A. Sasame. Metabolic activation of nitrofurantoin: possible implications for carcinogenesis. *Biochem. Pharmacol.* 1979; 28:601.

94. Hanzlik, P. J., and R. J. Collins. Hexamethyleneamine: the liberation of formaldehyde and the antiseptic efficiency under different chemical and biological conditions. *Arch. Intern. Med.* 1913;12:578.

95. Musher, D. M., and D. P. Griffith. Generation of formaldehyde from methenamine: effect of pH and

concentration, and antibacterial effect. *Antimicrob. Agents Chemother.* 1974;6:708.

96. Gleckman, R., S. Alvarez, D. W. Joubert, and S. J. Mathews. Drug therapy reviews: methenamine mandelate and methenamine hippurate. *Am. J. Hosp. Pharm.* 1979;36:1509.

97. Klinge, E., P. Mannisto, R. Mantyla, U. Lamminsivu, and P. Ottoila. Pharmacokinetics of methenamine in healthy volunteers. *J. Antimicrob. Chemother.* 1982;9:209.

98. Jackson, J., and T. A. Stamey. The Riker method for determing formaldehyde in the presence of methenamine. *Invest. Urol.* 1971;9:124.

99. Hamilton-Miller, J. M. T., and W. Brumfitt. Methenamine and its salts as urinary tract antiseptics. Variables affecting the antibacterial activity of formaldehyde, mandelic acid, and hippuric acid in vitro. *Invest. Urol.* 1977;14:287.

100. Harding, G. K. M., and A. R. Ronald. A controlled study of antimicrobial prophylaxis of recurrent urinary infection in women. *N. Engl. J. Med.* 1974;291:597.

101. Vainrub, B., and D. M. Musher. Lack of effect of methenamine in suppression of, or prophylaxis against, chronic urinary infection. *Antimicrob. Agents Chemother.* 1977;12:625.

102. Musher, D. M., D. P. Griffith, M. Tyler, and A. Woelfel. Potentiation of the antibacterial effect of methenamine by acetohydroxamic acid. *Antimicrob. Agents Chemother.* 1974;5:101.

103. Lipton, J. H. Incompatibility between sulfamethizole and methenamine mandelate. *N. Engl. J. Med.* 1963;268:92.

104. Barry, A., and S. Brown. Antibacterial spectrum

of fosfomycin trometamol. *J. Antimicrob. Chemother.* 1995;35:228.

105. Greenwood, D. Fosfomycin and fosmidomycin. In *Antibiotics and Chemotherapy: Anti-infective Agents and Their Use in Therapy*, ed. by F. O'Grady, A. P. Lambert, R. Finch, and D. Greenwood. New York: Churchill Livingstone, 1997, pp. 357–359.

106. Reeves, D. S. Fosfomycin trometamol. *J. Antimicrob. Chemother.* 1994;34:853.

107. Suarez, J., and M. Mendoza. Plasmid-encoded fosfomycin resistance. *Antimicrob. Agents Chemother.* 1991;35:791.

108. Bergan, T., S. Thorsteinsson, and E. Albini. Pharmacokinetic profile of fosfomycin trometamol. *Chemotherapy* 1993;39:297.

109. Kuhnen, E., G. Pfeifen, and C. Frenkel. Penetration of fosfomycin into cerebrospinal fluid across noninflamed and inflamed meninges. *Infection* 1987;15:422.

110. de Jong, Z., F. Pontonnier, and P. Plante. Single-dose fosfomycin trometanol (Monaril) versus multiple-dose norfloxacin: results of a multi-center study in females with uncomplicated lower urinary tract infections. *Urol. Int.* 1991;46:344.

111. Van Pienbroek, E., J. Hermans, A. Kaptein, and J. Mulder. Fosfomycin trometamol in a single-dose versus seven days nitrofurantoin in the treatment of acute uncomplicated urinary tract infections in women. *Pharm. World Sci.* 1993;15:257.

112. Elhanan, G., H. Tabenkin, R. Yahalom, and R. Raz. Single-dose fosfomycin trometamol versus 5-day cephalexin regimen for treatment of uncomplicated lower urinary tract infections in women. *Antimicrob. Agents Chemother.* 1994;38:2612.

The Fluoroquinolones

The fluoroquinolone antimicrobial drugs are synthetic compounds with greater potency and a broader antimicrobial spectrum of activity than their quinolone precursors, nalidixic acid and cinoxacin, which are used only as urinary tract antiseptics (see Chapter 9). The use and pharmacology of the quinolones have been reviewed by several authors.[1-3]

Discovery and Structure

The original quinolone, nalidixic acid, was discovered in the 1960s as a byproduct of the purification of the antimalarial drug, chloroquine.[4] Unfortunately, nalidixic acid has a narrow antibacterial spectrum, with activity mainly against gram-negative organisms. Nalidixic acid penetrates poorly into the tissues; thus it can be used only for the treatment of urinary tract infections. The study of nalidixic acid led, however, to the development of the fluoroquinolones[5] which have several advantages over the parent drug. The fluroroquinolones were introduced into therapy in the mid-1980s as orally administered antibiotics with activity that ranges from the Enterobacteriaceae and *Pseudomonas* to several gram-positive pathogens. The fluoroquinolones have revolutionized the management of a number of infections that were previously treatable only with parenteral therapy. The first group of fluoroquinolones are now referred to as the *second-generation quinolones* and are characterized by a fluorine on position 6 of the quinoline ring, as well as a carboxyl group at C-3, a keto at C-4 and a piperazinyl or methyl piperazinyl at C-7.[5] A third advance was made in the early 1990s with the synthesis of temafloxacin, which has greater activity against *Streptococcus pneumoniae* and good activity against anaerobes. Although temafloxacin itself produces serious toxicity, it has resulted in the development of the *third-generation compounds* sparfloxacin, trovafloxacin, grepafloxacin, clinafloxacin, and moxifloxacin, all of which have significantly improved activity against gram-positive bacteria, notably *Streptococcus pneumoniae*. Some of the third-generation fluoroquinolones have good activity against anaerobes and atypical pathogens and for some of them, enhanced potency is combined with improved pharmacokinetics, allowing them to be given once a day. The third-generation compounds are characterized by increasing structural complexity. Many of the effects of the quinolones can now be predicted by certain structural features, and it is hoped that additional modifications to the structure will improve their spectrum and activity while reducing adverse effects. Nine fluoroquinolones approved for clinical use in the United States include norfloxacin, ciprofloxacin, enoxacin, ofloxacin, lomefloxacin, levofloxacin, grepafloxacin, trovafloxacin, and sparfloxacin. Figure 10–1 shows the structures of selected quinolone compounds, classified by generation.

Mechanism of Action

Early studies of nalidixic acid showed that at bactericidal concentrations, the quinolone rapidly and reversibly inhibits DNA repli-

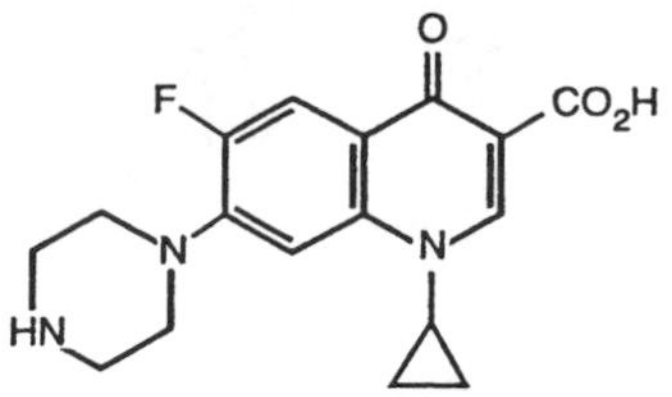

Ciprofloxacin

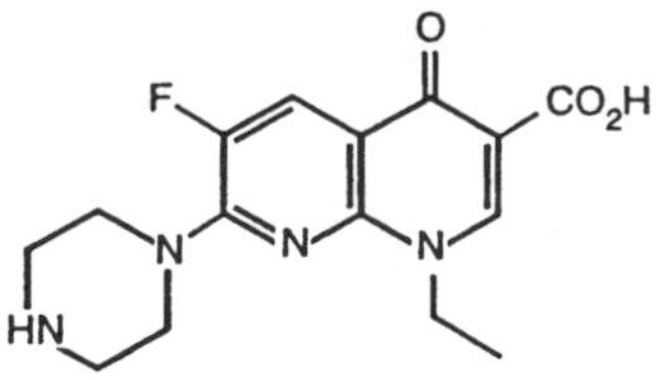

Enoxacin

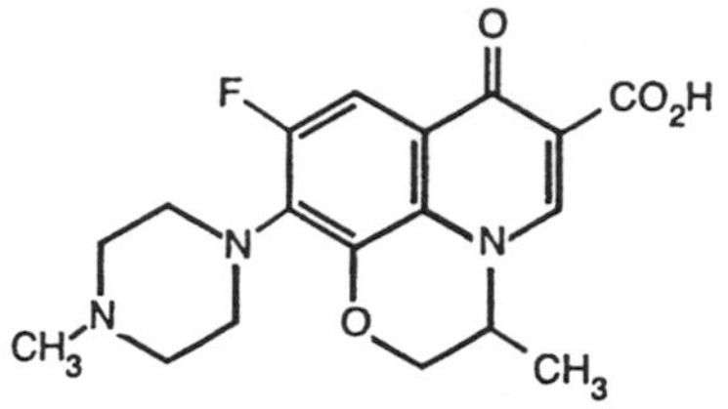

Ofloxacin

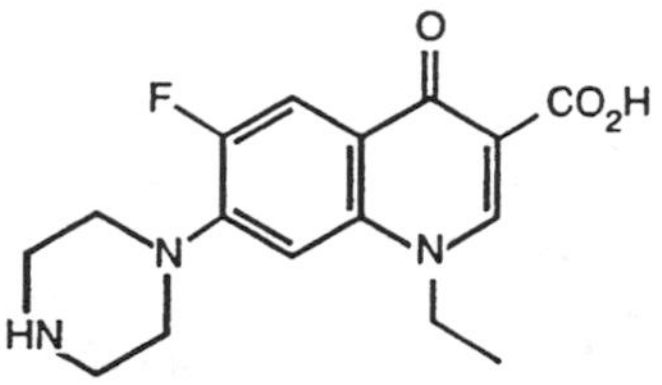

Norfloxacin

Second generation quinolones

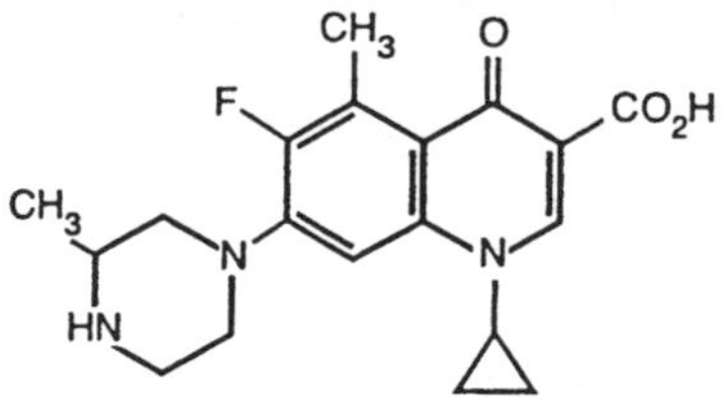

Grepafloxacin

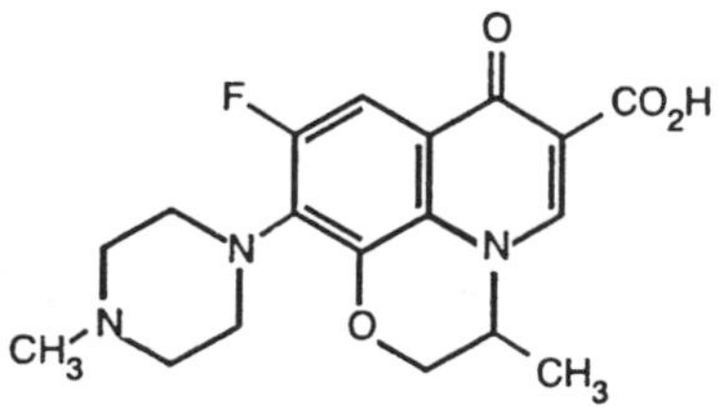

Levofloxacin

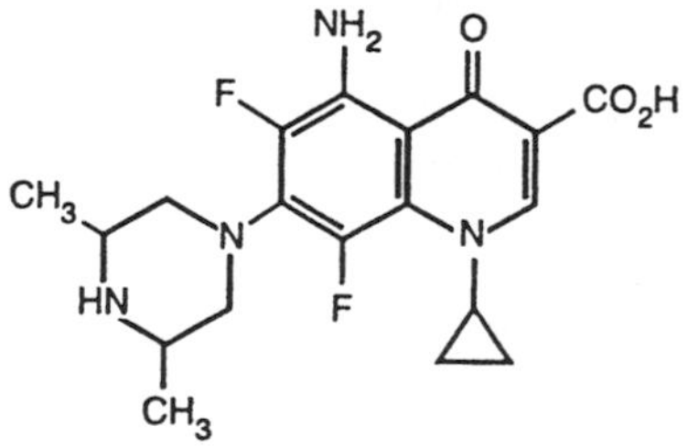

Sparfloxacin

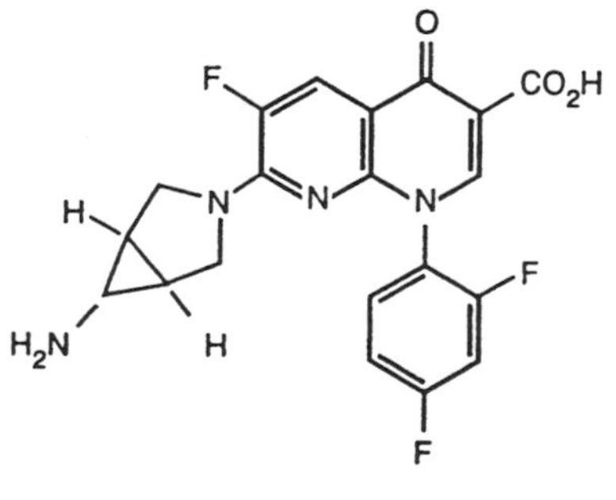

Trovafloxacin

Third generation quinolones

Figure 10–1. Selected second and third-generation quinolones available for clinical use in the United States.

cation in susceptible bacteria, while protein and RNA synthesis continue unabated for some time after exposure to the drug.[6,7] Semiconservative DNA replication is inhibited, but synthesis of DNA from a single-stranded DNA template is not.[8,9] Compared to bacteria, high concentrations of drug are required to inhibit nuclear DNA synthesis in eukaryotic cells.[10,11] In eukaryotes, nalidixic acid affects mainly the cytoplasmic organelles, such as mitochondria and chloroplasts.[10,12] Although it was rapidly established that inhibition of DNA replication is the initial event responsible for the bactericidal effect, early attempts to identify the molecular target of nalidixic acid largely served to rule out several potential sites of action, including interaction with the DNA template, effects on precursor synthesis, and effects on a number of enzymes involved in DNA metabolism.[10]

The target of nalidixic acid action was resolved when it was found that a crude extract from a nalidixic acid–sensitive strain of *Escherichia* coli conferred drug sensitivity on phage (øX174) DNA replication directed by enzymes from a nalidixic acid–resistant strain of *E. coli* (*nalA*r)[13] This assay system permitted the purification of the *nalA* gene product, a 105,000 dalton protein that is a subunit of DNA gyrase and the target of nalidixic acid action. DNA gyrase is one of a class of enzymes, called *topoisomerases*, that controls the amount of supercoiling in bacterial DNA.[14] As shown in the model presented in Figure 10–2, DNA gyrase converts relaxed closed-circular DNA to a superco-

iled form. The supercoiled DNA is twisted in the opposite direction of the double helix. This is called *negative supercoiling* and all super-coiled DNA isolated from natural sources is twisted in the negative direction with about one supercoil per 15 double-helical twists. Negative supercoiling of bacterial DNA is essential for DNA replication in the intact cell, and when DNA gyrase is inhibited, DNA replication is inhibited.

The gyrase enzyme of *E. coli* is a large molecule (400,000 daltons) composed of two 105,000-dalton A subunits and two 95,000-dalton B subunits.[14,15] In order to make a negative supercoil, the enzyme first binds to the DNA and the binding process itself generates a positive supercoil (see Fig. 10–2). The enzyme stabilizes the positively supercoiled node and then cuts both DNA strands. This nicking function is carried out by the A subunit, which is the *nalA* gene product. As diagrammed in Figure 10–2, a DNA segment is then passed through the transient double-strand break. This portion of the reaction requires the hydrolysis of ATP and is directed by the B subunit. The negative supercoil is completed by closing the double-strand break, a reaction that is again carried out by the A subunit. Nalidixic acid and the other drugs in its class bind tightly to the A subunit and inhibit both the nicking and the closing activity of the gyrase.[13,16] The physiological consequence is inhibition of DNA replication, followed ultimately by DNA degradation and cell death.[10,15]

The family of enzymes to which DNA gyr-

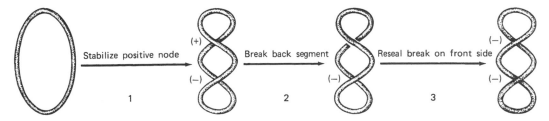

Figure 10–2. Model of the formation of negative DNA supercoils by DNA gyrase. The model presented here is the "sign inversion" model where the enzyme binds to two segments of DNA (1), creating a node of positive (+) superhelix. The enzyme then introduces a double-strand break in the DNA and passes the front segment through the break (2). The break is then resealed (3), creating a negative (−) supercoil. Nalidixic acid inhibits both the nicking and closing activity of the gyrase. (From Cozzarelli.[15])

ase belongs, DNA topoisomerases, can be classified into two types, I and II, which are characterized by reactions involving single- or double-stranded breaks in DNA, respectively.[17,18] Although all of the quinolones inhibit bacterial DNA gyrase, a type II topoisomerase, these drugs possess no activity against the mammalian type II enzyme, which is the target for several anticancer agents, such as etoposide. Several studies confirm that fluoroquinolones are highly selective against prokaryotic topoisomerase II.[19,20]

Although the evidence that gyrase is the intracellular target of the quinolones is strong, the existence of a second target, DNA topoisomerase IV (topo IV) has now been established.[21–23] Like the gyrase, topo IV is a bacterial type II DNA topoisomerase, but unlike the gyrase it cannot supercoil DNA.[24,25] Topoisomerase IV carries out the ATP-dependent relaxation of DNA and is a more potent decatenase than DNA gyrase.[26] It is composed of two subunits which in E. coli are encoded by the parC and parE genes. The parC gene is equivalent to GyrA and the parE gene is the equivalent of GyrB. The fluoroquinolones appear to have significant activity against topo IV–mediated decatenation of DNA.[26] Other evidence for a possible interaction between topo IV and the quinolones has come from studies with drug-resistant organisms. In clinical isolates of Staphylococcus aureus with high levels of fluoroquinolone resistance, mutations in both gyrA and grlA (the gene encoding the A subunit of topo IV) were found. Furthermore, clinical and laboratory isolates with low levels of flurroquinolone resistance were found to have mutations in only grlA.[27,28] These data suggest that topo IV is also a target of these drugs and that mutations in grlA may be a prerequisite for fluoroquinolone resistance before mutations in gyrA occur. There is also evidence that fluoroquinolones interact with GrlA in a manner similar to that with GyrA[27]

Although it is now well accepted that fluoroquinoline inhibition of DNA gyrase and topoisomerase IV are critical to their mechanism of action, it is not clear how quinolones bind to the topoisomerases or precisely how the enzyme inhibition causes cell death. Although quinolone molecules have been proposed to bind directly to the single-stranded DNA regions created by gyrase during formation of a cleavable complex,[29,30] these drugs probably bind efficiently only to a complex of the gyrase and DNA.[31] The interaction between fluoroquinolones and DNA gyrase stabilizes the cleavable complex.[5] The ternary complex between drug, enzyme, and DNA is reversible. Since fluoroquinolones stabilize the topoisomerase-DNA complex, the lethal event in the cell has been presumed to result from stabilization of the covalent bond between gyrase and DNA, a physical action that may lead to induction of DNA strand breaks, freezing of the replication fork, or both.[5,32–34]

Several physiological and growth conditions affect the bactericidal activity of the quinolones. The minimum inhibition concentrations (MICs) of quinolones are increased by elevated levels of magnesium in the 8–10 mM range,[35,36] concentrations that are often achieved in urine and that raise the quinolone MICs in some bacteria up to 64-fold.[37] Magnesium decreases penetration of quinolone into the bacterial cell or their accumulation after penetration.[38] When the pH is below 6–8, the bactericidal activity of some quinolones is antagonized, raising MICs several-fold.[39] This is particularly relevant to the treatment of urinary tract infections where urine pH values can be in the acidic range. This activity of the second-generation quinolones against anaerobes is poor, apparently because the decreased oxygen tension interferes with the killing activity of these compounds. However, the newer quinolones are bactericidal in an anaerobic environment and can be used to treat infections by anaerobic bacteria.

Resistance to the Quinolones

Resistance to the fluoroquinolones has been increasing with several mechanisms involved.[40] Resistance via mutations in the genes encoding topoisomerase II and IV is well established, and resistance due to increased drug efflux is common in clinical isolates.[41,42] Although resistance to these drugs was thought to be solely chromosomally encoded, the first natural plasmid carrying determinants for quinolone resistance has now been described.[40]

The supercoiling activity of gyrase involves the concerted action of two A subunits that mediate transient double-strand breakage and rejoining and two B subunits that provide energy by ATP hydrolysis for regeneration of enzyme conformation, thus initiating the next cycle of DNA cleavage, strand passage, and rejoining of the broken strands. In gram-negative bacteria, mutations in the *gyrA* subunit seem to be of primary importance for resistance to the fluoroquinolones, but mutations in topo IV can further increase the level of resistance. In gram-positive bacteria the reverse seems true, with topo IV being the primary target for the quinolones. In *E. coli* most of the mutations identified thus far are located in a small region of the gyrase A subunit, called the *quinolone resistance determining region* (QRDR). This region encodes amino acids 67 to 106,[43] the most common substitution being Ser 83 replaced by Leu, which results in a 40-fold increase in ciprofloxacin MICs. Higher increases are conferred by a double mutation at residues Ser 83 and Asp87.[44] In *E. coli*, topo IV has been identified as an additional target for quinolone action.[45] As with the gyrase, this enzyme is composed of two subunits, the *parC* and *parE* gene products. Among 15 clinical isolates of *E. coli* that were resistant to ciprofloxacin, all had topo IV mutations, whereas no mutations were detected in 12 clinical isolates from patients not resistant to ciporfloxacin.[46] Apparently, *parC* mutations occur mostly in highly quinolone-resistant strains and probably only in conjunction with *gyrA* mutations.[47,48]

Several efflux systems have been characterized in *E. coli*. and the multiple antibiotic resistance (*mar*) locus was found to be responsible for resistance to fluroroquinolones and other structurally unrelated antibiotics.[49,50] Mutations in the *mar* genes have pleiotropic effects, including decreased expression of the outer membrane protein OmpF, which could affect uptake of quinolones. However, *ompF* deletion mutants show only a twofold increase in quinolone MICs,[38,47] suggesting that the *acrAB* efflux system, which is overexpressed in *mar* mutants, plays the major role in decreasing quinolone accumulation.[51]

In gram-positive bacteria, such as *Staphylococcus aureus*, mutations in GrlA were present in isolates with a high level of quinolone resistance,[52] which is consistent with topo IV being the primary target of fluoroquinolones in *S. aureus* and other gram-positive bacteria.[53] However, chromosome-encoded membrane protein NorA also contributes to fluoroquinolone resistance in *S. aureus*. This protein acts as a reserpine-susceptible multidrug efflux transporter,[54] utilizing energy from the transmembrane proton gradient to actively pump out of the bacteria a number of structurally unrelated compounds, including several quinolones.

Several authors have described multi-drug resistance (MDR) efflux systems capable of extruding quinolones.[55,56] These systems are widely distributed and are probably essential in bacterial physiology. Most, if not all, bacterial species have several regulated MDR systems encoded chromosomally, which upon activation produce a quinolone-resistance phenotype. In some cases, the resistance is only low level, whereas in other cases clinically significant quinolone resistance develops.[57] For example, in vivo selection of *Klebsiella pneumoniae* strains with enhanced quinolone resistance due to drug efflux has been reported during fluoroquinoline treatment of patients, and the isolation of clinical strains of different species capable of extruding quinolones is being reported more frequently.[43,58,59] *Pseudomonas aeruginosa* has been the best studied system in terms of MDR. This organism possesses at least three different MDR pumps, whose activation produces a multiantibiotic-resistant phenotype.[60,61] Single-step mutants expressing MDR systems accounting for clinically relevant increased fluoroquinolone MIC values without mutations in topoisomerase genes have also been described in *Streptococcus pneumoniae*, *Staphylococcus aureus*, and *Stenotrophomonas maltophilia*.[57,62,63]

Since the MDR genes are widely distributed and the MDR phenotype is easily selectible by nonantibiotic compounds, it is very likely that quinolone-resistant bacteria can be selected in the environment without antibiotic-selective pressure. Thus, low-level quinolone resistance can be selected with compounds such as dyes, detergents, antiseptics, bile salts, or pine oil.[40] Some of these compounds are of common use in medical practice and some of them are present in the environment, either normally or as a consequence of industrial contamination. Certain environments might then be reservoirs of quinolone-resistance genes.

Another, mechansim of resistance to the quinolones is by decreased drug uptake, and this has been found only in gram-negative bacteria.[64–66] This resistance has been attributed mainly to mutations in OmpF, which is one of the major porins found in the outer membrane of bacteria such as *E. coli*. OmpF mutants show a reduced quinolone accumulation, but not complete blockage of drug entry.[67,68]

For some pathogens, fluoroquinolone resistance occurs frequently during clinical therapy: these include *Enterococcus* species, *Helicobacter pylori*, methicillin-resistant *Staphylococcus aureus* (MRSA), *Pseudomonas aeruginosa*, and *Streptococcus pneumoniae*.[69] Those organisms for which quinolone resistance is rare or occasional include *Acinetobacter* species, *E. coli,* methicillin-susceptible *S. aureus*, and *Shigella dysenteriae*. Great variations in quinolone resistance, exist between bacterial species and clinical settings, and with local epidemiology. Resistance is more commonly encountered in hospital acquired than community-acquired infections,[70–73] and is presently rare among the common pathogens causing infections in the community. However, this trend could change in the future with continued extensive use of fluoroquinolone drugs both in humans and as additives in animal feed.[74] There is a relationship between quinolone use and subsequent emergence of resistance, and several strategies for minimizing fluoroquinolone resistance have been suggested. These include administering adequate dosage, avoiding chelating medications, using appropriate antibiotic combinations, avoiding long-term treatment in hospitalized patients, avoiding the use of quinolones in trivial infections, and avoiding their use when therapeutic success in unlikely. Without practicing appropriate restraint, the use of this group of drugs will inevitably be threatened.

Antimicrobial Activity

As a group the fluoroquinolones have excellent in vitro activity against a wide range of both gram-positive and gram-negative bacteria.[75,76] They are bactericidal agents, and minimum bactericidal concentrations (MBCc) are usually one- or twofold higher than the MICs. Of the fluoroquinolones, norfloxacin is generally considered to be the least active, but this depends somewhat on the organism being tested. Significant differences in antibacterial activity exist among the different fluoroquinolones, some of which have broad-spectrum activity against both gram-negative and gram-positive species, while others, such as norfloxacin and lomefloxacin, are less effective against gram-positive pathogens.

In general, the fluoroquinolones are less active against staphylococci and streptococci than against the aerobic gram-negative rods. The newest fluoroquinolones are the most effective against staphylococci and streptococci, with clinafloxacin being the most active and trovafloxacin, grepafloxacin, and sparfloxacin also having good activity.[77,79] Ciprofloxacin and ofloxacin are less effective, but they have clinically useful activity against most *Staphylococcus aureus* isolates. Although quinolones demonstrated acceptable activity against methicillin-resistant *S. aureus* when they were first available, they are no longer reliable for treatment.[80,81] The older quinolones have only marginal activity against *Streptococcus pneumoniae* but most of the newer quinolones, including trovafloxacin, clinifloxacin, sparfloxacin, grepofloxacin, temofloxacin, and ofloxacin are very effective.

The quinolones traditionally have excellent activity against gram-negative aerobes, such as members of the family Enterobacteriaceae, *Pseudomonas aeruginosa, Haemophilus influenzae, Neisseria gonorrhoeae, Neisseria meningitidis,* and *Moraxella (Branhhamella) catarrhalis.*[80,82] All of the quinolones are highly effective, with the newer compounds clinafloxacin and ciprofloxacin being the most active. In addition to the Enterobacteriaceae, most of the common gram-negative bacteria that cause urinary tract infections are very sensitive to the fluoroquinolones in contrast to nalidixic acid. This includes *E. coli* and various species of *Salmonella, Shigella, Enterobacter, Campylabacter,* and *Neisseria.*

Several intracellular bacteria, including species of *Chlamydia, Mycoplasma, Legionella, Brucella,* and *Mycobacteria,* are inhibited by fluoroquinolones at concentrations that can be achieved in plasma. The newer fluoroquinolones, such as levofloxacin, sparfloxacin, grepafloxacin, and trovafloxacin, all have excellent activity against the atypical pathogens *Chlamydia trachomatis, Mycoplasma pneumoniae,* and *Legionella pneumophila.* Ciprofloxacin and ofloxacin are moderately active against *Mycobacterium tuberculosis, M. fortuitum,* and *M. kansasii.* Activity against the *M. avium* complex (MAC) is moderate, with growth of perhaps one-third of the MAC strains isolated from patients with AIDS being inhibited by some of the newly developed quinolones.[83,84]

In general, the fluoroquinolones are not effective against anaerobes, which limits their use in the treatment of intraabdominal infections.[3,85,86] Some of the newer quinolones, however, such as clinafloxacin and trovafloxacin, possess significant in vitro activity against *Bacteroides fragilis,* one of the most commonly encountered anaerobes in intraabdominal infections. Trovafloxacin is the most effective against anaerobes, with activity against *Bacteroides* species, being comparable to that of metronidazole. Trovafloxacin and clinafloxacin are effective against other anaerobes, including *Clostridium perfringens, C. difficile,* and *Peptostreptococci.*[3,82,87] The activity of these two compounds is from 16-to 64-fold greater than that of ciprofloxacin and is significantly greater than that of clindamycin, metronidazole, and cefoxitin, which are the standard drugs used to treat anaerobic infections. Table 10–1 summarizes the antibacterial activity of the clinically approved quinolones.[82,88]

Pharmacokinetics

The fluoroquinolones are well absorbed antimicrobial drugs that yield serum levels after oral administration that are well in excess of those required for efficacy against infections in the genitourinary tract, gynecological tissues, lung, skeletal muscle, and other important tissues and body fluids.[89] The fluoroquinlones differ from each other markedly with respect to their bioavailability, metabolism, and mode of elimination.

Absorption

The fluoroquinolones are rapidly but not always completely absorbed following oral administration. Oral bioavailability ranges from 30%–50% for norfloxacin to 70%–85% for ciprofloxacin, and for some newer members, such as oxfloxacin and fleroxacin, it approaches 100%.[79,90,91] This excellent bioavailability makes oral administrations preferable to parenteral administration. Peak serum concentrations of most of the quinolones are achieved in 1 to 3 h after an oral dose. The C_{max} and area under the serum concentration time curve (AUC) increase linearly with dose regardless of the route of administration. The presence of food in the gastrointestinal tract has little influence on the absorption of quinolones, causing a slight delay to peak serum levels that are moderately lower,[92] without changing the AUC and serum half-life. Concomitant administration of food may help minimize gastrointestinal distress associated with these drugs.[85]

Distribution

The fluoroquinolones penetrate well into various fluids and tissues of the body with the exception of the central nervous system. Their penetration into the cerebrospinal fluid is usually poor, although the cerebro-

Table 10–1. *Spectrum of in vitro activity of fluoroquinolones.*

Species	MIC$_{90}$ (μg/ml)								
	Ciprofloxacin	Enoxacin	Grepafloxacin	Levofloxacin	Lomefloxacin	Norfloxacin	Ofloxacin	Sparfloxacin	Trovafloxacin
Staphylococcus aureus	1.0	3.1	0.125	0.5	2.0	6.3	0.4	0.125	0.06
Coagulase-negative Staphylococcus	0.25	6.3	0.125	—	1.0	3.1	0.8	0.25	0.125
Methicillin-resistant *S. aureus*	>16	—	>8	>8	>16	>16	>16	>4	8
Groups A and B streptococcus	4.0	—	0.5	2.0	2.0	16.0	4.0	1.0	0.5
Streptococcus pneumoniae	2.0	16.0	0.5	3.13	8.0	16.0	3.1	0.25	0.125
Enterococcus	4.0	16.0	1	3.13	16.0	8.0	6.2	1	0.5
Escherichia coli	0.03	0.4	0.12	0.05	0.25	0.12	0.12	0.12	0.5
Salmonella or *Shigella*	0.02	0.12	0.12	0.12	0.25	0.06	0.12	0.06	0.12
Serratia marcescens	1.0	6.3	25	12.5	2.0	3.1	1.6	2.0	1.0
Klebsiella pneumophila	0.25	—	0.25	3.13	1.0	0.5	0.25	0.25	0.12
Pseudomonas aeruginosa	0.5	4.0	8	8	4.0	2.0	2.0	16	4
Xanthomonas maltophilia	2.0	8.0	—	—	8.0	4.0	3.1	—	—
Neisseria gonorrhoeae	0.01	0.25	0.06	0.1	0.12	0.06	0.06	0.008	0.016
Campylobacter jejuni	0.12	0.5	0.06	—	—	0.5	0.25	0.06	—
Haemophlus influenzae	0.01	0.12	0.06	0.015	0.12	0.06	0.03	0.016	0.016
Anaerobic cocci	8.0	16.0	—	—	—	64.0	8.0	—	—
Bacteroides fragilis	8.0	32.0	2	6.25	32.0	>128.0	8.0	2	8
Mycobacterium tuberculosis	1.0	>5.0	—	0.5	8.0	8.0	1.3	1.0	—
Chlamydia trachomatis	1.6	6.3	—	—	3.2	25.0	0.8	—	—
Mycoplasma pneumoniae	2.0	—	0.25	—	8	12	2.0	0.12	0.25
Legionella pneumophila	0.38	—	0.06	—	—	—	0.19	0.19	0.19

Source: Adapted from Schentag and Scully[88] and Phillips et al.[82]

spinal fluid levels of ofloxacin and ciprofloxacin reach 40% to 90% of serum levels when the meninges are inflamed.[80,93,94] Cerebrospinal fluid levels of fluoroquinolones do not reflect their concentrations in brain tissue. Ciprofloxacin, pefloxacin, and sparfloxacin reach high brain levels despite low cerebrospinal fluid concentrations.[95] Drug levels significantly higher than those in the serum are achieved in the kidney, prostate, liver, and lung, whereas the levels in saliva, bronchial secretions, and prostatic fluid are lower than in serum. [96–100] Fluoroquinolones produce excellent therapeutic ratios in the respiratory tract. For example, bronchial mucosal concentrations are 1.5–2 times those in serum, although ratios between sputum/bronchial secretion concentrations and those in serum after normal therapeutic doses range from 0.33–0.5 for ciprofloxacin and sparfloxacin to almost unity for pefloxacin, and lomefloxacin. Urine drug concentrations are high and remain above the MICs for most of the common urinary pathogens. Fecal levels are also high and sufficient to inhibit most intestinal patholgens. Ciprofloxacin and ofloxacin penetrate bone, where their concentrations are usually above the MICs for infecting bacteria. Biliary concentrations of the quinolones are five to eight times the simultaneous serum levels.[101] In contrast to nalidixic acid, which is 95% bound to serum protein, the newer fluoroquinolones are bound only about 30%.[102]

Metabolism and Excretion

The primary route of elimination of most fluoroquinolones is by the kidney,[103] but the degree of renal excretion versus hepatic metabolism varies widely. For example, for pefloxacin, trovafloxacin, grepafloxacin, clinafloxacin, and moxafloxacin, 10%–20% or less of the drug is recovered in the urine,[103,104] whereas other quinolones, notably ofloxacin, levofloxacin, and to a lesser extent, fleroxacin, are cleared almost exclusively by glomerular filtration and tubular secretion.[105] The tubular secretion of most fluoroquinolones is blocked by probenecid.[106] Fluoroquinolones excreted by the renal route require dosage modification when there is significant renal impairment.[107] In contrast, dose modification for ciprofloxacin, norfloxacin, and trovafloxacin is required only in patients with creatinine clearance of 20–30 ml/min or less, where halving the dose or extending the dosage interval is usually recommended. Pefloxacin requires no dose adjustment, as it is extensively metabolized. The fluoroquinolones are poorly cleared by both peritoneal dialysis and hemodialysis (<20%–30%).[85,92,107]

The fluoroquinolones are metabolized by the cytochrome P-450 system in the liver to metabolites with significantly less or no antibacterial activity. The metabolites then undergo enterohepatic recirculation.[108,109] Both the metabolites and unchanged drug are found in urine, bile, and feces. The different fluoroquinolones differ markedly in their degree of biotransformation. Ofloxacin and sparfloxacin are minimally metabolized and eliminated almost entirely unchanged in the urine. Pefloxacin, by contrast, is extensively converted to derivatives with reduced antibacterial activity. Ciprofloxacin, enoxacin, fleroxacin, lomefloxacin, and norfloxacin are eliminated partly by metabolism and partly by renal excretion.[91,92,110] Table 10–2 summarizes the effect of decreased renal function on the half-lives of the fluoroquinolones. The half-lives of both pefloxacin and norfloxacin are prolonged in severe liver disease, and even agents that are less extensively metabolized, such as ciprofloxacin, may accumulate in hepatic failure.[111,112] Transintestinal elimination of norfloxacin and ciprofloxacin is a minor excretory pathway that may be exploited in the treatment of some forms of infectious diarrhea. All of the quinolone drugs require major dose adjustments in patients with combined renal and hepatic failure.

Studies with fluoroquinolones in the elderly have shown that advancing age generally is associated with higher C_{max} and AUC values and slightly reduced total renal and nonrenal clearance.[113] With ciprofloxacin, norfloxacin, and trovafloxacin, differences in pharmacokinetics between the young and elderly are insignificant, however, markedly higher serum concentrations of en-

Table 10–2. Elimination half-lives of orally administered quinolones in patients with varying degrees (mild, moderate, severe) of renal dysfunction.

Drug	Elimination half-life in hours			
	Normal	Mild (CrCl 40–80 ml/min)	Moderate (CrCl 20–39 ml/min)	Severe (CrCl 5–19 ml/min)
Ciprofloxacin	3.3–6.9	4.5	4.5	6.9
Enoxacin	3.3–5.8	9.4	9.5	
Levofloxacin	6–8	9.1	27	35
Lomefloxacin	6.3–7.8	9.1	21	44
Norfloxacin	3.3–5.8	6.8	16.6	20.1
Ofloxacin	3.8–7.0	15.0	25.4	34.8
Sparfloxacin	16–22		35	39

CrCl, creatinine clearance rate.

Source: Data from Dahloff.[109]

oxacin and ofloxacin are achieved in the elderly.

Most diseases have minimal influence on quinolone pharmacokinetics. For example, cystic fibrosis and the gastrointestinal and other changes associated with AIDS do not seem to have any influence at all.[113] In burn patients the clearance of ciprofloxacin varies but is usually higher than expected on the basis of renal function.[114] Table 10–3 summarizes the pharmacokinetics of the fluoroquinolones.

Therapeutic Use

Their broad spectrum of activity, excellent bioavailability when given orally, good tissue penetration and a relatively low incidence of adverse effects account for the wide

Table 10–3. Pharmacokinetics of selected fluoroquinolones.

	Protein binding (%)	Serum C_{max}[a] (mg/liter)	Bioavailability (%)	Serum $t_{1/2}$ (hours)	Excretion (% of dose)		
					Urine		
					Parent drug	Metabolites	Bile/feces
Ciprofloxacin	35	2.0	85	3–6.9	30–60	10	<1/15–20
Enoxacin	43	2.5	90	4–6	50–55	15	NA[b]
Grepafloxacin	50	2.0	90	11–12	13	60	32
Levofloxacin	24–38	5.0	85–95	4–8	80–90	5	NA
Lomefloxacin	10	4.5	95	6–8	60–70	5–8	NA
Norfloxacin	15	2.0	80	3–7.4	20–40	10–20	30
Ofloxacin	8–30	8.5	85–95	3–7	70–90	5–10	3
Sparfloxacin	45	1.5	40–60	16–22	5–10	40	1.5/60
Trovafloxacin	70	6.0	70–90	10–11	8–10	>11	NA

[a] Oral dose of 500 mg. [b] NA, data not available.

Source: Adapted from Bergan.[113]

Table 10–4. *Dosage and therapeutic uses of selected fluoroquinolones.*

Fluoroquinolone	Common therapeutic uses	Daily dose
Ciprofloxacin	Gastroenteritis, travelers' diarrhea, UTIs, venereal diseases, osteomyelitis	500–750 mg bid, orally
Enoxacin	UTIs	200 mg bid, orally
Grepafloxacin	Community-acquired pneumonia, chronic bronchitis, venereal diseases	600 mg once/day, orally
Levofloxacin	Community-acquired pneumonia, UTIs	500 mg once/day orally or intravenously
Lomefloxacin	Acute diarrhea	400 mg once/day, orally
Norfloxacin	Travelers' diarrhea, UTIs	400 mg bid, orally
Ofloxacin	Community acquired pneumonia, gastroenteritis, travelers' diarrhea, UTIs, venereal diseases, osteomyelitis	400 mg bid, orally or intravenously
Sparfloxacin	Community-acquired pneumonia	400 mg on day 1, then 200 mg once/day, orally
Trovafloxacin	Community-acquired pneumonia	200 mg once/day, orally or intravenously

UTIs, urinary tract infections.

clinical use of the fluoroquinolones. Table 10–4 summarizes the therapeutic uses of several of the fluoroquinolones.

Urinary Tract Infections and Prostatitis

The fluoroquinolones are superior to nalidixic acid in their in vitro antibacterial spectrum and activity against virtually all potential bacterial urinary pathogens, with efficacy similar to or better than traditional antimicrobial agents, such as trimethoprim-sulfamethoxazole or amoxicillin.[115] The fluoroquinolones are therefore excellent drugs for the treatment of urinary tract infections of all types. The levels of fluoroquinolones achieved in the urine are many times the bactericidal concentrations for most pathogens, and their excellent tissue penetrability ensures adequate concentrations in kidney and prostate as well.[85] The fluoroquinolones are highly effective in treating uncomplicated urinary tract infections, and they are drugs of choice when the infecting organism is resistant to β-lactams. Excellent results have been obtained following standard regimens of both short-course and single-dose therapy.[116,117] In complicated infections and in the elderly, the quinolones were found to be at least as effective as β-lactams, amoxicillin-clavulanate, nitrofurantoin, and trimethoprim-sulfamethoxazole.[116,117] Cure rates of 50%–90% have been achieved in the treatment of prostatitis. The fluoroquinolones can be used to treat complicated urinary tract infections caused by *Pseudomonas aeruginosa* or other gram-negative bacteria that are multi-drug resistant, where they are as efficacious as standard parenteral aminoglycoside therapy.[118]

Gastrointestinal Tract Infections

As a group, the fluoroquinolones are potent inhibitors of the major bacterial enteropathogens except for *Clostridium difficile*, but at therapeutic dosage they have only a minimal effect on the normal anaerobic fecal flora. Because fluoroquinolones are excreted in the bile into the intestine, high concentrations of antibacterial activity are achieved in the bowel mucosa and in biliary fluid. In fact, fecal drug concentrations of ciprofloxacin are 10- to 100-fold greater than simultaneous serum concentrations, and they are not diminished by the presence of diarrhea.[119] The quinolones exert a strong suppressive effect on aerobic, gram-negative bacteria in the gut, whereas aerobic gram-positive organisms are only moderately affected.[120] Many of the quinolones have been used extensively for the prophylaxis and treatment of acute diarrhea.[121]

The treatment of choice for the oral management of typhoid fever in both adults and children is a 10-day course of fluoroquinolone therapy, which reduces associated complications and relapse rates to a greater extent than other antibiotics.[122,123] Fluoroquinolones, such as ciprofloxacin and norfloxacin, have also become the treatment of choice for eradicating the carrier state of this disease. In most cases of nontyphoid salmonellosis, antibiotics are usually not employed. However, when certain disorders (e.g., lymphoproliferative diseases, malignant disease, and AIDS, are complicated by salmonella gastroenteritis, fluoroquinolones, such as ciprofloxacin and norfloxacin, may be administered. Fluoroquinolones have become the drugs of choice in the management of invasive salmonellosis in AIDS patients.

The fluoroquinolones are effective therapy for shigellosis and have been used successfully in the treatment of patients with highly drug-resistant organisms, particularly those acquired in developing countries.[121] Ciprofloxacin has good efficacy in moderate to severe shigellosis,[124] where a single dose may be effective treatment. The fluoroquinolones are also highly effective treatment for cholera, where ciprofloxacin is as effective as the tetracyclines.[125]

Fluoroquinolones are effective for both the treatment and prophylaxis of travelers' diarrhea.[126,127] For those patients receiving chemoprophylaxis for travellers' diarrhea, fluoroqinolones taken once a day while in the area at risk produce the highest protection rate (up to 95%).[126,128] Most authorities do not recommend routine prophylaxis for travellers' diarrhea but administer quinolones as the drugs of choice for treatment when the patient becomes ill. Treatment with ciprofloxacin decreases the duration of diarrhea to about one episode per day, relieves associated abdominal cramps, and minimizes the number of liquid stools passed.[129]

In some cases, treatment of intestinal bacterial infections with fluoroquinolones is not appropriate. For example, in patients with diarrhea caused by *Campylobacter* species there is no clear effect on clinical outcome.[130] Although the fluoroquinolones have in vitro activity against *H. pylori*, their clinical use has been associated with a high failure rate and the rapid emergence of resistance.[79]

Sexually Transmitted Diseases

Because the fluoroquinolones are orally administered broad-spectrum agents that work against multiple genital pathogens, their role in the treatment of sexually transmitted diseases has been expanding.[85,131] They are very effective in the treatment of uncomplicated gonorrhea, including infections by penicillinase-producing strains. They also appear to be effective treatment for rectal and pharyngeal gonococcal infections.[132] Trovafloxacin is effective as a single dose against gonorrhea, but multiple dosing is required for chlamydial infections.[133,134] The fluoroquinolones are not effective in treating syphilis or granuloma inguinale.

Respiratory Tract Infections

The fluoroquinolones are very useful for the therapy of common respiratory infections, including community-acquired pneumonia, hospital-acquired pneumonia, and acute exacerbations of chronic bronchitis.[135-137] The major limitation for the use of the fluoroquinolones in respiratory infections has been their poor activity against *Streptoccus pneumoniae* and anaerobic bacteria. There have been several reports demonstrating therapeutic failures and serious life-threatening complications, including bacteremia and bacterial meningitis, in patients with *Streptococcus pneumoniae* while they were being treated with ciprofloxacin. The newer fluoroquinolones, however, such as sparfloxacin, levofloxacin, trovafloxacin, and grepafloxacin, are very active against *Streptococcus pneumoniae*, and they appear to be effective for the treatment of community-acquired pneumonia, including that caused by multidrug-resistant pathogens.[137,138] A major advantage of these newer fluoroquinolones is their good in vitro activity against the penicillin-resistant pneumococci.[136] The fluoroquinolones also appear to be useful agents in the management of pulmonary infections in patients with cystic fibrosis, and their use may obviate hospitalization and intravenous antibiotic therapy.[139]

Bone and Joint Infections

Treatment of osteomyelitis in adults requires prolonged therapy often lasting several weeks to months with agents active against *Staphylococcocus aureus* and gram-negative rods. Fluoroquinolones possess properties necessary for the treatment of bone and joint infections.[80,140] Several studies have now shown very satisfactory results for the fluoroquinolones (particularly ciprofloxacin) in treating osteomyelitis due to Enterobacteriaceae.[141,142] Good results have also been seen in staphylococcal and pseudomonal infections, but selection of resistant strains is more likely to occur in patients infected with these organisms.[143,144] The fluoroquinolones also appear to be very useful in infections due to multiresistant gram-negative bacilli and in clinical situations in which prolonged courses of therapy are indicated, such as infections of prosthetic joints.

Skin and Soft Tissue Infections

The fluoroquinolones are effective in the treatment of various kinds of skin and soft tissue infections, especially when these are caused by gram-negative organisms. When the primary pathogen is a gram-positive organism, β-lactams and macrolides are preferred. For those patients who require prolonged therapy and are infected with gram-negative organisms or mixed flora, the fluoroquinolones play a major role, either alone or in combination with other antibiotics. Fluoroquinolones, such as ciprofloxacin, ofloxacin and fleroxacin, achieve con-

centrations in the skin and soft tissues that are above the MBCs for susceptible bacteria.[85,145,146]

Mycobacterial Infections

Fluoroquinolones have excellent bactericidal activity against many mycobacteria.[147–149] Ofloxacin, ciprofloxacin, sparfloxacin, and pefloxacin all show good clinical efficacy in treatment of tuberculosis and leprosy.[150,151] The fluoroquinolones are also effectively used in combination regimens for the treatment of multiple drug–resistant tuberculosis. Disseminated infections caused by *Mycobacterium avium* complex (MAC) in patients with advanced AIDS are sometimes treated with fluoroquinolones in combination with a macrolide, ethambutol, rifampin, or amikacin. The fluoroquinolones appear to lack significant clinical efficacy when used alone, and it has been difficult to determine whether they contribute to the overall suppressive effect of these combinations.[150]

Prophylaxis and Treatment of Neutropenic Infections

Most pathogens causing sepsis in patients with severe neutropenia are aerobic gram-negative rods thought to originate from the patients own intestinal tract. Prophylactic antimicrobial therapy against these organisms is correlated with reduction in the incidence of gram-negative sepsis. Trimethoprim-sulfamethoxazole (TMP-SMX) has been used for several years for this purpose but it has been associated with both myelosuppression and fungal superinfections. In several studies, ciprofloxacin has been found to be preferable to TMP-SMX in prophylactic therapy of neutropenic patients, producing a lower incidence of infection, decreased colonization by resistant organisms, and less toxicity.[152] Similar results were obtained with norfloxacin and ofloxacin, and in studies comparing the efficacy of ciprofloxacin to norfloxacin directly, ciprofloxacin appears to be superior.[153–155] For treatment of neutropenic cancer patients with fever, the combination of a fluoroquinolone with an aminoglycoside has been found to be comparable to the β-lactam-aminoglycoside combination.[156] However, when used alone for this condition the quinolones were found to be less effective.[157]

Miscellaneous Infections

The fluoroquinolones are also effective in treating legionellosis and are now used alone and in combination as agents of choice for this disease, especially in cases where previous therapy with macrolide antibiotics has failed.[158] The fluoroquinolones may be useful in selected cases of bacterial meningitis caused by drug-resistant gram-negative bacilli.[80] Other infections where the the fluoroquinolones have been used in specific situations include prophylaxis of *Neisseria meningitidis* and treatment of *Brucella* infections, malignant external otitis caused by *Pseudomonas aeruginosa*, and selected cases of endocarditis.

Adverse Effects

In general, the fluoroquinolones are relatively safe drugs and severe toxic effects are rare. Even prolonged use of these compounds has been well tolerated. The different fluoroquinolones produce adverse effects at similar rates and it appears that the pattern of adverse reactions is comparable for all fluoroquinolones, although there are

Table 10–5.   Summary of type and frequency of adverse effects of the fluoroquinolones.

Site	Incidence (%)
Gastrointestinal	0.8–6.8
Central and peripheral nervous system	0.9–4.7
Serious reactions	<0.5
Skin/hypersensitivity	0.4–2.1
Phototoxicity/photoallergy	0.5–2
Cardiovascular	0.5–2
Renal/urogenital/hepatic	0.5–4.5
Blood disorders	0.5–5.3
Musculoskeletal/rheumatologoic	0.5–2
Cumulative incidences[a]	4.4–20

[a] During clinical trials the overall frequencies of adverse effects were reported to vary between 4.4% and 20%.

Source: From Stahlman and Lode.[161]

some differences in both the incidence and the type of reaction induced by certain compounds.[80,159] Serious adverse effects leading to cessation of treatment occur at frequencies between 0.7% and 4.6%.[160] Table 10–5 summarizes the type and incidence of adverse effects associated with the fluoroquinolones and Table 10–6 describes some of the problems arising from fluoroquinolone therapy.

The most common adverse effects, gastrointestinal upset (nausea, vomiting, and diarrhea), occur in 1%–5% of patients.[85] These effects tend to be mild, transient, and

Table 10–6.   Problems arising from quinolone therapy.

Problem	Implication(s) for clinical use
Arthropathies in young animals	Contraindicated for pregnant women, nursing mothers, children and adolescents (except in cystic fibrosis or other infections in which potential benefit outweighs risk)
Central nervous system toxicity	Special benefit/risk evaluation for patients at risk (appropriate benzodiazepines and psychoactive drugs)
Nephrotoxicity (and blood disorders)	Dose reduction for patients with impaired renal function and/or the elderly (age >65 years)
Adverse reactions to long-term treatment (arthropathies and ocular toxicity in adult dogs)	Periodic ophthalmologic examinations; long-term observation of patients
Theophylline	Monitoring of theophylline

Source: From Christ and Esch.[160]

dose dependent, and they are less common after intravenous administration. Grepafloxacin is especially likely to cause nausea. Because they lack activity against anaerobes, fluoroquinolone effects on the gut flora are less than with other broad-spectrum antimicrobials, including antibiotic-associated (pseudomembranous) colitis. Fluoroquinolones can cause reversible elevation of liver enzymes (usually transaminases), lactic dehydrogenase (LDH), alkaline phosphatase, and serum bilirubin.[162–164]

Fluoroquinolones have been associated with several neurotoxic effects. Although the mechanism of central nervous system toxicity is unknown, seizures induced either by quinolones such as those induced by magnesium deficiency, can be antagonized by MK-801 an NMDA-antagonist.[165,166]. Mild neurotoxic reactions in the form of headache, dizziness, tiredness, or sleeplessness, may occur, and abnormal vision, restlessness, and bad dreams have been reported. Severe neurotoxic side effects are seldom seen ($<0.5\%$), but they have occurred with most of the fluoroquinolones and include psychotic reactions, hallucinations, depression, and grand mal convulsions. Typically, these reactions start only a few days after the beginning of therapy and stop when the medication is stopped.[80,160] Central nervous system effects, particularly headaches, insomnia, and dizziness, occur more commonly with ofloxacin, lomefloxacin, and trovafloxacin than with other fluoroquinolones. Major psychiatric disturbances are also more common with ofloxacin and lomefloxacin. Convulsions have occurred significantly more frequently with lomefloxacin than with other fluoroquinolones, but all of the of the fluoroquinolones are contraindicated in patients with a history of convulsions. Elderly patients, especially those with pronounced arteriosclerosis, and patients with central nervous system lesions involving a lowered convulsion threshold, (e.g., after cerebrocranial injuries or stroke) are prone to neurologic complications and should be treated with quinolones only under close supervision.[161] Fluoroquinolones are associated with visual disturbances, including blurred and dimmed vision, disturbed vision, diplopia, change in color perception, flashing lights, decreased visual acuity, and cataracts.[160]

A variety of skin reactions have occurred with fluoroquinolone therapy, including both hypersensitivity and phototoxic reactions. Hypersensitivity reactions occur only occasionally, are generally mild to moderate in severity, and usually resolve after treatment is stopped. They include erythema, pruritus, urticaria, rash, and other cutaneous reactions.[80,160] Anaphylactic reactions have been reported rarely. Moderate to severe phototoxicity, manifested by an exaggerated sunburn reaction, has been seen in patients taking fluoroquinolones who are exposed to direct sunlight. This probably results from absorption of light by fluoroquinolones or their metabolites in the skin, following which transfer of photo energy releases oxygen radicals, causing damage to lipids in cell membranes.[167,168] Phototoxic reactions in association with quinolone therapy were first described with nalidixic acid,[169] but all the quinolones available today produce this effect. Among the fluoroquinolones, the potential for phototoxicity appears to be associated with fluorination at the 8-position and is predictably more common and potentially more severe with compounds such as lomefloxacin, fleroxacin, and sparfloxacin.[170] Because of the relatively high phototoxic potential of lomefloxacin and sparfloxacin, their clinical use has been limited in some countries. Lomefloxacin should be taken in the evening, as drug concentrations will have decreased by the next morning.[171] Patients should avoid excessive sunlight while taking the quinolones and should be advised to discontinue them if phototoxicity occurs. For unknown reasons more than 50% of patients with cystic fibrosis treated with ciprofloxacin experience a phototoxic reaction during therapy.[172]

When given to immature animals, fluoroquinolones can produce permanent damage to cartilage, manifest as erosions of cartilage in the major diarthridial joints and other signs of arthropathy.[173] Although the exact mechanism of this arthropathy is still unknown, some data indicate that fluoroquinolones bind magnesium, resulting in a magnesium deficiency. It has been proposed that depletion of free magnesium in joint cartilage leads to the production of reactive oxygen species that cause the damage.[174,175] Although no risk for humans has been demonstrated, on the basis of the animal data, fluoroquinolones are contraindicated in children and in pregnant or nursing women. Fluoroquinolones cause tendinitis, and occasionally rupture of the Achilles tendon occurs, even after short-term use.[176] Most of the reported tendon disorders have occurred with pefloxacin, the incidence being much lower with the other fluoroquinolones.[177]

Hypotension and tachycardia have been associated with most fluoroquinolones, but it is unclear if these are direct effects or if they are induced via histamine release.[178] Sparfloxacin and grepafloxacin, but not the other quinolones, were found to produce a moderate increase in the QT interval and associated ventricular arrhythmias. However, few serious adverse cardiovascular effects have been reported with these drugs, and all have occurred in patients with an underlying cardiac condition.[179] The fluoroquinolones should not be administered to patients with a known QT prolongation or preexisting rhythm disorders, or to patients being treated with antiarrhythmic agents, notably disopyramide, amiodarone, and sotalol. Fluoroquinolones are also contraindicated in patients receiving other drugs that can prolong the QT interval or cause torsade de pointes, such as terfenadine, astemizole, erythromycin, and cisapride. Rarely, acute interstitial nephritis or nephrotoxic reactions have occurred during fluoroquinolone therapy. There maybe crystalluria with elevation of plasma creatinine levels.[180]

Hematologic changes associated with fluoroquinolone therapy include both decreased and elevated platelet counts, leukopenia, leukocytosis, neutropenia, eosinophilia, elevated sedimentation rate, anemia, and hemolysis.[160,162,163] Temafloxacin produced a syndrome of hemolysis with uremia, coagulopathy, and hyperbilirubinemia[181] that resulted in its withdrawal from the market.

Although fluoroquinolones bind to DNA, it has been found that low to moderate doses of quinolones do not have genotoxic effects and do not present a mutagenic hazard to humans. Long-term studies in animals have shown no indication of carcinogenicity after life-long exposure to fluoroquinolones.[161]

Drug Interactions

The fluoroquinolones form chelates with metal ions, which reduces their absorption from the gastrointestinal tract, decreasing their therapeutic activity.[80,182–184] The fluoroquinolones should not be administered with antacids containing aluminum or magnesium, sucralfate (which contains aluminum),[185] multivitamin preparations containing minerals,[161] iron supplements, high-dose calcium supplements, or with dairy products (which are rich in calcium). The absorption of ciprofloxacin and norfloxacin seems to be more affected by metals than that of other fluoroquinolones.[186,187] Allowing a 4- to 6-h interval between the administration of antacids or sucralfate and fluoroquinolones avoids these interactions. Agents such as pirenzepine that affect gastric motility may prolong the absorption of the quinolones.[188]

One of the most significant interactions is that between certain fluoroquinolones and xanthine derivatives, such as theophylline and caffeine. Inhibition of the cytochrome P-450 system by certain fluoroquinolones and resulting reduction in plasma clearance of theophylline may result in nausea, vomiting, and convulsions when the two drugs are coadministered.[189,190] This effect is most pronounced with enoxacin, less so with pefloxacin and ciprofloxacin, and probably absent or insignificant with the other fluoroquinolones.[191–193] Fluoroquinolones also interfere with caffeine metabolism, and both sleep disturbances and upper gastrointestinal symptoms may result.[191] Thus, patients taking quinolones should be advised against an excessive caffeine intake. Ciprofloxacin can decrease phenytoin concentrations to subtherapeutic levels such that seizures occur.[194] Some quinolones (e.g., enoxacin, norfloxacin, or ofloxacin) enhance the effects of warfarin or its derivatives. Studies on the interactions between quinolones and warfarin indicate that enoxacin causes the prolongation of the elimination half-life of (R)-warfarin, while not affecting (S)-warfarin. Because the (R) enantiomer is much less active than the (S)-isomer, the overall enoxacin–warfarin interaction may be of little clinical significance.[195] However, it is generally recommended that patients have their prothrombin time monitored routinely when the two drugs are taken concurrently.[85]

Synergistic inhibition of central nervous system GABA receptors by fluoroquinolones and nonsteroidal anti-inflammatory drugs (NSAIDs) may cause neuroexcitatory phenomena. These effects are dose dependent and vary among the different fluoroquinolones.[196] Convulsions have been reported only in patients receiving enoxacin and fenbufen.[197]

REFERENCES

1. Andriole, V. T., ed. *The Quinolones*. New York: Academic Press, 1998.

2. Kuhlmann, J., A. Dalhoff, and H.-J. Zeiler, eds. *Quinolone Antibacterials*. New York: Springer-Verlag, 1998.

3. Gootz, T. D., and K. E. Brighty. Fluoroquinolone antibacterials: SAR, mechanism of action, resistance, and clinical aspects. *Med. Res. Rev.* 1996;16:433.

4. Lesher, G. Y., E. D. Froelich, M. D. Gruet, J. H. Bailey, and R. P. Brundage. 1,8 naphthyridine derivatives: a new class of chemotherapeutic agents. *J. Med. Pharmacol. Chem.* 1962;5:1063.

5. Gootz, T. D., and K. E. Brighty. Chemistry and mechanism of action of the quinolone antibacterials. In *The Quinolones*, ed. by V. T. Andriole. New York: Academic Press, 1998, pp. 29–80.

6. Goss, W. A., W. H. Deitz, and T. M. Cook. Mechanism of action of nalidixic acid on *Escherichia coli*. II. Inhibition of deoxyribonucleic acid synthesis. *J. Bacteriol.* 1965;89:1068.

7. Deitz, W. H., T. M. Cook, and W. A. Goss. Mechanism of action of nalidixic acid on *Escherichia coli*. III. Conditions required for lethality. *J. Bacteriol.* 1966;91:768.

8. Simon, T. J., W. E. Masker, and P. C. Hanawalt. Selective inhibition of semiconservative DNA synthesis by nalidixic acid in permeabilized bacteria. *Biochim. Biophys. Acta* 1974;349:271.

9. Schneck, P. K., W. L. Staudenbauer, and P. H. Hofschneider. Replication of bacteriophage M-13. Template specific inhibition of DNA synthesis by nalidixic acid. *Eur. J. Biochem.* 1973;38:130.

10. Pedrini; A. M. Nalidixic acid. In *Antibiotics V-1*, ed. by F. E. Hahn. New York: Springer-Verlag, 1979, pp. 154–175.

11. Mattern, M. R., and D. A. Seudiero. Dependence of mammalian DNA synthesis on DNA supercoiling. III. Characterization of the inhibition of replicative

and reapir-type DNA synthesis by novobiocin and nalidixic acid. *Biochim. Biophys. Acta* 1981;653:248.

12. Pienkos, P., A. Walfield, and C. L. Hershberger. Effect of nalidixic acid on *Euglena gracilis*: induced loss of chloroplast deoxyribonucleic acid. *Arch. Biochem. Biophys.* 1974;165:548.

13. Sugino, A., C. L. Peebles, K. N. Kreuzer, and N. R. Cozzarelli. Mechanism of action of nalidixic acid: purification of *Escherichia coli nalA* gene product and its relationship to DNA gyrase and a novel nicking-closing enzyme. *Proc. Natl. Acad. Sci. U.S.A.* 1977;74:4767.

14. Gellert, M. DNA topoisomerases. *Annu. Rev. Biochem.* 1981;50:879.

15. Cozzarelli, N. R. DNA gyrase and the supercoiling of DNA. *Science* 1980;207:953.

16. Gellert, M., K. Mizuuchi, M. H. O'Dea, T. Itoh, and J. Tomizawa. Nalidixic acid resistance: a second genetic character involved in DNA gyrase activity. *Proc. Natl. Acad. Sci. U.S.A.* 1977;74:4772.

17. Maxwell, A., and M. Gellert. The DNA dependence of the ATPase activity of DNA gyrase. *J. Biol. Chem.* 1984;259:14472.

18. Wigley, D. B. Structure and mechanism of DNA topoisomerase. *Annu. Rev. Biophys. Biomol. Struct.* 1995;24:185.

19. Hussy, P., G. Maass, B. Tümmler, F. Grosse, and U. Schomburg. Effect of 4-quinolones and novobiocin on calf thymus DNA polymerase α primase complex, topoisomerases I and II, and growth of mammalian lymphoblasts. *Antimicrob. Agents Chemother.* 1986;29:1073.

20. Barrett, J. F., T. D. Gootz, P. R. McGuirk, C. A. Farrell, and S. A. Sokolowski. Use of in vitro topoisomerase II assays for studying quinolone antibacterial agents. *Antimicrob. Agents Chemother.* 1989;33:1697.

21. Hooper, D. C., and J. S. Wolfson. Mode of action of the new quinolones: new data, *Eur. J. Clin. Microbiol. Infect. Dis.* 1991;10:223.

22. Palumbo, M., B. Gatto, Z. Zagotto, and G Palù, On the mechanism of action of quinolone drugs. *Trends Microbiol.* 1993;1:233.

23. Drlica, K., M. Malik, J.-Y. Wang, R. Levitz, and R. M. Burger. The fluoroquinolones as antituberculosis agents. *In Tuberculosis*, ed. by W. Rom and S. Garry. Boston: Little, Brown, 1995, pp. 817–827.

24. Kato, J., Y. Nishimura, R. Imamura, H. Niki, S. Hiraga, and H. Suzuki. New topoisomerase essential for chromosome segregation in *E. coli*. *Cell* 1990;63:393.

25. Kato, J., H. Suzuki, and H. Ikeda. Purification and characterization of DNA topoisomerase IV in *Escherichia coli*. *J. Biol. Chem.* 1992;267:25676.

26. Hoshino, K., A. Kitamura, I. Morrisey, K. Sato, J. Kato, and H. Ikeda. Comparison of inhibition of *Escherichia coli* topoisomerase IV by quinolones with DNA gyrase inhibition. *Antimicrob. Agents Chemother.* 1994;38:2623.

27. Ferrero, L., B. Cameron, B. Manse, D. Lagneaux, J. Crouzet, A. Famechon, and F. Blanche. Cloning and primary structure of *Staphylococcus aureus* DNA topoisomerase IV: a primary target of fluoroquinolones. *Mol. Microbiol.* 1994;13:641.

28. Ferrero, L., B. Cameron, and J. Crouzet. Anal-

ysis of *gyrA* and *grlA* mutations in stepwise-selected ciprofloxacin-resistant mutants of *Staphylococcus aureus. Antimicrob. Agents Chemother.* 1995;39:1554.

29. Shen, L., and A. G. Pernet. Mechanism of inhibition of DNA gyrase by analogues of nalidixic acid: the target of the drugs is DNA. *Proc. Natl. Acad. Sci. U.S.A.* 1985;82:307.

30. Shen, L. L., and D. T. W. Chu. Type II DNA topoisomerases as antibacterial targets. *Curr. Pharm. Design* 1996;2:195.

31. Willmott, C. J. R., and A. Maxwell. A single point mutation in the DNA gyrase A protein greatly reduces binding of fluoroquinolones to the gyrase DNA complex. *Antimicrob. Agents Chemother.* 1993;37:126.

32. Hiasa, H., D. O. Yousef, and K. J. Marians. DNA strand cleavage is required for replication fork arrest by a frozen topoisomerase-quinolone-DNA ternary complex. *J. Biol. Chem.* 1996;271:26424.

33. Drlica, K., and X. Zhao. DNA gyrase, topoisomerase IV, and the 4-quinolones. *Microbiol. Mol. Biol. Rev.* 1997;61:377.

34. Chen, C.-R., M. Malik, M. Snyder, and K. Drlica. DNA gyrase and topoisomerase IV on the bacterial chromosome: quinolone-induced DNA cleavage. *J. Mol. Biol.* 1996;258:627.

35. Lecomte, S., M. H. Baron, M. T. Chenon, C. Coupry, and N. J. Moreau. Effect of magnesium complexation by fluoroquinolones on their antibacterial properties. *Antimicrob. Agents Chemother.* 1994;38:2810.

36. Neu, H. C., A. Novelli, and N.-X. Chin. Comparative in vitro activity of a new quinolone, AM-1091. *Antimicrob. Agents Chemother.* 1989;33:1036.

37. Hirschhorn, L., and H. C. Neu. Factors influencing the in vitro activity of two new aryl-fluoroquinolone antimicrobial agents, difloxacin (A-56619) and A-56620. *Antimicrob. Agents Chemother.* 1986;30:143.

38. Chapman, J. S., and N. H. Georgopapadakou. Routes of quinolone permeation in *Escherichia coli. Antimicrob. Agents Chemother.* 1988;32:438.

39. Bauernfeind, A., and C. Petermuller. In vitro activity of ciprofloxacin, norfloxacin, and nalidixic acid. *Eur. J. Clin. Microbiol.* 1983;2:111.

40. Martinez, J. L., A. Alono, J. M. Gomez-Gomez, and F. Baquero. Quinolone resistance by mutations in chromosomal gyrase genes. Just the tip of the iceberg? *J. Antimicrob. Chemother.* 1998;42:683.

41. Weidemann, B., and P. Heisig. Mechanisms of quinolone resistance. *Infection* 1994;22(Suppl. 2):573.

42. Everett, M. J., and L. J. V. Piddock. Mechanisms of resistance to fluoroquinolones. In *Quinolone Antibacterials*, ed. by J. Kuhlmann, A. Dalhoff, and H.-J. Zeiler. New York: Springer-Verlag, 1998, pp. 260–296.

43. Yoshida, H., M. Bogaki, M. Nakamura and S. Nakamura. Quinolone resistance-determining region in the DNA gyrase *gyrA* gene of *Escherichia coli. Antimicrob. Agents Chemother.* 1990;34:1271.

44. Heisig, P. High-level fluoroquinolone resistance in a *Salmonella typhimurium* isolate due to alterations in both *gyrA* and *gyrB* genes. *J. Antimicrob. Chemother.* 1993;32:367.

45. Khodursky, A. B., E. L. Zechiedrich, and N. R. Cozzarelli. Topoisomerase IV is a target of quinolones in *Escherichia coli. Proc. Natl. Acad. Sci. U.S.A.* 1995; 92:11801.

46. Vila, J., J. Ruiz, P. Goni, A. Marcos, and T. J. Deanta. Detection of mutations in *parC* in quinolone-resistant clinical isolates of *Escherichia coli. Antimicrob. Agents Chemother.* 1996;40:491.

47. Heisig, P. Genetic evidence for a role of *parC* mutations in development of high-level fluoroquinolone resistance in *Escherichia coli. Antimicrob. Agents Chemother.* 1996;40:879.

48. Kumagai, Y., J. I. Kato, K. Hoshino, T. Akasaka, K. Sato, and H. Ikeda. Quinolone-resistant mutants of *Escherichia coli* DNA topoisomerase IV *parC* gene. *Antimicrob. Agents Chemother.* 1996;40:710.

49. Cohen, S. P., L. M. McMurry, D. C. Hooper, J. S. Wolfson, and S. B. Levy. Cross-resistance to fluoroquinolones in multiple-antibiotic-resistant (Mar) *Escherichia coli* selected by tetracycline or chloramphenicol: decreased drug accumulation associated with membrane changes in addition to OmpF reduction. *Antimicrob. Agents Chemother.* 1989;33:1318.

50. Maneewannakul, K., and S. B. Levy. Identification of *mar* mutants among quinolone-resistant clinical isolates of *Escherichia coli. Antimicrob. Agents Chemother.* 1996;40:1695.

51. Okusu, H., D. Ma, and H. Nikaido. AcrAB efflux pump plays a major role in the antibiotic resistance phenotype of *Escherichia coli* multiple-antibiotic-resistance (Mar) mutants. *J. Bacteriol.* 1996;178:306.

52. Ferrero, L., B. Cameron, B. Manse, D. Lagneaux, J. Crouzet, A. Famechon, and F. Blanche. Cloning and primary structure of *Staphylococcus aureus* DNA topoisomerase IV: a primary target of fluoroquinolones. *Mol. Microbiol.* 1994;13:641.

53. Yamagishi, J., T. Kojima, Y. Oyamada, K. Fujimoto, H. Hattori, S. Nakamura, and M. Inoue. Alterations in the DNA topoisomerase IV *grlA* gene responsible for quinolone resistance in *Staphylococcus aureus. Antimicrob. Agents Chemother.* 1996;40:1157.

54. Neyfakh, A. A., C. M. Borsch, and G. W. Kaatz. Fluoroquinolone resistance protein NorA of *Staphylococcus aureus* is a multidrug efflux transporter. *Antimicrob. Agents. Chemother.* 1993;37:128.

55. Paulsen, I. T., M. H. Brown, and R. A. Skurray. Proton-dependent multidrug efflux systems. *Microbiol. Rev.* 1996;60:575.

56. Saier, M. H., I. T. Paulsen, M. K. Sliwinski, S. S. Pao, R. A. Skurray, and H. Nikaido. Evolutionary origins of multidrug and drug-specific efflux pumps in bacteria. *FASEB J.* 1998;12:265.

57. Alonso, A., and J. L. Martinez. Multiple antibiotic resistance in *Stenotrophomonas maltophilia. Antimicrob. Agents Chemother.* 1997;41:1140.

58. Deguchi, T., M. Yasuda, M. Nakano, S. Ozeki, E. Kanematsu, Y. Nishino, S. Ishihara, and Y. Kawada. Detection of mutations in the *gyrA* and *parC* genes in quinolone-resistant clinical isolates of *Enterobacter cloacae. J. Antimicrob. Chemother.* 1997;40:543.

59. Ishii, H., K. Sato, K. Hoshino, M. Sato, A. Yamaguchi, T. Sawai, and Y. Osada. Active efflux of of-

loxacin by a highly quinolone-resistant strain of *Proteus vulgaris*. *J. Antimicrob. Chemother.* 1991;28:827.

60. Li, X. Z., D. M. Livermore, and H. Nikaido. Role of efflux pump(s) in intrinsic resistance of *Pseudomonas aeruginosa*: resistance to tetracycline, chloramphenicol, and norfloxacin. *Antimicrob. Agents Chemother.* 1994;38:1732.

61. Kohler, T., M. Michae-Hamzehpour, P. Plesiat, A. L. Kahr, and J. C. Pechere. Differential selection of multidrug efflux systems by quinolones in *Pseudomonas aeruginosa*. *Antimicrob. Agents Chemother.* 1997;41:2540.

62. Zeller, V., C. Janoir, M. D. Kitzis, L. Gutmann, and N. J. Moreau. Active efflux as a mechanism of resistance to ciprofloxacin in *Streptococcus pneumoniae*. *Antimicrob. Agents Chemother.* 1997;41:1973.

63. Kaatz, G. W., and S. M. Seo. Mechanisms of fluoroquinolone resistance in genetically related strains of *Staphylococcus aureus*. *Antimicrob. Agents Chemother.* 1997;41:2733.

64. Gutmann, L., R. Williamson, N. Moreau, M. D. Kitzis, E. Collatz, J. F. Acar, and F. W. Goldstein. Cross-resistance to nalidixic acid, trimethoprim and chloramphenicol associated with alterations in outer membrane proteins of *Klebsiella, Enterobacter* and *Serratia*. *J. Infect. Dis.* 1985;151:501.

65. Piddock, L. J. V. Mechanism of quinolone uptake into bacterial cells. *J. Antimicrob. Chemother.* 1991;27:399.

66. Mortimer, P. G., and L. J. V. Piddock. The accumulation of five antibacterial agents in porin-deficient mutants of *Escherichia coli*. *J. Antimicrob. Chemother.* 1993;32:195.

67. Cohen, S. P., L. M. McMurray, and S. B Levy. *marA* locus causes decreased expression of OmpF porin in multiple-antibiotic resistant (Mar) mutants of *Escherichia coli*. *J. Bacteriol.* 1988;170:5416.

68. Gambino, L. S., S. J. Gracheck, and P. F. Miller. Overexpression of the MarA positive regulator is sufficient to confer multiple antibiotic resistance in *Escherichia coli*. *J. Bacteriol.* 1993;175:2888.

69. Stratton, C. Avoiding fluoroquinolone resistance. *Postgrad. Med.* 1997;101:247.

70. Daum, T. E., D. R. Schaberg, M. S. Terpenning, W. S. Sottile, and C. A. Kauffman. Increasing resistance of *Staphylococcus aureus* to ciprofloxacin. *Antimicrob. Agents Chemother.* 1990;34:1862.

71. Schaefler, S. Methicillin-resistant strains of *Staphylococcus aureus* resistant to quinolones. *J. Clin. Microbiol.* 1989;27:335.

72. Yee, Y. C., R. R. Muder, M. H. Hsieh, and T. C. Lee. Molecular epidemiology of endemic ciprofloxacin-susceptible and -resistant Enterobacteriaceae. *Infect. Control Hosp. Epidemiol.* 1992;13:706.

73. Thornsberry, C. Susceptibility of clinical bacterial isolates to ciprofloxacin in the United States. *Infection* 1994;22(Suppl. 2):80.

74. Turnidge, J. Epidemiology of quinolone resistance. Eastern hemisphere. *Drugs* 1995;49(Suppl.2):43.

75. Eliopoulos, G. M. In vitro activity of new quinolone antimicrobial agents. In *Microbiology*, ed. by L. Leive. Washington, DC: American Society for Microbiology, 1986, pp. 219–221.

76. Wiedemann, B., and H. Grimm. Susceptibility to antibiotics: species incidence and trends. In *Antibiotics in Laboratory Medicine*, ed. by V. Lorian. Baltimore: Williams and Wilkins, 1996, pp. 900–1168.

77. Eliopoulos, G. M., C. B. Wennersten, and R. C. Moellering, Jr. Comparative in vitro activity of levofloxacin and ofloxacin against gram-positive bacteria. *Diagn. Microbiol. Infect. Dis.* 1996;25:35.

78. von Eiff, C., and G. Peters. In vitro activity of ofloxacin, levofloxacin and D-ofloxacin against staphylococci. *J. Antimicrob. Chemother.* 1996;38:259.

79. Wolfson, J. S., and D. C. Hooper. Fluoroquinolone antimicrobial agents. *Clin. Microbiol. Rev.* 1989;2:378.

80. Suh, B. and B. Lorber. Quinolones. *Med. Clin. North Am.* 1995;79:869.

81. Blumberg, H. M., D. Rimland, D. J. Carroll, P. Terry, and I. K. Wachsmuth. Rapid development of ciprofloxacin resistance in methicillin-susceptible and -resistant *Staphylococcus aureus*. *J. Infect. Dis.* 1991;163:1279.

82. Phillips, I., A. King, and K. Shannon. In vitro properties of the quinolones. In *The Quinolones*, ed. by V. T. Andriole. New York: Academic Press, 1998, pp. 81–116.

83. Gay, J. D., D. R. DeYoung, and G. D. Roberts. In vitro activities of norfloxacin and ciprofloxacin against *Mycobacterium tuberculosis, M. avium* complex, *M. cheloni, M. fortuitum* and *M. kansasii*. *Antimicrob. Agents Chemother.* 1984;26:94.

84. Fenion, C. H., and M. H. Cynamon. Comparative in vitro activities of ciprofloxacin and other 4-quinolones against *Mycobacterium tuberculosis* and *Mycobacterium intracellulare*. *Antimicrob. Agents Chemother.* 1986;29:386.

85. von Rosenstiel, N., and D. Adam. Quinolone antibacterials. An update of their pharmacology and therapeutic use. *Drugs* 1994;47:872.

86. Neu, H. C. Major advances in antibacterial quinolone therapy. *Adv. Pharmacol.* 1994;29A:227.

87. Spangler, S. K., M. R. Jacobs, and P. C. Appelbaum. Activity of CP 99, 219 compared with those of ciprofloxacin, grepafloxacin, metronidazole, cefoxitin, piperacillin, and piperacillin-tazobactam against 489 anaerobes. *Antimicrob. Agents Chemother.* 1994;38:2471.

88. Schentag, J. J., and B. E. Scully. Quinolones. In *Antimicrobial Therapy and Vaccines*, ed. by V. L. Lu, T. C. Merigan, and S. L. Barriere. Baltimore: Williams and Wilkins, 1999, pp. 875–901.

89. Gerding, D. N., and J. A. Hitt. Tissue penetration of the new quinolones in humans. *Rev. Infect. Dis.* 1989;11(Suppl. 5):S1046.

90. Brown, E. M., and D. S. Reeves. Quinolones. In *Antibiotic and Chemotherapy*, ed. by F. O'Grady, H. P. Lambert, R. G. Finch, and D. Greenwood. New York: Churchill Livingstone, 1997, pp. 419–452.

91. Schentag, J. J., D. E. Nix, and R. Wise. Pharmacokinetics and tissue penetration of quinolones. In *The New Generation of Quinolones*, ed. by C. Siporin, C. Heifetz, and J. Domagala. New York: Marcel Dekker, 1990, pp. 189–222.

92. Robson, R. A. Quinolone pharmacokinetics. *Int. J. Antimicrob. Agents* 1992;2:3.

93. Stahl, J. P., J. Croize, M. A. Lefebvre, J. P. Bru, A. Guyot, D. Leduc, J. B. Fourtillan, and M. Micoud. Diffusion of ofloxacin into the cerebrospinal fluid in patients with bacterial meningitis. *Infection* 1986; 14(Suppl):S254.

94. Wolff, M., L. Boutron, E. Singlas, B. Clair, J. M. Decazes, and B. Regnier. Penetration of ciprofloxacin into cerebrospinal fluid of patients with bacterial meningitis. *Antimicrob. Agents Chemother.* 1987;31:899.

95. Davey, P. G., M. Charter, S. Kelly, T. R. Varma, I. Jacobson, A. Freeman, E. Precious, and J. Lambert. Ciprofloxacin and sparfloxacin penetration into human brain tissue and their activity as antagonists of GABA_A receptor of rat vagus nerve. *Antimicrob. Agents Chemother.* 1994;38:1356.

96. Malmborg, A. S., and S. Rannikko. Enoxacin distribution in human tissues after multiple oral administration. *J. Antimicrob. Chemother.* 1988;21(Suppl. B): 57.

97. Duben, W., A. Student, M. Jablonski, and R. Malottke. Tissue concentration and effectiveness of ofloxacin in surgical patients. *Infection* 1986;14(Suppl. 1):S70.

98. Waldron, R., D. G. Arkell, R. Wise, and J. M. Andrews. The intraprostatic penetration of ciprofloxacin. *J. Antimicrob. Chemother.* 1986;17:544.

99. Rannikko, S., and A. S. Malmborg. Enoxacin concentration in human prostatic tissue after oral administration. *J. Antimicrob. Chemother.* 1986;17:123.

100. Naber, K. G., D. Adam, R. Wittenberger, and B. Bartosik-Wich. In vitro activity, serum, urine and prostatic adenoma concentrations of ofloxacin in urologic patients with complicated urinary tract infections. *Infection* 1986;14(Suppl. 1):S60.

101. Bergan, T. Pharmacokinetics of fluorinated quinolones. In *The Quinolones,* ed. by V. T. Andriole. New York: Academic Press, 1998, pp. 143–182.

102. Craig, W. A., and B. Suh. Protein binding and the antibacterial effects. Methods for the determination of protein binding. In *Antibiotics in Laboratory Medicine,* ed. by V. Lorian. Baltimore: Williams and Wilkins, 1991, pp. 367–402.

103. Fillastre, J. P., A. Leroy, B. Moulin, M. Dhib, F. Borsa-Lebas, and G. Humbert. Pharmacokinetics of quinolones in renal insufficiency. *J. Antimicrob. Chemother.* 1990;26(Suppl. B):51.

104. Stein, G. E. Pharmacokinetics and pharmacodynamics of newer fluoroquinolones. *Clin. Infect. Dis.* 1996;23(Suppl. 1):S19.

105. Fillastre, J. P., A. Leroy, and G. Humbert. Ofloxacin pharmacokinetics in renal failure. *Antimicrob. Agents Chemother.* 1987;31:156.

106. Wingender, W., K. H. Graefe, W. Gau, D. Forster, D. Beermann, and P. Schacht. Pharmacokinetics of ciprofloxacin after oral and intravenous administration in healthy volunteers. *Eur. J. Clin. Microbiol.* 1984;3: 355.

107. Ball, P. The quinolones. History and overview. In *The Quinolones,* ed. by V. T. Andriole. New York: Academic Press, 1998, pp. 1–28.

108. Rohwedder, R., T. Bergan, S. B. Thorsteinsson, and H. Scholl. Transintestinal elimination of ciprofloxacin. *Chemotherapy* 1990;36:77.

109. Dalhoff, A. Quinolones in antibiotics and chemotherapy. In *Pharmacokinetics of Selected Antibacterial Agents,* ed. by H. Schonfeld. New York: Karger, 1998, pp. 85–108.

110. Shimada, J., T. Mogita, and Y. Ishibashi. Clinical pharmacokinetics of sparfloxacin. *Clin. Pharmacokinet.* 1993;25:358.

111. Montay, G., and J. Gaillot. Pharmacokinetics of fluoroquinolones in hepatic failure. *J. Antimicrob. Chemother.* 1990;26(Suppl. B):61.

112. Eandi, M., I. Viano, F. Di Nola, L. Leone, and E. Genazzani. Pharmacokinetics of norfloxacin in healthy volunteers and patients with renal and hepatic damage. *Eur. J. Clin. Microbiol.* 1983;2:253.

113. Bergan, T. Pharmacokinetics of the fluoroquinolones. In *The Quinolones,* ed. by V. T. Andriole. New York: Academic Press, 1998, pp. 143–182.

114. Garrelts, J. C., G. Jost, S. F. Kowalsky, G. J. Krol, and J. T. Lettieri. Ciprofloxacin pharmacokinetics in burn patients. *Antimicrob. Agents Chemother.* 1996; 40:1153.

115. Childs, S. J. Quinolones for the urinary tract. In *The New Generation of Quinolones,* ed. by C. Siporin. New York: Marcel Dekker, 1990, pp. 223–242.

116. Naber, K. G. Use of quinolones in urinary tract infections and prostatitis. *Rev. Infect. Dis.* 1990; 11(Suppl.5):S1321.

117. Andriole, V. T. Use of quinolones in treatment of prostatitis and lower urinary tract infections. *Eur. J. Clin. Microbiol. Infect. Dis.* 1991;10:343.

118. Nicolle, L. E. Use of quinolones in urinary tract infection and prostatics. In *The Quinolones,* ed. by V. T. Andriole. New York: Academic Press, 1998, pp. 183–202.

119. Segreti, J., L. J. Goodman, R. M. Petrak, R. L. Kaplan, G. W. Parkhurst, and G. M. Trenholme. Serum and fecal levels of ciprofloxacin and trimethoprim-sulfamethoxazole in adults with diarrhea. *Rev. Infect. Dis.* 1988;10(Suppl. 1):S206.

120. Nord, C. E. Effect of the quinolones on the human intestinal microflora. *Drugs* 1995;49(Suppl. 2):81.

121. Hamer, D. H., and S. L. Gorbach. Use of the quinolones for the treatment and prophylaxis of bacterial gastrointestinal infections. In *The Quinolones,* ed. by V. T. Andriole. New York: Academic Press, 1998, pp. 267–285.

122. Gotuzzo, E., and C. Carrillo. Mini review: quinolones in typhoid fever. *Infect. Dis. Clin. Pract.* 1994; 3:345.

123. Green, S., and G. Tillotson. Use of ciprofloxacin in developing countries. *Pediatr. Infect. Dis. J.* 1997;16: 150.

124. Bennish, M. L., M. A. Salam, and W. A. Khan. Treatment of shigellosis: 111. Comparison of one or two dose ciprofloxacin with standard 5 day therapy. A randomized, blinded trial. *Ann. Intern. Med.* 1992;117: 727.

125. Gotuzzo, E., C. Seas, J. Echevarria, C. Carrillo, R. Mostorino, and R. Ruiz. Ciprofloxacin for the treatment of cholera: a randomized, double-blind, controlled

trial of a single daily dose in Peruvian adults. *Clin. Infect. Dis.* 1995;20:1485.

126. Caeiro, J. P., and H. DuPont. Management of travelers' diarrhea. *Drugs* 1988;56:73.

127. Wistrom, J., and R. Norrby. Antibiotic prophylaxis of travelers' diarrhoea. *Scand. J. Infect. Dis.* 1990; 22(Suppl. 70):111.

128. DuPont, H. L., and C. D. Ericsson. Prevention and treatment of travelers' diarrhea. *N. Engl. J. Med.* 1993;328:1821.

129. Salam, I., P. Katelaris, S. Leigh-Smith, and M. J. G. Farthing. Randomized trial of single-dose ciprofloxacin for travelers' diarrhea. *Lancet* 1994;344: 1537.

130. Ellis-Pegler, R. B., L. K. Hyman, R. J. H. Ingram, and M. McCarthy. A placebo controlled evaluation of lomefloxacin in the treatment of bacterial diarrhea in the community. *J. Antimicrob. Chemother.* 1995;36:259.

131. DiCarlo, R. P., and D. H. Martin. Use of the quinolones in sexually transmitted diseases. In *The Quinolones*, ed. by V. T. Andriole. New York: Academic Press, 1998, pp. 203–227.

132. Saavedra, S., C. R. Rivera-Vazquez, and C. H. Ramirez-Ronda. Quinolones and sexually transmitted diseases. In *The New Generation of Quinolones*, ed. by C. Sipporin, C. Heifetz, and J. Domagala. New York: Marcel Dekker, 1990, pp. 277–287.

133. Hook, E. W., G. B. Pinson, C. J. Blalock, and R. B. Johnson. Dose-ranging study of CP99,219 (trovafloxacin) for treatment of uncomplicated gonorrhea. *Antimicrob. Agents Chemother.* 1996;40:1720.

134. Haria, M., and H. M. Lamb. Trovafloxacin. *Drugs* 1997;54:435.

135. Niederman, M. S. Treatment of respiratory infections with quinolones. In *The Quinolones*, ed. by V. T. Andriole. New York: Academic Press, 1998, pp. 229–250.

136. Yu, V. L., and E. Vergis. New macrolides or new quinolones as monotherapy for patients with community acquired pneumonia. *Chest* 1998;113: 1159.

137. Stein, G., and D. Havlichek. Newer oral antimicrobials for resistant respiratory tract pathogens. Which show the most promise? *Postgrad. Med.* 1998; 103:67.

138. Grossman. R. F. The role of fluoroquinolones in respiratory tract infections. *J. Antimicrob. Chemother.* 1997;40(Suppl. A):59.

139. LeBel, M., Fluoroquinolones in the treatment of cystic fibrosis: a critical appraisal. *Eur. J. Clin. Microbiol. Infect. Dis.* 1991;10:316.

140. Lew, D. P., and F. A. Waldvogel. Quinolones and osteomyelitis. State-of-the-art. *Drugs* 49(Suppl. 2): 100 (1995).

141. Gentry, L. O., and G. Rodriguez-Gomez. Ofloxacin versus parenteral therapy for chronic osteomyelitis. *Antimicrob. Agents Chemother.* 1991;35:538.

142. Jauregui, L., and S. McInnes. Therapy of gastrointestinal, central nervous system, and bone infections with new quinolones. In *The New Generation of Quinolones*, ed. by C. Siporin, C. Heifetz, and J. Domagala. New York: Marcel Dekker, 1990, pp. 289–316.

143. Gentry, L. O. Oral antimicrobial therapy for osteomyelitis. *Ann. Intern. Med.* 1991;114:986.

144. Waldvogel, F. A. Use of quinolones for the treatment of osteomyelitis and septic arthritis. *Rev. Infect. Dis.* 1989;11(Suppl. 5):S1259.

145. Parish, L. C., and D. L. Jungkind. Systemic antimicrobial therapy for skin and skin structure infections: Comparison of fleroxacin and ceftazidime. *Am. J. Med.* 1993;94(Suppl. 3A):166.

146. Monk, J. P., and D. M. Campoli-Richards. Ofloxacin: a review of its antibacterial activity, pharmacokinetic properties and therapeutic use. *Drugs* 1987; 33:346.

147. Leysen, D. C., A. Haemers, and S. R. Pattyn. Mycobacteria and the new quinolones. *Antimicrob. Agents Chemother.* 1989;33:1.

148. Garcia-Rodriguez, J. A., and A. C. G. Garcia. In-vitro activities of quinolones against mycobacteria. *J. Antimicrob. Chemother.* 1993;32:797.

149. Gelber, R. H., A. Iranmanesh, L. Murray, P. Siu, and M. Tsang. Activities of various quinolone antibiotics against *Mycobacterium leprae* in infected mice. *Antimicrob. Agents Chemother.* 1992;36:2544.

150. Alangaden, G. J., and S. A. Lerner. The clinical use of fluoroquinolones for the treatment of mycobacterial diseases. *Clin. Infect. Dis.* 1997;25:1213.

151. Jacobs, M. R. Activity of quinolones against mycobacteria. *Drugs* 1995;49(Suppl. 2):67.

152. Dekker, A. W., M. Rozenberg-Arska, and J. Verhoef. Infection prophylaxis in acute leukemia: a comparison of ciprofloxacin with trimethoprim-sulfamethoxazole and colistin. *Ann. Intern. Med.* 1987; 107:7.

153. Bow, E. J., E. Rayner, and T. J. Louie. Comparison of norfloxacin with cotrimoxazole for infection prophylaxis in acute leukaemia: the trade-off for reduced gram-negative sepsis. *Am. J. Med.* 1988;84:847.

154. GIMEMA Infection Program. Prevention of bacterial infection in neutropenic patients with hematologic malignancies: a randomized, multicenter trial comparing norfloxacin with ciprofloxacin. *Ann. Intern. Med.* 1991;115:7.

155. Liang, R. H., R. W. Yung, T. K. Chan, P. Y. Chau, W. K. Lam, S. Y. So, and D. Todd. Ofloxacin versus co-trimoxazole for prevention of infection in neutropenic patients following cytotoxic chemotherapy. *Antimicrob. Agents Chemother.* 1990;34:215.

156. Meunier, F., S. H. Zinner, H. Gaya, T. Calandra, C. Viscoli, J. Klastersky, and M. Glauser. Prospective randomized evaluation of ciprofloxacin versus piperacillin plus amikacin for empiric antibiotic therapy of febrile granulocytopenic cancer patients with lymphomas and solid tumors. *Antimicrob. Agents Chemother.* 1991;35:873.

157. Davis, R., A. Markham, and J. A. Balfour. Ciprofloxacin: an updated review of its pharmacology, therapeutic efficacy and tolerability. *Drugs* 1996;51: 1019.

158. Meyer, R. D. Role of the quinolones in the treatment of legionellosis. *J. Antimicrob. Chemother.* 1991; 28:623.

159. von Keutz, E., and W. Christ. Toxicology and safety pharmacology of quinolones. In *Quinolone An-*

tibacterials, ed. by J. Kuhlmann, A. Dalhoff, and H.-J. Zeiler. New York: Springer-Verlag, 1998, pp. 297–337.

160. Christ, W., and B. Esch. Adverse reactions to fluoroquinolones in adults and children. *Infect. Dis. Clin. Pract.* 1994;3(Suppl. 3):S168–S176.

161. Stahlmann, R., and H. Lode. Safety overview. Toxicity, adverse effects, and drug interactions. In *The Quinolones,* ed. by V. T. Andriole. New York: Academic Press, 1998, pp. 369–415.

162. Wolfson, J. S. Quinolone antimicrobial agents: adverse effects and bacterial resistance. *Eur. J. Clin. Microbiol. Infect. Dis.* 1989;8:1080.

163. Paton, J. H., and D. S. Reeves. Clinical features and management of adverse effects of quinolone antibacterials. *Drug Safety* 1991;6:8.

164. Schacht, P., G. Arcieri, J. Branolte, H. Bruck, V. Chysky, E. Griffith, G. Gruenwaldt, R. Hullmann, C. A. Konopka, and B. O'Brien. World-wide clinical data on efficacy and safety of ciprofloxacin. *Infection* 1988; 16(Suppl. 1):29.

165. Nakamura, M., S. Abe, Y. Goto, A. Chishaki, K. Akazawa, and M. Kato. In vivo assessment of prevention of white-noise-induced seizure in magnesium-deficient rats by N-methyl-D-aspartate receptor blockers. *Epilepsy Res.* 1994;17:249.

166. Williams, P. D., and D. R. Helton. The proconvulsive activity of quinolone antibiotics in an animal model. *Toxicol. Lett.* 1991;58:23.

167. Takayama, S., M. Hirohashi, M. Kato, and H. Shimada. Toxicity of quinolone antibacterial agents. *J. Toxicol. Environ. Health* 1995;45:1.

168. Vassileva, S. G., G. Mateev, and L. C. Parish. Antimicrobial photosensitive reactions. *Arch. Intern. Med.* 1998;158:1993.

169. Brauner, G. J. Bullous photoreaction to nalidixic acid. *Am. J. Med.* 1975;58:576.

170. Domagala, J. M. Structure–activity and structure–side-effect relationships for the quinolone antibacterials. *J. Antimicrob. Chemother.* 1994;33:685.

171. Lowe, N. J., T. D. Fakouhi, R. S. Stern, T. Bourget, B. Roniker, and E. A. Swabb. Photoreactions with a fluoroquinolone antimicrobial: evening versus morning dosing.*Pharmacol. Ther.* 1994;56:587.

172. Burdge, D. R., E. M. Nakielna, and H. R. Rabin. Photosensitivity associated with ciprofloxacin use in adult patients with cystic fibrosis. *Antimicrob. Agents Chemother.* 1995;39:793.

173. Gough, A. W., O. B. Kasali, R. E. Sigler, and V. Baragi. Quinolone arthropathy–acute toxicity to immature cartilage. *Toxicol. Pathol.* 1992;20:436.

174. Forster, C., K. Kociok, M. Shakibaei, H. J. Merker, J. Vormann, T. Günther, and R. Stahlmann. Integrins on joint cartilage chondrocytes and alterations by magnesium deficiency in immature rats. *Arch. Toxicol.* 1996;70:261.

175. Stahlmann, R., J. Vormann, T. Günther, C. Forster, U. Zippel, E. Lozo, R. Schwabe, K. Kociok, M. Shakibaei and H. J. Merker. Effects of quinolones, magnesium deficiency or zinc deficiency on joint cartilage in rats. *Magnes. Bull.* 1977;19:7.

176. Royer, R. J., C. Pierfitte, and P. Netter. Features of tendon disorders with fluoroquinolones. *Therapie* 1994;49:75–76.

177. Carrasco, J. M., B. Gacia, C. Andujar, F. Garrote, P. de Juana, and T. Bermejo. Tendinitis associated with ciprofloxacin. *Ann. Pharmacother.* 1997;31:120.

178. Christ, W., and T. Lehnert. Toxicity of the quinolones. In *The New Generation of Quinolones,* ed. by C. Siporin, C. L. Heifetz, and J. M. Domagala. New York: Marcel Dekker, 1990, pp. 165–187.

179. Jaillon, P., J. Morganroth, I. Brumpt, G. Talbot, and the Sparfloxacin Safety Group. Overview of electrocardiographic and cardiovascular safety data for sparfloxacin. *J. Antimicrob. Chemother.* 1996; 37(Suppl. A): 161.

180. Thorsteinsson, S. B., T. Bergan, S. Oddsdottir, R. Rohwedder, and R. Holm. Crystalluria and ciprofloxacin, influence of urinary pH and hydration. *Chemotherapy* 1986;32:408.

181. Blum, M. D., D. J. Graham, and C. A. McCloskey. Temafloxacin syndrome. Review of 95 cases. *Clin. Infect. Dis.* 1994;18:946.

182. Polk, R. E., D. P. Healy, J. Sahai, L. Drwal, and E. Racht. Effect of ferrous sulfate and multivitamins with zinc on absorption of ciprofloxacin in normal volunteers. *Antimicrob. Agents Chemother.* 1989;33:1841.

183. Flor, S., D. R. P. Guay, J. A. Opsahl, K. Tack, and G. R. Matzke. Effects of magnesium-aluminum hydroxide and calcium carbonate antacids on bioavailability of ofloxacin. *Antimicrob. Agents Chemother.* 1990;34:2436.

184. Nix, D. E., J. H. Wilton, B. Ronald, L. Distlerath, V. C. Williams, and A. Norman. Inhibition of norfloxacin absorption by antacids. *Antimicrob. Agents Chemother.* 1990;34:432.

185. Parpia, S. H., D. E. Nix, L. G. Hejmanowski, H. R. Goldstein, J. H. Wilton, and J. J. Schentag. Sucralfate reduces the gastrointestinal absorption of norfloxacin. *Antimicrob. Agents Chemother.* 1989;33:99.

186. Neuvonen, P. J., and K. T. Kivisto. Milk and yogurt do not impair the absorption of ofloxacin. *Br. J. Clin. Pharmacol.* 1992;33:346.

187. Neuvonen, P. J., K. T. Kivisto, and P. Lehto. Interference of dairy products with the absorption of ciprofloxacin. *Clin. Pharmacol. Ther.* 1991;50:498.

188. Deppermann, K.-L., and H. Lode. Fluoroquinolones: Interaction profile during enteral absorption. *Drugs* 1993;45(Suppl. 3):65.

189. Wijnands, W. J. A., T. B. Vree, and C. L. A. van Heerwarden. The influence of quinolone derivatives on theophylline clearance. *Br. J. Clin. Pharmacol.* 1986;22: 677.

190. Maesen, F. P. V., P. Teengs, C. Baur, and B. I. Davies. Quinolones and raised plasma concentrations of theophylline. *Lancet* 1984;2:350.

191. Janknegt, R. Drug interactions with quinolones. *J. Antimicrob. Chemother.* 1990;26(Suppl. D):7.

192. Wijnands, W. J. A., C. L. A. van Heerwarden, and T. B. Vree. Enoxacin raises plasma theophylline concentration. *Lancet* 1984;2:108.

193. Radandt, J. M., C. R. Marchbanks, and M. N. Dudley. Interactions of fluoroquinolones with other drugs: mechanisms, variability, clinical significance and management. *Clin. Infect. Dis.* 1992;14:272.

194. Pollak, P. T., and K. L. Slayter. Hazards of doubling phenytoin dose in the face of an unrecognized in-

teraction with ciprofloxacin. *Ann. Pharmacother.* 1997; 31:61.

195. Toon, S., K. J. Hopkins, F. M. Garstang, L. Aarons, A. Sedman, and M. Rowland. Enoxacin–warfarin interaction: pharmacokinetic and stereochemical aspects. *Clin. Pharmacol. Ther.* 1987;42:33.

196. Akahane, K., M. Sekiguchi, T. Une, and Y. Osada. Structure-epileptogenic relationship of quinolones with special reference to their interaction with gamma-aminobutyric acid receptor sites. *Antimicrob. Agents Chemother.* 1989;331:1704.

197. Hori, S., J. Shimada, A. Saito, M. Matsuda, and T. Mitahara. Comparison of the inhibitory effects of new quinolones on gamma-aminobutyric acid receptor binding in the presence of anti-inflammatory drugs. *Rev. Infect. Dis.* 1989;11(Suppl. 5): 1397.

CHAPTER ELEVEN

Drugs that Act on Mycobacteria

Isoniazid, Rifampin, Ethambutol,
Streptomycin, and Pyrazinamide;
The Second-Line Antituberculosis Drugs;
Drugs Effective Against Leprosy; Drugs
Effective Against the *Mycobacterium
avium* Complex

The treatment of tuberculosis is a special problem within the field of chemotherapy. Some of the drugs used in treating this disease [streptomycin, para-aminosalicylic acid (PAS), cycloserine, kanamycin] have been presented in earlier chapters, since it was more convenient to consider them along with other agents having a similar mechanism of action. Many of the drugs employed in antituberculosis therapy are used only in treating infections caused by mycobacteria. The drugs used to treat tuberculosis may be divided into two groups according to their clinical usefulness. The primary, or first-line, agents have the greatest level of efficacy and an acceptable degree of toxicity. Drugs in this category include isoniazid, rifampin, ethambutol, pyrazinamide, and streptomycin.[1-3] The large majority of patients with tuberculosis can be treated successfully with these drugs. Excellent results are usually obtained with a 6-month course of treatment. Occasionally, because of resistance or patient-related factors (e.g., AIDS), it may be necessary to use the second-line agents in addition to the first-line drugs. Included among the second-line drugs are aminosalicylic acid, amikacin, capreomycin, ciprofloxacin, cycloserine, ethionamide, kanamycin, and ofloxacin.

Treatment of active tuberculosis virtually always includes simultaneous therapy with two or more of the primary drugs. It was observed some time ago that organisms resistant to a single drug are rather readily selected from populations of tubercle bacilli. Combinations of drugs are used to decrease the rate of emergence of resistance as well as increase the antibacterial effect. Combination chemotherapy has become a cornerstone of the treatment of tuberculosis.

The choice of drugs to be used in treating tuberculosis (see Table 11–1) depends on many factors, including the organ system involved, the severity of the disease, the state of the patient's renal and hepatic function, the in vitro sensitivity of the organism, and any history of relapse or failure to respond to previous therapy. The reader is referred to the therapeutic literature for specific recommendations regarding therapy. This introduction will be concerned only with brief mention of the therapeutic rationale behind the approaches used in treating pulmonary tuberculosis and the concept of preventive therapy.

Table 11–1. Drugs used to treat mycobacterial infections.

Infecting organism	Drug of choice	Alternatives
Mycobacterium tuberculosis	Isoniazid + rifampin + pyrazinamide ± ethambutol or streptomycin	Ciprofloxacin or oxafloxacin, para-aminosalicylic acid (PAS), cycloserine, ethionamide, kanamycin or amikacin
Mycobacterium kansasii	Isoniazid with rifampin with or without ethambutol or streptomycin	Clarithromycin, ethionamide, cycloserine
Mycobacterium avium complex (MAC)	Clarithromycin or azithromycin + one or more of the following: ethambutol, rifabutin, ciprofloxacin	Rifampin, clofazimine, amikacin
MAC prophylaxis	Rifabutin or clarithromycin	Azithromycin
Mycobacterim fortuitum complex	Amikacin and doxycyline	Rifampin, clarithromycin, a sulfonamide, ciprofloxacin or ofloxacin
Mycobacterium marinum (balnei)	Minocycline	Trimethoprim-sulfamethoxazole, clarithromycin, doxycycline
Mycobacterium leprae leprosy)	Dapsone with rifampin with or without clofazimine	Minocycline, ofloxacin, sparfloxacin, clarithromycin

Standard Therapy of Tuberculosis

Although treatment usually starts before the results of sensitivity testing are available, it is important that the physician always obtain appropriate cultures for determining drug susceptibility to ensure that therapy is continued with drugs that are active against the organism. There are two main principles of tuberculosis therapy: first, the treatment of tuberculosis must include at least two drugs to which the organism is susceptible, and second, treatment must continue long enough to sterilize the lesions and prevent relapse. Three populations of *Mycobacterium tuberculosis* are hypothesized to exist in the host: those in cavitary lesions, those in closed caseous lesions, and those within macrophages. Each of these populations varies in terms of rate of multiplication, level of metabolic activity, and oxygen concentration.[4] In cavities, the oxygen tension is high, the medium is neutral or slightly alkaline, and the multiplication is rapid. In the other two populations the oxygen tension is lower, the medium is neutral or acidic, and the replication is relatively slow. Antituberculosis drugs vary in their ability to kill bacteria in these three populations. The necessity of

having at least two bactericidal drugs present forms the basis for the currently recommended 6-month regimen of antituberculosis therapy consisting of isoniazid, rifampin, and pyrazinamide for two months followed by 4 months of isoniazid and rifampin.[4] Isoniazid and rifampin are the most efficacious antituberculosis drugs available. They are thought to be bactericidal for extracellular bacteria (including cavitary), intracellular (macrophages) bacteria, and bacteria in closed caseous lesions. Rifampin and pyrazinamide appear to be more active than isoniazid against slowly or intermittently replicating bacilli in macrophages and closed caseous lesions.

The standard 6-month course of therapy (isoniazid, rifampin, and pyrazinamide for 2 months followed by isoniazid and rifampin for four additional months) for drug-sensitive tuberculosis is the preferred treatment for both adults and children.[5] Pyridoxine also should be included to minimize adverse reactions to isoniazid.[6] This regimen is considered safe during pregnancy. Patients infected with HIV should receive more intensive therapy. Treatment should be initiated with at least a 4-drug regimen consisting of isoniazid, rifampin, pyrazinamide, and ethambutol or streptomycin. The combination of isoniazid and rifampin for 9 months is equally effective for fully susceptible organisms and may be more tolerable for some patients, particularly the elderly. Isoniazid plus ethambutol for 18 months is an alternative for patients who cannot tolerate rifampin.[2]

In areas where the rate of resistance to isoniazid is >4% or not well documented or when the patient has other risk factors for isoniazid-resistant tuberculosis, most experts recommend an initial four-drug combination of isoniazid, rifampin, pyrazinamide, and either ethambutol or streptomycin.[5,7] If susceptibility to all of the drugs is subsequently documented, the ethambutol or streptomycin can be stopped and pyrazinamide continued for only the first 2 months of treatment, with the isoniazid and rifampin being continued for a total of 6 months. If the tuberculosis is resistant only to isoniazid it can be treated with rifampin, pyrazinamide, and either ethambutol or streptomycin for 6 months, or with rifampin and ethambutol for 12 months.

If the treatment is appropriate, clinical improvement is readily seen. Within the first 2 weeks of therapy, there is a reduction of fever, decrease in cough, gain in weight, and an increase in the sense of well-being. There is also progressive radiological improvement. Over 90% of patients who receive optimal treatment will have negative cultures within 3 to 6 months, depending on the severity of the disease. Cultures that are still positive after 6 months are indicative of resistant organisms and alternative therapy should be considered.

Treatment of Drug-Resistant Tuberculosis

Compounding the resurgence in tuberculosis in recent years has been a substantial increase in resistance to both single-drug and multidrug treatment. Microbial resistance to the antituberculosis drugs may be either primary or secondary (acquired). Primary resistance occurs in patients who are not known to have had previous treatment with the antituberculosis drugs. Risk factors for primary resistance include exposure to a patient who has drug-resistant tuberculosis, being from a country with a high prevalence of drug resistance, and greater than 4% primary resistance to isoniazid in the community.[5] Resistance appears not to be distributed uniformly but is more prevalent in large urban areas and coastal or border communities. Some surveys in urban areas revealed that drug-resistant pulmonary tuberculosis occurred with about equal frequency in all ethnic groups, whereas others found the rates of resistance to be higher among Hispanics, Asians, and African-Americans than among whites.[8–10] Acquired resistance occurs in patients who have been treated in the past, and poor patient compliance is the primary reason that acquired drug resistance develops. To help prevent noncompliance and the development of drug-resistant tuberculosis, directly observed therapy (DOT) is advisable for most patients. Here, a health care worker observes the patient take the medication two to five times weekly.[11,12] The critical aim of treatment completion is to avoid the effects of nonadherence to therapy, such as persistent infectiousness on the part of the patient and higher rates of treatment failure, relapse, and drug resistance.

Management of patients with drug-resistant tuberculosis is complex and the best available expertise should be sought. Under no circumstances should a single drug be added to a failing regimen, as this creates ideal conditions for the development of resistance to the new medication. Treatment should be initiated with at least two effective drugs to which the patient has never been exposed. For the treatment of multiple drug–resistant tuberculosis (defined as M. tuberculosis resistant to isoniazid and rifampin, with or without resistance to other drugs) at least three or more drugs to which the organism is susceptible should be used. Therapy should be continued for 12–24 months after a negative culture. In some settings where multiple drug–resistant tuberculosis is likely, or in patients with a history of previous treatment of tuberculosis, some clinicians now start with combinations of five, six, or even seven drugs before susceptibility data are available.[13-15] The number of drugs used varies depending on the extent of disease and the potency of the available agents. A typical regimen for suspected multiple drug–resistant tuberculosis includes isoniazid, rifampin, ethambutol, pyrazinamide, an aminoglycoside or capreomycin, ciprofloxacin or ofloxacin, and either cycloserine, ethionamide, or aminosalicylic acid.

Intermittent Treatment

To improve compliance, the patient may be treated with intermittent high-dose, four-drug regimens in which two doses are administered per week following at least 2 weeks of daily therapy, or in which three doses per week are administered from the outset (see Table 11–2 for drug dosages under daily and twice-weekly therapy).[16,17]

Table 11–2. Usual dosages and most common side effects of the primary and secondary drugs used to treat tuberculosis.

	Dosage		Most comon side effects	Tests for side effects
	Daily	Twice weekly		
PRIMARY DRUGS				
Isoniazid	300 mg PO, IM	15 mg/kg up to 900 mg PO	Peripheral neuritis, hepatitis, hypersensitivity	Hepatic enzymes (not as a routine)
Ethambutol	15–25 mg/kg PO	50 mg/kg PO	Optic neuritis (reversible with discontinuation of drug; very rare at 15 mg/kg), skin rash	Red-green color discrimination and visual acuity
Rifampin	600 mg PO, IV	600 mg PO	Hepatitis, febrile reaction, rare purpura	Hepatic enzymes (not as a routine)
Pyrazinamide	1.5–2.5 g PO	2.5–3.5 g PO	Hyperuricemia, hepatotoxicity	Uric acid, SGOT/ SGPT
Streptomycin	15 mg/kg up to 1 g IM	20 mg/kg IM	Auditory, vestibular, and renal toxicity	Vestibular function, audiograms; BUN and creatinine
COMBINATIONS				
150 mg INH + 300 mg rifampin	2 tablets			
50 mg INH + 120 mg rifampin + 300 mg pyrazinamide	≤44 kg: 4 tablets 45–54 kg: 5 tablets ≥55 kg: 6 tablets			
SECONDARY DRUGS				
Capreomycin	15 mg/kg IM		Auditory, vestibular, and renal toxicity	Vestibular function, audiograms; BUN and creatinine
Kanamycin and amikacin	15 mg/kg IM, IV		Auditory and renal toxicity, rare vestibular toxicity	Vestibular function, audiograms; BUN and creatinine

(continued)

Table 11–2. Continued

	Dosage		Most comon side effects	Tests for side effects
	Daily	Twice weekly		
Ethionamide	250–500 mg bid PO		GI disturbance, hepatotoxicity, hypersensitivity	Hepatic enzymes
Para-aminosalicylic acid (PAS)	4–6 g bid PO		GI disturbance, hypersensitivity, hepatotoxicity, sodium load	Hepatic enzymes
Cycloserine	10–20 mg/kg up to 1 g PO		Psychosis, personality changes, convulsions, rash	Psychologic testing
Ciprofloxacin	500–750 mg bid PO		Nausea, abdominal pain, restlessness, confusion	
Ofloxacin	300–400 mg bid or 600–800 mg/day PO		Nausea, abdominal pain	

BUN, blood urea nitrogen; GI, gastrointestinal; IM, intramuscularly, IV, intravenously, PO, by mouth; SGOT/SGPT, serum glutamic-oxaloacetic/pyruvic transaminase.

Source: Modified from Bailey et al.[19] and The Medical Letter.[2]

These regimens are effective and relatively nontoxic. Most experts strongly recommend direct observation of all doses given intermittently.

Fixed-Dose Combinations

A combination of rifampin, isoniazid, and pyrazinamide has been approved by the Food and Drug Administration (FDA) for daily tuberculosis therapy during the initial 2 months of treatment. This combination simplifies compliance and prevents errors in self-administration and thus may decrease acquired drug resistance during unsupervised therapy.[18] Previously, a combination of isoniazid and rifampin had been available.

Atypical Mycobacterial Infections

Included among the atypical mycobacterial infections are *Mycobacterium kansasii, M. marinum, M. scrofulaceum,* and the *M. fortuitum* complex. These bacteria are frequently resistant to many of the commonly used antituberculosis drugs, and drug therapy is selected on the basis of their sensitivity in vitro.

Preventive Therapy of Tuberculosis

The term *chemoprophylaxis* is not appropriately applied with respect to tuberculosis.[2] In tuberculosis, instead of trying to prevent infection, a drug is given in order to prevent the development of clinically apparent disease in people who are already infected. Isoniazid is the only drug shown to be effective for preventing clinical symptoms of disease. It is usually given for 6 to 12 months (9 months for children) in a single daily dose of 300 mg for adults. At least 12 months is suggested for patients with AIDS or other immunosuppression or who have X-ray evidence of healed tubercular lesions. The risk of developing clinical tuberculosis is greatest in patients who are also infected with HIV, in those who have had close contact with patients having recent tuberculosis, and during the first 2 years after development of a positive tuberculin test. At the dosage used for preventive therapy, isoniazid can produce hepatitis. The likelihood that a person will develop hepatitis increases with age; because of this, all persons who are positive tuberculin reactors are not automatic candidates for preventive therapy. The following recommendations serve as guidelines for determining which patients with positive tuberculin tests should be considered for preventive therapy with isoniazid.[2]

Preventive therapy is recommended to age 35 (although in young adults who do not have associated risk factors, it is possible that the benefits of preventive therapy with isoniazid may not outweigh the risks.[21] Table 11–3 lists the high-priority candidates for preventive therapy. Infection with HIV is the most potent risk factor for the development of clinical tuberculosis in persons who are infected with tubercle bacilli.[5] In addition, even in the absence of any of the above risk factors, persons under 35 years of age in the following high-incidence groups are appropriate candidates for preventive therapy if they have a positive skin test: foreign-born persons from high-prevalence countries; medically undeserved low-income populations, including high-risk racial or ethnic minority populations, especially blacks, Hispanics, and Native Americans; and residents of facilities for long-term care (e.g., correctional institutions, nursing homes, and mental institutions).[5] Contraindications to preventive therapy include pregnancy, acute liver disease, and a history of previous isoniazid-associated hepatic injury or other severe reaction to the drug.

Table 11–3. Risk factors to be considered in determining candidates for preventive therapy with isoniazid.

Persons with HIV infection and persons with risk factors for HIV infection whose HIV infection status is unknown but who are suspected of having HIV infection
Household members and other close associates of persons with recently diagnosed tuberculous disease
Recent tuberculin skin test converters
Positive tuberculin reactors in the following special clinical situations:
  Diabetes mellitus
  Prolonged therapy with adrenocorticosteroids
  Immunosuppressive therapy
  Some hematological and reticuloendothelial diseases, such as leukemia or Hodgkin's disease
  Injection drug users known to be HIV seronegative
  End-stage renal disease
  Clinical situations associated with substantial rapid weight loss or chronic undernutrition (e.g., postgastrectomy)

Risk factors are according to guidelines presented by the American Thoracic Society.[5]

Isoniazid

Isoniazid was developed during a study of the tuberculostatic effects of pyridine car-

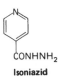
Isoniazid

boxylic acids.[22] Its structure is related to the vitamin nicotinamide which itself has a weak tuberculostatic action.

Antimicrobial Activity

Isoniazid is highly specific for mycobacteria. Concentrations of isoniazid of 600 µg/ml or greater are required to inhibit gram-positive and gram-negative bacteria, whereas the minimum inhibitory concentration for *Mycobacterium tuberculosis* is 0.05–0.25 µg/ml.[22] Isoniazid is also used to treat infection by *M. kansasii*, which is the most sensitive of the nontuberculous mycobacteria.

Mechanism of Action and Resistance

Isoniazid is bactericidal against actively growing tubercle bacilli; it is less effective against resting tubercle cells.[23] It has been reported to affect a number of cellular functions, and a variety of hypotheses have been advanced to explain the bactericidal action.[22,24,25] Any valid explanation of the mechanism of isoniazid action must account for its high specificity for mycobacteria. Although no proposal for a mechanism has been unequivocally linked to the bactericidal effect, the results of several studies suggest that the primary drug effect is to inhibit synthesis of mycolic acids.[26,27] *Mycolic acids*, which are β-hydroxy acids substituted at the α-position with a long aliphatic side chain, are important components of the cell walls of mycobacteria. When actively growing cultures of *Mycobacterium tuberculosis* are exposed to bactericidal concentrations of isoniazid, the cells rapidly lose their ability to incorporate precursors into mycolic acid.[28] The inhibition of mycolic acid synthesis is the earliest effect observed upon uptake of isoniazid into the bacterium, preceding the loss in cell viability by several hours. The mycolic acid–synthesizing system is inhibited at very low concentrations of the drug,[29], and isoniazid inhibits the production of very long–chain (greater than C_{26}) fatty acids that are precursors of the mycolic acids.[30] The first reaction specific to mycolic acid synthesis appears to be the desaturation of C_{24} and C_{26} fatty acids; this reaction, which is directed by a $\triangle^5$-desaturase, is inhibited by isoniazid.[31] It is not clear why the formation of a mycolate-deficient cell wall results in the loss of cell viability. Gross morphological changes are observed in isoniazid-treated cells by 24 h.[32] It is possible that mycolate-depleted cell walls are structurally weak, and distortion of cell architecture and finally cell rupture occur.[25]

A primary effect of isoniazid on mycolic acid synthesis would explain both the limited spectrum of action and the basis for the selective toxicity of the drug. The clinical usefulness of isoniazid is limited to *M. tuberculosis* and some atypical mycobacterial infections. Organisms of other genera and fungi are not affected unless extremely high concentrations are present in vitro. The mycolic acids are the major lipid components of the lipid-rich cell wall and other parts of the cell envelope of mycobacteria, and they appear to be unique to this class of organism. Since mycolic acids are not present in animal cells, there is selective toxicity with respect to the host.

Although it has been known for some time that inhibition of mycolic acid is an important factor in the mechanism of action of isoniazid, others remain unclear, including the question of what accounts for the lack of cell wall effect in some species of mycobacteria. Some evidence indicates that this is attributable to decreased permeability to the drug; however, no studies to date have demonstrated convincing differences in permeability to account for such great variations in susceptibility to the drug.[33] More important, the specific isoniazid target in the pathway of mycolate synthesis was unknown until recently, and the mechanism of inhibition is unknown. Recent evidence has shown that isoniazid specifically targets a long-chain enoyl-acyl carrier protein reductase (InhA), an enzyme essential for mycolic acid biosynthesis in *M. tuberculosis*. Data from X-ray crystallography and mass spectrometry reveal that an activated form of isoniazid attaches covalently to the nicotinamide ring of nicotinamide adenine dinucleotide that is bound within the active site of InhA.[34]

Isoniazid is a substrate for the endogenous mycobacterial enzyme KatG. Under normal conditions, KatG is the only catalase-peroxidase produced by *Mycobacterium tuberculosis*, and it is essential for growth of the organism inside macrophages but not in culture.[35] It has been proposed that KatG is required to activate isoniazid prior to exerting its bactericidal effect on a cellular target.[36] Isoniazid-resistant mutants frequently have an altered KatG gene producing a mutant protein, or they lack KatG altogether.[37] The most direct data suggest that KatG oxidizes isoniazid to a highly reactive acyldiimide or acyldiazonium ion that can then react with a cellular nucleophile and thereby inactivate a specific target.[38] This information compliments other observations indicating a role for mycobacterial catalase-peroxidase in the mechanism of action of isoniazid.[33]

RESISTANCE. Up to the 1980s, the incidence of primary resistance to isoniazid in the United States had remained stable at 4% of isolates of *M. tuberculosis*. By 1993, however, the incidence of resistance had doubled to about 9% and it may be much higher in certain populations, particularly among Asian and Hispanic immigrants to the United States.[14]

The larger the initial population of bacilli, the greater the likelihood that significant numbers of resistant cells exist before initiation of therapy. Selection of single-drug resistant mutants is discouraged by combination chemotherapy, but tubercle bacilli can acquire resistance to several drugs during therapy. This multiple drug resistance in mycobacteria is a consequence of multiple mutations and not multiple drug–resistance transfer as occurs with R factors in enterobacteria. It should be noted, however, that there is evidence for the occurrence of a plasmid for streptomycin resistance in M. smegmatis and that the resistance can be transferred by mycobacteriophage.[39] Both sensitivity and resistance to isoniazid have been transduced in another strain of the same organism.[40] Sensitivity is transduced at a higher frequency than resistance.

Several studies suggest that some mycobacteria resistant to isoniazid take up less drug than sensitive cells.[24] The mechanism of drug accumulation is not well understood. The drug becomes concentrated in the tubercle bacillus[41] and uptake is blocked by anoxia and metabolic poisons.[24] Under anaerobic conditions, the uptake of isoniazid is the same in drug-susceptible and drug-resistant strains.[33] Isoniazid is metabolized by the tubercle bacillus to the biologically inactive isonicotinic acid.[24] Resistance is not due to an increased rate of drug inactivation.[42]

The mechanism of resistance of M. tuberculosis to isoniazid is not known. Each of the hypotheses concerning the mechanisms of action of isoniazid attempts to deal with the problem of isoniazid resistance (see above). One hypothesis is that a lack of catalase-peroxidase is associated with isoniazid resistance, and the restoration of isoniazid susceptibility after transfer of the katG gene into isoniazid-resistant M. tuberculosis provides strong evidence to support this mechanism in some strains.[36,43] However, other studies indicate that the absence of catalase-peroxidase does not explain the mechanism of isoniazid resistance in most clinical isolates of M. tuberculosis. For example, one study in New York City showed that 35 (90%) of 39 isoniazid-sensitive and 31 (76%) of 41 isoniazid-resistant strains expressed the catalase-peroxidase enzyme.[44]

Mutations in the InhA gene may account for resistance. The InhA gene product has been shown to catalyze the NADH-specific reduction of a carrier protein, an essential step in fatty-acid elongation. Resistance to isoniazid in M. tuberculosis can be mediated by substitution of alanine for serine 94 in the InhA protein, and kinetic analysis has suggested that isoniazid resistance is due to a decreased affinity of the mutant protein for NADH.[45] This mutant InhA gene conferred resistance to isoniazid and ethionamide when it was transferred to isoniazid-sensitive strains of M. smegmatis and M. bovis.[46]

CONCENTRATION AND DURATION OF EXPOSURE. The effect of isoniazid in vitro and in vivo is related to both the concentration and duration of exposure to the drug.[47] This observation is of some clinical importance, since isoniazid levels rise and fall with each drug administration. At low concentration, the drug effect is bacteriostatic, and at higher levels, it is bactericidal. With multiple pulses of isoniazid there is a cumulative effect in vitro that is not observed if the pulses are too far apart.[47] When isoniazid is given to patients on an intermittent schedule, there are limits on how far apart the doses can be spaced and still retain the drug effect.[48] For example, with people who rapidly inactivate isoniazid (fast acetylators), therapeutic efficacy decreases sharply if the drug is given less often than twice a week.[49] This is, of course, what would be expected if the drug killed a certain percentage of the organisms and in the interval remaining before the next dose viable organisms multiplied sufficiently rapidly to restore the bacterial population. But there may be an additional explanation at the subcellular level. If M. tuberculosis, H37Ra strain, is exposed to isoniazid for 60 min in vitro (by this time there is virtually complete inhibition of mycolate synthesis)[28] and then permitted to grow in the absence of the drug, the mycolic acid–synthesizing capacity slowly returns to normal.[50] There is no recovery of activity if the exposure time is 10 h (by this time there is 90% loss of cell viability) or longer. Thus, the biochemical effect of isoniazid is reversible if exposure time is too short. Effective drug treatment may depend upon preventing the occurrence of this reversal.

Pharmacology of Isoniazid

ABSORPTION AND ADMINISTRATION. Isoniazid is provided in tablets for oral administration and in solution for intramuscular injection. It is rapidly absorbed from the gastrointestinal tract (primarily from the intestine)[51] and the plasma concentrations achieved after oral administration are equivalent to those achieved with intramuscular injection.[52] Peak plasma concentrations of 3–7 μg/ml are achieved 1–2 h after oral administration of usual doses to adults.[53] Lower peak plasma levels are obtained if gastric emptying is delayed by coadministration of antacids containing aluminum hydroxide.[53] Isoniazid does not bind to plasma protein and it is distributed throughout the body water.[54] Substantial levels of drug are found in pleural effusions and in the cerebrospinal fluid (20% of plasma levels) of both normal subjects and patients with tuberculous meningitis.[54] Isoniazid passes through the placenta, and concentrations in breast milk are similar to those in plasma. Studies of the distribution of radioactive isoniazid in humans have shown that the drug readily passes into, and is retained in, caseous tuberculous lesions.[54]

METABOLISM. The primary route of isoniazid metabolism in humans is by acetylation to acetyl isoniazid.[55] The enzyme responsible for the metabolism is an N-acetyltransferase that is located in the soluble fraction of liver cells.[56]

Two distinct human N-acetyltransferase gene loci exist—NAT1* and NAT2*. The hepatic enzyme responsible for the metabolism of isoniazid is NAT2. The genetic regulation of this enzyme is of fundamental clinical as well as basic importance (see Weber[57,58] for reviews). In the N-acetyltransferase reaction, an acetyl moiety from acetyl-Coenzyme A (acetyl-CoA) is first transferred to the enzyme, forming an acetylated enzyme intermediate (1). The acetyl group is then transferred to the drug, and the nonacetylated enzyme is regenerated (2). In humans, sulfamethazine and dapsone are acetylated by the same enzyme.[58]

(1) N-Acetyltransferase + acetyl-CoA ⇌ Acetyl N-acetyltransferase + CoA

(2) Acetyl-N-acetyltransferase + isoniazid ⇌ Acetyl isoniazid + N-acetyltransferase

The metabolism of isoniazid is noninducible, and the rate of metabolism is constant in any one patient. But there are large differences from one person to another in the rate of isoniazid acetylation. The isoniazid acetylator (NAT2) phenotype of the great majority of individuals can be characterized as either slow or rapid metabolism of the drug.[57,58] Slow acetylation is inherited as an autosomal recessive trait.[58] Thus, a slow acetylator is homozygous for two allelic genes, whereas rapid acetylators are either heterozygotes or homozygous for the rapid gene (see the table, below). The phenotype appears with varying frequency in populations of different racial origin. Estimates of the frequency of slow acetylators range from as low as 5% among Canadian Eskimos to as high as 83% among Egyptians and 90%

Genotype	Phenotype
slow-slow	Slow
slow-rapid	Rapid
rapid-rapid	Rapid

among Moroccans.[59] Forty-five to sixty percent of Caucasians are slow acetylators. Since acetylation is the primary route determining the rate at which isoniazid is elimi-

Isoniazid   Acetylated isoniazid

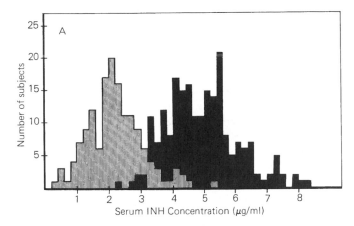

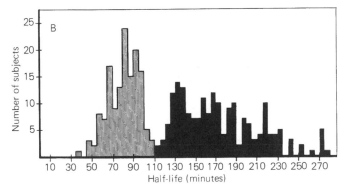

Figure 11–1. Bimodal distribution of serum isoniazid concentrations and half-lives in a large group of Finnish patients. More than 300 patients were given intravenous injections of 5 mg/kg of isoniazid (INH). Serum drug concentrations were assayed at multiple times after injection. (A) Distribution of the serum concentrations of isoniazid 180 min after injection; the stippled histograms represent rapid inactivators, and the solid histograms, slow inactivators. (B) Distribution of serum half-lives of isoniazid for patients of each group. (From Tiitinen.[61])

nated from the body,[57,60] slow acetylators will tend to have elevated levels of the drug in the plasma. This relationship is presented in Figure 11–1. In this study, isoniazid was given intravenously to over 300 Finnish patients, and serum drug levels and half-lives were determined.[61] The mean half-life for isoniazid in fast acetylators is about 80 min (range 40–110 mins), and it is 180 min (range from 110 to more than 270 min) in slow acetylators. The average serum concentration of active drug in rapid acetylators is 30–50% of that in the slow-metabolizing individuals.

Variability in NAT2 from person to person is due to mutation in the coding region of the *NAT2** gene. Of the more than 20 *NAT2** alleles that have been described, 3 or 4 account for greater than 95% of all human *NAT2** alleles discovered so far.[62–64] The *NAT2*4* allele is taken as the wild type, as it is found in individuals phenotyped as rapid acetylators. The other alleles are as-

sociated with reduced acetylation when any two of them are paired in an individual. Thus homozygosity in a mutant allele or compound heterozygosity of two different mutant alleles produces a slow acetylator. The mechanism of slow acetylation may involve reduced catalytic activity due to reduced protein production or stability or to decreased mRNA production or stability by the mutant allele.[65]

The distribution of *NAT2** alleles is neither uniform nor random across humans but varies with racial, ethnic, and geographic origin as noted earlier. In the future, individuals being treated with isoniazid will be genotyped as a guide to therapy. As a practical matter, such genotyping would not need to distinguish every known *NAT2** mutation, but would screen only for the three or four alleles that account for 95% of all alleles.

The genetic variations in the rate of isoniazid metabolism are of fundamental clinical importance, both in explaining limitations on the types of treatment schedules that can be employed in intermittent therapy and in the manifestation of drug toxicity. When isoniazid is given on a daily basis, as in standard therapy, the acetylator status of an individual does not affect the therapeutic result.[60] But the acetylator phenotype is very important in weekly, intermittent therapy in which rapid acetylators have fared considerably worse than slow acetylators.[60] Some untoward reactions are more likely to occur in slow-acetylating individuals. Peripheral neuropathy, a common adverse effect of isoniazid, is clearly dose related[66] and occurs more often in slow acetylators. Also, isoniazid hepatitis may occur with a higher frequency in slow acetylators[67] (see discussion of hepatitis in the next section for the mechanism). An interesting drug interaction between isoniazid and diphenylhydantoin occurs that is related to the acetylation polymorphism. Isoniazid is a noncompetitive inhibitor of diphenylhydantoin metabolism,[68] and when both drugs are given, patients who are slow acetylators are more likely to develop symptoms of diphenylhydantoin toxicity.[69] Diphenylhydantoin is metabolized by the microsomal mixed-function oxidase system,[57] which is inhibited in some manner by isoniazid.[70]

EXCRETION. Isoniazid and its metabolites are excreted in the urine. In humans, the major metabolites are acetylisoniazid and isonicotinic acid.[71,72] A small amount of unaltered drug is also excreted. The ratio of acetylisoniazid to free isoniazid in the urine of rapid acetylators is much greater than that of the slow acetylators.[72] The metabolites of isoniazid are less toxic and are more rapidly excreted by the kidney.[60] Although the principal limitation on the rate of excretion of isoniazid is the rate of its metabolism,[57] the drug will accumulate in patients with markedly impaired renal function (serum creatinine greater than 12), and isoniazid serum concentrations should be monitored in this group.[73] The effect of liver disease on isoniazid levels is not well documented. There is some evidence that serum concentrations of total isoniazid are higher in patients with chronic liver disease.[57,74] Isoniazid is removed by both peritoneal dialysis and hemodialysis.[57,75]

Adverse Effects of Isoniazid

NEUROTOXICITY. Isoniazid can produce a variety of effects in the central and peripheral nervous systems, the most common being peripheral neuritis. This dose-related effect[66] is more likely to occur in malnourished individuals, chronic alcoholics, and slow acetylators. The symptoms usually consist of numbness and tingling in the lower extremities.[76] Sometimes paresthesias occur in the hands and fingers as well. Frequently, there is also muscle aching, which is made worse by activity. Although sensory complaints dominate, weakness and, rarely, ataxia can occur. The syndrome reverses rapidly if the drug is withdrawn soon after the onset of symptoms, but if therapy is continued for more than a few weeks, residual difficulties may persist for as long as a year. The incidence is probably about 1% in patients taking 3 to 5 mg/kg of isoniazid daily but is considerably higher with larger doses. The peripheral neuritis results from pyridoxine deficiency. Isoniazid produces its neurotoxicity through inhibition of the activation of pyridoxine phosphokinase as well as by directly binding pyridoxine to enhance its urinary excretion.[77] The enzyme pyridoxine phosphokinase is responsible for the conversion of pyridoxine to pyridoxine 5' phosphate.[78] This active form of pyridoxine is a cofactor for the enzyme L-glutamic acid decarboxylase, which converts glutamic acid to gamma-aminobutyric acid. The hydrazine portion of isoniazid combines with pyridoxal phosphate (the active form of the vitamin) and inactivates its coenzyme action. The peripheral neuritis can be prevented by administration of 10 mg of pyridoxine with the isoniazid-containing regimen.[76,79] The pyridoxine does not affect the antibacterial action of isoniazid.[22]

Central nervous system side effects include symptoms of excitability, which extend from irritability and restlessness to seizures. Isoniazid overdosage (often as intentional ingestion)[80] can result in hyperglycemia, metabolic acidosis, and seizures. In the rabbit model, this acute central nervous system toxicity occurs more readily in slow acetylating animals (D. H. Hein and W. W. Weber, personal communication). Although the basis for the seizure activity is not clear, it is antagonized by pyridoxine and large doses of intravenous pyridoxine are administered to terminate seizures in patients with isoniazid overdosage.[80,81] Caution must be exercised when giving isoniazid to patients who are also receiving diphenylhydantoin. For reasons noted above, diphenylhydantoin toxicity (lethergy, incoordination) is more likely to occur in slow isoniazid inactivators receiving both drugs. A variety of psychological effects may be seen with isoniazid.[76] These range from complaints of depression and impairment of memory to the manifestation of acute toxic psychosis (more common in patients with a history of mental instability).[82] Other rare but serious neurological complications include toxic encephalopathy and optic neuritis.[76]

HEPATOTOXICITY. Hepatic toxicity is the most studied adverse effect of isoniazid. Although there were a few reports of hepatotoxicity in patients receiving isoniazid during the first two decades of its use, the extent of the problem was not clearly recognized until 1970 when it was reported that 19 of 2321 persons developed hepatitis while receiving the drug in a program of preventive therapy.[83] In response to this disclosure, the U.S. Public Health Service set up a nationwide program of surveillance of new recipients of isoniazid to identify the nature and extent of the risk associated with the drug. Several studies were also initiated to determine the pathophysiological and biochemical basis of the problem. The work carried out between 1971 and 1975 is reviewed in the proceedings of a conference held at the National Institutes of Health.[84]

From 10% to 20% of patients receiving isoniazid in preventive therapy develop evidence of subclinical hepatic injury as indicated by abnormal serum glutamic-oxaloacetic transaminase (SGOT) and bilirubin values.[85,86] Most patients who develop biochemical evidence of hepatic injury recover completely while continuing to take isoniazid. A few progress to the stage of clinically overt hepatitis. It is not clear why some patients are able to adapt to the liver injury while others progress. There is a definite relationship between the development of overt hepatitis and the age of the patient.[87] Progressive liver damage is rarely seen in patients under 20 years of age, but the incidence is 1.2% in patients aged 35 to 49 years and up to 2.3% in those 50 years and over.[88] Other factors that predispose to isoniazid-associated liver damage include excessive alcohol consumption, intravenous drug abuse, and a history of previous liver disease.[89] Women appear to have an increased risk for hepatotoxicity from isoniazid.[90,91] In one study, of 161 patients who died from isoniazid-associated hepatitis, 111 (69%) were female.[90] Patients on concurrent isoniazid and rifampin therapy have an increased incidence of hepatitis[92] that may result from a rifampin-mediated enzyme induction, causing an increased production of the toxic metabolites from mono-acetylhydrazine.[93,94]

Histological examination of liver biopsies from patients with clinical hepatitis revels mainly hepatocellular damage—in some cases there is submassive or massive necrosis.[95] Prior to the onset of jaundice, patients may complain of gastrointestinal symptoms (anorexia, nausea, vomiting, abdominal distress), weakness, and fatigue.[95] Hepatic injury may occur at any time during therapy. For example, in one study, 54% of the patients had received isoniazid for periods of 2–11 months before hepatic injury was noted.[95] Patients who are receiving isoniazid should be periodically evaluated for signs and symptoms of hepatitis. Periodic serum transaminase (SGOT) levels are probably not useful unless a patient is symptomatic.[86] Particular caution must be used when isoniazid must be administered to patients with preexisting liver disease.

Although individuals with isoniazid hepatitis have presented with features suggesting an allergic mechanism,[96] the liver injury is most likely caused by a toxic metabolite derived from the hydrazine moiety of the drug. As shown in the schema in Figure 11–2, acetylisoniazid is hydrolyzed to isonicotinic acid

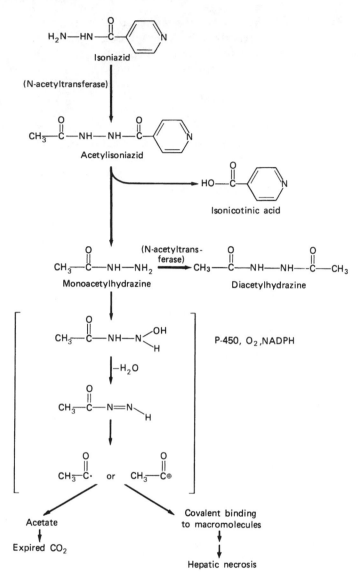

Figure 11–2. Proposed pathway by which isoniazid causes liver necrosis. Isoniazid is first converted to acetylisoniazid by *N*-acetyltransferase. Most of the acetylisoniazid is hydrolyzed to monoacetylhydrazine and isonicotinic acid (which is not hepatotoxic). There is evidence that monoacetylhydrazine is converted by the hepatic P-450 drug metabolizing system to one or more reactive intermediates that can covalently bind to components of liver cells. The compounds presented within brackets represent a suggested scheme for the production of the intermediates. The polymorphic *N*-acetyltransferase that converts isoniazid to acetylisoniazid also converts monoacetylhydrazine to diacetylhydrazine, which is nontoxic. (Prepared from Mitchell et al.[84] and Ellard and Gammon.[72])

and monoacetylhydrazine, a small amount of which can be recovered from human urine.[97] Monoacetylhydrazine has been shown to produce liver cell necrosis in rats.[84] The toxicity appears to result from metabolic activation of monoacetylhydrazine by the hepatic P-450 enzyme system to reactive species that link covalently to macromolecules in the liver. Pretreatment of rats with phenobarbital (a compound that induces P-450-dependent drug metabolizing activity) increases the extent of liver necrosis and the amount of covalent binding of hydrazine after administration of either acetylisoniazid

or acetylhydrazine.[84] It is clear that isonicotinic acid does not produce liver necrosis. If acetylisoniazid or isoniazid is radiolabeled in the pyridine ring and given to rats, no radioactivity becomes covalently associated with liver components. But if the animals are given acetylisoniazid labeled in the acetyl side chain, or labeled acetylhydrazine, there is significant covalent binding (as much as 0.5 nmoles/mg of hepatic protein).[84] These observations on metabolic activation and covalent binding have also been carried out with rat and human liver preparations in vitro.[98] The schema of events leading to isoniazid-mediated liver injury presented in Figure 11–2 is a reasonable proposal on the basis of the observations in humans and in animal models. The fact that older people are more likely to develop clinical hepatitis may simply reflect a decreased ability to rapidly repair hepatic damage with advancing age. At present, the model assumes that acylation of macromolecules in the liver leads to hepatic necrosis. This may be true, but the mechanism is not known.

Initial attempts to correlate hepatotoxicity with acetylator status led to the impression that rapid acetylators experience a higher incidence of isoniazid-induced liver injury than slow acetylators.[71,95] It is now clear that rapid acetylation is not a risk factor.[99,100] Indeed, in several controlled prospective studies it has been found that patients who are slow acetylators have a significantly higher incidence of hepatotoxicity than patients who are rapid acetylators.[67,101] Initially, it was reasoned that rapid acetylators would be at higher risk of hepatotoxicity because they produce more acetylisoniazid, the immediate precursor of monoacetylhydrazine. But in humans the major route for removal of monoacetylhydrazine from the body is by acetylation to diacetylhydrazine, which is not toxic (see Fig. 11–2). This second acetylation reaction is carried out by the same polymorphic N-acetyltransferase[102] and rapid acetylators convert monoacetylhydrazine to the nontoxic diacetyl form more rapidly than slow acetylators.[72,97] Using the measured rate constants for the various pathways shown in the schema of Figure 11–2, it has been calculated that, following a usual 300 mg dose of isoniazid, the same amount of monoacetylhydazine should be metabolized to potential hepatotoxic intermediates by both rapid and slow acetylators.[72] The relationship between acetylator status and isoniazid-induced hepatotoxicity is complex and theories linking the two are controversial; the reader is referred to a review for detailed discussion of the problem.[103]

ALLERGIC REACTIONS AND MISCELLANEOUS SIDE EFFECTS. Isoniazid occasionally causes allergic reactions including fever and a variety of rashes.[104] It is one of several drugs that can produce a syndrome very similar to lupus erythematosis.[105] The syndrome includes vasculitis and other clinical features of lupus as well as the serological abnormalities. Antinuclear antibodies have been found in a substantial percentage of tuberculosis patients treated with isoniazid.[106,107] The clinically manifest lupus syndrome occurs only rarely, however, and it usually disappears when therapy is stopped.

DRUG INTERACTIONS. Besides rifampin, a number of drugs can interact with isoniazid. Ethanol can increase the metabolism of isoniazid[77] and aluminum-containing antacids interfere with isoniazid absorption. Isoniazid can also increase the blood levels of phenytoin.[108]

Rifampin

Rifampin is one of a large number of semisynthetic derivatives of the antibiotic rifamycin B. The actions of the rifamycins have been reviewed by Wehrli and Staehelin[109] and by Hartmann.[110]

Mechanism of Action

The bactericidal effect of rifampin is due to inhibition of RNA synthesis.[111] The drug inhibits RNA synthesis by interacting directly with DNA-dependent RNA polymerase. Rifampin binds in a very tight[112] but noncovalent[113] manner to the enzyme from sensitive bacteria, but not to RNA polymerases from resistant strains.[112,114] Quantitative measurements have shown that one mole of rifampin is bound per mole of enzyme.[109]

Bacterial RNA polymerases are composed of several polypeptide chains. The core enzyme from Escherichia coli, for example, contains at least four subunits (2α, 1β, and $1\beta'$), and the enzyme core binds another unit, the σ factor. The σ factor effects recognition of the promoter regions of the DNA where transcription is initiated. The subunits of the core enzyme can be dissociated, separated from one another by electrophoresis, and then reassociated, to form a complex with enzyme activity.[115] This technique has been used to carry out recon-

Rifampin

stitution experiments in which components purified from rifampin-sensitive and rifampin-resistant RNA polymerases were employed. The effect of rifampin on the function of such reconstituted enzymes is shown in Table 11–4. The reconstituted enzymes are only about 20% as active as the original drug-sensitive and drug-resistant polymerases from which the subunits were derived, but it is clear that the β subunit must be derived from the drug-sensitive polymerase for substantial rifampin inhibition to take place.[115]

The β subunits of RNA polymerases from resistant bacterial strains have in some cases been found to have physical properties that are different from those of analogous drug-sensitive subunits.[116,117] Rifampin does not bind to the isolated β subunit, but it binds very tightly to the holo enzyme ($\alpha_2\beta\beta'$ σ) or to a partially reconstituted enzyme consisting of $\alpha_2\beta$.[118,119] Thus, the receptor for rifampin is the β subunit of bacterial, DNA-dependent RNA polymerase, but rifampin is bound tightly only when the β subunit is in the conformation it assumes when it is associated with two α subunits. The DNA polymerases are unaffected by the drug.

Until recently, the mechanism of rifampin resistance was studied exclusively in *E. coli* where it was found that single base pair changes occurred in the central region of the RNA polymerase beta β subunit gene (*rpoB*) (see above). The resurgence of tuberculosis has led to a renewed interest in the molecular basis of rifampin resistance in several species of *Mycobacterium*, including *M. smegmatis*, *M. leprae*, and *M. tuberculo-* sis.[120–123] It has been shown, for example, that rifampin-resistant *M. tuberculosis* has mutations in the *rpoB* equivalent of the *M. tuberculosis* β subunit gene that are very similar or identical to those in resistant *E. coli*.[121] The gene for the *rpoB* equivalent of resistant *M. tuberculosis* has been cloned and shown to confer rifampin resistance.[124] Thus the mechanisms of resistance in *E. coli* also apply to *M. tuberculosis*.

Rifampin inhibits the initiation of RNA synthesis, but synthesis in progress at the time of drug exposure is not affected.[125] If rifampin is added to RNA polymerase that has been preincubated with DNA template, the subsequent initiation of RNA chain synthesis is not inhibited.[126] The drug, however, does not block the formation of the complex between RNA polymerase and DNA.[127] The template-directed synthesis of a dinucleoside triphosphate is catalyzed by the enzyme even in the presence of rifampin, but the formation of a second phosphodiester bond does not take place.[128] Thus, neither the attachment of the enzyme to the promoter region of the DNA template nor the attachment of the first and second ribonucleoside triphosphates nor the formation of the first phosphodiester bond is significantly altered by the bound drug. This leaves three potential functions of the enzyme in initiation that could be affected by the drug: *(1)* the translocation of the enzyme to the next nucleoside residue on the DNA template; *(2)* the formation of the second diester bond; or *(3)* the binding of the newly synthesized RNA molecule to the site on the enzyme that accepts the RNA product after translocation.

Table 11–4.   *Demonstration that the β subunit is required for rifampin inhibition of bacterial RNA polymerase.* Purified polymerases from rifampin-sensitive and rifampin-resistant bacteria were dissociated, and the α, β, and β' subunits were separated by electrophoresis. The subunits were then mixed in stoichiometric ratio, σ factor was added, and the units were permitted to reassociate. The activity of the reconstituted enzymes was then assayed in the presence or absence of rifampin. The subscript r refers to subunits derived from the rifampin-resistant polymerase. Enzyme activity is expressed as milliunits per milligram enzyme protein.

	Specific activity of enzyme (mU/mg)		Inhibition by rifampin (%)
	Minus rifampin	Plus rifampin	
Original sensitive enzyme	242	1.5	99
Original resistant enzyme	124	120	3
Reconstituted enzyme			
$\alpha + \beta + \beta' + \sigma$	52	1.4	97
$\alpha_r + \beta_r + \beta'_r + \sigma$	27	25.6	5
$\alpha_r + \beta + \beta' + \sigma$	40	0.6	98
$\alpha + \beta_r + \beta' + \sigma$	88	69	22
$\alpha + \beta + \beta'_r + \sigma$	17.5	1.4	92

Source: From Heil and Zillig.[115]

The evidence available to date suggests that rifampin inhibits long-chain RNA synthesis by the third mechanism—that is, by preventing the binding of the initiated RNA molecule to the product-binding site on the enzyme.[129] In merodiploids, which contain roughly equal amounts of both drug-sensitive and drug-resistant β subunits, rifampin sensitivity is dominant.[130] It has been suggested that the drug-bound sensitive molecules may block the template so that the resistant polymerase cannot initiate RNA synthesis.[130]

Rifampin is selectively toxic because mammalian RNA polymerases are not affected by the drug. The RNA polymerases of sensitive bacteria are generally inhibited by concentrations in the range of 0.005–0.1 μg/ml. The RNA polymerase isolated from *Mycobacterium bovis* is inhibited 70% by rifampin at 0.1 μg/ml[131] whereas the enzyme from human placenta is not inhibited at 5 μg/ml.[132] Polymerase from rat liver nuclei is not affected until a concentration of 200 μg/ml is reached.[133] The same insensitivity has been found for nuclear polymerases from a variety of eukaryotic cells.[109]

There are several reports that RNA synthesis in mitochondria and chloroplasts is inhibited by rifampin.[134,135] The concentration of drug required for the effect, however, is more than 100 times that required to inhibit the bacterial enzymes. The fact that this RNA synthesis can be inhibited by rifampin has been used as an argument for these organelles resembling bacteria in their mechanism of RNA transcription. In view of the high concentrations required for inhibition, the rifampin effect may not provide good evidence for this proposal.[109]

Many rifamycin derivatives have been synthesized in the hope that greater activity against viral polymerases may be obtained. Some of these derivatives inhibit normal (and perhaps viral) RNA synthesis in mammalian cells, but only at high concentrations. In addition, synthesis of DNA and other biosynthetic processes are inhibited, so the specificity of the drug effect can be seriously questioned.[136] Recently, some very active semisynthetic derivatives of rifamycin have been developed which promise some hope in further shortening the duration of chemotherapy.[137]

Antimicrobial Activity and Clinical Use of Rifampin

Rifampin is very active against mycobacteria, gram-positive organisms, and *Neisseria* species.[138,139] There is less activity against gram-negative bacilli[139] because the drug does not readily penetrate the cell envelope. In vitro, the minimum bactericidal concentration of rifampin against *Mycobacterium tuberculosis* is 0.3–1.25 μg/ml.[138] Depending on the growth conditions, minimum inhibitory concentrations (MICs) can be in the range of 0.005–0.02 μg/ml.[138] The incidence of resistance to rifampin among *M. tuberculosis* isolates is low compared to that to streptomycin and isoniazid.[140] Resistance emerges by single-step mutation to a high-level resistance that is due to altered RNA polymerase,[131,141] and there is no cross-resistance with other antituberculosis drugs. The incidence of primary resistance among *M. tuberculosis* bacilli may be slowly increasing in the United States.[142] Rifampin is very effective at preventing emergence of resistance to isoniazid and streptomycin[143] and it has a very high sterilizing activity against *M. tuberculosis*. Rifampin is a better sterilizing drug than isoniazid. This may be because it is more effective at killing bacilli that are dormant much of the time but occasionally metabolize for short periods.[144]

Among the atypical mycobacteria, most isolates of *M. kansasii* (> 90%) and virtually all isolates of *M. marinum* are sensitive to rifampin at 0.78 μg/ml.[145] Isolates of the *M. avium-intracellulare-scrofulaceum* group are generally resistant, as are all isolates of *M. fortuitum*.[145,146] Rifampin has a rapid bactericidal action against *M. leprae*.[147]

In the United States, rifampin is used to treat mycobacterial infections and meningococcal carriers. Its efficacy in the treatment of tuberculosis is well established.[19,148,149] It is more active than ethambutol and it is as effective as isoniazid in the treatment of experimental tuberculosis in animal models.[150] Rifampin is useful in treating both pulmonary and extrapulmonary disease, including miliary tuberculosis and tuberculous meningitis.[151] When the drug is used alone, resistance develops readily, and the emergence of resistance is directly related to innoculum size.[152] Thus, rifampin is always used with other drugs in the treatment of tuberculosis. Pulmonary infections with *M. kansasii* and cutaneous infection with *M. marinum* have responded well to regimens containing rifampin.[153,154] The ability of rifampin to cause the rapid disappearance of *M. leprae* organisms from clinical specimens[155] has resulted in its inclusion in almost all drug regimens for initial treatment of leprosy.[147]

Rifampin is very active against *Neisseria meningitidis*, with MICs ranging from 0.004 to 0.125 μg/ml for sensitive organisms.[156] Rifampin is used to eliminate organisms from the nasopharynx of meningococcal carriers.[157] Drug-resistant meningococcal strains emerge readily,[158,159] even with treatment periods as short as 2 days.[160] Rifampin is recommended for the short-term treatment (adults, 600 mg daily for 4 days) of asymptomatic carriers of *Neisseria meningitidis*, but because of resistance, it is not indicated for the treatment of clinical infection.

In some countries, rifampin has been used to treat a rather wide variety of common gram-positive and gram-negative bacterial infections, a practice that is unwise because its use as a single drug in treating nontuberculous infection could promote the emergence of rifampin resistance in *M. tuberculosis*. A number of studies have shown that synergism may occur when rifampin is combined with certain other antibiotics, such as inhibitors of cell wall synthesis[161] or inhibitors of folate reductase.[162] Rifampin has been used on an investigative basis in combination with other antibiotics to treat selected severe infections by gram-positive and gram-negative bacteria,[163] and a fixed-ratio formulation containing trimethoprim and rifampin has been developed for treating urinary tract infections.[164]

The spectrum of rifampin's action against prokaryotic organisms with a sensitive polymerase appears to be determined by its ability to penetrate the cell envelope. Fungi, for example, are not susceptible to rifampin alone, but synergism may be observed with a combination of rifampin and amphotericin B in vitro.[165,166] This drug combination has also been shown to have an enhanced efficacy against fungal infections in animal models.[167,168] The combination is effective because amphotericin B alters the permeability of the fungal cell membrane, thus enabling increased rifampin entry and consequent inhibition of RNA synthesis (see discussion of amphotericin B action in Chapter 12).[165,166]

Pharmacology of Rifampin

Rifampin is well absorbed from the gastrointestinal tract, and peak serum levels of 7–9 μg/ml are achieved 2–3 h after oral administration of the usual 600 mg dose to an adult.[169,170] Peak serum levels of 9–12 µg/ml are achieved after oral administration of 10 mg/kg of rifampin suspension to infants or children.[171] Absorption is impaired if the drug is taken during or right after a meal[169,171] or if it is administered concomitantly with para-aminosalicylate (PAS).[170] Rifampin distributes widely in the tissues and body fluids[169] (see Table 11–5 for comparison of the pharmacokinetic properties of the major antituberculosis drugs).[172] Therapeutic levels of rifampin are achieved in the cerebrospinal[173,174] and pleural fluids.[175] Levels of drug exceeding the MICs for sensitive strains of N. meningitidis have been measured in saliva and tears.[171,177] Rifampin can penetrate into leukocytes and kill intracellular bacteria.[178] It also penetrates into nerves,[179] an important facet of its distribution in the treatment of lepromatous leprosy. About 85% of the drug in the serum is bound to plasma protein.[180]

Rifampin is metabolized in the liver by deacetylation and both the unaltered drug and the deacetylated metabolite are excreted in the bile.[181,182] The deacetylated metabolite is also biologically active. Unaltered drug is reabsorbed from the gastrointestinal tract in an enterohepatic cycle, but the deacetylated metabolite is very poorly reabsorbed. Thus, the drug is eliminated predominantly by the hepatic route. A small amount (10%–20%) of the drug and the metabolite are excreted in the urine, but the dosage of rifampin does not have to be modified in the presence of renal insufficiency. When hepatic function is impaired, however, the half-life is prolonged and serum levels of the drug increase.[74]

Rifampin is apparently taken into liver cells by an organic acid transport system. Rifampin can delay the clearance of bromsulfophthalein and unconjugated bilirubin from the plasma.[183] This effect is apparently due to its ability to compete for the uptake of these substances at the plasma membrane of liver cells.[184] The uptake of rifampin by the liver is significantly depressed by probenecid.[185] This results in a near doubling of the peak serum level.

The half-life and peak serum values of rifampin change during the course of therapy. After the first dose of 600 mg to an adult, the half-life is about 3.5 h. But after daily administration for a week or two, it is approximately 2 h [186] and remains constant thereafter.[107] The levels of rifampin in plasma assayed at 6 and 12 h after drug administration also fall during the first few days of therapy. This change in kinetics is apparently due to the fact that rifampin induces its own metabolizing enzymes in the liver.[182] The variation in the kinetics of rifampin during the initial period of daily administration is pharmacologically interesting, but it does not affect the therapeutic outcome, since the plasma levels achieved after prolonged daily administration are in the therapeutic range.

Adverse Effects of Rifampin

When given at the dosage recommended in Table 11-2, rifampin is a well-tolerated drug that rarely causes serious toxicity.[86] The adverse effects of rifampin are often divided into two groups—direct toxicity and immune system-mediated toxicity. Direct toxicity appears to be confined to the gastrointestinal tract and the liver. The most common side effects seen with daily rifampin administration are gastrointestinal reactions which usually consist of anorexia, nausea, mild abdominal discomfort, and occasionally diarrhea. Gastrointestinal distress can often be reduced by taking the drug during or immediately after a meal,[86] although lower peak serum levels will be achieved than when the drug is administered on an empty stomach.[169,171]. Some patients may experience cutaneous reactions consisting of flushing and itching with or without a rash. These reactions are usually short-lived and the drug regimen can be continued without interruption.[86] Headache, drowsiness, ataxia, dizziness, fatigue, and other central nervous system complaints occur occasionally. Rifampin and its metabolites may give a red-orange color to urine, feces, saliva, sweat, and tears (a special problem with patients wearing contact lenses). Patients should be warned of this to prevent unnecessary anxiety and expense.

Rifampin can cause hepatitis, especially in alcoholics and in patients with a history of previous liver disease.[86,188] Serum transami-

Table 11-5. Pharmacokinetic properties of the major antituberculosis drugs.

Drug	Solubility	Absorption from gastrointestinal tract	Protein binding (%)	Apparent volume of distribution (% body weight)	Tissue concentration	Half-life (min)	Metabolism
Isoniazid	Water slightly > lipid	Complete	None	60	Intracellular	80 fast acetylators 180 slow acetylators	Mostly metabolized
Rifampin	Lipid >> water	Almost complete	85	160	Intracellular	200 uninduced 120 induced	30%–60% deacetylated but active
Ethambutol	Water >> lipid	80%–95%	20–30	165[a]	Concentrated in lung tissue 5- to 10-fold over serum	240	10%–20% oxidized and inactive
Streptomycin	Water >> lipid	None	35	25	Very low	150	Not metabolized
Pyrazinamide	Not water-soluble	Complete	50	65	Intracellular	540–600	Mostly metabolized

[a] Steady-state volume of distribution calculated using a two-compartment model according to Lee et al.[176]

Source: Table prepared from data of Jenne and Beggs[172] and references cited in Chapters 5 and 11 under the pharmacology of each drug.

nase levels should be obtained periodically when the drug is administered to patients with chronic liver disease. Rifampin is usually administered with isoniazid, which is also hepatotoxic; some studies suggest that the rifampin-isoniazid combination produces hepatitis more frequently than isoniazid combined with other antituberculosis drugs. Rarely, fulminant hepatitis with hepatic encephalophathy has been reported with the isoniazid-rifampin combination.[189]

Immune-mediated toxicities appear to be related to immune system recognition of epitopes of rifampin. The intermittent or interrupted administration of rifampin seems to favor the development of immune system recognition of rifampin epitopes. A higher incidence of adverse reactions has been reported with bi-weekly and once-weekly intermittent therapy with rifampin in high dosage.[86,190] A flu-like syndrome consisting of fever and chills, sometimes accompanied by muscle aches, headache, and dizziness, occurs almost exclusively in patients receiving intermittent rifampin therapy. The syndrome appears most commonly during the third to sixth month of therapy and the symptoms start 1 to 2 h after each dose of rifampin and last for up to 8 h.[86] The syndrome is clearly dose related,[99,191] but most patients have circulating rifampin antibodies and there is considerable evidence that the syndrome has an immunological basis.[86,191] The syndrome can usually be stopped by changing from intermittent to daily rifampin administration.[86] Rarely, patients receiving high-dose, intermittent therapy have experienced shortness of breath and shock.[86] Hemolysis or thrombocytopenia occur rarely, and high titers of rifampin-dependent antibodies that bind complement to red cells and platelets have been identified in patients who experience acute hemolytic anemia or thrombocytopenic purpura.[86,191] Mild hemolysis may occur in conjunction with the flu-like syndrome.[192] If thrombocytopenic purpura occurs, the drug should be stopped immediately and should never be administered again. Acute renal failure has also occurred rarely, sometimes following shock or hemolysis. If renal failure occurs, rifampin should be withdrawn immediately. Renal function will almost always return to normal, but rifampin should never be administered again.[86] Severe reactions, such as shock or acute renal failure, may rarely occur when rifampin therapy is resumed after an interval, even in patients who have not previously experienced severe reactions.[86]

Rifampin has been shown to have immunosuppressive properties in various animal test systems.[154] Both cellular and humoral immune responses are reported to be affected after what have usually been quite high doses of drug. Rifampin binds to and activates the human glucocorticoid receptor, which regulates the expression of genes encoding the interleukins that regulate immune responses as well as genes encoding P-450 enzymes that metabolize drugs.[193] Conflicting evidence for an immunosuppressive effect has been obtained in human studies. Rifampin has been reported to attenuate the cutaneous reaction to purified protein derivative[194] and to depress the number of circulating T-lymphocyte (but not B-lymphocyte) rosettes in patients receiving the drug in therapeutic dosage,[195] but other studies have failed to show effects on a number of parameters of both humoral and cellular immunity.[196,197] In general, it can be said that if rifampin has an immunosuppressive effect at the doses used in the therapy of tuberculosis, the immunosuppression, when observed, has not impaired the therapeutic response or enhanced the susceptibility of patients to other infectious diseases.[154] Rifampin therapy has been associated with the production of light-chain proteinuria.[198] The mechanism is not known and it has not been of apparent clinical significance, except that a case of renal failure has been reported in one patient who also experienced prolonged dehydration.[199]

DRUG INTERACTIONS. Several interactions between rifampin and other drugs have been reported.[200] As mentioned above, the absorption of rifampin is inhibited by PAS, and these two drugs should be administered to a patient 8 to 12 h apart.[170] Early-phase hyperglycemia has been observed in some patients receiving rifampin therapy.[201] This is apparently due to an ability of rifampin to augment intestinal absorption of glucose.[201] Rifampin induces hepatic microsomal enzymes and reduces the serum half-life and plasma concentration of coumarin anticoagulants,[202] quinidine,[203] narcotics,[200] glucocorticoids,[204] thyroxin,[205] dapsone,[206] and oral contraceptives.[207] Because several women have become pregnant while taking oral contraceptives and rifampin,[207] alternative contraceptive measures should be considered. Other clinically relevant interactions include those with several drugs used for the treatment of human immunodeficiency virus infection (e.g., zidovudine, protease inhibitors, delaviridine), several anti-infective agents (e.g., itraconazole, fluconazole, and doxycycline), immunosuppressants (e.g., cyclosporine and tacrolimus), psychotropic agents (e.g., nortripyline and benzodiazepines), the calcium channel blocker nifedipine, and the sedatives midazolam and triazolam.[208] Apparently, rifampin induces several cytochrome P-450 isoenzymes.

Ethambutol

While screening randomly selected compounds for antimicrobial activity during the early 1960s, it was found that N,N'-diisopropyl ethylenediamine was active against some mycobacteria. Ethambutol is the most active of a series of congeners that was prepared to improve upon the activity of this new antimycobacterial structure.[209] Only the dextroisomer of ethambutol is active.[209]

$$H-\underset{\underset{C_2H_5}{|}}{\overset{\overset{CH_2OH}{|}}{C}}-NH-CH_2-CH_2-HN-\underset{\underset{C_2H_5}{|}}{\overset{\overset{CH_2OH}{|}}{C}}-H$$

Ethambutol

Antimicrobial Activity and Clinical Use

Ethambutol is active only against mycobacteria.[210] Ninety percent of strains of *M. tuberculosis* are sensitive to ethambutol at 2 µg/ml or less.[210,211] Most strains of *M.*

kansasii (MIC 0.4–3 µg/ml) and essentially all strains of *M. marinum* are sensitive to ethambutol in vitro, but isolates of the *M. avium-intracellulare-scrofulaceum* group are generally resistant, as are all isolates of *M. fortuitum*.[145,146]

Ethambutol has less sterilizing activity against *M. tuberculosis* than rifampin or isoniazid.[149] It suppresses the emergence of resistance to other antituberculosis drugs, but it is less active in this respect than rifampin, isoniazid, or streptomycin.[149] When ethambutol is used with isoniazid, rifampin, or streptomycin against *M. tuberculosis* in vitro, inhibition of growth is roughly additive.[212] The efficacy of ethambutol in the initial treatment of tuberculosis is well established.[213,214] Because ethambutol is usually bacteriostatic in clinical practice and since it has little activity against the slow-growing organisms, it is not as useful as the other major antituberculosis drugs for short-course chemotherapy.[215] As with the other antituberculosis drugs, tubercle bacilli can become resistant if ethambutol is used alone, so the drug is always given in combination with one or two other agents. The mechanism of the resistance is unknown, but there is no cross-resistance with other drugs.[216]

Mechanism of Action

Ethambutol is active against dividing mycobacteria but has no effect on nonproliferating cells.[217] Depending on the growth conditions and drug concentration, the response of mycobacteria to ethambutol in vitro may be bacteriostatic or bactericidal.[217] Ethambutol rapidly enters mycobacteria by passive diffusion, but growth inhibition is not apparent until many hours after addition of the drug to a culture. Both the association of radiolabeled ethambutol with mycobacteria and growth inhibition are prevented in a nonspecific manner by cations and polyamines.[218] The amount of growth inhibition obtained depends on length of exposure to the drug.[219]

The early effects of the drug are reversible, and when cells from inhibited cultures are resuspended in drug-free medium, growth

DRUGS THAT ACT ON MYCOBACTERIA 301

resumes after a prolonged lag period. There is no lag, however, if the cells had been exposed to the drug at low temperature. The lag period is thought to represent the time required for repair of the biochemical damage incurred during growth in the presence of the drug.[220]

Ethambutol has been reported to affect a wide variety of cellular functions, but most are probably secondary events (see review by Beggs[216]). As with isoniazid, any valid mechanism of ethambutol action must account for its unique specificity for mycobacteria. The drug is inactive against viruses, fungi, and bacteria of other genera. Ethambutol has been shown to inhibit the incorporation of mycolic acid into the cell wall of M. smegmatis.[221] This effect is rapid and it occurs at low drug concentrations. An effect on the transfer of mycolic acid to the cell wall would explain the very limited spectrum of action of this drug. Exposure of actively growing M. smegmatis to 3 μg/ml of ethambutol is followed by the rapid (within 1–12 min) accumulation of free mycolic acid and trehalose mycolates in the cell.[222] Subsequently, these components leak from the bacterium into the medium.[222]

Although these early studies suggested a target in the mycobacterial cell wall, they did not identify the specific target. The observation that ethambutol inhibited arabinose incorporation into the cell wall arabinogalactan led to the identification of arabinose decaprenylmonophosphate as the biogenetic source of arabinose in the cell wall arabinogalactan.[223,224] Arabinose incorporation into the cell wall was specifically inhibited by ethambutol, whereas arabinose incorporation into lipoarbinomannan was not as severely affected.[225] Chemical synthesis of the polyprenolphosphate arabinose donor then allowed a direct demonstration of the effect of ethambutol in cell-free assays of arabinose transfer.[226] It is now clear that arabinosyltransferase enzymes are the physiological target of ethambutol,[227] and a three-gene operon from M. avium has been identified (the emb region) that is sufficient to confer ethambutol resistance upon M. smegmatis when expressed from a high-copy vector.[228]

Two of the genes (embA and embB) encode arabinosyltransferases and are homologous to each other, while the third gene is homologous to transcriptional repressors and may play a role in regulating operon expression.

Pharmacology of Ethambutol

Ethambutol is rapidly and extensively (85%–95% of a dose) absorbed from the gastrointestinal tract.[229,230] Peak plasma levels of 3–6 ug/ml are achieved 2–4 h after oral administration of a 15 mg/kg dose.[231] Twenty to thirty percent of the drug is bound to plasma protein.[231] Using a two-compartment model, ethambutol was calculated to distribute into a central compartment volume of 0.36 liters/kg, with a steady-state distribution of 1.6 liters/kg.[176] Ethambutol enters the cerebrospinal fluid, where levels range from 10% to 50% of the simultaneous serum concentration.[232,233] Ethambutol penetrates into pulmonary parenchyma and caseous tuberculous lesions where the levels achieved are five to ten times and three times the simultaneous serum concentration, respectively.[234–236] Ethambutol readily passes across the human placenta.[237]

From 10% to 20% of a dose of ethambutol is metabolized in the liver by alcohol dehydrogenase to an aldehyde that is subsequently oxidized to the dicarboxylic acid.[230,238] Ethambutol and its metabolites are eliminated predominantly via the kidney,[230] with the parent drug being both filtered and secreted.[231] The mean half-life of ethambutol in normal adults is about 4 h[231] and this increases to 7 h in patients with complete renal failure.[239] The dosage should be reduced when the glomerular filtration rate is less than 30–50 ml/min.[75] Ethambutol is removed from the body by peritoneal dialysis and hemodialysis.[239] There is considerable controversy as to how the dosage of ethambutol should be adjusted in patients undergoing dialysis;[240–242] some experts feel that the drug should be avoided in the treatment of patients with severely impaired renal function.[86,243]

Adverse Effects

Ethambutol is generally well tolerated. It occasionally produces mild gastrointestinal upset, abdominal pain, allergic reactions (including dermatitis, pruritis, and rarely, anaphylaxis), joint pain, dizziness, mental confusion, fever, malaise, and headache. Clinically the most important adverse effect is retrobulbar neuritis. This is clearly a dose-related effect that was observed in 18% of patients receiving more than 35 mg/kg/day.[244] The incidence is about 1% in patients receiving the currently recommended regimens of daily or intermittent therapy (Table 11–2).[86,245] There are two types of retrobulbar neuritis.[244] In the most common type, the central fibers of the optic nerve are involved, and the signs are loss of central vision and disturbance in color discrimination. In the less common type, the peripheral fibers of the optic nerve are affected; here there may be no loss of visual acuity, but there is constriction of peripheral fields of vision. Vision may be unilaterally or bilaterally affected. The neuritis usually occurs after 2 months of therapy and is reversible on withdrawal of the drug, although isolated cases of persisting ocular damage have occurred in spite of prompt withdrawal.[246] The neuritis is retrobulbar; therefore the funduscopic appearance may be normal.[247] All patients should have a comprehensive ophthalmologic examination before initiation of therapy to establish an accurate baseline for reference. Routine testing of vision during therapy is usually not necessary because visual tests fail to detect ocular toxicity before symptoms (blurring of vision, loss of color discrimination) occur.[86,248,249] All patients should be advised to report any visual disturbances to the physician, and they should be questioned about their vision during each office visit. Some experts recommend routine visual testing if the patient is receiving a daily dosage greater than 15 mg/kg.[250]

Peripheral neuropathy occurs infrequently during ethambutol therapy. Patients experience symptoms of numbness and tingling in the extremities, which disappear when the drug is withdrawn.[251,252] Symptoms usually develop after 5–9 months of treatment,[251] and many of the patients who have been reported to have peripheral neuropathy have also had retrobulbar neuritis.[252,253] Only the sensory system is involved. Decreases in peripheral sensory nerve action potential and conduction velocity have been recorded in a small percentage of nonsymptomatic patients receiving ethambutol as well as in symptomatic patients.[253,254]

Ethambutol decreases the renal clearance of uric acid[255] and mild hyperuricemia occurs in 40%–5% of patients receiving the drug at conventional dosage.[256] Rarely, treatment with ethambutol has precipitated acute gouty arthritis.[257]

Ethambutol is not recommended for use in children because it is very difficult to assess the onset of visual disturbances. Because ethambutol readily passes across the human placenta[237] and because it is occasionally administered to pregnant women, there has been concern regarding potential teratogenicity. There is, however, no evidence of fetal abnormalities occurring in humans because of ethambutol treatment.[258,259]

Streptomycin

Streptomycin was the first drug shown to be effective against tuberculosis in humans.[54] It is an aminoglycoside antibiotic and its mechanism of bactericidal action, pharmacology, and toxicity have been discussed with the other aminoglycosides in Chapter 5. The great majority of strains of *M. tuberculosis* (95%), *M. kansasii* (88%), and *M. marinum* (100%) are sensitive to streptomycin at 10 ug/ml in vitro.[140,260] Streptomycin is bactericidal against *M. tuberculosis* in vitro at concentrations that are well below the peak concentrations of 25–30 μg/ml that are achieved in blood after administering a usual 1 g dose to an adult (see Table 5–5). In spite of its bactericidal effect in vitro, streptomycin has a relatively low sterilizing activity in vivo, because, like all of the aminoglycosides, streptomycin penetrates very poorly into cells and distributes essentially in the extracellular space (Chapter 5). Tuberculosis tends to be an intracellular infection and intracellular tubercle bacilli are not killed by streptomycin. Suter demonstrated this in vitro when he showed that extracellar tubercle bacilli were inhibited by streptomycin at 0.5 ug/ml, whereas 80–100 μg/ml were required to inhibit the same organisms located intracellularly in phagocytes.[261]

Streptomycin is the least nephrotoxic of the aminoglycosides, but it is quite ototoxic. Vestibular toxicity manifested by nausea, vomiting, tinnitus, and vertigo is more common than auditory toxicity, but hearing loss can occur. Patients should have their hearing and balance functions tested periodically during therapy and special caution must be taken to adjust the dosage of the drug when treating patients with impaired renal function. The toxic effects of streptomycin on eighth-nerve function and the necessity for parenteral administration make it less attractive than such potent oral drugs as isoniazid and rifampin. Accordingly, the use of streptomycin in the initial therapy of tuberculosis has declined markedly. It is used primarily in three-drug intensive therapy of severe disease.

Pyrazinamide

Pyrazinamide has become an important component of short-term multiple drug therapy. Pyrazinamide is the pyrazine analog of

Pyrazinamide

nicotinamide. It was synthesized following the finding that nicotinomide was tuberculostatic in animal models.[54]

Antimicrobial Activity and Use

The molecular mechanism of pyrazinamide action is not known. Pyrazinamide is bactericidal against human tubercle bacilli in vitro when the pH of the growth medium is acidic (pH 5.0–5.5), but there is little or no activity at neutral pH.[54,262] Blood withdrawn from human subjects after administration of pyrazinamide does not have antituberculosis activity in vitro.[263] However, like rifampin, pyrazinamide has a very high sterilizing activity in experimental animal models,[149,215] and this may imply that bacilli living in cavity walls are often in a very acidic environment.[264] Pyrazinamide readily enters cells and the growth of human tubercle bacilli cultured intracellularly in monocytes in vitro is inhibited by pyrazinamide at 12.5 μg/ml.[265] Some studies have shown the drug to be more effective against intracellular organisms than extracellular organisms.[54] In contrast to rifampin, pyrazinamide has little ability to prevent emergence of drug resistance.[149]

Like isoniazid, pyrazinamide is thought to be a pro-drug that requires deamidation by an endogenous mycobacterial enzyme, pyrazinamidase, to form pyrazinoic acid.[266,267] Pyrazinoic acid is considered a toxic metabolite, but the precise cellular functions inhibited by it have not been defined.[137] The gene that encodes pyrazinamidase, pncA, has been cloned from M. tuberculosis. The pncA genes from five clinical isolates resistant to pyrazinamide were found to be mutated, correlating with a loss of pyrazinamidase activity. Transformation of these resistant strains with a wild-type pncA gene restored both pyrazinamidase activity and pyrazinamide sensitivity.[268]

Pyrazinoic acid could also be produced intracellularly by hydrolysis of pyrazinoic acid esters by a non-specific cellular esterase.[269] Such esters have been shown to have potent activity against both M. tuberculosis and more difficult-to-treat atypical mycobacteria such as M. avium.[270] Some of these pyrazinoic acid esters have been shown to have 100-fold greater activity than pyrazinamide against M. tuberculosis.[271] These esters offer considerable promise as potent new antituberculosis agents.

Pyrazinamide is indicated for the initial treatment of active tuberculosis in adults and children and should be used only in combination with other antituberculosis agents. It is also indicated after treatment failure with other primary drugs in any form of active tuberculosis.

Pharmacology of Pyrazinamide

Pyrazinamide is well absorbed from the gastrointestinal tract. A peak serum concentration of 33 µg/ml is achieved 2 h after oral administration of 1.5 g to an adult.[272] The drug is widely distributed in the body and readily penetrates into cells. The major pathway of metabolism is by hydrolysis to pyrazinoic acid, which is oxidized to 5-hydroxypyrazinoic acid by xanthine oxidase.[273] The drug is excreted in the urine, with the major excretory product being 5-hydroxypyrazinoic acid.[273] Hydroxypyrazinoic acid is cleared more rapidly by the kidney than the parent drug[273] and most of the drug assayed in the serum is unchanged.[272] The mean half-life in humans is about 6 h.[272]

Adverse Effects of Pyrazinamide

Pyrazinamide commonly causes flushing and rarely causes hypersensitivity and photosensitivity reactions.[86] Mild nausea and anorexia are common and vomiting occurs less frequently. Renal failure also has been associated with pyrazinamide therapy, but the symptoms usually resolve upon discontinuation of the drug.[274,275] Clinically, the most important adverse reactions are liver injury and arthralgia.

Pyrazinamide causes a dose-related hepatotoxicity that is usually manifest by reversible increases in serum transaminase levels but may develop into symptomatic hepatitis.[86] In early studies, pyrazinamide therapy was associated with a high incidence of hepatotoxicity. Modern, short-course regimens containing both pyrazinamide and isoniazid, however, have not been associated with an unacceptable level of hepatotoxicity.[86] Serum transaminase levels (SGOT, SGPT) should be determined before therapy is begun and frequently monitored during therapy. The drug should not be administered to patients with preexisting liver disease and it should be stopped if significant evidence of liver damage occurs during treatment.

Pyrazinamide frequently causes hyperuricemia,[276] which results from the inhibition of renal excretion of uric acid by the pyrazinoic acid metabolite.[273] Rarely, high serum uric acid concentrations may precipitate acute gout in patients who have the disease.[86] Arthralgia occurs relatively frequently in patients receiving daily therapy (7%) but is much less frequent (1%) with twice-weekly regimens.[86] Arthralgia usually appears during the first 1 or 2 months of treatment, and both small and large joints are affected. The condition is usually self-limiting, it responds to aspirin,[277] and it rarely necessitates terminating therapy.

The Second-Line Antituberculosis Drugs

The second-line antituberculosis drugs are used primarily in the retreatment of patients in whom initial therapy failed because of the presence of resistant organisms. The frequency of primary resistance to one or more antituberculosis drugs in the United States is about 14% overall,[14] but as mentioned earlier, resistance is more prevalent in large urban areas, in coastal and border communities, and in certain racial and ethnic groups, such as Asians and Hispanics.[9] Thus, initial treatment of tuberculosis in certain groups of patients in restricted geographical locations would be more likely to require a four-drug regimen. Clearly, if sensitivity testing demonstrates that an organism is resistant to one or more of the initial drugs, or if they are not tolerated or are contraindicated, then the treatment regimen must be changed appropriately. The so-called minor or second-line drugs may have to be used in spite of a generally greater risk of toxicity.

Ethionamide

Ethionamide, a derivative of isonicotinic acid, inhibits the growth of human tubercle bacilli in vitro at 0.6–1.2 µg/ml.[278] It is equally effective in vitro against intracellular

Ethionamide

and extracellular bacilli.[54] Although it is structurally similar to isoniazid, there is no cross-resistance.[278] Ethionamide is used in combination with other drugs only to treat tuberculosis that is resistant to therapy with primary drugs,[279] or if therapy with the primary drugs is contraindicated.

Ethionamide is administered orally and a peak blood level of about 3 ug/ml is achieved after ingestion of a 500 mg dose of either ethionamide or its propyl derivative, prothionamide.[280] To minimize gastrointestinal effects, ethionamide is best taken with meals in divided doses. Ethionamide is distributed widely in the body and it enters the cerebrospinal fluid. The drug is extensively metabolized by sulfoxidation, N-methylation, desulfuration, and deaminataion; the metabolites are eliminated in the urine.[281] The half-life is about 2 h.[280]

The use of ethionamide is limited by gastrointestinal reactions, which occur frequently.[282,283] Gastrointestinal symptoms include anorexia, nausea, vomiting, abdominal pain, diarrhea, excessive salivation, and metallic taste. Ethionamide also frequently causes headache and a feeling of giddiness.[283] Hypersensitivity reactions and hepatitis can occur.[284] Serum transaminase levels should be assayed before therapy and then every 2 to 4 weeks during treatment. Rare reactions include alopecia, convulsions, deafness, diplopia, gynecomastia, hypotension, impotence, mental disturbances, hypoglycemia, and peripheral neuropathy.[86]

Cycloserine

Cycloserine is a structural analog of D-alanine that acts as an inhibitor of cell wall synthesis. Its structure and mechanism of action have been presented in Chapter 3. Cycloserine inhibits the growth of *M. tuberculosis* in vitro at concentrations of 10–20 µg/ml.[285] The great majority of strains of *M. kansasii* are sensitive to 10 µg/ml.[286] Cycloserine is used for the treatment of *M. tuberculosis* that is resistant to the primary agents[287] and, occasionally, for the treatment of infection by atypical mycobacteria (see Table 11–1).

Cycloserine is completely absorbed from the gastrointesinal tract,[288] and a peak blood level of 15 µg/ml is achieved 4 h after oral administration of 1 g to an adult.[289] The rate of excretion is relatively slow and higher blood levels are achieved with repeated administration.[289] Cycloserine distributes widely in the body tissues and fluids; it readily passes into the cerebrospinal fluid where the concentration is close to that in the blood.[285] The drug is excreted into the urine, and about 50% is eliminated in the first 12 h.[288] About 35% of the drug is unaccounted for and this may reflect some metabolism to unknown products.[288]

Adverse reactions to cycloserine are common.[86] The drug is neurotoxic and may cause dizziness, headache, slurred speech, tremors, insomnia, confusion, and potentially serious episodes of depression, anxiety, and psychosis.[285,290] At high serum concentrations, convulsions may occur.[285,290] The drug should not be given to patients with a history of epilepsy or psychiatric disease.[86] Hypersensitivity reactions and hepatitis occur rarely.

Para-Aminosalicylic Acid

Para-aminosalicylic acid (PAS) is a former primary antituberculosis agent whose importance in the treatment of tuberculosis has declined since more active and better tolerated drugs have become available. It is a structural analog of para-aminobenzoic acid and, like the sulfonamides, it inhibits the synthesis of folic acid. Unlike the sulfonamides, which have a broad spectrum of antibacterial activity, the action of PAS is quite specific for *M. tuberculosis*. The mechanism of action of PAS and the proposed basis for its restricted activity are discussed in detail with the mechanism of sulfonamide action in Chapter 7. The growth of most strains of *M. tuberculosis* is inhibited by PAS at 1 µg/ml in vitro. It is bacteriostatic against *M. tuberculosis* in vivo.[264] Para-aminosalicylic acid is indicated for the treatment of active pulmonary and extrapulmonary tuberculosis when the infecting organisms are known or strongly suspected to be susceptible to this drug and resistant to the first-line drugs. When used alone it is not very effective and resistance may develop rapidly. Therefore, it should be used only in combination therapy.

COOH

NH$_2$

para-Aminobenzoic acid

Para-aminosalicylic acid is well absorbed from the gastrointestinal tract and peak plasma levels of 75–100 μg/ml are achieved 1–2 h after ingestion of a 4 g dose.[291] It distributes widely in the body and readily enters caseous tissue.[292] Levels of drug in the cerebrospinal fluid are low. Like the penicillins, PAS is actively transported out of the cerebrospinal fluid into the blood by a weak carboxylic acid transport system.[293] It is metabolized in the liver, primarily by acetylation. Isoniazid is acetylated by a different enzyme and PAS is a weak competitive inhibitor of human isoniazid N-acetyltransferase in vitro.[294] This may account for the rather weak inhibition of isoniazid metabolism observed in tuberculosis patients also receiving large doses of PAS.[295] The half-life of PAS is 1–2 h and 85% of a dose of the drug is excreted in the urine within 10 h, predominantly as acetylated metabolites.[291]

Para-aminosalycylic acid is bulky and unpleasant to take and it commonly causes nausea, vomiting, diarrhea, and epigastric distress.[282] Gastrointestinal reactions are less common in children. A wide variety of allergic reactions can occur. Prolonged administration can lead to decreased iodine uptake and thyroid gland enlargement. Hepatitis and hypokalemia occur occasionally. Rare reactions include hemolytic anemia, thrombocytopenia, mild hypoprothrombinemia, and acute renal failure.[86] If possible, PAS should be avoided in patients with renal failure because it exacerbates acidosis. The drug is provided as the free acid and as the sodium, potassium, and calcium salts. The sodium salt should not be given to patients who are on a restricted sodium intake. It is unstable in aqueous solution and solutions should not be used if they are darker in color than a freshly prepared solution.[86]

Kanamycin and Amikacin

In addition to streptomycin, two other aminoglycosides are employed in the treatment of tuberculosis. Most strains of M. tuberculosis are inhibited by kanamycin at 10 μg/ml or less in vitro, but toxic effects are common with kanamycin. Amikacin is very active against several mycobacteria in vitro, with 99% of M. tuberculosis strains being inhibited by 3.2 μg/ml[296] and essentially all strains of M. fortuitum being inhibited by 1 μg/ml.[297] Both of these drugs must be administered intramuscularly and peak serum levels of 15–30 μg/ml are achieved about 1 h after administration of a standard dose (see Table 5–5). The mechanism of action, pharmacology, and toxicity of the aminoglycoside antibiotics are discussed in Chapter 5.

Viomycin and Capreomycin

Viomycin and capreomycin are closely related antibiotics possessing a complex cyclic peptide core structure.[298] Viomycin is now very rarely used and is of limited availability. The commercial preparation of capreomycin consists of four active cyclic peptide components.[298] Like the aminoglycosides, these are strongly basic antibiotics. Viomycin and capreomycin probably have very similar mechanisms of action but only that of viomycin has been examined in detail. Viomycin is a potent inhibitor of protein synthesis.[299] At low concentration, the antibiotic inhibits protein chain elongation by preventing translocation of the peptidyl-tRNA from the A site to the P site (see Figure 5–3).[300,301] At higher concentration, it inhibits formation of the initiation complex by preventing the binding of fMet-tRNA to the 30S ribosomal subunit (see Fig. 5–2).[300] Viomycin binds to both the 30S and the 50S ribosomal subunits,[302,303] and binding to both sites is important for the drug action. This is inferred from the observation that a mutant strain of M. smegmatis possessing a low level of viomycin resistance (20 μg/ml) con-

Viomycin

tained altered 30S ribosomal subunits, whereas another mutant that was highly resistant (1 mg/ml) had altered 50S subunits.[304] The resistance in both mutants is due to an alteration in the RNA component of the ribosomal subunits.[305] A similar mechanism of resistance based on modification (methylation) of ribosomal RNA is discussed for erythromycin in Chapter 6. Viomycin binds with higher affinity to the 50S ribosomal subunit than to the 30S subunit, and it is reasonable to propose that binding to the large ribosomal subunit results in inhibition of translocation and binding to the smaller unit is responsible for inhibition of initiation.[302]

Susceptible strains of *M. tuberculosis* respond to 10 µg/ml or less of capreomycin in vitro.[306,307] Capreomycin is used only in conjunction with other appropriate antitubercular drugs in the treatment of pulmonary tuberculosis when the first-line agents cannot be tolerated or when resistance occurs.[308,309]

Capreomycin is administered intramuscularly (see Table 11–2). Peak serum concentrations following a 1 g dose of capreomycin to an adult range from 20 to 47 µg/ml (manufacturer's data). Capreomycin is excreted in high concentration in the urine.

Like the aminoglycosides, capreomycin is both nephrotoxic and ototoxic.[54,308,309] Abnormal urine sediments are observed in a high percentage of patients receiving these drugs. Renal function studies (blood urea nitrogen and creatinine) should be made be-

fore therapy is started and on a weekly basis thereafter. Renal function usually improves when the drug is stopped. Ototoxicity may be manifest by disturbance in balance, tinnitus, or hearing loss. Assessment of balance and hearing should be performed at regular intervals during therapy. Hypersensitivity reactions (including urticaria, rashes, fever, and eosinophilia) occur occasionally and leukocytosis and leukopenia occur rarely.

Quinolones

A surprisingly large number of fluoroquinolones are being developed and studied as inhibitors of mycobacteria. Their bioavailability after oral administration, penetration into human macrophages, and concentration in the respiratory tract are advantages against mycobacteria.[1,310] Ofloxacin and ciprofloxacin are the best studied of the quinolones and have good activity against many mycobacteria, including *Mycobacterium tuberculosis*.

Drugs Effective Against Leprosy

Although leprosy is rarely encountered by physicians practicing in Europe and North America, it is a major health problem in some tropical and subtropical countries. For many years, dapsone has been the principal drug used for control of the disease. A number of surveys have shown, however, that

Table 11–6. Potency and pharmacokinetic characteristics of the major antileprosy drugs. Minimal inhibitory concentrations (MICs) against *M. leprae* were determined in the mouse footpad system. Corresponding data for clofazimine are not presented because its accumulation in reticuloendothelial cells makes it impossible to estimate an MIC against *M. leprae.*

Drug	MIC (μg/ml)	Dosage (mg)	Peak serum level (μg/ml)	Ratio of peak serum level to MIC	Calculated duration for which serum concentration exceeds MIC (days)	Nature of drug effect
Dapsone	0.003	100	1.5	500	10	Cidal (+)
Rifampin	0.3	600	10	30	1	Cidal (+++)
Ethionamide	0.05	500	3	60	1	Cidal (++)

+, relative degree of bactericidal activity.

Source: The table was constructed from a table of Colston et al.[280] and from other data and calculations reviewed in references[280] and [316].

dapsone resistance is increasing and that it is already widespread.[311,312] In order to prevent the emergence of resistance and to try to reduce the infectiousness of the patient more rapidly, two or three drugs are now used simultaneously for the initial treatment of multibacillary, lepromatous, and borderline lepromatous leprosy.[313,314] After the initial period of intensive therapy, treatment is continued with daily administration of dapsone for many years to life. Most two-drug regimens for initial therapy include the daily administration of dapsone (100 mg) plus daily rifampin (600 mg) or clofazimine (100 mg). Patients with dapsone-resistant *M. leprae* may be treated with rifampin in combination with clofazimine and ethionamide. On the basis of promising results from preliminary studies, the World Health Organization is conducting a large-scale trial comparing the combination of rifampin and ofloxacin with the conventional regimen of dapsone, rifampin, and colfazimine for the treatment of multibacillary disease.[315] It is hoped that the duration of treatment can be shortened from the current minimum of 24 months to fewer than 6 months with this regimen. The minimal inhibitory concentrations of several drugs against *M. leprae* determined in the mouse footpad system are presented in Table 11–6.[280,316]

Sulfones (Dapsome)

The sulfones, like the sulfonamides, are structural analogs of para-aminobenzoic acid, and they interfere with folic acid metabolism by acting as competitive inhibitors of

Dapsone

dihydropteroate synthetase. The mechanism of action of the sulfones is discussed with the mechanism of sulfonamide action in Chapter 7.

ANTIMICROBIAL ACTIVITY AND USE IN LEPROSY. The minimal inhibitory concentration of dapsone for sensitive strains of *M. leprae* is about 0.003 μg/ml,[317] and at the concentrations of drug achieved in daily therapy, the effect is bactericidal in both the mouse footpad infection[318] and in leprosy patients undergoing treatment.[319] The sulfonamides and sulfones have been reported to have beneficial effects in a variety of dermatologic disorders (e.g., dermatitis herpetiformis) in which their efficacy cannot be ascribed to an antibacterial action.[320] It is possible that the sulfones have significant anti-inflammatory[320] and immune regulatory[321,322] actions that contribute to their effectiveness in the treatment of leprosy. It is clear, however, that strains of *M. leprae* become resistant to sulfone therapy and that they maintain this resistance when transferred from the patient to the mouse model.[323] This finding argues strongly for a direct antibacterial action being the primary factor that accounts for the therapeutic efficacy of sulfones in leprosy patients.

The most important sulfone currently used to treat leprosy is dapsone. Dapsone is administered orally (100 mg) in daily therapy.

PHARMACOLOGY OF DAPSONE. Dapsone is well absorbed from the gastrointestinal tract and a single 100 mg oral dose yields peak plasma levels of 1.1–1.5 μg/ml in 2–4 h.[324] In patients receiving 225 mg of acedapsone every 11 weeks, the blood levels of free dapsone average 0.05 μg/ml, or about what would be expected for the absorption of 2.4 mg of dapsone per day.[325] Dapsone readily distributes into the body fluids and tissues and it is 70%–80% bound to plasma protein.[326] Dapsone is acetylated to monoacetyl dapsone by the same polymorphic N-acetyl-transferase that acetylates isoniazid.[327] The acetylated drug is deacetylated and a ratio of monoacetylated dapsone to dapsone is rapidly established in the plasma. Although this ratio is higher in patients who are rapid acetylators than in slow acetylators (1.1 versus 0.2 at 4 h after drug administration),[327] the acetylation phenotype does not affect the overall half-life of the drug.[327,328] Dapsone is ultimately excreted in the urine, predominantly as glucuronide and sulfate conjugates.[327] The average serum half-life of dapsone is 25–27 h, but there is a rather wide variation between different individuals (13–53 h).[280] The half-life is reduced in patients who are also receiving rifampin,[206] but this interaction does not appear to affect the therapeutic outcome.

ADVERSE EFFECTS OF THE SULFONES. With the doses used to treat leprosy, adverse reactions to the sulfones are usually mild and occur infrequently. The most common adverse reactions to dapsone are hemolytic anemia and methemoglobinemia.[329] The young, the old, and those with glucose-6-phosphate dehydrogenase deficiency are at increased risk of developing anemia. Most patients who are receiving the higher doses of dapsone that are used in treating dermatologic disorders (200–300 mg daily) experience a loss of 1–2 g of hemoglobin and a mild reticulocytosis, but at the usual dosage (100 mg daily) used in the treatment of leprosy, hemolysis is uncommon. Methemoglobinemia can be detected in most patients receiving dapsone.[329] The methemoglobinemia is caused by N-oxidation products of dapsone that are produced by microsomal metabolism.[330] The most serious hematologic side effect is marrow suppression, which is rare, but deaths due to agranulocytosis and aplastic anemia have been reported.

Peripheral neuropathy, predominantly involving motor function, is an unusual complication of sulfone therapy.[331] Oral administration of sulfones may be accompanied by anorexia, nausea, and vomiting. Other adverse effects include vertigo, blurred vision, tinnitus, fever, headache, psychosis, hematuria, pruritis, and a variety of skin rashes. Patients who have lepromatous leprosy may develop erythema nodosum leprosum during the first year of chemotherapy. The reaction is characterized by fever and tender erythematous skin nodules, sometimes accompanied by malaise, neuritis, joint swelling, and albuminuria. The syndrome is thought to result from increased circulating immune complexes with accompanying vasculitis and inflammatory reaction. Occasional patients with borderline or tuberculoid leprosy may experience a so-called reversal reaction, characterized by swelling of existing skin and nerve lesions, that occurs soon after chemotherapy is started. If proper precautions are taken, dapsone can be administered for many years in therapeutic doses. Treatment should be initiated with a small dose and the dosage then increased gradually. Patients must be under consistent and prolonged laboratory and clinical supervision.

Rifampin

Rifampin produces the most profound bactericidal response of any of the antileprosy drugs.[314] The minimum inhibitory concentration of rifampin for *M. leprae* in the mouse footpad assay is about 0.3 μg/ml.[332] Rifampin produces a rapid bactericidal effect in patients with lepromatous leprosy, but when the drug is used alone, a few viable organisms persist and it alone cannot significantly shorten the duration of treatment.[147] Rifampin is used in initial, combined drug therapy of the disease. It has generally been given in a daily regimen of therapy, which is very expensive, but it can also be given once monthly in higher dosage (1200 mg) along with daily dapsone.[333] The mechanism of action, pharmacology, and adverse effects of rifampin were presented earlier in this chapter.

Clofazimine

Clofazimine is a substituted phenazine quinoneimine that is red in color and very hydrophobic. It was originally used to treat tu-

Clofazimine

berculosis and was first shown to be useful for the treatment of leprosy in 1962.[334]

ANTIMICROBIAL ACTIVITY AND USE. Clofazimine has a wide spectrum of antibacterial action in vitro. Its effect on *M. leprae* in the mouse model is bactericidal.[335] Because it accumulates in the tissues, it is not possible to accurately determine a minimum inhibitory concentration against *M. leprae*. From clinical experience, the bactericidal activity of clofazimine in humans is similar to that of dapsone.[333,335] The mechanism of clofazim-

ine action has not been clearly defined. It can act as an electron acceptor and inhibit essential energy-yielding reactions in respiration.[336] Clofazimine also forms stable complexes with nucleic acids, but no direct relationship between the binding and the antimycobacterial action has been demonstrated.[337] No resistant strains of leprosy bacilli have been reported to date.[333]

Clofazimine is used to treat dapsone-resistant leprosy[338] and to treat patients who experience immune complex reactions during sulfone therapy. The drug clearly has beneficial effects that are unrelated to its antibacterial action. Clofazimine has been shown to inhibit neutrophil motility and lymphocyte transformation in normal adults.[339] Its antiinflammatory effects have been exploited in the treatment of some noninfectious conditions, such as discoid lupus erythematosis.[340] Clofazimine controls the neuritic complications of leprosy[341] and suppresses erythema nodosum leprosum (ENL) reactions that occur in patients with lepromatous leprosy during treatment with other antileprosy drugs.[342,343] Its ability to suppress ENL reactions is unique among the antileprosy drugs and it probably represents an anti-inflammatory (or immune modulating) activity. Clofazimine is apparently not effective in treating the "reversal" reaction experienced by patients with borderline or tuberculous leprosy during the early phase of chemotherapy.[344] Clofazimine is also effective in treating skin ulceration due to *Mycobacterium ulcerans*.[345]

PHARMACOKINETICS. Because clofazimine is very hydrophobic, it is administered in capsules as a microcrystalline suspension in an oil-detergent base. The usual dose for treating leprosy is 100 mg given daily or three times weekly. The drug is apparently incompletely absorbed from the gut. About 50% of a dose is recovered in the feces unchanged.[346] High concentrations of drug are found in the bile, indicating that some of the drug recovered in the feces represents excretion by the biliary route.[347] In addition to the bile and gall bladder, very high concentrations are achieved in adipose tissue and there is considerable concentration of the drug in liver, lung, kidney, spleen, and skin.[347] Clofazimine accumulates in reticuloendothelial cells, where deposits of drug crystals have been detected in mesenteric lymph nodes nearly 4 years after the drug was stopped.[348] Because it is retained in the tissues, clofazimine is excreted very slowly and the half-life in humans is about 70 days.[349] Very small amounts of dehalogenated and deaminated metabolites have been identified as glucuronide conjugates in the urine.[350]

ADVERSE EFFECTS. Clofazimine causes a red-brown pigmentation of the skin and conjuctiva and darkening of skin lesions. The drug also imparts a red color to urine, feces, sputum, and sweat.[348,351] Many patients with ligher skin find clofazimine unacceptable because of the skin discoloration. Skin pigmentation is more of a problem in patients who are receiving higher dosage for treatment of erythema nodosum leprosum reactions. Patients may experience dryness of the skin, particularly of the forearms and lower legs, which may progress to icthiosis.[348] Some patients who are receiving 200 mg a day or more have experienced diarrhea and abdominal pain, which clear on cessation of therapy.[348,352] At the lower dosage used to treat dapsone-resistant leprosy, clofazimine is quite well tolerated. At higher doses, more drug deposits as crystals in the tissues and unusual reactions like eosinophilic enteritis[353] and splenic infarction[354] may result.

Ethionamide

This drug has not been approved by the FDA for the treatment of leprosy but it is sometimes used in the United States in combination with rifampin to treat dapsone-resistant leprosy in patients who cannot accept the skin-depigmentation effect of clofazimine.[315] Resistance to ethionamide can develop quickly when the drug is used alone, so it must be used with other effective agents. Patients taking ethionamide should be monitored closely for hepatotoxicity. Prothionamide is a congener of ethionamide that is widely used throughout the world but

not in the United States. Its pharmacology is similar to that of ethionamide.

Thalidomide

Thalidomide is the treatment of choice for severe or recurrent erythema nodosum leprosum (ENL) which develops in 10%–50% of patients treated for lepromatous leprosy. It is characterized by painful skin nodules, fever, malaise, wasting, vasculitis, and peripheral neuritis. Thalidomide is usually given at a daily dose of 400 mg until the reaction is controlled and then reduced gradually to 50 mg daily. Relief of symptoms is rapid and reliable and seems to be associated with a decrease in elevated concentrations of tumor necrosis factor-α. If taken during the first trimester of pregnancy, teratogenicity is common even with small doses. Sedation occurs in most patients, and constipation and dry mouth or skin are common. Peripheral neuropathy can occur with chronic use.

Drugs Effective Against the Mycobacterium avium *Complex*

Before the AIDS epidemic, *Mycobacterium avium* complex (MAC) infection was uncommon and occurred primarily as a slowly progressive pneumonitis in elderly patients with chronic pulmonary disorders. Disseminated MAC infection was rarely found in immunocompromised patients. With the onset of the AIDS epidemic, the incidence of MAC infection, principally disseminated disease, has increased dramatically. This infection is now the most common systemic bacterial infection in patients with AIDS. It is seen in perhaps one-fifth of patients who have not received prophylaxis, and the incidence appears to be rising as patients live longer.[355] These patients usually are in the advanced stages of AIDS, they have T-lymphocyte counts below 100 cells/mm,[3] and they have symptoms of fever, night sweats, weight loss, and anemia at the time of diagnosis.[356] By the time symptoms appear, MAC infection is usually widely disseminated to multiple organs, including lymphoid tissues, spleen, liver, the gastrointestinal tract, and bone marrow. In persons who do not have AIDS, MAC infection is usually limited to the lungs, and patients have a chronic productive cough and chest X-rays showing showing evidence of limited, diffuse, and/or cavitary disease.[357]

Drugs are now available for both the prevention and treatment of MAC infection in patients with AIDS. Because M. avium and M. intracellulare are common throughout the environment and the immunocompromised state of AIDS patients makes them more prone to acquiring MAC disease, prophylactic measures to prevent this disease in these patients is an important goal. Past recommendations suggested initiation of MAC prophylaxis in patients with absolute CD4 counts of less than 75 cells; however, many clinicians use a count of less than 50 cells as a more reasonable level for initiating prophylaxis. The three drugs now approved for prophylaxis are clarithromycin, azithromycin, and rifabutin.[358]

To prevent the emergence of resistance, all prophylactic drug regimens should include at least two drugs. Four or five drug combinations are no longer recommended,[359] and prophylaxis is now carried out with a two-drug regimen consisting of either clarithromycin or azithromycin combined with ethambutol or rifabutin.[360] No treatment regimen surpasses a 90% response rate. Ciprofloxacin, amikacin, and rifampin have been included in salvage therapy, although this combination is less effective. Clofazimine, which was often used in past treatment strategies, is now thought to be of little or no benefit against MAC infection.[361]

Rifabutin

Rifabutin is a semisynthetic derivative of rifamycin S. Like rifampin, it inhibits mycobacterial RNA polymerase, but rifabutin has better activity against the MAC organisms than rifampin. It has good activity against most mycobacteria including the MAC and some strains of M. tuberculosis. The MAC isolates are inhibited at concentrations ranging from 0.25 to 1.0 µg/ml, and many strains of M. tuberculosis are inhibited at con-

centrations of around 0.125 µg/ml. There is cross-resistance between rifampin and rifabutin with both M. avium and M. tuberculosis.

Rifabutin now has proven value in preventing or delaying mycobacterial infections in immunocompromised patients, and it has been approved in the United States for the prevention of MAC infections in AIDS patients. Rifabutin is generally well tolerated, with the most common complaints being rash, gastrointestinal intolerance, and neutropenia.[362,363] The drug should be discontinued if visual symptoms occur. Like rifampin, it causes an orange-tan discoloration of skin, urine, feces, saliva, tears, and contact lenses, and it induces microsomal enzymes, decreasing the half-life of a number of drugs. Among the drugs that have been affected by rifabutin are clarithromycin, azoles, protease inhibitors, methadone, theophylline, dilantin, corticosteroids, oral contraceptives, warfarin, oral hypoglycemics, and some antiarrhythmics.[363]

Macrolides

Azithromycin and clarithromycin have become major drugs used to prevent MAC infection. Their pharmacology and adverse effects were discussed in Chapter 6. Clarithromycin is about fourfold more active than azithromycin against MAC bacteria in vitro and is active against most nontuberculous mycobacteria. Azithromycin has a greater intracellular penetration, with tissue levels generally exceeding plasma levels by two orders of magnitude.

Azithromycin persists for an extended time inside macrophages and tissues and thus can be given once a week, which is a considerable advantage for many patients.[364] However, clarithromycin appears to be slightly more effective for prophylactic monotherapy, being roughly equivalent to the azithromycin-rifabutin combination. These macrolides are used at relatively high doses to treat MAC infections, and tinnitus, dizziness, and reversible hearing loss have occurred occasionally.

Quinolones

Ciprofloxacin, ofloxacin, fleroxacin, and sparfloxacin all have inhibitory activity against *M. tuberculosis* and MAC bacteria in vitro.

Amikacin

Amikacin may have a role as a third or fourth agent in a multiple drug regimen for MAC treatment. Its pharmacology and adverse effects were discussed in Chapter 5. Most isolates of MAC are inhibited in vitro by 8 to 32 μg/ml of amikacin.

REFERENCES

1. Houston, S., and A. Fanning: Current and potential treatment of tuberculosis. *Drugs* 1994;48:689.

2. The Medical Letter. Drugs for tuberculosis in handbook of antimicrobial therapy. New York: The Medical letter, Inc., 1998, pp. 60–66.

3. Brausch, L., and J. Bass. The treatment of tuberculosis. *Med. Clin. North Am.* 1993;77:1277.

4. American Medical Association. Antimycobacterial drugs. In *Drug Evaluations Annual*, ed. by D. R. Bennett. American Medical Association, 1994, pp. 1627–1657.

5. A joint statement of the American Thoracic Society and the Centers for Disease Control and Prevention. Treatment of tuberculosis and tuberculosis infection in adults and children. *Am. J. Respir. Crit. Care Med.* 1994;149:1359.

6. Snider, D. E., Jr. Pyridoxine supplementation during isoniazid therapy. *Tubercle* 1980;61:191.

7. Committee on Infections Diseases. Chemotherapy for tuberculosis in infants and children. *Pediatrics* 1992;89:161.

8. Ben-Dor, I., and G. Mason. Drug-resistant tuberculosis in a Southern California hospital: trends from 1969 to 1984. *Am. Rev. Respir. Dis.* 1987;135:1307.

9. Barnes, P. F. The influence of epidemiologic factors on drug resistance rates in tuberculosis. *Am. Rev. Respir. Dis.* 1987;136:325.

10. Carpenter, J., A. Obnibene, E. Gorby, R. Neimes, J. Koch, and W. Perkins. Antituberculosis drug resistance in South Texas. *Am. Rev. Respir. Dis.* 1983; 128:1055.

11. Barnes, P., and S. Barrons. Tuberculosis in the 1990's. *Ann. Intern. Med.* 1993;119:400.

12. Chaulk, C., and V. Kazadjian for the Public Health Tuberculosis Guidelines Panel. Directly observed therapy for treatment completion of pulmonary tuberculosis. *JAMA* 1998;279:943.

13. Goble, M., M. Iseman, L. Madsen, D. Waite, L. Ackerson, and C. Horsburgh. Treatment of 171 patients with pulmonary tuberculosis resistant to isoniazid and rifampin. *N. Engl. J. Med.* 1993;328:527.

14. Iseman, M. D. Treatment of multidrug-resistant tuberculosis. *N. Engl. J. Med.* 1993;329:784. Erratum in 1993;329:1435

15. O'Brien; R. J. Drug-resistant tuberculosis: etiology, management and prevention. *Semin. Respir. Infect.* 1994;9:104.

16. Cohn, D., B. Catlin, K. Peterson, F. Judson, and J. Sbarbaro. A 62-dose, 6-month therapy for pulmonary and extrapulmonary tuberculosis—A twice-weekly, directly observed, and cost-effective program. *Ann. Intern. Med.* 1990;112:407.

17. Hong Kong Chest Service/British Medical Research Council. Controlled trial of 2, 4, and 6 months of pyrazinamide in 6-month, three-times-weekly regimens for smear-positive pulmonary tuberculosis, including an assessment of a combined preparation of isoniazid, rifampin, and pyrazinamide. *Am. Rev. Respir. Dis.* 1991;143:700.

18. Moulding, T., A. Dutt, and L. Reichman. Fixed-dose combinations of antituberculosis medications to prevent drug resistance. *Ann. Intern. Med.* 1995;122: 951.

19. Bailey, W. C., J. W. Raleigh, and J. A. Turner. Treatment of mycobacterial disease. *Am. Rev. Respir. Dis.* 1977;115:185.

20. Johnson, R. F., and K. H. Wildrick. "State of the art" review. The impact of chemotherapy on the care of patients with tuberculosis. *Am. Rev. Respir. Dis.* 1974;109:636.

21. Taylor, W. C., M. D. Aronson, and T. L. Delbanco. Should young adults with a positive tuberculin test take isoniazid? *Ann. Intern. Med.* 1981;94:808.

22. Krishna Murti, C. R. Isonicotinic acid hydrazide. In *Antibiotics III*, ed. by J. W. Corcoran and F. E. Hahn. New York: Springer-Verlag, 1975, pp. 623–652.

23. Schaefer, W. B. The effect of isoniazid on growing and resting tubercle bacilli. *Am. Rev. Tuberc.* 1954; 69:125.

24. Youatt, J. A review of the action of isonizid. *Am. Rev. Respir. Dis.* 1969;99:729.

25. Takayama, K., and L. A. Davidson. Isonicotinic acid hydrazide. In *Antibiotics V-I*, ed. by F. E. Hahn. New York: Springer-Verlag, 1979, pp. 98–119.

26. Winder, F. G., and S. A. Rooney. The effects of isoniazid on the carbohydrates of *Mycobacterium tuberculosis* BCG. *Biochem. J.* 1970;117:355.

27. Winder, F. G., and P. B. Collins. Inhibition by isoniazid of synthesis of mycolic acids in *Mycobacterium tuberculosis*. *J. Gen. Microbiol.* 1970;63:41.

28. Takayama, K., L. Wang, and H. L. David. Effect of isoniazid on the in vivo mycolic acid synthesis, cell growth, and viability of *Mycobacterium tuberculosis*. *Antimicrob. Agents Chemother.* 1972;2:29.

29. Wang, L., and K. Takayama. Relationship between the uptake of isoniazid and its action on in vivo mycolic acid synthesis in *Mycobacterium tuberculosis*. *Antimicrob. Agents Chemother.* 1972;2:438.

30. Takayama, K., H. K. Schnoes, E. L. Armstrong, and R. W. Boyle. Site of inhibitory action of isoniazid in the synthesis of mycolic acids in *Mycobacterium tuberculosis*. *J. Lipid Res.* 1975;16:308.

31. Davidson, L. A., and K. Takayama. Isoniazid inhibition of the synthesis of monosaturated long-chain fatty acids in *Mycobacterium tuberculosis* H37Ra. *Antimicrob. Agents Chemother.* 1979;16:104.

32. Takayama, K., L. Wang, and R. S. Merkal. Scanning electron microscopy of the H37RA strain of *Mycobacterium tuberculosis* exposed to isoniazid. *Antimicrob. Agents Chemother.* 1973;4:62.

33. Riley, L. W. Isoniazid chemistry, metabolism and mechanism of action. In *Tuberculosis*, ed. by W. Rom and S. Gavat. Boston: Little Brown 1996, pp. 763–771.

34. Rozwarski, D., G. Grant, D. Barton, W. Jacobs, and J. Sacchettini. Modification of the NADH of the isoniazid target (InhA) from *Mycobacterium tuberculosis. Science* 1998;27:98.

35. Wilson, T., G. deLisle, and D. Collins. Effect of inhA and katG on isoniazid resistance and virulence of *Mycobacterium bovis. Mol. Microbiol.* 1995;15:1009.

36. Zhang, Y., B. Heym, B. Allen, D. Young, and S. Cole. The catalase-peroxidase gene and isoniazid resistance of *Mycobacterium tuberculosis. Nature* 1992;358:591.

37. Musser, J., V. Kapar, D. Williams, B. Kreiswirth, D. Van Soolinen and J. von Embden. Characterization of the catalase-peroxidase gene (katG) and inhA locus in isoniazid resistant and susceptible strains of *Mycobacterium tuberculosis* by automated DNA sequencing: restricted array of mutations associated with drug resistance.*J. Infect. Dis.* 1996;173:196.

38. Johnson, K., and P. Schultz. Mechanistic studies of the oxidation of isoniazid by the catalase peroxidase from *Mycobacterium tuberculosis. J. Am. Chem. Soc.* 1994;116:7425.

39. Jones, W. D., and H. L. David. Preliminary observations on the occurrence of a streptomycin R-factor in *Mycobacterium smegmatis. Tubercle* 1972;53:35.

40. Saroja, D., and K. P. Gopinathan. Transduction of isoniazid susceptibility-resistance and streptomycin resistance in mycobacteria. *Antimicrob. Agents Chemother.* 1973;4:643.

41. Beggs, W. H., and J. W. Jenne. Capacity of tubercle bacilli for isoniazid accumulation. *Am. Rev. Respir. Dis.* 1970;102:94.

42. Fishbain, D., G. Ling, and D. J. Kushner. Isoniazid metabolism and binding by sensitive and resistant strains of *Mycobacterium smegmatis. Can. J. Microbiol.* 1972;18:783.

43. Zhang, Y., T. Garbe, and D. Young. Transformation with katG restores isoniazid-sensitivity in *Mycobacterium tuberculosis* isolates resistant to a range of drug concentrations. *Mol. Microbiol.* 1993;8:521.

44. Stoeckle, M., L. Guan, N. Riegler, I. Weitzman, B. Kreiswirth, J. Kornblum, F. Laraque, and L. Riley. Catalase-peroxidase gene sequences in isoniazid-sensitive and resistant strains of *Mycobacterium tuberculosis* from New York City. *J. Infect. Dis.* 1993;168:1063.

45. Dessen, A., A. Quemard, J. Blanchard, W. Jacobs, and J. Sacchettini. Crystal structure and function of the isoniazid target of *Mycobacterium tuberculosis. Science* 1995;267:1638.

46. Banerjee, A., E. Dubnau, A. Quemard, V. Balasubramanian, K. Um, T. Wilson, D. Collins, G. deLisle, and W. Jacobs. *inhA*, a gene encoding a target for isoniazid and ethionamide in *Mycobacterium tuberculosis. Science* 1994;263:227.

47. Armstrong, A. R. Further studies on the time concentration relationships of isoniazid on tubercle bacilli in vitro. *Am. Rev. Respir. Dis.* 1965;91:440.

48. Vivien, J. H., R. Thibier, and A. Lepeuple. Recent studies on isoniazid. *Adv. Tuberc. Res.* 1972;18:148.

49. Tuberculosis Chemotherapy Centre, Madras. A controlled comparison of a twice-weekly and three once-weekly regimens in the initial treatment of pulmonary tuberculosis. *Bull. WHO* 1970;43:143.

50. Takayama, K., E. L. Armstrong, and H. L. David. Restoration of mycolate synthetase activity in *Mycobacterium tuberculosis* exposed to isoniazid. *Am. Rev. Respir. Dis.* 1974;110:43.

51. Barley, J. F., D. F. Evered, and S. M. Tromon. Transport of isoniazid in rat small intestine in vitro. *Biochem. Parmacol.* 1972;21:2660.

52. Olson, W. A., A. W. Pruitt, and P. G. Dayton. Plasma concentrations of isoniazid in children with tuberculous infections. *Pediatrics* 1981;67:876.

53. Hurwitz, A., and D. L. Schlozman. Effects of antacids on gastrointestinal absorption of isoniazid in rat and man. *Am. Rev. Respir. Dis.* 1974;109:41.

54. Robson, J. M., and F. M. Sullivan. Antituberculosis drugs. *Pharmacol. Rev.* 1963;15:169.

55. Peters, J. H., K. S. Miller, and P. Brown. Studies on the metabolic basis for the genetically determined capacities for isoniazid inactivation in man. *J. Pharmacol. Exp. Ther.* 1965;150:298.

56. Jenne, J. W. Partial purification and properties of the isoniazid transacetylase in human liver. Its relationship to the acetylation of p-aminosalicylic acid. *J. Clin. Invest.* 1965;44:1992.

57. Weber, W. W. *The Acetylator Genes and Drug Response.* New York: Oxford University Press, 1987.

58. Weber, W. W., and D. W. Hein. Acetylation pharmacogenetics. *Pharmacol. Rev.* 1985;37:1.

59. Karim, A. K. M. B, M. S. Elfellah, and D. A. P. Evans. Human acetylator polymorphism: estimate of allele frequency in Lybia and details of global distribution. *J. Med. Genet.* 1981;18:325.

60. Ellard, G. A. Variations between individuals and populations in the acetylation of isoniazid and its significance for the treatment of pulmonary tuberculosis. *Clin. Pharmacol. Ther.* 1976;19:610.

61. Tiitinen, H. Isoniazid and ethionamide serum levels and inactivation in Finnish subjects. *Scand. J. Respir. Dis.* 1969;50:110.

62. Vatsis, K. P., W. W. Weber, D. A. Bell, J. M. Dupret, D. A. P. Evans, D. M. Grant, D. W. Hein, H. J. Lin, U. A. Meyer, M. V. Relling, E. Sim, T. Suzuki, and Y. Yamazoe. Nomenclature for N-acetyltransferases. *Pharmacogenetics* 1995;5:1.

63. Grant, D. M., M. Blum, M. Beer, and U. A. Meyer. Monomorphic and polymorphic human arylamine N-acetyltransferases: a comparison of liver isozymes and expressed products of two cloned genes. *Mol. Pharmacol.* 1991;39:184.

64. Levy, G. N., and W. W. Weber. Interindividual

variability of N-acetyltransferases in man. In *Interindividual Variability in Drug Metabolism in Man*, ed. by G. M. Pacifici and O. Pelkonen. London: Taylor and Francis, in press.

65. Grant, D. M., K. Morike, D. Eichelbaum, and U. A. Meyer. Acetylation pharmacogenetics: the slow acetylator phenotype is caused by decreased or absent arylamine N-acetyltransferase in human liver. *J. Clin. Invest.* 1990;85:968.

66. Devadatta, S., P. R. J. Gangadharam, R. H. Andrews, W. Fox, C. V. Ramakrishnan, J. B. Selkon, and S. Velu. Peripheral neuritis due to isoniazid. *Bull. WHO* 1960;23:587.

67. Musch, E., M. Eichelbaum, J. K. Wang, W. von Sassen, M. Castro-Parra, and H. J. Dengler. Die Häufigkeit hepatotoxisher Nebenwirkungen der tuberkulostatischen Kombinationstherapie (INH, RMP, EMB) in Abhängigkeit vom Acetyliererphänotyp. *Klin. Wochenschr.* 1982;60:513.

68. Kutt, H., K. Verebely, and F. McDowell. Inhibition of diphenylhydantoin metabolism in rats and rat liver microsomes by antitubercular drugs. *Neurology* 1968;18:706.

69. Kutt, H., W. Winters, and F. H. McDowell. Depression of parahydroxylation of diphenylhydantoin by antituberculous chemotherapy. *Neurology* 1966;16:594.

70. Muakkassah, S. F., W. R. Bidlack, and W. C. T. Yang. Mechanism of the inhibitory action of isoniazid on microsomal drug metabolism. *Biochem. Pharmacol.* 1981;30:1651.

71. Mitchell, J. R., U. P. Thorgeirsson, M. Black, J. A. Timbrell, W. R. Snodgrass, W. Z. Potter, D. J. Jollow, and H. R. Keiser. Increased incidence of isoniazid hepatitis in rapid acetylators: possible relation to hydrazine metabolites. *Clin. Pharmacol. Ther.* 1975;18:70.

72. Ellard, G. A., and P. T. Gammon. Pharmacokinetics of isoniazid metabolism in man. *J. Pharmacokinet. Biopharm.* 1976;4:83.

73. Bowersox, D. W., R. H. Winterbauer, G. L., Stewart, B. Orme, and E. Barron. Isoniazid dosage in patients with renal failure. *N. Engl. J. Med.* 1973;289:84.

74. Acocella, G., L. Bonollo, M. Garimoldi, M. Mainardi, L. T. Tenconi, and F. B. Nicolis. Kinetics of rifampicin and isoniazid administered alone and in combination to normal subjects and patients with liver disease. *Gut* 1972;13:47.

75. Bennett, W. M., R. S. Muther, R. A. Parker, P. Feig, G. Morrison, T. A. Golper, and I. Singer. Drug therapy in renal failure: dosing guidelines for adults. *Ann. Intern. Med.* 1980;93:62.

76. Goldman, A. L., and S. S. Braman. Isoniazid: a review with emphasis on adverse effects. *Chest* 1972;1:62.

77. Stork, C., and R. Hoffman. Toxicology of antituberculosis drugs. In *Tuberculosis*, ed. by W. Rom and S. Garat. Boston: Little Brown, 1996, pp. 829–841.

78. Holtz, P., and D. Palm. Pharmacological aspects of vitamin B-6. *Pharmacol. Rev.* 1964;16:113.

79. Tuberculosis Chemotherapy Centre, Madras. The prevention and treatment of isoniazid toxicity in the therapy of pulmonary tuberculosis. 2. An assessment of the prophylactic effect of pyridoxine in low dosage. *Bull. WHO* 1963;29:457.

80. Sievers, M. L., and R. N. Herrier. Treatment of acute isoniazid toxicity. *Am. J. Hosp. Pharm.* 1975;32:202.

81. Wason, S., P. G. Lacouture, and F. H. Lovejoy. Single high-dose pyridoxine treatment for isoniazid overdose. *JAMA* 1981;246:1102.

82. Weidorn, W. S., and F. Ervin. Schizophrenic-like psychotic reaction with administration of isoniazid. *Arch. Neurol. Psychiat.* 1954;72:321.

83. Garibaldi, R. A., R. E. Drusin, S. H. Ferebee, and M. B. Gregg. Isoniazid-associated hepatitis: report of an outbreak. *Am. Rev. Respir. Dis.* 1972;106:357.

84. Mitchell, J. R., H. J. Zimmerman, K. G. Ishak, U. P. Thorgeirsson, J. A. Timbrell, W. R. Snodgrass, and S. D. Nelson. Isoniazid liver injury: clinical spectrum, pathology, and probable pathogenesis. *Ann. Intern. Med.* 1976;84:181.

85. Mitchell, J. R., M. W. Long, U. P. Thorgeirsson, and D. J. Jollow. Acetylation rates and monthly liver function tests during one year of isoniazid preventive therapy. *Chest* 1975;68:181.

86. Girling, D. J. Adverse effects of antituberculosis drugs. *Drugs* 1982;23:56.

87. Kopanoff, D., D. Snider and G. Caras. Isoniazid related hepatitis. *Am. Rev. Respir. Dis.* 1992;145:494.

88. A joint statement of the American Thoracic Society, American Lung Association, and the Center for Disease Control. Preventive therapy of tuberculous infection. *Am. Rev. Respir. Dis.* 1974;110:371.

89. Felton, C., and H. Shah. Isoniazid: clinical use and toxicity. In *Tuberculosis*, ed. by W. Rom and S. Garat. Boston: Little Brown and Co., 1996, pp. 773–778.

90. Snider, D., and G. Caras. Isoniazid-associated hepatitis deaths. A review of available information. *Am. Rev. Respir. Dis.* 1992;145:494.

91. Moulding, T., A. Redecker, and G. Kanel. Twenty isoniazid associated deaths in one state. *Am. Rev. Respir. Dis.* 1989;140:700.

92. Steele, M., R. Burk, and R. DesPrez. Toxic hepatitis with isoniazid and rifampin. A meta-analysis. *Chest* 1991;99:465.

93. Jenner, P., and G. Ellard. Isoniazid-related hepatotoxicity: a study of the effect of rifampicin administration on the metabolism of acetylisoniazid in man. *Tubercle* 1989;70:93.

94. Ellard, G., and P. Gammon. Pharmacokinetics of isoniazid metabolism in man. *J. Pharmacokinet. Biopharm.* 1976;4:83.

95. Black, M., J. R. Mitchell, H. J. Zimmerman, K. G. Ishak, and G. R. Epler. Isoniazid-associated hepatitis in 114 patients. *Gastroenterology* 1975;69:289.

96. Maddrey, W. C., and J. K. Biotnott. Isoniazid hepatitis. *Ann. Intern. Med.* 1973;79:1.

97. Timbrell, J. A., J. M. Wright, and T. A. Baillie. Monoacetylhydrazine as a metabolite of isoniazid in man. *Clin. Pharmacol. Ther.* 1977;22:602.

98. Nelson, S. D., J. R. Mitchell, J. A. Timbrell, W. R. Snodgrass, and G. B. Corcoran. Isoniazid and

iproniazid: activation of metabolites to toxic intermediates in man and rat. *Science* 1976;193:901.

99. Singapore Tuberculosis Service/British Medical Research Council. Controlled trial of intermittent regimens of rifampin plus isoniazid for pulmonary tuberculosis in Singapore; the results of up to 30 months. *Am. Rev. Respir. Dis.* 1977;116:807.

100. Ellard, G. A., and D. J. Girling. The hepatotoxicity of isoniazid among the three acetylator phenotypes. *Am. Rev. Respir. Dis.* 1981;123:568.

101. Dickinson, D. S., W. C. Bailey, B. I. Hirschowitz, S. J. Soong, L. Eidus, and M. M. Hodgkin. Risk factors for isoniazid (INH)-induced liver dysfunction. *J. Clin. Gastroenterol.* 1981;3:271.

102. Hein, D. W., and W. W. Weber. Polymorphic N-acetylation of phenelzine and monoacetylhydrazine by highly purified rabbit liver isoniazid N-acetyltransferase. *Drug Metab. Disp.* 1982;10:225.

103. Weber, W. W., D. W. Hein, A. Litwin, and G. M. Lower: Relationship of acetylator status to isoniazid toxicity, lupus erythematosus, and bladder cancer. *Fed. Proc.* 1983;42:3086.

104. Berté, S. J., J. D. DiMase, and C. S. Christianson. Isoniazid, PAS, and streptomycin intolerance in 1744 patients. An analysis of reactions to single drugs and drug groups plus data on multiple reactions, type and time of reactions, and desensitization. *Am. Rev. Respir. Dis.* 1964;90:598.

105. Alarcon-Segovia, D. Drug-induced lupus syndromes. *Mayo Clin. Proc.* 1969;44:664.

106. Alarcon-Segovia, D., E. Fishbein, and H. Alcala. Isoniazid acetylation rate and development of antinuclear antibodies upon isoniazid treatment. *Arthritis Rheum.* 1971;14:748.

107. Rothfield, N. F., W. F. Bierer, and J. W. Garfield. Isoniazid induction of antinuclear antibodies. *Ann. Intern. Med.* 1978;88:650.

108. Miller, R., J. Porter, and D. Greenblatt. Clinical importance of the interaction of phenytoin and isoniazid. *Chest* 1979;75:356.

109. Wehrli, W., and M. Staehelin. Actions of the rifamycins. *Bacteriol. Rev.* 1971;35:290.

110. Hartmann, G. R. Molecular mechanism of action of rifamycins. In *Drug Receptor Interactions in Antimicrobial Chemotherapy*, ed. by J. Drews and F. E. Hahn. New York: Springer-Verlag, 1975, pp. 295–300.

111. Lancini, G., R. Pallanza, and L. G. Silvestri. Relationships between bactericidal effect and inhibition of ribonucleic acid nucleotidyltransferase by rifampicin in *Escherichia coli* K-12. *J. Bacteriol.* 1969;97:761.

112. Wehrli, W., F. Knüsel, K. Schmid, and M. Staehelin. Interaction of rifamycin with bacterial RNA polymerase. *Proc. Natl. Acad. Sci. U.S.A.* 1968;61:667.

113. Lill, U. I., and G. R. Hartmann. On the binding of rifampicin to the DNA-directed RNA polymerase from *Escherichia coli. Eur. J. Biochem.* 1973;38:336.

114. di Mauro, E., L. Synder, P. Marino, A. Lamberti, A. Coppo, and G. P. Tocchini-Valentini. Rifampicin sensitivity of the components of DNA-dependent RNA polymerase. *Nature* 1969;222:533.

115. Heil, A., and W. Zillig. Reconstitution of bacterial DNA-dependent RNA-polymerase from isolated subunits as a tool for the elucidation of the role of the subunits in transcription. *FEBS Lett.* 1970;11:165.

116. Rabussay, D., and W. Zillig. A rifampicin resistant RNA-polymerase from *E. coli* altered in the β-subunit. *FEBS Lett.* 1969;5:104.

117. Linn, T., R. Losick, and A. L. Sonenschein. Rifampin resistance mutation of *Bacillus subtilis* altering the electrophoretic mobility of the beta subunit of ribonucleic acid polymerase. *J. Bacteriol.* 1975;122:1387.

118. Stetter, K. O., and W. Zillig. Transcription in Lactobacillaceae. DNA-dependent RNA polymerase from *Lactobacillus curvatus. Eur. J. Biochem.* 1974;48:527.

119. Lill, U. I., and G. R. Hartmann. Formation of RNA polymerase sub-assembly composed of subunit α from *Escherichia coli* and of subunit β from *Micrococcus luteus. Hoppe-Seyler's Z. Physiol. Chem.* 1977;358:1605.

120. Cole, S. Rifamycin resistance in mycobacteria. *Res. Microbiol.* 1996;147:48.

121. Telenti, A., P. Imboden, F. Marchesi, T. Schidheini, and T. Bodmer. Detection of rifampicin-resistance mutations in *Mycobacterium tuberculosis. Lancet* 1993;341:647.

122. Levin, M., and G. Hatfull. *Mycobacterium smegmatis* RNA polymerase: DNA supercoiling, action of rifampicin and mechanism of rifampicin resistance. *Mol. Microbiol.* 1993;8:277.

123. Honore, N., and S. Cole. Molecular basis of rifampin resistance in *Mycobacterium leprae. Antimicrob. Agents Chemother.* 1993;37:414.

124. Donnabella, V., F. Martiniuk, D. Kinney, M. Bacerdo, S. Bonk, B. Hanna, and W. Rom. Isolation of the gene for the beta-subunit of RNA polymerase from a clinical isolate of rifampin resistanct *Mycobacterium tuberculosis* and identification of new mutants. *Am. J. Respir. Mol. Cell Biol.* 1994;11:639.

125. Sippel, A., and G. Hartman. Mode of action of rifamycin on the RNA polymerase reaction. *Biochim Biophys. Acta* 1968;157:218.

126. Sippel, A. E., and G. R. Hartmann. Rifampicin resistance of RNA polymerase in the binary complex with DNA. *Eur. J. Biochem.* 1970;16:152.

127. Hinkle, D. C., W. F. Mangel, and M. J. Chamberlin. Studies of the binding of *Escherichia coli* RNA polymerase to DNA. IV. The effect of rifampicin on binding and on RNA chain initiation. *J. Mol. Biol.* 1972;70:209.

128. McClure, W. R., and C. L. Cech. On the mechanism of rifampicin inhibition of RNA synthesis. *J. Biol. Chem.* 1978;53:8949.

129. Kessler, C., M. I. Huaifeng, and G. R. Hartmann. Competition of rifampicin with binding of substrate and RNA to RNA polymerase. *Eur. J. Biochem.* 1982;122:515.

130. Austin, S. J., I. P. B Tittawella, R. S. Hayward, and J. G. Scaife. Amber mutations of *Escherichia coli* RNA polymerase. *Nature N. Biol.* 1971;232:133.

131. Konno, K., K. Oizumi, and S. Oka. Mode of action of rifampin on mycobacteria. II. Biosynthetic studies on the inhibition of ribonucleic acid polymerase

of *Mycobacterium bovis* BCG by rifampin and uptake of rifampin-^{14}C by *Mycobacterium phlei*. *Am. Rev. Respir. Dis.* 1973;107:1006.

132. Voigt, H. P., R. Kaufmann, and H. Matthei. Solubilized DNA-dependent RNA polymerase from human placenta; a magnesium-dependent enzyme. *FEBS Lett.* 1970;10:257.

133. Wehrli, W., J. Nüesch, F. Knüsel, and M. Staehelin. Action of rifamycins on RNA polymerase. *Biochim. Biophys. Acta* 1968;157:215.

134. Reid, B. D., and P. Parsons. Partial purification of mitochondrial RNA polymerase from rat liver. *Proc. Natl. Acad. Sci. U.S.A.* 1971;68:2830.

135. Armstrong, J. J., S. J. Surzycki, B. Moll, and R. P. Levine. Genetic transcription and translation specifying chloroplast components in *Chlamydomonas reinhardi*. *Biochemistry* 1971;10:692.

136. Busiello, E., A. D. Girolamo, L. Fisher-Fantuzzi, and C. Vesco. Multiple effects of rifamycin derivatives on animal-cell metabolism of macromolecules. *Eur. J. Biochem.* 1973;35:251.

137. Barry, C. E. New horizons in the treatment of tuberculosis. *Biochem. Pharmacol.* 1997;54:1165.

138. Lorian, V., and M. Finland. In vitro effect of rifampin of mycobacteria. *Appl. Microbiol.* 1969;17:202.

139. Atlas, E., and M. Turck. Laboratory and clinical evaluation of rifampicin. *Am. J. Med. Sci.* 1968;256:247.

140. Kopanoff, D. E., J. O. Kilburn, J. L. Glassroth, D. E. Snider, L. S. Farer, and R. C. Good. A continuing survey of tuberculosis primary resistance in the United States: March 1975 to November 1977. *Am. Rev. Respir. Dis.* 1978;118:835.

141. White, R. J., G. C. Lancini, and L. G. Silverstri. Mechanism of action of rifampin on *Mycobacterium smegmatis J. Bacteriol.* 1971;108:737.

142. Stottmeier, K. D. Emergence of rifampin-resistant *Mycobacterium tuberculosis* in Massachusetts. *J. Infect. Dis.* 1976;133:88.

143. Hobby, G. L., and T. F. Lenert. Observations on the action of rifampin and ethambutol alone and in combination with other antituberculosis drugs. *Am. Rev. Respir. Dis.* 1972;105:292.

144. Dickinson, J. M., and D. A. Mitchison. Experimental models to explain the high sterilizing activity of rifampin in the chemotherapy of tuberculosis. *Am. Rev. Respir. Dis.* 1981;123:367.

145. Kuze, F., T. Kursawa, K. Bando, Y. Lee, and N. Maekawa. In vitro and in vivo susceptibility of atypical mycobacteria to various drugs. *Rev. Infect. Dis.* 1981;3:885.

146. Yates, M. D., and C. H. Collins. Sensitivity of opportunist mycobacteria to rifampicin and ethambutol. *Tubercle* 1981;62:117.

147. Waters, M. F. R., R. I. W. Rees, J. M. H. Pearson, A. B. G. Laing, H. S. Helmy, and R. H. Gelber. Rifampicin for lepromatous leprosy: nine years' experience. *BMJ* 1978;1:133.

148. Fox, W. The chemotherapy of tuberculosis: a review. *Chest* 1979;76:785.

149. Mitchison, D. A. Basic mechanisms of chemotherapy. *Chest* 1979;76(Suppl):771.

150. Grumbach, F. Experimental in vivo studies of new antituberculosis drugs; capreomycin, ethambutol, rifampicin. *Tubercle* 1969;50(Suppl.):12.

151. Visudhiphan, P., and S. Chiemchanya. Evaluation of rifampicin in the treatment of tuberculous meningitis in children. *J. Pediatr.* 1975;87:983.

152. Kradolfer, F., and R. Schnell. Incidence of resistant pulmonary tuberculosis in relation to initial bacterial load. *Chemotherapy* 1970;15:242.

153. Pezzia, J., J. W. Raleigh, M. C. Bailey, E. A. Toth, and J. Silverblatt. Treatment of pulmonary disease due to *Mycobacterium kansasii*: recent experience with rifampin. *Rev. Infect. Dis.* 1981;3:1035.

154. Sanders, W. E. Rifampin. *Ann. Intern. Med.* 1976;85:82.

155. Leprosy Chemotherapy Committee of the U.S. Leprosy Panel and the Leonard Wood Memorial. Rifampin therapy of lepromatous leprosy. *Am. J. Trop. Med. Hyg.* 1975;24:475.

156. Devine, L. F., and C. R. Hagerman. Spectra of susceptibility of *Neisseria meningitidis* to antimicrobial agents in vitro. *Appl. Microbiol.* 1970;19:329.

157. Deal, W. B., and E. Sanders. Efficacy of rifampin in treatment of meningococcal carriers. *N. Engl. J. Med.* 1969;281:641.

158. Beam, W. E., N. R. Newberg, L. F. Devine, W. E. Pierce, and J. A. Davies. The effect of rifampin on the nasopharyngeal carriage of *Neiseseria meningitidis* in a military population. *J. Infect. Dis.* 1971;124:39.

159. Sivonen, A., O. Renkonen, P. Weckstrom, K. Koskenvuo, V. Raunio, and P. H. Makela. The effect of chemoprophylactic use of rifampin and minocycline on rates of carriage of *Neisseria meningitidis* in army recruits in Finland. *J. Infect. Dis.* 1978;137:238.

160. Devine, L. F., D. P. Johnson, S. L. Rhode, C. R. Hagerman, W. E. Pierce, and R. D. Peckinpaugh. Rifampin: effect of two-day treatment of the meningococcal carrier state and the relationship to the levels of drug in sera and saliva. *Am. J. Med. Sci.* 1971;261:79.

161. Tuazon, C. U., M. Y. C. Lin, and J. N. Sheagren. In vitro activity of rifampin alone and in combination with nafcillin and vancomycin against pathogenic strains of *Staphylococcus aureus*. *Antimicrob. Agents Chemother.* 1978;13:759.

162. Kerry, D. W., J. M. T. Hamilton-Miller, and W. Brumfitt. Trimethoprim and rifampicin: in vitro activities separately and in combination. *J. Antimicrob. Chemother.* 1975;1:417.

163. Simmons, N. A. Synergy and rifampicin. *J. Antimicrob. Chemother.* 1977;3:109.

164. Brumfitt, W., and J. M. T. Hamilton-Miller. Rifaprim (rifamycin plus trimethoprim): pharmacokinetics and effects on the normal flora of man. *Biopharm. Drug Dispos.* 1981;2:157.

165. Medoff, G., G. S. Kobayashi, C. N. Kwan, D. Schlessinger, and P. Venkov. Potentiation of rifampicin and 5-fluorocytosine as antifungal antibiotics by amphotericin B. *Proc. Natl. Acad. Sci. U.S.A.* 1972;69:196.

166. Kobayashi, G. S., S. C. Cheung, D. Schlessinger, and G. Medoff. Effects of rifamycin derivatives, alone and in combination with amphotericin B, against *His-*

toplasma capsulatum. Antimicrob. Agents Chemother. 1974;5:16.

167. Kitahara, M., G. S. Kobayashi, and G. Medoff. Enhanced efficacy of amphotericin B and Rifampicin combined in treatment of murine histoplasmosis and blastomycosis. *J. Infect. Dis.* 1976;133:663.

168. Arroyo, J., G. Medoff, and G. S. Kobayashi. Therapy of murine aspergillosis with amphotericin B in combination with rifampin or 5-fluorocytosine. *Antimicrob. Agents Chemother.* 1977;11:21.

169. Furesz, S., R. Scotti, R. Pallanza, and E. Mapelli. Rifampicin: a new rifamycin III: absorption, distribution, and elimination in man. *Arzneimittelforschung* 1967;17:534.

170. Boman, G. Serum concentration and half-life of rifampicin after simultaneous oral administration of aminosalicylic acid or isoniazid. *Eur. J. Clin. Pharmacol.* 1974;7:217.

171. McCracken, G. H., C. M. Ginsburg, T. C. Zweighaft, and J. Clahsen. Pharmacokinetics of rifampin in infants and children: relevance to prophylaxis against *Haemophilus influenzae* type b disease. *Pediatrics* 1980;66:17.

172. J. W. Jenne and W. H. Beggs. Correlation of in vitro and in vivo kinetics with clinical use of isoniazid, ethambutol and rifampin. *Am. Rev. Respir. Dis.* 1973; 107:1013.

173. Oliveira, J. J. G. Cerebrospinal fluid concentrations of rifampin in meningeal tuberculosis. *Am. Rev. Respir. Dis.* 1972;106:432.

174. Sippel, J. E., I. A. Mikhail, N. I. Girgis, and H. H. Youssef. Rifampin concentrations in cerebrospinal fluid of patients with tuberculous meningitis. *Am. Rev. Respir. Dis.* 1974;109:579.

175. Boman, G., and A.-S. Malmborg. Rifampicin in plasma and pleural fluid after single doses. *Eur. J. Clin. Pharmacol.* 1974;7:51.

176. Lee, C. S., D. C. Brater, J. G. Gambertoglio, and L. Z. Benet. Disposition kinetics of ethambutol in man. *J. Pharmacokinet. Biopharm.* 1980;8:335.

177. Hoeprich, P. D. Prediction of antimeningococcic chemoprophylactic efficacy. *J. Infect. Dis.* 1971;123:125.

178. Mandel, G. L. Interaction of intraleukocytic bacteria and antibiotics. *J. Clin. Invest.* 1973;52:1673.

179. Allen, S. W., G. A. Ellard, P. T. Gammon, R. C. King, A. C. McDougall, R. J. W. Rees, and A. G. M. Weddell. The penetration of dapsone, rifampicin, isoniazid and pyrazinamide into peripheral nerves. *Br. J. Pharmacol.* 1975;55:151.

180. Boman, G., and V.-A. Ringberger. Binding of rifampicin by human plasma proteins. *Eur. J. Clin. Pharmacol.* 1974;7:369.

181. Acocella, G., F. B. Nicholis, and A. Lamarina. A study on the kinetics of rifampicin in man. *Chemotherapy* 1967;5:87.

182. Furesz, S. Chemical and biological properties of rifampicin. *Antibiot. Chemother.* 1970;16:316.

183. Cohn, H. D. Clinical studies with a new rifamycin derivative. *J. Clin. Pharmacol.* 1969;9:118.

184. Kenwright, S., and A. J. Levi. Sites of competition in the selective hepatic uptake of rifamycin-SV, fla-

vaspidic acid, bilirubin, and bromsulphthalein. *Gut* 1974;15:220.

185. Kenwright, S., and A. J. Levi. Impairment of hepatic uptake of rifamycin antibiotics by probenecid, and its therapeutic implications. *Lancet* 1973;2:1401.

186. Acocella, G., V. Pagani, M. Marchetti, G. C. Baroni, and F. B. Nicholis. Kinetic studies on rifampicin. I. Serum concentration analysis in subjects treated with different oral doses over a period of two weeks. *Chemotherapy* 1971;16:356.

187. Nitti, V., F. Delli Veneri, A. Ninni, and G. Meola. Rifampicin blood serum levels and half-life during prolonged administration in tuberculosis patients. *Chemotherapy* 1972;17:121.

188. Gronhagen-Riska, C., P. E. Helstrom, and B. Froseth. Predisposing factors in hepatitis induced by isoniazid-rifampin treatment of tuberculosis. *Am. Rev. Respir. Dis.* 1978;118:461.

189. Pessayre, D., M. Bentata, C. Degott, O. Nouel, J.-P. Miguet, B. Rueff, and J.-P. Benhamou. Isoniazid-rifampin fulminant hepatitis. *Gastroenterology* 1977; 72:284.

190. Aquinas, M., W. G. L. Allan, P. A. L. Horsfall, P. K. Jenkins, W. Hung-Yan, D. Girling, R. Tall, and W. Fox. Adverse reactions to daily and intermittent rifampicin regimens for pulmonary tuberculosis in Hong Kong. *BMJ* 1972;1:765.

191. Pujet, J.-C., J.-C. Homberg, and G. Decroix. Sensitivity to rifampin: incidence, mechanism, and prevention. *BMJ* 1974;2:415.

192. Mattson, K., and J. Janne. Mild intravasal haemolysis associated with flu-syndrome during intermittent rifampicin treatment. *Eur. J. Respir. Dis.* 1982;63: 68.

193. Calleja, C., J. Pascussi, J. Mani, P. Maureland, and M. Vilarem. The antibiotic rifampin is a nonsteroidal ligand and activator of the human glucocorticoid receptor. *Nat. Med.* 1998;4:92.

194. Mukerjee, P., S. Schuldt, and J. E. Kasik: Effect of rifampin on cutaneous hypersensitivity to purified protein derivative in humans. *Antimicrob. Agents Chemother.* 1973;4:607.

195. Supta, S., M. H. Grieco, and I. Siegel. Suppression of T-lymphocyte rosettes by rifampin. Studies in normals and patients with tuberculosis. *Ann. Intern. Med.* 1975;82:484.

196. Albert, R. K., and S. Lakshminaryan. Long-term therapy with rifampin and the secondary antibody response to killed influenza vaccine. *Am. Rev. Respir. Dis.* 1978;117:605.

197. Humber, D. P., H. Nsanzumuhire, J. A. Alouch, A. D. B. Webster, V. A. Aber, D. A. Mitchison, D. J. Girling, and A. J. Nunn. Controlled double-blind study of the effect of rifampin on humoral and cellular immune responses in patients with pulmonary tuberculosis and in tuberculosis contacts. *Am. Rev. Respir. Dis.* 1980;122:425.

198. Graber, C. D., J. Jebaily, R. L. Galphin, and E. Doering. Light chain proteinuria and humoral immunoincompetence in tuberculosis patients treated with rifampin. *Am. Rev. Respir. Dis.* 1973;107:713.

199. Warrington, R. J., G. R. Hogg, F. Paraskevas, and K. S. Tse. Insidious rifampin-associated renal fail-

ure with light-chain proteinuria. *Arch. Intern. Med.* 1977;137:927.

200. Acocella, G., and R. Conti. Interaction of rifampicin with other drugs. *Tubercle* 1980;61:171.

201. Takasu, N., T. Yamada, H. Miura, S. Sakamoto, M. Korenaga, K. Nakajima, and M. Kanayama. Rifampicin-induced early phase hyperglycemia in humans. *Am. Rev. Respir. Dis.* 1982;125:23.

202. O'Reilly, R. A. Interaction of chronic daily warfarin therapy and rifampin. *Ann. Intern. Med.* 1975;83:506.

203. Twum-Barima, Y. Quinidine-rifampin interaction. *N. Engl. J. Med.* 1981;304:1466.

204. Buffington, G. A., J. H. Dominguez, W. F. Piering, L. A. Hebert, M. Kauffman, and J. Lemann. Interaction of rifampin and glucocorticoids. Adverse effect on renal allograft function: *JAMA* 1976;236:1958.

205. Ohnhaus, E. E., H. Burgi, A. Burger, and H. Studer. The effect of antipyrine, phenobarbital and rifampicin on throid hormone metabolism in man. *Eur. J. Clin. Invest.* 1981;11:381.

206. Gelber, R. H., and J. W. Rees. Dapsone metabolism in patients with dapsone-resistant leprosy. *Am. J. Trop. Med. Hyg.* 1975;24:963.

207. Skolnick, J. L., B. S. Stoler, D. B. Katz, and W. H. Anderson. Rifampin, oral contraceptives, and pregnancy. *JAMA* 1976;236:1382.

208. Strayhorn, V., A. Baciewicz, and T. Self. Update on rifampin drug interactions, III. *Arch. Intern. Med.* 1997;157:2453.

209. Shepherd, R. G., C. Baughn, M. L. Cantrall, B. Goodstein, J. P. Thomas, and R. G. Wilkinson. Structure-activity studies leading to ethambutol, a new type of antituberculous compound. *Ann. N.Y. Acad. Sci.* 1966;133:686.

210. Karlson, A. The in vitro activity of ethambutol (dextro-2,2'-[ethyl-ethylenediimino]-di-1-butanol) against tubercle bacilli and other microorganisms. *Am. Rev. Respir. Dis.* 1961;84:905.

211. Lucchesi, M., and P. Mancini. The antimycobacterial activity of ethambutol (ETB). *Antibiot. Chemother.* 1970;16:230.

212. Beggs, W. H. Growth inhibition of tubercle bacilli after pulsed exposures to combinations of antituberculous drugs. *Res. Commun. Chem. Pathol. Pharmacol.* 1975;11:487.

213. Doster, B., F. J. Murray, R. Newman, and S. F. Woolpert. Ethambutol in the initial treatment of pulmonary tuberculosis: U.S. Public Health Service tuberculosis therapy trials. *Am. Rev. Respir. Dis.* 1973;107:177.

214. Bobrowitz, I. D. Ethambutol-isoniazid versus streptomycin-ethambutol-isoniazid in original treatment of cavitary tuberculosis. *Am. Rev. Respir. Dis.* 1974;109:548.

215. Fox, W. Whither short-course chemotherapy? *Br. J. Dis. Chest* 1981;75:331.

216. Beggs, W. H. Ethambutol. In *Antibiotics V-1*, ed. by F. E. Hahn. New York: Springer-Verlag, 1979, pp. 43–66.

217. Forbes, M., N. A. Kuck, and E. A. Peets. Mode of action of ethambutol. *J. Bacteriol.* 1962;84:1099.

218. Beggs, W. H., and F. A. Andrews. Nonspecific ionic inhibition of ethambutol binding by *Mycobacterium smegmatis*. *Antimicrob. Agents Chemother.* 1973;4:115.

219. Beggs, W. H. and J. W. Jenne. Growth inhibition of *Mycobacterium tuberculosis* after single-pulsed exposures to streptomycin, ethambutol, and rifampin. *Infect. Immunol.* 1970;2:479.

220. Forbes, M., N. A. Kuck, and E. A. Peets. Effect of ethambutol on nucleic acid metabolism in *Mycobacterium smegmatis* and its reversal by polyamines and divalent cations. *J. Bacteriol.* 1965;89:1299.

221. Takayama, K., E. L. Armstrong, K. A. Kanugi, and J. O. Kilburn. Inhibition by ethambutol of mycolic acid transfer into the cell wall of *Mycobacterium smegmatis*. *Antimicrob. Agents Chemother.* 1979;16:240.

222. Kilburn, J. O., and K. Takayama. Effects of ethambutol on accumulation and secretion of trehalose mycolates and free mycolic acid in *Mycobacterium smegmatis*. *Antimicrob. Agents Chemother.* 1981;20:401.

223. Takayama, K., and J. Kilburn. Inhibition of synthesis of arabinogalactan by ethambutol in *Mycobacterium smegmatis*. *Antimicrob. Agents Chemother.* 1989;33:1493.

224. Wolucka, B., M. McNeil, E. deHoffmann, T. Chojnacki, and P. Brennan. Recognition of the lipid intermediate for arabinogalactan/arabinomannan biosynthesis and its relation to the mode of action of ethambutol on mycobacterium. *J. Biol. Chem.* 1994;269:23328.

225. Deng, L., K. Mikusova, P. Brennan, and G. Besra. Recognition of multiple effects of ethambutol on metabolism of mycobacterial cell envelope. *Antimicrob. Agents Chemother.* 1995;39:694.

226. Lee, R., K. Mikusova, P. Brennan, and G. Besra. Synthesis of the mycobacerial arabinose donor β-O-arabinofuranosyl-1-monophosphoryl-decaprenol, development of a basic arabinosyl-transferase inhibitor. *J. Am. Chem. Soc.* 1995;117:11829.

227. Mikusova, K., R. Slayden, G. Besra, and P. Brennan. Biogenesis of the mycobacterial cell wall and the site of action of ethambutol. *Antimicrob. Agents Chemother.* 1995;39:2484.

228. Belanger, A., G. Besra, M. Ford, K. Mikusova, J. Belisle, P. Brennan, and J. M. Inamine. The embAB genes of *Mycobacterium avium* encode an arabinosyl transferase involved in cell wall arabinan biosynthesis that is the target for the antimycobacterial drug ethambutol. *Proc. Natl. Acad. Sci. U.S.A.* 1996;93:11919.

229. Place, V. A., and J. P. Thomas. Clinical pharmacology of ethambutol. *Am. Rev. Respir. Dis.* 1963;87:901.

230. Peets, E. A., W. M. Sweeney, V. A. Place, and D. A. Buyske. The absorption, excretion, and metabolic fate of ethambutol in man. *Am. Rev. Respir. Dis.* 1965;91:51.

231. Lee, C. S., J. G. Gambertoglio, D. C. Brater, and L. Z. Benet. Kinetics of oral ethambutol in the normal subject. *Clin. Pharmacol. Ther.* 1977;22:615.

232. Gundert-Remy, U., M. Klett, and E. Weber. Concentration of ethambutol in cerebrospinal fluid in man as a function of non-protein-bound drug fraction in serum. *Eur. J. Clin. Pharmacol.* 1973;6:133.

233. Bobrowitz, I. D. Ethambutol in tuberculous meningitis. *Chest* 1972;61:529.

234. Djurovic, V., G. Delacroix, and P. Daumet. L'éthambutol chez l'homme. Etude comparative de taux sériques érythrocytaires et pulmonaires. *Nouv. Presse Med.* 1973;2:2815.

235. Kelly, R. G., E. Kaleita, and H. J. Eisner. Tissue distribution of [^{14}C]ethambutol in mice. *Am. Rev. Respir. Dis.* 1981;123:689.

236. Liss, R. H., R. J. Letourneau, and J. P. Schepis. Distribution of ethambutol in primate tissues and cells. *Am. Rev. Respir. Dis.* 1981;123:529.

237. Shneerson, J. M., and R. S. Francis. Ethambutol in pregnancy—foetal exposure. *Tubercle* 1979;60:167.

238. Peets, E. A., and D. A. Buyske. Comparative metabolism of ethambutol and its L-isomer. *Biochem Pharmacol.* 1964;13:1403.

239. Dume, T., C. Wagner, and E. Wetzels. Zur Pharmakokinetik von Ethambutol bei Gesunden und Patienten mit terminaler Niereninsuffizienz. *Dtsch. Med. Wochenschr.* 1971;96:1430.

240. Lee, C. S., T. C. Marbury, and L. Z. Benet. Clearance calculations in hemodialysis: application to blood, plasma and dialysate measurements for ethambutol. *J. Pharmacokinet. Biopharm.* 1980;8:69.

241. Leading Article. Tuberculosis in patients having dialysis. *BMJ* 1980;280:349.

242. Mitchison, D. A., and G. A. Ellard. Tuberculosis in patients having dialysis. *BMJ* 1980;280:1186.

243. Mitchison, D. A., and G. A. Ellard. Tuberculosis in patients having dialysis. *BMJ* 1980;280:1533.

244. J. E. Leibold: The ocular toxicity of ethambutol and its relation to dose. *Ann. N. Y. Acad. Sci.* 1966;135:904.

245. Barron, G. J., L. Tepper, and G. Iovine. Ocular toxicity from ethambutol *Am. J. Opthalmol.* 1974;77:256.

246. Boman, G., and B. Calissendorff. A case of irreversible bilateral optic damage after ethambutol therapy. *Scand. J. Respir. Dis.* 1974;55:176.

247. Alvarez, K., and L. Krop. Ethambutol-induced ocular toxicity revisited. *Ann. Pharmacother.* 1993;27:102.

248. Nasemann, J., E. Zrenner, and K. Riedel. Recovery after severe ethambutol intoxication—psychophysical and electrophysiological correlation. *Doc. Ophthalmol.* 1989;71:279.

249. Citron, K. M. Ethambutol: a review with special reference to ocular toxicity. *Tubercle* 1969;50(Suppl.):32.

250. Addington, W. W. The side effects and interactions of antituberculosis drugs. *Chest* 1979;76:782.

251. Tugwell, P., and S. L. James. Peripheral neuropathy with ethambutol. *Postgrad. Med. J.* 1972;48:667.

252. Nair, V. S., M. LeBrun, and I. Kass. Peripheral neuropathy associated with ethambutol. *Chest* 1980;77:98.

253. Takeuchi, H., M. Takahshi, J. Kang, S. Ueno, S. Tarui, Y. Nakao, and T. Otori. Ethambutol neuropathy: clinical and electroneuromyographic studies. *Folia Psychiatr. Neurol. Jpn.* 1980;34:45.

254. Takeuchi, H., M. Takahashi, S. Tarui, S. Sanagi, and H. Takenaka. Peripheral nerve conduction function

in patients treated with antituberculotic agents, with special reference to ethambutol and isoniazid. *Folia Psychiatr. Neurol. Jpn.* 1980;34:57.

255. Poslethwaite, A. E., and W. N. Kelley. Studies on the mechanism of ethambutol-induced hyperuricemia. *Arthritis Rheum.* 1972;15:403.

256. Postlethwaite, A. E., A. G. Bartel, and W. N. Kelley. Hyperuricemia due to ethambutol. *N. Engl. J. Med.* 1972;286:761.

257. Khanna, B. K. Acute gouty arthritis following ethambutol therapy. *Br. J. Dis. Chest* 1980;74:409.

258. Lewit, T., L. Nebel, S. Terracina, and S. Karman. Ethambutol in pregnancy: observations on embryogenesis. *Chest* 1974;66:25.

259. Bobrowitz, I. D. Ethambutol in pregnancy. *Chest* 1974;66:20.

260. Van Scoy, R. E. Antituberculous agents: isoniazid, rifampin, streptomycin, ethambutol. *Mayo Clin. Proc.* 1977;52:694.

261. Suter, E. Multiplication of tubercle bacilli within phagocytes cultivated in vitro, and effect of streptomycin and isonicotinic acid hydrazide. *Am. Rev. Tuberc.* 1952;65:775.

262. Dickinson, J. M., and D. A. Mitchison. Observations in vitro on the suitability of pyrazinamide for intermittent chemotherapy of tuberculosis. *Tubercle* 1970;51:389.

263. McDermott, W., L. Ormond, C. Muschenheim, K. Deuschle, R. M. McCune, and R. Tompsett. Pyrazinamide-isoniazid in tuberculosis. *Am. Rev. Tuberc.* 1954;69:319.

264. Jindani, M., V. R. Aber, E. A. Edwards, and D. A. Mitchison. The early bactericidal activity of drugs in patients with pulmonary tuberculosis. *Am. Rev. Respir. Dis.* 1980;121:939.

265. Mackaness, G. B. The intracellular activation of pyrazinamide and nicotinamide. *Am. Rev. Tuberc.* 1956;74:718.

266. Konno, K., F. Feldman, and W. McDermott. Pyrazinamide susceptibility and amidase activity of tubercle bacilli. *Am. Rev. Respir. Dis.* 1967;95:461.

267. Butler, W., and J. Kilburn. Susceptibility of mycobacterium tuberculosis to pyrazinamide and its relationship to pyrazinamidase activity. *Antimicrob. Agents Chemother.* 1983;24:600.

268. Scorpio, A., and Y. Zhang. Mutations in *pncA*, a gene encoding pyrazinamide/nicotinamidase, cause resistance to the antituberculosis drug pyrazinamide in tubercle bacillus. *Nat. Med.* 1996;2:662.

269. Cynamon, M., S. Klemens, T. Chou, R. Gimi, and J. Welch. Antimycobacterial activity of a series of pyrazinoic acid esters. *J. Med. Chem.* 1992;35:1212.

270. Cynamon, M., R. Gimi, F. Gyenes, C. Sharpe, K. Bergmann, H. Han, L. Gregor, R. Rapola, G. Luciano, and J. Welch. Pyrazinoic acid esters with broad spectrum in vitro antimycobacterial activity. *J. Med. Chem.* 1995;38:3902.

271. Bergmann, K., M. Cynamon and J. Welch. Quantitative structure-activity relationships for the in vitro antimycobacterial activity of pyrazinoic acid esters. *J. Med. Chem.* 1996;39:3394.

272. Ellard, G. A. Absorption, metabolism and excretion of pyrazinamide in man. *Tubercle* 1969;50:144.

273. Weiner, I. M., and J. P. Tinker. Pharmacology of pyrazinamide: metabolic and renal function studies related to the mechanism of drug-induced urate retention. *J. Pharmacol. Exp. Ther.* 1972;180:411.

274. Namba, S., T. Igari, K. Nishiyana, K. Hasimoto, T. Takemura, and K. Kimura. A case of pyrazinamide associated myoglobinuric renal failure. *Jpn. J. Med.* 1991;30:468.

275. Sanwikarja, S., R. Kauffmann, J. Velde, and J. Serlie. Tubulointerstitial nephritis associated with pyrazinamide. *Neth. J. Med.* 1989;34:40.

276. Ellard, G. A., and R. M. Haslam. Observations on the reduction of the renal elimination of urate in man. *Tubercle* 1976;57:97.

277. Horsfall, P. A. L., J. Plummer, W. G. L. Allan, D. J. Girling, A. J. Nunn, and W. Fox. Double blind controlled comparison of aspirin, allopurinol and placebo in the management of arthralgia during pyrazinamide administration. *Tubercle* 1979;60:13.

278. Rist, N., F. Grumbach, and D. Libermann. Experiments on the antituberculosis activity of alpha-ethylthioisonicotinamide. *Am. Rev. Tuberc.* 1959;79:1.

279. Lees, A. W. Ethionamide, 500 mg daily, plus isoniazid, 500 mg or 300 mg daily, in previously untreated patients with pulmonary tuberculosis. *Am. Rev. Respir. Dis.* 1967;95:109.

280. Colston, M. J., G. A. Ellard, and P. T. Gammon. Drugs for combined therapy: experimental studies on the antileprosy activity of ethionamide and prothionamide. *Lepr. Rev.* 1978;49:115.

281. Bieder, A., P. Brunel, and L. Mazeau. Identification de trois métabolites de l'éthionamide: chromatographie, spectrophotométrie, polarographie. *Anal. Pharm. Fr.* 1966;24:493.

282. Verbist, L., J. Prignot, J. Cosemans, and A. Gyselen. Tolerance to ethionamid and PAS in original treatment of tuberculosis patients. *Scand. J. Respir. Dis.* 1967;47:225.

283. Fox, W., D. K. Robinson, and R. Tall. A study of acute intolerance to ethionamide, including a comparison with prothionamide, and of the influence of a vitamin B–complex additive in prophylaxis. *Tubercle* 1969;50:125.

284. Simon, E., E. Veres, and G. Banki. Changes in SGOT activity during treatment with ethionamide. *Scand. J. Respir. Dis.* 1969;50:314.

285. Storey, P. B., and R. L. McLean. A current appraisal of cycloserine. *Antibiot. Med.* 1957;4:223.

286. Gernez-Rieux, C., and B. Devulder. Comparative investigation in vitro of the sensitivity of atypical mycobacteria to cycloserine and to other antibacterial substances. *Scand. J. Respir. Dis.* 1970;71(Suppl.):22.

287. Horsfall, P. A. Treatment of resistant pulmonary tuberculosis in Hong Kong with regimens of second-line drugs. *Tubercle* 1972;53:166.

288. Conzelman, G. M. The physiologic disposition of cycloserine in the human subject. *Am. Rev. Respir. Dis.* 1956;74:739.

289. Welch, H., L. E. Putnam, and W. A. Randall. Antibacterial activity and blood and urine concentrations of cycloserine, a new antibiotic, following oral administration. *Antibiot. Med.* 1955;1:72.

290. Nair, S., W. Maguire, H. Baron, and R. Imbruce. The effect of cycloserine on pyridoxine-dependent metabolism in tuberculosis. *J. Clin. Pharmacol.* 1976;16:439.

291. Way, E. L., P. K. Smith, D. L. Howie, R. Weiss, and R. Swanson. The absorption, distribution, excretion and fate of para-aminosalicylic acid. *J. Pharmacol.* 1948;93:368.

292. Heller, A., R. H. Ebert, D. Koch-Weser, and L. J. Roth. Studies with C^{14}-labelled para-aminosalicylic acid and isoniazid. *Am. Rev. Tuberc.* 1957;75:71.

293. Spector, R., and A. V. Lorenzo. The active transport of para-amino-salicylic acid from the cerebrospinal fluid. *J. Pharmacol. Exp. Ther.* 1973;185:642.

294. Jenne, J. W. Partial purification and properties of the isoniazid transacetylase in human liver. Its relationship to the acetylation of para-aminosalicylic acid. *J. Clin. Invest.* 1965;44:1992.

295. Jenne, J. W., F. M. MacDonald, and E. Mendoza. A study of the renal clearances, metabolic inactivation rates, and serum fall-off interaction of isoniazid and para-aminosalicylic acid in man. *Am. Rev. Respir. Dis.* 1961;84:371.

296. Gangadharam, P. R. J., and E. R. Candler. In vitro anti-mycobacterial activity of some new aminoglycoside antibiotics. *Tubercle* 1977;58:35.

297. Dalovisio, J. R., and G. A. Pankey. In vitro susceptibility of *Mycobacterium fortuitum* and *Mycobacterium chelonei* to amikacin. *J. Infect. Dis.* 1978;137:318.

298. Bycroft, B. W., D. Cameron, L. R. Croft, A. Hassanali-Walji, A. W. Johnson, and T. Webb. Total structure of capreomycin 1B, a tuberculostatic peptide antibiotic. *Nature* 1971;231:301.

299. Davies, J., L. Gorini, and B. D. Davis. Misreading of RNA codewords induced by aminoglycoside antibiotics. *Mol. Pharmacol.* 1965;1:93.

300. Liou, Y.-F., and N. Tanaka. Dual actions of viomycin on the ribosomal functions. *Biochem. Biophys. Res. Commum.* 1976;71:477.

301. Modolell, J., and D. Vazquez. The inhibition of ribosomal translocation by viomycin. *Eur. J. Biochem.* 1977;81:491.

302. Misumi, M., and N. Tanaka. Binding of [^{14}C] tuberactinomycin O, an antibiotic closely related to viomycin, to the bacterial ribosome. *Biochem. Biophys. Res. Commun.* 1978;82:971.

303. Choi, E. C., M. Misumi, T. Nishimura, N. Tanaka, S. Nomoto, T. Teshima, and T. Shiba. Viomycin resistance: alterations of either ribosomal subunit affect the binding of the antibiotic to the pair subunit and the entire ribosome becomes resistant to the drug. *Biochem. Biophys. Res. Commun.* 1979;87:904.

304. Yamada, T., K. Masuda, K. Shoji, and M. Hori. Analysis of ribosomes from viomycin-sensitive and resistant strains of *Mycobacterium smegmatis.* *J. Bacteriol.* 1972;112:1.

305. Yamada, T., Y. Mizugichi, K. H. Nierhaus, and H. G. Wittmann. Resistance to viomycin conferred by RNA of either ribosomal subunit. *Nature* 1978;275:460.

306. Hobby, G. L., T. F. Lenert, M. Donikian, and D. Pikula. The activity of viomycin against *Mycobac-*

terium tuberculosis and other microorganisms in vitro and in vivo. *Am. Rev. Tuberc.* 1951;63:17.

307. McClatchy, J. K., W. Kanes, P. T. Davidson, and T. S. Moulding. Cross-resistance in *M. tuberculosis* to kanamycin, capreomycin and viomycin. *Tubercle* 1977;58:29.

308. Donomae, I. The combined use of capreomycin and ethambutol in retreatment of pulmonary tuberculosis. *Am. Rev. Respir. Dis.* 1968;98:699.

309. Wilson, T. M. Capreomycin and ethambutol. *Practitioner* 1967;199:817.

310. Leysen, D., A. Haemers, and S. Pattyn. Mycobacteria and the new quinolones. *Antimicrob. Agents Chemother.* 1989;33:1.

311. Pearson, J. M. H., R. J. W. Rees, and M. F. R. Waters. Sulfone resistance in leprosy. A review of one hundred proven cases. *Lancet* 1975;2:69.

312. Pearson, J. M. H. The problem of dapsone-resistant leprosy. *Int. J. Lepr.* 1981;49:417.

313. Waters, M. F. R. The diagnosis and management of dapsone-resistant leprosy. *Lepr. Rev.* 1977;48:95.

314. Ellard, G. A. Combined treatment for lepromatous leprosy. *Lepr. Rev.* 1980;51:199.

315. Wright, P. and R. Wallace. Antimycobacterial agents. In *Harrison's Principles of Internal Medicine*, 14th ed., ed. by A. Fauci, E. Braunweld, K. Isselbacher, J. Wilson, J. Martin, D. Kasper, S. Hawer, and D. Long, New York: McGraw Hill, 1998, pp. 997–1003.

316. Colston, M. J., G. R. F. Hilson, G. A. Ellard, P. T. Gammon, and R. J. W. Rees. The activity of thiacetazone, thiambutosine, thiocarlide and sulfamethoxypyridazine against *Mycobacterium leprae* in mice. *Lepr. Rev.* 1978;49:101.

317. Levy, L., and J. H. Peters. Susceptibility of *Mycobacterium laprae* to dapsone as a determinant of patient response to acedapsone. *Antimicrob. Agents Chemother.* 1976;9:102.

318. Levy; L. Bactericidal action of dapsone against *Mycobacterium leprae* in mice. *Antimicrob. Agents Chemother.* 9:614 (1976).

319. Shepard, C. C., L. Levy, and P. Fasal. The death of *Mycobacterium leprae* during treatment with 4,4'-diaminodiphenylsulfone (DDS). *Am. J. Trop. Med. Hyg.* 1968;17:769.

320. Bernstein, J. E., and A. L. Lorincz. Sulfonamides and sulfones in dermatologic therapy. *Int. J. Dermatol.* 1981;20:82.

321. Stendahl, O., L. Molin, and C. Dahlgren. The inhibition of polymorphonuclear leukocyte cytotoxicity by dapsone. *J. Clin. Invest.* 1978;62:214.

322. Anderson, R., E. M. S. Gatner, C. E. van Rensburg, G. Grabow, F. M. G. H. Imkamp, S, K. Kok, and A. J. van Rensburg. In vitro and in vivo effects of dapsone on neutrophil and lymphocyte functions in normal individuals and patients with lepromatous leprosy. *Antimicrob. Agents Chemother.* 1981;19:495.

323. Shepard, C. C., L. Levy, and P. Fasal. The sensitivity to dapsone (DDS) of *Mycobacterium leprae* from patients with and without previous treatment. *Am. J. Trop. Med. Hyg.* 1969;18:258.

324. Glazko, A. J., W. A. Dill, R. G. Montalbo, and E. L. Holmes. A new analytical procedure for dapsone.

Application to blood-level and urinary-excretion studies in normal men. *Am. J. Trop. Med. Hyg.* 1968;17:465.

325. Ozawa, T., C. C. Shepard, and A. B. A. Karat. Application of spectrophotofluorometric procedures to some problems in *Mycobacterium leprae* infections in mice and man treated with dapsone (DDS), diacetyl-DDS (DADDS), and di-formyl-DDS (DFD). *Am. J. Trop. Med. Hyg.* 1971;20:274.

326. Riley, R. W., and L. Levy. Characteristics of the binding of dapsone and monoacetyldapsone by serum albumin. *Proc. Soc. Exp. Bio. Med.* 1973;142:1168.

327. Gelber, R., J. H. Peters, R. Gordon, A. J. Glazko, and L. Levy. The polymorphic acetylation of dapsone in man. *Clin. Pharmacol. Ther.* 1971;12:227.

328. Peters, J. H., G. R. Gordon, and J. F. Murray. Metabolic disposition of dapsone in African leprosy patients. *Lepr. Rev.* 1979;50:7.

329. Editorial. Adverse reactions to dapsone. *Lancet* 1981;2:184.

330. Cucinell, S. A., Z. H., Israili, and P. G. Dayton. Microsomal N-oxidation of dapsone as a cause of methemoglobin formation in human red blood cells. *Am. J. Trop. Med. Hyg.* 1972;21:322.

331. Rapoport, A. M., and S. B. Guss. Dapsone-induced peripheral neuropathy. *Arch. Neurol.* 1972;27:184.

332. Holmes, I. B. Minimum inhibitory and bactericidal dosages of rifampicin against *Mycobacterium leprae* in the mouse foot-pad: relationship to serum rifampicin concentration. *Int. J. Lepr.* 1974;42:289.

333. Yawalkar, S. J., A. C. McDougall, J. Languillon, S. Ghosh, S. K. Hajra, D. V. A Opromolla, and C. J. S. Tonello. Once-monthly rifampicin plus daily dapsone in initial treatment of lepromatous leprosy. *Lancet* 1982;1:1199.

334. Browne, S. G., and L. M. Hogerzeil. "B663" in the treatment of leprosy. *Lepr. Rev.* 1962;33:6.

335. Colston, M. J., G. R. F. Hilson, and D. K. Banerjee. The "proportional bactericidal test": a method for assessing bactericidal activity of drugs against *Mycobacterium leprae* in mice. *Lepr. Rev.* 1978;49:7.

336. Rhodes, P. M., and D. Wilkie. Antimitochondrial activity of Lampren in *Saccharomyces cerevisiae*. *Biochem. Pharmacol.* 1973;22:1047.

337. Morrison, N. E., and G. M. Marley. Clofazimine binding studies with deoxyribonucleic acid. *Int. J. Lepr.* 1976;44:475.

338. Levy, L., C. C. Shepard, and P. Fasal. Clofazimine therapy of lepromatous leprosy caused by dapsone-resistant *Mycobacterium leprae*. *Am. J. Trop. Med. Hyg.* 1972;21:315.

339. Gatner, E. M. S., R. Anderson, C. E. van-Rensburg, and F. M. J. H. Imkamp. The in vitro and in vivo effects of clofazimine on the motility of neutrophils and transformation of lymphocytes from normal individuals. *Lepr. Rev.* 1982;53:85.

340. Mackey, J. P., and J. Barnes. Clofazimine in the treatment of discoid lupus erythematosis. *Br. J. Dermatol.* 1974;91:93.

341. Pfaltzgraff, R. E. The control of neuritis in leprosy with clofazimine. *Int. J. Lepr.* 1972;40:392.

342. Schulz, E. J. Forty four months' experience in the treatment of leprosy with clofazimine (Lamprene(Geigy)). *Lepr. Rev.* 1972;42:178.

343. Browne, S. G., D. J. Harman, H. Waudby, and A. C. McDougall. Clofazimine (Lamprene, B663) in the treatment of lepromatous leprosy in the United Kingdom. A 12 year review of 31 cases, 1966–1978. *Int. J. Lepr.* 1981;49:167.

344. Imkamp, F. M. J. H. Clofazimine (Lamprene or B663) in lepra reactions. *Lepr. Rev.* 1981;52:135.

345. Lunn, H. F., and R. J. W. Rees. Treatment of mycobacterial skin ulcers in Uganda with a riminophenothiazine derivative (B.663). *Lancet* 1964;1:247.

346. Banerjee, D. K., G. A. Ellard, P. T. Gammon, and M. F. R. Waters. Some observations on the pharmacology of clofazimine (B663). *Am. J. Trop. Med. Hyg.* 1974;23:1110.

347. Mansfield; R. E. Tissue concentrations of clofazimine (B663) in man. *Am. J. Trop. Med. Hyg.* 1974;23:1116.

348. Jopling, W. H. Complications of treatment with clofazimine (Lamprene:B663). *Lepr. Rev.* 1976;47:1.

349. Levy, L. Pharmacologic studies of clofazimine. *Am. J. Trop. Med. Hyg.* 1976;23:1097.

350. Feng, P. C., C. C. Fenslau, and R. R. Jackobson. Metabolism of clofazimine in leprosy patients. *Drug Metab. Disp.* 1981;9:521.

351. Levy, L., and H. P. Randall. A study of skin pigmentation by clofazimine. *Int. J. Lepr.* 1970;38:404.

352. Plock, H., and D. L. Leiker. A long-term trial with clofazimine in reactive lepromatous leprosy. *Lepr. Rev.* 1976;47:25.

353. Mason, G. H., R. B. Ellis-Pegler, and J. F. Arthur. Clofazimine and eosinophilic enteritis. *Lepr. Rev.* 1977;48:175.

354. McDougall, A. C., W. R. Horsfall, J. E. Hede, and A. J. Chaplin. Splenic infarction and tissue accumulation of crystals associated with the use of clofazimine (Lamprene; B663) in the treatment of pyodrema gengrenosum. *Br. J. Dermatol.* 1980;102:227.

355. Havlik, J., C. Horsburgh, B. Metchock, P. Williams, S. Fann, and S. Thompson. Disseminated *Mycobacterium avium* complex infection: clinical identification and epidemiologic trends. *J. Infect. Dis.* 1992;165:577.

356. Masur, H., and the PHS Task Force on Prophylaxis and Therapy for *Mycobacterium avium* complex. Recommendations on prophylaxis and therapy for disseminated *Mycobacterium avium* complex disease in patients infected with the human immunodeficiency virus. *N. Engl. J. Med.* 1993;329:898.

357. Havur, D., and J. Ellner. *Mycobacterium avium* complex. In *Mandell, Douglas and Bennett's Principles and Practice of Infectious Diseases*, 4th ed., ed. by C. L. Mandell, R. Dolin, and J. E. Bennett. New York: Churchill Livingstone, 1995, pp. 2250–2264.

358. Cavert, W. Preventing and treating major opportunistic infections in AIDS. *Postgrad. Med.* 1997;102:125.

359. Canadian HIV Trials Network Protocol 010 Study Group. A comparison of two regimens for the treatment of *Mycobacterium avium* complex bacteria in AIDS: rifabutin, ethambutol, and clarithromycin versus rifampin, ethambutol, clofazimine and ciprofloxacin. *N. Engl. J. Med.* 1996;335:377.

360. AIDS Clinical Trials Group Protocol 157 Study Team. Clarithromycin therapy for bacteremic *Mycobacterium avium* complex disease: a randomized, double-blind, dose-ranging study in patients with AIDS. *Ann. Intern. Med.* 1994;121:905.

361. Chaisson, R., P. Keiser, M. Pierre, W. Fessel, J. Ruskin, C. Lahart, C. Benson, K. Meek, N. Siepman, and J. Craft. Clarithromycin and ethambutol with or without clofazimine for the treatment of bacteremic *Mycobacterium avium* complex disease in patients with HIV infection. *AIDS* 1997;11:311.

362. Nightingale, S., D. Cameron, F. Gordin, P. Sullam, D. Cohn, R. Chaisson. Two controlled trials of rifabutin prophylaxis against *Mycobacterium avium* complex infections in AIDS. *N. Engl. J. Med.* 1993;329:828.

363. French, A., D. Benatom, and F. Gordin. Nontuberculous mycobacterial infections. *Med. Clin. North Am.* 1997;81:361.

364. California Collaborative Treatment Group. Prophylaxis against disseminated *Mycobacterium avium* complex with weekly azithromycin, daily rifabutin, or both. *N. Engl. J. Med.* 1996;335:392.

Drugs Employed in the Treatment of Fungal Infections

CHAPTER TWELVE

Antifungal Drugs

The Polyene Antibiotics, Flucytosine, Azoles, Iodide, Griseofulvin, and Topical Agents

The treatment of fungal disease can be divided into two quite different problems according to the location of the infection. The most common fungal infections are superficial and are either treated with one of several topical drugs or with oral drugs, such as ketoconazole, terbinafine, or griseofulvin. The systemic mycoses constitute quite a different therapeutic problem. These infections are often very difficult to treat and long-term, parenteral therapy with potentially toxic drugs may be required. The systemic mycoses are sometimes considered in two groups according to the infecting organism. The *opportunistic infections* refer to those mycoses—candidiasis, aspergillosis, cryptococcosis, and phycomycosis—that commonly occur in debilitated and immunosuppressed patients. These infections are a particular problem in patients with leukemias and lymphomas, in people who are receiving immunosuppressive therapy, and in patients with such predisposing factors as AIDS and diabetes mellitus. Other systemic mycoses—for example, blastomycosis, histoplasmosis, coccidioidomycosis, and sporotrichosis—tend to have a relatively low incidence that may vary considerably according to geographical area. It should be noted, however, that both histoplasmosis and coccidioidomycosis have presented with increasing frequency as AIDS-associated opportunistic infections.[1] In many cases, systemic fungal infections are self-

limited and treatment is not required. In the case of progressive systemic infection, however, therapeutic intervention is required, and at this time, only five drugs are employed in treatment: amphotericin B (a polyene antibiotic), flucytosine, and three imidazole compounds (ketoconazole, fluconazole, and itraconazole).[1-4] Two significant areas of progress in the treatment of fungal diseases are the introduction of the newer azole antifungals, which have improved antifungal efficacy and have largely replaced ketoconazole, and the introduction of the lipid formulations of amphotericin B, which have improved the pharmacokinetics and decreased the toxicity of the drug.

The Polyene Antibiotics

Structures and Physical Properties

The polyene antibiotics are a large group of compounds, but many of them are too toxic to be used in therapy. Amphotericin B and nystatin, the only compounds used clinically in the United States, are produced by soil actinomycetes.

The polyenes are large molecules with a hydroxylated portion, which is hydrophilic, and a portion containing four to seven conjugated double bonds, which is lipophilic.[5] The unsaturated chromophore region is subject to photooxidation, and this contributes to the instability of these compounds in solution. This lipophilic portion also dictates a poor solubility in aqueous media.

Mechanism of Action

EFFECT ON CELL PERMEABILITY. Research on the mechanism of action of the polyene antibiotics has been reviewed by Kinsky[6] and by Holz.[7] Early experiments demonstrated that exposure of intact sensitive yeast cells to nystatin or amphotericin B affected a number of biochemical functions including respiration and glycolysis. Investigators found that adding K^+ or NH_4^+ to the buffer solution in which the yeast cells were suspended prevented inhibition of glycolysis occurring at neutral pH.[8] The amount of nystatin taken up by the yeast cell was not altered by NH_4^+ or K^+, and nystatin treatment rapidly depleted intracellular K^+. These observations suggested that glycolysis inhibition was secondary to the loss of K^+, resulting from a nystatin-induced change in membrane permeability. The demonstration that polyenes did not inhibit glycolysis by yeast extracts or respiration by yeast mitochondrial suspensions supported this conclusion.[9]

Liras and Lampen[10] examined the sequence of events occurring after addition of a polyene to yeast cells at a concentration sufficient to inhibit growth. There was an immediate and rapid loss of K^+, followed about 10 min later by a loss of Mg^{2+}, decreased amino acid transport, and inhibition of protein synthesis. After 20 min, RNA synthesis and glucose comsumption declined. The loss of K^+, and perhaps also Mg^{2+}, is thought to be the critical event occurring at minimal inhibitory concentrations of drug. This is inferred from the observation that inhibition of fungal growth by low concentrations of amphotericin B or candicidin can be prevented by addition of both K^+ and Mg^{2+} to the growth medium.[11,12] It is clear that these ions do not affect the binding of the antibiotics to yeast cell membranes.[13] Observations such as these have led to the proposal that low concentrations of amphotericin B, nystatin, and candicidin increase the permeability of fungal cell membranes to small cations (most importantly K^+, thereby leading to an alteration in the intracellular milieu and eventually to cell death.[7] The killing effect of the polyenes does not require growth of the organism.

THE SITE OF ACTION—THE CELL MEMBRANE. The polyene antibiotics are bound only to cells sensitive to their killing effect.[14] These drugs are bound by isolated cell walls and protoplast membranes derived from yeasts, and virtually all of the antibiotic bound by intact protoplasts is found in the cell membrane.[15] The binding to membranes is tight but reversible.[13] As will become clear, the specificity of polyene action is defined by the association of the drug with the membranes of sensitive cells. These drugs inhibit the growth of fungi, protozoa, and algae, but bacteria neither bind the drugs nor are they sensitive to them. This difference in the sensitivity of different organisms is determined by the presence of sterols in their cell membranes. In sensitive yeast cells, for example, nystatin is distributed in various subcellular fractions in direct proportion to sterol content.[15] The higher algae contain sterols in their membranes and are sensitive

Amphotericin B

to the polyenes. The blue-green algae do not contain sterols and are insensitive. There are no sterols in bacterial cell membranes, and even bacterial protoplasts will not bind polyenes.[16]

The sterol requirement for polyene sensitivity has been demonstrated even more directly. If membranes from sensitive cells that bind nystatin are extracted with ethanol-ace-tone, the membranes' ability to bind nystatin is abolished (see Table 12–1). The binding capacity can be partially restored by incubating the extracted particles with ergosterol. One of the clearest demonstrations of the correlation between sterol in the cell membrane and sensitivity to the polyene antibiotics was carried out with *Acholeplasma laidlawii*. In contrast to most mycoplasma, this saprophytic organism does not require sterols for growth.[17] In a sterol-free medium, these organisms are resistant to polyene antibiotics, but when they are grown in a cholesterol-containing medium, they incorporate sterol into the membrane and are sensitive to amphotericin B (see Table 12–2).[18]

Some of the most fundamental information regarding the mechanism of polyene action has been derived from the study of the drug effects in synthetic membrane systems. De Kruijff and co-workers[19] have shown, for example, that nystatin and amphotericin B cause a selective permeability change in cholesterol-containing liposomes, with the membranes becoming more permeant to K^+ than to glucose. This suggests that aqueous pores of a specific size are created.[20] The concept that amphotericin B and nystatin form aqueous channels is supported by several observations made with black lipid membranes. The experimental system consists of two chambers connected by a small hole that is covered by a lipid membrane. Aqueous solutions are placed in the chambers on either side of the membrane and changes in electrical conductance between the solutions can be recorded as a function of antibiotic effects on the permeability of the lipid barrier.[21] When nystatin or amphotericin B is added to only one side of the membrane, the conductances are small and variable and they are cation selective.[22]

Table 12–1. *The effect of sterol on the ability of a particulate fraction from* Neurospora crassa *to bind nystatin.* A particulate fraction was prepared from pulverized, lyophylized, mycelial mats of *Neurospora crassa* by high-speed centrifugation. A portion was extracted with ethanol-acetone, and reconstituted particles were prepared by adding the ethanol-acetone extract or ergosterol back to the extracted particulate fraction. The reconstituted particles were then dried, suspended in buffer, and assayed for their capacity to bind nystatin at a concentration of 10 μg/ml. Values represent micrograms of nystatin bound by equivalent 0.4 ml aliquots of particulate fraction per hour.

Particle treatment	Addition	Nystatin bound
None	None	13.3
Extracted	None	0
Extracted	Extract	10.1
Extracted	Ergosterol	6.8

Source: Data from Kinsky.[16]

When the antibiotic is added to both sides of the membrane, the conductance is markedly increased and it is anion selective.[22] The effects on conductance are sterol dependent, and when the antibiotic is present on both sides of the membrane, stepwise conductance changes are observed that result from the transient formation of single ion channels.[23] A model portraying the formation of such a transmembrane channel is presented in Figure 12–1.[24]

The model of Figure 12–1 portrays the transmembrane channels that are formed when amphotericin B or nystatin is added to two sides of a black lipid membrane. It differs from the channels formed in liposomes made from egg phosphatidylcholine or in biomembranes in that addition of drug to only one side of a liposome bilayer or biomembrane is sufficient to produce characteristic permeability changes that are cation rather than anion selective.[25] An important difference between the different membranes is the thickness of the bilayer, the black lipid membrane being thicker than the liposomal or biomembrane bilayer.[25] If the black lipid membrane is made with phospholipids containing 18 carbons or less in the fatty acid

Table 12–2. Interconversion of Acholeplasma laidlawii *between sensitivity and resistance to amphotericin B by growth in the presence and absence of cholesterol. Acholeplasma laidlawii* were grown in medium with (sensitive, S cells) and without (resistant, R cells) 20 *μg/ml* cholesterol. Both types of cells were harvested, washed, suspended in cholesterol-free medium, and assayed for viability with and without *25 μg/ml* of amphotericin B. Cholesterol was then added to the R cells, and each parent culture was divided in half for further incubation at either 4° or 37°C. At the end of this second incubation, viability tests were performed as before. *Acholeplasma laidlawii* has a generation time of about 2 hr; therefore, if the drug had no effect on growth during the 2-hr incubation in the presence of amphotericin B, the number of cells would be expected to double and approach 200% of the initial viability assay. If the drug had a killing effect, then the percentage of survivors would be less than 100% (that is, less than the initial viability assay carried out before exposure to the drug). Growing the R cells at 37°C in cholesterol medium makes them drug sensitive, whereas the S cells are made drug insensitive by growth at 37°C without cholesterol.

Cell type	Survivors after a 2-hr exposure to amphotericin B (%)
S cells	2
R cells	200
S cells incubated in cholesterol-free medium for 2 hrs at	
37°C	150
4°C	5
R cells incubated in cholesterol-containing medium for 2 hr at	
37°C	3
4°C	180

Source: From Feingold.[18]

side chain (membrane thickness 24 Å or less), then nystatin in the presence of ergosterol will span the membrane and create a one-sided pore.[26] If the fatty acid side chain is longer, the membrane is thicker and it is necessary to add the drug to both sides to achieve pore formation. Thus, it has been shown that the thickness of the membrane as well as the presence of sterol is important for polyene action.[25,26]

THE CHANNEL MODEL AND THE KILLING EFFECT. The difference between the two-sided channel formed by adding the drug to both sides of a lipid bilayer and the one-sided channels formed in membranes 24 Å or less in thickness is presented in the model of Figure 12–2[22] The one-sided channel shown in parts B and C of the figure is thought to be analogous to the channels that are formed in fungal cell membranes. The channel is composed of several polyene-sterol units which form a ring with a pore in the center.[27] The diameter of the pore is estimated to be about 8 Å, as it has been shown that molecules larger than this size are excluded from pores created in black lipid membranes.[28] A number of organic compounds with a molecular size of 6–8 Å can enter the pore and interact with the channel walls, blocking the passage of inorganic ions.[29] The one-sided, cation selective pore model accounts for many observations that have been made on amphotericin B and nystatin effects both in intact fungi and in model membrane systems.

It is probably an oversimplification to say that the killing effect of amphotericin B and nystatin is entirely explained by the formation of one-sided, cation-selective channels that lead to loss of K⁺ and a subsequent derangement of cellular metabolism that is lethal. It is likely that amphotericin B disrupts cells through multiple mechanisms, one of which may reflect some pore formation resulting from specific interactions of amphotericin B with phospholipids[30–32] Oxidative damage to cells may even be as important a factor in cell death as channel formation.[33,34] Amphotericin B undergoes autooxidation with concomitant formation of free radicals

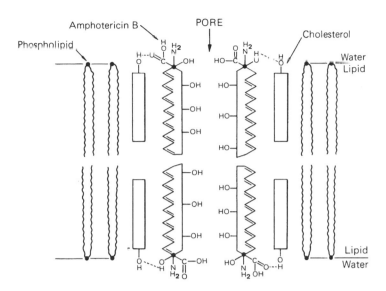

Figure 12–1. A hypothetical model of a pore formed by amphotericin B in a lipd bilayer membrane. Considerable evidence supports the hypothesis that amphotericin B and nystatin can form pores in artificial lipid bilayer membranes. When the antibiotic is added to both sides of the membrane, the pores are quite anion selective. Since sucrose (radius = 5.2 Å) is not permitted to pass through, the radius of the pore is thought to be less than 4–5Å. The pore is formed by several polyene molecules packed side by side in a cylinder formation. The principal interactions between the antibiotic and the membrane involve hydrophobic bonds between the lipophilic heptaene segment of the antibiotic and the sterols. The dashed lines represent possible hydrogen bonds. The solid circles oriented at the membrane surfaces represent the polar head groups of the phospholipids, and the wavy lines denote the hydrophobic fatty acid chains. In this configuration, amphotericin B is 20–24 Å long and extends into but does extend across the distance of the bilayer. The ion conductance of artificial bilayer membranes is markedly potentiated when the antibiotic is added to both sides, presumably because continuous pores passing from one membrane surface to the other can be readily formed.[21] (Adapted from Andreoli,[24] Fig. 11.)

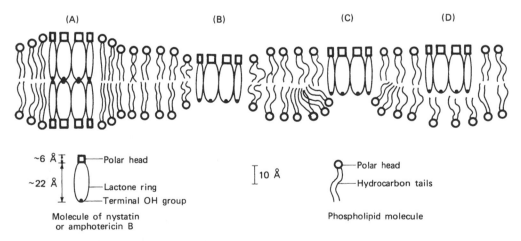

Figure 12–2. Diagram of one-sided pores (B,C) and a two-sided pore (A) formed by amphotericin B or nystatin; (D) one-sided pore precursor. A region of unmodified bilayer is depicted between (A) and (B). Note that the phospholipids lengthen to accommodate the long two-sided pore (A). They also can deform somewhat to allow the one-sided pore (B) to span the membrane. (From Marty and Finkelstein.[22])

that induce lipid peroxidation in the membranes of target cells (see scheme in Fig. 9–2).[33,35] Because of extensive binding to serum components, in particular lipoproteins,[36,37] the amount of free amphotericin B in plasma that is available to form transmembrane channels is small. Some of the drug is brought into cells by endocytosis through a process in which LDL receptors are thought to play a role.[38] Binding of the drug to LDL and of the complex to LDL receptors could explain both the increased toxicity of the amphotericin B/LDL complex and the correlation between inhibition of the amphotericin B lipoprotein interaction and decreased toxicity for amphotericin B bound to surfactants.[39,40] Indeed, these observations support the design of amphotericin B derivatives or lipid formulations that decrease the drug binding to LDL.[37] One effect of the polyenes that is potentially of great therapeutic importance is their ability to promote the entry of antimetabolites and other antibiotics into the cell. This effect forms the rationale for some combined drug approaches to the treatment of some fungal infections and perhaps also to some cancers, and it cannot be explained by the formation of cation-selective pores that permit only the passage of small ions.

EFFECTS OF POLYENES ON MAMMALIAN CELL MEMBRANES. If the presence of sterols in a membrane is a determinant for sensitivity to the polyene antibiotics, then, since mammalian cell membranes contain sterols, one might expect that these drugs would affect the permeability of host cells. This is indeed the case. Polyenes have been shown to affect a variety of cells from higher organisms. One cell system in which polyene effects have been studied in some detail is the human red blood cell. Erythrocytes suspended in isotonic saline rupture on exposure to high concentrations of amphotericin B,[41] an effect that can be inhibited by serum—probably because of polyene binding to the cholesterol in lipoprotein.[42] Upon exposure to amphotericin B, human erythrocytes lose potassium at a rate that is related to the drug concentration.[43] The interaction of the polyenes with the red cell membrane also seems to be sterol dependent. This is suggested by the observation that erythrocytes from patients with spur-cell anemia are especially sensitive to amphotericin B.[44] These cells have abnormally high amounts of membrane cholesterol. The precise mechanism of amphotericin B–induced hemolysis is not well defined. It is clear that, since the permeability to small ions is altered, there is a substantial shift of water into the erythrocyte and cell rupture occurs.[45] Thus it would seem that rupture results from osmolysis and is not a function of massive disruption of the erythrocyte membrane by the amphotericin B molecule itself.

When present at a high enough concentration, amphotericin B inhibits the growth of mammalian cells in culture. At lower drug concentrations K^+ efflux occurs.[46] The membrane permeability changes induced by low concentrations of polyenes are reversible, and it has been suggested that cells are able to repair or compensate for polyene-induced changes in membrane permeability when the drug is present at concentrations lower than those that lead to growth inhibition.[46] At higher concentrations of drug, the cell may not be able to repair the permeability defect and it is possible that inhibition of animal cell growth occurs by mechanisms that are similar to those that lead to the death of fungal cells.

Amphotericin B clearly facilitates the entry of relatively large molecules into mammalian cells. This has been demonstrated with actinomycin D–resistant tumor cells, for example. Resistance to the anticancer drug actinomycin D can result from decreased entry into tumor cells.[47–49] But when amphotericin B was added to cultured human cells (HeLa), which had been selected for this type of resistance, the cells were again sensitive to the actinomycin D.[50] In this study it was also demonstrated that amphotericin B treatment resulted in the increased entry of radioactive actinomycin D into the cells. Actinomycin D has a molecular weight of 1255 and facilitation of its entry cannot be explained by the creation of small channels 8 Å in diameter that exclude molecules the size of glucose (molecular weight 129). Amphotericin B has been shown to enhance the uptake of bacterial DNA into HeLa cells,[51] an observation that suggests that it may stimulate other mechanisms by which molecules enter cells, such as by endocytosis.[7]

STIMULATION OF THE IMMUNE RESPONSE. Amphotericin B stimulates both humoral and cell-mediated immunity in mice.[52] Contact sensitivity to 2,4 dinitro-fluorobenzene was augmented in mice by amphotericin B, and humoral immunity was enhanced with a potency comparable to complete Freund's adjuvant. Amphotericin B also enhances phagocytic activity, but it has adverse effects on natural killer cell function in vitro.[53,54] These effects on the immune response suggest that amphotericin B may have therapeutic value apart from its antibiotic activity and they may contribute to the synergism of amphotericin B with antitumor compounds (see below).

BASIS FOR SELECTIVE TOXICITY. When administered parenterally, the polyenes are very toxic drugs. These drugs do not exhibit the high degree of selective toxicity found with most antibiotics that are useful in therapy. Much of the basis for the limited selective toxicity of amphotericin B and nystatin lies in the different sterol compositions of animal and fungal membranes. Ergosterol is the principal sterol in fungal membranes and cholesterol is the principal sterol in animal membranes. Amphotericin B binds to ergosterol with a higher affinity than to cholesterol.[55] When added to the growth medium, ergosterol is more effective than cholesterol at antagonizing the K^+-releasing and growth inhibitory effects of amphotericin B on fungi.[56,57] Both *Mycoplasma mycoides* organisms and egg lecithin liposomes were found to be much more sensitive to amphotericin B methyl ester when the membranes contained ergosterol than when they contained cholesterol.[58] It is possible that other differences between the membranes of fungal and mammalian cells also contribute to the rather limited selective toxicity of these drugs.

Potentiation and Antagonism of the Effects of Other Drugs by Amphotericin B

The combination of amphotericin B and flucytosine can be synergistic in a few fungi growing in vitro, including species of *Cryptococcus* and *Candida* that are sensitive to both drugs.[59-61] When a low concentration of amphotericin B is present, *Candida* organisms growing in culture take up much more radioactive flucytosine into the acid-precipitable fraction.[60] Thus, it is reasonable to suggest that synergism is due to the ability of amphotericin B to facilitate the entry of flucytosine into the organism. It is difficult to conceive how increased uptake of flucytosine occurs. Synergism has been observed at concentrations of amphotericin B that are well below its minimal inhibitory concentration for the test organism. Flucytosine is transported into fungal cells and one could speculate that at low concentrations of amphotericin B, the uptake mechanism is somehow enhanced. Amphotericin B and flucytosine used together have produced at least additive, and possibly synergistic, effects in experimental cryptococcal and candidal infections in mice.[62-64] The combination of amphotericin B and flucytosine has been used successfully to treat patients with cryptococcal meningitis.[65,66] The combination cured or improved more patients and produced more rapid sterilization of the cerebrospinal fluid than more extended treatment with a higher daily dose of amphotericin B alone. As the combined approach permits a smaller dosage of amphotericin B to be used for a shorter period of time, there is less nephrotoxicity.[66]

The action of rifampin in vitro is also potentiated by amphotericin B. By itself, rifampin is not particularly effective against fungi, apparently because it cannot readily enter these organisms. In the presence of low concentrations of amphotericin B, however, rifampin has antifungal activity in vitro.[60] This potentiation has been shown in several species of fungi including *Candida albicans*, *Histoplasma capsulatum*, and *Coccidioides immitis*.[67-69] Synergism has been shown with amphotericin B and minocycline against *Candida* species, *Torulopsis glabrata*, and *Cryptococcus neoformans* in vitro[70]; however, no survival benefit was noted in vivo in a murine model of cryptococcosis.[71] It should not be assumed that the combination of amphotericin B and another antifungal drug will necessarily produce an additive or synergistic effect in vitro. Antagonism has been found with the combination of amphotericin B and the imidazole drugs against *Candida albicans* in vitro, against *Aspergillus* in mice,[73] and after administration to humans.[74] This antagonism may occur because the imidazoles inhibit the synthesis of ergosterol, which is required for the action of amphotericin B.[75] However, other studies, for example, with the triazole SCH 39304 and amphotericin B, have shown no such antagonism in animal models of coccidioidomycosis and candidiasis.[76,77] Indeed, the results of some studies have suggested a beneficial effect of imidazole plus amphotericia B regimes,[78] and clinical experience in treatment of certain human mycoses has supported the simultaneous use of these two classes of antifungal drugs.[79]

The possibility that a drug might be used to allow another drug to achieve an effective intracellular concentration is in itself an intriguing concept. The use of agents that alter cell permeability in combination therapy could prove to be particularly useful in the treatment of cancer. Amphotericin B has been shown to potentiate the uptake of several drugs into tumor cells in vitro and to enhance the cytotoxic action of several drugs (including tetracycline and a nitrosourea) as determined by inhibition of macromolecular synthesis in cultured animal and human cells.[50,80,81] Potentiation of cytotoxicity of several anticancer agents in vivo has been demonstrated against the transplantable AKR leukemia in mice.[82,83] The mechanism of the amphotericin B effect in vivo appears to be more complex than that seen in cell culture systems. Amphotericin B has an immunopotentiating effect in mice,[52,84–86] and its effect in potentiating the cytotoxicity of anticancer drugs in vivo may largely reflect its immunoadjuvant activity. Even though the effects of amphotericin B in the intact animal may reflect more than one action, the possibility of a new therapeutic approach using membrane-active antibiotics is certainly attractive.[87]

Antimicrobial Activity and Resistance

Amphotericin B is not active against bacteria. Most fungi that cause systemic mycoses are sensitive to amphotericin B in vitro at concentrations (1–2 µg/ml) that are achieved in the bloodstream during intravenous therapy with the usual dosage (see Table 12–3).[88,89] The drug is also active against some protozoa, and, by intravenous administration, it is effective in the treatment of mucocutaneous leishmaniasis (*Leishmania brasiliensis*).[90] Amphotericin B administered intravenously in liposomes has been shown to have activity in a mouse model of visceral leishmaniasis.[91] The selectivity for *Leishmania* is thought to result from the presence of certain ergosterol precursors in their membranes, an unusual situation outside of fungi. Amphotericin B is now used as a second-line therapeutic agent for *Leishmania brasiliensis* and *L. mexicana*[37] where it may be especially promising for treatment of T cell–deficient individuals.[92]

There are also reports that amphotericin B and some of its derivatives have antiviral and specifically anti-HIV activity. Amphotericin B, amphotericin B methyl ester, a more soluble derivative, MS8209, and nystatin have all been shown to inhibit cellular infection by HIV in vitro.[93,94] It has been speculated that this activity is related to the 2.5-fold higher cholesterol:lipid ratio of HIV virions as compared with the host.[95] It has been shown that the derivative MS8209 blocks virus-host fusion or uptake but does not affect cell–cell fusion.[94] Since many HIV

Table 12–3. *Minimal inhibitory concentrations of amphotericin B for selected fungi.*

Organism	Minimal inhibitory concentration (µg/ml)	
	Average	Range
Candida albicans	1.9	0.05–3.25
Cryptococcus neoformans	0.2	
Histoplasma capsulatum	0.04	
Blastomyces dermatitidis	0.1	
Coccidioides immitis	0.5	
Paracoccidioides brasiliensis	0.1	
Torulopsis glabrata	0.25	
Sporothrix schenkii	0.07	
Candida tropicalis	3.5	0.2–25

Source: Data taken from Rippon,[89] Table 29–3.

patients undergo antibiotic therapy for persistent fungal infections, this possible action against HIV could confer a double benefit. Amphotericin B has also been found to have some activity against prions, the cause of scrapie and other neurodegenerative diseases.[96] In addition, amphotericin B may enhance resistance to microbial infections, most likely a result of immune stimulatory effects.[97]

The sensitivity of *Candida albicans* to amphotericin B methyl ester varies markedly with the phase of growth—organisms harvested during exponential growth were found to be sensitive to 0.2 μg of amphotericin methyl ester per ml, but organisms harvested during the stationary phase required much higher concentrations of drug to achieve the same rate of K^+ release.[57] Removal of the wall from stationary-phase organisms creates protoplasts that have the same sensitivity as that of exponential phase organisms, demonstrating that the composition of the cell wall can affect the sensitivity to the drug.[98] A high degree of intrinsic resistance can be achieved under certain growth conditions. Treatment of stationary-phase cells with sulfhydryl-reactive reagents and reducing reagents alters the sensitivity in a way that suggests that the cell wall of starved cells contains a factor that does not produce resistance when it is in the reduced form.[99] If the cell wall impedes drug entry to its site of action at the cell membrane, this could contribute to intrinsic differences in amphotericin B sensitivity observed among the various fungi.

There are some species of fungi with intrinsic resistance to amphotericin B. For instance, *Trichosporon beigelii*, *Pseudallescheria boydii*, and some of the dematiaceous fungi exhibit marked intrinsic resistance to this drug.[100] The development of resistance to the polyenes during therapy of fungal infection is uncommon, but when resistance does occur, it is related to a poor clinical outcome.[101–103] Polyene-resistant yeasts cause infections primarily in high-risk cancer patients.[100] It is uncertain whether this unique epidemiology is due to a certain immunocompromised state, exposure to cytotoxic cancer chemotherapy, or frequent administration of amphotericin B. Under clinical conditions of relapse of disease after a course of amphotericin B therapy, the more recent isolate is usually of the same order of susceptibility as initial specimens. In a survey of 1372 yeast isolates from 308 patients, 55 isolates were found to be resistant to amphotericin B as defined by growth at or above 2 μg/ml.[104] All of the resistant isolates came from six cancer patients who had experienced long-term therapy with amphotericin B.[104] These resistant isolates, as well as others reported on a case-by-case basis, have decreased amounts or a complete lack of ergosterol in the cell membrane.[104–106] Polyene-resistant strains of fungi that have been selected in vitro also have decreased levels of or a lack of ergosterol.[107,108] Some resistant strains have been shown to have high levels of ergosterol precursors that have a lower affinity for polyenes than ergosterol. For example, a nystatin-resistant strain of *Saccharomyces cerevisiae* was found to have 5,6-dihydroergosterol, rather than ergosterol, as its main sterol component. Membrane sterol analysis of a *Cryptococcus neoformans* isolate recovered from the cerebrospinal fluid of an AIDS patient who failed therapy with fluconazole and amphotericin B revealed only 4% of the membrane sterols to be ergosterol compared with 71% in the pretreatment isolate. Researchers suggested that there was a lack of sterol $\Delta^{8,7}$ isomerase in the relapse isolate.[109,110] It appears that the emergence of polyene-resistant fungi usually represents a selection for organisms with impaired enzymatic functions required for ergosterol synthesis. Resistant strains grow more slowly than the parent strain and there is cross-resistance between the polyenes but not with other antifungal drugs.[5]

Polyene Preparations and Therapeutic Uses

Amphotericin B has undergone somewhat of a resurgence over the past few years despite the popularity of the newer, less-toxic azole antifungal agents. This has occurred for several reasons, including the introduction of new, less-toxic liposomal delivery systems for the drug, an increase in fungal disease worldwide, a better understanding of the mechanism of action of the drug, and an expansion of the spectrum of activity to include select virus, parasite, and possibly, prion infections.[37] Despite the availability of new azole antifungal agents, amphotericin B remains the cornerstone of therapy for most disseminated and deep organ fungal infections.[111] Most experts in infectious disease consider amphotericin B the drug of choice in the treatment of life-threatening fungal infections. Amphotericin B also can be useful in selected patients with profound neutropenia and fever that is unresponsive to broad-spectrum antibiotics, and it is still considered the treatment of choice for empirical therapy of suspected fungal infections in neutropenic patients.

TOPICAL ADMINISTRATION. Amphotericin B and nystatin are available as creams, lotions, and ointments for topical treatment of superficial *Candida* infections (see Table 12–4 for drugs of choice against fungal infections). The polyenes are not useful in treating superficial infections caused by the common dermatophytes. The topical preparations are applied two to four times daily.

Nystatin and amphotericin B are pro- vided as tablets and suspensions for treatment of intestinal candidiasis. Since there is very little absorption of these drugs from the intestinal tract, oral administration constitutes a local use of the drug analogous to local topical therapy. *Candida albicans* is the fungus most commonly involved in superinfection in patients receiving antibacterial therapy. There are tetracycline preparations that also contain nystatin for the purpose of preventing fungal overgrowth in the bowel. The use of these fixed-ratio combinations has not been proven effective and does not reflect rational therapy. (See Chapter 6 for discussion of the nystatin-tetracycline preparations.) Although treatment with an oral imidazole is preferred, oropharyngeal candidiasis may be treated by sluicing an oral suspension of polyene around the mouth and swallowing it or by sucking on a vaginal suppository.

PARENTERAL ADMINISTRATION. Amphotericin B is the only polyene available for parenteral use. It is administered by slow intravenous infusion for the treatment of deep fungal infections. The tolerance to ampho-

Table 12–4. *Drugs employed in the treatment of selected fungal infections.*

Infecting fungus	Drugs of choice	Alternatives
SUPERFICIAL INFECTIONS		
Dermatophytes	Topical agents	Topical agents
Epidermophyton	Clotrimazole	Tolnaftate, haloprogin
Microsporon		Oral therapy
Trichophyton		Griseofulvin or ketoconazole
Candida albicans		
Superficial	Nystatin (topical)	An azole (topical)
Intestinal	Fluconazole	Ketoconazole or itraconazole
SYSTEMIC INFECTIONS		
Aspergillus	Amphotericin B	Itraconazole
Blastomyces dermatitidis	Amphotericin B or itraconazole	Ketoconazole or fluconazole
Candida spp.	Amphotericin B (with or without flucytosine)	Ketoconazole or itraconazole
Coccidioides immitis	Fluconazole or amphotericin B	Ketoconazle or itraconazole
Cryptococcus neoformans	Amphotericin B (with or without flucytosine)	Ketoconazole, fluconazole, or itraconazole
Histoplasma capsulatum	Itraconazole or amphotericin B	Ketoconazole or fluconazole
Mucor	Amphotericin B	None
Paracoccidioides brasiliensis	Itraconazole or amphotericin B	Ketoconazole
Sporothrix schenkii	Amphotericin B or itraconazole	Fluconazole

tericin B varies substantially from patient to patient, and because some patients experience fever, chills, hypotension, and dyspnea, a small test dose is administered initially to determine the patient's tolerance. A test dose of 1 mg is administered to adults in 20 ml of 5% dextrose over a 10 to 30-min time interval and the patient's pulse, blood pressure, temperature, and respiration rate are then monitored every 30 min for 4 hr.[112] The amount of drug administered on the next dose depends on the severity of the reaction. In patients with rapidly progressing fungal infections, it is desirable to administer the first day's dose in the therapeutic range. Patients with good cardiopulmonary function who experience only mild reaction to the test dose may receive 0.3 mg/kg by slow intravenous administration over a period of 2–4 hr. Hydrocortisone hemisuccinate (0.7 mg/kg) is often added to the infusion in an effort to decrease the severity of reaction. A smaller dose of amphotericin B is administered to patients who have a marked reaction to the test dose. In time, patients usually become tolerant to the febrile reaction, the dosage of hydrocortisone may be reduced, and the steroid can subsequently be discontinued. In patients with normal renal function, the dosage of amphotericin B is increased progressively to 0.5 mg/kg by the third to fifth day of therapy.[112] The daily maintenance dosage in progressive systemic infections is 0.5 to no more than 0.7 mg/kg and the duration of therapy is usually 6–12 weeks. In patients who have indolent fungal infections, a lower initial dosage is administered following the test dose and the dosage is increased by 5 or 10 mg increments up to 0.4–0.6 mg/kg daily. Patients should be carefully monitored for drug toxicity with bi-weekly determinations of hematocrit and serum creatinine, potassium, and bicarbonate.

Attempts have been made to adjust the maintenance dosage of amphotericin B to the sensitivity of the infecting organism. Drutz et al.[113] published a study in which they treated patients daily with enough amphotericin B to provide peak serum levels at least twice those required to inhibit the fungal isolate. This method has not been widely applied because the concentration of amphotericin B required to inhibit a fungus depends greatly on assay technique, and this varies considerably among different laboratories. Also, it is not clear that the blood level of amphotericin B reflects appropriate fungicidal levels in infected tissues. The distribution and pharmacokinetic properties of the drug are not well understood.

When the daily maintenance dosage has been achieved, some patients can be gradually changed to a schedule in which a double dose is given every other day. It has been shown that such alternate-day therapy maintains appropriate serum concentrations, and it is more convenient and usually well tolerated by the patient.[114] This is an important consideration, since systemic fungal infections require many weeks of intravenous amphotericin B therapy.

The levels of amphotericin B in the cerebrospinal fluid after intravenous administration are very low compared to the blood levels,[114] and intrathecal as well as intravenous administration of amphotericin B is required for treatment of coccidioidal meningitis and refractory cases of cryptococcal meningitis. For intrathecal administration, 0.2–0.5 mg of the drug is dissolved in 5 ml of cerebrospinal fluid and injected into either the lumbar area or directly into the cisterna magna. The drug is administered intrathecally two or three times a week. In monkeys, it has been shown that higher concentrations of drug are achieved in the cisternal fluid after injection in the lumbar area if amphotericin B is dissolved in 10% dextrose in water and the animal is placed in the Trendelenburg position (the body at a 30° tilt with the head downward).[115] The specific gravity of the dextrose solution is greater than that of the cerebrospinal fluid and it migrates downhill to the cisterna magna, carrying the amphotericin B with it. Intrathecal administration may be accompanied by such side effects as radiculitis, paresthesias, paresis, headache, and visual impairment. Addition of 5–15 mg of hydrocortisone to the injection may reduce effects due to local irritation. In some cases the drug is delivered directly into the ventricular cerebrospinal fluid by injection into a subcutaneous dome of siliconized rubber (Ommaya reservoir)[116] that is connected via a burr hole to a catheter in the lateral cerebral ventricle. This method of administration is useful in some patients, but it is accompanied by a high incidence of complications related to technical problems of insertion and maintenance of the reservoir and the production of arachnoiditis and bacterial infection.[117]

LIPID FORMULATIONS. Three lipid-based formulations of amphotericin B are available in the United States.[118–120] These preparations have reduced the toxicity of this drug toward humans while retaining its excellent antifungal action. Amphotericin B colloidal dispersion (ABCD) contains roughly equimolar amounts of amphotericin B and cholesteryl sulfate that form a colloidal suspension when dispersed in aqueous solution.[1]

A small unilamellar vesicle (SUV) formulation of liposomal amphotericin B is available in which 50 mg of amphotericin B is combined with 350 mg of lipid to yield an approximately 10% molar ratio.[118] The SUV formulation is supplied as a lyophilized powder that is rehydrated with 5% glucose to yield a particle size of about 80 nm after complete dispersion. Because of its size and in vivo stability, this liposomal preparation has physiochemical properties and a pharmacokinetic profile that are considerably different from those of the other lipid-complexed amphotericin B formulations, with greatly increased area under the plasma concentration–time curve and a much lower clearance at equivalent doses.[121] The third formulation available is amphotericin B lipid complex (ABLC). This is a preparation of dimyristoylphosphatidylcholine and dimyristoylphosphatidylglycerol in 7;3 mixture with approximately 35 mol% amphotericin B, and it forms ribbon-like sheets that range in size from 1.5 to 11 µm[1] All of these formulations are aggregations of drug and lipid with little if any amphotericin B entrapped in solution inside, and the success of these systems most likely involves the favorable disposition and release of the drug.[37]

In most cases, amphotericin B in lipid formulations retains all or part of its antifungal activity, whereas toxicity is greatly reduced or abolished. Nephrotoxicity has been diminished markedly, and infusion-related toxicities, such as fever, chills, and nausea, occur at a rate less than that seen with conventional amphotericin B.[119,122] Of the three lipid formulations, the liposomal preparation is the least hepatotoxic and nephrotoxic.[121] Two hypotheses have been formulated to explain the increased in vitro selectivity of the lipid formulations of amphotericin B. According to the first, selective transfer of the drug occurs to fungal but not mammalian cells. The second hypothesis is based on the idea that only free amphotericin B damages cells and that amphotericin B is gradually released from a liposomal formulation.[123,124] Because Fungi are more sensitive to amphotericin B than mammalian cells, they are susceptible at low amphotericin B concentrations and mammalian cells are affected only by higher free-amphotericin B concentrations that are never attained with the liposomal formulations.[125] Amphotericin B lipid formulations can be engulfed by macrophages, which may subsequently release free amphotericin B, and macrophages can, therefore, be considered reservoirs from which amphotericin B is slowly released.[126] Table 12–5 summarizes the properties of the lipid formulations of amphotericin B.

Animal studies have demonstrated that the lipid formulations of amphotericin B are similar to the parent compound in antifungal activity, and preliminary trials in humans show similar efficacy.[128,129] At this time, the major drawback to the use of the lipid formulations of amphotericin B is their high cost. Several investigators have advocated mixing amphotericn B with 'Intralipid', a product used for total parenteral nutrition.[130] This combination is much less costly and it is more readily available than the commercially prepared lipid preparations. However, these "home-made" lipid formulations are not standardized, they have undergone no quality-control testing, they appear to be less stable, and they may be more nephrotoxic than standard amphotericin B.[131,132]

Table 12–5. Properties of lipid formulations of amphotericin B.

	Amp B	ABLC	ABCD	Amp B[a] Liposomal
Drug form	Micelles	Ribbons, sheets	Disks	Unilamellar vesicles
Mol% Amp B	34	35	50	<10
Maximum plasma concentration	—	Lower than Amp B	Lower than Amp B	Higher than Amp B
Infusion-related toxicity	High	Moderate	Moderate	Mild
Relative nephrotoxicity				
Increase in creatinine level	++++	+/−	+/−	+/−
Decrease in potassium level	++++	+/−	+/−	++
Anemia	++++	Trace	Trace	Trace

ABCD, amphotericin B colloidal dispersion; ABLC, amphotericin B lipid complex; Amp B, amphotericin B deoxycholate.

[a]Several forms have been used, but here only the unilamellar liposomes produced by Vestar (San Dimas, CA), with amphotericin B in the lipid membrane surrounding the central aqueous core, are considered.

Source: Data are from de Marie *et al.*[127] and Graybill.[1]

USE IN NONFUNGAL INFECTIONS. The liposomal preparation of amphotericin has been found to be effective treatment for visceral leishmaniasis, especially in immunocompetent adults and children.[118] Amphotericin B also has potential utility in AIDS and in certain prion-caused diseases. Amphotericin B has been shown to significantly delay the onset of the encephalopathy symptoms of the prion-caused disease scrapie in hamster and mouse models. Amphotericin B may interact directly with the normal PrPC (cellular isoform of prion protein) brain protein and delay its interaction with the scrapie pathological protease-resistant protein, which accumulates in the brain.[133] This accumulation is linked to the spongiform encephalopathy associated with this disease.

Pharmacokinetics of the Polyenes

ABSORPTION AND ADMINISTRATION. Amphotericin B is poorly absorbed from the gastrointestinal tract. Several attempts have been made to use amphotericin B orally, but blood levels of drug achieved are low and inconsistent.[134] Amphotericin B is essentially insoluble in water; therefore, in preparing the drug for intravenous administration it is brought into a colloidal dispersion with sodium deoxycholate. The drug-deoxycholate mix is supplied as a dry powder, which is first suspended in sterile water and then added to a 5% solution of dextrose in water. The final concentration of the drug in the infusion fluid should be 0.1 mg/ml. Since the drug will precipitate from saline solutions and solutions containing preservatives, they should never be employed. The personnel administering this drug must be cautioned to watch for precipitate formation. If a precipitate forms, the solution should be immediately discarded.

Amphotericin B should be administered slowly over a period of 2–4 hrs. Rapid infusion of therapeutic doses is dangerous because cardiotoxicity may result. Perhaps by virtue of its effect on cell membranes, amphotericin B is very irritating, and it is associated with a high incidence of thrombophlebitis. The risk of this complication is lowered by using a small needle and a slow drip. Since the course of therapy is often long, the physicain can preserve the maximum amount of vein for future infusion by alternating therapy between extremities and by starting the infusion site distally and moving it proximally if necrosis or occlusion of the veins occurs.

Amphotericin B is slowly degraded by light. When stored in the powder form, it should be kept in the dark. The intravenous solution should be administered promptly after preparation. It has been recommended that amphotericin B be kept from light during the infusion, but when the infusion bottle is covered with a paper bag or tinfoil, it is awkward to monitor the rate of drug administration. It has been shown that there is no significant loss in biological activity over the course of 8 h at room temperature under normal lighting conditions.[135,136] Thus, it is not necessary to cover the infusion bottle during drug administration.

DISTRIBUTION AND EXCRETION. The data available on distribution of amphotericin B in both humans and animals are very limited. The pharmacokinetics of amphotericin B appear to be largely determined by its ability to be sequestered in membranes. Immediately at the end of an infusion, no more than 10% of the injected dose can be accounted for in the serum and no more than 40%, by calculation, in the extracellular fluid.[114] More than 90% of the drug in the plasma is bound to β-lipoprotein (probably to the sterol component).[137] After infusion of conventional doses, peak serum concentrations measured by bioassay are in the range of 1–2 μg/ml and the concentration falls to a trough of 0.2–0.6 μg/ml just before the next infusion 24 hr later.[114] As shown in Table 12–6,[138] the concentration of drug achieved in the cerebrospinal fluid is very low and concentrations in aqueous humor and in peritoneal, pleural, and joint fluids are approximately one-half that in the blood.

The distribution kinetics of amphotericin B can be described by a three-compartment model in which the drug is distributed from the intravascular compartment to two peripheral compartments, one of which equilibrates rapidly and the other slowly.[139] Initially, the drug is rapidly eliminated from the intravascular compartment and the rapidly equilibrating peripheral compartments ($t^{1/2} =$ 24 hr for this elimination phase) as it is taken up by the slowly equilibrating storage compartment. These kinetics may reflect concentration of the drug in cell membranes which that act as a storage depot that slowly releases the drug back into the body fluids. Amphotericin B has a very high volume of

Table 12–6. *Concentration of amphotericin B in body fluids of humans compared with the simultaneous serum concentration.* Amphotericin B was injected intravenously and concentrations were determined by bioassay.

Source	Concentration of amphotericin B (μg/ml)	
	Body fluid	Serum
Cerebrospinal fluid	0.05	1.0–2.12
Peritoneal fluid	0.22–0.32	0.4–1.7
Pleural fluid	0.66	1.02
Joint fluid	0.29	0.78
Bronchial secretion	0–0.16	1.36
Aqueous humor	0.5	0.6–1.3
Uterine tissue	1.26	1.26
Cord blood	0.37	1.26
Amniotic fluid	0.16	1.26

Source: Data are from several sources as summarized by Polak,[138] Table 1.

distribution (4 liters/kg), which is consistent with extensive binding in the tissues.[139] The terminal elimination phase has a half-life of about 15 days.[139] Thus, the drug is retained in the body for a long time. Amphotericin B was detected in the renal tissue of a patient who had completed a course of therapy 12 months previously.[140]

It is not known if amphotericin B is metabolized in the body nor how the great majority of the drug is eliminated. In humans, only 3% of a dose is eliminated in the urine as biologically active drug and blood levels are not affected by renal failure.[139,141] The dosage of amphotericin B does not have to be modified in patients with preexisting renal failure and the drug is not removed by hemodialysis or by peritoneal dialysis.[137,141,142] Some drug must be eliminated in the bile. In a study of radiolabeled amphotericin B distribution in monkeys, the highest concentration of radiolabel was found in the bile;[143] but in the dog only 3% of a dose was accounted for by excretion of bioactive compound in the bile.[144] No metabolites of the drug have been identified, but it is possible that conversion to metabolites without fungal activity occurs.

Toxicity of the Polyenes

When given orally for the treatment of intestinal candidiasis, nystatin and amphotericin B may cause nausea, vomiting, and diarrhea. When given topically, there are essentially no side effects, other than occasional irritation.

During intravenous infusion of amphotericin B, patients frequently experience fever, chills, nausea, and headache.[145] Shaking chills and fever respond to meperidine hydrochloride (45 mg) and discontinuation of the infusion.[146] Occasionally, patients experience dyspnea, hypotension, and delirium during infusion. As discussed above, an initial test dose is administered to determine the patient's tolerance to the drug and subsequent dosage is determined by the response. If therapy is resumed after the patient has been off the drug for more than a week, the initial dosage procedure should be followed. Rapid infusion of amphotericin B may cause cardiotoxicity and severe acute reactions, so the drug is always infused over a period of at least 2 hr. Infusion of amphotericin B is associated with a high incidence of thrombophlebitis.

Virtually all patients who receive a therapeutic course of intravenous amphotericin B demonstrate some degree of nephrotoxicity during therapy.[147–149] For example, in one study of 56 patients, elevated blood urea nitrogen values were observed in 93% of the patients, and 83% had high serum creatinine values.[147] The degree of permanent impairment of renal function is related to the total dosage of the drug received. When a course of therapy is completed, renal function gradually improves, but with a total dosage greater than 4 g in an adult, significant permanent renal damage occurs.[147] Some experts recommend that the dosage of amphotericin B be reduced during therapy if the serum creatinine rises above 3.5 mg/dl in order to reduce complications (nausea, vomiting, dehydration) arising from uremia.[112] The results of animal studies suggested that it might be possible to reduce the extent of azotemia by simultaneous administration of bicarbonate or mannitol.[150,151] A careful study has shown, however, that mannitol infusion does not protect against nephrotoxicity in humans.[152] It is important to ensure that the patient is well hydrated in order to minimize azotemia.[112]

Amphotericin B affects renal function in two ways: by acutely reducing renal blood flow and by a direct toxic action on the renal tubular cells. It has been shown that infusion of amphotericin B into the renal artery of a dog causes vasoconstriction,[153] and an acute reduction in renal blood flow and glomerular filtration rate has been observed in humans.[147,154,155] The toxic action on renal tubular cells probably reflects an action of amphotericin B on membrane permeability. Specimens of renal tissue obtained at biopsy or postmortem examination show tubular degenerative changes with intratubular and interstitial calcium deposits.[156] Amphotericin B nephropathy is manifested by abnormal urine sediment, azotemia, and renal tubular acidosis.[155] Hypokalemia develops in a significant number of patients who require potassium replacement. Hypomagnesemia can also occur. Renal potassium wasting and nephrocalcinosis may both result from a tubular defect in acid excretion.[155] Studies of the nephrotoxicity in animal models also support the concept that amphotericin B affects the renal tubule, modifying its ability to acidify the urine.[150,157] It is clear that amphotericin B can interact with mammalian cell membranes and alter their permeability to small cations like potassium (see Mechanism of Action for detailed discussion). A significant part of the nephrotoxicity of amphotericin B may be due to a similar effect on the membranes of the cells of the distal tubule. Patients receiving amphotericin B should have bi-weekly determination of serum creatinine, potassium, and bicarbonate, and special caution should be exercised in patients who are receiving other nephrotoxic drugs such as aminoglycosides. Loading with sodium chloride has decreased the nephrotoxicity associated with amphotericin B in both patients and experimental animals. Administration of 1 liter of saline intravenously on the day that amphotericin B is to be given has been recommended for adults who are able to tolerate the sodium load and who are not already receiving that amount in intravenous fluids.[158]

Amphotericin B causes a normochromic, normocytic anemia with a normal red cell life span.[159] The hematocrit frequently falls to a stable value of 22%–35%.[160] The drug apparently causes the anemia by inhibiting erythropoietin production (either directly or indirectly as a result of renal failure) rather than by suppressing the bone marrow directly.[161] The hemolysis discussed earlier in this chapter occurs only at concentrations higher than those achieved during therapy.[43] The anemia should be monitored with biweekly hematocrits during the first 4 weeks of treatment and weekly thereafter.

Rare side effects include leukopenia, severe abdominal pain, and anaphylaxis. The safety of amphotericin B during the first trimester of pregnancy has not been established, but several patients treated with the drug during the last two trimesters of pregnancy have given birth to normal infants.[162] Serious pulmonary reactions have been reported in patients receiving both amphotericin B and leukocyte transfusions.[163] The reactions are characterized by sudden dyspnea, hypoxemia, hemoptysis, and the appearance of persistent interstitial infiltrates on chest roentgenograms. The mechanism of the reaction is unknown, but it is 10 times more frequent in leukocyte recipients who are also receiving amphotericin B than in leukocyte recipients who are not receiving the drug.[163] The pulmonary reaction may be fatal.

The water-soluble methyl ester of amphotericin B is available in the United States for investigational use. Amphotericin B methyl ester was found to have about the same antifungal activity as amphotericin B in vitro,[164,165] but studies in animal models show that it is much less nephrotoxic.[166,167] Early clinical trials indicate that amphotericin B methyl ester is less nephrotoxic than amphotericin B in humans, but that either the methyl ester or other contaminating polyenes in the preparation produce leukoencephalopathy.[168,169]

The lipid formulations of amphotericin B are tolerated better than conventional amphotericin B.[170,171] This seems to be especially true for the liposomal preparations where patients have experienced fewer adverse effects, including renal tubular damage, potassium wasting, mild anemia, and infusion-related reactions such as fever, chills, rigors, nausea, and vomiting.[118,121] Even patients who had previously experienced adverse effects with the conventional formulation have been able to tolerate the liposomal preparation.[122]

Flucytosine

Flucytosine, the 5-fluoro-substituted analog of cytosine, was originally synthesized as a potential anticancer drug. And although it

5-Fluorocytosine   cytosine deaminase   5-Fluorouracil

was found not be to cytotoxic for mammalian cells, it was active against some fungi. Flucytosine has been reviewed by Scholer.[172]

Mechanism of Action

Flucytosine is transported into fungal cells where it is deaminated by cytosine deaminase to 5-fluorouracil (Figure 12–3). The uptake of 5-fluorocytosine, and thus the inhibition of growth, can be blocked by cytosine.[173] The anticancer drug cytosine arabinoside will also block the flucytosine effect by competing for uptake of the drug.[174] The conversion of flucytosine to 5-fluorouracil is an absolute requirement for drug activity; mutant fungi with no cytosine deaminase activity are resistant to flucytosine.[175,176]

As can be seen from Figure 12–3, 5-fluorouracil is converted to 5-fluorouracilribose monophosphate. This reaction in fungi seems to depend primarily on uridinemonophosphate (UMP) pyrophosphorylase.[177] Mutant fungi that are resistant to very high concentrations of both 5-fluorocytosine and 5-fluorouracil have been

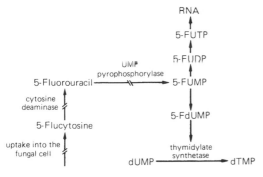

Figure 12–3. Action of flucytosine in fungi. 5-Flucytosine is transported into the fungal cell where it is deaminated to 5-fluorouracil (5-FU). The 5-FU is then converted to 5-fluorouracil-ribose monophosphate (5-FUMP), which can either be converted to 5-FUTP and incorporated into RNA or be converted by ribonucleotide reductase to 5-FdUMP, which is a potent inhibitor of thymidylate synthetase. The arrows with break marks represent those reactions that have been shown to be absent in various flucytosine-resistant fungi.

isolated.[178] Their resistance is often the result of a mutation that affects the production of UMP pyrophosphorylase. The product of the UMP pyrophosphorylase reaction, 5-fluorouracil-ribose monophosphate (FUMP), enters two pathways that are potentially important for the cytotoxic effect. It is clear that a significant amount of the FUMP is converted to the triphosphate (FUTP), which is incorporated into RNA and replaces as much as 50% of the uracil in fungal RNA.[179,180] The production of "faulty" RNA containing the uracil analog may contribute to the action of the drug, but it does not explain the early inhibition of DNA and RNA synthesis observed after addition of flucytosine to fungal cultures.[181]

Like mammalian cells, fungi can reduce the sugar on FUMP, converting it to 5-fluoro-2'-deoxyuridine-5'-monophosphate (FdUMP).[182] FdUMP is a potent inhibitor of thymidylate synthetase in both fungi and mammalian cells.[182,183] As shown in Figure 12–4, FdUMP binds covalently to a cysteinyl residue in the active site of thymidylate synthetase,[184,185] forming a stable covalent ternary complex involving the enzyme,

FdUMP, and the methylenetetrahydrofolate cofactor.[186,187] It has been proposed that a similar ternary covalent complex is formed as an intermediate in the normal enzymatic reaction with dUMP.[186,187] Apparently the analog behaves as a quasi-substrate capable of participating in the reaction process up to the stage of the one-carbon transfer from the cofactor, but the reaction cannot be completed and the enzyme is essentially irreversibly inactivated. By inhibiting thymidylate synthetase, FdUMP blocks the production of thymidine monophosphate and consequently inhibits DNA synthesis. In some tumor cells growing in vitro, inhibition of DNA synthesis is the principal event responsible for the cytotoxicity of fluorouracil,[188] and this may be the case in flucytosine-sensitive fungi as well.

The selective toxicity of flucytosine is explained by the difference in the abilities of the host cells and the fungal cells to convert the drug to fluorouracil. Sensitive fungi have cytosine deaminase and this enzyme has not been found in mammalian cells. For a long time it was thought that deamination to 5-fluorouracil did not occur in humans,[189] but it has now been demonstrated that serum from humans receiving therapeutic doses of flucytosine does contain some fluorouracil.[190] Less than 4% of a dose of flucytosine is converted to fluorouracil[190] and it is probable that this deamination is carried out by

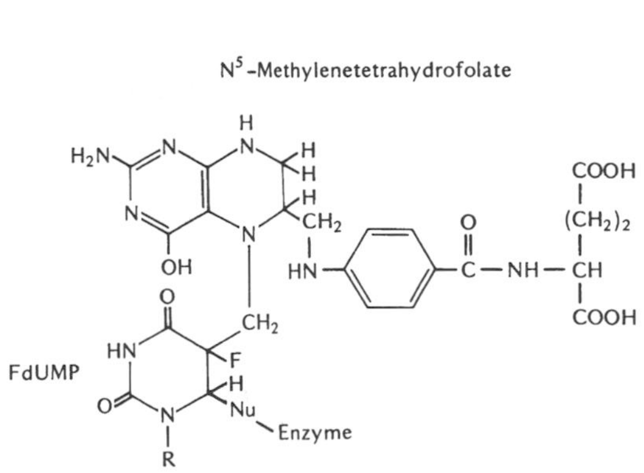

N^5–Methylenetetrahydrofolate

Figure 12–4. Proposed structure for the complex of thymidylate synthetase, FdUMP, and methylenetetrahydrofolate. Nu, nucleophilic site on the enzyme; R, deoxyribose 5'-phosphate moiety of FdUMP. (Adapted from Langenbach et al.[186])

the intestinal flora.[189] The production of fluorouracil may be sufficient to account for some of the toxicity observed clinically with flucytosine.

Antimicrobial Activity and Clinical Use

The spectrum of flucytosine activity is limited to only a few fungi that are clinically important. The fungicidal activity of flucytosine is highest in yeasts, including species of *Candida, Torulopsis,* and *Cryptococcus* (see Table 12–7). Flucytosine has fungistatic activity against *Aspergillus fumigatus* and the fungi that cause chromomycosis (species of *Phialophora* and *Cladosporium*).[172] Most other fungal pathogens are highly resistant. Ninety-eight percent of strains of *Cryptococcus neoformans*, 92% of *Candida albicans,* and 79% of *Candida* species other than *C. albicans* are initially sensitive to flucytosine.[172] An organism with a minimum inhibitory concentration greater than 15–20 μg/ml is usually considered resistant. Resistance can develop during treatment and this is a major problem when the drug is used alone in therapy.[172,191]

There are many possible mechanisms of resistance to flucytosine, several of which have been demonstrated in resistant strains isolated from patients. These include (see Fig. 12–3) a decrease in the activity of the cytosine-specific permease responsible for drug entry into the fungus,[178] a loss of cytosine deaminase activity,[192] or a decrease in UMP pyrophosphorylase activity.[178,193–195] Mutant organisms created in the laboratory have been shown to be resistant by all these mechanisms and also by the absence of a feedback inhibition of pyrimidine synthesis.[175] This last mechanism is especially interesting. Normally, aspartic transcarbamylase, the first enzyme in the pyrimidine biosynthetic pathway, is under feedback inhibitory control by UTP. A mutation resulting in a loss of this regulation leads to increased endogenous synthesis of uridine nucleotides, which compete with the fluorine-containing uridine analogs created from the drugs to overcome the antifungal effect.

As discussed earlier in this chapter, the combination of amphotericin B and flucytosine is sometimes additive or slightly synergistic both in vitro and in laboratory animals infected with sensitive fungi. In serious mycoses due to sensitive strains, flucytosine should be combined with amphotericin B for therapy.[191] The use of the combination may have several advantages: (*1*) there may be a more potent antifungal effect than with either drug alone; (*2*) it may permit a lower dose of amphotericin B to be used, thus avoiding some of the toxicity inherent to this drug;[66] and (*3*) the rate of emergence of resistance to therapy should be much lower than with flucytosine alone. Flucytosine is used in combination with amphotericin B to

Table 12–7. Minimal inhibitory concentrations of flucytosine for selected fungi.

Organism	Minimal inhibitory concentration (μg/ml)	
	Approximate mean or median	Range
Candida albicans	0.1–1.0	0.02–20
Candida tropicalis	0.3–6.0	0.10–400
Torulopsis glabrata	0.1–1.0	0.03–3
Cryptococcus neoformans	0.4–2.0	0.05–15
Aspergillus fumigatus	1.0–12.0	0.25–200
Phialophora verrucosa	1.0–12.0	
Cladosporium trichoides	2.0–3.0	

Source: Data collected from several reports in the literature cited by Scholer.[172]

treat cryptococcal meningitis and systemic candidiasis.[191] The combined therapy is also highly effective in the treatment of cryptococcosis in patients with AIDS; in two studies the response rate to the combination was 100% in contrast to 40%–65% in patients given amphotericin B alone.[196,197] There is no advantage to using the combination against flucytosine-resistant organisms, and the minimal inhibitory concentration (MIC) for the infecting organism should be determined. High concentrations of flucytosine are achieved in the urine and the drug may be used alone to treat candidiasis and chromoblastomycosis in the urinary tract.[198,199] Flucytosine is the only drug reported to be really effective in treating chromomycosis.[200]

New prospects for flucytosine therapy are now emerging that are based not only on an improved understanding of its applications but also on its possible combination with new companion drugs such as itraconazole and fluconazole.[199,201] These azoles are not only highly effective against susceptible fungi but are also well tolerated, and combining them with flucytosine may have advantages over more conventional regimens. In the initial treatment of cryptococcal meningitis in patients with AIDS, the two combined regimens (flucytosine with itraconazole or fluconazole) have increased the cure rate and have shortened the time to remission.[202,203] In candidosis, the flucytosine–amphotericin B combination is still the treatment of choice. But the combination of flucytosine with one of the two triazoles is synergistic both in vitro and in vivo,[204] and these combinations could be indicated for the treatment of systemic candidosis in premature infants who tolerate amphotericin B poorly, or when prolonged antifungal treatment is required in adults.[199] This approach may also reduce the risk of clinical resistance developing to these drugs.

Pharmacokinetics

Flucytosine is rapidly and almost completely absorbed from the gastrointestinal tract and it is routinely administered orally. The usual dosage is 150 mg/kg of body weight per day given in divided doses every 6 h. After oral administration of a single 30 mg/kg dose to patients with normal renal function, peak serum levels of 30–50 μg/ml are achieved in about 2 h.[205] With repeated administration of 37.5 mg/kg every 6 h, the steady-state concentration maximum in serum should not exceed 100 μg/ml and the minimum should not fall below 20 μg/ml.[172] Flucytosine is not bound to plasma protein.[137,206] The volume of distribution (0.68 liters/kg) approximates the total body water.[206,207] Concentrations of flucytosine that are above fungistatic levels are achieved in most body fluids.[172] Concentrations in cerebrospinal fluid average 75% of the simultaneous serum concentration.[208] Concentrations in bile (rat),[172] bronchial secretion (dog),[209] and peritoneal fluid (human)[172] approximate the simultaneous serum concentration, whereas concentrations in human saliva, joint fluid,[210] and aqueous humor[211] are one-fourth to one-half the serum concentration. Penetration into blood clots and fibrin clots is apparently poor.[212]

Flucytosine is excreted via the kidney by means of glomerular filtration and 90% of a dose is recovered in the urine as unchanged drug within 48 h.[206] Very high concentrations (1000–3000 μg/ml) are achieved in the urine of patients with normal renal function.[205] The rate of flucytosine excretion is linearly related to the rate of creatinine clearance,[137,205] and the half-life in patients with normal renal function is 3–5 h.[206,207] The half-life is not affected by hepatic failure,[213] but it is markedly increased with renal failure[205,207] and dosage adjustment is necessary. Several methods of calculating a dosage based on creatinine clearance rate or serum creatinine have been published.[112,205,206] One recommended method is to increase the dosage interval, using the creatinine clearance as a guide to renal function—one 35 mg/kg dose every 6 h for a creatinine clearance over 40 ml/min, every 12 h for a clearance of 20–40 ml, and every 24 h for a clearance between 10 and 20.[205] Such a schedule does not substitute for dosage adjustment based on serum levels of the drug. Flucytosine levels may be determined by both bioassay[214] and chemical assay.[215] Peak levels should be measured 1–2 h after ingestion of a dose and trough levels should be measured just before the next dose. If the peak level is higher than 100 µg/ml, a reduction in dosage is indicated. The elimination kinetics of flucytosine differ greatly from those of amphotericin B, which is eliminated very slowly and does not require dosage modification in patients with renal failure. It must be remembered that, when the two drugs are used together, amphotericin B is a nephrotoxic drug and serum levels of flucytosine should be determined periodically. Flucytosine is rapidly eliminated by hemodialysis at a rate that is similar to that of creatinine, and a normal dose of 35 mg/kg should be administered for replacement after dialysis.[137,207] Flucytosine is also eliminated by peritoneal dialysis.[216] The only metabolism that has been detected in humans is a small amount (0.1%–3.5%) of conversion to 5-fluorouracil[190] that probably represents deamination by intestinal flora.[189]

Adverse Effects of Flucytosine

When administered alone to patients with good renal function, flucytosine is well tolerated.[172] About 5% of patients experience nausea, diarrhea, and, less commonly, vomiting.[172,217] There have been isolated reports of enterocolitis occurring during therapy with both flucytosine and amphotericin B.[218] Skin rashes occur occasionally. Reversible hepatic dysfunction, manifested by mild elevations in serum transaminases and alkaline phosphatase, occurs in about 5% of patients.[172,219] Rarely, more severe liver damage occurs. Patients receiving flucytosine should have their serum transaminase and alkaline phosphatase levels monitored weekly.

The major complication associated with flucytosine therapy is bone marrow depression, which is usually manifest as a reversible neutropenia, with occasional thrombocytopenia.[66,172] A few cases of fatal bone marrow aplasia have been reported.[220,221] Bone marrow toxicity is associated with serum levels of flucytosine greater than 100 µg/ml.[66,222] Patients with renal failure are at higher risk of developing this complication.

Concomitant therapy with amphotericin B may increase the risk of bone marrow depression by two mechanisms: by enhancing the uptake of flucytosine (or fluorouracil) into the cells of the marrow or by causing renal impairment and reducing the rate of flucytosine elimination. Because of the marrow toxicity, the blood levels of flucytosine should be carefully monitored and leukocyte and platelet counts should be obtained twice a week.[112]

Since patients who are treated with flucytosine have detectable levels of fluorouracil in their serum, it has been suggested that the bone marrow depression, and possibly also the diarrhea, might be due to fluorouracil.[190] Bone marrow depression caused by fluorouracil, like that occurring during flucytosine therapy, is manifested by leukopenia and less often by thrombocytopenia.[223] After rapid intravenous administration of a therapeutic dose (15 mg/kg) of fluorouracil, peak levels of 0.1 to 1 mM are seen in the plasma and the drug is rapidly cleared with a plasma half-life of 10–20 min.[224,225] Maximum fluorouracil levels in the range of 1–3 µg/ml (0.008–0.023 mM) have been assayed in the serum of patients with clinical toxicity who were receiving therapeutic doses of flucytosine.[190] Although the levels of fluorouracil assayed during flucytosine administration are only 8%–23% of the lower limit of peak levels achieved by administering fluorouracil in therapeutic amounts (0.1 mM), patients receiving flucytosine every 6 h are exposed to quite constant low levels of fluorouracil.[190] It is conceivable that continuous exposure to these low concentrations of fluorouracil could produce the bone marrow depression observed during flucytosine therapy.

The Azoles (Imidazoles and Triazoles)

The azole antifungals are categorized into two broad classes, imidazoles and triazoles, according to whether they have two or three nitrogens in the five-membered azole ring. Both groups have similar antifungal spectra and mechanisms of action, but the triazoles are more slowly metabolized and have less effect on human sterol synthesis than the imidazoles.

Systemic antifungal therapy has made considerable strides since the 1960s and 1970s, a time that could be considered the amphotericin B era.[226] At that time, opportunistic infections were not nearly as common as they are now, treatment of major systemic mycoses always involved hospitalization, and therapy was associated with significant toxic effects. The introduction of ketoconazole in the early 1980s allowed outpatient therapy for several endemic mycoses, notably histoplasmosis, blastomycosis, and coccidioidomycosis. Ketoconazole could have considerable toxicity at higher doses but overall it was a safer drug than amphotericin B.[227,228] Introduction of triazole's in the 1990s enabled outpatient therapy for most endemic mycoses with a low incidence of toxicity.[226] The two major drugs in the triazole class are fluconazole and itraconazole. These drugs are less toxic and more easily administered, but resistance emerges readily, especially during treatment of patients with AIDS.[226,229–231]

The imidazole structure has been used in a variety of ways to develop some very useful chemotherapeutic agents. The benzimi-

Fluconazole

Miconazole

Ketoconazole

Itraconazole

dazole derivatives thiabendazole and mebendazole have a broad-spectrum anthelminthic activity. The 5-nitroimidazole, metronidazole, is very active against several protozoa and a variety of anaerobic bacteria that are human pathogens. Several imidazole derivatives were found to be active against fungi and have been introduced for the chemotherapy of fungal infections. Some antifungal imidazoles, such as clotrimazole, miconazole, and and econazole, are available only for topical therapy. Ketoconazole is a water-soluble imidazole that can be administered orally for the treatment of both superficial and deep fungal infections. The newest drugs, the triazoles, include itraconazole and fluconazole for systemic therapy and terconazole, which is available only for topical administration. The antifungal imidazoles have been the subject of several comprehensive reviews (clotrimazole,[232] miconazole,[232,233] ketoconazole,[234,235] fluconazole,[226,236] and itraconazole.[226,237]

Mechanism of Action and Resistance

At low concentrations the azoles are fungistatic and at higher concentrations they are fungicidal. The azoles inhibit the synthesis of ergosterol, the principal sterol in fungal cell membranes, through inhibition of lanosterol 14α demethylase, a cytochrome P-450. Azoles bind to the heme of fungal cytochrome P-450 and inhibit the binding of lanosterol (as well as molecular oxygen) to the enzyme.[100] This prevents hydroxylation of the 14α-methyl group of lanosterol, thus blocking the formation of ergosterol.[110] The depletion of ergosterol alters membrane fluidity, with concomitant reduction in the activity of membrane-associated enzymes, increased membrane permeability, and inhibition of cell growth and replication. The azoles also inhibit, either directly or indirectly, 3-ketosteroid reductase, the enzyme that catalyses the synthesis of 4,4-demethylated 14-methylsterols that function much like ergosterol.[238] When the azoles inhibit lanosterol demethylase, 14α-methyl fecosterol accumulates[239] and subsequent desaturation of this compound by the enzyme Δ⁵,⁶ sterol desaturase results in the accumulation of 14α-

methyl-3,6-diol, which causes growth arrest. Other consequences of azole action include inhibition of respiration,[240] toxic interaction with membrane phospholipids,[240,241] and inhibition of the morphogenetic transformation of yeasts to the mycelium form.[242]

Alterations in the the activity or amount of lanosterol demethylase and sterol desaturase enzymes account for some of the clinical resistance to azoles,[239,243,244] but alterations in permeability of the fungal cell membrane to azoles also occurs.[245] Active drug efflux may be an important mechanism of resistance to azoles.[100,246,247] A number of *mdr* (*m*ultidrug *r*esistance) genes that encode energy, dependent efflux pumps called *MDR transporters* have been identified in drug-resistant fungi.[248,249] Amplification of *mdr* genes with increased expression of transporter leading to low intracellular concentrations of drug would account for cross-resistance to azoles and other metabolic inhibitors.[250]

Antifungal Activity

The antifungal imidazoles have a broad spectrum of in vitro activity against a variety of fungi that are pathogenic to humans. The dermatophytes such as *Microsporum*, *Trichophyton*, and *Epidermophyton* species are susceptible. The yeasts such as *Cryptococcus neoformans*, *Candida* species, and *Torulopsis glabrata* are generally susceptible as are a variety of dimorphic fungi that cause deep infections such as *Coccidioides immitis*, *Histoplasma capsulatum*, *Blastomyces dermatitidis*, and *Paracoccidioides brasiliensis*.[233,235] The in vitro activity of itraconazole, fluconozole and ketoconazole against several yeasts is presented in Table 12–8.

In animal models, the azoles are active against most of the organisms that cause systemic or deep-seated fungal infections, such as *Cryptococcus neoformans*, *Candida albicans*, and the common dimorphic fungi, such as *Coccidioides immitis*, *Histoplasma capsulatum*, *Blastomyces dermatitidiis*, *Paracoccidioides brasiliensis*, and *Sporothrix schenckii*.[237,252–254] The azoles are less active against many non *albicans* species of *Candida* and related yeasts, including *Candida*

Table 12–8.   In vitro activity of antifungal agents against 177 vaginal yeast isolates.

Organism (no. of isolates)	MIC$_{50}$[b] (MIC$_{90}$)[c] mg/liter at 48 h		
	Itraconazole	Ketoconazole	Fluconazole
Candida albicans (100)	0.02 (0.02)	0.02 (0.02)	1.25 (2.5)
Candida glabrata (39)	0.05 (0.39)	0.2 (0.78)	20 (40)
Candida parapsilosis (26)	0.02 (0.02)	0.02 (0.1)	2.5 (5)
Candida tropicalis (7)	0.02	0.05	2.5
Saccharomyces cerevisiae (5)	0.78	0.78	20

[a] Antifungal susceptibility tests were performed using a macrobroth dilution method prior to the introduction of U.S. National Committee for Clinical Laboratory Standards (NCCLS) guidelines. Some isolates were subsequently tested using the NCCLS method with little variability in results. [b] Minimum inhibitory concentrations were at or below the given value for 50% of the isolates. [c] Minimum inhibitory concentrations were at or below the given value for 90% of the isolates.

Source: Data from Haria et al. and Lynch and Sobel.[237, 251]

krusei and *Candida glabrata* (*Torulopsis glabrata*). Itraconazole is more active than the other azole drugs against *Aspergillus* species.[254]

In vitro susceptibility testing of antifungal drugs has not been of great value because of the limited correlation of the results with the clinical response. Comparisons of minimal inhibitory concentrations from laboratory to laboratory and from study to study must be made with caution because the results are influenced by a variety of factors, including the growth medium. Standardization of testing parameters, such as inoculum preparation, medium composition, incubation conditions, and end point criteria, by the U.S. National Committee for Clinical Laboratory Standards[255,256] has resulted in increased interlaboratory reproducibility for broth dilution methods. Although broth dilution techniques generally produce more reproducible end points and minimum inhibitory concentration values, clinical response remains the most reliable guide to choosing the appropriate therapy.[257]

Until the 1990s, the development of clinically important resistance to azoles was quite rare even after prolonged courses of therapy.[258,259] Treatment failures have increased, however, among patients infected with HIV who are receiving intermittent or continuous fluconazole therapy for oropharyngeal or esophageal candidiasis, and laboratory and epidemiologic data confirm that both in vitro and clinical resistance have emerged.[260,261] The antifungal efficacy of the azoles could be markedly compromised if resistance to fluconazole and other azoles becomes widespread, especially with the increasing use of fluconazole in patients with and without AIDS.

Azole Preparations and Clinical Use

Miconazole, clotrimazole and newer imidazoles, such as econazole, terconazole, butoconazole, tioconazole, oxiconazole, and sulconazole, are available in creams and lotions for the topical treatment of common fungal infections on the skin. The imidazoles are very effective in the treatment of *Candida* and dermatophyte infections of the skin.[262,263] Dermatophyte infections of the nails are more difficult to treat and may require oral therapy with griseofulvin, terbinafine, or ketoconazole. Miconazole and clotrimazole creams applied once a day at bedtime for 14 days are as effective as nystatin cream in the treatment of vaginal candidiasis.[264,265] Clotrimazole is also available as a vaginal tablet which, when inserted at bedtime for seven nights, is as effective as treatment with the creams.[264]

Much of the clinical experience with ketoconazole in systemic mycoses has been derived from multicenter studies in which many of the patients had previously been treated unsuccessfully with other antifungal drugs. It is clear that ketoconazole is effective in the treatment of paracoccidioidomycosis,[266,267] and patients with histoplasmosis have responded well to ketoconazole therapy,[267,268]where the response rate for chronic cavitary, pulmonary, and disseminated disease is around 85%.[228] For blastomycosis the response rate is close to 90% and in coccidioidomycosis the results are comparable to those with amphotericin B, although not as good as in the treatment of histoplasmosis.[269] Ketoconazole has some drawbacks, however. For example, the slow response to therapy makes it inappropriate for treatment of patients with severe or rapidly progressive mycoses. In addition, the efficacy of ketoconazole is poor in immunosupressed patients and in meningitis. Ketoconazole suppresses but does not necessarily eradicate *Coccidioides immitis*. Thus, many patients with coccidioidomycosis respond to ketoconazole, but when therapy is stopped, the disease may recur.[270,271] Ketoconazole is not useful in treating patients with aspergillosis, mucormycosis, or sporotrichosis.

Ketoconazole clearly has a role in the oral therapy of some superficial mycoses. It is very effective in treating chronic mucocutaneous candidiasis,[234,272] a condition that frequently does not respond to other antifungal drugs. More than 50% of patients with *Candida* infection of the oropharynx are clinically cured within 1 week and the rest within 3 weeks after initiation of ketoconazole therapy.[273] Most skin infections caused by *Candida* species respond to ketoconazole.[273] Ketoconazole is effective in patients with dermatophyte infections,[234,274] including those with griseofulvin-resistant dermatophytosis,[275] but the problem of recurrence of infection after termination of therapy remains.

Itraconazole has become the treatment of choice for most patients with mild to moderate histoplasmosis, blastomycosis, and sporotrichosis, and fluconazole has become the treatment of choice for coccidioidal meningitis. Fluconazole is also useful for treatment of patients with candidemia, localized forms of mucocutaneous and visceral candidiasis, and cryptococcal meningitis. Coccidioidomycosis is effectively treated with either itraconazole or fluconazole. As noted previously, for several of these infections it is recommended that patients with severe disease receive amphotericin B.[226]

Pharmacokinetics of the Azoles

ABSORPTION. Ketoconazole is the first azole for which the pharmacology was studied in detail. Ketoconazole is well absorbed from the gastrointestinal tract. After administration of a single 200 mg tablet to an adult, peak serum levels of 2–4 μg/ml are achieved in 1–2 h and are maintained for 2–3 h.[276,277] The manufacturer's recommended dosage of ketoconazole for an adult is 200 mg, or at most 400 mg, taken once daily. It has been found that a dosage of 400 or 800 mg/day is frequently required for maximal clinical response in the treatment of systemic fungal infection.[278] A 400 mg oral dose yields a peak plasma level of 6–7 μg/ml.[277] Ketoconazole is a dibasic compound and the pH must be acid for both dissolution and absorption. Concomitant administration of drugs that reduce gastric acidity, such as cimetidine or antacids, results in lower peak plasma concentrations.[279] If these drugs must be given, it is best to administer them 2 h after the daily dose of ketoconazole. In patients with achlorhydria, it may be necessary to dissolve the drug in 0.2N HCl and administer it through a glass or plastic straw. Food impairs the absorption of ketoconazole and higher plasma levels will be obtained if the drug is administered 1 to 2 h before a meal.[280]

Like ketoconazole, itraconazole is available only for oral administration and requires an acidic environment for optimal solubilization and absorption.[281,282] Whereas food decreases the absorption and bioavailability of ketoconazole, the bioavailability of itraconazole is two to three times higher when taken with food than when taken on an empty stomach.[281] After a single dose, the plasma concentrations of itraconazole and ketoconazole are similar, however, after 7 to 14 days of treatment (steady state), the peak plasma concentrations of itraconazole are three to five times higher.[253,283] A loading dose of 200 mg of itraconazole administered three times daily for 3 days is recommended in patients with serious infections to reduce the time until steady-state concentrations are attained.

Fluconazole is available as both an oral and intravenous formulation. Unlike ketoconazole and itraconazole, its absorption is not altered by the presence of food or gastric acidity.[284] Peak plasma concentrations are proportional to the dose and occur within 2 to 4 h after oral administration. Plasma concentrations at steady state are 2 to 2.5 times higher than after a single dose, and administration of a loading dose of fluconazole is recommended in patients with serious infections.

DISTRIBUTION. Ketoconazole and itraconazole are both extensively bound (>99%) to plasma proteins,[285] predominantly to albumin,[235] and the unbound drug distributes well throughout most tissues. Fluconazole, by contrast, is highly water-soluble and minimally bound to plasma proteins, and distributes in a volume that approximates that of total body water.[4,236] Ketoconazole does not pass into the cerebrospinal fluid in the absence of meningeal disease and only low and unreliable levels are achieved in the presence of meningeal inflammation. In one study the average cerebrospinal fluid concentration in patients receiving a 400 mg dose of ketoconazole was 0.39 μg/ml (range 0–0.85 μg/ml).[276] Some investigators have found somewhat higher cerebrospinal fluid levels,[235] but poor penetration into the cerebrospinal fluid may explain reported failures of ketoconazole therapy in cryptococcal and coccidioidal meningitis.[286] Significant concentrations of ketoconazole are achieved in joint fluid and possibly also in saliva.[276] After oral administration, a high level of ketoconazole has been detected in human skin.[276] In rats the drug was found to be distributed throughout the subcutaneous tissue and the animals' fur showed antifungal activity for at least 48 h after a single oral dose.[287] This distribution is consistent with the clinical observation that oral ketoconazole is effective in treating superficial fungal infections in the skin and hair. In rats receiving radiolabeled ketoconazole, the highest levels of radioactivity were found in liver, adrenal gland, and connective tissue.[235]

Body fluids (cerebrospinal fluid, aqueous humor, saliva, sputum, sweat, and vaginal fluid) contain less than half the concentration of itraconazole present in plasma, whereas itraconazole accumulates in body tissues and pus in concentrations up to 19 times the plasma concentration.[288] The concentrations of fluconazole in most body tissues and fluids usually exceed 50% of the corresponding plasma concentrations and are especially high in cerebrospinal fluid and urine.[289] The peak cerebrospinal fluid concentrations of fluconazole in patients with fungal meningitis are 80% to 90% of peak plasma concentrations, and urinary concentrations of fluconazole usually exceed those of other oral azoles.[290]

METABOLISM AND ELIMINATION. Ketoconazole is extensively metabolized by O-dealkylation and aromatic hydroxylation to a large number of metabolites that do not have antifungal activity.[235] The serum half-life of ketoconazole is approximately 3 h[276,277] and the half-life is apparently determined entirely by the rate of metabolism in the liver. The half-life of the drug is not affected by renal failure and dosage modification is not necessary in patients with impaired renal function.[276] In a patient with hepatic insufficiency the half-life was prolonged.[276] The peak levels achieved with repeated doses of ketoconazole appear to be lower than those obtained at the initiation of therapy,[276] suggesting that ketoconazole may induce its own hepatic metabolism. Induction of hepatic enzymes was not observed in rats, however.[291] Rifampin, a drug that induces the hepatic microsomal metabolizing system, decreased the peak serum concentration of ketoconazole by an order of magnitude in a patient who received both of these drugs as well as isoniazid.[276]

Like ketoconazole, itraconazole is extensively metabolized in the liver and excreted almost exclusively as metabolites in both the feces and urine. More than 30 metabolites of itraconazole have been identified, but only dihydroxyitraconazole has been found to have antifungal activity.[237] Because relatively

Table 12–9. Pharmacokinetic properties of systemic antifungal agents.

	Amphotericin B	Flucytosine	Ketoconazole	Itraconazole	Fluconazole
Oral bioavailability (%)	<5	≥80	75[a]	>70[a]	>80
Protein binding (%)	91–95	4	99	>99	11
Apparent volume of distribution (liters/kg)	4.0	0.6–0.7	—[b]	—[b]	0.7–0.8
Peak plasma concentration (μg/ml)	1.2–2.0	30–45	1.5–3.1	0.2–0.4	10.2
Terminal elimination half-life	15 days	3–6 h	20–24 h[c]	7–10 h[c]	24–42 h
Unchanged drug in urine (%)	3	>75	2–4	<1	80
Cerebrospinal fluid concentration (% of plasma concentration)	2–4	>75	<10	<1	>70

[a]The absolute bioavailability of ketoconazole and itraconazole has not been determined because of the absence of a form suitable for intravenous use. The values represent the bioavailability of these agents relative to that of an oral solution in normal subjects. [b]The apparent volume of distribution was not assessed in humans because of the absence of a form suitable for intravenous use. In dogs, the apparent volumes of distribution of ketoconazole were 9.7 and 17 liters/kg, respectively. [c]Itraconazole and ketoconazole exhibit dose-dependent elimination. Longer terminal elimination half-lives are possible with large daily doses.

Source: Data are from Como and Dismukes,[4] Gallis et al.,[294] Daneshmend and Warnock,[295] Saag and Dismukes,[253] Grant and Glissold,[288] Van Peer et al.,[281] Hardin et al.,[282] Barone et al.,[283] Tucker et al.,[295] Humphrey et al.,[297] Brammer et al.,[292] and Francis and Walsh.[298]

little itraconazole is excreted in the urine, reduction in dosage is not required in patients with renal impairment.[4] Very little itraconazole or ketoconazole is removed by hemodialysis. In contrast to ketoconazole and itraconazole, fluconazole is minimally metabolized and 80% of dose is excreted unchanged in the urine.[292] The terminal elimination half-life increases from approximately 30 h in patients with normal renal function to 98 h in patients with severe renal impairment,[293] and the dose should be reduced in patients with glomerular filtration rates below 50 ml/min. Fluconazole is removed during hemodialysis and to a lesser extent during peritoneal dialysis. Table 12–9 summarizes the pharmacokinetic properties of the systemic imidazoles as well as those of amphotericin B and flucytosine.

Adverse Effects of Imidazoles and Triazoles

Clotrimazole, miconazole, and other imidazoles are well tolerated on topical application to the skin and vagina. Occasional patients experience burning sensations and irritation during treatment of vaginal candidiasis.[232] There have been a few reports of contact dermatitis with miconazole.[299,300]

Ketoconazole, fluconazole, and itraconazole (particularly the latter two) are much better tolerated than the older antifungal drugs. The most common side effects of ketoconazole are gastrointestinal reactions, with nausea occurring in about 3% of patients and abdominal pain in about 1%.[235] Itching occurs in about 2% of patients and headache, diarrhea, rashes, dizziness, and somnolence occur at an incidence of less than 1%. Reversible increases in serum transaminases and alkaline phosphatase occur occasionally.[235] Rarely (about 1 in 15,000 courses of therapy), patients have developed clinical hepatitis, and if the drug is not discontinued immediately, *fatal hepatic necrosis can occur.*[272,301]

Fluconazole and itraconazole produce the same adverse effects. The incidence of adverse effects with fluconazole is 16%, about half of them being gastrointestinal complaints and headache and skin rash being the next most frequent.[236] These effects are rarely severe enough to require termination of treatment. Elevations in hepatic enzymes occur in less than 5% of the general population receiving fluconazole, with a somewhat higher incidence occurring in immunocompromised patients.[302]

Treatment with itraconazole is accompanied by gastrointestinal disturbances, dizziness, pruritus, and headache in approximately 7% of patients treated for 4 weeks, with the incidence increasing to 17.7% in patients treated for more than a month.[303] The adverse effects are generally transient and of mild to moderate severity. Itraconazole treatment is accompanied by transient increases in hepatic enzymes in 1%–7% of patients[304] receiving continuous therapy, and rarely hepatic toxicity requires drug discontinuation.

The main difference between the toxicity of ketoconazole and the newer triazole drugs relates to the effect on steroid synthesis. Inasmuch as the interaction of azoles with C-14 alpha demethylase in fungal cells accounts for their fungicidal activity, a similar interaction with mammalian P-450s accounts for some major toxicities associated with this group of drugs.

A number of male patients receiving ketoconazole have developed gynecomastia with breast pain.[305] The breast pain abates despite continuation of therapy, although gynecomastia persists. Gynecomastia results from inhibition of testosterone synthesis. In male volunteers it has been shown that a therapeutic dose of ketoconazole is followed by a reversible drop in circulating testosterone (to 14% of baseline by 8 h after a 600 mg dose) and a rise in luteinizing hormone (to 145% of baseline by 8 h).[306] It has also been shown that therapeutic concentrations of ketoconazole markedly inhibit testosterone synthesis by Leydig cells isolated from rat testes.[306] Ketoconazole inhibits 14-demethylation of lanosterol, thus preventing its conversion to ergosterol in fungi and to cholesterol in mammalian cells.[307] Given such a mechanism, the synthesis of a variety of steroids should be affected. In humans the cortisol response to adrenocorticotropic hormone (ACTH) is significantly inhibited by 4 h after a 400 or 600 mg dose of ketoconazole.[308] At 1 µg/ml, ketoconazole inhibits ACTH-stimulated corticosterone production by isolated rat adrenal cells.[308] Although ketoconazole interferes with ACTH tests, the drug has not been associated with the production of addisonian symptoms. Some patients may complain of decreased libido and it is possible that long-term therapy with higher doses will produce oligospermia as a result of decreased androgen synthesis. By contrast, fluconazole and itraconazole, when given in recommended doses, do not inhibit steroidogenesis.[309,310] Although several patients have noted impotence, usually reversible, while receiving 200–600 mg of itraconazole daily, their plasma testosterone concentrations were normal. A few patients taking itraconazole have had hypertension, hypokalemia, or pedal edema.[304] The basis for these effects is unknown but, like impotence, they usually resolve after stopping the drug.

New Azole Agents

Several new azole antifungal drugs are under development,[2] and it is hoped that these new derivatives will be more potent at inhibiting the target enzyme, have an expanded antifungal spectrum, and have improved oral availability. Voriconazole (UK-109496) is a triazole with antifungal activity against many opportunistic fungi, including *Aspergillus* spp., *Candida krusei*, and *Candida glabrata*, that are resistant to fluconazole,[311] and preliminary studies have shown efficacy against serious fungal infections, including aspergillosis. Saperconazole is a lipophilic, poorly water-soluble, fluorinated triazole with a structure very similar to that of itraconazole. It has potent broad spectrum antifungal activity, with in vitro activity against *Aspergillus* spp. greater than that of itraconazole and at least equivalent to that of amphotericin B.[312] ZD-0870 is a triazole that is effective against fluconazole-resistant *Candida* spp. and other opportunistic fungi, and it has been effective in the treatment of experimental *Trypanosoma cruzi* infections.[313,314]

Drug Interactions

Most drug interactions with the azoles occur by one of two mechanisms: either inhibition of absorption of the azole, leading to decreased bioavailability, or interference with the activity of hepatic microsomal enzymes, which alters the metabolism of the azole, the interacting drug, or both. Concomitant administration of drugs that reduce gastric acidity, such as cimetidine, antacids, proton pump inhibitors (e.g., omeprazole), and didanosine, results in lower concentrations of the azoles because of decreased absorption.[315] Drugs that increase the metabolism of azoles include isoniazid, phenytoin, and rifampin.[4] The azoles increase the plasma concentrations of cyclosporine, digoxin, phenytoin, terfenadine, astemizole, and warfarin by inhibiting their metabolism.[4] All three of the systemically administered azoles are potent inhibitors of P-450s. Although ketoconazole has a greater in vitro inhibitory effect than itraconazole and fluconazole on P-4503A4, the enzyme that catalyzes the conversion of cyclosporine to its major metabolites, all three azoles have caused clinically important increases in plasma cyclosporine concentration.[316]

Iodide

Potassium iodide has been used for many years to treat lymphocutaneous sporotrichosis.[317] It is not useful in treating extracutaneous sporotrichosis, for which amphotericin B or itraraconazole are the drugs of choice. In tropical countries iodide is also used to treat subcutaneous phycomycosis caused by *Basidiobolus haptosporus* or *B. meristosporus*. The mechanism of the antifungal action of iodide is unknown. A solution of potassium iodide (1 g/ml) is taken orally three times a day. Adults begin with 3 ml/day and increase the amount slowly to 9 to 12 ml/day, as tolerance permits.[317] The most common adverse effects are bitter taste, gastrointestinal discomfort, excessive lacrimation, swelling of the salivary glands, and acneiform rash.

Griseofulvin

The dermatophytes and yeasts, such as *Candida albicans*, are responsible for most superficial fungal infections. The dermophytic infections are treated either with topical drugs or with one of three oral agents, ketoconazole, griseofulvin, or terbinafine. Griseofulvin has been isolated from a number

Griseofulvin

of molds of the genus *Penicillium*. The drug is inactive against bacteria and against yeasts and fungi that cause systemic disease. Its use in chemotherapy is limited to the chemotherapy of infections of the skin, hair, and nails caused by the dermatophytes. These fungi include members of the genera *Microsporum*, *Epidermophyton*, and *Trichophyton*. The antifungal action and pharmacology of griseofulvin has been reviewed by Davies.[318]

Mechanism of Action

Although it is not clear whether the therapeutic use of griseofulvin has a predominantly fungistatic or fungicidal action, experiments with cultured fungi demonstrate that it can act as a fungicide. For griseofulvin to exert a killing effect, the organism must be growing.[319] The drug is concentrated as much as 100-fold by *Microsporum gypseum*.[320] The uptake of griseofulvin by fungi is energy dependent, and correlated with the sensitivity of the organism to the drug.[321] When growing fungi are exposed to griseofulvin, the total DNA and phosphorus content increases, but there is no change in protein, carbohydrate, lipid, and RNA content.[322] The drug causes gross morphological changes in the fungus, including the production of binucleate and multinucleate cells.[323] Thus, one of the major cellular effects of griseofulvin is inhibition of fungal mitosis.

At high concentrations, griseofulvin causes metaphase arrest in mammalian cells growing in vitro. Much of the information on the mechanism of action of griseofulvin has come from studies of the effect of the drug on mammalian cells. The gross effect of griseofulvin is similar to that of colchicine; the mitotic spindle is disrupted.[324,325] Upon entering the cell, griseofulvin binds to soluble protein.[326] The principle cellular receptors for griseofulvin are the microtubules, the proteins that form the mitotic spindle. These spindle fibers are long strands consisting of bundles of microtubules that connect the two centrioles of the dividing cell; some spindle fibers connect the kinetochores of the chromosomes to the centrioles. The spindle fibers determine the appropriate segregation of the sister chromatids to opposite poles during anaphase. In telophase, the microtubules disappear when the nuclear envelope forms. Several drugs, including colchicine, vinblastine, and vincristine, bind to the microtubules to inhibit mitosis.[327]

Microtubules are polymers made up of a 120,000 molecular-weight protein called *tubulin* (Fig. 12–5).[328] Tubulin consists of two nonidentical protomeric subunits, α-tubulin and β-tubulin, each having a molecular weight of approximately 54,000. In addition to polymerized tubulin dimers, other proteins are associated with the microtubule to make a complex unit that participates in a variety of cellular functions, such as cell locomotion and the movement of intracellular organelles, in addition to mitosis. It is clear that griseofulvin can interact with tubulin that has been purified free of microtubule-associated proteins and block the polymerization of tubulin into microtubules.[329–331] This implies that griseofulvin may act in a manner similar to that of other drugs that block microtubule assembly, although it is clear that the griseofulvin binding site on tubulin is different from those occupied by colchicine or the Vinca alkaloids.[332]

In addition to blocking microtubule assembly, griseofulvin may also affect microtubule function. During the contraction of spindle fibers in mitosis, for example, it may be necessary for adjacent microtubules to

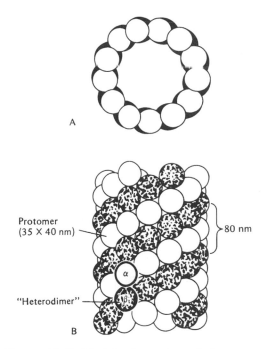

Figure 12–5. Model of a microtubule, cross-sectional (A) and longitudinal (B) views. There are 13 protofilaments in each microtubule. The protofilaments are made up of heterodimers, and each heterodimer, in turn, consists of 35 × 40 nm globular protein subunits (protomers) of α- and β-tubulin. (From Bryan.[328])

slide over one another in order to segregate the chromosomes in opposite poles of the cell.[333] It has been suggested that this sliding process, which would require the action of microtubule-associated proteins, is also inhibited by griseofulvin.[334] There is evidence that griseofulvin binds to a microtubule-associated protein[335] in addition to its binding to tubulin itself. Mutant Chinese hamster ovary cells have been isolated that are resistant to griseofulvin and that contain altered β-tubulin.[336] These mutants are cross-resistant to colchicine and vinblastine, suggesting that the mutation may affect a critical interaction between β-tubulin and some other component of microtubule assembly such as α-tubulin or microtubule-associated protein.

Although we have focused on the effect of griseofulvin on mitosis in this discussion, inhibition of microtubule assembly can interfere with other cellular functions as well. The first effects of griseofulvin reported in fungi were gross changes in the morphology of hyphae which curled in the presence of the drug; before the drug structure was identified, this was referred to as *curling factor*.[337] Microtubules are involved in the maintenance of cell shape and it is likely that the morphological changes caused by the drug are a direct result of the drug-microtubule interaction.

Dermatophytes that are resistant to griseofulvin have been selected in vitro, but the mechanism of resistance has not been determined and it is not known if resistance develops during therapy.[318] In some cases, therapeutic failure has correlated with the presence of a high minimum inhibitory concentration in vitro[338] but, in general, sensitivity testing of dermatophytes has not proven to be a useful guide in therapy.[318]

Pharmacokinetics

The usual dosage of griseofulvin for adults is 500 mg of the microsize preparation per day taken as two or four divided doses. With widespread lesions, therapy may begin with 1 g/day with subsequent reduction to 500 mg/day. Griseofulvin is essentially insoluble in water and absorption of the drug from the gastrointestinal tract is improved as the size of the drug particles is made smaller. The ultrafine particle form is more rapidly, completely, and uniformly absorbed and it is administered at one-half the dosage (250 mg/day) of the microsize form.[339] The absorption of griseofulvin is increased when the drug is taken with a fatty meal.[340,341] In animals, much higher plasma levels are obtained when the drug is given in an oil water emulsion.[342] It is not known whether the drug itself passes through the mucosa of small intestine by diffusion or whether it is taken up in the form of a mixed micelle with fat. At least 50% of the ultrafine particle form of the drug is absorbed from the intestine.[343] Griseofulvin, applied topically, penetrates into all levels of the stratum corneum, but (for unknown reasons) it is only effective in treating fungal infection of the skin when given orally.[344]

The dermatophytic fungi reside in superficial keratinized tissue, and it is the distribution of the drug into this compartment that is particularly important with regard to its therapeutic effect. Griseofulvin binds to keratin and high concentrations of the drug occur in the stratum corneum, the outermost layer of the epidermis that contains the keratinized cells. There are apparently two routes by which the drug reaches the skin surface: *(1)* by passive diffusion in the epidermal fluid and *(2)* by secretion in the sweat.[345] After repeated administration of 500 mg of griseofulvin every 12 h, the plasma level is about 1.4 µg/ml and levels in the skin of the palm vary from 12 to 22 µg/g tissue.[346] The minimal inhibitory concentration for common sensitive dermatophytes in vitro is less than 2 µg/ml.[89,318] Griseofulvin binding by keratin is of high enough affinity to account for selective localization in the skin, but it is clearly reversible. As the blood concentration of the drug decreases, the concentration of the drug in the stratum corneum declines at roughly the same rate.[346] The average course of therapy for tinea of the body is 3–6 weeks. Infections of intertriginous areas and the thick skin of the palms and the soles require 4–8 weeks of therapy.

Two other sites of dermatophyte infection of special interest are the hair and the nails. Researchers discovered some time ago that when guinea pigs with ringworm infection were treated for a few days with oral griseofulvin, the fungus was eradicated from the hair follicle and the base of the hair shaft but the tips of the hair remained infected.[347] Subsequently, it was shown that orally administered griseofulvin became associated with hair.[348] Thus it seems that the griseofulvin becomes associated with keratin in the hair follicle, and as the hair grows, fungi are not able to grow in the griseofulvin-containing region. This unique aspect of the drug distribution is an important component of its clinical effectiveness in treating infection by dermatophytic fungi.

In addition to the action on microtubules, there is another biological effect of griseofulvin that may contribute to its clinical effectiveness. Some dermatophytes produce enzymes that digest keratin,[349] and these keratinases may be important in helping the fungus penetrate and parasitize keratinous structures. Some data suggest that griseofulvin-containing hair may not be as good a substrate for these enzymes as normal hair.[350]

Dermatophyte infection of the nails requires long-term griseofulvin therapy. The duration of drug administration is in part determined by the time required for complete growth of the nail. The drug probably becomes associated with keratin as the nail is being formed. Apparently, griseofulvin cannot diffuse through the nail structure in the same way that it can pass through the layers of the skin, and fungi continue to infect the portion of the nail that was formed before initiation of therapy. Infection of the fingernails requires therapy for 3–6 months and infection of the toe nails, 6–12 months and sometimes longer.

The distribution properties of griseofulvin are uniquely appropriate to its clinical use in dermatophyte infections. Chemotherapy requires a minimum of several weeks (this varies with the location of the infection), but the patient's symptoms are usually relieved within a few days.

The half-life of orally administered radiolabeled griseofulvin is 22 h.[343] About 40% of the radioactivity is excreted in the feces and the remainder in the urine.[351] About 50% of a dose of griseofulvin is excreted in the urine within 5 days, mostly as 6-demethylgriseofulvin and its glucuronide, with a minor amount as other metabolites.[351] Griseofulvin is metabolized by microsomal enzymes in the liver; in the rat, the rate of metabolism is increased by coadministration of phenobarbital.[351] In humans, concomitant administration of clinically usual doses of phenobarbital also reduces blood levels of griseofulvin, but this may not be due to an increased rate of metabolism. Studies in subjects receiving griseofulvin intravenously or orally indicate that the major effect of phenobarbital in humans is to decrease the gastrointestinal absorption of griseofulvin.[352] Griseofulvin itself apparently increases the rate of metabolism of the coumarin anticoagulants and diminishes the effect of these drugs.[353] Adjustment of the anticoagulant dosage may be required.

Adverse Effects of Griseofulvin

A common side effect of griseofulvin therapy is headache. This may occur in as many as 10% of patients. The headache usually disappears within a few days despite continuation of therapy. Rarely, lapses of memory, impairment of judgment, and impairment of performance of routine duties have been reported, and for this reason, other agents should be used to treat pilots and bus drivers. Griseofulvin occasionally causes gastrointestinal distress, skin rashes, and paresthesias. Superinfection with *Candida* can occur during therapy. Leukopenia has been reported, and occasional blood counts are advisable during the first few weeks of therapy. Griseofulvin is reported to potentiate the effect of alcohol.[318]

Griseofulvin increases porphyrin excretion in humans[354] and the porphyrogenic effect has been studied in a mouse model. The increased level of porphyrins results from the induction of increased levels of δ-aminolevulinic acid (ALA) synthetase, the rate-limiting enzyme in porphyrin metabolism.[355] The exact site of griseofulvin action in the heme pathway is not completely clear. It has been shown that administration of griseofulvin to mice and rats causes the accumulation of N-methylprotoporphyrins, which inhibit ferrochetalase, the terminal enzyme in the pathway.[356] Other porphyrogenic compounds also cause the accumulation of inhibitory N-methylporphyrins.[357] It has been proposed that inhibition of ferrochetalase results in decreased heme formation and less heme-mediated feedback repression of ALA synthetase.[358] As the end of the heme pathway is inhibited and the beginning is stimulated, porphyrin intermediates accumulate. Griseofulvin-induced protoporphyria in mice is similar to human protoporphyria in that there is cutaneous photosensitivity, liver damage, and accumulation of protoporphyrin in the liver.[339] Although the effect of griseofulvin on porphyrin metabolism in humans is not usually of clinical consequence,[360] in patients with porphyria, the drug can increase urinary pyrrole excretion and precipitate acute episodes of symptomatology.[318] Griseofulvin rarely produces hepatotoxicity and occasionally photosensitivity in patients without a history of porphyria. The drug is contraindicated in patients with porphyria or hepatocellular failure.

As mentioned earlier, griseofulvin in high doses causes metaphase arrest in mammalian cells growing in vitro. Like colchicine, griseofulvin has an anti-inflammatory effect, and it has been shown to produce some relief in patients with acute gouty arthritis and the shoulder-hand syndrome of rheumatoid arthritis. As with any drug inhibiting mammalian cell division, there was initially some concern over the possibility that griseofulvin might have an adverse effect on rapidly dividing systems like the cells of the bone marrow and spermatogonia. The available evidence, however, supports the conclusion that griseofulvin at the doses used clinically does not affect spermatogenesis.[361] At very high doses, the drug is teratogenic in mice and cats.[362,363] Although there is no evidence of teratogenicity in humans, it is prudent to withhold the drug from pregnant women. Mice fed griseofulvin form hepatocellular aggregates composed of intermediate filaments which resemble the Mallory bodies that occur in human alcoholic liver disease.[364,365] Prolonged exposure to very high levels of griseofulvin is associated with a significant incidence of hepatomas in mice and thyroid tumors in rats.[366,367]

New Systemic Antifungal Agents

Several new antifungal drugs are being developed; these include the pneumocandins and papulocandins, which are echinocandin analogs that are very potent antifungals in vitro and seem to be fungicidal in vivo.[1,368] These fungicidal drugs inhibit cell wall synthesis by inhibiting β-1,3-glucan synthetase,

and because this enzyme is not present in mammalian cells, the effect of these drugs is highly specific. The compounds developed to date are much less effective when given orally than when given parenterally, and they are not effective against *Cryptococcus neoformans*, which could be a major limitation.[1] Another class of antifungals, the nikkomycins, are potent inhibitors of chitin synthase, which is crucial to fungal cell wall synthesis. Both in vitro and animal studies have shown that nikkomycin Z has excellent activity against *Coccidioides immitis, Blastomyces dermatitidis,* and *Histoplasma capsulatum,* and it may be synergistic when administered in combination with other drugs active against *Candida* spp.[119,369] The pradimicins are another class of antifungals, that act through calcium-dependent binding to mannans in the fungal cell wall and are fungicidal against *Candida* and *Aspergillus* spp.[370,371]

Topical Drugs Used to Treat Superficial Fungal Infection

Several compounds are employed for the topical treatment of superficial fungal infections in addition to those already discussed (nystatin, amphotericin B, and azoles).

Undecylenic Acid

Undecylenic acid is one of a number of fatty acids possessing antifungal activity. The reason for this activity is not known. Undecylenic acid is sold in various proprietary preparations for the treatment of tinea pedis. The only side effect is a transient burning sensation on application. A 6-week course of therapy with 2% undecylenic acid powder produces clinical and mycological cures in about 50% of cases of tinea pedis.[372] It is not as effective in treating tinea pedis as tolnaftate, haloprogin, or imidazoles.[373]

Tolnaftate

Tolnaftate is used in the treatment of a wider spectrum of dermatophytic infections than is undecylenic acid. It is quite effective in the

Tolnaftate

treatment of infection with *Trichophyton rubrum*, a fungus that is often resistant to other topical agents and to griseofulvin. *Candida* spp. are not sensitive. The mechanism of action of tolnaftate is unknown. There are no known adverse effects. Treatment of dermatophytic infections for 4 weeks yielded a cure rate of 93% with tolnaftate and 95% with clotrimazole.[374]

Haloprogin

Haloprogin is a halogenated phenolic ether with in vitro and in vivo activity against dermatophytes that is equivalent to that of tolnaftate.[375] Unlike tolnaftate, haloprogin is active against *Candida* species but it is less active in vitro than clotrimazole or miconazole.[376] In a double-blind clinical trial, topi-

Haloprogin

cal therapy with haloprogin was found to be as effective as topical miconazole in treating pityriasis versicolor and dermatophyte and *Candida* infections.[377] Haloprogin was not tolerated as well as miconazole; the chief side effects are irritation, burning sensations, and peeling of the skin.[377] The mechanism of action is not known. Haloprogin is used principally to treat tinea pedis.

Imidazoles and Triazoles for Topical Use

Indications for the topical use of the azoles include ringworm, tinea versicolor, and mucocutaneous candidiasis. Resistance to imidazoles or triazoles is very rare among the fungi that cause these superficial mycoses. Among the topical azoles are econazole, terconazole, butoconazole, tioconazole, oxi-

conazole, and sulconazole, and selection of one of these drugs is largely based on cost and availability. Their mechanism of action is similar to that of the other imidazoles, and they are available in creams, lotions, and solutions for the topical treatment of candidiasis and dermatophyte infections.[378]

Ciclopirox Olamine

Ciclopirox is a broad spectrum antifungal agent that is fungicidal to *Candida albicans*, *Epidermophyton floccosum*, *Microsporum canis*, *Trichphyton mentagrophytes*, and *Trichophyton rubrum*.[379] After application to the skin, it penetrates into hair follicles and sebaceous glands and it also penetrates through the epidermis into the systemic circulation. It is available as a cream and lotion for the treatment of cutaneous candidiasis and dermatophyte infections, and it occasionally causes hypersensitivity reactions.

Allylamines

The allylamines are a group of synthetic agents effective in the topical and oral treatment of dermatophytoses and superficial forms of candidiasis. Like the azoles, the allylamines inhibit fungal ergosterol bosynthesis but act through inhibition of squalene-2,3-epoxidase, which is not a P-450. These drugs are fungicidal for most filamentous fungi and they concentrate in the nails and stratum corneum.[380,381] Three members of this group—naftifine, terbinafine and butenafine—are clinically useful. Naftifine is used for the topical treatment of dermatophytoses, including tinea corporis and tinea cruris, but it is less effective in the treatment of cutaneous candidiasis. Terbinafine is effective in tinea corporis, tinea cruris, and tinea pedis. Terbinafine is less active against *Candida* spp. and *Malassezia furfur*. The allylamines are available for topical administration as creams and terbinafine is available for oral use in the treatment of nail infections by dermatophytes. Adverse effects with oral terbinafine appear to be minimal and include most commonly taste perversion and gastrointestinal disturbances and rarely hepatitis and rash.[119] Allergic contact dermatitis has been reported with the topical preparations.

Nystatin

Nystatin is a polyene antifungal like amphotericin B and has the same mechanism of action. However, nystatin is more toxic and is not used systemically. Nystatin is not absorbed from the gastointestinal tract, skin, or vagina. It is used only for treating candidiasis, and it is supplied in preparations intended for cutaneous, vaginal, or oral administration for this purpose.

REFERENCES

1. Graybill, J. The future of antifungal therapy. *Clin Infect. Dis.* 1996;22(Suppl. 2):5166.
2. Groll, A., S. Piscitelli, and T. Walsh. Clinical pharmacology of systemic antifungal agents: A comprehensive review of agents in clinical use, current investigational compounds, and putative targets for antifungal drug development. *Adv. Pharmacol.* 1998;44:343.
3. Kauffman, C., and P. Carver. Antifungal agents in the 1990s: current status and future developments. *Drugs* 1997;53:539.
4. Como, J., and W. Dismukes. Oral azole drugs as systemic antifungal therapy. N. Engl. J. Med. 1994; 330:263.
5. Hamilton-Miller, J. M. T. Chemistry and biology of the polyene macrolide antibiotics. *Bacterial Rev.* 1973;37:166.
6. Kinsky, S. C. Antibiotic interactions with model membranes. *Annu. Rev. Pharmacol.* 1970;10:119.
7. Holz, R. W. Polyene antibiotics: nystatin, amphotericin B, and filipin. In *Antibiotics V-2*, ed. by F. E. Hahn. New York: Springer-Verlag, 1979, pp. 313–340.
8. Marini, F., P. Arnow, and J. O. Lampen. The effect of monovalent cations on the inhibition of yeast metabolism by nystatin. *J. Gen. Microbiol.* 1961;24:51.
9. Lampen, J. O. Interference by polyenic antifungal antibiotics (especially nystatin and filipin) with specific membrane functions. In *Biochemical Studies of Antimicrobial Drugs*, ed. by B. A. Newton and P. E. Reynolds. London: Cambridge University Press, 1966, pp. 111–130.
10. Liras, P., and J. O. Lampen. Sequence of candicidin action on yeast cells. *Biochim. Biophys. Acta* 1974;372:141.
11. Liras, P., and J. O. Lampen. Protection by K$^+$ and Mg^{2+} of growth and macromolecule synthesis in candicidin-treated yeast. *Biochim. Biophys. Acta* 1974; 374:159.
12. Brajtburg, J., G. Medoff, G. S. Kobayashi, and S. Elberg. Influence of extracellular K$^+$ or Mg^{2+} on the stages of the antifungal effects of amphotericin B and filipin. *Antimicrob. Agents Chemother.* 1980;18:593.
13. Kerridge, D., T. Y. Koh, and A. M. Johnson.

The interaction of amphotericin B methyl ester with protoplasts of *Candida albicans*. *J. Gen. Microbiol.* 1976;96:117.
14. Lampen, J. O., and P. M. Arnow. Significance of nystatin uptake for its antifungal action. *Proc. Soc. Exp. Biol. Med.* 1959;101:792.
15. Lampen, J. O., P. M. Arnow, Z. Borowska, and A. I. Laskin. Location and role of sterol at nystatin-binding sites. *J. Bacteriol.* 1962;84:1152.
16. Kinsky, S. C. Nystatin binding by protoplasts and a particulate fraction of *Neurospora crassa*, and a basis for the selective toxicity of polyene antifungal antibiotics. *Proc. Natl. Acad. Sci. U.S.A.* 1962;48: 1049.
17. Razin, S., M. Argaman, and J. Avigan. Chemical composition of Mycoplasma cells and membranes. *J. Gen. Microbiol.* 1963;33:477.
18. Feingold; D. S. The action of amphotericin B on *Mycoplasma laidlawii*. *Biochem. Biophys. Res. Commun.* 1965;19:261.
19. De Kruijff, B., W. J. Gerritsen, A. Oerlemans, R. A. Demel, and L. L. M. van Deenen. Polyene antibiotic-sterol interactions in membranes of *Acholeplasma laidlawii* cells and lecithin liposomes. I. Specificity of the membrane permeability changes induced by the polyene antibiotics. *Biochim. Biophys. Acta* 1974; 339:30.
20. De Kruijff, B., and R. A. Demel. Polyene antibiotic-sterol interactions in membranes of *Acholeplasma laidlawii* cells and lecithin liposomes. III. Molecular structure of the polyene antibiotic-cholesterol complexes. *Biochim. Biophys. Acta* 1974;339:57.
21. Cass, A., A. Finkelstein, and V. Krespi. The ion permeability induced in thin lipid membranes by the polyene antibiotics nystatin and amphotericin B. *J. Gen. Physiol.* 1970;56:100.
22. Marty, A., and A. Finkelstein. Pores formed in lipid bilayer membranes by nystatin. Differences in its one-sided and two-sided action. *J. Gen. Physiol.* 1975; 65:515.
23. Ermishkin, L. N., K. M. Kasumov, and V. M. Potzeluyev. Single ionic channels induced in lipid bilayers by polyene antibiotics amphotericin B and nystatine. *Nature* 1976;262:698.
24. Andreoli, T. E. The structure and function of amphotericin B-cholesterol pores in lipid bilayer membranes. *Ann. N.Y. Acad. Sci.* 1974;235:448.
25. Van Hoogevest, P., and B. De Kruijff. Effect of amphotericin B on cholesterol-containing liposomes of egg phosphatidylcholine and didocosenoyl phosphatidylcholine. A refinement of the model for the formation of pores by amphotericin B in membranes. *Biochim. Biophys. Acta* 1978;511:397.
26. M. E. Kleinberg: One-sided pores formed by nystatin in lipid bilayer membranes. Ph.D. Thesis, Yeshiva University, 1983.
27. Finkelstein, A., and R. Holz. Aqueous pores created in thin lipid membranes by the polyene antibiotics nystatin and amphotericin B. In *Membranes*, Vol. 2, ed. by G. Eisenman. New York: Marcel Dekker, 1973, pp. 377–408.
28. Holz, R., and A. Finkelstein. The water and nonelectrolyte permeability induced in thin lipid mem-

branes by the polyene antibiotics nystatin and amphotericin B. *J. Gen. Physiol.* 1970;56:125.

29. Borisova, M. P., L. N. Ermishkin, and A. Y. Silberstein. Mechanism of blockage of amphotericin B channels in a lipid bilayer. *Biochim. Biophys. Acta* 1979;553:450.

30. Perkins, W. R., S. Minchey, L. Boni, C. Swenson, M. Popescu, R. Pasternack, and A. Janoff. Amphotericin B phospholipid interactions responsible for reduced mammalian cell toxicity. *Biochem. Biophys. Acta* 1992;1107:271.

31. Legrand, P., E. A. Romero, B. I. Cohen, and J. Bolard. Effects of aggregation and solvent on the toxicity of amphotericin B to human erythrocytes. *Antimicrob. Agents Chemother.* 1992;36:2518.

32. Lambing, H. E., B. D. Wolf, and S. C. Hartsel. Temperature effects on the aggregation state and activity of amphotericin B. *Biochem. Biophys. Acta* 1993;1152:185.

33. Brajtburg, J., S. Elberg, D. Schwartz, A Vertut-Croquin, D. Schlesinger, G. Kobayashi, and G. Medoff. Involvement of oxidative damage in erythrocyte lysis induced by amphotericin B. *Antimicrob. Agents Chemother.* 1985;27:172.

34. Georgeopapadakou, N. H., and T. Walsh. Antifungal agents: chemotherapeutic targets and immunologic targets. *Antimicrob. Agents Chemother.* 1996; 40:279.

35. Lamy-Freund, M. T., V. F. N. Ferreira, and S. J. Schreier. Mechanism of inactivation of the polyene antibiotic amphotericin B. Evidence for radical formation in the process of autioxidation. *J. Antibiot.* 1985;38:753.

36. Brajtburg, J., S. Elberg, J. Boland, G. Kobayashi, R. Levy, R. Ostlund, D. Schlessinger, and G. Medoff. Interaction of plasma proteins and lipoproteins with amphotericin B. *J. Infect. Dis.* 1984;149:986.

37. Hartsel, S., and J. Bolard. Amphotericin B: new life for an old drug. *Trends Pharmacol. Sci.* 1996;17:445.

38. Verdut-Doi, A., S. I. Ohnishi, and J. Bolard. The endocytic process in CHO cells, a toxic pathway of the polyene antibiotic amphotericin B. *Antimicrob. Agents Chemother.* 1994;38:2373.

39. Koldin, M. H., G. S. Kobayashi, J. Brajtburg, and G. Medoff. Effects of elevation of serum cholesterol and administration of amphotericin B complexed to lipoproteins on amphotericin B-induced toxicity in rabbits. *Antimicrob. Agents Chemother.* 1985;28:144.

40. Barwicz, J., S. Christian, and I. Gruda. Effects of the aggregation state of amphotericin on its toxicity to mice. *Antimicrob. Agents Chemother.* 1992;36:2310.

41. Kinsky, S. C. Comparative responses of mammalian erythrocytes and microbial protoplasts to polyene antibiotics and vitamin A. *Arch. Biochem. Biophys.* 1963;102:180.

42. Klimov, A. N., A. A. Nikiforova, and A. M. Tchistiakova. Inhibition of cholesterol esterification by polyene antibiotics in blood plasma. *Biochim. Biophys. Acta* 1975;380:76.

43. Butler, W. T., and E. Cotlove. Increased permeability of human erythrocytes induced by amphotericin B. *J. Infect. Dis.* 1971;123:341.

44. McBride, J. A., and H. S. Jacob. Abnormal kinetics of red cell membrane cholesterol in acanthocytes: studies in genetic and experimental abetalipoproteinemia and in spur cell anemia. *Br. J. Hematol.* 1970;18:383.

45. Butler, W. T., D. W. Alling, and E. Cotlove. Potassium loss from human erythrocytes exposed to amphotericin B. *Proc. Soc. Exp. Biol. Med.* 1965;118:297.

46. Malewicz, B., H. M. Jenkin, and E. Borowski. Dissociation between the induction of potassium efflux and cytostatic activity of polyene macrolides in mammalian cells. *Antimicrob. Agents Chemother.* 1980;17:699.

47. Kessel, D., and H. B. Bosmann. On the characteristics of actinomycin D resistance in L5178Y cells. *Cancer Res.* 1970;30:2695.

48. Peterson, R. H. F., J. A. O'Neil, and J. L. Biedler. Some biochemical properties of Chinese hamster cells sensitive and resistant to actinomycin D. *J. Cell Biol.* 1974;63:773.

49. H. Polet: Role of the cell membrane in the uptake of ^{3}H-actinomycin D by mammalian cells in vitro. *J. Pharmacol. Exp. Ther.* 1975;192:270.

50. Medoff, J., G. Medoff, M. N. Goldstein, D. Schlessinger, and G. S. Kobayashi. Amphotericin B-induced sensitivity to actinomycin D in drug-resistant HeLa cells. *Cancer Res.* 1975;35:2548.

51. Kumar, V. K., G. Medoff, G. S. Kobayashi, and D. Schlessinger. Amphotericin B enhances uptake of *Escherichia coli* DNA into HeLa cells. *Nature* 1974;250:323.

52. Little, J. R., S. H. Stein, and K. D. Little. Amphotericin B-a model murine immunostimulant. In: *Antibiotics and Host Immunity*, ed. by H. Szentivany, H. Friedman, G. Gillissen. New York: Plenum Press, 1987, pp. 253–263.

53. Lin, S. H., G. Medoff and G. S. Kobayashi. Effects of amphotericin B on macrophages and their precursor cells. *Antimicrob. Agents Chemother.* 1977;111:154–158.

54. Hauser, W. E., and J. S. Remington. Effect of amphotericin B on natural cell activity in vitro. *J. Antimicrob. Chemother.* 1983;11:257–262.

55. Readio, J. D., and R. Bittman. Equilibrium binding of amphotericin B and its methyl ester and borate complex to sterols. *Biochim. Biophys. Acta* 1982;685:219.

56. Kotler-Brajtburg, J., H. D. Price, G. Medoff, D. Schlessinger, and G. S. Kobayashi. Molecular basis for the selective toxicity of amphotericin B for yeast and filipin for animal cells. *Antimicrob. Agents Chemother.* 1974;5:377.

57. Gale, E. F. The release of potassium ions from *Candida albicans* in the presence of polyene antibiotics. *J. Gen. Microbiol.* 1974;80:451.

58. Archer, D. B. Effect of the lipid composition of *Mycoplasma mycoides* subspecies *capri* and phosphatidyl choline vesicles upon the action of polyene antibiotics. *Biochim. Biophys. Acta* 1976;436:68.

59. Medoff, G., M. Comfort, and G. S. Kobayashi. Synergistic action of amphotericin B and 5-fluorocytosine against yeast-like organisms. *Proc. Soc. Exp. Biol. Med.* 1971;138:571.

60. Medoff, G., G. S. Kobayashi, C. N. Kwan, D. Schlessinger, and P. Venkov. Potentiation of rifampicin and 5-fluorocytosine as antifungal antibiotics by amphotericin B. *Proc. Natl. Acad Sci. U.S.A.* 1972;69: 196.

61. Montgomerie, J. Z., J. E. Edwards, and L. B. Guze: Synergism of amphotericin B and 5-fluorocytosine for *Candida* species. *J. Infect. Dis.* 1975; 132:82.

62. Block, E. R., and J. E. Bennett. The combined effect of 5-fluorocytosine and amphotericin B in the therapy of murine cryptococcosis. *Proc. Soc. Exp. Biol. Med.* 1973;142:476.

63. Titsworth, E., and E. Grunberg. Chemotherapeutic activity of 5-fluorocytosine and amphotericin B against *Candida albicans* in mice. *Antimicrob. Agents Chemother.* 1973;4:306.

64. Rabinovich, S., B. D. Shaw, T. Bryant, and S. T. Donta. Effect of 5-fluorocytosine and amphotericin B on *Candida albicans* infection in mice. *J. Infect. Dis.* 1974;130:28.

65. Utz, J. P., I. L. Garriques, M. A. Sande, J. F. Warner, G. L. Mandel, R. F. McGehee, R. J. Duma, and S. Shadomy. Therapy of cryptococcosis with a combination of flucytosine and amphotericin B. *J. Infect. Dis.* 1975;132:368.

66. Bennett, J. E., W. E. Dismukes, R. J. Duma, G. Medoff, M. A. Sande, H. Gallis, J. Leonard, B. T. Fields, M. Bradshaw, H. Haywood, Z. A. McGee, T. R. Cate, G. C. Cobbs, J. F. Warner, and D. W. Alling. A comparison of amphotericin B alone and combined with flucytosine in the treatment of cryptococcal meningitis. *N. Engl. J. Med.* 1979;301:126.

67. Edwards, J. E., J. Morrison, D. K. Henderson, and J. Z. Montgomerie. Combined effect of amphotericin B and rifampin on *Candida* species. *Antimicrob. Agents Chemother.* 1980;17:484.

68. Kobayashi, G. S., S. C. Cheung, D. Schlessinger, and G. Medoff. Effects of rifamycin derivatives, alone and in combination with amphotericin B, against *Histoplasma capsulatum. Antimicrob. Agents Chemother.* 1974;5:16.

69. Rifkind, D., E. D. Crowder, and R. N. Hyland. In vitro inhibition of *Coccidoides immitis* strains with amphotericin B plus rifampin. *Antimicrob. Agents Chemother.* 1974;6:783.

70. Lew, M. A., K. M. Beckett, and M. J. Levin. Combined activity of minocycline and amphotericin B in vitro against medically important yeasts. *Antimicrob. Agents Chemother.* 1978;14:465.

71. Graybill, J. R., and L. Mitchell. Treatment of murine cryptococcosis with minocycline and amphotericin B. *Sabouraudia* 1980;18:137.

72. Schacter, L. P., R. J. Owellen, H. K. Rathbun, and B. Buchanan: Antagonism between miconzaole and amphotericin B. *Lancet* 1976;2:318.

73. Schaffner, A., and P. G. Frick. The effect of ketoconazole on amphotericin B in a model of disseminated aspergillosis. *J. Infect. Dis* 1985;151:902.

74. Dupont, B., and E. Drouhet. In vitro synergy and antagonism of antifungal agents against yeast-like fungi. *Postgrad. Med. J.* 1979;55:683.

75. Borgers, M. Mechanism of action of antifungal drugs, with special reference to the imidazole derivatives. *Rev. Infect. Dis* 1980;2:520.

76. Albert, M. M., J. R. Graybill, and M. G. Rinaldi. Treatment of murine cryptococcal meningitis with an SCH 39304-amphotericin B combination. *Antimicrob. Agents Chemother.* 1991;35:1721.

77. Sugar, A. M. Interactions of amphotericin B and SCH 39304 in the treatment of experimental murine candidiasis: lack of antagonism of a polyene-azole combination. *Antimicrob. Agents Chemother.* 1991;35: 1669.

78. Sugar, A. M., M. Salibian, and L. Z. Goldani. Saperconazole therapy of murine disseminated candidiasis: efficacy and interactions with amphotericin B. *Antimicrob. Agents Chemother.* 1994;38:371.

79. Sugar, A. M. Use of amphotericin B with azole antifungal drugs: what are we doing? *Antimicrob. Agents Chemother.* 1995;39:1907.

80. Medoff, G., C. N. Kwan, D. Schlessinger, and G. S. Kobayashi. Potentiation of rifampicin, rifampicin analogs, and tetracycline against animal cells by amphotericin B and polymyxin B. *Cancer Res.* 1973;33: 1146.

81. Medoff, G., C. N. Kwan, D. Schlessinger, and G. S. Kobayashi. Permeability control in animal cells by polyenes: a possibility. *Antimicrob. Agents Chemother.* 1973;3:441.

82. Valeriote, F., G. Medoff, and J. Dieckman. Potentiation of anticancer agent cytotoxicity against sensitive and resistant AKR leukemia by amphotericin B. *Cancer Res.* 1979;39:2041.

83. Medoff, G., F. Valeriote, and J. Dieckman. Potentiation of anticancer agents by amphotericin B. *J. Natl. Canc. Inst.* 1981;67:131.

84. Thomas, M. Z., G. Medoff, and G. S. Kobayashi. Changes in murine resistance to *Listeria monocytogenes* infection induced by amphotericin B. *J. Infect. Dis.* 1973;127:373.

85. Shirley, S. F., and J. R. Little. Immunopotentiating effects of amphotericin B. I. Enhanced contact sensitivity in mice. *J. Immunol.* 1979;123:2878.

86. Shirley, S. F., and J. R. Little. Immunopotentiating effects of amphotericin B. II. Enhanced in vitro proliferative responses of murine lymphocytes. *J. Immunol.* 1979;123:2883.

87. Presant, C. A. Amphotericin B. New perspectives. *Arch. Intern. Med.* 1980;140:469.

88. Hoeprich, P. D. Chemotherapy of systemic fungal diseases. *Annu. Rev. Pharmacol. Toxicol.* 1978;18: 205.

89. Rippon, J. W. Pharmacology of actinomycotic drugs. In *Medical Mycology, The Pathogenic Fungi and the Pathogenic Actinomycetes,* 2nd ed. Philadelphia: W. B. Saunders, 1982, pp. 723–737.

90. Sampaio, S. A. P., J. T. Godoy, L. Paiva, N. L. Dillon, and C. Da Silva Lucaz. The treatment of American (mucocutaneous) leishmaniasis with amphotericin B. *Arch. Dermatol.* 1960;82:627.

91. New, R. R. C., M. L. Chance, and S. Heath. Anti-leishmanial activity of amphotericin and other antifungal agents entrapped in liposomes. *J. Antimicrob. Chemother.* 1981;8:371.

92. Murray, H. W., J. Hariprashad, and R. Fichtl.

Treatment of experimental visceral leischmaniasis in a T-cell deficient host: response to amphotericin B and pentamidine. *Antimicrob. Agents Chemother.* 1993;37: 1504.

93. Selvan, M. P., R. Blay, S. Geyer, S. Buck, L. Pollock, R. Mayner, and J. Epstein. Inhibition of HIV-1 replication in H9 cells by nystatin-A compared with other antiviral agents. *AIDS Res. Hum. Retrovirusus* 1993;9:475.

94. Pleskoff, O., M. Seman, and M. Alizon. Amphotericin B derivative blocks human immunodeficiency virus type 1 entry after CD4 binding: effect on virus–cell fusion but not in cell–cell fusion. *J. Virol.* 1995;69: 570.

95. Aloia, R. C., H. Tian, and F. C. Jensen. Lipid composition and fluidity of the human immunodeficiency virus envelope and host cell plasma membranes. *Proc. Natl. Acad. Sci. U.S.A.* 1993;90:5181.

96. McKenzie, D., D. Kaczkowski, R. Marsh, and J. Aiken. Amphotericin B delays both scrapie agent and *prp-res* accumulation early in infection. *J. Virol.* 1994; 68:7534.

97. Bolard, J. In *Recent Progress in Antifungal Chemotherapy*, ed. by H. Yamaguchi, G. S. Kobayashi, and H. Takahashi. New York: Marcel Dekker, 1991, pp. 293–305.

98. Gale, E. F., A. M. Johnson, D. Kerridge, and T. Y. Koh. Factors affecting the changes in amphotericin sensitivity of *Candida albicans* during growth. *J. Gen. Microbiol.* 1975;87:20.

99. Gale, E. F., A. M. Johnson, D. Kerridge, and E. A. Miles. Phenotypic resistance to amphotericin B in *Candida albicans*: the role of reduction. *J. Gen. Microbiol.* 1978;109:191.

100. Alexander, B., and J. Perfect. Antifungal resistance trends towards the year 2000. *Drugs* 1997;54: 657.

101. Guinet, R., J. Chanas, A. Gouiller, G. Bonnefoy, and P. Ambroise-Thomas. Fatal septicemia due to amphotericin B-resistant *Candida susitaniae*. *J. Clin. Microbiol.* 1983;18:443.

102. Dick, J. D., B. R. Rosengard, W. G. Merz, R. K. Stuart, G. M. Hutchins, and R. Saval. Fatal disseminated candidiasis due to amphotericin B-resistant *Candida lusitaniae*. *Ann. Intern. Med.* 1985;102:67.

103. Powderly, W. G., G. S. Kobayashi, G. P. Herzig, and G. Medoff. Amphotericin B–resistant yeast infection in severely immunocompromised patients. *Am. J. Med.* 1988;84:826.

104. Dick, J. D., W. G. Merz, and R. Saral. Incidence of polyene-resistant yeasts recovered from clinical specimens. *Antimicrob. Agents Chemother.* 1980;18:158.

105. Woods, R. A., M. Bard, I. E. Jackson, and D. J. Drutz. Resistance to polyene antibiotics and correlated sterol changes in two isolates of *Candida tropicalis* from a patient with an amphotericin B-resistant funguria. *J. Infect. Dis.* 1974;129:53.

106. Merz, W. G. and G. R. Sandford. Isolation and characterization of a polyene-resistant variant of *Candida tropicalis*. *J. Clin. Microbiol.* 1979;9:677.

107. Fryberg, M., A. C. Oehlschlager, and A. M. Unrau. Sterol biosynthesis in antibiotic-resistant yeast: nystatin. *Arch. Biochem. Biophys.* 1974;160:83.

108. Pierce, A. M., H. D. Pierce, A. M. Unrau, and A. C. Oehlschlager. Lipid composition and polyene resistance of *Candida albicans* mutants. *Can. J. Biochem.* 1978;56:135.

109. Kelly, S., D. Lamb, and M. Taylor. Resistance to amphotericin B associated with defective sterol Δ^{8-7} isomerase in a *Cryptococcus neoformans* strain from an AIDS patient. *FEMS Microbiol. Lett.* 1994;122:39.

110. Van den Bossche, H. Anti-candida drugs: the biochemical basis for their activity. *Crit. Rev. Microbiol.* 1987;15:57.

111. Gallis, H. A. Amphotericin B: a commentary on its role as an antifungal agent and as a comparative agent in clinical trials. *Clin. Infect. Dis.* 1996;22(Suppl. 2):S145.

112. Bennett, J. E. Antifungal agents. In *Principles and Practice of Infectious Diseases*, ed. by G. L. Mandell, R. G. Douglas, and J. E. Bennett. New York: Wiley, 1979, pp. 243–253.

113. Drutz, D. J., A. Spickard, D. E. Rogers, and M. G. Koenig. Treatment of disseminated mycotic infections. *Am. J. Med.* 1968;45:405.

114. Bindschadler, D. D., and J. E. Bennett. A pharmacologic guide to the clinical use of amphotericin B. *J. Infect. Dis.* 1969;120:427.

115. Alazraki, N. P., J. Fierer, S. E. Halpern, and R. W. Becker. Use of a hyperbaric solution for administration of intrathecal amphotericin B. *N. Engl. J. Med.* 1974;290:641.

116. Ratcheson, R. A., and A. K. Ommaya. Experience with the subcutaneous cerebrospinal-fluid reservoir: preliminary report of 60 cases. *N. Engl. J. Med.* 1968;279:1025.

117. Diamond, R. D., and J. E. Bennett. A subcutaneous reservoir for intrathecal therapy of fungal meningitis. *N. Engl. J. Med.* 1973;228:186.

118. Coukell, A. J., and R. N. Brogden. Liposomal amphotericin B. Therapeutic use in the management of fungal infections and visceral leishmaniasis. *Drugs* 1988;55:585.

119. Kauffman, C. A., and P. L. Carver. Antifungal agents in the 1990s. Current status and future developments. *Drugs* 1997;53:539.

120. Abu-Salah, K. M. Amphotericin B: an update. *Br. J. Biomed. Sci.* 1996;53:122.

121. Boswell, G., D. Buell, and I. Bekevsky. Ambisome (liposomal amphotericin B): a comparative review. *J. Clin. Pharmacol.* 1998;38:583.

122. Meunier, F., H. G. Prentice, and O. Ringden. Liposomal amphotericin B (Ambisome): safety data from a phase II/III clinical trial. *J. Antimicrob. Chemother.* 1991;28(Suppl. B):83.

123. Jullien, S., J. Brajtburg, and J. Bolard. Affinity of amphotericin B for phosphatidyl choline vesicles a determinant of the in vitro cellular toxicity of liposomal preparations. *Biochem. Biophys. Acta* 1990;1021:39.

124. Joly, V., J. Bolard, L. Saint-Julien, C. Carbon, and P. Yéni. Influence of phospholipid/amphotericin B ratio and phospholipid type on in vitro renal cell toxicities and fungicidal activities of lipid-associated amphotericin B formulations. *Antimicrob. Agents Chemother.* 1996;36:262.

125. Adler-Moore, J., and R. T. Profitt. Develop-

ment, characterization, efficacy and mode of action of ambisome, a unilamellar liposomal formulation of amphotericin B. *J. Liposome Res.* 1993;3:429.

126. Legrand, P., A. Vertut-Doï, and J. Bolard. Comparative internalization and recycling of different amphotericin B formulations by a macrophage-like cell line. *J. Antimicrob. Chemother.* 1996;37:519.

127. de Marie, S., R. Janknegt, and I. Bakker-Woudenberg. Clinical use of liposomal and lipid-complexed amphotericin B. *J. Antimicrob. Chemother.* 1994;37:907.

128. Anaissie, E. J., M. White, and O. Uzun. Amphotericin B lipid complex (ABLC) versus amphotericin B for treatment of hematogenous and invasive candidiasis: a prospective, randomized, multicenter trial. Abstracts of 35th Interscience Conference on Antimicrobial Agents and Chemotherapy, San Francisco, September, 1995.

129. Sharkey, P. K., J. R. Graybill, E. S. Johnson, S. Hawrath, R. Pollard, A. Kolokathis, D. Mildran, P. Fan-Havard, R. Eng, T. Patterson, J. Pottage, M. Simberkoff, J. Wolf, R. Meyer, R. Gupta, L. Lee, and D. Gordon. Amphotericin B lipid complex compared with amphotericin B in the treatment of cryptococcal meningitis in patients with AIDS. *Clin. Infect. Dis.* 1996; 22:315.

130. Meunier, F. Alternative modalities of administering amphotericin B: current issues. *J. Infect. Dis.* 1994;28(Suppl. 1):51.

131. Ranchère, J. Y., J. F. Latour, C. Fuhrmann, C. Lagallarde, and F. Loveuil. Amphotericin B intralipid formulation: stability and particle size. *J. Antimicrob. Chemother.* 1996;37:1165.

132. Joly, V., P. Aubry, A. Ndayiragide, I. Carrière, E. Kacna, N. Mlika-Cabanne, J.-P. Abaulker, J.-P. Coulaud, B. Larouze, and P. Yeni. Randomized comparison of amphotericin B deoxycholate dissolved in dextrose or intralipid for the treatment of AIDS-associated cryptococcal meningitis. *Clin. Infect. Dis.* 1996;23:556.

133. Demaimay, R., K. Adjou, C. Lasmezas, F. Lazarini, K. Cheriti, M. Senaw, J.-P. Deslys, and D. Dormont. Pharmacological studies of a new derivative of amphotericin B, M5-8209, in mouse and hamster scrapie. *J. Gen. Virol.* 1994;75:2499.

134. Kravetz, H. M., V. T. Andriole, M. A. Huber, and J. P. Utz. Oral administration of solubilized amphotericin N. *Engl. J. Med.* 1961;265:183.

135. Shadomy, S., D. L. Brummer, and A. V. Ingroff. Light sensitivity of prepared solutions of amphotericin B. *Am Rev. Respir. Dis.* 1973;107:303.

136. Block, E. R., and J. E. Bennett. Stability of amphotericin B in infusion bottles. *Antimicrob. Agents Chemother.* 1973;4:648.

137. Block, E. R., J. E. Bennett, L. G. Livotti, W. J. Klein, R. R. MacGregor, and L. Henderson. Flucytosine and amphotericin B: Hemodialysis effects on the plasma concentration and clearance. *Ann. Intern Med.* 1974; 80:613.

138. Polak, A. Pharmacokinetics of amphotericin B and flucytosine. *Postgrad. Med. J.* 1979;55:667.

139. Atkinson, A. J., and J. E. Bennett. Amphotericin B pharmacokinetics in humans. *Antimicrob. Agents Chemother.* 1978;13:271.

140. Reynolds, E. S., Z. M. Tomkiewicz, and G. T. Dammin. The renal lesion related to amphotericin B treatment for coccidioidomycosis. *Med. Clin. North Am.* 1963;47:1149.

141. Feldman, H. A., J. D. Hamilton, and R. A. Gutman. Amphotericin B in an anephric patient. *Antimicrob. Agents Chemother.* 1973;4:302.

142. Muther, R. S., and W. M. Bennett. Peritoneal clearance of amphotericin B and 5-fluorocytosine. *West. J. Med.* 1980;133:157.

143. Lawrence, R. M., P. D. Hoeprich, F. A. Jagdis, N. Monji, A. C. Huston, and C. P. Schaffner. Distribution of doubly radiolabelled amphotericin B methyl ester and amphotericin B in the non-human primate, *Macaca mulatta. J. Antimicrob. Chemother.* 1980;6: 241.

144. Craven, P. C., T. M. Ludden, D. J. Drutz, W. Rodgers, K. A. Haegele, and H. B. Skrdlant. Excretion pathways of amphotericin B. *J. Infect. Dis.* 1979;140: 329.

145. Seabury, J. H., and H. E. Dascomb. Experience with amphotericin B. *Ann. N.Y. Acad. Sci.* 1960;89: 202.

146. Burks, C., J. Aisner, C. L. Fortner, and P. H. Wiernik. Meperidine for the treatment of shaking chills and fever. *Arch. Intern. Med.* 1980;140:483.

147. Butler, W. T., J. E. Bennett, D. W. Alling, P. T. Wertlake, J. P. Utz, and G. J. Hill. Nephrotoxicity of amphotericin B; early and late effects in 81 patients. *Ann. Intern. Med.* 1964;61:175.

148. Wilson, R., and S. Feldman. Toxicity of amphotericin B in children with cancer. *Am. J. Dis. Child.* 1979;133:731.

149. Carlson, M. A., and R. E. Condon. Nephrotoxicity of amphotericin B. *J. Am. Coll. Surg.* 1994;179: 361.

150. Gouge, T. H., and V. T. Andriole. An experimental model of amphotericin B nephrotoxicity with renal tubular acidosis. *J. Lab. Clin. Med.* 1971;78:713.

151. Hellebusch, A. A., F. Salama, and E. Eadie. The use of mannitol to reduce the nephrotoxicity of amphotericin B. *Surg. Gynecol. Obstet.* 1972;134:241.

152. Bullock, W. E., R. G. Luke, C. E. Nuttall, and D. Bhathena. Can mannitol reduce amphotericin B nephrotoxicity? Double-blind study and description of a new vascular lesion in kidneys. *Antimicrob. Agents. Chemother.* 1976;10:555.

153. Butler, W. T., G. J. Hill, C. F. Szwed, and V. Knight. Amphotericin B renal toxicity in the dog. *J. Pharmacol. Exp. Ther.* 1964;143:47.

154. Burgess, J. L., and R. Birchall. Nephrotoxicity of amphotericin B with emphasis on changes in tubular function. *Am. J. Med.* 1972;53:77.

155. McCurdy, D. K., M. Frederic and J. R. Elkinton. Renal tubular acidosis due to amphotericin B. *N. Engl. J. Med.* 1968;278:124.

156. Wertlake, P. T., W. T. Butler, G. J. Hill, and J. P. Utz. Nephrotoxic tubular damage and calcium deposition following amphotericin B therapy. *Am. J. Pathol.* 1963;43:449.

157. Steinmetz, P. R., and L. R. Lawson. Defect in uninary acidification induced in vitro by amphotericin B. *J. Clin. Invest.* 1970;49:596.

158. Branch, R. A. Prevention of amphotericin-B-induced renal impairment. A review on the use of sodium supplementation. *Arch. Intern. Med.* 1988;148:2389.

159. Brandriss, M. W., S. M. Wolff, R. Moores and F. Stohlman. Anemia induced by amphotericin B. *JAMA* 1964;189:663.

160. Medoff, G., and G. S. Kobayashi. Strategies in the treatment of systemic fungal infections. *N. Engl. J. Med.* 1980;302:145.

161. MacGregor, R. R., J. E. Bennett, and A. J. Erslev. Erythropoietin concentration in amphotericin B-induced anemia. *Antimicrob. Agents Chemother.* 1978;14:270.

162. Silberfarb, P. M., G. A. Sarosi, and F. E. Tosh. Cryptococcosis and pregnancy. *Am. J. Obstet. Gynecol.* 1972;112:714.

163. Wright, D. G., K. J. Robichaud, P. A. Pizzo, and A. B. Deisseroth. Lethal pulmonary reactions associated with the combined use of amphotericin B and leukocyte transfusions. *N. Engl. J. Med.* 1981;304:1185.

164. Howarth, W. R., R. P. Tewari, and M. Solatorovsky. Comparative in vitro antifungal activity of amphotericin B and amphotericin B methyl ester. *Antimicrob. Agents Chemother.* 1975;7:58.

165. Huston, A. C., and P. D. Hoeprich. Comparative susceptibility of four kinds of pathogenic fungi to amphotericin B and amphotericin B methyl ester. *Antimicrob. Agents Chemother.* 1978;13:905.

166. Keim, G. R., P. L. Sibley, Y. H. Yoon, J. S. Kulesza, I. H. Zaidi, M. M. Miller, and J. W. Poutsaika. Comparative toxicological studies of amphotericin B methyl ester and amphotericin B in mice, rats, and dogs. *Antimicrob. Agents Chemother.* 1976;10:687.

167. Jagdis, F. A., P. D. Hoeprich, R. M. Lawrence, and C. P. Schaffner. Comparative pharmacology of amphotericin B and amphotericin B methyl ester in the nonhuman primate, *Macaca mulatta. Antimicrob. Agents Chemother.* 1977;12:582.

168. Ellis, W. G., R. A. Sobel, and S. L. Nielsen. Leukoencephalopathy in patients treated with amphotericin B methyl ester. *J. Infect. Dis.* 1982;146:125.

169. Balmaceda, C., R. Walker, H. Castro-Malaspina, and J. Dalman. Reversal of amphotericin-B-related encephalopathy. *Neurology* 1994;44:1183.

170. Leenders, A., and S. de Marie. The use of lipid formulations of amphotericin B for systemic fungal infections. *Leukemia* 1996;10:1570.

171. Brogden, R., K. Goa, and A. Coukell. Amphotericin B colloidal dispersion. A review of its use against systemic fungal infections and visceral leishaniasis. *Drugs* 1998;56:365.

172. Scholer, H. J. Flucytosine. In *Antifungal Chemotherapy*, ed. by D. C. E. Speller. New York: Wiley, 1980, pp. 35–106.

173. Polak, A., and H. J. Scholer. Fungistatic activity, uptake and incorporation of 5-fluorocytosine in *Candida albicans* as influenced by pyrimidines and purines. I. Reversal experiments. *Pathol. Microbiol.* 1973;39:148.

174. Holt, R. J., and R. L. Newman. The antimycotic activity of 5-fluorocytosine. *J. Clin. Pathol.* 1973;26:167.

175. Jund, R., and F. Lacrute. Genetic and physiological aspects of resistance to 5-fluoropyrimidines in *Saccharomyces cerevisiae. J. Bacteriol.* 1970;102:607.

176. Giege, R., and J. H. Weil. Étude des tRNA de levure ayant incorporé du fluorouracile provenant de la désamination in vivo de la 5-fluorocytosine. *Bull. Soc. Chim. Biol.* 1970;52:135.

177. Grenson, M. The utilization of exogenous pyrimidines and the recycling of uridine-5'-phosphate derivatives in *Saccharomyces cerevisiae*, as studied by means of mutants affected in pyrimidine uptake and metabolism. *Eur. J. Biochem.* 1969;11:249.

178. Block, E. R., A. E. Jennings, and J. E. Bennet. 5-fluorocytosine resistance in *Cryptococcus neoformans. Antimicrob. Agents Chemother.* 1973;3:649.

179. Polak, A., and H. J. Scholer. Fungistatic activity, uptake and incorporation of 5-fluorocytosine in *Candida albicans* as influenced by pyrimidines and purines. II. Studies on distribution and incorporation. *Pathol. Microbiol.* 1973;39:334.

180. Polak, A., and H. J. Scholer. Mode of action of 5-fluorocytosine and mechanisms of resistance. *Chemotherapy* 1975;21:113.

181. Polak, A., and W. H. Wain. The influence of 5-fluorocytosine on nucleic acid synthesis in *Candida albicans, Cryptococcus neoformans*, and *Aspergillus fumigatus. Chemotherapy* 1997;23:243.

182. Diasio, R. B., J. E. Bennett and C. E. Myers. Mode of action of 5-fluorocytosine. *Biochem. Pharmacol.* 1978;27:703.

183. Heidelberger, C. Fluorinated pyrimidines. In *Progress in Nucleic Acid Research,* Vol. 14, ed. by J. N. Davidson and W. E. Cohen. New York: Academic Press, 1965, pp. 1–50.

184. Bellisario, R. L., G. F. Maley, J. H. Galivan, and F. Maley. Amino acid sequences at the FdUMP binding site of thymidylate synthetase. *Proc. Natl. Acad. Sci. U.S.A.* 1976;73:1848.

185. Pagolotti, A. L., K. M. Ivanetich, H. Sommer, and D. V. Santi. Thymidylate synthetase: studies on the peptide containing covalently bound 5-fluoro-2'-deoxyuridylate and 5,10-methylenetetrahydrofolate. *Biochem. Biophys. Res. Commun.* 1976;70:972.

186. Langenbach, R. J., P. V. Danenberg, and C. Heidelberger. Thymidylate synthetase: mechanism of inhibition by 5-fluoro-2'-deoxyuridylate. *Biochemistry* 1974;13:471.

187. Santi, D. V., C. S. McHenry, and H. Sommer. Mechanism of interaction of thymidylate synthetase with 5-fluorodeoxyuridylate. *Biochemistry* 1974;13:471.

188. Heidelberger, C. Fluorinated pyrimidines and their nucleosides. In *Antineoplastic and Immunosuppressive Agents*, Part II, ed. by A. C. Sartorelli and D. G. Johns. Berlin: Springer-Verlag, 1975, pp. 193–231.

189. Koechlin, B. A., F. Rubio, S. Palmer, T. Gabriel, and R. Duschinsky. The metabolism of 5-fluorocytosine-2^{14}C and of cytosine-^{14}C in the rat and the disposition of 5-fluorocytosine-2^{14}C in man. *Biochem. Pharmacol.* 1966;15:435.

190. Diasio, R. B., D. E. Lakings, and J. E. Bennett. Evidence for conversion of 5-fluorocytosine to 5-

fluorouracil in humans: possible factor in 5-fluorocytosine clinical toxicity. *Antimicrob. Agents Chemother.* 1978;14:903.

191. J. E. Bennett: Flucytosine. *Ann. Intern Med.* 1977;86:319.

192. Hoeprich, P. D., J. L. Ingraham, E. Kleker, and M. J. Winship. Development of resistance to 5-fluorocytosine in *Candida parapsilosis* during therapy. *J. Infect. Dis.* 1974;130:112.

193. Normark, S., and J. Schönebeck. In vitro studies of 5-fluorocytosine resistance in *Candida albicans* and *Torulopsis glabrata. Antimicrob. Agents Chemother.* 1972;2:114.

194. Fasoli, M., and D. Kerridge. Isolation and characterization of fluoropyridine-resistant mutants in two *Candida* species. *Ann. N.Y. Acad. Sci.* 1988;544:260.

195. Kerridge, D., M. Fasoli, and F. J. Wayman. Drug resistance in *Candida albicans* and *Candida glabrata. Ann. N.Y. Acad. Sci.* 1988;544:245.

196. Larsen, R. A., M. A. E. Leal, and L. S. Chang. Fluconazole compared with amphotericin B plus flucytosine for cryptococcal meningitis in AIDS. A randomized trial. *Ann. Intern. Med.* 1990;113:183.

197. de Gans, J., P. Portegies, G. Tiessens, J. K. M. Eeftinck, C. J. van Buttel, and R. J. van Ketel. Itraconazole compared with amphotericin B plus flucytosine in AIDS patients with cryptococcal meningitis. *AIDS* 1997;6:185.

198. Wise, G. J., P. J. Kozinn, and P. Goldberg. Flucytosine in the management of genitourinary candidiasis: 5 years of experience. 1980; *J. Urol.* 124:70.

199. Viviani, M. A. Flucytosine—what is its future? *J. Antimicrob. Chemother.* 1995;35:241.

200. Mauceri, A. A. Flucytosine. An effective oral treatment for chromomycosis. *Arch. Dermatol.* 1974; 109:873.

201. Larsen R. A., S. A. Bozzette, D. Jones, D. Haghighat, M. A. Leal, D. Forthal, M. Bauer, J. G. Tilles, J. A. McCutchan, and J. M. Leedom. Fluconazole combined with flucytosine for treatment of cryptococcal meningitis in patients with AIDS. *Clin. Infect. Dis.* 1994;9:211.

202. Viviani, M. A., A. M. Tortorano, A. Pagano, G. M. Vigevani, G. Gubertini, S. Cristina, M. Assaisso, F. Suter, C. Farina, and B. Minetti. European experience with itraconazole in systemic mycoses. *J. Am. Acad. Dermatol.* 1990;23:587.

203. Larsen, R. A. Fluconazole combined with flucytosine. In: *Program and Abstracts of the Second International Conference on Cryptococcus and Cryptococcosis.* Milan, 1993, Abstract L43, p. 100.

204. Polak, A. Combination therapy for systemic mycoses. *Infection* 1989;17:203.

205. Schönebeck, J., A. Polak, M. Fernex, and H. J. Scholer. Pharmacokinetic studies on the oral antimycotic agent 5-fluorocytosine in individuals with normal and impaired kidney function. *Chemotherapy* 1973;18:321.

206. Wade, D. N., and G. Sudlow. The kinetics of 5-fluorocytosine elimination in man. *Aust. N. Z. J. Med.* 1972;2:153.

207. Cutler, R. E., A. D. Blair, and M. R. Kelley. Flucytosine kinetics with normal and impaired renal function. *Clin. Pharmacol. Ther.* 1978;24:333.

208. Block, E. R., and J. E. Bennett. Pharmacological studies with 5-Fluorocytosine. *Antimicrob. Agents Chemother.* 1972;1:476.

209. Pennington J. E., E. R. Block, and H. Y. Reynolds. 5-Fluorocytosine and amphotericin B in bronchial secretions. *Antimicrob. Agents. Chemother.* 1974;6:324.

210. Levinson, D. J., D. C. Silcox, J. W. Rippon, and S. Thomsen. Septic arthritis due to non-encapsulated *Cryptococcus neoformans* with coexisting sarcoidosis. *Arthritis Rheum.* 1974;17:1037.

211. Richards, A. B., B. R. Jones, J. Whitwell, and Y. M. Clayton. Corneal and intra-ocular infection by *Candida albicans* treated with 5-fluorocytosine. *Trans. Ophthalmol. Soc. U.K.* 1970;89:867.

212. Rubinstein, E. Amphotericin B and 5-fluorocytosine penetration into blood and fibrin clots. *Chemotherapy* 1979;25:249.

213. Block, E. R., Effect of hepatic insufficiency on 5-fluorocytosine concentrations in serum. *Antimicrob. Agents Chemother.* 1973;3:141.

214. Kasper, R. L., and D. J. Drutz. Rapid, simple bioassay for 5-fluorocytosine in the presence of amphotericin B. *Antimicrob Agents Chemother.* 1975;7:462.

215. Bury, R. W., M. L. Mashford, and H. M. Miles. Assay of flucytosine (5-fluorocytosine) in human plasma by high-pressure liquid chromatography. *Antimicrob. Agents Chemother.* 1979;16:529.

216. Holdsworth, S. R., R. C. Atkins, D. F. Scott, and R. Jackson. Management of candida peritonitis by prolonged peritoneal lavage containing 5-FC. *Clin. Nephrol.* 1975;4:157.

217. Vandevelde, A. G., A. A. Mauceri, and J. E. Johnson. 5-Fluorocytosine in the treatment of mycotic infections. *Ann. Intern. Med.* 1972;77:43.

218. Harder, E. J., and P. E. Hermans. Treatment of fungal infections with flucytosine. *Arch. Intern. Med.* 1975;135:231.

219. Steer, P., M. J. Marks, P. D. Klite, and T. C. Eickhoff. 5-fluorocytosine, an oral antifungal compound. *Ann. Intern. Med.* 1972;76:15.

220. Meyer, R., and J. L. Axelrod. Fatal aplastic anemia resulting from flucytosine. *JAMA* 1974;228:1573.

221. Bryan, C. S., and J. A. McFarland. Cryptococcal meningitis. Fatal marrow aplasia from combined therapy. *JAMA* 1978;239:1068.

222. Kauffman, C. A., and P. T. Frame. Bone marrow toxicity associated with 5-fluorocytosine therapy. *Antimicrob. Agents Chemother.* 1977;11:244.

223. Pratt, W. B., and R. W. Ruddon. The antimetabolites. In *The Anticancer Drugs.* New York: Oxford University Press, 1979, pp. 98–147.

224. Clarkson, B., A. O'Conner, L. Winston, and D. Hutchison. The physiologic disposition of 5-fluorouracil and 5-fluoro-2'-deoxyuridine in man. *Clin. Pharmacol. Ther.* 1965;5:581.

225. Meyers, C. E., R. Diasio, H. M. Eliot, and B. A. Chabner. Pharmacokinetics of the fluoropyrimidines: implications for their clinical use. *Cancer Treat. Rev.* 1976;3:175.

226. Kauffman, C. A. Role of azoles in antifungal therapy. *Clin. Infect. Dis.* 1996;22(Suppl. 2):5148.

227. Dismukes, W. E., A. M. Stamm, J. R. Graybill, P. Craven, D. Stevens, R. Stiller, G. Sarosi, G. Medoff, C. Gregg, H. Gallis, B. Fields, R. Marier, T. Kerkering, L. Kaplowitz, G. Cloud, C. Bowles, and S. Shadomy. Treatment of systemic mycoses with ketoconazole: emphasis on toxicity and clinical resistance in 52 patients. National Institute of Allergy and Infectious Diseases Collaborative Antifungal Study. *Ann Intern. Med.* 1983;98:13.

228. National Institute of Allergy and Infectious Diseases Mycoses Study Group. Treatment of blastomycosis and histoplasmosis with ketoconazole: results of a prospective randomized clinical trial. *Ann. Intern. Med.* 1985;103:861.

229. Sangeorzan, J. A., S. F. Bradley, X. He, L. Zaving, G. Ridenour, R. Tiballi, and C. Kauffman. Epidemiology of oral candidiasis in HIV-infected patients: colonization, infection, treatment, and emergence of fluconazole resistance. *Am. J. Med.* 1994;97:339.

230. Rex, J. H., M. G. Rinaldi, and M. A. Pfaller. Resistance of Candida species to fluconazole. *Antimicrob. Agents Chemother.* 1995;39:1.

231. White, A., and M. B. Goetz. Azole-resistant *Candida albicans*: report of two cases of resistance to fluconazole and review. *Clin. Infect. Dis.* 1994;19:687.

232. Holt, R. J. The imidazoles. In *Antifungal Chemotherapy*, ed. by D. C. E. Speller. New York: Wiley, 1980, pp. 108–147.

233. Heel, R. C., R. N., Brogden, G. E. Pakes, T. M. Speight, and G. S. Avery. Miconazole: a preliminary review of its therapeutic efficacy in systemic fungal infections. *Drugs* 1980;19:7.

234. Symposium (various authors). First international symposium on ketoconazole. *Rev. Infect. Dis.* 1980;2: 519–699.

235. Heel, R. C., R. N. Brogden, A. Carmine, P. A. Morley, T. M. Speight, and G. S. Avery. Ketoconazole: a review of its therapeutic efficacy in superficial and systemic fungal infections. *Drugs* 1982;23:1.

236. Goa, K. L., and L. B. Barradell. Fluconazole: an update of its pharmacodynamic and pharmacokinetic properties. *Drugs* 1995;50:658.

237. Haria, M., H. M. Buyston, and K. L. Goa. Itraconazole. A reappraisal of its pharmacological properties and therapeutic use in the management of superficial fungal infection. *Drugs* 1996;51:585.

238. Van den Bossche, H., P. Marichal, L. LeJeane, M.-C. Coene, J. Gorrens, and W. Cools. Effects of itraconazole on cytochrome P-450 dependant sterol 14-demethylation and reduction of 3-ketosteroids. *Antimicrob. Agents Chemother.* 1993;37:2101.

239. Watson, P. F., M. E. Rose, S. W. Ellis, H. England, and S. Kelly. Defective sterol C5-6 desaturation and azole resistance: a new hypothesis for the mode of action of azole antifungals. *Biochem. Biophys. Res. Commun.* 1989;164:1170.

240. Van den Bossche, H., G. Willemsens, W. Cools, P. Marichal, and W. Lauwers. Hypothesis on the molecular basis of the antifungal activity of N-substituted imidazoles and triazoles. *Biochem. Soc. Trans.* 1983;11: 665.

241. Sud, I. J., D. L. Chou, and D. S. Feingold. Effect of free fatty acids on liposome susceptibility to imidazole antifungals. *Antimicrob. Agents Chemother.* 1979;16:660.

242. deBrabander, M., F. Aerts, J. van Cutsem, H. Van den Bossche, and M. Borgers. The activity of ketoconazole in mixed cultures of leukocytes and *Candida albicans. Sabouraudia* 18:197 (1980).

243. White, T. C., The presence of an RYG7K amino acid substitution and loss of allelic variation correlate with an azole-resistant lanosterol demethylase in *Candida albicans. Antimicrob. Agents Chemother.* 1997;41: 1488.

244. Sanglard, D., K. Kuchler, F. Ischer, F. J.-L. Pagani, M. Monod, and J. Bille. Mechanisms of resistance to azole antifungal agents in *Candida albicans* isolates from AIDS patients involve specific multidrug transporters. *Antimicrob. Agents Chemother.* 1995;39:2378.

245. Hitchcock, C. A., K. J. Barrett-Bee, and N. J. Russell. The lipid composition and permeability to azole of an azole-and polyene-resistant mutant of *Candida albicans. J. Med. Vet. Mycol.* 1987;25:29.

246. Albertson, G. D., M. Niimi, R. D. Cannon, and H. Jenkinson. Multiple efflux mechanisms are involved in *Candida albicans* fluconazole resistance. *Antimicrob. Agents Chemother.* 1996;60:2835.

247. Venkateswarlu, K., D. W. Denning, N. J. Manning, and S. Kelly. Reduced accumulation of drug in *Candida krusei* accounts for itraconazole resistance. *Antimicrob. Agents Chemother.* 1996;40:2443.

248. Balzi, E., and A. Goffeau. Genetics and biochemistry of yeast multidrug resistance. *Biochem. Biophys. Acta* 1994;1187:152.

249. Fling, M. E., J. Kopf, A. Tarmarkin, J. Gorman, H. Smith, and Y. Koltin. Analysis of a *Candida albicans* gene that encodes a novel mechanism for resistance to benomyl and methotrexate. *Mol. Gen. Genet.* 1991; 227:318.

250. Sanglard, D., F. Ischer, M. Monod, and J. Bille. Susceptibility of *Candida albicans* multidrug transporter mutants to various antifungal agents and other metabolic inhibitors. *Antimicrob. Agents Chemother.* 1996; 40:2300.

251. Lynch, M., and J. Sobel. Comparative in vitro activity of antimycotic agents against pathogenic vaginal yeast isolates. *J. Med. Vet. Mycol.* 1994;32:267.

252. Grant, S. M., and S. P. Clissold. Fluconazole: a review of its pharmacodynamic and pharmacokinetic properties, and therapeutic potential in superficial and systemic mycoses. *Drugs* 1990;39:877.

253. Saag, M. S., and W. E. Dismukes. Azole antifungal agents: emphasis on new triazoles. *Antimicrob. Agents Chemother.* 1998;32:1.

254. Schmitt, H. J., F. Edwards, J. Andrade, Y. Niki, and D. Armstrong. Comparison of azoles against aspergilli in vitro and in an experimental model of pulmonary aspergillosis. *Chemotherapy* 1992;38:118.

255. National Committee for Clinical Laboratory Standards. Reference method for broth dilution antifungal susceptibility testing of yeasts-M27. *Villanova (PA): NCCLS,* 1996.

256. Pfaller, M., and M. Rinaldi. Antifungal susceptibility testing: current state of technology, limitations,

and standardization. *Infect. Dis. Clin. North Am.* 1993; 7:435.

257. Rex, J. H., Pfaller, M. A., M. G. Rinaldi, A. Polak, and J. Galgiani. Antifungal susceptibility testing. *Clin. Microbiol. Rev.* 1993;6:367.

258. Fan-Havard, P., D. Capano, S. M. Smith, A. Mangia, and R. H. K. Eng. Development of resistance in *Candida isolates* from patients receiving prolonged antifungal therapy. *Antimicrob. Agents Chemother.* 1991;35:2302.

259. Odds, F. C. Resistance of yeasts to azole-derivative antifungals. *J. Antimicrob. Chemother.* 1993; 31:463.

260. Cameron, M. L., W. A. Schell, S. Bruch, J. A. Bartlett, H. A. Waskin, and J. R. Perfect. Correlation of in vitro fluconazole resistance of *Candida* isolates in relation to therapy and symptoms of individuals seropositive for human immunodeficiency virus type 1. *Antimicrob. Agents Chemother.* 1993;37:2449.

261. Sandren, P., A. Bjørneklett, and A. Maeland. Norwegian Yeast Study Group: susceptibilities of Norwegian *Candida albicans* strains to fluconazole: emergence of resistance. *Antimicrob. Agents Chemother.* 1993;37:2443.

262. Clayton, Y. M., and B. L. Connor. Clinical trial of clotrimazole in the treatment of superficial fungal infections. *Postgrad. Med. J.* 1974;50(Suppl. 1):66.

263. Mandy, S. J., and T. C. Garrott. Miconazole treatment for severe dermatophytoses. *JAMA* 1974; 230:72.

264. Sawyer, P. R., R. N. Brogden, R. M. Pinder, T. M. Speight, and G. S. Avery. Clotrimazole: a review of its antifungal activity and therapeutic efficacy. *Drugs* 1975;9:424.

265. Proost, J. M., F. M. Maes-Dockx, M. O. Nelis, and J. M. van Cutsem. Miconazole in the treatment of mycotic vulvovaginitis. *Am. J. Obstet. Gynecol.* 1972; 112:688.

266. Restrepo, A., D. A. Stevens, I. Gomez, E. Leiderman, R. Angel, J. Fuentes, A. Arana, G. Mejia, A. C. Vanegas, and M. Robledo. Ketoconazole: a new drug for the treatment of paracoccidioidomycosis. *Rev. Infect. Dis.* 1980;2:633.

267. Negroni, R., A. M. Robles, A. Arechavala, M. A. Tuculet, and R. Galimberti. Ketoconazole in the treatment of paracoccidioidomycosis and histoplasmosis. *Rev. Infect. Dis.* 1980;2:643.

268. Hawkins, S. S., D. W. Gregory, and R. H. Alford. Progressive disseminated histoplasmosis: favorable response to ketoconazole. *Ann. Intern. Med.* 1981;95: 446.

269. Galgiani, J. N., D. A. Stevens, J. R. Graybill, W. E. Dismukes, and G. A. Cloud. Ketoconazole therapy of progressive coccioidomycosis: comparison of 400-and 800-mg doses and observations at higher doses. *Am. J. Med.* 1988;84:603.

270. Catanzaro, A., H. Einstein, B. Levine, J. B. Ross, R. Schillaci, J. Fierer, and P. J. Friedman. Ketoconazole for treatment of disseminated coccidioidomycosis. *Ann. Intern. Med.* 1982;96:436.

271. DeFelice, R., J. N. Galgiani, S. C. Campbell, S. D. Palpant, B. A. Friedman, R. R. Dodge, M. G. Weinberg, L. J. Lincoln, P. O. Tennican, and R. A. Bar-

bee. Ketoconazole treatment of nonprimary coccidioidomycosis. Evaluation of 60 patients during three years of study. *Am. J. Med.* 1982;72:681.

272. Petersen, E. A., D. W. Alling, and C. H. Kirkpatrick. Treatment of chronic mucocutaneous candidiasis with ketoconazole. *Ann. Intern. Med.* 1980;93:791.

273. Symoens, J., M. Moens, J. Dom, H. Schiejgrond, J. Dony, V. Schuermans, R. Legendre, and N. Finestine. An evaluation of two years of clinical experience with ketoconazole. *Rev. Infect. Dis* 1980;2:674.

274. Degreef, H., M. van de Kerckhove, D. Grevers, J. van Cutsem, H. van der Bossche, and M. Borgers. Ketoconazole (R41400) in the treatment of dermatophyte infections. *Int. J. Dermatol.* 1981;20:662.

275. Robertson, M. H., P. Rich, F. Parker, and J. M. Hanifin. Ketoconazole in griseofulvin-resistant dermatophytosis. *J. Am. Acad. Dermatol.* 1982;2:224.

276. Brass, C., J. N. Galgiani, T. F. Blaschke, R. Defelice, R. A. O'Rielly, and D. A. Stevens. Disposition of ketoconazole, an oral antifungal, in humans. *Antimicrob. Agents Chemother.* 1982;21:151.

277. Daneshmend, T. K., D. W. Warnock, A. Turner, and C. J. C. Roberts. Pharmacokinetics of ketoconazole in normal subjects. *J. Antimicrob. Chemother.* 1981;8: 299.

278. Graybill, J. R., P. C. Craven, W. Donovan, and E. B. Matthew. Ketoconazole therapy for systemic fungal infections. Inadequacy of standard dosage regimens. *Am. Rev. Respir. Dis.* 1982;126:171.

279. van der Meer, J. W. M., J. J. Keuning, H. W. Scheijgrond, J. Heykants, J. van Cutsem, and J. Brugmans. The influence of gastric acidity on the bioavailability of ketoconazole. *J. Antimicrob. Chemother.* 1980;6:552.

280. Mannisto, P. T., R. Mantyla, S. Nykanen, U. Lamminsivu, and P. Ottoila. Impairing effect of food on ketoconazole absorption. *Antimicrob. Agents Chemother.* 1982;21:730.

281. van Peer, A., R. Woestenborghs, J. Heykants, R. Gasparni, and G. Gauwenbergh. The effects of food and dose on the oral systemic availability of itraconazole in healthy subjects. *Eur. J. Clin. Pharmacol.* 1989;36:423.

282. Hardin, T. C., J. R. Graybill, R. Fetchick, R. Woestenborghs, M. G. Rinaldi, and J. G. Kuhn. Pharmacokinetics of itraconazole following oral administration to normal volunteers. *Antimicrob. Agents Chemother.* 1988;32:1310.

283. Barone, J. A., J. G. Koh, R. H. Bierman, J. Colaizzi, K. Swanson, M. Gaffar, B. Moskovitz, W. Mechlinski, and V. Van de Velde. Food interaction and steady-state pharmacokinetics of itraconazole capsules in health male volunteers. *Antimicrob. Agents Chemother.* 1988;32:1310.

284. Blum, R. A., D. T. D'Andrea, B. M. Florentino, J. Wilton, D. Hilligess, M. Gavolner, E. Henry, H. Goldstein, and J. Schentag. Increased gastric pH and the bioavailability of fluconazole and ketoconazole. *Ann. Intern. Med.* 1991;114:755.

285. Heykants, J., A. VanPeer, V. Van de Velde, P. Van Rooy, W. Meuldermans, K. Laurijson, R. Woestenborghs, J. Van-Cutjem, and G. Cauwenbergh. The clinical pharmacokinetics of itraconazole: an overview. *Mycoses* 1989;2(Suppl. 1):67.

286. Brass, C., J. N. Calgiani, S. C. Campbell, and D. A. Stevens. Therapy of disseminated or pulmonary coccidiodomycosis with ketoconazole. *Rev. Infect. Dis.* 1980;2:656.

287. van Cutsem, J., M. van der Flaes, M. Thienpont, J. Dony, and C. Horig. Quantitative Bestimmung von Ketoconazole in den Haaren oral behandelter Ratten und Meerschweinchen. *Mycosen* 1980;23:418.

288. Grant, S. M., and S. P. Clissold. Itraconazole. A review of its pharmacodynamic and pharmacokinetic properties, and therapeutic use in superficial and systemic mycoses. *Drugs* 1989;37:310.

289. Grant, S. M., and S. P. Clissold. Fluconazole: a review of its pharmacodynamic and pharmacokinetic properties, and therapeutic use in superficial and systemic mycoses. *Drugs* 1990;39:877. [Erratum *Drugs* 1990;40:867].

290. Lazar, J. D., and D. M. Hilligoss. The clinical pharmacology of fluconazole. *Semin. Oncol.* 1990;17: (Suppl. 6):14.

291. Niemegeers, C. J. E., J. C. Levron, F. Awouters, and P. A. J. Janssen: Inhibition and induction of microsomal enzymes in the rat. A comparative study of four antimycotics: miconazole, econazole, clotrimazole, and ketoconazole. *Arch. Int. Pharmacodyn.* 1981;251: 26.

292. Brammer, K. W., A. J. Coakley, S. G. Jezequel, and M. H. Tarbit. The disposition and metabolism of [^{14}C]fluconazole in humans. *Drug Metab. Dispos. Biol. Fate Chem.* 1991;19:764.

293. Toon, S., C. E. Ross, R. Gokal, and M. Rowland. An assessment of the effects of impaired renal function and hemodialysis on the pharmacokinetics of fluconazole. *Br. J. Clin. Pharmacol.* 1990;29:221.

294. Gallis, H., R. Drew, and W. Pickard. Amphotericin B: 30 years of clinical experience. *Rev. Infect. Dis.* 1990;12:308.

295. Daneshmend, T., and D. Warnock. Clinical pharmacokinetics of systemic antifungal drugs. *Clin. Pharmacol.* 1983;8:17.

296. Tucker, R. M., P. L. Williams, E. G. Arathoon, B. E. Levine, A. I. Hartstein, L. H. Hanson, and D. A. Stevens. Pharmacokinetics of fluconazole in cerebrospinal fluid and serum in human coccoidiodal meningitis. *Antimicrob. Agents Chemother.* 1988;32: 369.

297. Humphrey, M. J., S. Jerons, and M. Tarbit. Pharmacokinetic evaluation of UK-49,858, a metabolically stable triazole antifungal drug in animals and humans. *Antimicrob. Agents Chemother.* 1985;28:648.

298. Francis, P., and T. J. Walsh. Evolving role of flucytosine in immunocompromised patients: new insights into safety, pharmacokinetics, and antifungal therapy. *Clin. Infect. Dis.* 1993;15:1003.

299. van Hecke, E., and S. van Brabant. Contact sensitivity to imidazole derivatives. *Contact Dermatitis.* 1981;7:348.

300. E. K. Foged and O. Hammershoy. Contact dermatitis due to miconazole nitrate. *Contact Dermatitis* 1982;8:284.

301. Heiberg, J. K., and E. Svejgaard. Toxic hepatitis during ketoconazole treatment. *BMJ.* 1981;283:825.

302. Perfect, J. R., M. H. Lindsay, and R. N. Drew. Adverse drug reactions to systemic antifungals. Prevention and management. *Drug Safety* 1992;7:323.

303. Cauwenberg, G., R. Legendre, and N. Blatchford. Itraconazole, a novel oval antifungal: its efficacy and safety profile. Presented at 8th Regional Conference of Dermatology, Bali, June 16–20, 1995.

304. Tucker, R. M., Y. Haq, D. W. Denning, and D. A. Steven. Adverse effects associated with itraconazole in 189 patients on chronic therapy. *J. Antimicrob. Chemother.* 1990;26:561.

305. De Felice, R., D. G. Johnson, and J. N. Calgiani. Gynecomastia with ketoconazole. *Antimicrob. Agents Chemother.* 1981;19:1073.

306. Pont, A., P. L. Williams, S. Azhar, E. Reaven, D. I. Spratt, E. R. Smith, R. E. Reitz, C. Bochra, and D. A. Stevens. Ketoconazole blocks testosterone synthesis. *Clin. Res.* 1982;30:274A.

307. van den Bossche, H., G. Willemsens, W. Cools, F. Cornelissen, W. F. Lauwers, and J. M. van Cutsem. In vitro and in vivo effects of the antimycotic drug ketoconazole on sterol synthesis. *Antimicrob. Agents Chemother.* 1980;17:922.

308. Pont, A., P. L. Williams, D. S. Loose, D. Feldman, R. E. Reitz, C. Bochra, and D. A. Stevens. Ketoconazole blocks adrenal steroid synthesis. *Ann. Intern Med.* 1982;97:370.

309. Hanger, D. P., S. Jerons, and J. T. B. Shaw. Fluconazole and testosterone: in vivo and in vitro studies. *Antimicrob. Agents Chemother.* 1988;32:646.

310. Phillips, P., J. R. Graybill, R. Fetchick, and J. F. Dunn. Adrenal response to corticotropin during therapy with itraconazole. *Antimicrob. Agents Chemother.* 1987;31:647.

311. Barry, A. L., and S. D. Brown. In vitro studies of two triazole antifungal agents (voriconazole [UK-109,496] and fluconazole) against *Candida* species. *Antimicrob. Agents Chemother.* 1996;40:1948.

312. van den Bossche, H., P. Marichal, G. Willemsens, D. Bellens, J. Gorrens, I. Ruels, M. Coene, L. Le Jeane, and P. Janssen. Saperconazole: a selective inhibitor of the cytochrome P450 dependent ergosterol synthesis in *Candida albicans, Aspergillus fumigatus* and *Trichophyton mentagrophytes*. *Mycoses* 1990;33:335.

313. Urbina, J. A., K. Lazardi, T. Aguirre, M. Pivas, and R. Pivas. Antiproliferative effects and mechanisms of action of ICI 195, 739, a novel bis-triazole derivative, on epimostigotes and amastigotes of trypanosoma (schizothrypanum) cruzi. *Antimicrob. Agents Chemother.* 1991;35:730.

314. Cartledge, J. D., D. Denning, and B. Dupont. Treatment of fluconazole resistant oral candidiasis with D0870 in patients with AIDS [Abstract M89]. 34th Intersience Conference on Antimicrobial Agents and Chemotherapy, Orlando, October 1994.

315. Pattick, M. P. E., and P. Phillips. Itraconazole: precautions regarding drug interactions and bioavailability. *Can. J. Infect. Dis.* 1994;5:179.

316. Back, D. J., and J. F. Tija. Comparative effects of the antimycotic drugs ketoconazole, itraconazole and terbinafine on the metabolism of cyclosporin by human liver microsomes. *Br. J. Clin. Pharmacol.* 1991;32:624.

317. Bennett, J. E. Chemotherapy of systemic mycoses. *N. Engl. J. Med.* 1974;290:320.

318. Davies, R. R., Griseofulvin. In *Antifungal Chemotherapy,* ed. by D. C. E. Speller. New York: Wiley, 1980, pp. 149–182.

319. Foley, E. J., and G. A. Greco. Studies on the mode of action of griseofulvin. *Antibiotics Annual* 1959–60, p. 670.

320. El-Nakeeb, M. A., and J. O. Lampen. Uptake of griseofulvin by the sensitive dermatophyte, *Microsporum gypseum. J. Bacteriol.* 1965;89:564.

321. El-Nakeeb, M. A., and J. O. Lampen. Uptake of griseofulvin by microorganisms and its correlation with sensitivity to griseofulvin. *J. Gen. Microbiol.* 1965;39:285.

322. Huber, F. M., and D. Gottlieb. The mechanism of action of griseofulvin. *Can. J. Microbiol.* 1968;14:111.

323. Gull, K., and A. P. J. Trinci. Griseofulvin inhibits fungal mitosis. *Nature* 1973;244:292.

324. Malawista, S. E., H. Sato, and K. G. Bensch. Vinblastine and griseofulvin reversibly disrupt the living mitotic spindle. *Science* 1968;160:770.

325. Weber, K., J. Wehland, and W. Herzog. Griseofulvin interacts with microtubules both in vivo and in vitro. *J. Mol. Biol.* 1976;102:817.

326. Creasey, W. A., K. G. Bensch, and S. E. Malawista. Colchicine, vinblastine and griseofulvin: pharmacological studies with human leukocytes. *Biochem. Pharmacol.* 1971;20:1579.

327. Pratt, W. B., and R. W. Ruddon. Plant alkaloids, enzymes and miscellaneous anticancer drugs. In *The Anticancer Drugs.* New York: Oxford University Press, 1979, pp. 221–272.

328. Bryan, J. Biochemical properties of microtubules. *Fed. Proc.* 1974;33:152.

329. Wehland, J., W. Herzog, and K. Weber. Interaction of griseofulvin with microtubules, microtubule protein and tubulin. *J. Mol. Biol.* 1977;111:329.

330. Keates, R. A. B. Griseofulvin at low concentration inhibits the rate of microtubule polymerization in vitro. *Biochem. Biophys. Res. Commun.* 1981;102:746.

331. Sloboda, R. D., G. Van Blaricom, W. A. Creasey, J. L. Rosenbaum, and S. E. Malawista. Griseofulvin: association with tubulin and inhibition of in vitro microtubule assembly. *Biochem. Biophys. Res. Commun.* 1982;105:882.

332. Wilson, L. Properties of colchicine binding protein from chick embryo brain. Interactions with vinca alkaloids and podophyllotoxin. *Biochemistry* 1970;9:4999.

333. McIntosh, J. R., P. K. Helper, and D. G. Van Wie. Model for mitosis. *Nature* 1969;224:659.

334. Grisham, L. M., L. Wilson, and K. Bensch. Antimitotic action of griseofulvin does not involve disruption of microtubules. *Nature* 1973;244:294.

335. Roobol, A., K. Gull, and C. I. Pogson. Evidence that griseofulvin binds to a microtubule associated protein. *FEBS Lett.* 1977;75:149.

336. Cabral, F., M. E. Sobel, and M. M. Gottesman. CHO mutants resistant to colchicine, colcemid or griseofulvin have altered β-tubulin. *Cell* 1980;20:29.

337. Brian, P. W., P. J. Curtis, and H. G. Hemming. A substance causing abnormal development of fungal hyphae produced by *Penicillium janczewski* ZAL. I. Biological assay, production, and isolation of "curling factor." *Trans. Br. Mycol. Soc.* 1946;29:173.

338. Artis, W. M., B. M. Olde, and H. E. Jones. Griseofulvin-resistant dermatophytosis correlates with in vitro resistance. *Arch. Dermatol.* 1981;117:16.

339. Straughn, A. B., M. C. Meyer, G. Raghow, and K. Rotenberg. Bioavailability of microsize and ultramicrosize griseofulvin products in man. *J. Pharmacokin. Biopharma.* 1980;8:347.

340. Crounse, R. G. Effective use of griseofulvin. *Arch. Dermatol.* 1963;87:86.

341. Khalafalla, N., Z. A. Elgholm, and S. A. Khalil. Influence of high fat diet on gastrointestinal absorption of griseofulvin tablets in man. *Pharmazie* 1981;36:692.

342. Carrigan, P. J., and T. R. Bates. Biopharmaceutics of drugs administered in lipid-containing dosage forms. I: GI absorption of griseofulvin from an oil-in-water emulsion in the rat. *J. Pharm. Sci.* 1973;62:1476.

343. Lin, C. C., J. Magat, R. Chang, J. McGlotten, and S. Symchowicz. Absorption, metabolism and excretion of ^{14}C-griseofulvin in man. *J. Pharmacol. Exp. Ther.* 1973;187:415.

344. Epstein, W. L., V. P. Shah, H. E. Jones, and S. Riegelman. Topically applied griseofulvin in prevention and treatment of *Trichophyton mentagrophytes. Arch. Dermatol.* 1975;111:1293.

345. Shah, V. P., W. L. Epstein, and S. Riegelman. Role of sweat in accumulation of orally administered griseofulvin in skin. *J. Clin. Invest.* 1974;53:1673.

346. Epstein, W. L., V. P. Shah, and S. Riegelman. Griseofulvin levels in stratum corneum. Study after oral administration in man. *Arch. Dermatol.* 1972;106:344.

347. Gentles, J. C. Experimental ring worm in guinea pigs: oral treatment with griseofulvin. *Nature* 1958;182:476.

348. Gentles, J. C., M. J. Barnes, and K. H. Fantes. Presence of griseofulvin in hair of guinea pigs after oral administration. *Nature* 1959;183:256.

349. Collins, J. P., S. F. Grappel, and F. Blank. Role of keratinases in dermatophytosis. II. Fluorescent antibody studies with keratinase II of *Trichophyton mentagrophytes. Dermatologica* 1973;146:95.

350. Yu, R. J., and F. Blank. On the mechanism of action of griseofulvin in dermatophytosis. *Sabouraudia* 1973;11:274.

351. Lin, C., and S. Symchowicz. Absorption, distribution, metabolism, and excretion of griseofulvin in man and animals. *Drug Metab. Rev.* 1975;4:75.

352. Riegelman, S., M. Rowland, and W. L. Epstein. Griseofulvin-phenobarbital interaction in man. *JAMA* 1970;213:426.

353. Cull, S. I., and P. M. Catalano. Griseofulvin-warfarin antagonism. *JAMA* 1967;199:582.

354. Rimington, C., P. N. Morgan, K. Nicholls, J. D. Everall, and R. R. Davies. Griseofulvin administration and prophyrin metabolism. *Lancet* 1963;2:318.

355. Granick, S. Induction of the synthesis of δ-aminolevulinic acid synthetase in liver parenchyma cells in culture by chemicals that induce acute porphyria. *J. Biol. Chem.* 1963;238:2247.

356. De Matteis, F., and A. H. Gibbs. Drug-induced conversion of liver haem into modified porphyrins. *Biochem. J.* 1980;187:285.

357. Tephly, T. R., A. H. Gibbs, and F. De Matteis. Studies on the mechanism of experimental porphyria produced by 3,5-diethoxycarbonyl-1,4-dihydrocollidine. *Biochem. J.* 1979;180:241.

358. De Matteis, F., and A. H. Gibbs. Stimulation of the pathway of porphyrin synthesis in the liver of rats and mice by griseofulvin, 3,5-diethoxycarbonyl-1,4-dihydrocollidine and related drugs: evidence for two basically different mechanisms. *Biochem. J.* 1975;146:285.

359. Sandberg, S., and I. Romslo. Phototoxicity of protoporphyrin as related to its subcellular localization in mice livers after short-term feeding with griseofulvin. *Biochem. J.* 1981;198:67.

360. Watson, C. J., F. Lynch, I. Bossenmaier, and R. Cardinal. Griseofulvin and porphyrin metabolism. Special reference to normal fecal porphyrin excretion. *Arch. Dermatol.* 1968;98:451.

361. Goldman, L. Griseofulvin. *Med. Clin. North Am.* 1970;54:1339.

362. Klein, M. F., and J. R. Beall. Griseofulvin: a teratogenic study. *Science* 1972;175:1483.

363. Scott, F. W., A. de La Hunta, R. D. Schultz, S. I. Bistner, and R. C. Riis. Teratogenesis in cats associated with griseofulvin therapy. *Teratology* 1975;11:79.

364. Denk, H., and W. W. Franke. Rearrangement of the hepatocyte cytoskeleton after toxic damage: involution, dispersal and peripheral accumulation of Mallory body material after drug withdrawal. *Eur. J. Cell Biol.* 1981;23:241.

365. Tinberg, H. M. Intermediate filaments: analysis of filamentous aggregates induced by griseofulvin, and antitubulin agent. *Biochem. Biophys. Res. Commun.* 1981;99:458.

366. Epstein, S. S., J. Andrea, S. Joshi, and N. Mantel. Hepatocarcinogenicity of griseofulvin following parenteral administration to infant mice. *Cancer Res.* 1967;27:1900.

367. Rustia, M., and P. Shubik. Thyroid tumors in rats and hepatomas in mice after griseofulvin treatment. *Br. J. Cancer* 1978;38:237.

368. Bartizal, K., G. Abruzzo, T. D. Krupa, K. Nollstadt, D. Schmatz, R. Schwartz, M. Hammond, J. Balkovec, and F. Vanmiddlesworth. In vitro antifungal activities and in vivo efficacies of 1,3-β-D-glucan synthesis inhibitors L-671,329, L-646,991, tetrahyroechino candin B, and I-687,781, a papulocandin. *Antimicrob. Agents Chemother.* 1992;36:1648.

369. Hector, R. F., B. L. Zimmer, and D. Pappagianis. Evaluation of nikkomycins X and Z in marine models of coccidioidomycosis, histoplasmosis, and blastomycosis. *Antimicrob. Agents Chemother.* 1990;34:587.

370. Oakley, K. L., C. B. Moore, and D. W. Denning. Activity of pradimicin BMS-181184 against *Aspergillus* spp. [Abstract No. F180]. Abstracts 36th Interscience Conference on Antimicroial Agents and Chemotherapy, New Orleans, September 1996.

371. Wardle, H. M., D. Law, and D. W. Denning. In vitro activity of GMS-181184 compared with those of fluconazole and amphotericin B against various *Candida* spp. *Antimicrob. Agents Chemother.* 1996;40:2229.

372. Smith, E. B., R. F. Powell, J. L. Graham, and J. A. Ulrich. Topical undecylenic acid in tinea pedis: a new look. *Int. J. Dermatol.* 1977;16:52.

373. Clayton, Y. M. Dermatophyte infections. *Postgrad. Med. J.* 1979;55:605.

374. Keczkes, K., I. Leighton, and C. S. Good. Topical treatment of dermatophytoses and candidoses. *Practitioner* 1975;214:412.

375. Harrison, E. F., P. Zwadyk, R. J. Bequette, E. E. Hamlow, P. A. Tavormina, and W. A. Zygmunt. Haloprogin: a topical antifungal agent. *Appl. Microbiol.* 1970;19:746.

376. Langsadl, L., and Z. Jedlickova. Sensitivity of strains of *Candida albicans* to jaritin, haloprogin, clotrimazole and miconazole. *Postgrad. Med. J.* 1979;55:695.

377. Clayton, Y. M., R. W. Gange, D. M. MacDonald, and J. A. Carruthers. A clinical double-blind trial of topical haloprogin and miconazole against superficial fungal infections. *Clin. Exp. Dermatol.* 1979;4:65.

378. Gupta, A., T. Einarson, R. Summerbell, and N. Shear. An overview of topical antifungal therapy in dermatomycoses. A North American perspective. *Drugs* 1998;55:645.

379. Bennett, J. E. Antifungal agents. In *Goodman and Gilman's The Pharmacological Basis of Therapeutics*, 9th ed., ed. by J. Hardman, L. Limbird, P. Molinoff, and R. Ruddon. New York: McGraw-Hill, 1996, pp. 1175–1190.

380. Schmitt, H. J., E. M. Bernard, J. Andrade, F. Edwards, B. Schmitt, and D. Armstrong. MIC and fungicidal activity of terbinafine against clinical isolates of *Aspergillus* spp. *Antimicrob. Agents Chemother.* 1988;32:780.

381. Ryder, N. S. Terbinafine: mode of action and properties of the squalene epoxidase inhibition. *Br. J. Dermatol.* 1992;126(Suppl. 39):2.

Drugs Employed in the Treatment of Parasitic Disease

The parasitic diseases, which are prevalent under conditions of crowding, poverty, and poor sanitation, constitute one of the major health problems of humankind. Parasitic infections generally are not responsible for producing a fulminant, life-threatening situation; rather, they are often chronic in nature, and in hyperendemic areas where there is substantial undernutrition as well, the chronic disability may have far-reaching effects on the society. In many areas of the world, chronic parasitic infection is accepted as a part of life by the rural population. Large numbers of people living under conditions of poor sanitation in tropical areas may be infected simultaneously with a number of different parasites. Children are, as a rule, more frequently affected than adults. Because they lack acquired humoral and tissue immunity, the morbidity and mortality is also greater in children. Particularly in the developing countries in the tropics, the constant infection and accompanying anemia and malnutrition may result in decreased intellectual function in the people who grow up under these conditions. This, in turn, may affect the rate at which the people in these areas can acquire the education and the technical skills that are necessary to provide better living standards that would contribute greatly to the solution of the problem of parasitic disease. The successful control of parasitic disease is dependent on a variety of public health measures, including vector control, improvement of sanitation, health education, and drug administration. Although there has been some encouraging progress in the development of vaccines, chemotherapy is still the most effective, efficient and inexpensive way to control most parasitic infections. Drugs are now available that are especially effective in treating human infections caused by flukes and intestinal parasites. However, better drugs are needed to treat some of the systemic parasitic infections and to counteract the development of drug resistance seen especially in *Plasmodium falciparum* malaria and certain other protozoan parasites. Resistance is more common in protozoa than helminths, probably because of their more rapid proliferation. As many of the parasitic diseases are not major health problems in scientifically advanced countries, the development of antiparasitic drugs for human use has not proven to be as economically attractive as the development of other antimicrobial drugs. As a result, the number of investigators engaged in fundamental aspects of antiparasitic drug research is relatively small. Because there has been less basic research in this area and it is often very difficult to develop good experimental systems in which to study antiparasitic drug effects, both the mechanisms of action and the pharmacology of many antiparasitic drugs are not well understood.

CHAPTER THIRTEEN

Chemotherapy of Malaria

Malaria is one of the major health concerns of the world. Many researchers consider malaria to be the most important infectious disease, with an estimated 2.1 billion people living in areas where malaria is transmitted. Every year, there are 100 to 300 million new cases of malaria, and 1 to 2 million people die, mostly in Africa.[1] In endemic malarial areas young children are at greatest risk because their natural immunity to the disease is weakest.[2] In recent years the severity of the malaria problem has worsened in many parts of the world because of resistance of the parasites to antimalarial drugs, resistance of the mosquito vectors to insecticides; socioeconomic declines that have led to a decreased capacity to combat the disease, and movement of nonimmune populations into areas where malaria is transmitted.[1] In the future, global warning may induce circumstances favorable for malaria transmission in wider geographical areas.[3] Although malaria exerts its greatest effects in the developing countries of the tropics and subtropics, increase in international travel has caused malaria to become a problem for many individuals who normally live outside the transmission area. As many as 30,000 American and European travelers probably contract malaria every year. Currently, Malaria diagnoses in the United States consist primarily of imported cases in travelers, military personnel, and immigrants from malaria-endemic countries.[4] Very infrequently, infection is acquired locally by the bite of an infected mosquito entering the country in an aircraft coming from a malarious area or is transmitted congenitally from an infected mother or through blood transfusion.

In the past, the greatest contribution to controlling malaria has been the effort to control the mosquito vector, and it is likely that control of the disease will ultimately be achieved through immunization.[5] In the near future, however, the major mechanisms of combating the disease will continue to be a combination of vector control and chemotherapy, with disease prevention assuming a more important role.[4] *Disease prevention* refers to the rapid diagnosis and treatment of symptomatic persons (and not the prevention of malarial infection and/or interruption of transmission). This includes treatment and prevention of malaria-related anemia, and prevention of severe and fatal outcomes through the effective treatment of simple, uncomplicated malaria. Effective disease prevention should also facilitate the acquisition of effective immunity.

For centuries the mainstay of antimalarial therapy was quinine. The fascinating history of this drug is well worth reading.[6] The access to and control of quinine production has had considerable influence on world history over the past 400 years; malaria has literally determined the fates of nations. The possession of antimalarial drugs and the development of new, more effective antimalarials has been and still is intimately bound up with the establishment of national spheres of influence, which have risen and declined over the past 200 years. It is perhaps for this reason that a large proportion of the research on antimalarial drugs is still funded or carried out by the military.

The field of malariology is highly specialized, and many aspects of antimalarial chemotherapy will not be discussed in this chapter. Instead the emphasis will be on the mechanisms of drug action and on pharmacology. Treatment of malaria differs greatly from one region to another depending on the type of plasmodium and the degree of drug resistance. For more extensive information, the reader is referred to specialized texts and reviews.[1,7–10]

The Disease

Malaria is characterized clinically by paroxysms of severe chills, fever, and profuse sweating. These episodes sometimes occur at reasonably well-defined intervals determined by the life cycle of the invading plasmodium (Fig. 13–1). Other frequent symptoms of a malarial attack include malaise, headache, delirium, aching muscles, abdominal discomfort, vomiting, and diarrhea. In some cases, the disease can become chronic with repeated relapses. It is the result of infection with protozoa of the genus *Plasmodium*. There are more than 40 species of this genus, of which only four affect humans—*P. vivax, P. falciparum, P. malariae,* and *P. ovale.* Malaria caused by the last organism is rare. The organisms are transmitted to humans in the saliva of the female *Anopheles* mosquito. The lapse between the invasion time and the onset of clinical symptoms varies according to the species of the plasmodium, as does the frequency of the febrile paroxysms. As summarized in Table 13–1, the most common type of malaria is that caused by *P. falciparum,* which causes most cases and nearly all the deaths.[1] This form is called *malignant tertian malaria*, and it is characterized by paroxysms of somewhat longer duration than every other day, occurring at irregular intervals. The second most common form is the tertian variety caused by *P. vivax,*

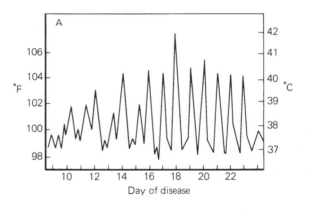

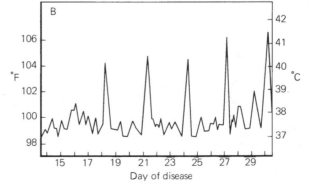

Figure 13–1. (A) Temperature chart of a patient with vivax malaria. Both tertian (every other day) and quotidian (every day) fever patterns can be seen. (B) Temperature chart of a patient with quartan malaria demonstrating fever spikes with 2 days between each episode. (From Coggeshall.[11])

Table 13–1. Some characteristics of the three common malarias.

Common name	Agent	Frequency of occurrence	Latency after infection	Frequency of febrile paroxysms	Severity
Malignant tertian (estivoautumnal)	*Plasmodium falciparum*	Most common	12 days	Irregular	Severe
Tertian malaria	*Plasmodium vivax*	Less common	26 days	Every 2 days	Mild
Quartan malaria	*Plasmodium malariae*	Least common	18–40 days	Every 3 days	Intermediate

which is distinguished by febrile paroxysms occurring every other day. *Quartan malaria* is caused by *P. malariae*. This is the least common of the three and is generally characterized by fever spikes occurring every 72 h.[12] About four-fifths fifths of all malaria cases are caused by *P. falciparum*, and this organism is responsible for about two-thirds of the deaths due to malaria.[1,12] Malaria caused by other species is rarely fatal, but it is more difficult to cure completely and, particularly in the case of *P. vivax*, may be accompanied by severe debilitation.

The Life Cycle of the Parasite

In order to understand the rationale behind the therapy of malaria, it is necessary to understand the life cycle of the plasmodium. The various stages are presented in schematic form in Figure 13–2. The vector for this disease, the female *Anopheles* mosquito, becomes a carrier of the plasmodium by ingesting the blood of a host that contains the male and female sexual forms of the parasite. In the stomach of the mosquito, the male gametocyte produces hairlike bodies that detach and fertilize the female gametocyte—to form the zygote. The parasite then penetrates the stomach wall and forms a cyst on its outer surface. Numerous cell divisions take place to produce an oocyst containing thousands of sporozoites. The cyst bursts, releasing the sporozoites into the body cavity. The sporo-

zoites migrate to the salivary glands, and, when the mosquito bites a suitable host, some of the sporozoites are injected into the bloodstream of the host. The sporozoites rapidly disappear from the blood and appear within the parenchymal cells of the liver. They divide inside the liver cells to form a hepatic (exoerythrocytic) schizont containing numerous merozoites. The different latency times for the disease are defined by variations in the length of this hepatic phase. The patient is asymptomatic during this time. After this latent period, the affected hepatic cells burst, releasing merozoites into the bloodstream. Some of these may reinvade the liver cells, producing secondary hepatic schizonts, but the vast majority invade the erythrocytes where they again multiply asexually. A mature erythrocytic schizont is formed, which then ruptures, and again merozoites are released. The rupture of the parasitized erythrocyte is accompanied by the release of pyrogenic substances, which cause the rapid rise in body temperature. The released merozoites have two fates. The asexual forms can reinvade erythrocytes to give rise to continued cycles of division and rupture. In those cases in which the fever becomes periodic, the length of the interval between fever paroxysms is determined by the rate at which this synchronized intraerythrocytic growth takes place. A few of the merozoites produced with each erythrocyte cycle undergo a sexual division to form the male and female gametocytes, which are then ingested by the mosquito, and the life cycle in the vector is continued.

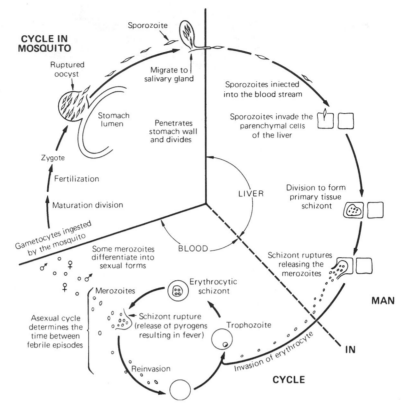

Figure 13–2. Schematic diagram of the life cycle of the malarial parasite.

The Therapeutic Rationale

The erythrocytic stages of the plasmodium cycle are the most sensitive to antimalarial drugs. The exoerythrocytic (liver) stage is more difficult to treat, and, unfortunately, the sporozoites injected by the mosquito into the bloodstream are not sensitive to any of the antimalarial drugs. Since the sporozoite is not affected, it is not possible to prevent viable plasmodia from reaching the liver. Therefore, therapy must be directed toward the hepatic or the erythrocytic stages of the parasite cycle. Unfortunately, effective treatment of the erythrocytic stage of the cycle, although it will make the person asymptomatic, often does not get rid of the parasite completely. When therapy is stopped, symptoms can resume because merozoites are released into the bloodstream from the liver. To completely rid the body of *P. vivax* or *P. ovale* it is necessary to administer drugs that are effective against the hepatic forms of the

parasite. Often, however, when a person remains in an area where malaria is endemic and continual reinvasion is a virtual certainty, it is not reasonable to attempt complete eradication of the parasite from the body. In such a case, therapy is aimed at suppressing the symptomatology by inhibiting the erythrocytic stages of the cycle.

There are two characteristics of *P. falciparum* that modify treatment. On rupture of the hepatic schizont, the merozoites of this organism do not reinvade the liver and cause secondary tissue schizonts; thus, successful treatment of the initial acute attack results in complete eradication of the organism from the patient. A second characteristic of *P. falciparum* is that it becomes resistant to drug therapy much more readily than the other strains.

There is a marked correlation between the development of drug resistance in *P. falciparum* and the extent to which a drug has been used in a particular area.[7,13,14] During the 1950s and 1960s, chloroquine was used for suppressive therapy on a mass scale where every member of a population was treated. The purpose of such mass drug administration was to eliminate the disease in a local area. In this case, mass drug administration was carried out in conjunction with a comprehensive program to eliminate the mosquito vector. Unfortunately, such eradication programs accelerated the selection of resistant parasites.[13] Resistance to chloroquine was first reported in South America in 1961, and the incidence of resistance has increased such that in some regions of Southeast Asia and South America, virtually all strains of *P. falciparum* are chloroquine resistant. In Africa most malaria cases are caused by *P. falciparum*[15] and now chloro-

quine resistance is widespread on that continent, necessitating a revision in the recommendations for prevention of malaria in travelers to this area.[16]

The choice of drugs for the treatment of malaria is dictated by several factors, including the severity of the infection, the patient's age, the degree of background immunity (if any), the likely pattern of sensitivity of the parasites in the area, and the cost and availability of such drugs. For this reason, recommendations vary according to geographic region and should be reviewed constantly. Several drug regimens employed in the treatment and prophylaxis of malaria are presented in Table 13–2. The therapeutic goals include prophylaxis, treatment of the acute attack (clinical cure), and radical cure. Pro-

Table 13–2. Drugs of choice for the treatment of malaria. Dosage regimens used for antimlarial prophylaxis in nonimmune travelers are presented in Table 13–3 and dosages used for treating acute malarial attacks are presented in Table 13–4.

Therapeutic goal	Drug regimen of choice	Alternative
PROPHYLAXIS		
Prophylaxis of disease in an area where chloroquine-resistant malaria has not been reported	Chloroquine phosphate	
Prophylaxis of disease in regions with chloroquine-resistant *P. falciparum* malaria	Mefloquine or doxycycline	Chloroquine phosphate plus either pyrimethamine-sulfadoxine or proguanil
TREATMENT OF ACUTE ATTACK		
Chloroquine-sensitive Strains		
Oral therapy	Chloroquine phosphate	
Parenteral therapy	Quinidine gluconate or quinine dihydrochloride	Artemether
Chloroquine-resistant *P. falciparum*	Quinidine gluconate plus either doxycycline or pyrimethamine-sulfadoxine	Mefloquine, halofantrine
Chloroquine-resistant *P. vivax*	Quinine sulfate plus either doxycycline or pyrimethamine-sulfadoxine, or mefloquine	Atovaquone plus either proguanil or doxycycline Artesunate plus mefloquine
RADICAL CURE		
Eradication of persistent exoery-throcytic parasites after clinical cure of acute attack by *P. vivax* or *P. ovale*	Primaquine phosphate	

phylaxis and chemotherapy of human malaria have become progressively more complex and less satisfactory, primarily because drug-resistant strains of *P. falciparum* have developed in areas of extensive antimalarial use. Increasing the dose of the antimalarial drugs to combat the resistance is dangerous because of the risk of toxicity from most of the available antimalarial drugs, and resistance to the newer antimalarial agents may eventually develop.

Prophylaxis

The risk of malaria can be reduced by using personal protection measures and by regular use of effective chemoprophylaxis. The objective of chemoprophylaxis is to prevent the clinical effect of malaria infection by the use of medication. The drugs used for prophylaxis must be very well tolerated because they are used by millions of travelers. Whether antimalarial chemoprophylaxis should be recommended depends on the risk of infection. Guidelines have to be simple, accurate, comprehensible, and applicable to most travelers at risk. In areas where malaria is endemic, chloroquine is the drug of choice for prophylaxis of infections due to *P. vivax*, *P. ovale*, *P. malariae*, and chloroquine-sensitive strains of *P. falciparum*.[17] In areas with chloroquine-resistant *P. falciparum*, weekly mefloquine is recommended to most travelers. Mefloquine is contraindicated only for those with hypersensitivity to the drug and it is currently not recommended for persons with underlying seizure or neuropsychiatric disorders. Daily doxycycline is recommended for those who cannot use mefloquine, except children younger than 8 years and pregnant women, and it is the drug of choice for travelers to western Cambodia and the few who might spend the night at the Thai-Myanmar or Thai-Cambodia borders where mefloquine resistance has emerged.[4,17] Weekly chloroquine is an alternative for those who can use neither mefloquine nor doxycycline, but it is much less effective. Weekly chemoprophylaxis (mefloquine and chloroquine) should be started preferably 1 to 2 weeks before travel so that potential adverse effects can be as-

sessed. Daily prophylaxis (doxycycline and proguanil) can be started 1 to 2 days before arriving in the malaria area. Prophylaxis with mefloquine, doxycycline, and chloroquine must be continued for 4 weeks after leaving the malaria area.

In areas where chloroquine-resistant *P. falciparum* is endemic, pyrimethamine-sulfadoxine is no longer recommended for prophylaxis because of its potential toxicity. Instead, travelers are advised to take chloroquine weekly and carry a single dose of the pyrimethamine-sulfadoxine combination to treat a presumed malarial attack until help from a physician becomes available. In certain parts of Africa south of the Sahara, chloroguanide is used with chloroquine for prophylaxis of chloroquine-resistant *P. falciparum* malaria. Chemoprophylaxis, along with personal protection to prevent infection, may have a role in the protection of selected high-risk groups, such as young children and pregnant women who reside in malaria-endemic areas.[18,19] In nonimmune women, contracting malaria during pregnancy poses a severe risk to both mother and fetus. Chloroquine has a good record of safe use in pregnancy, but due to widespread chloroquine resistance, it cannot be recommended for either prophylaxis or treatment. Mefloquine appears to be safe and effective when given in the second and third trimesters of pregnancy, but recommendations for prophylaxis in the first trimester are still under consideration.[20]

Treatment of Acute Attack

The clinical attack of malaria is treated with drugs effective against the erythrocytic stage of the plasmodium. With *P. vivax*, *P. ovale*, and *P. malariae* the drug of choice is chloroquine, which is also used together with other antimalarials to control mixed infections with *P. vivax* and chloroquine-resistant strains of *P. falciparum*. Recent studies have shown that the traditional 3-day course of chloroquine treatment of 25 mg/kg of body weight can be compressed into 36 h for convenience.[21]

The treatment of *P. falciparum* depends on the parasites' sensitivity to antimalarial drugs in the area where the infection was acquired. Infections known to be sensitive to chloroquine (e.g., those from North Africa, Central America north of the Panama Canal, Haiti, or the Middle East) should be treated with oral chloroquine. *P. falciparum* infections in areas with known chloroquine resistance should be treated with the combination of quinine and tetracycline, if the infection is mild (parasite density in the blood is less than 5%), there are no complications, and the patient can take oral medications. Pyrimethamine-sulfadoxine as a single oral dose may be substituted for tetracycline except for infections that have been acquired in Southeast Asia or the Amazon basin. Although sporadic resistance to pyrimethamine-sulfadoxine has been reported from parts of Africa, this combination may still be used. If the patient cannot take oral medications, if there is evidence of complications, or if the estimated parasite density is greater than 5%, the patient should be treated with intravenous quinidine gluconate. Quinidine is more active than quinine but it is also more cardiotoxic and more expensive. The patient still requires treatment with a second drug for chloroquine-resistant *P. falciparum*, and either tetracycline or pyrimethamine-sulfadoxine may be given when the patient can take oral therapy.[16] Mefloquine is an alternative for the treatment of *P. falciparum* malaria resistant to chloroquine, but because of more serious toxicities compared to the other agents, it is usually not recommended. During administration of quinidine gluconate, blood pressure (for hypotension) and electrocardiogram (for alterations in the QRS complex and QT interval) should be monitored continuously and total blood glucose (for hypoglycemia) periodically. Quinidine and quinine should be used with extreme caution if the patient has previously received mefloquine.[22]

Because of increased travel and a resurgence of malaria in many areas of the world, physicians in technically advanced countries are treating an increasing number of acute malarial attacks among civilians who have traveled abroad,[23] including attacks caused by multiple drug–resistant strains of *P. falciparum*.[24] In endemic areas, the problem of malarial treatment is sometimes complicated by the presence of simultaneous infection with two types of plasmodia. Such mixed infections may require different drug combinations for successful therapy.[25]

A malarial attack should be viewed as a medical emergency, especially for nonimmune individuals such as travelers, pregnant women, or young children. If *P. falciparum* malaria is suspected as a result of travel history and clinical findings, treatment must be instituted promptly with a rapidly acting blood schizonticide, otherwise the patient's clinical status may deteriorate rapidly. When chloroquine is called for, the oral route is used whenever possible, but it can also be given parenterally (intravenously or intramuscularly) if suitable precautions are taken. If given intravenously, it should be given by controlled rate intravenous infusion. Usually within 48 to 72 h of initiating therapy patients show marked clinical improvement and a substantial decrease in parasitemia. Lack of response or failure to clear the parasites from the blood by 7 days usually indicates drug resistance.

Attacks of malaria may recur during or after a course of antimalarial chemotherapy, even in the absence of reinfection. Recurrent attacks caused by *P. vivax*, *P. ovale,* or *P. malariae* usually are well controlled by another course of chlorquine, combined or followed with a course of primaquine in the case of *P. vivax* or *P. ovale*. Some patients with *P. vivax* infection may require more than one course of treatment to effect a radical cure. *P. falciparum* malarial attacks or parasitemia after appropriate treatment with chloroquine usually indicates infection with chloroquine-resistant plasmodia. Treatment with quinine usually solves this problem, but some multidrug-resistant strains fail to respond adequately to the usual doses of quinine. Quinine has been successfully combined with a slower-acting schizontocide such as doxycycline in Southeast Asia or with antifolates in most of Africa. Mefloquine is a good alternative to quinine in areas where resistance to it has not been encountered. Derivatives of artemisinin (qinghaosu), obtained from qinghao or sweet wormwood (*Artemisia annua*) and developed as pharmaceutical agents in China, are the most rapidly acting of all antimalarial drugs. They have been used extensively for the treatment of drug-resistant *P. falciparum* malaria in China and Southeast Asia.

Treatment is a special problem in children and pregnant women. The treatment for children is usually the same as for adults but with appropriate dose adjustments and safety precautions. Tetracyclines, however, should not be given to children under 8 years old except in an emergency. There are no pediatric formulations of mefloquine, primaquine, or in many countries, quinine or chlorquine. Quinine, and particularly chlorquine, are dangerous in overdoses, and should be stored in childproof containers. When treating children, particular care should be taken to ensure that the correct doses are given and retained. Early vomiting is common, particularly after the administration of mefloquine or quinine to infants, and is more likely in children with high fever.[9] *P. falciparum* malaria is particularly severe in children and pregnant women, and pregnant women should avoid travel to endemic areas if at all possible. Chloroquine and quinine can be used during pregnancy, but antifolates, tetracyclines, and primaquine should be avoided. Primaquine should not be given to pregnant women or newborn babies because of the risk of hemolyis.

Although infections with *P. vivax, P. ovale,* or *P. malariae* are very rarely fatal, an infection with *P. falciparum* may progress rapidly to a lethal multisystem disease. The clinical manifestations of severe malaria depend on age.[26] Hypoglycemia, convulsions, and severe anemia are relatively more common in adults.[27,28] Cerebral malaria (with coma), shock, and acidosis, which often terminate in respiratory arrest, may occur at any age.

Radical Cure

In order to prevent relapse after a clinical attack of *P. vivax* or *P. ovale* has been treated, it is necessary to administer a drug that is effective against the hepatic forms of the parasite. A 2-week course of primaquine is usually employed to eradicate forms of the parasite that survive in the liver. This prevents relapse in most cases. As mentioned above, radical cure of *P. falciparum* is usually achieved with successful treatment of the acute attack. In people who might have become infected with *P. falciparum* while receiving suppressive therapy, radical cure is ensured by continuing the medication for 6 weeks after the last exposure.

Antimalarials Effective Against Erythrocytic Forms of the Plasmodium

4-Aminoquinolines (Chloroquine and Amodiaquine)

PREPARATIONS AND THERAPEUTIC USE. The most widely used 4-aminoquinolines are chloroquine, hydroxychloroquine, and amodiaquine. These drugs are effective against the asexual erythrocytic forms of human plasmodia, but are inactive against the hepatic forms and have little or no activity against the sexual forms.[29] Hydroxychloroquine is a N-ethylhydroxy derivative of chloroquine that is essentially equivalent to the

Chloroquine

Amodiaquine

parent compound against *P. falciparum* malaria. However, this analog is preferred for treatment of mild rheumatoid arthritis and lupus erythematosus because the high doses required may cause less ocular toxicity than chloroquine.[30,31] Amodiaquine is similar to chloroquine in its mode of action and dosage requirements, but it is active against some *P. falciparum* strains that are no longer susceptible to chloroquine.[32] It is no longer recommended for prophylaxis of *P. falciparum* malaria because it is associated with hepatic toxicity and agranulocytosis.[22] The 4-aminoquinolines are used both for prophylaxis and for treatment of acute attacks of malaria. Successful treatment of the acute attack of P. falciparum results in radical cure, but as these drugs are not effective against hepatic forms, they do not produce radical cure of P. vivax or P. ovale. As chloroquine is employed more commonly than the other 4-aminoquinoline compounds, this discussion will focus on its mechanism of action, pharmacology, and side effects.

Chloroquine phosphate and chloroquine sulfate are available for oral administration, but only the former is marketed in the United States. The dosage regimens used for prophylaxis and for treatment of acute attacks are presented in Tables 13–3 and 13–4, respectively. The 4-aminoquinolines are also used to treat patients with rheumatoid arthritis, discoid lupus erythematosis, and some idiopathic light sensitivity disorders.[33,34] The mechanisms for the beneficial effects in these conditions are not known.

Table 13–3. *Prophylactic dosages of antimalarial drugs.* All people receiving primaquine should first be tested for glucose-6-phosphate dehydrogenase deficiency. Dosage information is from the Centers for Disease Control.

Generic name	Usage	Oral adult dose	Oral pediatric dose
Chloroquine phosphate	In areas where chloroquine-resistant malaria has not been reported	300 mg base (500 mg salt) orally, once per week	5 mg/kg base (8.3 mg/kg salt) orally, once per week, maximum dose of 300 mg base
Hydroxychloroquine		310 mg base (400 mg salt) orally, once per week	5 mg/kg base (6.5 mg/kg salt) orally, once per week up to a maximum dose of 310 mg base
Mefloquine	In areas where chloroquine-resistant malaria has been reported	228 mg base (250 salt) orally, once per week	<15 kg: 4.6 mg/kg base, once per week 15–19 kg: 1/4 tablet, once per week 20–30 kg; ½ tablet, once per week 31–45 kg: 3/4 tablet, once per week >45 kg: 1 tablet, once per week
Doxycycline	An alternative to mefloquine	100 mg orally, once per day	>8 years of age: 2 mg/kg, orally, once per day, maximum dose of 100 mg/day
Proguanil[a]	Used simultaneously with chloroquine as an alternative to mefloquine or doxycycline	200 mg orally, once per day, in combination with weekly chloroquine	<2 years: 60 mg/day 2–6 years: 100 mg/day 7–10 years: 150 mg/day >10 years: 200 mg/day
Primaquine	Traveler must be tested before use. Postexposure prevention for relapsing malaria	15 mg base (26.3 mg salt), orally, once per day for 14 days	0.3 mg/kg base (0.5 mg/kg salt) orally, once per day for 14 days

[a] Not available in the United States.

Table 13–4. Drug regimens used to treat acute malarial attacks.

Condition	Drug	Adult dose	Pediatric dose
Attacks due to all plasmodia except chloroquine-resistant *P. falciparum* and chloroquine-resistant *P. vivax*			
Oral therapy	Chloroquine phosphate	1 g (600 mg base), then 500 mg (300 mg base) 6 h later, then 500 mg (300 mg base) at 24 and 48 h	10 mg base/kg (max. 600 mg base) then 5 mg base/kg 6 h later, then 6 mg base/kg at 24 and 48 h
Parenteral therapy	Chloroquine HCl	250 mg (200 mg base) IM q6h	Not recommended
Attacks due to chloroquine-resistant *P. falciparum*	Quinine sulfate plus either	650 mg q8h × 3–7 days	25 mg/kg/day in 3 doses × 3–7 days
	doxycycline or	100 mg bid × 7 days	2 mg/kg/day × 7 days
	pyrimethamine-sulfadoxine	3 tablets at once on last day of quinine	<1 year: 1/4 tablet 1–3 years: 1/2 tablet 4–8 years: 1 tablet 9–14 years: 2 tablets
	Mefloquine hydrochloride	15 mg/kg salt orally, single dose, up to a maximum of 1000–1250 mg	15 mg/kg orally, single dose
All plasmodia-parenteral therapy	Quinidine gluconate	10 mg/kg loading dose (max 600 mg) in normal saline slowly over 1 to 2 h, followed by continuous infusion of 0.02 mg/kg/min until oral therapy can be started	Same as adult dose
	Artemether[a]	2.2 mg/kg IM, then 1.6 mg/kg every day	Same as adult dose
Prevention of relapses: *P. vivax* and *P. ovale* only	Primaquine phosphate	26.3 mg (15 mg base) per day × 14 days or 89 mg (45 mg base) per week × 8 weeks	0.3 mg base/kg/day × 14 days

[a] Not available in the United States.

MECHANISM OF ACTION. Chloroquine is taken up by human cells in culture and, as with plasmodia, it has been suggested that some of the drug may be trapped in the low pH environment of the lysosomes.[35] A lot of the chloroquine is also bound to tissue constituents. Drug distribution studies in animals have demonstrated extensive tissue binding, particularly in the kidney, liver, and lung.[36] The drug binds to protein and to RNA[37] as well as to DNA. The amount of chloroquine bound by some tissues is nearly as high as that found in parasitized red blood cells. This argues strongly against any hypothesis of selective toxicity based purely on preferential concentration of the drug in the infected red cell.

Despite significant advances in the understanding of chloroquine action over the past few years, the precise mechanism of parasite killing by chloroquine is still not completely known. The complex interplay between the malarial parasite and its erythrocytic host partially contributes to this difficulty. It is likely that chloroquine inhibits parasite growth by a number of additive or synergistic effects that are difficult to reproduce in studies in vitro using parasite components. The mechanism of action of chloroquine and other aminoquinolines and methanolquinolines has been reviewed by O'Neill et al.[38] and Foley and Tilley.[39] Chloroquine is toxic to many cells. This is manifest by the range of adverse effects experienced even when chloroquine is given at a moderate dose. The multiple actions of chloroquine have inhibited efforts to establish the molecular basis for its inhibitory activity against the malaria parasite. A major effect of chloroquine and related drugs is interference with hemoglobin digestion in the blood stages of the malaria parasite's life cycle. Chloroquine accumulates at high concentrations in the acidic food vacuole where it is believed to interfere with the polymerization of heme or in the detoxification of the reactive oxygen species, resulting in death of the parasite. The following mechanisms have all been proposed for the action of chloroquine.

Interaction of chloroquine with DNA. Early studies of chloroquine effects in parasitized erythrocytes showed that parasite nucleic acid synthesis is inhibited earlier than protein synthesis and that inhibition occurs when the drug is present at 10^{-6} to $10^{-5} M$.[40,41] This observation spawned a number of studies that were carried out in bacteria to try to determine a mechanism for inhibition of nucleic acid synthesis. Since it is difficult to work with parasite systems, it is not surprising that investigators chose to examine the mechanism of chloroquine inhibition of DNA synthesis in bacteria. When a culture of *Bacillus megaterium* is exposed to chloroquine at high concentrations, there is a rapid killing effect preceded by inhibition of nucleic acid and protein synthesis.[42] This effect is observed at about 100 times the concentration of drug required for inhibition of nucleic acid synthesis in the parasitized erythrocyte. The ability of chloroquine to inhibit nucleic acid synthesis can be demonstrated in purified systems in which DNA or RNA synthesis is carried out under the direction of DNA template and a purified polymerase enzyme from *Escherichia coli*.[43] Again, high concentrations of drug are required for inhibition. The effect of chloroquine in the purified polymerase system is reversed as larger amounts of DNA template are added to the enzyme reaction, suggesting that the drug inhibits nucleic acid synthesis by affecting the ability of DNA to act as a template. The interaction of chloroquine with DNA has been demonstrated by a number of physical methods[44] and it is clear that the aromatic part of the drug intercalates between the base pairs of the double-stranded DNA helix.[45,46] However, it is highly unlikely that association of chloroquine with the DNA of the parasite is responsible for its antimalarial effect.[10]

Since the basic structure of DNA is quite similar in different types of cells, it is not surprising that at the high concentrations of drug that affect nucleic acid synthesis in bacteria, chloroquine inhibits cell replication and nucleic acid synthesis in cultured mammalian cells.[47] It has been shown that the binding affinity of chloroquine for DNA isolated from mammalian tissues is the same as that for purified plasmodial DNA.[48] Since significant DNA binding occurs at approximately 100 times the serum concentration required for the schizontocidal effect, chloroquine does not produce side effects due to cytotoxic action on rapidly dividing cell systems (bone-marrow depression, hair loss, gastrointestinal ulceration, etc.).

Accumulation in the acidic food vacuole. Parasitized erythrocytes concentrate chloroquine approximately 100-fold more than unparasitized erythrocytes.[49] This accumulation of chloroquine to a high concentration is considered essential to its ability to inhibit parasite growth.[50–52] Although the accumulation of chloroquine is clearly related to its activity,[53] the mechanism by which chloroquine interferes with parasite metabolism is not clear. The mechanism of the accumulation is a matter of some controversy, but electon microscopic studies indicate that the main site for 4-aminoquinoline drug accumulation in *P. falciparum* is within the acid food vacuole of the parasite.[38] Upon treatment with chloroquine, parasites show lysosomal disruption, and this acidic organelle is thought to be the site at which the drug exerts its effects.

Originally, it was assumed that the accumulated chloroquine might interfere with normal lysosomal function. Quinoline compounds are known to disrupt biochemical processes in the lysosomes of mammalian cells, and this led to the idea that inhibition of lysosomal function might cause an inhibition of hemoglobin digestion and starvation of the parasite.[54,55] Chloroquine has also been shown to inhibit phospholipases from plasmodia and other sources. Inhibition of phospholipase action could prevent the degradation of endocytic vesicles in the food vacuole, thereby preventing hemoglobin degradation. Indeed, chloroquine causes the accumulation of vesicles within the food vacuole,[52] an observation that is consistent with the inhibition of phospholipase activity. None of these effects, however, explain the selective activity of chloroquine against plasmodia. While the inhibition of hemoglobin digestion by protease inhibitors is reversible upon removal of the inhibitor,[56] the inhibition of parasite growth by quinolines is irreversible.[57] Thus while chloroquine can directly inhibit hemoglobin digestion, it appears to have additional irreversible effects.

Heme polymerization. Degradation of hemoglobin produces free heme (ferriprotoporphyrin IX) as a byproduct. If the released heme were allowed to accumulate within the food vacuole of the parasite, the heme level could reach 200–500 mM. The parasite cannot degrade these potentially lytic heme molecules and is thus faced with a huge toxic waste problem, which it resolves by polymerizing the heme into nontoxic crystals of hemozoin.[39] The molecular mechanism of hemozoin formation is complex, but some of the process has been worked out. Demonstration of a "heme polymerizing" activity in extracts of malaria-infected erythrocytes[58] led some researchers to propose that the parasite encodes a "heme polymerase" enzyme.[59] Subsequently, it was shown that this polymerizing activity can survive extensive boiling and protease treatments, and that the activity in parasite extracts is the result of preformed heme polymers that apparently act as nucleation centers, allowing the efficient addition of further heme monomers.[60,61] This template effect promotes heme polymerization in the later stages of hemoglobin digestion and heme disposal. In the initial stages of heme polymerization, heme sequestration must occur in the absence of performed nucleation sites and thus additional polymerization-enhancing factors must facilitate the initial phase of heme sequestration in the food vacuole. It has been proposed that both lipid components[62] and histidine-rich proteins[63] promote heme polymerization in the early stages of parasite growth.[63] However, there may be additional enzymic or chemical catalysts that have yet to be characterized.[39]

Several early observations indicated that the process of hemozoin formation was in some way involved with the action of chloroquine. For example, ultrastructural studies showed that chloroquine caused morphological alterations of pigment granules in murine *Plasmodium* species, and biochemical studies showed that chloroquine formed a tight complex with free heme.[39] This led to the proposal that chloroquine interferes with pigment formation by forming a complex with a transiently available form of heme,[64] and it was shown that the polymerization of heme in vitro was inhibited by chloroquine at concentrations in the high-micromolar to low-millimolar range.[58] These observations suggested that a chloroquine-induced inhibition of heme sequestration may lead to a buildup of toxic heme molecules and heme-chloroquine complexes within the parasite. Thus, inhibiton of heme polymerization is believed to poison the parasite with its own metabolic debris. Several workers have now confirmed that chloroquine inhibits both spontaneous heme polymerization and parasite extract–catalysed heme polymerization.[59,60,65,66] The mechanism probably involves competition for the heme substrate, although chloroquine can also prevent elongation of hemozoin polymers and depolymerize preformed complexes.[67,68] Inhibition of heme polymerization apparently occurs through binding of chloroquine and other quinoline antimalarials to the dimeric form of heme,[69] and additional data suggest that the quinoline–heme complex binds to the polymer.[70]

The idea that quinolines act by inhibiting heme polymerization is supported by a number of structure–function studies in which the antimalarial activities of a range of compounds have been shown to be correlated with their abilities to inhibit heme polymerization.[66,71] Despite these data, there is still some debate as to whether heme polymerization is the primary target of quinolines in vivo.[72] For example, some workers have found only a small reduction in the amount of hemozoin that is formed, and others have suggested that inhibition of hemozoin formation is secondary to parasite killing.[73,74] There is also debate regarding which parasite component is the final target of the buildup of free heme. For example, moderate heme concentrations have been shown to inhibit parasite enzymes and disrupt membranes, presumably on account of the detergent-like properties of this hydrophobic molecule.[75,76] In chloroquine-resistant strains of *P. berghei*, which produce less visible pigment than chloroquine-sensitive strains, the level of hemoglobin is not decreased.[77] This suggests that the presence of free heme per se is not fatal, at least in the case of *P. berghi*. Therefore, the toxic event may reflect the formation of heme–chloroquine complexes, which may be more toxic than heme itself.

Free radical–dependent mechanism. Apart from its inhibitory effects on enzymes, heme is toxic to cells by free radical–dependent mechanisms.[78] Upon degradation of hemo-

globin, heme is released from the protein, and the heme iron underoes oxidation to the ferric state. This results in the production of reactive oxygen species (superoxide anion, H_2O_2, and hydroxyl radicals) that react with lipids and proteins.[79] The malaria parasite utilizes the oxidant defense enzymes superoxide dismutase, glutathione peroxidase, and possibly catalase to protect itself against reactive oxygen species.[80,81] Nevertheless, the malaria parasite is quite sensitive to oxidant stress[82,83] and oxidative mechanisms are thought to be important in killing of the parasite by the host.[84] In the food vacuole where the oxidative stress is generated, host-derived catalase and peroxidase activities probably contribute to H_2O_2 breakdown, although parasite-derived proteases will rapidly destroy the host enzymes. In addition, free heme displays both catalase and peroxidase activities,[85] and chloroquine is an efficient inhibitor of the catalase activity.[86] This suggests that formation of chloroquine–heme complexes in the food vacuole could inhibit the catalase activity of heme, thereby prolonging the half-life of any H_2O_2 that is produced. The build-up of H_2O_2 would be expected to cause peroxidative damage to both proteins and lipids; indeed, there is direct evidence that chloroquine enhances the ability of heme to catalyze lipid peroxidation,[87] as well as supporting evidence that reactive oxygen species are involved in the mechanism of chloroquine action.[88,89] If peroxidative damage to membranes and/or enzymes is the final target of chloroquine action, it would explain the irreversible nature of chloroquine activity against the parasite.

CHLOROQUINE RESISTANCE. The response of *P. falciparum* to antimalarial drugs ranges from a high degree of sensitivity to complete resistance to clinically achievable concentrations of drug. In the past 40 years, resistance to chloroquine has steadily spread from two origins, one in South America and one in Southeast Asia. Chloroquine resistance now exists in nearly every country where malaria is endemic, and currently there are only a few effective and affordable drugs that can take its place.[90,91] Although chloroquine resistance developed 20 years later in Africa,

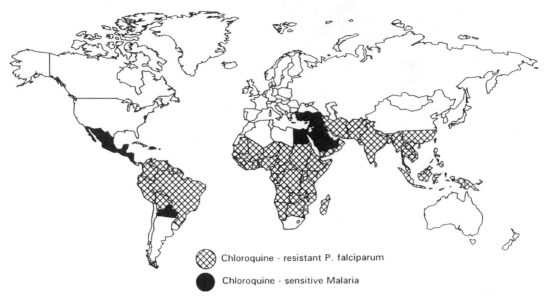

Figure 13–3. Distribution of malaria and chloroquine-resistant *Plasmodium falciparum*, 1993. (From Zucker and Campbell.[16])

it has now spread to all parts of sub-Saharan Africa.[92] Figure 13–3 shows the world distribution of malaria and of chloroquine-resistant *P. falciparum*. Once established, the chloroquine-resistance phenotype; appears to be stable and persists even in the absence of the selective pressure of drug use.[93] Chloroquine resistance emerged much later in *P. vivax* than in *P. falciparum*, but it has been reported in both Southeast Asia and South America.[94,95]

Chloroquine-resistant parasites accumulate chloroquine in their acidic food vacuoles much less efficiently than chloroquine-sensitive strains,[57,96,97] which suggests that drug resistance results mainly from exclusion of the drug from the site of action. But in some cases, a decreased sensitivity of the target may also be involved.[98,99] Several membranes have to be crossed for the drug to reach the hematin in the food vacuole, and three molecular mechanisms have been proposed to explain the decreased accumulation of chloroquine by resistant parasites.

Originally it was thought that the lack of drug accumulation was the result of increased drug efflux from the resistant parasite, and a P-glycoprotein was implicated as the pump responsible for the efflux. Drug-resistant parasites were reported to release accumulated chloroquine almost 50 times faster than chloroquine-sensitive isolates, and verapamil was shown to reduce the apparent rate of drug efflux from chloroquine-resistant parasites.[50] Since verapamil is known to reverse the P-glycoprotein–mediated efflux of drugs in multidrug-resistant tumor cells, it was proposed that efflux of chloroquine by a plasmodial P-glycoprotein is responsible for chloroquine resistance.[100] However, the biochemical data indicating an increased level of drug efflux in chloroquine-resistant parasites have since been questioned,[57] and a number of other studies have indicated that the decreased steady-state levels of chloroquine are due to a diminished rate of drug accumulation rather than an increased rate of drug export.[99,101–104]

Most evidence now indicates that chloroquine resistance involves decreased drug uptake rather than enhanced drug efflux. Reduced chloroquine uptake could result from altered pH gradients across the food vacuole membrane or between the parasite cytosol and the erythrocyte cytosol, from an alteration in membrane permeability or in the activity of a permease or transporter, or from an alteration in some molecule, such as a protein associated with hematin in the food vacuole that compromises drug access to hematin. The factors responsible for reduced chloroquine uptake have a degree of structural specificity, as minor changes in chloroquine's structure can yield compounds with good activity against chloroquine-resistant strains.[104] This is consistent with the involvement of either a specific permease/transporter or a molecule associated with hematin in the food vacuole.

If the level of chloroquine accumulation by parasitized erythrocytes is due simply to an ion-trapping mechanism, then the intravacuolar concentration of chloroquine will be determined by the difference in pH between the medium and the food vacuole. This proposal led to the idea that the decreased accumulation of chloroquine in resistant parasites could result from a modified vacuolar pH.[99,102] For example, an increase in vacuolar pH of 0.5 would be sufficient to decrease chloroquine accumulation by 10-fold.[101,105] Because chloroquine-resistant parasites were found to be more sensitive to the protein pump inhibitor bofilomycin A, it was suggested that an increased vacuolar pH could be caused by a "weakened proton pump."[102] Although the genes for two of the eight subunits of the plasmodial $[H^+]$ATPase have been cloned, no mutations have been found that could account for chloroquine resistance,[106,107] and studies on digitonin-permeabilized infected erythrocytes did not reveal large differences in the vacuole pH of sensitive and resistant parasites.[108] Additional studies using intact parasitized erythrocytes are needed to further assess the theory that modified vacuolar pH can account for chloroquine resistance.

Other proposed mechanisms for the decreased steady-state chloroquine concentration in resistant parasites are loss or alteration of a protein involved in chloroquine uptake[109] or the loss of an intracellular "receptor."[110] The precise mechanism of chloroquine uptake remains unknown. Because amiloride derivatives, which are Na^+/H^+ exchanger inhibitors, inhibit chloroquine uptake by the parasite, and from evidence that chloroquine itself stimulates Na^+/H^+ exchange activity, a Na^+/H^+ exchanger is thought to be linked to chloroquine uptake.[111] Such an exchanger may not necessarily play a primary role in chloroquine uptake, rather it could play a secondary role in maintaining cellular pH subsequent to chloroquine uptake. Thus, it is possible that no specific transporters are required for chloroquine uptake and that the drug crosses the necessary membranes into the food vacuole by diffusion, driven primarily by concentration gradients, pH gradients, and its binding to hematin. Genetic studies suggest that resistance can be caused by mutation in a single gene that has been mapped to a region of chromosome 7 that clearly does encode a P-glycoprotein homolog.[112,113] The leading candidate for the chloroquine resistance mediator is cg2, a gene that encodes a highly polymorphic protein that is apparently located at both the space separating the parasite from the erythrocyte host and in the food vacuole, the proposed site of chloroquine-hematin interaction. Although it has been postulated that this protein may actually be an integral membrane Na^+/H^+ exchanger,[114] this appears not to be the case,[115] and other investigators have suggested that the cg2 protein transports chloroquine out of the parasite or blocks drug influx.[116] Cg2 polymorphism appears to be necessary but not sufficient for chloroquine resistance, an observation that is consistent with the view that chloroquine resistance is a multigene phenomenon.

Resistance to multiple antimalarial drugs has been observed in clinical isolates[117–119] and has been generated in vitro.[120] Substantial evidence from both field and laboratory studies indicates that there is cross-resistance between chloroquine and amodiaquine or its metabolites,[121–123] between quinine and mefloquine, and between these quinolinemethanols and halofantrine.[117–119,124] However cross-resistance between the 4-aminoquinolines and the quinolinemethanols does not develop readily. Resistance to mefloquine, quinine, and halofantrine appears to be inversely correlated with resistance to chloroquine and amodiaquine, which suggests that the development of a high level of resistance to chloroquine renders the parasites more sensitive to the quinolinemethanols.[125]

PHARMACOKINETICS OF CHLOROQUINE. Chloroquine and amodiaquine are both absorbed rapidly from the gastrointestinal tract. When given orally chloroquine has a high bioavailability of between 80% and 90%. The pharmacokinetic properties of chloroquine are complex. It has a very long terminal elimination phase ($t\frac{1}{2}$ of around 1–2 months)[126] and it is distributed relatively slowly into a very large apparent volume (100–1000 liter/kg).[127] This is due to extensive sequestration of chloroquine in tissues, particularly liver, spleen, kidney, lung, melanin-containing tissues, and to a lesser extent, brain and spinal cord. As a result of the complex pharmacokinetics, the plasma levels of the drug shortly after dosing are determined primarily by the rate of distribution rather than the rate of elimination.[127,128] After parenteral administration, rapid entry together with slow exit of chloroquine from a small central compartment can result in transiently high and potentially lethal concentrations of the drug in plasma. Thus, chloroquine is given either slowly by constant intravenous infusion or in small divided doses by the subcutaneus or intramuscular routes.[129] Chloroquine is safer when given orally because the rates of absorption and distribution are more closely matched, with peak plasma levels being attained in about 3–5 h.

The slow release of chloroquine from tissue binding sites is responsible for the long half-life of the drug (the serum half-life is about 4 days when 300 mg of drug is given weekly[130]), permitting administration on a weekly basis for prophylaxis. When initiating prophylactic therapy with chloroquine, one either administers the drug (300 mg of the base) for 1 or 2 weeks prior to entering the endemic malarial area or one starts therapy with 600 mg of drug per week and subsequently reduces the dose to 300 mg weekly. These loading doses are administered in order to occupy tissue binding sites and achieve therapeutic concentrations of free drug in the blood. About 45% of the drug in the plasma is bound to protein.[131] Because of tissue binding, small amounts of chloroquine can be recovered from the urine many weeks after termination of therapy.

The principal metabolite of chloroquine in humans is desethylchloroquine.[132] This metabolite contributes to the drug's efficacy when it is used prophylactically, but is probably unimportant in determining the response to therapy in acute malaria.[127] The drug is excreted slowly in the urine, 70% as chloroquine, 23% as desethylchloroquine, and the remainder as other metabolites.[133] The rate of chloroquine excretion is directly related to the rate of creatinine clearance,[134] and in patients who are receiving the drug for long-term prophylaxis, it is recommended that the dose be reduced by 50% if the glomerular filtration rate is less than 30 ml/min.[134,135] The renal status of the patient does not affect the dosage used on an acute basis for treatment of a malarial attack. Because of its binding in the tissues, chloroquine is not removed by hemodialysis.[136] It is excreted more rapidly in acid urine.[137]

Chloroquine is metabolized by the liver microsomal drug metabolizing system. In the presence of an inhibitor of this metabolizing process, SKF-525A, the plasma half-life of the drug is prolonged.[138] Experiments in animals have shown that primaquine inhibits the metabolism of chloroquine, leading to higher and more prolonged chloroquine plasma levels.[138] This may be another reason (besides unnecessary risk of primaquine toxicity) why the fixed-ratio primaquine-chloroquine combination should not be given for routine prophylaxis during the time that a person remains in an endemic malarial area.

ADVERSE EFFECTS OF CHLOROQUINE. Chloroquine is a safe drug if taken in the correct doses. Most adverse effects from antimalarial doses of chloroquine are relatively mild, since the amounts used for clinical prophylaxis are small and the larger doses employed to treat acute attacks are given only for short periods. Acute chloroquine toxicity is most frequently seen when the drug is administered too rapidly by the intravenous route. At the dosage used for oral treatment of acute malarial attacks, chloroquine can cause dizziness, headache, difficulty in visual accommodation, nausea, vomiting, itching, and skin rashes. When oral therapy is not possible, chloroquine hydrochloride is administered parenterally, and respiratory depression, cardiovascular collapse, convulsions, and death have been reported with overdosage by parenteral routes. Chloroquine should never be administered by intravenous injection as a bolus but should be given by controlled rate intravenous infusion. Provided it does not enter the circulation too rapidly, either because the infusion is too fast or the dose given in an intramuscular or subcutaneous injection is too large, hypotension will not occur and parenteral chloroquine is well tolerated. The physician should take special caution to ensure that the dosage has been correctly calculated on the basis of body weight if the drug must be administered intramuscularly to infants or children. Chloroquine is one of the drugs that can cause hemolysis in patients with glucose-6-phosphate dehydrogenase deficiency.[139] It does not have significant toxicity at the low levels of drug employed for prophylactic therapy. With the use of high doses of chloroquine for prolonged periods in the treatment of rheumatoid arthritis, lupus erythematosis, and discoid lupus, toxic effects in the eye, ear, heart, and central nervous system occur.[36] In this type of nonmalarial therapy, 250 mg of chloroquine base are usually administered daily and this yields trough serum concentrations that generally fall in the range of 0.2–0.4 μg/ml. At trough concentrations of 0.8 μg/ml, side effects occur in 80% of patients.[140] Occasionally, arthritis or lupus patients have experienced photosensitivity, skin pigmentation, alopecia, bleaching of the hair, myasthenia, and leukopenia.[36] In endemic malarial areas some people self-administer the drug on a daily basis for a variety of reasons. In the few instances where ocular damage or heart block has been reported during prophylactic therapy of malaria, such excessive dosage is evident.[141,142]

At the doses recommended for antimalarial therapy, chloroquine may cause visual disturbances such as blurring of vision or difficulty in focusing or accommodation.[36]

These changes disappear when therapy is discontinued. When the drug is administered in higher dosage for the treatment of rheumatoid diseases, it can cause a characteristic retinopathy that may lead to severe visual damage. Serious visual impairment rarely occurs if the daily dosage does not exceed 250 mg of base.[143] The retinal lesion appears as a hyperpigmentation of the macula surrounded by a zone of depigmentation that in turn is encircled by another ring of pigment.[144] This bull's-eye lesion is most commonly seen in patients who have received chloroquine, but similar lesions have been observed rarely in patients who have never received the drug.[145] In a few cases the retinopathy has not become apparent until months after cessation of chloroquine therapy.[146] The cause of the retinopathy resulting from chloroquine treatment is not known. The drug is localized in the melanin-containing areas of the eye,[147] and it binds extensively to preparations of choroidal melanin both in vivo and in vitro.[148] The drug binds to melanin in the skin as well,[149] and studies of the binding of iodoquine (the iodine-containing analog of chloroquine) to purified melanin and DNA suggest that it binds more strongly to melanin than to nucleic acid.[150] The binding is due primarily to electrostatic interactions between the positively charged drug molecules and negatively charged groups of the melanin polymer.[151] It is often assumed that the avid association of the drug with the retinal pigment is in some way responsible for the retinopathy. Because some other drugs with a high affinity for melanin do not cause retinopathy[152] and since chloroquine is retinotoxic in albino animals,[153,154] the retinopathy may not be a direct result of binding to the retinal pigment, although the pigment may serve as a reservoir that maintains a high concentration of drug that is toxic to other retinal or neural components. In addition to retinopathy, prolonged high-dose administration of chloroquine can produce hazy vision that results from deposition of the drug in the cornea.[36]

Prolonged high-dose therapy with chloroquine is rarely accompanied by ototoxicity.[155] Again, a careful study of the distribution of chloroquine in the inner ear of rats demonstrates that the drug is located in the melanin-containing tissues of the stria vascularis and the planum semilunatum.[156] The importance of melanin in localization of the drug was confirmed by the absence of radioactive chloroquine in the inner ear tissue of albino rats. In contrast to the aminoglycosides, which are also ototoxic drugs (Chapter 5), chloroquine is not concentrated in the fluids of the inner ear.[156] Chloroquine is safe when used during pregnancy in the low doses employed for malaria chemoprophylaxis. Less than 5% of the maternal dose is found in breast milk.

PRECAUTIONS AND CONTRAINDICATIONS. Physicians should be aware that chloroquine is one of several antimalarials that can cause hemolysis in patients with glucose-6-phosphate dehydrogenase deficiency. Chloroquine should be used cautiously (or not at all) in patients having hepatic disease or severe gastrointestinal, neurological, or blood disorders.[22] For patients receiving long-term high-dose therapy, ophthalmological and neurological evaluation is recommended every 3 to 6 months.

DRUG INTERACTIONS. In controlled studies, cimetidine (but not ranitidine) decreased the clearance and metabolism of chloroquine and increased the elimination half-life, all by about 50%.[157] Concomitant use of gold or phenylbutazone with chloroquine should be avoided because of the tendency of all three drugs to produce dermatitis.[22]

Mefloquine

Mefloquine is a 4-quinolinemethanol derivative that is chemically related to quinine.

Mefloquine

This compound was developed in the U.S. Army Drug Development Program.[158,159] Mefloquine is effective in the treatment of *P. falciparum* that is resistant to other drugs and it is being used in high-risk groups in regions where drug-resistant *P. falciparum* poses a serious problem. Mefloquine is a generally well tolerated, safe, and effective antimalarial drug.[159]

ANTIMALARIAL ACTIVITY AND THERAPEUTIC USE. Mefloquine is a highly active blood schizontocide, especially against mature trophozoite and schizont forms of malarial parasites, but it is not active against the liver stages of *P. vivax* or against gametocytes.[160] A single oral dose of mefloquine is curative against chloroquine-resistant falciparum malaria in semi-immune patients and nonimmune volunteers.[160,161] The drug is also effective in suppressive prophylaxis of both *P. falciparum* and *P. vivax*.[162] The major ultrastructural abnormality produced by mefloquine in *P. falciparum* is swelling of the parasitic food vacuoles.[163] Like chloroquine, low extracellular concentrations of mefloquine raise the intravacuolar pH of plasmodia in excess of that predicted from passive distribution of a weak base.[164] This suggests that mefloquine is concentrated in plasmodia by an unknown mechanism.

Mefloquine is active against strains of *P. berghei* that have been selected for resistance to chloroquine, primaquine, pyrimethamine, or sulfonamides.[165] Like quinine, mefloquine does not cause clumping of pigment in *P. berghei*, it competitively inhibits clumping caused by chloroquine,[165] and it binds to hemin.[166] Mefloquine accumulates to an equivalent degree in erythrocytes parasitized either with chloroquine-susceptible *P. berghei* or with a chloroquine-resistant subline that accumulates little chloroquine.[167] The undiminished accumulation by erythrocytes infected with the resistant strain may account for the effectiveness of mefloquine against chloroquine-resistant malaria.

Some authors have suggested that the mechanism of action of mefloquine and other quinolinemethanols may be similar to that of chloroquine,[168] However, while the evidence that heme interactions underpin the mode of action of the 4-aminoquinolines is quite compelling, it is not clear that heme is the only, or even the major, target for the antimalarial action of the quinolinemethanols. Mefloquine interacts relatively weakly with free heme and has been shown to inhibit heme polymerization in vitro with a similar or lower efficiency than chloroquine.[58,66,168,169] Given the lower basicity of mefloquine, it seems unlikely that it would attain the intravacuolar concentration required to inhibit heme polymerization. Furthermore, mefloquine and quinine do not cause a decrease in hemozoin production as chloroquine does.[73] Mefloquine is also a much less potent enhancer of the peroxidase activity of heme than chloroquine, and it has been shown to interfere with the ability of chloroquine to enhance heme-induced cell lysis.[87] Thus mefloquine seems to interfere with a different step in the parasite-feeding process than chloroquine.[170] Mefloquine may act by forming toxic complexes with free heme that damage membranes and interact with other plasmodial components.[171] The orientation of the hydroxyl and amine groups with respect to each other in mefloquine may be essential for its hydrogen bonding and antimalarial activity.[172] Two high-affinity mefloquine binding proteins with molecular masses of 22-23 kDa and 36 kDa have been demonstrated by photoaffinity labeling in P. falciparum–infected erythrocytes.[173] Although the binding proteins have not been identified, they are believed to be involved in mefloquine uptake or action. There is also evidence to suggest a role for the plasmodial P-glycoprotein (P-glycoprotein homolog-1, Pgh-1) in mefloquine resistance, raising the possibility that Pgh-1 may also bind mefloquine. In contrast to chloroquine, mefloquine binds to phospholipids, it associates with the membranes of unparasitized erythrocytes,[166] it does not bind to DNA,[174] and its uptake apparently does not require energy.[167]

A great deal has been learned from the development of clinical resistance to antimalarial drugs in P. falciparum, and as a consequence, the use of mefloquine is being restricted by public health authorities. Although mefloquine is effective for the treatment and prophylaxis of all species of human malaria, the restricted indication for its use is in the treatment of patients infected with chloroquine-resistant P. falciparum, particularly those infected with strains resistant to many drugs. It should not be used for therapy when chloroquine resistance is not a problem. Mefloquine is especially useful as a prophylactic agent for nonimmune travelers who stay for only brief periods in areas where these infections are endemic.

It has been shown that plasmodia can develop resistance to mefloquine,[175] and the most careful effort is being made to minimize the chance of resistance emerging in P. falciparum. Still, some isolates of P. falciparum exhibit resistance to mefloquine, especially those obtained from people who have been exposed to the drug. Those who have resistant parasites generally will require larger than the usual doses of mefloquine to control the malaria, but increased toxicity may then result. Many of the isolates also display multidrug-resistant (MDR) phenotypes, with the frequency of MDR depending on the geographic origin and exposure to antimalarial drugs. Mefloquine resistance in isolates of P. falciparum is associated with amplification of the pfmdr1 gene,[119,120,176] and selection for mefloquine resistance in vitro leads to pfmdr gene amplification. Thus, it appears that P-glycoprotein homolog-1 is responsible for at least some forms of mefloquine resistance, and as resistance to halofantrine and quinine is also increased by mefloquine selection, amplification of the pfmdr1 gene may yield cross-resistance.[120,176,177]

PHARMACOKINETICS. Mefloquine is slowly and incompletely absorbed from the gastrointestinal tract.[178] It is usually given orally because parenteral preparations cause severe local reactions. Food increases the oral absorption, and a peak blood concentration of 0.8 µg/ml is achieved about 36 h after a single ingestion of 1000 mg as four 250 mg tablets.[178] When the drug is given in an aqueous suspension, it is more rapidly and completely absorbed, and probably because of extensive enterogastric and enterohepatic circulation, plasma levels of mefloquine rise in a biphasic manner to a peak in about 17 h. The mean plasma half-life of mefloquine is about 14 days[178] and effective drug levels may persist for 30 days or more.[159] The long half-life permits treatment with a single dose, but the half-life is variable (range 6–23 days), suggesting that occasional treatment failures may be anticipated as a result of host factors if the drug is used for single-dose therapy on a large scale.[178] After a single 1000 mg dose, the time required for clearance of *P. falciparum* parasitemia has been reported to be 50 and 103 h in two separate studies.[160,179]

Mefloquine is 99% bound to plasma protein.[180] The drug is widely distributed in the body and it has a high volume of distribution (13.3 liters/kg), consistent with extensive tissue binding.[178] Mefloquine is partially metabolized in the liver and is excreted predominantly in the feces.[180,181] This is consistent with evidence that mefloquine undergoes biliary excretion and extensive enterohepatic circulation in animals. One of the metabolites is a carboxylic acid derivative that is present in relatively high concentrations in the plasma.[180] The carboxylic acid is not bioactive but it has the same toxicity as the parent drug in animal studies. The relatively higher levels of the metabolite in plasma are due to the fact that it has a much smaller volume of distribution than the parent drug.[180] Age and ethnicity of the patient can cause alterations in the pharmacokinetics of mefloquine, as do pregnancy and malarial illness; however, dosing regimens are not substantially altered by these factors.[127,182,183]

ADVERSE EFFECTS. Side effects of mefloquine therapy have been generally mild and transient.[159,160] They include nausea, vomiting, diarrhea, and bradycardia. Sinus bradycardia may occur in about 7% of patients, with the onset being 4–7 days after drug administration; the pulse rate returns to normal within 2 weeks.[160] There has been no evidence of myocardial damage on electrocardiograms and no symptoms have accompanied slowing of the pulse rate.

Central nervous system toxicity occurs in about 50% of patients taking mefloquine. Dizziness, ataxia, headache, alterations in motor function or the level of consciousness, and visual or auditory disturbances occur but are self-limiting and usually mild. The use of mefloquine has been associated with adverse neuropsychiatric effects, including anxiety, depression, hallucinations, acute psychosis, and seizures.[184–186] Serious side effects occur at a rate of 1 in 13,000 in prophylactic use and 1 in 250 with therapeutic use.[187] The ability of mefloquine to interact with and modulate the function of human P-glycoprotein has been suggested as a possible explanation for the neurotoxic side effects of mefloquine.[188] P-glycoprotein is thought to play an important role in detoxification, particularly at the blood-brain barrier,[189] and an inhibitory effect of the drug on human P-glycoprotein could allow mefloquine to exacerbate the neurotoxicity of other compounds.[39]

PRECAUTIONS AND CONTRAINDICATIONS. High doses of mefloquine cause developmental abnormalities in rodents. Therefore, mefloquine should be used during pregnancy only if the potential benefit justifies the potential risk.[171] Mefloquine is contraindicated in patients with a history of seizures, severe neuropsychiatric disturbances, or adverse reactions to quinoline antimalarials, such as quinine, quinidine, and chloroquine.

DRUG INTERACTIONS. Patients taking mefloquine while also taking valproic acid had loss of seizure control and lower than expected blood levels of valproic acid.[22] In patients taking both drugs, the blood levels of valproic acid should be monitored and the dosage adjusted appropriately. Mefloquine generally should not be given with the quinoline antimalarials because of an increased risk of convulsions and cardiotoxicity. Caution is also advised in taking mefloquine along with drugs that can alter cardiac conduction such as beta blockers and calcium channel blockers.[1]

Cinchona Alkaloids (Quinine and Quinidine)

ANTIPLASMODIAL ACTIVITY AND THERAPEUTIC USE. The cinchona alkaloids are all compounds isolated from the bark of the cin-

Quinine

chona tree.[190] The most important member of the group is quinine. Until the 1920s, when more potent synthetic antimalarials were first introduced, the cinchona alkaloids were the only specific antimalarial drugs available in the Western World. The use of quinine in antimalarial therapy would probably be merely of historical interest if it were not for the development of resistance to the more potent drugs in *P. falciparum*. For reasons that are still unknown, resistance has not readily developed to quinine, and, in spite of its lesser potency, the drug again has a role in the treatment of malaria. Although pure quinine can be produced by chemical synthesis, many of the preparations available for antimalarial use in less developed nations are obtained by extracting cinchona alkaloids from natural sources. Quinine is the principal alkaloid present in such mixtures, but variable amounts of quinidine (the dextrostereoisomer of quinine), cincocin, cinchonidin, and other alkaloids are also present.

Quinine is an effective blood schizontocide but it is not active against the liver stages of *P. vivax* or *P. ovale*. There is some gametocidal activity against *P. vivax*, *P. malariae,* and *P. ovale.*[29] Quinine is used to treat acute attacks of malaria caused by chloroquine-resistant and multidrug-resistant *P. falciparum* (see Table 13–4 for dosage). The preferred regimen for severe infections is intravenous quinidine gluconate, which has supplanted quinine for this indication.[191] Oral medication to maintain therapeutic concentrations is then given as soon as it can be tolerated. Quinine is not used for prophylaxis of malaria because of its short half-life, toxicity, and lack of patient compliance.

Clinical resistance to quinine formerly was uncommon but reports of quinine resistance are increasing and efficacy with quinine treatment has fallen below 50% in some parts of Southeast Asia where quinine has been used to treat chloroquine-resistant parasites.[192,193] In these areas, quinine is now prescribed in combination with tetracycline in an effort to increase cure rates.[194] There is abundant evidence for cross-resistance between quinine and mefloquine and between these quinolinemethanols and halofantrine.[119,195] As mentioned previously, it appears that cross-resistance between the 4-aminoquinolines and the quinolinemethanols does not develop readily and that resistance to mefloquine, quinine, and halofantrine may be inversely correlated with resistance to chloroquine and amodiaquine.[117,118,196,197]

Quinine has a mechanism of action similar to that of both chloroquine and mefloquine, but it is not known whether its mechanism is more like one than the other. It interacts rather weakly with heme and has been shown to inhibit heme polymerization[73,168] and heme catalase activity.[86] In the absence of a specific transporter, quinine is likely to be accumulated less efficiently in the food vacuole than chloroquine. Like chloroquine, quinine binds to DNA[198] but the biological significance of this interaction is not known.

PHARMACOKINETICS OF QUININE AND QUINIDINE. In the United States, pure quinine is available as the sulfate for oral administration and quinidine is available as the gluconate for intravenous administration. Quinine for injection is no longer available in the United States. The intravenous injection of quinidine is preferred in patients with severe attacks of malaria when absorption of quinine sulfate cannot be assured. Preparations of quinine in alkaloid mixtures are available for intramuscular administration in many countries. Quinine passes unchanged through the stomach and is rapidly and completely absorbed from the small intestine. A mean plasma quinine level between 3 and 5 $\mu g/ml$ is required to control parasitemia and higher levels are associated with toxic effects.[10] After oral administration of 650 mg of quinine sulfate (540 mg base) every 8 h for 3 days, a steady-state level of about 4 μg quinine per ml is achieved in the plasma in 48 h in afebrile, adult volunteers.[199]

The pharmacokinetic properties of the cinchona alkaloids are altered considerably in malaria, with a contraction in the volume of distribution and a reduction in clearance that is proportional to the severity of disease.[200] Consequently, doses should be reduced by 30% to 50% after the third day of treatment to avoid accumulation of the drugs in patients who remain seriously ill. Binding to plasma proteins, principally to α1-acid glycoprotein, is increased in malaria (approximately 80%–90% for quinine).[201,202] This explains why plasma quinine levels that have been associated with blindness and deafness after self-poisoning do not cause such adverse effects in the patient undergoing treatment of severe malaria. The therapeutic range for the unbound drug, which depends on the sensitivity of the infecting malaria parasites to the drug, has not been defined precisely, but it probably lies between 0.8 and 2 mg/liter, corresponding to total plasma concentrations of approximately 4 to 8 mg/liter for quinidine and 8 to 20 mg/liter for quinine.

Dosage regimens for quinidine are similar to those for quinidine, although quinidine binds less to plasma proteins and has a larger apparent volume of distribution, faster systemic clearance, and a shorter terminal elimination half-life than quinine.[127,191,203] Patients with acute falciparum malaria have significantly higher (approximately twofold) plasma quinine levels when they are febrile than when they are afebrile.[204,205] Quinine is extensively metabolized in the liver, primarily by hydroxylation, and the hydroxylated products are excreted principally by the kidney.[206] Quinine is widely distributed in the body, but it does not accumulate in the tissues like chloroquine. The renal excretion of quinine is enhanced when the urine is acidic, and only small amounts of the drug are removed from the body during hemodialysis or peritoneal dialysis.[207]

ADVERSE EFFECTS OF QUININE. Both quinine and quinidine have low therapeutic ratios; although serious cardiovascular or nervous system toxicity is unusual during antimalarial treatment. The adverse reactions associated with quinine also occur with the other cinchona alkaloids, although there may be quantitative differences in the various responses. Quinine produces a curare-like effect on skeletal muscle that is exploited clinically in the treatment of nocturnal recumbancy leg muscle cramps. Because of its curare-like action, quinine may potentiate the effects of neuromuscular blocking agents and it can cause respiratory distress in patients with myasthenia gravis. When quinine is given in full therapeutic doses, a typical dose-related cluster of symptoms occurs. In mild form this consists of ringing in the ears, headache, nausea, and disturbed vision. If the drug is continued or if large individual doses are given, gastrointestinal, cardiovascular, and dermal effects are seen. This symptom complex is similar to salicylism and is called *cinchonism*. The visual disturbances, which are generally transient, may be confused with the prodromal visual manifestations of thrombotic cerebrovascular disease.[208] Hearing and vision are particularly affected by these drugs. Tinnitus, decreased auditory acuity, and vertigo result from functional impairment of the eighth cranial nerve. Visual signs consist of blurred vision, disturbed color perception, photophobia, diplopia, night blindness, constricted visual fields, mydriasis, and even blindness.[209] Gastrointestinal symptoms are also prominent in cinchonism. Nausea, vomiting, abdominal pain, and diarrhea can result from the local irritant action of quinine and the nausea and vomiting may also arise from some central nervous system effect. In high concentrations, quinine, like its dextroisomer quinidine, can directly depress the myocardium. Quinine also causes vasodilitation by a direct effect on vascular smooth muscle. The cardiovascular symptoms are apparently due to an effect on myocardial calcium flux and an α-adrenergic blocking action.[210,211] During intravenous therapy, high blood levels of quinine may be achieved; as a result of the myocardial depression and vasodilitation, the patient can go into shock. The drug therefore must be given slowly when the intravenous route is employed, and oral quinine sulfate must be substituted as soon as possible. Hyperinsulinemia and severe hypoglycemia can occur even at therapeutic doses. This results from a powerful stimulatory effect on pancreatic β cells and may occur with either quinine or quinidine. Even if treated with glucose infusions, this complication can be serious and possibly life threatening, especially in pregnant patients and in those with prolonged, severe infections.[195]

Quinine can cause contraction of uterine muscle, and it has been used to stimulate contraction during labor. It does not have significant effect until labor has begun. At toxic doses, quinine can cause abortion. The drug crosses the placenta, and it is unclear whether the abortifacient effect is due to its action on the uterus or to fetal poisoning. If other antimalarial drugs can be used, quinine should not be given to pregnant women. Quinine may cause hemolysis in glucose-6-phosphate dehydrogenase–deficient patients and it is associated with the production of drug-induced immune thrombocytopenia.[212] Quinine may cause hypersensitivity reactions characterized by skin rashes, flushing of the skin, and pruritis. Sometimes massive hemolysis and hemoglobinuria occur in association with malaria, a condition that is referred to as *blackwater fever*. Some cases of blackwater fever may occur as a result of hypersensitivity to quinine.[29] Of all the antimalarial drugs, quinine has the poorest ratio between therapeutic potency and toxicity.

PRECAUTIONS AND CONTRAINDICATIONS. Parenteral solutions of quinine are highly irritating, therefore the drug should not be given subcutaneously.[30] Concentrated solutions may cause abscesses when injected intramuscularly or thrombophlebitis when infused intravenously. Patients who have a history of episodes of hemolysis, hypersensitivity, cardiac arrythmia, tinnitus, or optic neuritis should be treated with other drugs whenever possible.

DRUG INTERACTIONS. Absorption of quinine from the gastrointestinal tract can be delayed by antacids containing aluminum. Quinine and quinidine can delay the absorption of digoxin and related cardiac glycosides. Quinine also increases the half-life and consequently the plasma levels of digoxin.[213] Quinine may raise plasma levels of warfarin and related anticoagulants.[30] The renal clearance of quinine can be increased by acidification of the urine.

Halofantrine

Halofantrine was the most promising antimalarial of several phenanthrene methanols developed by the Walter Reed Army Institute of Research to combat drug-resistant malaria. It is now used as an alternative to quinine and mefloquine to treat acute malarial attacks caused by chloroquine-resistant and multidrug-resistant strains of *P. falciparum*. Its use is limited by significant toxicity and because it is not readily available.

ANTIMALARIAL ACTIVITY AND MECHANISM OF ACTION. Halofantrine is an orally administered blood schizontocide that is active against both chloroquine-sensitive and chloroquine-resistant plasmodia. The racemic form acts only against asexual erythrocytic stages of *Plasmodium* spp., including multidrug-resistant strains of *P. falciparum*. Halofantrine has no activity against gametocytes or against the pre-erythrocytic hepatic stages. The mechanism of halofantrine action is unknown. There is some evidence to suggest that halofantrine interacts with ferriprotoporphyrin IX, although the data are conflicting,[214,215] and an alternative proposal is that halofantrine inhibits a proton pump present at the host–parasite interface.[216]

CLINICAL USES. Halofantrine is administered as an alternative to quinine and mefloquine for treatment of acute attacks of malaria due to chloroquine-resistant or multidrug-resistant strains of *P. falciparum*. Because of variable drug absorption, the clinical response can vary. Halofantrine is intrinsically more active than mefloquine and is better tolerated,[217] but it has the disadvantages of multiple dose administration and erratic oral bioavailability. An intravenous preparation is available to circumvent the problem of variable drug absorption. Clinical resistance is limiting the drug's usefulness, and if it is used prophylactically, its prolonged elimination may promote selection of resistant strains of the malaria parasite. Both the variable peak plasma halofantrine concentrations and possible cross-resistance with mefloquine may accelerate the emergence of resistance. To preserve the efficacy of halofantrine, it is important that the drug be used only for treatment of acute attacks in areas where there is established resistance to chloroquine and pyrimethamine-sulfadoxine.

PHARMACOKINETICS. Upon oral administration, absorption of halofantrine is slow, erratic, and dose limited. Absorption is augmented considerably by coadministration with fats or fatty food, and micronized preparations also increase bioavailability.[218] In experimental animals, the drug is well distributed and extensively metabolized to unidentified compounds that are eliminated in the feces. In humans, halofantrine is converted to N-desbutyl halofantrine, a major metabolite with potent antimalarial activity.[219,220] Due to erratic absorption, the pharmacokinetics of the parent drug and this metabolite are highly variable.

ADVERSE EFFECTS. The most common adverse effects associated with halofantrine include nausea, vomiting, abdominal pain, a dose-related diarrhea, pruritis, headache, and rash, although sometimes it is difficult to distinguish between the disease and treatment-related effects.[221] Pruritus and rash have occurred primarily in dark-skinned people who have reacted similarly to chloroquine.[222] The adverse effects are usually self-limited, but halofantrine can produce cardiac conduction abnormalities that are potentially fatal and limit its usefulness.[223,224] Like quinidine, it delays ventricular repolarization, producing a prolongation of the QT interval that can be proarrhythmic. Occasionally, there are atrioventricular conduction abnormalities and, rarely, second-degree block occurs. The cardiac effects of halofantrine are augmented by previous treatment with mefloquine, and halofantrine should not be given to patients who have received mefloquine in the previous month, to patients with prolongation of the QT interval, or to those receiving other drugs known to prolong the QT interval. Ideally, an electrocardiogram should be performed before starting treatment to exclude a baseline long QT interval. Because high doses can produce embryo toxicity in rats and rabbits and decrease longevity in rat pups ingesting the drug in maternal milk,[219] halofantrine is not recommended for pregnant or lactating women.

Artemisinin

Artemisinin and its derivatives possess potent antimalarial activity and have proved to be remarkably effective alternatives to quinine for the treatment of severe chloroquine-resistant *P. falciparum* malaria.[225] Artemisinin is extracted from the herb *Artemisia annua*, which has been used in traditional Chinese medicine for the treatment of febrile diseases. Reduction of the parent lactone, artemisinin, yields dihydroartemisinin, which is itself a potent antimalarial compound. From dihydroartemisinin other active derivatives can be synthesized. Artemisinin, dihydroartemisinin, the water-soluble artesunate, and the lipophilic alkylether artemether are all being used for the treatment of malaria.[225] These drugs are being used in Asia, but they are presently not available in Europe, the United States, and several other countries. They are used for treating uncomplicated and severe infections by chloroquine-resistant *P. falciparum* where they have given consistently faster parasite and fever clearance times than quinine, and have proved to be rapidly effective against cerebral malaria.[226–228]

MECHANISM OF ACTION. Artemisinin and its derivatives exert their antimalarial activity by iron-mediated cleavage of the peroxide bridge in artemesinin and generation of a short-lived but highly reactive organic free radical.[229] Essential to their activity is the interaction of artemisinin with heme in the parasite, which seems to be catalysed by both heme-bound and free iron.[230] The artemisinin radical subsequently binds to membrane proteins and alkylation reactions eventually cause destruction of the parasite.

Uptake studies with radiolabeled artemisinin and dihydroartemisinin have shown that these compounds are concentrated in food vacuoles and mitochondria.[231] Morphological changes in parasite membranes can be observed after 2 h of drug exposure,[232] and the onset of growth inhibition by artemisinin starts after an exposure of 4 to 5 h. Early and late trophozoites show the most prominent effects.

PHARMACOKINETICS. The pharmacokinetics of artemisinin and its derivatives are not yet known in detail, because a sensitive and specific assay for measuring concentrations in biological fluids has not been available. In general, absorption of orally administered artemisinin or its derivatives is rapid but incomplete,[225] and substantial hydrolysis of artesunate (probably complete) and artemether into dihydroartemisinin probably occurs even before absorption. Artesunate, artemether, arteether, and probably also artemisinin are transformed into dihydroartemisinin, which is subsequently converted into inactive metabolites.[225] Artesunate is unstable in solution and is therefore dispensed together with an ampule of 5% sodium bicarbonate solution.[9] The two are mixed immediately before injection (intravenous or intramuscular) and the resulting sodium artesunate is hydrolyzed rapidly in vivo to the biologically active metabolite dihydroartemisinin. Artemether is more stable and is formulated in peanut oil and given by intramuscular injection. In clinical studies, rectal suppositoreis of artemisinin have proved to be as effective as the parenteral drugs,[233] permitting drug treatment for severe malaria in rural settings where administration by injection is not possible. Artesunate is the most rapidly acting of the available compounds, both because of rapid absorption and rapid conversion to dihydroartemisinin. Elimination is mainly by hepatic metabolism,[234] with all of the compounds being transformed into dihydroartemisinin, which is subsequently converted into inactive metabolites.

ADVERSE EFFECTS. Clinical studies have shown that the toxicity of artemisinin, artemether, or artesunate is much less than that of chloroquine. Studies in dogs and rats have shown that administration of an acute lethal dose is accompanied by signs of both neurotoxicity and cardiotoxicity. In these animal studies, artemether, the closely related compound arteether, and the metabolite dihydroartemisin have induced a consistent and selective pattern of damage to some of the brain stem nuclei.[235] The relevance of these findings to their use in humans is unresolved but remains a cause of concern. In treatment of patients with malaria, adverse effects are minimal, and signs and symptoms usually cannot be differentiated from malaria-related effects. Indeed, careful observations in small numbers of volunteers showed no adverse drug effects. It is possible that neurotoxic effects occur upon long-term accumulation in brain tissue. Cardiotoxic effects in patients were limited to a prolongation of the QT interval. From a clinical point of view, the cardiac effects are not very important, except that combination with other drugs that prolong the QT interval should be avoided. A decrease in reticulocyte count has been observed in monkies, and hemolysis occurs in vitro when erythrocytes are exposed to 1 mM artemether, with artemesinin, dihydroartemisinin, and artesunate also causing hemolysis but less so than artemether.[225] Local reactions after intramuscular injection of these compounds are rare and much less frequent than after intramuscular injection of quinine. Mutagenicity studies in animals showed that artemisinin is not mutagenic, and no serious congenital defects have been reported after the few occasions these compounds were taken by pregnant women.

Antimalarials Effective Against Exoerythrocytic Forms of the Plasmodium

8-Aminoquinolines (Primaquine)

ANTIMALARIAL ACTIVITY AND THERAPEUTIC USE. The only commonly employed member of the 8-aminoquinoline group is primaquine. Other drugs in this group include pamaquine and quinocide. The ring structure of these drugs is the same as that of chloroquine, and as one might expect, they also bind to DNA.[236] But the similarity between

CH₃O—[quinoline ring structure]
NH—CH—(CH₂)₃—NH₂
CH₃
Primaquine

the two groups of compounds seems to end here. The 8-aminoquinolines are effective against the exoerythrocytic stages of the parasite. As shown in Table 13–5, 8-aminoquinolines such as primaquine have the ability to destroy gametocytes, including those of P. falciparum strains that are multidrug resistant.[28] At higher doses, some activity is obtained against the asexual blood forms of P. vivax but not those of P. falciparum. Because of its tissue schizontocidal activity, primaquine is used primarily to obtain radical cure of P. vivax and P. ovale malaria. Primaquine is given along with a blood schizonticide, usually chloroquine, to eradicate erythrocytic stages of these plasmodia and reduce the possibility of emerging drug resistance. The usual adult dose is 15 mg of the base taken daily for 14 days. Southeast Asian strains of P. vivax have exoerythrocytic stages that are more resistant to primaquine than strains from other regions.[237] It has been shown that the tissue schizontocidal activity of primaquine is a function of total dose rather than duration of administration,[238] and higher dose regi-

mens (30 mg daily for 14 days or 60 mg for 7 days) are recommended for eliminating these resistant strains in patients with normal glucose-6-phosphate dehydrogenase activity.[239]

MECHANISM OF ACTION. The mechanism of action of the 8-aminoquinolines is unknown. There is evidence that primaquine may become associated with the mitochondria of the exoerythrocytic forms of plasmodia growing in culture[240] and that exposure to primaquine causes the mitochondria to swell and become vacuolated.[241] The mechanism of action of the 8-aminoquinolines may be related to the action of naphthoquinones such as atovaquone, which has been shown to inhibit the cytochrome bc1 complex of the mitochondrial respiratory chain and collapse the mitochondrial membrane potential.[242-244] Primaquine at high concentration inhibits the growth of B. megaterium, and protein synthesis is inhibited early in the time course of the drug effect.[245] The interpretation of this observation is subject to the same reservations as the inhibition of bacterial nucleic acid synthesis by chloroquine. Inhibition of protein synthesis at high primaquine concentrations has been demonstrated in a subcellular system from rat liver that incorporates amino acids into polypeptide under the direction of synthetic mRNA.[246,247] Chloroquine in high concentration also inhibits protein synthesis in this

Table 13–5. Activity of the major antimalarial drugs against different forms of P. vivax *and* P. falciparum.

Drug	Blood schizontocidal activity		Tissue schizontocidal activity P. vivax	Gametocidal activity	
	P. falciparum	P. vivax		P. falciparum	P. vivax
Chloroquine	+	+	−	−	−
Mefloquine	+	+	−	−	−
Quinine	+	+	−	−	±
Primaquine	−	±	+	+	+
Pyrimethamine	+	+	−	−	−
Sulfonamides and sulfones	+	±	−	−	−
Tetracyclines	±	?	?	?	?

Source: Prepared from information reviewed in Dietrich and Kern.[29]

system. These experiments are not definitive, and there is no suggestion that the primary effect of the drug is either in the mitochondrion or at the level of protein synthesis.

There is good reason to believe that much of the antimalarial effect of 6-methoxy-8-aminoquinolines like primaquine may be due to products of metabolism and not to the drugs themselves.[248] This possibility injects an element of doubt into the meaning of in vitro studies of the biochemical effects of primaquine. The reader is referred to a review by Grewal[249] for a detailed discussion of studies concerned with the mechanism of primaquine action.

PHARMACOKINETICS OF PRIMAQUINE. Primaquine is rapidly absorbed from the gastrointestinal tract and peak concentrations of the drug are achieved in the plasma 1–2 h after an oral dose.[250] It is usually given orally as it causes marked hypotension after parenteral administration. The concentration of unaltered drug in the plasma declines rapidly the (half-life is about 4 h) and less than 1% of a dose is excreted as unaltered drug in the urine in 24 h.[250] The apparent volume of distribution is several times that of total body water. Studies in animals indicate that the rapid plasma half-life of the drug is due largely to rapid metabolism.[250,251] It is clear that, at least for pamaquine and pentaquine, some of the metabolites are more potent antimalarials than the parent compounds.[252,253] This would also seem to be the case with primaquine. The prophylactic effect of a single dose of primaquine is maximal when it is administered 12 h before infection.[253] The difference between the time of peak plasma levels of the unaltered drug and peak therapeutic effect may be due to the fact that more active forms of the drug are being produced by metabolism in the patient. Several metabolites of primaquine have been identified in the urine of animals, including the 5-hydroxy, 6-hydroxy, and 5,6-dihydroxy derivatives.[254] The carboxyl derivative is the major metabolite found in human plasma.[255] This nontoxic metabolite is eliminated more slowly and accumulates with multiple doses.[256] The metabolites of primaquine seem to have greater hemolytic activity than the parent drug.[257]

ADVERSE EFFECTS OF PRIMAQUINE (GLUCOSE-6-PHOSPHATE DEHYDROGENASE DEFICIENCY). At the doses usually employed to prevent recurrence of malaria, primaquine is generally well tolerated.[258] Occasionally, patients may experience abdominal discomfort, nausea, or headache. Leukopenia occurs rarely and agranulocytosis very rarely. Like several other oxidant drugs, primaquine promotes the conversion of hemoglobin to methemoglobin, producing cyanosis when the methemoglobin level is about 10% of the normal level of hemoglobin.[258] A primaquine metabolite is probably responsible for the hemoglobin oxidation.[259] Cyanosis is unusual with the dosage regimens that are commonly recommended for malaria therapy. The most important side effect of primaquine is hemolytic anemia, which occurs in people with glucose-6-phosphate dehydrogenase (G6PD) deficiency. This condition has been called *primaquine sensitivity*, and it is due to metabolites of primaquine that undergo redox cycling in the erythrocytes.[260]

Although most patients tolerate primaquine well, therapeutic doses can precipitate acute intravascular hemolysis in patients who have a deficiency of G6PD in their red cells (for a review see Beutler[261]). Males are more likely to experience hemolysis than females, since the gene determining the G6PD deficiency is carried on the X chromosome.[262] The severity of hemolysis is directly related to the degree of enzyme deficiency and the primaquine dosage. A number of G6PD variants exist and the degree of enzyme deficiency varies widely. G6PD deficiency occurs in about 10% of black males who possess the African variant (A⁻) which is characterized by a mild deficiency. People of eastern Mediterranean and west Asian descent possessing the Mediterranean variant (B⁻) and east Asian populations possessing Asian variants have more severe enzyme deficiency.[263,264] In blacks with the A⁻ variant only erythrocytes older than 55 days are hemolyzed,[265] but in people with B⁻ and Asian variants, younger erythrocytes are en-

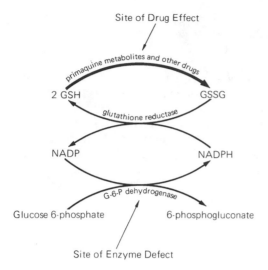

Figure 13–4. Scheme of the principal reactions related to the hemolysis that occurs in primaquine-sensitive patients. In the presence of primaquine metabolites and a number of other drugs, reduced glutathione (GSH) is converted to oxidized glutathione (GSSG). In erythrocytes from normal individuals the GSH level is maintained at a constant amount by the glutathione reductase reaction, which requires NADPH. The principal source of NADPH in the cell is the glucose-6-phosphate dehydrogenase (G6PD) reaction. In primaquine-sensitive individuals, G6PD activity is low, and the cell consequently cannot provide enough NADPH to keep up the levels of GSH in the presence of hemolyzing drugs. The depressed levels of GSH apparently render the erythrocyte unable to inactivate hydrogen peroxide. Oxidative damage to erythrocyte membranes by hydrogen peroxide renders the cells susceptible to mechanical breakage.

zyme deficient and more severe hemolysis occurs.[258]

Hemolysis may be precipitated by a variety of oxidant drugs in G6PD-deficient patients, including several antimicrobial agents such as other 8-aminoquinolines, 4-aminoquinolines (chloroquine), quinine, sulfonamides, sulfones, and nitrofurantoin.[261] Hemolysis is due to mechanical breakage, which is thought to occur because red cell membranes become fragile as a result of oxidative damage. The G6PD-deficient red cell has a low reducing capacity and cannot pre-

vent the membrane damage. As shown in Figure 13–4, glucose-6-phosphate dehydrogenase is responsible for the oxidation of glucose-6-phosphate to 6-phosphogluconic acid. This reaction is necessary to produce NADPH, which functions as a proton donor in the glutathione reductase reaction. In this second reaction, reduced glutathione is produced from oxidized glutathione. Reduced glutathione is necessary for the maintenance of red cell integrity. A metabolite of primaquine acts in the erythrocyte as an oxidizing agent and converts reduced glutathione to oxidized glutathione.[266] With a deficiency of G6PD, the cell is unable to produce enough NADPH to regenerate the reduced form of glutathione, and hemolysis takes place.

There is evidence that in the red cell, glutathione peroxidase is the major mechanism of defense against oxidative damage.[267] This enzyme catalyzes the reduction of hydrogen peroxide with the generation of water and oxidized glutathione. In addition, it can catalyze the reduction of lipid peroxides. It has been suggested that the action of glutathione peroxidase may break the autocatalytic chain reaction of lipid peroxidation and thus protect the red cell membrane from oxidative damage.[268] In the presence of primaquine, the G6PD-deficient patient may not produce enough reduced glutathione to provide adequate reducing equivalents for this reaction, and the resulting oxidative damage to the membrane may predispose the red cell to lysis.

The effect of an oxidizing agent on the glutathione content of normal and G6PD-deficient red cells is presented in Figure 13–5.[269] The glutathione content in erythrocytes was measured after incubation with acetylphenylhydrazine, one of the most effective hemolytic compounds. Before exposure to acetylphenylhydrazine, the erythrocytes from normal controls and G6PD-deficient individuals contain the same amount of reduced glutathione. After 2 h of incubation in the presence of the oxidant, the erythrocytes from the G6PD-deficient individuals have a much lower level of reduced glutathione. Rapid clinical tests are now routinely available for identifying the G6PD-deficient patient.[270]

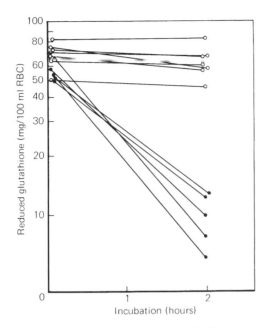

Figure 13–5. Reduced glutathione (GSH) content of normal and G6PD-deficient red blood cells. Assays for GSH were performed on blood samples from seven nonsensitive (○-○) and five primaquine-sensitive subjects (●-●). The erythrocytes were then incubated in the presence of acetylphenylhydrazine for 2 h, and the GSH assay was repeated. (From Beutler.[269])

Patients of appropriate ethnic origin should be tested for G6PD deficiency. High-dose daily regimens of primaquine should be avoided in G6PD-deficient patients. For radical cure of *P. vivax,* patients with the African A⁻ variant may be treated with 45 mg of base weekly for 8 weeks, and those with the Mediterranean B⁻ variant should receive 30 mg weekly for 30 weeks.[258]

PRECAUTIONS AND CONTRAINDICATIONS. Although it has not been established conclusively that primaquine causes teratogenic effects in humans, use of this drug probably should be postponed until after delivery. Patients should be tested for G6PD deficiency before they receive primaquine because of the possibility of the hemolytic reaction described above. At daily doses exceeding 30 mg of primaquine base, repeated blood counts and at least a gross examination of the urine for hemoglobin should be carried out.

DRUG INTERACTIONS. Primaquine should not be used in patients who are receiving other potentially hemolytic drugs. The same applies for compounds that can depress the myeloid elements of the bone marrow.

Inhibitors of Folate Metabolism and Antibiotics

The Inhibitors of Folic Acid Synthesis

ANTIMALARIAL ACTIVITY AND THERAPEUTIC USE. Several compounds that inhibit the synthesis of folic acid have been developed for antimalarial use; these include pyrimethamine, chloroguanide, and cycloguanil pamoate. Pyrimethamine is the most potent of these drugs and is most widely used clinically. Chloroguanide (proguanil) is not sold

Pyrimethamine

in the United States but is available in other countries under the trade name *Paludrine.* Chloroguanide itself is not the active form of the drug. It was demonstrated some time ago that chloroguanide has no effect on the exoerythrocytic forms of *P. gallinaceum* in vitro. When the drug was incubated with minced liver tissue, however, it proved to be very effective.[271] The active dihydrotriazine metabolite produced by the body tissues is a closed ring form that has a structure similar to that of pyrimethamine (Fig. 13–6). Chloroguanide together with chloroquine is used as a safe alternative to mefloquine or other regimens for the prophylaxis of *P. falciparum* malaria or mixed *P. vivax* and *P. falciparum* infections in parts of eastern, southern, and central Africa. Prophylaxis is recommended during exposure and for 4 weeks afterward.[272] Although not available in the United States, chloroguanide is widely available in Canada and overseas. It is in-

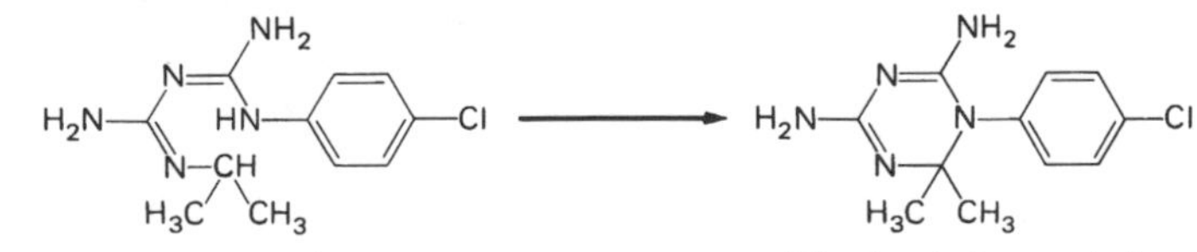

Figure 13–6. Chloroguanide is inactive as an antimalarial compound until it is altered by ring closure in the body to form the active dihydrotriazine metabolite.

Chloroguanide

Dihydrotriazine metabolite
(active form of drug)

effective against multidrug-resistant strains of *P. falciparum* in Thailand and New Guinea. Cycloguanil pamoate is a repository form of the active triazine metabolite of chloroguanide that has been used in combination with acedapsone to obtain suppressive prophylaxis by injection at intervals of 3 months or more. This repository drug is not available in the United States. The combination of trimethoprim and sulfamethoxazole (see Chapter 7) may also be used to treat malaria when conventional antimalarial agents are not available.[273]

Pyrimethamine and the other drugs in this class are active against the erythrocytic forms of *P. falciparum* and they are used in combination with a sulfonamide or a sulfone to treat acute attacks of chloroquine-resistant falciparum malaria.[29] Because the onset of antiplasmodial action is slow, the rapid-acting blood schizontocide quinine is usually administered simultaneously (see Table 13–4 for dosage regimens). Pyrimethamine alone is rarely used for the prophylaxis or treatment of malaria because resistance is widespread. Although the pyrimethamine-sulfonamide combination has some activity against the erythrocytic forms of *P. vivax*, it has not proven to be effective therapy for treatment of the acute attack of vivax malaria, where chloroquine is the drug of choice.[274] Pyrimethamine and the other folate inhibitors are active against the primary hepatic schizont formed by *P. falciparum*. Prophylactic use of the combination is no longer recommended because of the potential for serious sulfonamide toxicity.[275] The combination of pyrimethamine, a sulfonamide, and quinine is a regimen of choice in the treatment of an acute attack of malaria due to a chloroquine-resistant organism where resistance to the combination is not known to occur. Pyrimethamine is also used for the suppressive treatment of chloroquine-resistant *P. falciparum* malaria in parts of Africa where resistance to antifolates has not yet fully developed. Travelers to these areas are told to carry a treatment dose of pyrimethamine-sulfadoxine to take in case of a presumed malarial illness. Medical attention should be obtained as soon as possible after that. Pyrimethamine and chlorguanide do not diminish gametocytemia or sterilize gametocytes in mosquitos that feed on the patient subsequent to medication.[276]

MECHANISM OF ACTION. Early investigations carried out in bacteria demonstrated that pyrimethamine, like trimethoprim, inhibits the synthesis of reduced forms of folic acid.[277] Since the mechanism of action of this type of dihydrofolate reductase inhibitor has been discussed in detail in Chapter 7, the effect of pyrimethamine will be reviewed here only briefly. It is suggested that both descriptions be read for a comprehensive understanding of the drug effect.

It has been shown that plasmodia synthesize dihydrofolate de novo in much the same way that bacteria do (Fig. 13–7)[278,279] Dihydrofolate is then reduced in the presence of dihydrofolate reductase to tetrahydrofolate. This is the form of the compound that can function as the one-carbon carrier molecule required for the synthesis of methionine, glycine, thymidine, and the purines. Pyrimethamine inhibits the dihydrofolate reductase enzyme isolated from *P. berghei* in a manner that is competitive with the natural substrate dihydrofolate.[280] In Figure 13–8, the structure of pyrimethamine is redrawn to show the similarity between the drug and the pteridine moiety of dihydrofolate.

The reduction of folic acid compounds is a necessary step in the normal biochemistry of the host as well as the plasmodium (Fig.

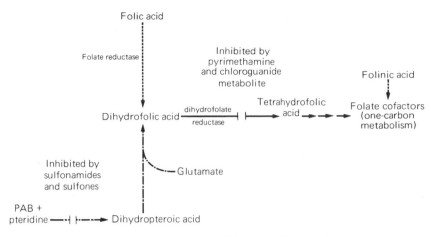

Figure 13–7. Schematic representation of sites of action for inhibitors of dihydrofolate synthesis and reduction. Reactions occurring in parasite only (—·—·—), humans only (–––––––), and parasite and humans (——).

13–7). Inhibition of this enzyme by the drug would be expected to have a severe adverse effect in the patient (easily demonstrated with other antifolates, such as methotrexate). This is not the case, however. The selective toxicity of pyrimethamine is based on the fact that it binds very strongly to the dihydrofolate reductase from plasmodia and very weakly to the human enzyme.[281–283] This relationship is presented in Table 13–6.

The concentration of the pyrimethamine required to inhibit the enzyme from *P. berghei* is only about 5×10^{-10} *M*, whereas a concentration of 1.8×10^{-6} *M* is required to inhibit human dihydrofolate reductase. This amounts to a 3600-fold difference in the sensitivity of the two enzymes to the drug. The different sensitivities probably reflect differences in the amino acid composition at or near the active site of the enzyme. The dif-

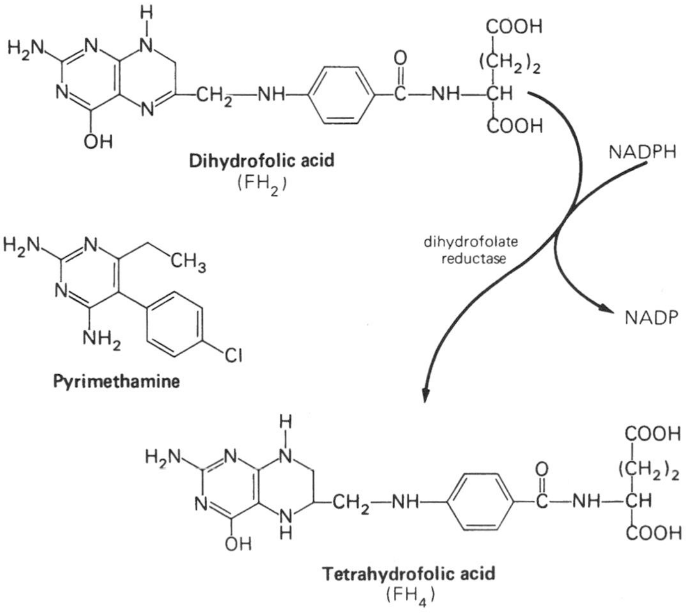

H₂N — ... Dihydrofolic acid (FH₂)

Pyrimethamine

Tetrahydrofolic acid (FH₄)

NADPH

NADP

dihydrofolate reductase

Figure 13–8. Dihydrofolate reductase reaction. This enzyme converts FH_2 to FH_4. It is inhibited by pyrimethamine, which is presented here to demonstrate the structural similarity to the pteridine portion of the normal substrate FH_2.

Table 13–6. Inhibition of dihydrofolate reductases by pyrimethamine and trimethoprim. Dihydrofolate reductase was purified from several sources. The concentration of drug (nanomolar) required to inhibit the activity of each enzyme preparation by 50% is shown.

Source of enzyme	50% inhibitory concentration (nM)	
	Pyrimethamine	Trimethoprim
Protozoal		
Plasmodium berghei	0.5	70
Bacterial		
Escherichia coli	2500	5
Mammalian		
Human liver	1800	300,000

Source: Data compiled from Ferone et al.[282] and Burchall and Hitchings.[283]

ference between the spectrum of enzyme inhibition by pyrimethamine and that of trimethoprim can also be appreciated from the data in Table 13–6. Pyrimethamine acts quite selectively on the plasmodial enzyme. Trimethoprim is most active against the bacterial enzyme, but it also has considerable selective toxicity for the plasmodial reductase.

COMBINATION THERAPY WITH SULFONES AND SULFONAMIDES. Since the plasmodium must synthesize dihydrofolic acid, such drugs as the sulfonamides and sulfones, which compete for the utilization of para-aminobenzoic acid in that synthetic pathway, should be active as antimalarial agents. This is the case. The antifolate compounds act at three stages in the parasite life cycle; the pre-erythrocytic (hepatic) phase; the asexual (blood) stage, where their main effect is; and they also inhibit sporozoite development in the mosquito.[127] Inhibition by antifolates occurs relatively late in the life cycle of malarial parasites as a result of failure of nuclear division at the time of schizont formation in erythrocytes and liver. This mechanism is consistent with the slow onset of action of the antifolates as compared to that of chloroquine and other quinoline antimalarials. When used alone sulfonamides and sulfones have a relatively poor efficacy against *P. vivax* and a good but slow action against *P. falciparum*.[284] When sulfonamides or sulfones are administered with a dihydro-

folate reductase inhibitor like pyrimethamine, a synergistic effect may be obtained in antimalarial therapy.[285] This can be seen in the experiment presented in Figure 13–9, which demonstrates that the presence of very low concentrations of sulfadiazine markedly reduces the amount of pyrimethamine required for the therapeutic effect. The combination of a sulfonamide and trimethoprim is used in the treatment of a variety of bacterial infections. The biochemical basis for the synergism often observed with combinations of a dihydrofolate reductase inhibitor and a sulfonamide or sulfone is discussed in detail in Chapter 7.

RESISTANCE TO PYRIMETHAMINE. Malarial organisms can develop resistance to pyrimethamine and cross-resistance to other antifolate drugs usually occurs.[286,287] Resistance to pyrimethamine may develop in regions of prolonged or extensive drug use. Dihydrofolate reductase genes have been cloned and sequenced in strains of *P. falciparum* that are either sensitive or resistant to pyrimethamine. Single base pair mutations in the dihydrofolate reductase gene confer reduced affinity to the drugs and thus resistance.[288] There may be resistance to pyrimethamine and not the biguanides, and vice versa, depending on the site of the point mutation.

PHARMACOKINETICS OF PYRIMETHAMINE. Pyrimethamine is provided in 25 mg tablets,

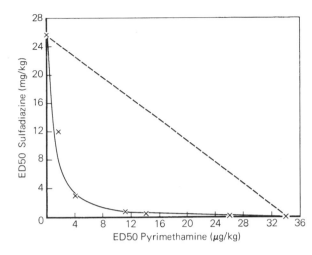

Figure 13-9. Synergism observed with sulfadiazine and pyrimethamine in chicks infected with *P. gallinaceum.* The figure presents the doses of pyrimethamine and sulfadiazine, administered both singly and together in various proportions, which were required to reduce parasitemia to 50% of controls. If the effect of the two drugs had been additive rather than synergistic, the data points would have described the dashed line. (Modified from Rollo.[285])

either alone or in combination with 500 mg sulfadoxine (*Fansidar*) or 100 mg dapsone (*Maloprim*). The drug is well absorbed from the gastrointestinal tract. Average peak levels of about 225 nanograms per ml are achieved in the plasma of adult volunteers 4 h after ingestion of a single 25 mg tablet (Table 13-7).[289,290] The half-life of pyrimethamine is about 4 days, and after a single 50 mg dose, suppressive levels are maintained in the blood for at least 2 weeks.[291] Neither the absorption of pyrimethamine nor its half-life is affected by the presence of sulfadoxine or dapsone in the combined preparations.[289,290] Pyrimethamine is bound in the tissues to a much greater extent than chloroguanide and its apparent volume of distribution is about 3 liters/kg.[290] It accumulates mainly in the kidneys, lungs, liver, and spleen. Pyrimethamine is extensively metabolized, with only about 1%–2% of a dose being recov-

ered in the urine unchanged in 24 h.[292] Blood concentrations of pyrimethamine are lower in patients with malaria than in healthy subjects, reflecting either incomplete absorption or an expanded volume of distribution.[293] Chloroguanide is excreted in the urine, 60% as unchanged drug, 30% as the bioactive traizine metabolite, and the remainder as other metabolites.[294] Because tissue binding is less and excretion by the kidneys is more rapid, chloroguanide is shorter acting than pyrimethamine and it is given daily for prophylaxis (the adult dose is usually 100 mg). Because of its longer half-life and higher potency, pyrimethamine is now the more popular drug. Pyrimethamine is secreted in human milk and sufficient drug passes into the breast milk of a woman receiving 25 mg weekly to yield suppressive levels in the nursing infant.[295]

The preparation of sulfonamide or sulfone

Table 13-7.   Pharmacokinetic characteristics of pyrimethamine, sulfadoxine, and dapsone as they are administered in the combined preparation containing 25 mg pyrimethamine and either 500 mg sulfadoxine or 100 mg dapsone. The pharmacology of the sulfonamides and sulfones is presented in detail in Chapters 7 and 11, respectively.

Drug	Time to peak plasma concentration (hours)	Mean peak plasma concentration after administration of one tablet to an adult (μg/ml)	Mean plasma half-life (hours)
Pyrimethamine	4.2	0.225 (range 0.150–0.300)	90 (range 50–140)
Sulfadoxine	3.7	63.2	184
Dapsone	2 to 4	1.55	27

Source: Table prepared from data of Weidekamm et al.[289] and Ahmad and Rogers.[290]

that is used in conjunction with pyrimetham-ine is determined by the frequency of admin-istration. When pyrimethamine is adminis-tered twice a day for treatment of the acute attack of malaria, a short-acting drug like sulfadiazine is administered. When pyrime-thamine is administered once weekly for prophylaxis, it is combined with the longer-acting drugs sulfadoxine or dapsone (see Ta-ble 13–7). Sulfadoxine is very slowly ex-creted in the urine, almost entirely as the unchanged drug,[296] and it has a half-life of 7–9 days.[289,297]

ADVERSE EFFECTS OF PYRIMETHAMINE. When pyrimethamine is used alone in antimalarial doses it causes little toxicity except occa-sional skin rashes and hematopoietic depres-sion. When 25 mg is administered daily, as in the treatment of toxoplasmosis, megalo-blastic anemia of the folate deficiency type may occur. Patients who may have a pro-pensity to folate deficiency, such as alcohol-ics, the aged, pregnant women, malnour-ished patients, and those with chronic intestinal diseases, are at risk of developing hematological complications. At concentra-tions of pyrimethamine that are achieved in the plasma of adults receiving 25 mg weekly, the drug partially inhibits folate reductase in primary cultures of human marrow cells.[298] When daily therapy is continued for more than a few days, folinic acid (10 mg/kg daily) may be administered to prevent the anemia. As can be seen in Figure 13–7, fol-inic acid cannot be utilized by the plasmo-dium,[278] but it is taken into the mammalian cell and shunts around the drug-blocked re-action. The marrow-depressant effect of pyr-imethamine has been exploited with the use of higher doses in the treatment of polycy-themia rubra vera. Although animal studies suggest that pyrimethamine may have tera-togenic potential, the drug has been admin-istered to pregnant women, and teratogenic-ity has not been reported in humans. Fansidar should not be administered to per-sons who are allergic to sulfonamides, and it should not be administered to children un-der 2 months of age, as sulfonamides may induce neonatal jaundice. Routine hemo-grams should be obtained from persons who are on Fansidar prophylaxis for longer than 6 months.

When the combination of pyrimethamine-sulfadoxine is used in malaria it is the sul-fonamide that accounts for the toxicity as-sociated with this drug combination. In most countries it is no longer used for antimalarial prophylaxis because in about 1/5000 to 1/8000 people there are severe and even fatal cutaneous reactions such as erythema mul-tiforme, Stevens-Johnson syndrome, and toxic epidermal necrolysis. This drug com-bination has also been associated with serum sickness–type reactions, urticaria, exfoliative dermatitis, and hepatitis.[275]

Antibiotics

It has been known for many years that some antibiotics (e.g., the tetracyclines, chloram-phenicol) have antimalarial activity. Studies with infected animals suggest an effect on both the erythrocytic and tissue forms of or-ganisms. When tetracyclines are given alone, the rate of clearance of P. falciparum is slow.[299] Although the tetracyclines are not optimal antimalarial agents, the emergence of multidrug-resistant strains of P. falcipa-rum has given them a role in therapy. Tet-racyclines are particularly useful for the treatment of the acute malarial attack due to multidrug-resistant strains of P. falciparum that also show partial resistance to qui-nine.[300] Because the infection usually does not respond for 3 or 4 days, it is essential to administer a rapid-acting blood schizonto-cide, like quinine, at the beginning of the course of therapy.[301–303] Several tetracylines appear to be equivalent, but tetracycline or doxycycline is usually recommended. Since there is a risk of changing the drug sensitiv-ity of pathogenic bacteria, the tetracyclines should not be used on a long-term basis. In-stead, doxycycline is used alone by travelers for short-term prophylaxis of multidrug-resistant strains. Clindamycin is another an-tibiotic that can affect a radical cure of P. falciparum.[304] It also acts slowly, and a rapid-acting drug such as quinine must be given initially. The possibility of developing colitis should be remembered if clindamycin is being considered for therapy (see Chapter 6.)

REFERENCES

1. Hoffman, S. Diagnosis, treatment and prevention of malaria. *Med. Clin. North Am.* 1992;76:1327.
2. Karunakaran, C. S. A clinical trial of malaria prophylaxis using a single dose of chloroquine at different intervals in an endemic malarious area. *J. Trop. Med. Hyg.* 1980;83:195.
3. Stone; R. Global warming: if mercury soars, so may health hazards. *Science* 1995;267:957.
4. Olliaro, P., J. Cattani, and D. Wirth. Malaria, the submerged disease. *JAMA* 1996;275:230.
5. Wernsdorfer, W. H. Prospects for the development of malaria vaccines. *Bull. WHO* 1981;59:335.
6. Kreig, M. B. The incredible history of quinine. In *Green Medicine.* New York: Rand McNally, 1964, pp. 165–206.
7. Barat, L., and P. Bloland. Drug resistance among malaria and other parasites. *Infect. Dis. Clin. North Am.* 1997;11:969.
8. Krogstad, D. J., *Plasmodium* species (malaria). In *Mandell, Douglas and Bennett's Principles and Practice of Infectious Diseases*, ed. by G. Mandell, J. Bennett, and R. Dolin. New York: Churchill-Livingstone, 1995, pp. 2415–2427.
9. White, N. J. The treatment of malaria. *N. Engl. J. Med.* 1996;335:800.
10. Peters, W. Chemotherapy of malaria. In *Malaria*, Vol. 1, ed. by J. P. Kreier. New York: Academic Press, 1980, pp. 145–283.
11. Coggeshall, L. T. Malaria. In *Textbook of Medicine*, ed. by P. B. Beeson and W. McDermott. Philadelphia: W. B. Saunders, 1963, pp. 383–389.
12. Population Information Program. Community-based health and family planning. *Popul. Rep. L* 1982; 3:L–77.
13. Wernsdorfer, W. H., and R. L. Kouznetsov. Drug-resistant malaria—occurrence, control, and surveillance. *Bull. WHO* 1981;58:341.
14. Thaithong, S., G. H. Beale, and M. Chutmongkonkul. Susceptibility of *Plasmodium falciparum* to five drugs: an in vitro study of isolates mainly from Thailand. *Trans. R. Soc. Trop. Med. Hyg.* 1983;77:228.
15. Wernsdorfer; W. H., The importance of malaria in the world. In *Malaria*, Vol. 1, ed. by J. P. Kreier. New York: Academic Press, 1980, pp. 1–93.
16. Zucker, J. R., and C. C. Campbell. Malaria: principles of prevention and treatment. *Infect. Dis. Clin. North Am.* 1993;7:547.
17. Lobel, H., and P. Kozarsky. Update on prevention of malaria for travelers. *JAMA* 1997;278:1767.
18. Greenwood; B. Malaria chemoprophylaxis in endemic regions. In: *Malaria—Waiting for the Vaccine*, ed. by G.A.T. Target. London: Long School of Hygiene and Tropical Medicine; First Annual Public Health Forum, 1991, pp. 83–104.
19. Fryauff, D., J. Baird, H. Basri, I. Sumawinata, Purnomo, T. Richie, C. Ohrt, E. Mouzin, C. Church, A. Richards, B. Subianto, B. Sandjaja, F. Wignall, and S. Hoffman. Randomized placebo-controlled trial of primaquine for prophylaxis of falciparum and vivax malaria. *Lancet* 1995;346:1190.
20. Malaria. In: *International Travel and Health: Vaccination Requirements and Health Advice: Situations as of January 1995.* Geneva, Switzerland: World Health Organization 67, 1994.
21. Pussard, E., J. P. Lepers, F. Clavier, L. Raharimalala, J. LeBras, M. Frisk-Holmberg, Y. Bergqvist, and F. Verdier. Efficacy of a loading dose of oral chloroquine in a 36-hour treatment schedule for uncomplicated *Plasmodium falciparum* malaria. *Antimicrob. Agents Chemother.* 1991;35:406.
22. Tracy, J. W., and L. T. Webster. Chemotherapy of parasitic infections. In *Goodman and Gilman's The Pharmacological Basis of Therapeutics*, ed. by J. G. Hardman, L. E. Limbird, P. B. Molinoff, R. W. Ruddon, and A. G. Gilman. New York: McGraw-Hill, 1995, pp. 955–985.
23. Centers for Disease Control. Occurrence of malaria acquired during travel abroad among civilians, 1970–1976. *J. Infect. Dis.* 1979;139:255.
24. Centers for Disease Control. *Plasmodium falciparum* malaria contracted in Thailand resistant to chloroquine and sulfonamide-pyrimethamine—Illinois. *MMWR Morb. Mortal Wkly. Rep.* 1980;29:493.
25. Miller, M. B., J. L. Bratton, J. P. Hanson, M. Cohen, R. D. Reynolds, D. C. Lohr, J. Hunt, and D. Jilek. Experience with mixed infections of *Plasmodium falciparum* and *vivax*. *Mil. Med.* 1973;138:567.
26. World Health Organization, Division of Control of Tropical Diseases. Severe and complicated malaria. *Trans. R. Soc. Trop. Med. Hyg.* 1990;84(Suppl.2):1.
27. Molyneux, M. E., T. E. Taylor, J. J. Wirima, and A. Borgstein. Clinical features and prognostic indicators in paediatric cerebral malaria: a study of 131 comatose Malawian children. *Q. J. Med.* 1989;71: 441.
28. Marsh, K., D. Forster. C. Waruiru, I. Mwangi, M. Winstanley, V. Marsh, C. Newton, P. Winstanley, P. Warn, N. Peshu, G. Pasvol, and R. Snow. Indicators of life-threatening malaria in African Children. *N. Engl. J. Med.* 1995;332:1399.
29. Dietrich, M., and P. Kern. Malaria. *Antibiot. Chemother.* 1981;30:224.
30. Easterbrook, M. Ocular effects and safety of antimalarial agents. *Am. J. Med.* 1988;85(Suppl. 4A):23.
31. Rynes, R. I., and H. N. Bernstein. Ophthalmologic safety profile of antimalarial drugs. *Lupus* 1993; 2:S17.
32. Schmidt, L. H., D. Vaughan, D. Mueller, R. Crosby, and R. Hamilton. Activities of various 4-amino-quinolines against infections with chloroquine-resistant strains of *Plasmodium falciparum*. *Antimicrob. Agents Chemother.* 1977;11:826.
33. Dubois, E. L., Antimalarials in the management of discoid and systematic lupus erythematosis. *Semin. Arthritis Rheum.* 1978;8:33.
34. Tanenbaum, L. and D. L. Tuffanelli. Antimalarial agents. *Arch. Dermatol.* 1980;116:587.
35. Polet, H. Influence of sucrose on chloroquine-3-H^3 content of mammalian cells in vitro: the possible role

of lysosomes in chloroquine resistance. *J. Pharmacol. Exp. Ther.* 1970;173:71.

36. Berliner, R. W., D. P. Earle, J. V. Taggart, C. G. Zubrod, W. J. Welch, N. J. Conan, E. Bauman, S. T. Scudder, and J. A. Shannon. Studies on the chemotherapy of human malarias: VI. The physiological disposition, anti-malarial activity, and toxicity of several derivatives of 4-aminoquinoline. *J. Clin. Invest.* 1948; 27(Suppl.):98.

37. Irvin, J. L., E. M. Irvin, and F. S. Parker. The interaction of antimalarials with nucleic acids. *Science* 1949;110:426.

38. O'Neill, P. M., P. G. Bray, S. R. Hawley, S. A. Ward, and B. K. Park. 4–aminoquinolines—past, present and future: a chemical perspective. *Pharmacol. Ther.* 1998;77:29.

39. Foley, M., and L. Tilley. Quinoline antimalarials: mechanisms of action and resistance and prospects for new agents. *Pharmacol. Ther.* 1998;79:55.

40. Polet, H. and C. F. Barr. Chloroquine and dihydroquinine: In vitro studies of their antimalarial effect upon *Plasmodium knowlesi. J. Pharmacol. Exp. Ther.* 1968;164:380.

41. Schellenberg, K. A., and G. R. Coatney. The influence of antimalarial drugs on nucleic acid synthesis in *Plasmodium gallinaceum* and *Plasmodium berghei. Biochem. Pharmacol.* 1961;6:143.

42. Ciak, J., and F. E. Hahn. Chloroquine: mode of action. *Science* 1966;151:347.

43. Cohen, S. N., and K. L. Yielding. Inhibition of DNA and RNA polymerase reactions by chloroquine. *Proc. Nat. Acad. Sci. U.S.A.* 1965;54:521.

44. Cohen, S. N., and K. L., Yielding. Spectrophotometric studies of the interaction of chloroquine with deoxyribonucleic acid. *J. Biol. Chem.* 1965;240:3123.

45. Waring, M. Variation of the supercoils in closed circular DNA by binding of antibiotics and drugs: evidence for molecular models involving intercalation. *J. Mol. Biol.* 1970;54:247.

46. Bolte, J., C. Demuynck, J. Lhomme, M. C. Fournie-Zaluski, and B. P. Roques. Synthetic models of deoxyribonucleic acid complexes with antimalarial compounds. Comparative ultraviolet and proton magnetic resonance study of quinoline-base, quinoline-quinoline, and base-base stacking interactions. *Biochemistry* 1979;18:4928.

47. Gabourel, J. D. Effects of hydroxychloroquine on the growth of mammalian cells in vitro. *J. Pharmacol. Exp. Ther.* 1963;141:122.

48. Gutteridge, W. E., P. I. Trigg, and P. M. Bayley. Effects of chloroquine on *Plasmodium knowlesi* in vitro. *Parasitology* 1972;64:37.

49. Macomber, P. B., R. L. O'Brien, and F. E. Hahn. Chloroquine: physiological basis of drug resistance in *Plasmodium berghei. Science* 1966;152:1374.

50. Krogstad, D. J., I. Y. Gluzman, D. E. Kyle, A. M. Oduola, S. K. Martin, W. K. Milhous, and P. H. Schlesinger. Efflux of chloroquine from *Plasmodium falciparum*: mechanism of chloroquine resistance. *Science* 1987;238:1283.

51. Yayon, A., Z. I. Cabantchik, and H. Ginsburg. Identification, of the acidic compartment of *Plasmodium falciparum*—infected human erythrocytes as the target of the antimalarial drug chloroquine. *EMBO J.* 1984;3:2695.

52. Yayon, A., R. Timberg, S. Friedman, and H. Ginsburg. Effects of chloroquine on the feeding mechanism of the intraerythrocytic human malarial parasite *Plasmodium falciparum. J. Protozool.* 1984;31:367.

53. Yayon, A., Z. I. Cabantchik, and H. Ginsburg. Susceptibility of human malaria parasites to chloroquine is pH dependent. *Proc. Natl. Acad. Sci. U.S.A.* 1985;82:2784.

54. Goldberg, D. E., A. F. G. Slater, A. Cerami, and G. B. Henderson. Haemoglobin degradation in the malaria parasite *Plasmodium falciparum*: an ordered process in a unique organelle. *Proc. Natl. Acad. Sci. U.S.A.* 1990;87:2931.

55. Gabay, T., M. Krugliak, G. Shalmaeiv, and H. Ginsburg. Inhibition by antimalarial drugs of haemoglobin denaturation and iron release in acidified erythrocytes: possible mechanism of their antimalarial effect. *Parasitology* 1994;108:371.

56. Rosenthal, P. J., J. H. McKerrow, M. Aikawa, H. Nagasawa and J. H. Leech. A malarial cysteine proteinase is necessary for haemoglobin degradation by *Plasmodium falciparum. J. Clin. Invest.* 1988;82: 1560.

57. Ginsburg, H., and M. Krugliak. Quinoline-containing antimalarials mode of action: drug resistance and its reversal. *Biochem. Pharmacol.* 1992;43:63.

58. Slater, A. F. G., and A. Cerami. Inhibition by chloroquine of a novel haem polymerase enzyme activity in malaria trophozoites. *Nature* 1992;355:167.

59. Chou, A. C., and C. D. Fitch. Heme polymerase: modulation by chloroquine treatment of a rodent malaria. *Life Sci.* 1992;51:2073.

60. Dorn, A., R. Stoffel, H. Matile, A. Bubendorf, and R. G. Ridely. Malarial haemozoin/β-haematin supports haem polymerization in the absence of protein. *Nature* 1995;374:269.

61. Ridley, R. G. Haemozoin formation in malaria parasites: is there a haem polymerase? *Trends Microbiol.* 1996;4:253.

62. Bendrat, K., B. J. Berger, and A. Cerami. Haem polymerization in malaria. *Nature* 1995;378:138.

63. Sullivan, D. J., I. Y. Gluzman, and D. E. Goldberg. *Plasmodium* hemozoin formation mediated by histidine-rich proteins. *Science* 1996;271:219.

64. Fitch, C. D. Antimalarial schizonticides: ferriprotoporphyrin IX intercalation hypothesis. *Parasitol. Today* 1986;2:330.

65. Egan, T. J., D. C. Ross, and P. A. Adams. Quinoline antimalarial drugs inhibit spontaneous formation of β-haematin (malaria pigment). *FEBS Lett.* 1994;352: 54.

66. Raynes, K., M. Foley, L. Tilley, and L. Deady. Novel bisquinoline antimalarials: synthesis, antimalarial activity and inhibition of haem polymerization. *Biochem. Pharmacol.* 1996;52:551.

67. Sullivan, D. J., I. Y. Gluzman, D. G. Russell, and D. E. Goldberg. On the molecular mechanism of chloroquine's antimalarial action. *Proc. Natl. Acad. Sci. U.S.A.* 1996;93:11865.

68. Pandey, A. V. and B. L. Tekwani. Depolymerisation of malarial hemozoin: a novel reaction initiated

by blood schizonticidal antimalarials. *FEBS Lett.* 1977; 402:236.

69. Dorn, A., S. R. Vippagunta, H. Matile, C. Jaquet, J. L. Vennerstrom, and R. G. Ridley. An assessment of drug-hematin binding as a mechanism for inhibition of haematin polymerisation by quinoline antimalarials. *Biochem. Pharmacol.* 1998;55:727.

70. Sullivan, D. J., H. Matile. R. G. Ridley, and D. E. Goldberg. A common mechanism for blockade of heme polymerization by antimalarial quinolines. *J. Biol. Chem.* 1998;273:31103.

71. Goldberg, D. E., V. Sharma, A. Oksman, I. Y. Gluzman, T. E. Wellems, and D. Piwnica-Worms. Probing the chloroquine resistance locus of *Plasmodium falciparum* with a novel class of multidentate metal (III) coordination complexes. *J. Biol. Chem.* 1997;272: 6567.

72. Meshnick, S. R. Is haemozoin a target for antimalarial drugs? *Ann. Trop. Med. Parasitol.* 1996;90: 367.

73. Chou, A. C., and C. D. Fitch. Control of heme polymerase by chloroquine and other quinoline derivatives. *Biochem. Biophys. Res. Commun.* 1993;195: 422.

74. Asawamahasakda, W., I. Ittarat, C. C. Chang, P. McElroy, and S. R. Meshnick. Effects of antimalarials and protease inhibitors on plasmodial hemozoin production. *Mol. Biochem. Parasitol.* 1994;67:183.

75. Menting, J. G. T., L. Tilley, Deady, L. W., K. Ng, A. F. Cowman, and M. Foley. The antimalarial drug, chloroquine, interacts specifically with lactate dehydrogenase from *Plasmodium falciparum.* *Mol. Biochem. Parasitol.* 1997;88:215.

76. Vander Jagt, D. L., L. A. Hunsaker, and N. M. Campos. Characterization of haemoglobin degrading, low molecular weight protease from *Plasmodium falciparum.* *Mol. Biochem. Parasitol.* 1986;18:389.

77. Wood, P. A., and J. W. Eaton. Hemoglobin catabolism and host-parasite heme balance in chloroquine-sensitive and chloroquine-resistant *Plasmodium berghei* infections. *Am. J. Trop. Med. Hyg.* 1993;48:465.

78. Meshnick, S. R., K. P. Chang, and A. Cerami. Heme lysis of the bloodstream forms of *Trypanosoma brucei.* *Biochem. Pharmacol.* 1977;26:1923.

79. Atamna, H., and H. Ginsburg. Origin of reactive oxygen species in erythrocytes infected with *Plasmodium falciparum.* *Mol. Biochem. Parasitol.* 1993;61: 231.

80. Fairfield, A. S., S. R. Meshnick, and J. W. Eaton. Malaria parasites adopt host cell superoxide dismutase. *Science* 1983;221:764.

81. Becuwe, P., C. Slomianny, D. Camus, and D. Dive. Presence of an endogenous superoxide dismutase activity in three rodent malaria species. *Parasitol. Res.* 1993;79:349.

82. Vennerstrom, J. L., and J. W. Eaton. Oxidants, oxidant drugs, and malaria. *J. Med. Chem.* 1988;31: 1269.

83. Vial, H., Recent developments and rationale towards new strategies for malarial chemotherapy. *Parasite* 1996;3:3.

84. Hunt, N. H., and R. Stocker. Oxidative stress and the redox status of malaria-infected erythrocytes. *Blood Cells* 1990;16:499.

85. Green, M. D., L. Xiao, and A. A. Lal. Formation of hydroxyeicosatetraenoic acids from hemozoincatalyzed oxidation of arachidonic acid. *Mol. Biochem. Parasitol.* 1996;83:183.

86. Ribeiro, M. C. de A., O. Augusto, and A. M. da C. Ferreira. Influence of quinoline-containing antimalarials in the catalase activity of ferriprotoporphyrin 1X. *J. Inorg. Biochem.* 1997;65:15.

87. Sugioka, Y., and M. Suzuki. The chemical basis for the ferriprotoporphyrin 1X-chloroquine complex induced lipid peroxidation. *Biochim. Biophys. Acta* 1991; 1074:19.

88. Malhotra, K., D. Salmon, J. Le Bras, and J. L. Vilde. Potentiation of chloroquine activity against *Plasmodium falciparum* by the peroxidase-hydrogen peroxide system. *Antimicrob. Agents Chemother.* 1990;34: 1981.

89. Dubois, V. L., D. F. Platel, G. Pauly, and J. Tribouley-Duret. *Plasmodium berghei*: implication of intracellular glutathione and its related enzyme in chloroquine resistance in vivo. *Exp. Parasitol.* 1995;81:117.

90. Ridley, R. G., Dissecting chloroquine resistance. *Curr. Biol.* 1998;8:346.

91. Foote, S. J. and A. F. Cowman. The mode of action and mechanism of resistance to antimalarial drugs. *Acta Trop.* 1994;56:157.

92. Bjorkman, A., and P. A. Phillips-Howard. Drug-resistant malaria: mechanisms of development and inferences for malaria control. *Trans. R. Soc. Trop. Med. Hyg.* 1990;84:323.

93. Le Bras, J., P. Deloron, A. Ricour, B. Andrieu, J. Savel, and J. P. Couland. *Plasmodium falciparum*: drug sensitivity in vitro of isolates before and after adaptation to continuous culture. *Exp. Parasitol.* 1983;56: 9.

94. Schuurkamp, G. J., P. E., Spicer, R. K. Kereu, P. K. Bulungol, and K. H. Rieckmann. Chloroquine-resistant *Plasmodium vivax* in Papua New Guinea. *Trans. R. Soc. Trop. Med. Hyg.* 1992;86:121.

95. Myat-Phone-Kyaw, Myint-Oo, Myint-Lwin, Thaw-Zin, Kyin-Hla-Aye and Nwe-Nwe-Yin. Emergence of chloroquine-resistant *Plasmodium vivax* in Myanmar (Burma). *Trans. R. Soc. Trop. Med. Hyg.* 1993;87:687.

96. Bray, P. G., M. Mungthin, R. G. Ridley, and S. A. Ward. Access to haematin: the basics of chloroquine resistance. *Mol. Pharmacol.* 1998;54:170.

97. Saliba, K. J., P. I. Folb, and P. J. Smith. Role for the *Plasmodium falciparum* digestive vacuole in chloroquine resistance. *Biochem. Pharm.* 1998;56:313.

98. Geary, T. G., J. B. Jensen, and H. Ginsburg. Uptake of [3H]chloroquine by drug-sensitive and -resistant strains of the human malaria parasite *Plasmodium falciparum.* *Biochem. Pharmacol.* 1986;35:3805.

99. Geary, T. G., A. D. Divo, J. B. Jensen, M. Zangwill, and H. Ginsburg. Kinetic modeling of the response of *Plasmodium falciparum* to chloroquine and its experimental testing in vitro. Implications for mechanism of action of and resistance to the drug. *Biochem. Pharmacol.* 1990;40:685.

100. Martin, S. K., A. M. J. Oduola, and W. K. Mil-

hous. Reversal of chloroquine resistance in *Plasmodium falciparum* by verapamil. *Science* 1990;235:899.

101. Ginsburg, H., and W. D. Stein. Kinetic modeling of chloroquine uptake by malaria-infected erythrocytes. Assessment of the factors that may determine drug resistance. *Biochem. Pharmacol.* 1991;41:1463.

102. Bray, P. G., R. E. Howells, G. Y. Ritchie, and S. A. Ward. Rapid chloroquine efflux phenotype in both chloroquine-sensitive and chloroquine-resistant *Plasmodium falciparum*. A correlation of chloroquine sensitivity with energy-dependent drug accumulation. *Biochem. Pharmacol.* 1992;44:1317.

103. Bray, P. G., M. K. Boulter, G. Y. Ritchie, R. E. Howells, and S. A. Ward. Relationship of global chloroquine transport and reversal of resistance in *Plasmodium falciparum*. *Mol. Biochem. Parasitol.* 1994;63:87.

104. Ridley, R. G., and A. T. Hudson. Quinoline antimalarials. *Exp. Opin. Ther. Patents* 1998;8:121.

105. Krogstad, D. J., and P. H. Schlesinger. A perspective on antimalarial action: effects of weak bases on *Plasmodium falciparum*. *Biochem. Pharmacol.* 1986;35:547.

106. Karcz, S. R., V. R. Herrmann, and A. F. Cowman. Cloning and characterization of a vacuolar ATPase. A subunit homologue from *Plasmodium falciparum*. *Mol. Biochem. Parasitol.* 1993;58:333.

107. Karcz, S. R., V. R. Herrmann, F. Trottein, and A. F. Cowman. Cloning and characterization of the vacuolar ATPase B subunit from *Plasmodium falciparum*. *Mol. Biochem. Parasitol.* 1994;65:123.

108. Krogstad, D. J., P. H. Schlesinger, and I. Y. Gluzman. Antimalarials increase vesicle pH in *Plasmodium falciparum*. *J. Cell Biol.* 1985;101:2301.

109. Warhurst, D. C., Antimalarial schizonticides: why a permease is necessary. *Parasitol. Today* 1986;4:211.

110. Hawley, S., P. Bray, K. Park, and S. Ward. Amodiaquine accumulation in *Plasmodium falciparum* as a possible explanation for its superior antimalarial activity over chloroquine. *Mol. Biochem. Parasitol.* 1996;80:15.

111. Wunsch, S., C. P. Sanchez, M. Gekle, L.-G. Wortmann, J. Wiesner, and M. Lanzer. Differential stimulation of the Na^+/H^+ exchanger determines chloroquine uptake in *Plasmodium falciparum*. *J. Cell Biol.* 1998;140:2645.

112. Su, X., L. A. Kirkman, H. Fujoka, and T. E. Wellems. Complex polymorphisms in a 330 kDa protein are linked to chloroquine-resistant *P. falciparum* in Southeast Asia and Africa. *Cell* 1997;91:593.

113. Wellems, T. E., L. A. Panton, I. Y. Gluzman, V. E. do Rosario, R. W. Geadz, A. Walker-Jonah, and D. J. Krogstad. Chloroquine resistance not linked to *mdr*-like genes in a *Plasmodium falciparum* cross. *Nature* 1990;345:253.

114. Sanchez, C. P., P. Horrocks, and M. Lanzer. Is the putative chloroquine resistance mediator cg2 the Na^+/H^+ exchanger of *Plasmodium falciparum*? *Cell* 1996;92:601.

115. Wellems, T. E., J. C. Wootton, H. Fujoka, X. Su, R. Cooper, D. Barach, and D. A. Fidock. *P. falciparum* CG2, linked to chloroquine resistance, does not resemble Na^+/H^+ exchangers. *Cell* 1998;94:285.

116. O'Brien, C. Beating the malaria parasite at its own game. *Lancet* 1997;350:192.

117. Webster, H. K., E. F. Boudreau, K. Pavanand, K. Yongvanitchit and L. W. Pang. Antimalarial drug susceptibility testing of *Plasmodium falciparum* in Thailand using a microdilution radioisotope method. *Am. J. Trop. Med. Hyg.* 1985;34:228.

118. Webster, H. K., S. Thaithong, K. Pavanand, K. Yongvanitchit, C. Pinswasdi, and E. F. Boudreau. Cloning and characterization of mefloquine-resistant *Plasmodium falciparum* from Thailand. *Am. J. Trop. Med. Hyg.* 1895;34:1022.

119. Wilson, C. M., S. K. Volkman, S. Thaithong, R. K. Martin, D. E. Kyle, W. K. Milhous and D. F. Wirth. Amplification of *pfmdr1* associated with mefloquine and halofantrine resistance in *P. falciparum* from Thailand. *Mol. Biochem. Parasitol.* 1993;57:151.

120. Cowman, A. F, D. Galatis, and J. K. Thompson. Selection for mefloquine resistance in *Plasmodium falciparum* is linked to amplification of the *pfmdr* 1 gene and cross-resistance to halofantrine and quinine. *Proc. Natl. Acad. Sci. U.S.A.* 1994;91:1143.

121. Peters, W. Chemotherapy and drug resistance. In *Malaria*. London: Academic Press, 1987.

122. Bray, P. G., S. R. Hawley, M. Mungthin, and S. A. Ward. Physicochemical properties correlated with drug resistance and the reversal of drug resistance in *Plasmodium falciparum*. *Mol. Pharmacol.* 1996;50:1559–1566.

123. Bray, P. G., S. R. Hawley, and S. A. Ward. 4-Aminoquinoline resistance of *Plasmodium falciparum*: insights from the study of amodiaquine uptake. *Mol. Pharmacol.* 1996;50:1551.

124. Nateghpour, M., S. A. Ward, and R. E. Howells. Development of halofantrine resistance and determination of cross-resistance patterns in *Plasmodium falciparum*. *Antimicrob. Agents Chemother.* 1993;37:2337.

125. Ward, S. A., P. G. Bray, M. Mungthin, and S. R. Hawley. Current views on the mechanisms of resistance of quinoline-containing drugs in *Plasmodium falciparum*. *Ann. Trop. Med. Parasitol.* 1995;89:121.

126. Frisk-Holmberg, M., Y. Bergqvist, E. Termond, and B. Domej-Nyberg. The single dose kinetics of chloroquine and its major metabolite desethylchloroquine in healthy subjects. *Eur. J. Clin. Pharmacol.* 1984;26:521.

127. White, N. J. Antimalarial pharmacokinetics and treatment regimens. *Br. J. Clin. Pharmacol.* 1992;34:1.

128. Edwards, G., P. A. Winstanley, and S. A. Ward. Clinical pharmacokinetics in the treatment of tropical diseases. Some applications and limitations. *Clin. Pharmacokinet.* 1994;27:150.

129. White, N. J., K. D. Miller, F. C. Churchill, C. Berry, J. Brown, S. B. Williams, and B. M. Greenwood. Chloroquine treatment of severe malaria in children. Pharmacokinetics, toxicity, and new dosage recommendations. *N. Engl. J. Med.* 1988;319:1493.

130. Brohult, J., L. Rombo, V. Sirleaf, and E. Bengtsson. The concentration of chloroquine in serum during short and long term malaria prophylaxis with standard and double dosage in non-immunes: clinical implications. *Ann. Trop. Med. Parasitol.* 1979;73:401.

131. Adelusi, S. A., and L. A., Salako. Protein bind-

ing of chloroquine in the presence of aspirin. *Br. J. Clin. Pharmacol.* 1982;13:451.

132. McChesney, E. W., W. D. Conway, W. F. Banks, J. E. Rogers, and J. M. Shekosky. Studies of the metabolism of some compounds of the 4-amino-7-chloroquinoline series. *J. Pharmacol. Exp. Ther.* 1966; 151:482.

133. McChesney, E. W., M. J. Fasco, and W. F. Banks. The metabolism of chloroquine in man during and after repeated oral dosage. *J. Pharmacol. Exp. Ther.* 1967;158:323.

134. Fabre, J., J. DeFreudenreich, A. Duckert, J. S. Pitton, M. Rudhardt, and C. Virieux. Influence of renal insufficiency on the excretion of chloroquine, phenobarbital, phenothiazines and methacycline. *Helv. Med. Acta* 1979;33:307.

135. Bennett, W. M., R. S. Muther, R. A. Parker, P. Feig, G. Morrison, T. A. Golper, and I. Singer. Drug therapy in renal failure: dosing guidelines for adults. Part I: Antimicrobial agents, analgesics. *Ann. Intern. Med.* 1980;93:62.

136. Van Stone, J. C. Hemodialysis and chloroquine poisoning. *J. Lab. Clin. Med.* 1976;88:87.

137. Price Evans, D. A., K. A. Fletcher, and J. D. Baty. The urinary excretion of chloroquine in different ethnic groups. *Ann. Trop. Med. Parasitol.* 1979;73:11.

138. Gaudette, L. E., and G. R. Coatney. A possible mechanism of prolonged antimalarial activity. *Am. J. Trop. Med. Hyg.* 1961;10:321.

139. Choudhry, V. P., N. Madan, and S. K. Sood. Intravascular hemolysis and renal insufficiency in children with glucose-6-phosphate dehydrogenase deficiency, following antimalarial therapy. *Ind. J. Med. Res.* 1980; 71:561.

140. Frisk-Holmberg, M., Y. Bergkvist, B. Domeij-Nyberg, L. Hellstrom, and F. Jansson. Chloroquine serum concentration and side effects: evidence for dose-dependent kinetics. *Clin. Pharmacol. Ther.* 1979;25: 345.

141. Oli, J. M., H. N. C. Ihenacho, and R. S. Talwar. Chronic chloroquine toxicity and heart block. A report of two cases. *East Afri. Med. J.* 1980;57:505.

142. Trojan, H. J., Augenschäden bei Langzeitprophylaxe der Malaria mit Chloroquin. *Klin. Monatsbl. Augenheilk.* 1982;180:232.

143. Marks, J. S. Chloroquine retinopathy: Is there a safe daily dose? *Ann. Rheum. Dis.* 1982;41:52.

144. Scherbel, A. L., A. H. Mackenzie, J. E. Nousek, and M. Atdjian. Ocular lesions in rheumatoid arthritis and related disorders with particular reference to retinopathy. *N. Engl. J. Med.* 1965;273:360.

145. Weise, E. E., and L. A. Yanuzzi. Ring maculopathies mimicking chloroquine retinopathy. *Am. J. Ophthalmal.* 1974;78:204.

146. Burns, R. P. Delayed onset of chloroquine retinopathy. *N. Engl. J. Med.* 1966;275:693.

147. Berstein, H., N. Zvaifler, M. Rubin, and A. M. Mansour. The ocular deposition of chloroquine. *Invest. Ophthalmol.* 1963;2:384.

148. Potts, A. M. The reaction of uveal pigment in vitro with polycyclic compounds. *Invest. Ophthalmol.* 1964;3:405.

149. Sams, W. M., and J. E. Epstein. The affinity of melanin for chloroquine. *J. Invest. Dermatol.* 1965;45: 482.

150. Blois, M. Melanin binding properties of iodoquine. *J. Invest. Dermatol.* 1968;50:250.

151. Tjalve, H., M. Nilsson, and B. Larsson. Studies on the binding of chlorpromazine and chloroquine to melanin in vivo. *Biochem. Pharmacol.* 1981;30: 1845.

152. Kuhn, H., P. Keller, E. Kovacs, and A. Steiger. Lack of correlation between melanin affinity and retinopathy in mice and cats treated with chloroquine or flunitrazepam. *Albrecht von Graefes Arch. Klin. Ophthalmol.* 1981;216:177.

153. Reinert, H., and D. A. Rutty. Mechanisms of chloroquine and phenothiazine retinopathies. *Toxicol. Appl. Pharmacol.* 1969;14:635.

154. Hodgkinson, B. J., and H. Kolb. A preliminary study of the effect of chloroquine on the rat retina. *Arch. Ophthalmol.* 1970;84:509.

155. Toone, E. C., G. D. Hayden, and H. M. Ellman. Ototoxicity of chloroquine. *Arthritis Rheum.* 1965;8: 475.

156. Dencker, L., and N. G. Lindquist. Distribution of labeled chloroquine in the inner ear. *Arch. Otolaryngol.* 1975;101:185.

157. Ette, E. I. Effect of ranitidine on chloroquine disposition. *Drug Intel. Clin. Pharmacol.* 1987;21:732.

158. Sweeney, T. R. The present status of malaria chemotherapy: mefloquine, a novel antimalarial. *Med. Res. Rev.* 1981;1:281.

159. Development of mefloquine as an antimalarial drug. *Bull. WHO* 1983;61:169.

160. Harinasuta, T., D. Bunnag, and W. H. Werndorfer. A phase II clinical trial of mefloquine in patients with chloroquine-resistant falciparum malaria in Thailand. *Bull. WHO* 1983;61:299.

161. Trenholme, G. M., R. L. Williams, R. E. Dejardins, H. Frischer, P. E. Carson, K. H. Rieckmann, and C. J. Canfield. Mefloquine (WR 142,490) in the treatment of human malaria. *Science* 1975;190:792.

162. Pearlman, E. J., E. B. Doberstyn, S. Sudsok, W. Thiemanun, R. S. Kennedy, and C. J. Canfield. Cheomo-suppressive field trials in Thailand. IV. The suppression of *Plasmodium falciparum* and *Plasmodium vivax* parasitemias by mefloquine. *Am. J. Trop. Med. Hyg.* 1980;29:1131.

163. Jacobs, G. H., M. Aikawa, W. K. Milhous, and J. R. Rabbege. An ultra structural study of the effects of mefloquine on malaria parasites. *Am. J. Trop. Med. Hyg.* 1987;36:9.

164. Schlesinger, P. H., D. J. Krogstad, and B. L. Herwaldt. Antimalarial agents: mechanisms of action. *Antimicrob. Agents Chemother.* 1988;32:793.

165. Peters, W., R. E. Howells, J. Portus, B. L. Robinson, S. Thomas, and D. C. Warhurst. The chemotherapy of rodent malaria. XXVII. Studies on mefloquine (WR 142,490) *Ann. Trop. Med. Parasitol.* 1977;71: 407.

166. Chevli, R., and C. D. Fitch. The antimalarial drug mefloquine binds to membrane phospholipids. *Antimicrob. Agents Chemother.* 1982;21:581.

167. Fitch, C. D., R. L. Chan, and R. Chevli. Chloroquine resistance in malaria: accessibility of drug re-

ceptors to mefloquine. *Antimicrob. Agents Chemother.* 1979;15:258.

168. Slater, A. F. G. Chloroquine: mechanism of drug action and resistance in *Plasmodium falciparum. Pharmacol. Ther.* 1993;57:203.

169. Chevli, R., and C. D. Fitch. The antimalarial drug mefloquine binds to membrane phospholipids. *Antimicrob. Agents Chemother.* 1982;21:581.

170. Geary, T. G., L. C. Bonanni, J. B. Jensen, and H. Ginsburg. Effects of combinations of quinoline-containing antimalarials on *Plasmodium falciparum* in culture. *Ann. Trop. Med. Parasitol.* 1986;80:285.

171. Palmer, K. J., S. M. Holliday, and R. N. Brogden. Mefloquine. A review of its antimalarial activity, pharmacokinetic properties and therapeutic efficacy. *Drugs* 1993;45:430.

172. Karle, J. M., and I. L. Karle. Crystal structure and molecular structure of mefloquine methylsulfonate monohydrate: implications for a malaria receptor. *Antimicrob. Agents Chemother.* 1991;35:2238.

173. Desneves, J., G. Thorn, A. Berman, D. Galatis, N. La Greca, J. Sinding, M. Foley, L. W. Deady, A. F. Cowman, and L. Tilley. Photoaffinity labeling of mefloquine-binding proteins in human serum, uninfected erythrocytes and *Plasmodium falciparum* infected erythrocytes. *Mol. Biochem. Parasitol.* 1996;82:181.

174. Davidson, M. W., B. G. Griggs, D. W. Boykin, and W. D. Wilson. Mefloquine, a clinically useful quinoline-methanol antimalarial which does not significantly bind to DNA. *Nature* 1975;254:632.

175. Peters, W., J. Portus, and B. L. Robinson. The chemotherapy of rodent malaria. XXVIII. The development of resistance to mefloquine (WR 142,490). *Ann. Trop. Med. Parasitol.* 1977;71:419.

176. Peel, S. A., S. C. Merritt, J. Handy, and R. S. Baric. Derivation of highly mefloquine-resistant lines from *Plasmodium falciparum* in vitro. *Am. J. Trop. Med. Hyg.* 1993;48:385.

177. Peel, S. A., P. Bright, B. Yount, J. Handy, and R. S. Baric. A strong association between mefloquine and halofantrine resistance and amplification, overexpression, and mutation in the P-glycoprotein gene homolog *(pfmdr)* of *Plasmodium falciparum* in vitro. *Am. J. Trop. Med. Hyg.* 1994;51:648.

178. Dejardins, R. E., C. L. Pamplin, J. von Bredow, K. G. Barry, and C. J. Canfield. Kinetics of a new antimalarial, mefloquine. *Clin. Pharmacol. Ther.* 1979;26:372.

179. Jiang, J. B., G. Q. Li, X. B. Guo, Y. C. Kong, and K. Arnold. Antimalarial activity of mefloquine and qinghaosu. *Lancet* 1982;2:285.

180. Schwartz, D. E., W. Weber, D. Richard-Lenoble, and M. Gentilini. Kinetic studies of mefloquine and of one of its metabolites, Ro 21-5104, in the dog and man. *Acta Trop.* 1980;37:238.

181. Jauch, R., E. Griesser, and G. Oesterhelt. Metabolismus von Ro 21-5998 (Mefloquin) bei der Ratte. *Arzneimittelforschung* 1980;30:60.

182. Karbwang, J., and N. J. White. Clinical pharmacokinetics of mefloquine. *Clin. Pharmacokinet.* 1990;19:264.

183. Palmer, K. J., S. M. Holliday, and R. N. Brogden. Mefloquine. a review of its antimalarial activity, pharmacokinetic properties and therapeutic efficacy. *Drugs* 1993;45:430.

184. Hennequin, C., P. Bourée, N. Bazin, F. Bisaro, and A. Feline. Severe psychiatric side effects observed during prophylaxis and treatment with mefloquine. *Arch. Intern. Med.* 1994;154:2360.

185. Schlagenhauf, P., R. Steffen, H. Lobel, R. Johnson, R. Letz, A. Tschopp, N. Vranjes, Y. Bergqvist, O. Ericsson, U. Hellgren, L. Rombo, S. Mannino, J. Handschin, and D. Sturchler. Mefloquine tolerability during chemoprophylaxis: focus on adverse event assessments, stereochemistry and compliance. *Trop. Med. Int. Health* 1966;1:485.

186. Barrett, P. J., P. D. Emmins, P. D. Clarke, and D. J. Bradley. Comparison of adverse events associated with use of mefloquine and combination of chloroquine and proguanil as antimalarial prophylaxis: postal and telephone survey of travelers. *BMJ* 1996;313:525.

187. Weinke, T., M. Trautmann, T. Held, G. Weber, D. Eichenlaub, K. Fleischer, W. Kern, and H. D. Pohle. Neuropsychiatric side effects after the use of mefloquine. *Am. J. Trop. Med. Hyg.* 1991;45:86.

188. Riffkin, C., R. Chung, D. Wall, J. R. Zalcberg, A. F. Cowman, M. Foley, and L. Tilley. Modulation of the function of human MDR1 P-glycoprotein by the antimalarial drug mefloquine. *Biochem. Pharmacol.* 1996;52:1545.

189. Cordon-Cardo, C., J. P. O'Brien, D. Casals, L. Rittman-Grauer, J. L. Biedler, M. R. Melamed, and J. R. Bertino. Multidrug-resistance gene (P-glycoprotein) is expressed by endothelial cells at bloodbrain barrier sites. *Proc. Natl. Acad. Sci. U.S.A.* 1989;86:695.

190. Guerra, F. The introduction of cinchona in the treatment of malaria. *J. Trop. Med. Hyg.* 1977;80:112.

191. Miller, K. D., A. E. Greenberg, and C. C. Campbell. Treatment of severe malaria in the United States with a continuous infusion of quinidine gluconate and exchange transfusion. *N. Engl. J. Med.* 1989;321:65.

192. Watt, G., L. Loesuttivibool, G. D. Shanks, E. F. Bordreau, A. E. Brown, K. Pavanand, K. Webster, and S. Wechgrityaya. Quinine with tetracycline for the treatment of drug-resistant falciparum malaria in Thailand. *Am. J. Trop. Med. Hyg.* 1992;47:108.

193. Giboda, M. and M. B. Denis. Response of Kampuchean strains of *Plasmodium falciparum* to antimalarials: in vivo assessment of quinine and quinine plus tetracycline; multiple drug resistance in vitro. *J. Trop. Med. Hyg.* 1988;91:205.

194. Bunnag, D., J. Karbwang, K. Na-Bangchang, A. Thanavibul, S. Chittamas, and T. Harinasuta. Quinine-tetracycline for multidrug resistant falciparum malaria. *Southeast Asian J. Trop. Med. Public Health.* 1996;27:15.

195. White, N. J. Antimalarial drug resistance: the pace quickens. *J. Antimicrob. Chemother.* 1992;30:571.

196. Knowles, G., W. L. Davidson, D. Jolley, and M. P. Alpers. The relationship between the in vitro response of *Plasmodium falciparum* to chloroquine, quinine and mefloquine. *Trans. R. Soc. Trop. Med. Hyg.* 1984;78:146.

197. Lambros, C., and J. D. Notsch. *Plasmodium fal-*

ciparum: mefloquine resistance produced in vitro. *Bull. WHO* 1984;62:433.

198. Hahn; F. E. Quinine. In *Antibiotics V-2*, ed. by F. E. Hahn. New York: Springer-Verlag, 1979, pp. 353–362.

199. Hall, A. P., A. W. Czerwinski, E. C. Madonia, and K. L. Evensen. Human plasma and urine quinine levels following tablets, capsules, and intravenous infusion. *Clin. Pharmacol. Ther.* 1973;14:580.

200. White, N. J., S. Looareesuwan, D. A. Warrell, M. J. Warrell, D. Bunnag, and T. Harinasuta. Quinine pharmacokinetics and toxicity in cerebral and uncomplicated falciparum malaria. *Am. J. Med.* 1982;73:564.

201. Silamut, K., P. Molunto, M. Ho, T. M. Davis, and N. J. White. Alpha 1-acid glycoprotein (orosomucoid) and plasma protein binding of quinine in falciparum malaria. *Br. J. Clin. Pharmacol.* 1991;32:311.

202. Winstanley, P., C. Newton, W. Watkins, E. Mberu, S. Ward, P. Warn, I. Mwangi, C. Waruiru, G. Pasvol, D. Warrell, and K. Marsh: Towards optimal regimens of parenteral quinine for young African children with cerebral malaria: the importance of unbound quinine concentration. *Trans. R. Soc. Trop. Med. Hyg.* 1993;87:201.

203. White, N. J. Drug treatment and prevention of malaria. *Eur. J. Clin. Pharmacol.* 1988;34:1.

204. Trenholme, G. M., R. L. Williams, K. H. Rieckmann, H. Frisher, and P. E. Carson. Quinine disposition during malaria and during induced fever. *Clin. Pharmacol. Ther.* 1976;19:459.

205. Sabchareon, A., T. Chongsuphajaisiddhi, and P. Attanath. Serum quinine concentrations following the initial dose in children with falciparum malaria. *Southeast Asian J. Trop. Med. Public Health* 1982;13:556.

206. Brodie, B. B., J. E. Baer, and L. C. Craig. Metabolic products of the cinchona alkaloids in human urine. *J. Biol. Chem.* 1951;188:567.

207. Sabto J., R. M. Pierce, R. H. West, and F. W. Gurr: Hemodialysis, peritoneal dialysis, plasmapheresis and forced diuresis for the treatment of quinine overdose. *Clin. Nephrol.* 1981;16:264.

208. Fisher, C. M. Visual disturbances associated with quinidine and quinine. *Neurology* 1981;31:1569.

209. Bateman, D. N., and E. H. Dyson. Quinine toxicity. *Adverse Drug React. Acute Poisoning Rev.* 1986; 5:215.

210. Gattass, G. R., and L. De Meis. The mechanism by which quinine inhibits the Ca^{++} transport of sarcoplasmic reticulum. *Biochem. Pharmacol.* 1978;27:539.

211. Mecca, T. E., J. T. Elam, C. B. Nash, and R. W. Caldwell. α-Adrenergic blocking properties of quinine HCl. *Eur. J. Pharmacol.* 1980;63:159.

212. Pfueller, S. L., P. K. Hosseinzadeh, and B. G. Firkin. Requirement of factor VIII-related antigen for platelet damage and for in vitro transformation of lymphocytes from patients with drug-induced thrombocytopenia. *J. Clin. Invest.* 1981;67:907.

213. Wandell, M., J. R. Powell, D. Hager, P. E. Fenster, P. E. Graves, K. A. Conrad, and S. Goldman. Effect of quinine on digoxin kinetics. *Clin. Pharmacol. Ther.* 1980;28:425.

214. Warhurst, D. C. Antimalarial interaction with ferriprotoporphyrin 1X monomer and its relationship

to activity of the blood schizonticides. *Ann. Trop. Med. Parasitol.* 1987;81:65.

215. Blauer, G. Interaction of ferriprotoporphyrin 1X with the antimalarials amodiaquine and halofantrine. *Biochem. Int.* 1988;17:729.

216. Warhurst, D. C., and C. O. Diribe. Effect of halofantrine on the proton pump of intraerythocytic *Plasmodium berghei* [Abstract TuP1-8]. *Excerpta Medica International Congress Series* 1988;810:129.

217. ter Kuile, F. O., G. Dolan, F. Nosten, M. D. Epstein, C. Luxemburger, L. Phaipun, T. Chongsuphajaisiddhi, H. K. Webster, and N. J. White. Halofantrine versus mefloquine in the treatment of multidrug resistant falciparum malaria. *Lancet* 1993;341:1044.

218. Gillespie, S. H., E. P. Msaki, A. Ramsay, F. I. Ngowi, and R. Fox. A new micronized formulation of halofantrine hydrochloride in the treatment of acute *Plasmodium falciparum* malaria. *Trans. R. Soc. Trop. Med. Hyg.* 1993;87:467.

219. Schuster, B. G., and C. J. Canfield. Preclinical studies with halofantrine. *Parasitol. Today* 1989; 5(Suppl.):3.

220. Basco, L. K., and J. Le Bras. In vitro activity of halofantrine and its relationship to other standard antimalarial drugs against African isolates and clones of *Plasmodium falciparum*. *Am. J. Trop. Med. Hyg.* 1992; 47:521.

221. Bryson, H., and K. Goa. Halofantrine: a review of its antimalarial activity, pharmacokinetics, properties and therapeutic potential. *Drugs* 1992;43:236.

222. Sowunmi, A., O. Walker, and L. A. Salako. Pruritus and antimalarial drugs in Africans. *Lancet* 1989; 2:213.

223. Karbwang, J., and K. N. Bangchang. Clinical pharmacokinetics of halofantrine. *Clin. Pharmacokinet.* 1994;27:104.

224. Nosten, F., F. ter Kuile, C. Luxemburger, C. Woodson, D. E. Kyle, T. Chongsuphajaisiddhi, and N. J. White. Cardiac effects of antimalaria treatment with halofantrine. *Lancet* 1993;341:1054.

225. de Vries, P. J., and T. K. Dien. Clinical pharmacology and therapeutic potential of artemisinin and its derivatives in the treatment of malaria. *Drugs* 1996; 52:818.

226. Hien, T., and N. White. Qinghaosu. *Lancet* 1993;341:603.

227. Hien, T. T., N. P. J. Day, N. H. Phu, N. T. H. Mai., T. T. H. Chau, P. P. Loc, D. X. Sinh, L. V. Chuong, H. Vinh, D. Waller, T. E. A. Peto, and N. J. White. A controlled trial of artemether or quinine in Vietnamese adults with severe falciparum malaria. *N. Engl. J. Med.* 1996;335:76.

228. van Hensbroek, M. B., E. Onyiorah, S. Jaffar, G. Schneider, A. Palmer, J. Frenkel, G. Enwere, S. Forck, A. Nusmeijer, S. Bennett, B. Greenwood, and D. Kwiatkowski. A trial of artemether or quinine in children with cerebral malaria. *N. Engl. J. Med.* 1996;335: 69.

229. Meshnick, S. R., T. E. Taylor, and S. Kamchongwongpaisan. Artemisinin and the antimalarial endoperoxides: from herbal remedy to targeted chemotherapy. *Microbiol. Rev.* 1996;60:301.

230. Meshnick, S. R., Y.-Z. Yang, V. Lima, F. Kuy-

pers, S. Kamchonwongpaisan, and Y. Yuthavong. Iron-dependent free radical generation and the antimalarial artemisinin (qinghaosu). *Antimicrob. Agents Chemother.* 1993;37:1108.

231. Gu, H. M., D. C. Warhurst, and W. Peters. Uptake of [³H]dihydroartemisinin by erythrocytes infected with *Plasmodium falciparum* in vitro. *Trans. R. Soc. Trop. Med. Hyg.* 1984;78:265.

232. Kaiwa, S., S. Kano, and M. Suzuki. Morphologic effects of artemether on *Plasmodium falciparum* in *Aotus trivirgatus. Am. J. Trop. Med. Hyg.* 1993;49:812.

233. Hien, T. T., K. Arnold, H. Vinh, B. M. Cuong, N. H. Phu, T. T. H. Chau, N. T. M. Hoa, L. Y. Chuono, N. T. H. Mai, N. N. Vinh, and T. T. M. Trang: Comparison of artemisinin suppositories with intravenous artesunate and intravenous quinine in the treatment of cerebral malaria. *Trans. R. Soc. Trop. Med. Hyg.* 1992;86:582.

234. Leskovac, V., and A. D. Theoharides. Hepatic metabolism of artemisinin drugs: I. Drug metabolism in rat liver microsomes. *Comp. Biochem. Physiol C.* 1996;99:391.

235. Brewer, T. G., J. O. Peggins, S. J. Grate, J. M. Petras, B. S. Levine, P. J. Weina, J. Swearengen, M. H. Heiffer, and B. G. Schuster. Neurotoxicity in animals due to arteether and artemether. *Trans. R. Soc. Trop. Med. Hyg.* 1994;88(Suppl. 1):S33.

236. Whichard, L. P., C. R. Morris, J. M. Smith, and D. J. Holbrook. The binding of primaquine, pentaquine, pamaquine, and plasmocid to deoxyribonucleic acid. *Mol. Pharmacol* 1968;4:630.

237. Krotoski, W. A. Frequency of relapse and primaquine resistance in Southeast Asian vivax malaria. *N. Engl. J. Med.* 1980;303:587.

238. Schmidt, L. H., R. Fradkin, D. Vaughan, and J. Rasco. Radical cure of infections with *Plasmodium cynomolgi*: a function of total 8-aminoquinoline dose. *Am. J. Trop. Med. Hyg.* 1977;26:1116.

239. Clyde, D. F., and V. C. McCarthy. Radical cure of Chesson strain vivax malaria in man by 7, not 14, days of treatment with primaquine. *Am. J. Trop. Med. Hyg.* 1977;26:562.

240. Aikawa, M., and R. L. Beaudoin. *Phasmodium fallax*: high-resolution autoradiography of exoerythrocytic stages treated with primaquine in vitro. *Exp. Parasitol.* 1970;27:454.

241. Aikawa, M., and R. L. Beaudoin. Morphological effects of 8-aminoquinolines on the exoerythrocytic stages of *Plasmodium fallax. Mil. Med.* 1969;134:986.

242. Fry, M., and M. Pudney; Site of action of the antimalarial hydroxynaphthoquinone, 2[trans-4-(4' chlorophenyl)cyclohexyl]-3-hydroxy-1,4-naphthoquinone (566C80). *Biochem Pharmacol.* 1992;43:1545.

243. Vaidya, A. B., M. S. Lashgari, L. G. Pologe, and J. Morrisey. Structural features of *Plasmodium* cytochrome b that may underlie susceptibility to 8-aminoquinolines and hydroxynaphthoquinones. *Mol. Biochem. Parasitol.* 1993;58:33.

244. Srivastava, I. K., H. Rottenberg, and A. B. Vaidya. Atovaquone, a broad spectrum antiparasitic drug, collapses mitochondrial membrane potential in a malarial parasite. *J. Biol. Chem.* 1997;272:3961.

245. Olenick, J. G., and F. E. Hahn. Mode of action of primaquine: Preferential inhibition of protein biosynthesis in *Bacillus megaterium. Antimicrob. Agents Chemother.* 1972;1:259.

246. Roskoski, R. and S. R. Jaskunas. Chloroquine and primaquine inhibition of rat liver cell-free polynucleotide-dependent polypeptide synthesis. *Biochem. Pharmacol.* 1972;21:391.

247. Lefler, C. F., H. S. Lilja, and D. J. Holbrook. Inhibitions of aminoacylation and polypeptide synthesis by chloroquine and primaquine in rat liver in vitro. *Biochem. Pharmacol.* 1973;22:715.

248. Greenberg, J., D. J. Taylor, and E. S. Josephson. Studies on *Plasmodium gallinaceum* in vitro. II. The effects of some 8-aminoquinolines against the erythrocytic parasites. *J. Infect. Dis.* 1951;88:163.

249. Grewal, R. S. Pharmacology of 8-aminoquinolines. *Bull. WHO* 1981;59:397.

250. Greaves, J., D. A. P. Evans, H. M. Gilles, K. A. Fletcher, D. Bunnag, and T. Harinasuta. Plasma kinetics and urinary excretion of primaquine in man. *Br. J. Clin. Pharmacol.* 1980;10:399.

251. Holbrook, D. J., J. B. Griffin, L. Fowler, and B. R. Gibson. Tissue distribution of primaquine in the rat. *Pharmacology* 1981;22:330.

252. Taylor, D. J., E. S. Josephson, J. Breenberg, and G. R. Coatney. The in vitro activity of certain antimalarials against erythrocytic forms of *Plasmodium gallinaceum. Am. J. Trop. Med. Hyg.* 1952;1:132.

253. Alving, A. S., R. D. Powell, G. J. Brewer, and J. D. Arnold. Malaria, 8-aminoquinolines and haemolysis. In *Drugs, Parasites and Hosts,* ed. by L. G. Goodwin and R. H. Nimmo-Smith. Boston: Little, Brown, 1962, pp. 83–111.

254. Strother, A., I. M. Fraser, R. Allahyari, and E. B. Tilton. Metabolism of 8-aminoquinoline antimalarial agents. *Bull. WHO* 1981;59:413.

255. Mihaly, G. W., S. A. Ward, G. Edwards, M. L. Orme, and A. M. Breckenridge. Pharmacokinetics of primaquine in man: identification of the carboxylic acid derivative as a major plasma metabolite. *Br. J. Clin. Pharmacol.* 1984;17:441.

256. Ward, S. A., G. W. Mihaly, G. Edwards, S. Looareesuwan, R. E. Phillips, P. Chanthavanich, D. A. Warrell, M. L. Orme, and A. M. Breckenridge. Pharmacokinetics of primaquine in man. II. Comparison of acute vs. chronic dosage in Thai subjects. *Br. J. Clin. Pharmacol.* 1985;19:751.

257. Symposium (various authors). Primaquine. In *Pharmacokinetics, Metabolism, Toxicity, and Activity. Proceedings of a meeting of the Scientific Working Group on the Chemotherapy of Malaria,* ed. by W. H. Wernsdorfer and P. I. Trigg. New York: John Wiley & Sons, 1987,

258. Clyde, D. F. Clinical problems associated with the use of primaquine as a tissue schizontocidal and gametocidal drug. *Bull. WHO* 1981;59:391.

259. Fletcher, K. A., D. A. Price Evans, H. M. Gilles, J. Greaves, D. Bunnag, and T. Harinasuta. Studies on the pharmacokinetics of primaquine. *Bull. WHO* 1981; 59:407.

260. Fletcher, K. A., P. F. Barton, and J. A. Kelly. Studies on the mechanisms of oxidation in the eryth-

rocyte by metabolites of primaquine. *Biochem. Pharmacol.* 1988;37:2683.

261. Beutler; E. Drug-induced hemolytic anemia. *Pharmacol. Rev.* 1969;21:73.

262. La Du, B. N. Pharmacogenetics: defective enzymes in relation to reactions to drugs. *Annu. Rev. Med.* 1972;23:453.

263. Salvidio, E., I. Pannacciulli, A. Tizianello, and F. Ajmar. Nature of hemolytic crisis and the fate of G6PD deficient, drug-damaged erythrocytes in Sardinians. *N. Engl. J. Med.* 1967;276:1339.

264. Chan, T. K., D. Todd, and S. C. Tso: Drug-induced haemolysis in glucose-6-phosphate dehydrogenase deficiency. *BMJ* 1976;2:1227.

265. Beutler, E., R. J. Dern, and A. S. Alving. The hemolytic effect of primaquine. IV. The relationship of red cell age to hemolysis. *J. Lab. Clin. Med.* 1954;44:439.

266. Fraser, I. M., and E. S. Vessel. Effects of metabolites of primaquine and acetanilid on normal and glucose-6-phosphate dehydrogenase deficient erythrocytes. *J. Pharmacol. Exp. Ther.* 1968;162:155.

267. Cohen, G., and P. Hochstein. Glutathione peroxidase: the primary agent for the elimination of hydrogen peroxide in erythrocytes. *Biochemistry* 1963;2:1420.

268. Awasthi, Y. C., E. Beutler, and S. K. Srivastava. Purification and properties of human erythrocyte glutathione peroxidase. *J. Biol. Chem.* 1975;250:5144.

269. Beutler, E. The glutathione instability of drug sensitive red cells; A new method for the in vitro detection of drug sensitivity. *J. Lab. Clin. Med.* 1957;49:84.

270. Beutler, E., K. G. Blume, J. C. Kaplan, G. W. Lohr, B. Ramot, and W. N. Valentine. International committee for standardization in hematology: recommended screening test for glucose-6-phosphate dehydrogenase (G-6-PD) deficiency. *Br. J. Hematol.* 1979; 43:469.

271. Hawking, F., and W. L. M. Perry. Activation of paludrine. *Br. J. Pharmacol.* 1948;3:320.

272. Drugs for parasitic infections. In *Handbook of AntiMicrobial Therapy.* New York: Medical Letter, 1998, pp. 101–121.

273. Hutchinson, D. B. A., and J. A. Farquhar. Trimethoprim-sulfamethoxazole in the treatment of malaria, toxoplasmosis, and pediculosis. *Rev. Infect. Dis.* 1982;4:419.

274. Doberstyn, E. B., C. Teerakiartkamjorn, R. G. Andre, P. Phintuyothin, and S. Noeypatimanondh. Treatment of vivax malaria with sulfadoxine-pyrimethamine and with pyrimethamine alone. *Trans. R. Soc. Trop. Med. Hyg.* 1979;73:15.

275. Miller, K. D., H. O. Lobel, R. F. Satriale, J. N. Kuritsky, J. N. Stern, and C. C. Campbell. Severe cutaneous reactions among American travellers using pyrimethamine-sulfadoxine (Fansidar) for malaria prophylaxis. *Am. J. Trop. Med. Hyg.* 1986;35:451.

276. Rieckmann, K. H., J. V. McNamara, H. Frischer, T. A. Stockert, P. E. Carson, and R. D. Powell. Gametocytocidal and sporontocidal effects of primaquine and of sulfadiazine with pyrimethamine in a chloroquine-resistant strain of *P. falciparum. Bull. WHO* 1968;38:625.

277. Wood, R. C., and G. H. Hitchings. Effect of pyrimethamine on folic acid metabolism in *Streptococcus faecalis* and *Escherichia coli. J. Biol. Chem.* 1959; 234:2377.

278. Ferone, R., and G. H. Hitchings. Folate cofactor biosynthesis by *Plasmodium berghei.* Comparison of folate and dihydrofolate as substrates. *J. Protozool.* 1966; 13:504.

279. Ferone, R. Folate metabolism in malaria. *Bull. WHO* 1977;55:291.

280. Ferone, R. Dihydrofolate reductase from pyrimethamine-resistant *Plasmodium berghei. J. Biol. Chem.* 1970;245:850.

281. Burchall, J. J. Comparative biochemistry of dihydrofolate reductase. *Ann. N.Y. Acad. Sci.* 1971;186:143.

282. Ferone, R., J. J. Burchall, and G. H. Hitchings. *Plasmodium berghei* dihydrofolate reductase; isolation, properties, and inhibition by antifolates. *Mol. Pharmacol.* 1969;5:49.

283. Burchall, J. J. and G. H. Hitchings. Inhibitor binding analysis of dihydrofolate reductases from various species. *Mol. Pharmacol.* 1965;1:126.

284. Rozman, R. S. Chemotherapy of malaria. *Annu. Rev. Pharmacol.* 1973;13:127.

285. Rollo, I. M. The mode of action of sulfonamides, proguanil and pyrimethamine on *Plasmodium gallinaceum. Br. J. Pharmacol.* 1955;10:208.

286. Hitchings, G. H. Pyrimethamine: the use of an antimetabolite in the chemotherapy of malaria and other infections. *Clin. Pharmacol. Ther.* 1960;1:570.

287. Knowles, G. Genetics of cross-resistance between antifolate drugs in *Plasmodium yoelii. J. Parasitol.* 1982;68:157.

288. Peterson, D. A., W. K. Milhous, and T. E. Wellems. Molecular basis of differential resistance to cycloquanil and pyrimethamine in *Plasmodium falciparum* malaria. *Proc. Natl. Acad. Sci. U.S.A.* 1990;87:3018.

289. Weidekamm, E., H. Plozza-Nottebrock, I. Forgo, and U. C. Dubach. Plasma concentrations of pyrimethamine and sulfadoxine and evaluation of pharmacokinetic data by computerized curve fitting. *Bull. WHO* 1982;60:115.

290. Ahmad, R. A., and H. J. Rogers. Pharmacokinetics and protein binding interactions of dapsone and pyrimethamine. *Br. J. Clin. Pharmacol.* 1980;10:519.

291. Brooks, M. H., J. P. Malloy, P. J. Bartelloni, T. W. Sheehy, and K. G. Barry. Quinine, pyrimethamine, and sulphorthodimethoxine: clinical response, plasma levels, and urinary excretion during the initial attack of naturally acquired falciparum malaria. *Clin. Pharmacol. Ther.* 1969;10:85.

292. Stickney, D. R., W. S. Simmons, R. L. DeAngelis, R. W. Rundles, and C. A. Nichol. Pharmacokinetics of pyrimethamine (PRM) and 2,4-diamino-5-(3',4'-dichlorophenyl)-6-methyl pyrimidine (DMP) relevent to meningeal leukemia. *Proc. Am. Assoc. Cancer Res.* 1973;14:52.

293. Winstanley, P. A., W. M. Watkins, C. R. Newton, J. C. Nevill, E. Mberu, P. A. Warn, C. M. Waruiva, I. N. Mwangi, D. A. Warrell, and K. Marsh. The dis-

position of oral and intramuscular pyrimethamine/sulphadoxine in Kenyan children with high parasitaemia but clinically non-severe falciparum malaria. *Br. J. Clin. Pharmacol.* 1992;33:143.

294. Smith, C. G., J. Ihrig, and R. Menne. Antimalarial activity and metabolism of biguanides. *Am. J. Trop. Med. Hyg.* 1960;10:694.

295. Clyde, D. F. Prolonged malaria prophylaxis through pyrimethamine in mother's milk. *East Afr. Med. J.* 1960;37:659.

296. Bohni, E., B. Fust, J. Rieder, K. Schaerer, and L. Havas. Comparative toxicological, chemotherapeutic and pharmacokinetic studies with sulformethoxine and other sulfonamides in animals and man. *Chemotherapy* 1969;14:195.

297. Peck, C. C., A. N. Lewis, and B. E. Joyce. Pharmacokinetic rationale for a malarial suppressant administered once monthly. *Ann. Trop. Med. Parasitol.* 1975; 69:141.

298. Wrickramasinghe, S. N., and R. A. C. Litwinczuk. Effects of low concentrations of pyrimethamine on human bone marrow cells in vitro: possible implications for malaria prophylaxis. *J. Trop. Med. Hyg.* 1981;84:233.

299. Colwell, E. J., R. L. Hickman, and S. Kosakal. Quinine-tetracycline and quinine-bacterim treatment of acute falciparum malaria in Thailand. *Ann. Trop. Med. Parasitol.* 1973;67:125.

300. Chongsuphajaisiddhi, T., C. H. M. Gilles, D. J. Krogstad, L. A. Salako, D. A. Warrell, N. J. White, R. E. Beales, J. A. Najera, U. K. Sheth, H. C. Spencer, and W. H. Wernsdorfer. Severe and complicated malaria. *Trans. R. Soc. Trop. Med. Hyg.* 1986;80(Suppl.): 1.

301. Reacher, M., C. C. Campbell, J. Freeman, E. B. Doberstyn, and A. D. Brandling-Bennet. Drug therapy for *Plasmodium falciparum* malaria resistant to pyrimethamine-sulfadoxine (Fansidar). A study of alternate regimens in eastern Thailand, 1980. *Lancet* 1981; 2:1066.

302. Colwell, E. J., R. L. Hickman, and S. Kosakal. Tetracycline treatment of chloroquine-resistant falciparum malaria in Thailand. *JAMA* 1972;220:684.

303. Colwell, E. J., R. L. Hickman, R. Intraprasert, and C. Tirabutana. Minocycline and tetracycline treatment of acute falciparum malaria in Thailand. *Am. J. Trop. Med. Hyg.* 1972;21:144.

304. Miller, L. H., R. H. Glew, D. J. Wyler, W. A. Howard, W. E. Collins, P. G. Contacos, and F. A. Neva. Evaluation of clindamycin in combination with quinine against multidrug-resistant strains of *Plasmodium falciparm. Am. J. Trop. Med. Hyg.* 1974;23:565.

CHAPTER FOURTEEN

Chemotherapy of Protozoal Diseases

Most protozoal and helminthic infections occur in impoverished populations living under poor sanitary conditions. Because parasitic infections occur largely in residents of developing tropical nations, physicians in the United States and many other temperate zone nations generally have little knowledge of and often little interest in parasitic diseases.[1] Some parasitic infections, like amebiasis, occur in North America and Europe, but the incidence is not high and they occur predominantly in economically poor rural settings, like Indian reservations, and in poor inner city areas populated by recent immigrants from regions where parasitic diseases are endemic. Large-scale programs of chemotherapy are important in controlling some of these parasitic diseases in the tropics, but they have less impact than efforts devoted to the control of vectors, elimination of reservoirs of infection, and amelioration of the poor sanitary and living conditions responsible for transmission of parasites. It has been said that the frequency of intestinal parasitism can be used as an indicator of the level of development of a community and that the control of these parasitic infections is not only a public health task but a matter of economic development.[2] Until such time as the living standards are raised, however, chemotherapy will pay a major role in the management of most parasitic diseases.

The problem of the chemotherapy of parasitic diseases in the developing regions of the world is complicated by a number of factors. First, the size of the population infected with parasites or living in areas where parasitic diseases are endemic is huge. Second, therapy is complicated by the fact that quite often individuals are infected with several organisms simultaneously. To provide such people with appropriate medical care it is sometimes necessary to carry out numerous diagnostic and follow-up laboratory tests and institute multiple-drug therapy. After this is done in a careful way, the person often returns to an environment in which multiple parasites are endemic, and optimum conditions for recurrent infection exist. Third, many people are used to being infected and are not well enough educated to understand and be conscientious in following the treatment recommended by the physician. This is linked to the fact that health workers (often from an alien culture) are sometimes considered outsiders whose efforts are felt as threatening to well-established life patterns.[3]

At present, there are no immunization procedures for protection against protozoal and helminthic disease. The physician must rely on drugs that are discussed in this chapter and in the following one, for treatment of these conditions. Not a great deal is known about the mechanisms of action or mechanisms behind the toxic effects and the side effects of many of these drugs.

Drugs Used to Treat Amebiasis and Other Protozoal Infections Occurring in North America and Europe

Amebiasis

Amebiasis results from infection by the protozoan *Entamoeba histolytica*. Distinct species of *Entamoeba* that are morphologically identical are involved in human infection.[4] *Entamoeba dispar*, the more prevalent species, is associated solely with the asymptomatic carrier state, whereas the pathogenic species, *E. histolytica*, invades tissues and causes symptomatic disease. Amebiasis occurs in all parts of North America and throughout the world. As with malaria and many other parasitic diseases, it is important to know the life cycle of the protozoan and the normal progression of the disease process in order to understand the therapy. Humans are the principal host and main source of infection by *E. histolytica*. The patient becomes infected by ingesting mature cysts, which are resistant to the acidic environment of the stomach and pass to the small intestine (Fig. 14–1). The cyst disintegrates in the small intestine, releasing four amebas, which divide to form eight trophozoites. The trophozoites pass into the large intestine where they may live and multiply for a time in the crypts of the bowel. Some of the trophozoites are able to invade the intestinal epithelium and encystation and ulceration of the intestinal wall takes place. The presence of bacteria is required for survival of the protozoan in the intestine of the host. Although diarrhea is often seen, ulceration does not usually result in prolonged diarrhea or abdominal pain. Indeed, many affected patients have no complaints. The cysts formed from the trophozoites on the surface of the colon are passed in formed stools. Upon excretion, cysts remain viable for weeks to months, depending on environmental conditions. Thus, people readily become asymptomatic carriers of the disease by passing cysts in the stool for long periods of time. Infection may result from ingestion of as little as a single cyst in contaminated food or water, and larger amounts may be associated with a shorter incubation period (days instead of 1–2 weeks) until the onset of symptomatic intestinal disease. Patients with active diarrhea do not spread the disease because the trophozoites are not able to mature into the active cyst forms in the hyperactive bowel. The lesions produced by *E. histolytica* are primarily located in the large bowel, although secondary systemic invasion can occur. The organisms may pass up the

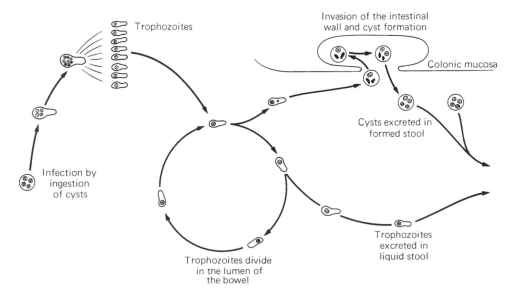

Figure 14–1. Life cycle of *Entamoeba histolytica*.

Table 14–1. Drugs used to treat intestinal protozoa and protozoal infections that occur in North America and Europe. Dehydroemetine and pentamidine are not marketed in the United States but they may be obtained from the Parasitic Disease Division of the Centers for Disease Control. Diloxanide and spiramycin are not available in the United States.

Infecting organism	Drug of choice	Alternative
Entamoeba histolytica		
Asymptomatic cyst passer	Paromomycin or diiodohydroxyquin	Diloxanide
Mild intestinal disease[a]	Metronidazole[b]	
Severe intestinal disease[a]	Metronidazole[b]	
Hepatic abscess[a]	Metronidazole[b]	Chloroquine phosphate
Balantidium coli	Tetracycline	Diiodohydroxyquin and metronidazole
Cryptosporidium	Paromomycin	
Cyclospora	Trimethoprim-sulfamethoxazole	
Dientamoeba fragilis	Diiodohydroxyquin or paromomycin or tetracycline	
Giardia lamblia	Metronidazole	Furazolidone or paromomycin
Isospora spp. *(coccidiosis)*	Trimethoprim-sulfamethoxazole	
Pneumocystis carinii	Trimethoprim-sulfamethoxazole	Pentamidine
Toxoplasma gondii	Pyrimethamine plus sulfadiazine	Spiramycin
Trichomonas vaginalis	Metronidazole[b]	

[a] Treatment should be followed by paromomycin or diiodohydooxyquin. [b] Tinidazole, a nitroimidazole similar to metronidazole, appears to be as effective but better tolerated. It is not available in the United States.

portal vein to the liver producing hepatitis and abscesses. Encystation rarely occurs in organs other than the liver.

Treatment of amebiasis is complex, as the clinician must prescribe multiple drugs to eradicate the parasite in the bowel lumen and in tissues. Further complicating the situation is the lack of availability of some drugs in many developing countries, multiple toxic effects of different drugs, and disagreement regarding whether asymptomatic intestinal infections should be treated. Metronidazole is effective against all forms of the parasite—the intestinal cysts, the trophozoites in the intestinal lumen, and the extraintestinal cysts. At low doses, it is effective in the treatment of liver abscess,[5,6] and at higher doses, it is effective in treating amebic dysentery.[7,8] It is now considered the drug of choice for both these forms of the disease (Table 14–1).[9,10] Metronidazole is also used to treat patients who are asymptomatic cyst passers, but in about 10% of such patients, the usual course of therapy fails to eradicate intestinal infection.[11] Three

luminal drugs are available for treating the carrier state. Diloxanide furoate, a bisubstituted acetanilid, is relatively nontoxic and was formerly in wide use worldwide but it is no longer available in the United States. The treatment of choice is now either paromomycin or diiodohydroxyquin (iodoquinol), with diloxanide being an alternative where available. Paromomycin is a nonabsorbable aminoglycoside that is highly effective. It may cause a mild increase in stool frequency but has advantages for use in situations where systemic therapy should be avoided, such as with children or during pregnancy. Diiodohydroxyquin is a halogenated hydroxyquinoline that can cause a variety of toxic effects; however, little toxicity has been associated with its use in amebiasis. A 20-day course of this drug is required for treatment to be effective.

Complicated intestinal disease is best treated with metronidazole or another nitroimidazole Only metronidazole is available in the United States; elsewhere, tinidazole and ornidazole are used and have fewer toxic effects than metronidazole. Tetracycline or erythromycin combined with an intraluminal agent is effective treatment for mild amebic colitis in patients who cannot tolerate metronidazole, but this combination therapy will not eradicate trophozoites in the liver. The role of the antibiotics is interesting since, with the exception of paromomycin (Chapter 5), which has been demonstrated to have a direct amebicidal effect in vitro,[12] the antibiotics do not affect the amebae directly but inhibit the growth of amebas by reducing the bacterial population of the bowel. The amebas are dependent upon bacteria in the bowel for growth.[13]

Chloroquine is only active against *E. histolytica* in the liver, but is usually not recommended for treatment of hepatic amebiasis unless treatment with metronidazole is unsuccessful or contraindicated. Patients treated with tetracycline must be carefully followed for evidence of hepatic involvement. Dehydroemetine is also available from the Parasite Division of the Centers for Disease Control (CDC) but has many toxic effects associated with its use. It must be administered in a controlled, monitored hospital setting. There is no objective evidence that the combination of emetine or dehydroemetine and metronidazole improves the outcome in the treatment of invasive amebiasis. Emetines are thus not recommended except under extraordinary circumstances. Metronidazole alone is adequate initial therapy for amebic liver abscess, but a luminal cysticidal agent must be administered following metronidazole therapy for the treatment of intestinal infection (Table 14–2).[14]

Table 14–2. The site of action of the antiamebic drugs.

| Drug | Effective against: | |
	Intestinal disease	Hepatic abscess
Metronidazole	+	+
Diiodohydroxyquin	+	−
Antibiotics	+	−
Diloxanide furoate	+	−
Chloroquine	−	+

The drugs used to treat amebiasis and other protozoal infections encountered in North America and Europe are presented in Table 14–1. Some of the drugs have been discussed in previous chapters (tetracyclines, Chapter 6; trimethoprim-sulfamethoxazole, Chapter 7; pyrimethamine and chloroquine, Chapter 13). Paromomycin, an aminoglycoside antibiotic that is also used to treat cestodiasis (tapeworm infection), is discussed in Chapter 15. The macrolide antibiotic spiramycin has been widely used in Europe to treat toxoplasmosis.[15,16] This drug is not available in the United States.

Metronidazole

Several 5-nitroimidazole compounds are active against a variety of bacteria that metabolize anaerobically. Metronidazole was the first of these compounds demonstrated to have trichomonicidal and amebicidal activity and it is the only 5-nitroimidazole that is

Metronidazole

Tinidazole

marketed in the United States. Tinidazole is a close structural analog of metronidazole that is used in many countries to treat amebiasis. The pharmacology and clinical use of metronidazole and tinidazole have been the subject of several symposia and reviews.[17–21] Other members of the 5-nitroimidazole class include nimorazole and ornidazole, both of which are marketed in some regions of the world for treating amebiasis. The following discussion will focus on metronidazole.

ANTIMICROBIAL ACTIVITY AND THERAPEUTIC USE. Metronidazole was first used for the treatment of trichomoniasis and it has been the drug of choice for treating that infection since 1960.[22] Cure rates of about 95% are achieved with the standard regimen of 250 mg three times daily for 7 days.[20] A single-dose regimen of 2 g is almost as effective as the 7-day course of therapy.[23,24] Cure rates of approximately 85% are achieved with the 7-day regimen in the treatment of giardiasis.[25] Higher daily doses are required for the treatment of amebic dysentery or liver abscess (750 mg three times daily for 5–10 days).[26] Occasionally, beneficial results have been reported with metronidazole therapy in other protozoal infections, but with the exception of giardiasis and possibly balantidiasis, the efficacy of the drug has not been established.[27]

Metronidazole has a bactericidal action that is specific for obligate anaerobes. The in vitro activity of metronidazole against selected protozoa and anaerobic bacteria is presented in Table 14–3.[28–32] At concentrations that are readily achieved in the serum after oral or intravenous administration, metronidazole is active against *Bacteroides fragilis* and other *Bacteroides* species, *Fusobacterium* species, *Clostridium perfringens*, and other *Clostridium* species. It is less active against anaerobic gram-positive cocci but most strains of *Peptococcus* and *Peptostreptococcus* and many strains of *Viellonella* species are susceptible.[17] Against susceptible organisms, metronidazole is bactericidal at concentrations equal to or only slightly higher than the minimal inhibitory concentration.[21]

Metronidazole is an alternative to clindamycin for treatment of serious anaerobic infections, particularly those caused by *B. fragilis*. Compared with clindamycin, metronidazole has the advantages of a potent bactericidal activity and lower potential for *C. difficile* overgrowth. It has the disadvantage of a more narrow spectrum, specifically the absence of activity against gram-positive cocci such as microphilic streptococci.[33] For *B. fragilis* infections, the drug is usually administered intravenously, and the recommended adult dosage is 15 mg/kg as a loading dose followed by maintenance doses of 7.5 mg/kg every 6 h. The

Table 14–3. *Activity of metronidazole against selected protozoa and anaerobic bacteria in vitro.* The minimum concentration of metronidazole required for lethality against protozoa or anaerobic bacteria in vitro depends on the time of drug exposure and the assay conditions. The minimum lethal concentrations are presented as ranges with the higher value representing a concentration of drug where 90% or more of strains are killed.

Organism	Minimum lethal concentration (range in μg/ml)
PROTOZOA	
Entamoeba histolytica	0.6–4
Giardia lamblia	2–4
Trichomonas vaginalis	0.5–5
BACTERIA	
Bacteroides fragilis	0.5–8
Bacteroides spp.	0.5–4
Clostridium perfringens	0.5–8
Other *Clostridium* spp.	0.1–8
Fusobacterium spp.	0.1–1
Gardnerella vaginalis (in anaerobic culture)	4–16
Peptococcus spp.	0.5–16
Peptostreptococcus spp.	0.1–8

Source: The data were compiled from Gillin and Diamond,[28] Muller et al.,[29] Sutter and Finegold,[30] Appelbaum and Chatterton,[31] and Ralph and Amatnieks.[32]

drug is infused slowly over 1 h. There has been considerable experience in the treatment of a variety of anaerobic infections, and the drug has been shown to be effective in the treatment of intraabdominal, pelvic, pleuropulmonary, central nervous system, and bone and joint infections.[21] Metronidazole is particularly useful in treating susceptible anaerobic cerebral infections (usually in combination with other antibiotics) and anaerobic meningitis because of its bactericidal activity and good penetration into cerebrospinal fluid and brain, including abscess contents. Many of these infections are mixed in that both aerobic and anaerobic organisms are present, and it is often necessary to combine metronidazole with an appropriate antibiotic that is active against aerobic bacteria. Several controlled clinical trials have shown that metronidazole, either alone or in combination with another antibiotic, is effective as prophylaxis in surgical operations in which the risk of postoperative anaerobic infection is high (e.g., colon surgery and vaginal or abdominal hysterectomy).[20,21] Metronidazole administered orally is effective for acute dental infections, such as Vincent's gingivostomatitis.[17] Metronidazole is nearly as effective as oral vancomycin in the treatment of antibiotic-associated, pseudomembranous colitis caused by *Clostridium difficile*.[34] The high cost of vancomycin and the increase in the incidence of vancomycin-resistant enterococcal infections during the last few years make the use of metronidazole more desirable. It should be noted, however, that pseudomembranous colitis has been reported to occur as a side effect of metronidazole therapy.[35] Metronidazole is used to treat peptic ulcer disease due to *Helicobacter pylori* along with tetracycline, amoxicillin, and clarithromycin.

Although resistance can develop to metronidazole, it has not proven to be a clinical problem. The primary causes of failure of metronidazole therapy in trichomoniasis are reinfection and failure to take the medication. A few isolates of *T. vaginalis* that are no longer susceptible to the usual dosage have been identified but they have responded to higher-dose therapy.[29] Rarely, failure of therapy may occur in trichomoniasis because of metabolism of metronidazole by vaginal bacteria.[36] Resistance among anaerobic bacteria has not been reported with the usual course of treatment, but a strain of metronidazole-resistant *B. fragilis* has been selected during long-term therapy.[37] No plasmid-mediated resistance has been reported.

In addition to its usefulness in treating some protozoal and bacterial infections, it has been found that metronidazole has a beneficial effect in the treatment of patients with guinea worm infection (*Dracunculus medinensis*).[38,39] The drug does not affect the worm directly, but patients report marked relief, perhaps as a result of an immunosuppressant effect.[40] Metronidazole has been found to have some efficacy in the treatment of Crohn's disease[41] and it has been used on an investigational basis as a radiosensitizing agent in the treatment of certain malignancies.[27,42]

MECHANISM OF ACTION OF METRONIDAZOLE. The common characteristic of organisms that are sensitive to metronidazole is that they are anaerobic and contain electron transport proteins with a low redox potential (ferridoxin-like and flavodoxin-like). Anaerobic organisms possess unique mechanisms of energy production and electron transfer that permit their survival in the absence of oxygen. It has been shown that metronidazole inhibits hydrogen production in cultures of the anaerobic bacterium. *C. perfringens* and the protozoan *Trichomonas vaginalis*.[43,44] The principal mechanism of hydrogen evolution in these organisms is by the pyruvate phosphoroclastic reaction. In this complex reaction, pyruvate is converted to acetyl phosphate with the evolution of carbon dioxide and hydrogen. There are two enzymes systems involved:

(1) Pyruvate + phosphate $\rightarrow$
$\qquad$ acetyl phosphate + CO_2
$\qquad$ + $2H^+$
(2) $2H^+ + 2e \rightarrow H_2$

Metronidazole inhibits the generation of H_2 without affecting the rate of acetyl phosphate synthesis.[45] Thus, it is the second reaction that is inhibited by the drug. This reaction requires the participation of an electron transfer protein (ferredoxin in clostridia), which has a redox potential of about -460 mV. The redox potential of metronidazole is -415 mV, and it acts as an electron sink, drawing off electrons from the reduced electron transfer protein. The resulting nitro group reduction of metronidazole is required for biological activity. Both the spectrum of action and the selective toxicity of the 5-nitroimidazoles are explained to a large extent by the fact that only anaerobes have redox systems of sufficiently negative potential to interact with the drugs.

In addition to its ability to kill sensitive anaerobic organisms, metronidazole is mutagenic[46] and it radiosensitizes hypoxic cells.[47] All three of these effects may be caused by chemically reactive reduction products of the drug. The degree of drug resistance expressed by a series of metronidazole-resistant mutants of B. fragilis is inversely proportional to the activity of pyruvate dehydrogenase, an enzyme that is required for the phosphoroclastic reaction and drug reduction in this organism.[48,49] Similarly, it has been shown that a strain of Salmonella typhimurium that is deficient in nitro reductase activity does not respond to the mutagenic action of metronidazole.[50,51] Structure–activity studies have shown that the electron affinity of a nitroimidazole is correlated with both its cytotoxicity and radiosensitization potential.[52,53] Taken together, these observations support a model in which drug reduction is required to produce all three biological effects of metronidazole.

Both protozoa (E. histolytica and T. vaginalis) and bacteria metabolize metronidazole to N-(2-hydroxyethyl)oxamic acid and acetamide (see Fig. 14–2).[54–56] A relatively metronidazole-resistant strain of B. fragilis has been shown to have a decreased capacity to metabolize the drug to the stable acetamide product.[57] Lethality is enhanced if the resistant bacterium is cultured in the presence of a different organism possessing nitro reductase activity. This suggests that the second bacterium has produced a diffusible drug product that can interact with and kill the resistant B. fragilis. These observations are consistent with the proposal (diagrammed in Fig. 14–2) that nitro-group reduction produces a partially reduced reactive intermediate of metronidazole that can either interact with the susceptible organism to produce a lethal effect or react with water to form the stable acetamide metabolite.[57] The biologically important reactive form (or forms) of metronidazole has not been identified, but it is clear that the drug becomes covalently bound to macromolecular com-

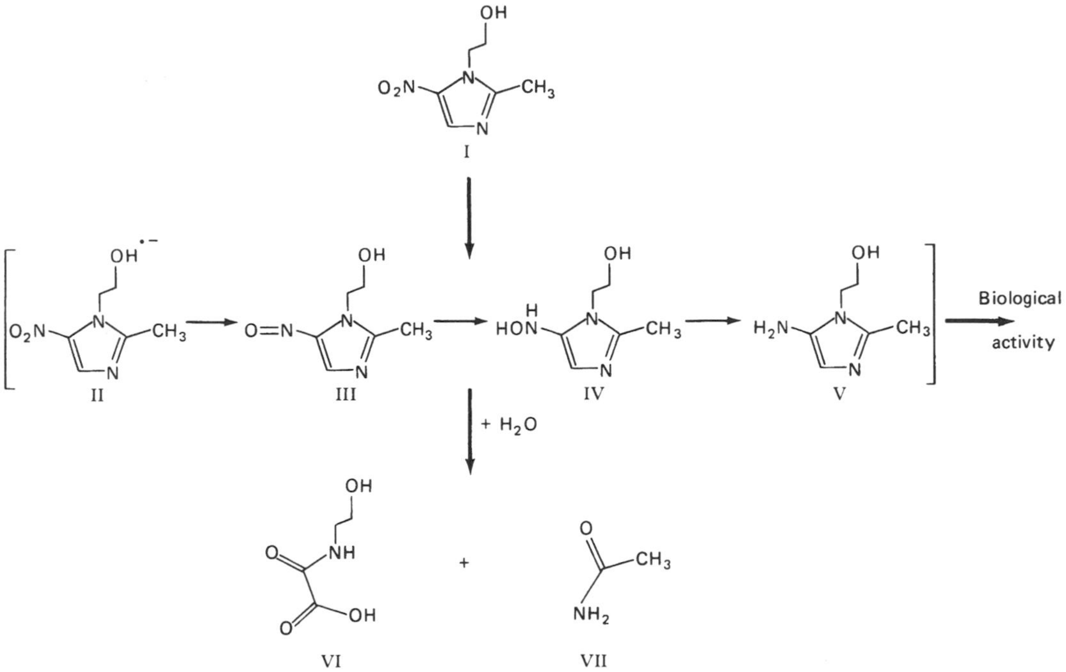

Figure 14–2. Bacterial metabolism of metronidazole. Metronidazole (I) is reduced to form N-(2-hydroxyethyl)oxamic acid (VI) and acetamide (VII). Potential reactive intermediates include the radical anion (II), nitroso (III), hydroxylamine (IV), and amino (V) derivatives. The interaction of one or more of the reactive intermediates with DNA is likely to be the primary event responsible for the cell-killing, mutagenic, and radiosensitization effects of metronidazole. (From Beaulieu et al.[55])

ponents of the cell, including DNA.[58–60] The interaction with DNA is likely to account for the killing, mutagenic, and radiosensitization effects of metronidazole.

PHARMACOLOGY OF METRONIDAZOLE. Metronidazole is well absorbed (90%–95%) from the gastrointestinal tract.[61] Peak plasma levels of the unmetabolized drug are achieved within 1 h after oral administration; the peak level is 3.7 µg/ml after a 250 mg dose, 9.8 µg/ml after 500 mg, and 11.8 µg/ml after 1 g.[62] Similar peak concentrations are achieved 4 h after administration of suppositories containing 500 mg, 1 g, and 2 g, respectively.[62] The absorption of metronidazole is not decreased if the drug is ingested with food, although the time to peak concentration may be somewhat delayed.[63] When administered intravenously, metronidazole is infused slowly over a period of 1 h. After a loading dose of 15 mg/kg followed by maintenance doses of 7.5 mg/kg given intravenously every 8 h, the peak levels at steady state average 26 µg/ml and trough levels average 18 µg/ml.[21] Since the minimum inhibitory concentrations for most anaerobes including *Bacteroides fragilis* are less than 6 µg/ml, these concentrations are highly effective in therapy.

Very little metronidazole is bound to plasma protein; reports have ranged between 1% and 11%, depending upon the assay method.[64,65] Metronidazole distribtues widely in the body[66] and its apparent volume of distribution is about 80% of the body weight.[65] The drug penetrates well into body tissues and fluid compartments, including vaginal secretions,[66] seminal fluid,[67] bile,[68]

hepatic abscess,[66] saliva,[66] empyema fluid,[69] synovial fluid,[70] bone,[21] and pelvic tissues.[21] In the absence of meningeal inflammation, the concentration of metronidazole in the cerebrospinal fluid is about one-half the simultaneous serum concentration.[71] In patients with meningitis the cerebrospinal fluid concentration of metronidazole is the same as the simultaneous serum concentration.[64,72] Tinidazole is more lipophilic than metronidazole and cerebrospinal fluid concentrations in normal volunteers are 88% of the simultaneous serum concentration.[71] Metronidazole penetrates into brain abscesses in concentrations that are equivalent to those in serum.[73] Metronidazole crosses the placenta[74,75] and it is secreted in breast milk.[67,76]

The pharmacokinetic characteristics of metronidazole and tinidazole[77–79] are summarized in Table 14–4. The elimination half-life of metronidazole in adults is 8–9 h,[61,64,65] and in infants the half-life is inversely related to the gestational age.[75] Metronidazole is extensively metabolized in the liver by side-chain oxidation and conjugation.[80] The two major oxidative metabolites are a hydroxy metabolite [1-(2-hydroxyethyl)-2-hydroxymethyl-5-nitroimidazole] and an acid metabolite [1-acetic acid-2-methyl-5-nitroimidazole]. The hydroxy metabolite appears in substantial concentrations in the plasma[61] and has about 30% of the bioactivity of the unchanged drug.[32,51,81] The acid metabolite does not appear in the serum[61,79] and it is only 2%–5% as bioactive as the unchanged drug. In people with normal renal function, most (80%) of a dose of metronidazole is ultimately excreted in the urine,[65] with only

Table 14–4. *Pharmacokinetic characteristics of metronidazole and tinidazole.*

Drug	Elimination half-life (hours)	Protein binding (%)	Apparent volume of distribution (% of body weight)	Ratio of cerebrospinal fluid to serum concentration with normal meninges	Extent of metabolism
Metronidazole	8–9	1–11	~80	0.43	Extensive
Tinidazole	9.5–12	20	60–80	0.88	Little or none

Source: Table constructed from data in Houghton et al.,[61] Ralph et al.,[64] Schwartz and Jeunet,[65] Jokipii et al.,[71] Taylor et al.,[77] Welling and Munro,[78] and Stambaugh et al.[80]

about 15% being excreted unchanged.[64] The capacity for ultimate excretion via the hepatic route is high, however, and the elimination half-life is not altered by renal failure.[82] If there is significant hepatic failure, the dosage should be reduced and serum levels should be monitored. Metronidazole is removed by hemodialysis and a replacement dose is necessary after the dialysis procedure to regain therapeutic levels.[83]

ADVERSE EFFECTS OF METRONIDAZOLE. At the dosage regimens that are used for the treatment of T. vaginalis infection, metronidazole has been well tolerated. Occasionally, patients experience nausea, a metallic taste in the mouth, epigastric distress, and diarrhea.[74] Patients receiving a single 2 g dose may experience vertigo and headache.[24] Rarely, nervous system toxicity, including weakness, vertigo, and ataxia, has been observed. Peripheral neuropathy is more common and is occasionally not reversible even with the discontinuation of the drug. This reaction has been noted mainly with prolonged use in patients with Crohn's disease or with high doses.[33] Metronidazole can also produce unpleasant sensations in some patients when they drink alcoholic beverages. Because of this disulfiram-like effect, metronidazole was at one time tried for the treatment of alcoholism but it was not found to be useful. Metronidazole inhibits liver alcohol dehyrogenase, but since this inhibition occurs at concentrations approximately 100 times those found in the serum during therapy, it is unlikely that this is related to the effect.[84,85] In the course of evaluating its usefulness in the therapy of alcoholism, it was found that the simultaneous administration of metronidazole and disulfiram can produce psychosis.[86] The basis of this drug interaction is not known. Convulsions and encephalopathy have been reported with high doses of metronidazole,[87] as has transient leukopenia. Metronidazole increases the plasma half-life and the hypoprothrombinemic effect of warfarin.[88]

As metronidazole has been shown to be carcinogenic in mice and rats and mutagenic in bacteria, there has been considerable concern regarding possible long-term effects in humans. Long-term, high-dose feeding of metronidazole produces lung tumors in mice and hepatomas and mammary tumors in rats.[89,90] Tumorigenicity has not been observed in hamsters.[74] As discussed previously, metronidazole is mutagenic in bacteria that have nitro reductase activity.[50,51] Concern regarding possible genetic effects in humans increased when it was found that histidine auxotrophs of Salmonella typhimurium show a marked increase in mutation rate when exposed to urine from patients receiving doses of the drug that are normal for treatment of trichomoniasis.[91] The hydroxy metabolite is 10 times more active in the Salmonella assay than metronidazole.[92] It is possible that humans are exposed to products of metronidazole nitro group reduction. It is important to note that small amounts of the acetamide and N-(2-hydroxyethyl)oxamic acid products that are produced on reductive activation of metronidazole (compounds VI and VII in the metabolic scheme of Fig. 14–2) have been detected in the urine of humans taking the drug in therapeutic dosage.[93] Acetamide has been shown to be a liver carcinogen for rats and the presence of acetamide in the urine of rats taking metronidazole is entirely due to metabolism of the drug by intestinal flora.[94] Under anaerobic conditions, mammalian liver microsomes can both reduce metronidazole to its nitro anion radical[95] and activate it to a mutagen.[50] In the presence of oxygen, however, the drug is reoxidized, inactivating it as a potential carcinogen.

From the above observations, it would seem that the use of metronidazole is accompanied by a theoretical risk to humans. There is, however, no direct evidence of carcinogenic, mutagenic, or teratogenic effects in humans. Two small retrospective studies have found no increase in the incidence of cancer in patients who were previously treated with metronidazole.[96,97] Tests for mutagenicity in mammalian systems have been negative,[98] and the drug has been administered to pregnant patients without evidence of fetal malformation.[99] It is nevertheless prudent to avoid use of metronidazole during pregnancy whenever possible.

PRECAUTIONS. The dosage of metronidazole should be reduced in patients with severe obstructive liver disease, alcoholic cirrhosis, or severe renal dysfunction.[100] It should also be used with caution in patients with active central nervous system disease because of its neurological toxicity.

Chloroquine

Chloroquine has a direct toxic effect against trophozoites of E. histolytica and it is concentrated in the liver. Thus, chloroquine has been used as a systemic amebicide to treat hepatic amebiasis when therapy with metronidazole is contraindicated or unsuccessful. It is used in an adult dose of 1 g daily for 2 days, followed by 500 mg daily for at least 2 to 3 weeks. This dose can be repeated if necessary. The complete pharmacology of chloroquine is discussed in Chapter 13.

Diloxanide Furoate

Diloxanide is one of a series of substituted acetanilides found to be amebicidal both in vitro and in vivo in rats.[101] In early clinical

Diloxanide furoate

studies it was shown that diloxanide is well tolerated and effective at eradicating amebic cysts.[102] Several esters of diloxanide were subsequently tested and the furoate ester was found to be 10 times more active than the parent compound in vitro (active at 10^{-8} vs. $10^{-7}M$), but less toxic in animal models.[101,103] Diloxanide furoate is presently not available in the United States. The mechanism of action of these compounds is unknown.

Diloxanide furoate yields cure rates of 90%–95% in the treatment of asymptomatic cyst carriers.[104,105] Somewhat lower cure rates (83%) are achieved in nondysenteric, symptomatic intestinal amebiasis.[105] Although the drug is effective at clearing stools

of cysts of E. histolytica, it is not very effective in the treatment of acute dysentery where trophozoites are present in the stool.[106] Diloxanide furoate has no activity against liver abscess, but as a luminal amebicide it has achieved wide and successful use for the treatment of symptomless and mildly symptomatic cyst-passers.[107] It is considered an alternative to paromomycin and diiodohydroxyquin for this purpose.[10,105]

Diloxanide furoate is administered orally and the usual adult dosage is 500 mg taken three times daily for 10 days. Studies in rats show that the ester is hydrolyzed by intestinal esterases and the drug is absorbed as diloxanide, which is excreted in the urine.[108] Some of the greater effectiveness of diloxanide furoate versus diloxanide in vivo may reflect slower absorption from (and thus longer retention in) the intestinal tract.[108] Diloxanide furoate is very well tolerated. The principal side effect is excessive flatulence, which is experienced by nearly all patients.[104,105] Occasional patients may experience nausea, anorexia, diarrhea, or abdominal cramps.[105]

Diiodohydroxyquin (Iodoquinol)

Several iodinated 8-hydroxyquinolines are effective in the treatment of intestinal amebiasis; these include diiodohydroxyquin, iodochlorhydroxyquin, and chiniofon. Diiodohydroxyquin (iodoquinol) is the only one

Diiodohydroxyquin

of these compounds available in the United States for oral administration. Iodochlorhydroxyquin (clioquinol) was formerly available for the treatment of intestinal protozoal infections but the oral preparation was removed from the U.S. market when it became clear that it could cause subacute myelooptic neuropathy. The 8-hydroxyquinolines have limited antibacterial and antifungal activity and some topical formulations of io-dochlorhydroxyquin are available for treating localized dermatophytic and bacterial infections of the skin. The 8-hydroxy-quinolines are amebidicidal, and their mechanism of action is not known.

THERAPEUTIC USE. Diiodohydroxyquin is used alone (650 mg three times a day for 20 days) to treat asymptomatic cyst passers, where the cure rate is at least 80%.[109] Diiodohydroxyquin and paromomycin are now considered co-drugs of choice for the treatment of asymptomatic cyst passers. Diiodohydroxyquin may be administered in combination with metronidazole to provide additional luminal amebicidal activity when treating intestinal and hepatic amebiasis. The drug is a luminal amebicide and has no effect on hepatic abscesses. This lack of effectiveness against E. histolytica in the liver probably reflects the low concentration of the drug in this organ. Amebae in the gut would be exposed to much higher concentrations.

Diiodohydroxyquin is considered by many specialists to be one of the drugs of choice for the treatment of Dientamoeba fragilis infection and an alternative to the tetracyclines in Balantidium coli infection (balantidiasis). The dosage here is the same as for treating amebiasis, but the duration of therapy is half as long (10 days). Diiodohydroxyquin, at high dosage and upon chronic administration, is reputed to be useful in the treatment of acrodermatitis enteropathica, a hereditary disease characterized by vesiculobullous and eczematoid skin lesions and diarrhea.[110] The condition has been linked to zinc deficiency and it has been suggested that the beneficial effect of diiodohydroxyquin is related to its ability to act as a zinc ionophore.[111]

PHARMACOKINETICS AND ADVERSE EFFECTS. Diiodohydroxyquin is not readily absorbed from the gastrointestinal tract. About 5% of a single oral dose can be recovered in the urine as the glucuronide conjugate and a small amount is excreted as the sulfate.[112] Considerably more iodochlorhydroxyquin than diiodohydroxyquin is absorbed—about 25% of an oral dose.[113]

At normally prescribed doses, adverse effects of diiodohydroxyquin are mild. Diiodohydroxyquin occasionally causes headaches, diarrhea, nausea, vomiting, skin rashes, and anal pruritis. Although the systemic absorption of this iodinated drug is limited, slight enlargement of the thyroid gland is occasionally observed. The drug can interfere with some thyroid function tests. It should not be given to people who have a known iodine sensitivity. The most important untoward effect with the 8-hydroxyquinolines is subacute myelo-optic neuropathy. This syndrome includes dysesthesia, weakness, and other manifestations of peripheral neuropathy; it is sometimes accompanied by loss of visual acuity and even optic atrophy with permanent blindness. The mechanism of the toxicity is unknown. It was first noticed in Japan where iodochlorhydroxyquin was being sold without prescription.[114] Although the bulk of the cases have involved iodochlorhydroxyquin, blindness can result from diiodohydroxyquin administration as well.[115] Before this effect was recognized, the halogenated hydroxyquinolines were used to treat chronic nonspecific diarrhea in children and to prevent, as well as treat, "traveler's" diarrhea.[116] Such nonspecific use of these drugs is clearly unwarranted. The adverse visual effects are rare when the drug is used to treat amebiasis.

Paromomycin

The pharmacology of paromomycin was discussed along with that of the other aminoglycosides in Chapter 5. After oral administration, little of the drug is absorbed into the systemic circulation; thus, side effects are limited to gastrointestinal upset and diarrhea. Paromomycin acts directly on amebae, but also has antibacterial activity against normal and pathogenic microorganisms in the gastrointestinal tract. It is administered in a dose of 25–35 mg/kg/day in 3 doses for 7 days. In addition to being used in amebiasis, paromomycin is used to treat other protozoal infections. It has been found to be effective in some cases of visceral leishmaniasis,[117] and it is presently the treatment of choice for cryptosporidiosis (25–35 mg/kg/day in 3 or 4 doses).

Emetine and Dehydroemetine

THERAPEUTIC USE. Emetine was the mainstay of treatment of severe intestinal and extraintestinal amebiasis for many years. Now the

Emetine

emetines are used only as alternative agents when metronidazole has failed to achieve a cure. The emetines kill the trophozoite forms of the amebas directly, but they are not very active against the cyst form of *E. hystolytica* in the intestinal wall.

ADVERSE EFFECTS. Emetines have multiple adverse effects. They are irritating compounds and care should be taken in handling the drug solution to ensure that it does not contact the eyes and mucous membranes. Because of their irritating properties, the administration of emetines is virtually always accompanied by pain and tenderness at the site of injection.[118] Nausea occurs quite frequently (31% of patients) even though the drug is administered parenterally.[118] This is probably due to a central action, and vomiting and dizziness may also occur. Emetine can also induce diarrhea. This effect, as well as the hypotensive effect of emetines, may occur as a result of a blockade of the sympathetic nervous system.[119,120] The fact that the drug itself causes diarrhea can complicate assessment of the response to therapy in the patient who has amebic dysentery. The emetines can produce a reversible generalized muscle weakness and aching. It has

been suggested that this side effect is due to a neuromuscular block,[120,121] but other investigators have concluded that the weakness is due to a direct effect on the muscle fiber that occurs at a subcellular level.[122] Emetine also has an effect when applied directly to the nerve axon,[123] however, and at this time, it is is not possible to provide a clear statement of the mechanism, of the muscle weakness.

The major adverse effects of emetine are on the heart, and the signs and symptoms of cardiotoxicity include tachycardia, abnormalities in the electrocardiogram, dyspnea, and sometimes precordial pain.[118] Electrocardiographic abnormalities, such as lengthening of the P-R and Q-T intervals and flattening or inversion of the T waves, occurred in approximately 50% of the patients in one large study.[118] Changes in cardiac rhythm are unusual. The electrocardiographic abnormalities rarely regress unless the drug is discontinued. Both electrocardiographic changes and signs of myopathy may appear after cessation of therapy. The side effects of dehydroemetine are similar to those of emetine, although dehydroemetine appears to be less cardiotoxic.[124,125] The difference is not large, however, and it should be noted that electrocardiographic changes occur only slightly less frequently in patients receiving dehydroemetine than in those receiving an equivalent dose of emetine.[126] It is thought that the cardiotoxicity of emetine is related to its slow rate of elimination, which favors drug accumulation.[124] Dehydroemetine may be less cardiotoxic simply because it is more rapidly eliminated and tissue levels are lower.[124]

It is clear that certain precautions in patient management are warranted in view of the toxicity of the emetines. An electrocardiogram should be taken before therapy is initiated and repeatedly thereafter. The drugs should be stopped when significant electrocardiographic changes develop. In order to decrease symptoms associated with cardiotoxicity, the patient should remain sedentary during therapy and for a while thereafter. Emetines should not be used in patients with heart disease, in children, or in pregnant women unless absolutely necessary—that is, if metronidazole and chloroquine are ineffective.

Drugs Used to Treat Leishmaniasis and Trypanosomiasis

The Diseases

There are three principal diseases caused by *Leishmania:* visceral leishmaniasis (kala-azar), the result of infection with *L. donovani*; cutaneous leishmaniasis, *L. tropica* and *L. mexicana*; and American mucocutaneous leishmaniasis, *L. braziliensis*. The *Leishmania* organisms, which assume the flagellated form in the insect vector and in culture, are ovid unflagellated organisms in humans. The unflagellated form (amastigote) is an intracellular parasite of macrophages and reticuloendothelial cells. The *Leishmania* are transmitted from a reservoir of numerous species of small animals and rodents to the human host by the bite of sandflies of the genus *Phlebotomus*. Visceral leishmaniasis is a disease of gradual onset characterized by fever, weight loss, hepatosplenomegaly, lymphadenopathy, hemorrhage, and hepatic malfunction. Cutaneous leishmaniasis is characterized by a superficial ulceration of the skin at the site of the bite. The organism can be identified in scrapings from the edge of the ulcerations, which are prone to bacterial infection. The degree of involvement depends largely on the cell-mediated immunity of the host, varying from single lesions that heal with scarring to spreading ulcers that never heal. The self-healing form is often called *Oriental sore*. American mucocutaneous leishmaniasis occurs in several different forms. There may be extensive ulceration of the mucous membrane of the mouth, palate, pharynx, and nose. Progressive and grossly disfiguring erosion may take place.

The diseases caused by *Leishmania* and their treatment have been reviewed by several authors.[117,127–129] The treatment of choice for all three forms of leishmaniasis is a pentavalent antimonial, such as sodium stibogluconate (see Table 14–5). In areas where lesions of cutaneous leishmaniasis heal spontaneously, specific treatment is not necessary, but with long-lasting or disfiguring lesions, drug treatment is advisable.[127] In the case of mucocutaneous or visceral leishmaniasis, the host must have a competent immune response for chemotherapy to be curative. Cases of mucocutaneous leishmaniasis that do not respond to antimonials may respond to a course of intravenous therapy with amphotericin B,[130] an antifungal drug that is reviewed in Chapter 12. Pentamidine is useful for treating visceral leishmaniasis caused by strains of *L. donovani*, which are relatively resistant to antimonial drugs.[131]

Treatment with these second-line agents is less satisfactory because of their toxicity at therapeutic doses. However, liposomal encapsulated amphotericin and other amphotericin B formulations have been used successfully to treat multiple drug–resistant visceral leishmaniasis.[132,133] Other drugs that are being tried include interferon gamma to boost the immune response, allopurinol, which inhibits the growth of *Leishmania* spp. in vitro, paromomycin, an aminoglycoside antibiotic with broad antimicrobial activity, pentamidine, and ketoconazole. These agents are in various stages of testing.[117,134] Preliminary studies indicate that topical treatment with paromomycin ointment may be effective in the treatment of cutaneous Old World leishmaniasis.[135]

Trypanosomiasis also occurs in three forms. African trypanosomiasis (sleeping sickness) is caused by *Trypanosoma brucei gambiense* or *Trypanosoma brucei rhodesiense*. Both are transmitted to humans by the bite of dipteran flies of the genus *Glossina* (tsetse flies). The Gambian form is characterized by a slow onset with low morbidity and the classical symptoms of sleeping sickness don't appear until the late stages of the disease, often 4 or more years after the initial infection.[136] In contrast, the Rhodesian form is an acute disease with rapid onset, high morbidity, and almost 100% mortality in untreated cases.[136] The first stage of African trypanosomiasis (the hemolymphatic stage) is characterized by invasion of the lymphatic system, with lymphadenopathy, hepatosplenomegaly, intermittent febrile attacks, dyspnea, and tachycardia. The chronic, sleeping-sickness stage is initiated by inva-

Table 14–5.   Drugs used to treat leishmaniasis and trypanosomiasis. Sodium stiboglucoate, suramin, melarsoprol, and nifurtimox are not marketed in the United States but they may be obtained from the Parasitic Disease Division of the Centers for Disease Control. Tryparasamide and benznidazole are not available in the United States.

Infecting organism	Drug of choice	Alternative
LEISHMANIASIS		
Leishmania donovani (kala-azar, visceral leishmaniasis)	Sodium stibogluconate	Amphotericin B, lipid-encapsulated amphotericin B, pentamidine, or paromomycin
Leishmania tropica (Oriental sore, cutaneous leishmaniasis)	Sodium stibogluconate	
Leishmania brazilliensis (American mucocutaneous leishmaniasis)	Sodium stibogluconate	
AFRICAN TRYPANOSOMIASIS		
Trypanosoma brucei gambiense or *T. brucei rhodesiense*		
Hemolymphatic stage	Suramin or eflornithine	Pentamidine
Late disease with central nervous system involvement	Melarsoprol or eflornithine	Tryparsamide plus suramin[a]
SOUTH AMERICAN TRYPANOSOMIASIS		
Trypanosoma cruzi (Chagas' disease)	Nifurtimox	Benznidazole

[a] *Trypanosoma brucei gambiense* only.

sion of the central nervous system. This stage is marked by headache, increasing mental dullness and apathy, and disturbances in coordinate neurological functions. In the final stages, the patient sleeps continually, emaciation becomes profound, and coma and death result. African trypanosomiasis in the hemolymphatic stage is effectively treated with suramin. Pentamidine is also useful in the early stage of infection, especially in the Gambian form of the disease.[136] After the parasite has invaded the central nervous system, melarsoprol or eflornithine are the drugs of choice.

The third form of trypanosomiasis, South American trypanosomiasis (Chagas' disease), is caused by *Trypanosoma cruzi* and is transmitted to humans by reduviid bugs. These organisms evoke a symptom complex quite unlike the African trypanosomes.[137] Myocarditis, leading to cardiomyopathy in the chronic stage, is a prominent feature of Chagas' disease. Nifurtimox is currently considered to be the drug of choice. Benz-

nidazole also appears to be clinically useful in controlling the infection, as determined by elimination of the parasite from the blood.[137] Both nifurtimox and benznidazole have been shown to destroy the tissue forms of *T. cruzi*.[137] *Trypanosoma cruzi* is especially vulnerable to drugs that form intracellular free radicals, and both nifurtimox and benznidazole have this ability. Both these agents are effective in reducing the duration and severity of acute and congenital Chagas' disease, but they achieve parasitologic cures in only about 50% of treated patients, can cause severe side effects, and must be taken for extended periods.[138] These drugs have also not been demonstrated to alter the clinical courses of patients with chronic *T. cruzi* infections, and many chronic-phase patients remain infected despite vigorous treatment.

Sodium Stibogluconate

A number of antimonial compounds have been used to treat leishmaniasis and schistosomiasis. The trivalent compound antimony potassium tartrate (tartar emetic) was the first antimonial shown to produce a leishmanicidal effect. Other trivalent antimonials, such as stibophen, a drug that has been used to treat schistosomiasis, were subsequently found to be effective leishmanicides and to be less toxic than tartar emetic. Trivalent antimonials were used widely for the treatment of leishmaniasis until the introduction of the pentavalent antimonials sodium stibogluconate and meglumine antimoniate (not available in the United States), which have become the drugs of choice because of equivalent efficacy and decreased toxicity.

Clinical formulations of sodium stibogluconate consist of multiple uncharacterized molecular forms, some of which have high molecular masses (1000–4000).[128] Typical preparations contain 30% to 34% pentavalent antimony by weight. Clinical formulations of sodium stibogluconate may be described as an unknown number of uncharacterized complexes of Sb with carbohydrates derived from gluconic acid. In the United States, sodium stibogluconate is available only from the Centers for Disease Control as an aqueous solution containing an equivalent of 100 mg of Sb^{+5}/ml.

The mechanism of the leischmanicidal effect of the pentavalent antimonials has not been defined. The trivalent antimonials are active against both leishmania[139] and schistosomes[140] in vivo and in vitro. Their schistosomicidal activity is due to selective inhibition of parasite phosphofructokinase. The flagellate form of leishmanial organisms in culture can grow in the presence of high concentrations of pentavalent antimonials, and it is possible that the metal must be reduced to the trivalent form before these drugs are active against the parasite in vivo.[141] It is also possible that the pentavalent antimonials act in a manner that is different from the trivalent compounds and that the flagellated form of the parasite in culture is not sensitive to the pentavalent drugs.

Inhibition of amastigote bioenergetics appears to be part of the mechanism of action of sodium stibogluconate.[128] Exposure of the amastigotes to this drug for 4 h results in

Sodium stibogluconate
(a pentavalent antimonial)

Antimony potassium tartrate
(a trivalent antimonial)

both a dose-dependent decrease in viability and decrease in CO_2 production from certain substrates. Both glycolysis and fatty-acid oxidation, processes primarily localized in unusual organelles termed *glycosomes*, are inhibited. This is accompanied by a net reduction in the generation of ATP and GTP. Other mechanisms may be involved in the action of this drug, such as nonspecific binding of antimony to the sulfhydryl groups of amastigote proteins having molecular weights of 14,000–68,000.[128]

In vivo, *Leishmania* organisms are rapidly taken up by mononuclear phagocytic cells where they reside chronically. As liposomes are also removed from the circulation by these cells, there have been several attempts to improve therapeutic efficacy by entrapping antileishmanial drugs in liposomes. Liposome-encapsulated stibogluconate administered intravenously to mice infected with *L. donovani* has been shown to be more effective than the free drug alone.[117,142,143] Enhanced antileishmanial activity has also been shown with lisosome-encapsulated trivalent antimonials,[142,143] 8-aminoquinolines,[144] and amphotericin B.[145]

PHARMACOKINETICS. Sodium stibogluconate is administered intramuscularly or by slow intravenous infusion. It appears to distribute into the extracellular fluid and it is cleared by the kidney at a rate that approximates that of inulin.[146] Six hours after intravenous administration, plasma antimony levels are less than 1% of peak values. Lower and more sustained plasma antimony levels are achieved with intramuscular administration, but nevertheless, more than 80% of the drug is excreted in 6 h.[146] Sodium stibogluconate is eliminated in two phases, with the first phase having a half-life of about 2 h and the second a half-life of 33 to 76 h. This slow phase may reflect conversion of the pentavalent antimonial to the trivalent form, which is taken up and retained by the liver. This conversion may account for accumulation and slow release of the drug during multiple dosing schedules of administration.[147] The rapid first-phase clearance of most of the drug suggests that it will not accumulate in patients with normal renal function and that courses of therapy longer than 10 days may be administered without substantial increase in the frequency of toxic symptoms. Patients with decreased glomerular filtration rate will accumulate the drug and toxicity may occur.[146]

CLINICAL USES. In the United States, sodium stibogluconate is available only from the Centers for Disease Control. Sodium stibogluconate is still the drug of choice for leishmaniasis despite an increased incidence of resistance. Its main disadvantages are the long course of therapy, the necessity for parenteral administration, and the relatively high cost of treatment. For cutaneous leishmaniasis, a daily dose of sodium stibogluconate (20 mg of pentavalent antimony per kg) for 20 days is administered. Different species of *Leishmania* may respond differently to the drug, but for mucocutaneous and systemic leishmaniasis (kala-azar) 30-day therapy is used. Similar doses are used for children as they seem to tolerate the drug well. If unfavorable reactions occur in particularly debilitated individuals, the drug may be given on alternate days or for longer intervals. Cure rates are generally high when the above recommendations are followed. In endemic areas the incidence of treatment failures with this drug in visceral, mucocutaneous, and some forms of cutaneous leishmaniasis has increased dramatically.[148] Resistance to sodium stibogluconate has now been well documented in both laboratory-derived strains and clinical isolates.[149,150] Drug resistance may be a result of decreased drug transport, but there is conflicting evidence for this.[149,150]

ADVERSE EFFECTS. The pentavalent antimonials are much less toxic than the trivalent compounds and are generally well tolerated. Side effects include pain at the injection site, rashes, pruritis, abdominal pain, diarrhea, weakness, dizziness, jaundice, albuminuria, and electrocardiographic changes. The electrocardiographic changes are reversible, and interruption of treatment is usually not required. The electrocardiographic changes may be delayed and include T-wave flattening and inversion and prolongation of the Q-T interval. If possible, the antimonials should not be administered to patients with cardiac disease, liver disease, or renal failure. Acute symptoms resembling serum sickness may occur during the treatment of visceral leishmaniasis. These symptoms appear to result from parasite destruction, which leads to high levels of circulating immune complexes.[151] In cases of visceral leishmaniasis, it is often difficult to determine whether the electrocardiographic changes are a consequence of infection or of drug toxicity.[152]

Pentamidine

Pentamidine is one of a number of diamidine compounds, including propamidine and stilbamidine, that have trypanocidal activity.

Pentamidine

Another diamidine, hydroxystilbamidine, was formerly used in the treatment of North American blastomycosis.

THERAPEUTIC USE. As mentioned above, pentamidine isethionate is used as an alternative to sodium stibogluconate in the treatment of visceral leishmaniasis. It is also useful in the treatment of early trypanosomiasis before central nervous system involvement and in chemoprophylaxis against Gambian trypanosomiasis. In the treatment of Gambian trypanosomiasis, pentamidine is given in an intravenous dose similar to that used to treat *Pneumocystis carinii* pneumonia (PCP) (see below) along with suramin. Alternatively, a series of 7 intramuscular doses of pentamidine alone can be administered.[153] Pentamidine is not used to treat *T. b. rhodesiense*, which affects the brain early in the course of infection. Pentamidine has been successfully used to treat visceral leishmaniasis (kala-azar caused by *L. donovani*). The physician practicing in Europe or North America does not come into contact with these diseases, although very rarely they are diagnosed in travelers who become symptomatic after returning home.[154] The experience of the European or North American physician with this drug has been primarily in the treatment of infection by *Pneumocystis carinii*.[155] *Pneumocystis carinii* is an opportunistic organism, since it produces pneumonitis almost exclusively in the compromised host, most commonly in patients with human immunodeficiency virus (HIV) and patients with malignant disease or organ transplants who are receiving immunosuppressive therapy.[156,157] For a number of years, pentamidine was the drug of choice for treatment of *Pneumocystis carinii* pneumonitis,[157,158] but this infection also responds well to trimethoprim-sulfamethoxazole,[155,159] which is less toxic and has replaced pentamidine as the drug of choice (Table 14–1).

Pentamidine is one of a number of drugs that have been used extensively for the prophylaxis and treatment of mild to moderate PCP. Prophlaxis has decreased the incidence of the disease and delayed the onset of PCP, and increased the median survival of patients with AIDS.[160] Prophylaxis is indicated for any HIV-infected adult or adolescent with a CD4 count less than 200 cells/mm[3] including pregnant women.[161] For prophylaxis against PCP, aerosolized pentamidine, oral trimethoprim-sulfamethoxazole, and oral dapsone are all effective. Trimethoprim-sulfamethoxazole (TMP-SMX) is the drug of choice despite its high incidence of adverse effects, as it is less expensive and some patients prefer oral medication. When pentamidine is used prophylactically, it is inhaled as an aerosol directly into the lungs to minimize systemic toxicity. It is usually given in a monthly dose of 300 mg of a 5% to 10% nebulized aqueous solution of pentamidine isethionate delivered over 30 to 45 min via Respirgard nebulizer.[162] In HIV-infected patients with CD4+ cell counts of 100–200/mm[3], pentamidine is better tolerated than, but is just as effective as, trimethprim-sulfamethoxazole or dapsone in preventing PCP. In more debilitated patients having lower CD4 counts, pentamidine is less effective than the other drugs, which also have the advantage of efficacy against *T. gondii* infection.[163]

For treatment of mild to moderate PCP, TMP-SMX is the treatment of choice. Intravenous pentamidine isethionate is an alternative for patients with severe PCP who are intolerant or unresponsive to TMP-SMX. The usual dosage is 4 mg/kg given parenterally each day for 14 days. A lower 2 to 3 mg/kg daily dose may be equally effective and produce substantially less toxicity.[164] Clinical improvement usually occurs 4 to 6 days after the first injection if therapy is successful. A high proportion of cures is usually seen even though toxicity may force stoppage of therapy. Results are less favorable in debilitated patients with altered immunity or cancer.

MECHANISM OF ACTION. The mechanism of action of pentamidine is not yet defined. Dicationic compounds like pentamidine may display multiple effects on a given parasite or act by different mechanisms in various parasites. The diamidines are taken up by a transporter that is selective for adenine and adenosine, purines that are needed for survival of the parasites.[165] Melamine-based arsenicals use a similar purine (P-2) transporter, which accounts for the cross-resistance to diamidines exhibited by certain arsenical resistant strains of *T. brucei*. Diamidines interfere with polyamine biosynthesis in trypanosomes by reversible inhibition of S-adenosyl-L-methionine decarboxylase,[166] and another major target for the diamidines may be DNA. The diamidines bind to DNA at sequences composed of at least four consecutive A-T base pairs.[167] Other trypanocidal diamidines with structures analogous to pentamidine (hydroxystilbamidine, berenil) have been shown to bind to DNA and polynucleotides in a nonintercalative manner.[168,169] In the case of the diamidines, it is possible that the DNA binding may be related to the trypanocidal action. When diamidines are added to trypanosomes growing in culture, they interact selectively with kinetoplast DNA.[170,171] The kinetoplast is a specialized structure that contains its own DNA (as opposed to the nuclear DNA), and in trypanosomes, this prominent body is a part of the mitochondrial system. The diamidines cause a disorganization of the kinetoplast DNA and the organelle eventually loses its nucleic acid. It has been proposed that the bound drug may interfere with kinetoplast DNA replication.[172] The effects of pentamidine on trypanosome kinetoplast DNA were found to be consistent with its being a type II topoisomerase inhibitor.[173] It also inhibits ATP-dependent topoisomerases in extracts of *Pneumocystis carinii*.[174]

PHARMACOKINETICS. Pentamidine is not well absorbed from the gastrointestinal tract and it is routinely administered by intramuscular injection. Following a single intravenous dose to patients with AIDS, pentamidine disappears from plasma with an apparent half-life of about 6 h;[175] however, it is eliminated much more slowly in urine as the unchanged drug, with renal clearance accounting for only about 2% of plasma clearance.[176] In patients receiving multiple injections of the drug over a 13-day period, drug accumulation occurred and no steady-state plasma concentration was attained.[176] In many patients, pentamidine could still be detected in plasma after 6 weeks. The extensive accumulation of pentamidine in tissues and its slow rate of excretion may account for both its therapeutic and prophylactic efficacy against African trypanosomiasis.[153] The highest concentrations of drug are achieved in the liver, kidney, adrenal gland, and spleen of patients with AIDS, with intermediate concentrations being achieved in lung.[177] Higher pulmonary concentrations can be attained with inhalation of pentamidine aerosol, either for prophylaxis or as adjunctive treatment for mild to moderate PCP. The size of particles generated by the nebulizer and the patient's ventilatory patterns will determine the actual dose delivered deep in the lung tissue.

In mice, pentamidine is stored in the tissues and slowly excreted in the urine, predominantly or totally as the unchanged drug.[178,179] The highest levels of pentamidine are found in the kidney, a localization that may contribute to its renal toxicity.[179] Pentamidine does not enter the central nervous system to any extent. Therefore, it cannot be used to treat trypanosomiasis during the later phases of the disease, which are marked by central nervous system involvement.

ADVERSE EFFECTS. The administration of pentamidine sometimes causes pain at the injection site, and this can be followed by abscess formation and tissue necrosis. The drug is quite toxic. About 50% of the patients treated with therapeutic doses of pentamidine experience toxicity, regardless of whether they have AIDS. Intravenous injection of pentamidine can be followed by several alarming and sometimes dangerous reactions, including breathlessness, tachycardia, dizziness or fainting, headache, and vomiting. These reactions are believed to be related to the sharp fall in blood pressure that follows too rapid intravenous administration of the drug and may be related in part to the release of histamine.[164,180] Pancreatitis and hypoglycemia and, paradoxically, hyperglycemia and insulin-dependent diabetes have been documented following administration of pentamidine. The hypoglycemia may be life threatening or even fatal if not recognized. Other adverse effects include skin rashes, thrombophlebitis, thrombocytopenia, anemia, neutropenia, elevation of liver enzymes, and nephrotoxicity. Since adverse reactions are more severe after intravenous administration, the intramuscular route is preferred.[155] Particular care must be taken when pentamidine is administered to patients with diabetes, hypertension, malnutrition, or hepatic or renal disease. The renal dysfunction caused by pentamidine is reversible and has been seen in about 24% of patients receiving the drug. It is a significant problem in HIV-infected individuals with PCP. It is possible that the nephrotoxicity is due to inhibition of renal dihydrofolate reductase by the drug. Pentamidine is a potent inhibitor of purified rat kidney dihydrofolate reductase, and the activity of this enzyme is markedly reduced in extracts prepared from kidneys of rats that had been administered a single dose (20 mg/kg) of pentamidine 24 h earlier.[178] Renal dysfunction is also a frequent complication of high-dose therapy with the anticancer drug methotrexate, which is also a potent inhibitor of mammalian dihydrofolate reductase.[181]

Suramin

Suramin is a compound developed from a group of nonmetallic dyes, such as trypan blue, that are known to have trypanocidal activity. In the United States, suramin is available only from the Centers for Disease Control. It is used in the treatment of both types of African trypanosomiasis in the early stages of the disease, prior to involvement of the central nervous system.[136] Although suramin is used to treat African trypanosomiasis, it is of no value in treating South American trypanosomiasis caused by *T. cruzi*. Because only small amounts of the drug enter the cerebrospinal fluid, suramin is considered to be more effective against West African trypanosomiasis than against the East African infection. Because of the relatively high incidence of treatment failures, some clinicians recommend combining suramin with pentamidine for the treatment of early-stage West African infection.[153] Suramin is given by slow intravenous injection as a 10% aqueous solution. A 100 to 200 mg test dose is given initially to assess the patient's tolerance, as the drug can occasionally cause serious immediate reactions (nausea, vomiting, shock, and loss of consciousness). If the test dose is not attended by a severe reaction, a dose of 1 g is given adults on days 1, 3, 7, 14, and 21 in the therapy of African trypanasomiasis. If there is intolerance to the test dose, therapy should not be initiated. The cause of the intolerance is not known. Because suramin does not penetrate into the central nervous system, for treatment of trypansosomiasis with central nervous system involvement an arsenical must also be employed. Suramin will clear the hemolymphatic system of trypanosomes even in late-stage disease, so it is sometimes administered before starting melarsoprol to reduce the risk of reactive encephalopathy associated with the administration of that arsenical. Suramin is also effective for the prophylaxis of African trypanosomiasis. However, chemoprophylaxis is not recommended for travelers on occasional brief visits to endemic areas, because the risk of serious toxicity outweighs the risk of acquiring the disease. For chemoprophylaxis, a single dose of 1 g is usually repeated weekly for 5 or 6 weeks. Suramin in a dose of 1 g weekly for 4 weeks, is also effective in the treatment of infection by one of the filaria, *Onchocerca vovlulus*,[182] although it has now been largely replaced by ivermectin for treatment of this disease. Suramin has been reviewed by several authors.[183,184]

MECHANISM OF ACTION. The primary mechanism of action of suramin is not yet defined. At concentrations in the range of 1–10 μM the drug inhibits a wide variety of enzymes,[183,185] often in a manner that is competitive with one of the components of the reaction. Suramin is, for example, a potent inhibitor of several enzymes in the complement system, where inhibition is competitive with the substrates.[186] Inhibition of viral reverse transcriptase is competitive with the template-primer,[187] whereas inhibition of the lactate dehydrogenase from *O. volvulus* is competitive with respect to the NADH cofactor.[188] It has been suggested that the large, negatively charged drug just binds nonspecifically to cationic sites on proteins, and in the case of some enzymes, the binding is sufficient to produce a reversible inactivation. Suramin does not diffuse across mammalian cell membranes, but it forms tight complexes with serum proteins and the drug protein complexes are taken up by phagocytic cells of the reticuloendothelial

Suramin

system. The drug may accumulate in lysosomes and inhibit intralysosomal enzymes.[183,189] If it could readily pass through host cell membranes, the drug would be too toxic to be useful in therapy. That the poor permeability property of the drug is critical to limiting its toxicity is exhibited by the effect of suramin on the sodium pump in red blood cells. Exposure of intact red cells to low concentrations of suramin does not affect the activity of (Na^+-K^+)–activated ATPase. But when the red cell membrane is ruptured and suramin is allowed to enter the cell, it is a potent inhibitor of the ATPase at the inside surface of the membrane.[190]

Given that a number of enzymes are inhibited by suramin, it is perhaps not surprising that the mechanism for its selective toxicity has not been defined. Trypanosomes take up only small amounts of suramin in vivo, and selective toxicity is probably not due solely to selective uptake by the parasite.[191] The drug appears to be taken into the parasite by endocytosis, and once inside the organism, suramin progressively inhibits respiration and glycolysis. There is evidence that the drug inhibits production of ATP in *Trypanosoma brucei* in vivo by inhibiting glycerol-3-phosphate oxidase and glycerol-3-phosphate dehydrogenase, both of which are important enzymes in metabolic pathways that are unique to the parasite.[191] The inhibition of several trypanosomal glycolytic enzymes was much more effective than on the homologous enzymes of mammalian origin.[184] The energy supply of *O. volvulus* depends mainly on glycolysis, and the tricarboxylic acid cycle is absent or of minor importance. It has been suggested that the

critical targets of suramin action in this filarial organism may be lactic dehydrogenase and malic dehydrogenase, both of which serve to generate NADPH in the absence of the citric acid cycle.[188,192]

PHARMACOKINETICS. Suramin is administered by slow intravenous injection to avoid local inflammation and necrosis associated with subcutaneous or intramuscular injections. Suramin, displays complex pharmacokinetics. The plasma concentration falls fairly rapidly for a few hours after administration, then more slowly for a few days, with a half-life of about 48 h for this second phase, and finally, very slowly, with a terminal elimination half-life of about 50 days. The persistence in plasma is probably due to the drug's extremely tight binding to plasma proteins (>99.7% after a typical 1-g dose)[153,183,193] The slow release from plasma protein and the slow excretion by the kidney permit the drug to be administered on a weekly or even a bi-monthly basis for chemoprophylaxis of sleeping sickness. One day after intravenous administration of 1 g of suramin to an adult the plasma concentration was found to be 40 µg/ml; after 10 days, it was 8 µg/ml.[183] Because it accumulates in the body, intervals of several days are maintained between doses, as described above. Suramin is not metabolized to any extent, and renal clearance accounts for elimination of about 80% of the drug from the body. The distribution of suramin is not known, although clearly some of the drug is taken into the cells of the reticuloendothelial system.[183] Since suramin does not enter the central nervous system, it cannot be used to treat trypanosomiasis during the later phases of the disease, which are marked by central nervous system involvement.

ADVERSE REACTIONS. Suramin can cause several types of adverse reactions, which vary in intensity and frequency and tend to be more severe in debilitated patients. The most serious immediate reactions are nausea, vomiting, shock, and loss of consciousness, but fortunately, the incidence is low. Malaise and fatigue are common. The incidence of severe, immediate reactions to suramin has been estimated at 1 in 2000–4000 cases.[183] The basis for the hypotensive response is unknown, but the risk is minimized by administering a small test dose to determine the patient's sensitivity and by infusing the drug slowly. Later reactions, occurring 3–24 h after drug administration, include fever, rashes, photophobia, lachrymation, abdominal distention, and, in certain groups of people (e.g., the Kissi people of Sierra Leone), cutaneous hyperesthesia of the soles or palms.[183] The most common delayed reaction (occurring after several days) is renal dysfunction, and frequent urinalyses should be performed to monitor for the proteinuria that often occurs during therapy. Hematuria and cylinduria occur when renal damage is extensive, and if they occur, further treatment with suramin should be postponed or abandoned. Special caution must be exercised when administering suramin to patients with preexisting renal disease. Other delayed reactions include exfoliative dermatitis, stomatitis, debility, and weakness. Jaundice is a rare but dangerous complication and suramin is contraindicated in patients with preexisting liver disease. Rarely, blood dyscrasias and hemolytic anemia have been reported with therapy.

In addition to reactions that are caused by the drug directly, treatment of onchocerciasis may precipitate allergic reactions due to the death of adult worms and microfilariae.[183] Optic atrophy may also occur following treatment of ocular onchocerciasis. This complication probably results from death of microfilariae in the optic nerve which initiates an inflammatory reaction leading to subsequent atrophy.[194]

In spite of the impressive list of potential reactions, suramin is a reasonably safe drug if administered carefully. In one series, for example, suramin was administered to 26,963 onchocerciasis patients in Venezuela with no deaths.[195] Suramin is known to be teratogenic in animal models[196] and it should not be administered to pregnant women (especially those in the first trimester).

The Arsenicals

There are several organic arsenical drugs that have been employed in treating trypanosomiasis. Because of toxicity, their use in all but the meningoencephalitic stages of sleeping sickness has been discontinued, and pentamidine and suramin are used instead. The arsenicals are produced in trivalent (melarsoprol) and pentavalent (tryparsamide) forms. Becuase tryparsamide is more toxic than melarsoprol, the former drug is no longer widely employed.

The arsenicals interact with sulfhydryl (SH) groups in proteins, and they have been shown to inactivate a wide variety of enzymes. The integrity of SH groups is essential in maintaining the appropriate structure and consequently the function of a number of enzymes. Many of the toxic effects, as well as the trypanocidal action of organic arsenicals, are probably due to inactivation of SH groups.

Melarsoprol
(trivalent)

Tryparsamide
(pentavalent)

Given a nonspecific mechanism of action such as this, one could predict that the arsenicals are very toxic drugs, which is indeed the case; side effects are common. The basis of the selective toxicity of these agents is not completely clear, but a differential permeability between the host cells and trypanosomes may be important. Susceptible African trypanosomes actively concentrate melarsoprol via an unusual purine transporter, and resistance seems to result from altered drug uptake via this transporter.[165,197] Cross-resistance between arsenicals and diamidines (e.g., pentamidine) in cloned lines of *T. brucei* suggests that both drugs are concentrated by the same transport system.[198] The nonmetallic moiety of the drug probably contributes to some specificity of action. Of the many enzymes that can be affected, the terminal glycolytic enzyme pyruvate kinase has long been thought to be the primary site of the trypanocidal action.[199] There are differences between pyruvate kinases of mammalian and trypanosomal origin.[200] Some of the selective toxicity of the organic arsenical drugs may be attributable to the special sensitivity of this critical enzyme in the trypanosome. Studies by Fairlamb and co-workers, however, suggest that a major target of melarsoprol may be trypanothione, a dithiol spermidine-glutathione adduct.[201] Apparently, trypanothione substitutes for glutathione in trypanosomes to maintain a reducing environment inside the parasite. Irreversible binding of melarsoprol to trypanothione results in formation of a compound (MelT) that is a potent competitive inhibitor of trypanothione reductase, the enzyme responsible for maintaining trypanothione in its reduced form.[201] At concentrations of 0.5 to 10 μM, melarsoprol causes lysis of sensitive strains of *T. brucei* in vitro, whereas resistant strains are not lysed at concentrations exceeding 100 μM.[202] Despite the focus on trypanothione as a drug target, resistant trypanosomes do not contain increased levels of trypanothione, and the trypanothione reductases from both sensitive and resistant strains are equally inhibited by MelT.[198]

Melarsoprol and tryparsamide would not be used in therapy except for the fact that they penetrate into the cerebrospinal fluid. Melarsoprol is the drug of choice for the treatment of trypanosomal meningoencephalitis (Table 14–5). Melarsoprol is also active against the earlier stages of the disease, but it is not used before central nervous system involvement occurs because of its potential for causing encephalopathy. In the United States, melarsoprol is available only from the Centers for Disease Control. Patients who are severely debilitated are treated with suramin before initiation of melarsoprol therapy.[203,204] Relapse after a course of melarsoprol therapy occurs at a rate of about 5% in areas of *T. rhodesiense* and at slightly higher rates in areas of *T. gambiense*.[204] It appears likely that relapse is due to reseeding of the central nervous system by tissue parasites.[205] Patients with West African trypanosomnasis who relapse should be treated with eflornithine, whereas those with East African trypanosomiasis often respond favorably to a second course of melarsoprol.[153]

PHARMACOKINETICS. Melarsoprol is administered by slow intravenous injection. The drug is very irritating to tissues and special care must be taken to ensure that extravasation does not take place during injection. As with many of the drugs used in the treatment of parasitic infections, the dosage schedule is complex. Adults in good condition should be given up to 2.5 mg/kg of melarsoprol daily for 3 or 4 days; this course should be repeated after an interval of at least 7 days. A third course may be given, if required, after another 10 to 21 days. In children and underweight patients, even more cautious dosage regimens are employed.[206] Following such regimens, 80% to 90% of patients are cured. The concentration of drug achieved in cerebrospinal fluid is only 2%–20% of that in plasma, but this is sufficient for the trypanocidal effect.[207] The rate of drug elimination is fairly rapid—after a 3-day course of therapy, the plasma level of active drug in humans drops by 50% in about 24 h,[207] with 70% to 80% of the arsenic appearing in the feces.[153]

ADVERSE EFFECTS. Melarsoprol therapy is often accompanied by side effects, which include hypertension, abdominal pain, vomiting, albuminuria, peripheral neuropathy, arthralgia, angioneurotic edema, and rashes.[206] The first administration of drug is sometimes followed by an exacerbation of fever. This is thought to represent a Herxheimer-type reaction. The most serious complications of melarsoprol therapy involve the nervous system. A potentially fatal side effect is the development of reactive encephalopathy.[204,208] This usually occurs between the first two courses of therapy. It is more common in patients with East African sleeping sickness than in those with West African sleeping sickness and is more likely to develop in patients whose cerebrospinal fluid contains trypanosomes.[153] The first symptoms are headache and dizziness, followed by mental dullness, confusion, and ataxia. In more severe cases, incontinence, convulsions, and loss of consciousness occur. Reactive encephalopathy has been reported in 1%–5% of patients receiving melarsoprol.[208] This reaction may occur in the early hemolymphatic stages as well as in the later central nervous system stages of the disease. The cause is not known, but it may be an immune reaction elicited by the rapid release of trypanosomal antigens from dying parasites, rather than a direct toxic effect of the drug.[153] Hypersensitivity reactions to melarsoprol can also occur, particularly during the second or subsequent course of treatment. Prednisolone given simultaneously can reduce the frequency of reactive encephalopathy and can control the hypersensitivity reactions as well.[153] Albuminuria occurs frequently, and occasionally the appearance of numerous casts in the urine, or evidence of hepatic disturbances, may necessitate modification of treatment. Vomiting and abdominal colic also are common, but their incidence can be reduced by injecting the melarsoprol slowly into the supine, fasting patient. The patient should stay in bed and not eat for several hours after the injection. The drug should be given only in the hospital since the patient's condition must be closely monitored. This also allows for modification of the dosage regimen if necessary. In patients with leprosy, arsenicals may precipitate an erythema nodosum leprosum reaction. The use of the drug is contraindicated during epidemics of influenza. Severe hemolytic reactions have been reported in patients with deficiency of glucose-6-phosphate dehydrogenase.[209] In addition to causing the toxic reactions of other arsenicals, tryparsamide can cause blindness.

Nifurtimox

In contrast to the trypanosomes that cause African sleeping sickness, T. cruzi, the etiological agent of Chagas' disease, mutliplies

Nifurtimox
(Bayer 2502)

intracellularly as the amastigote form. Its intracellular location has contributed to the difficulty in finding therapeutically useful drugs against the disease. The development of a method of growing T. cruzi within cells in tissue culture facilitated the conduction of large-scale drug screening programs. With the help of cell cultures and animal screening models, a nitrofuran derivative, nifurtimox, was found to be active against both the intracellular amastigote and the extracellular trypomastigote stages of the parasite.[210,211] At a concentration of 10 µM, nifurtimox blocks the intracellular cycle of T. cruzi, and at 10–100 µM it inhibits penetration of vertebrate cells by trypomastigotes.[212] At concentrations above 100µM, the drug is toxic to the host cells. Nifurtimox-resistant strains of T. cruzi can be selected in vitro.[212]

Although nifurtimox is very effective against T. cruzi in vitro, when it is used clinically to treat Chagas' disease, the drug is suppressive, not curative.[213] Initially, it was thought that the drug eliminated the parasite from both patients with acute infection[214] and those with the chronic stage of the disease[215] (characterized by myocardiopathy and colonic and esophageal dilatation). When more sensitive xenodiagnostic and immune methods were used to detect T. cruzi in treated patients, however, it was found that nifurtimox reduced parasitemia to very low levels but it did not eliminate the organism completely.[213] Clinical improvement and negative serology are often obtained in the treatment of acute Chagas' disease, but treatment of chronic patients usually does not produce any clinical improvement and serology remains positive.[138,213] In the acute stage, therapy with nifurtimox results in disappearance of parasitemia, amelioration of symptoms, and a clinical cure in over 80% of patients treated with the drug. Strains of the disease present in different areas show different susceptibilities to nifurtimox.

The mechanism of action of nitrofurans has been discussed in some detail in Chapter 9 in the section describing the mechanism of action of nitrofurantoin. As occurs with other 5-nitrofuran derivatives, nifurtimox undergoes reductive activation to a nitroaromatic anion radical.[216,217] If molecular oxygen is present, the drug radical may react with it, producing active oxygen species, such as hydrogen peroxide and hydroxyl radicals.[218] The trypanosomal enzyme responsible for initial proximal nifurtimox reduction has not been demonstrated unequivocally, but trypanothione reductase has been implicated.[219] This reaction not only results in formation of electrophile drug products but also blocks reduction of the disulfide form of trypanothione to its biologically active dithiol form. Also, *T. cruzi* appears to be deficient in enzymatic defenses against reactive oxygen species.[218] Reaction of free radicals with cellular macromolecules results in cellular damage that includes lipid peroxidation and membrane injury, enzyme inactivation, damage to DNA, and mutagenesis. The intracellular amastigote form of *T. cruzi* appears to have a higher nifurtimox reducing activity than the extracellular forms of the parasite.[216] Reductive activation of nifurtimox also occurs in mammalian cells where the reducing enzyme is NADPH-cytochrome P-450 reductase.[217]

PHARMACOKINETICS AND ADVERSE EFFECTS. Nifurtimox is well absorbed from the gastrointestinal tract and it is administered orally to adults at a dose of 8 to 10 mg/kg daily in 4 divided doses for 120 days. Some patients experience gastric upset and weight loss upon treatment. If the latter occurs, the dosage should be reduced. Peak plasma levels of nifurtimox are seen after about 3.5 h.[220] Serum concentrations of the drug are low in relation to the doses administered, probably as a result of a marked first-pass effect. Less than 0.5% of a dose is excreted in the urine. The elimination half-life of nifurtimox is only about 3 h. Nifurtimox is rapidly and almost completely metabolized and the metabolites are excreted predominantly by the kidney—there is virtually no unaltered drug in the urine.[221,222] One pathway of metabolism is via nitro group reduction by microsomal NADPH-cytochrome P-450 reductase in liver, kidney, and other tissues.[217,223]

Side effects are common during nifurtimox therapy. In one study, for example, 69% of adults receiving standard dosage complained of one type of reaction or another.[214] The exact incidence of nifurtimox-induced side effects is uncertain, however, because many placebo-treated Chagas' disease patients have the same complaints.[214] Side effects appear to be more common in adults than children. The most commonly reported untoward reactions (complaint by more than 10% of adults under treatment) are anorexia, nausea, and vomiting; stomach pain; nervous excitation; vertigo; headache; myalgia; insomnia; and skin rashes.[214] The ingestion of alcohol should be avoided during treatment because the incidence of side effects may increase. Like many other nitrofuran derivatives, nifurtimox is mutagenic in bacterial test systems.[224]

Eflornithine (α-Difluoromethylornithine)

$$H_2NCH_2CH_2CH_2 - \overset{\overset{\displaystyle CHF_2}{|}}{\underset{\underset{\displaystyle NH_2}{|}}{C}} - COOH$$

Eflornithine

Eflornithine was originally designed as an anticancer drug. It is a selective and irreversible inhibitor of ornithine decarboxylase, the enzyme that catalyzes the conversion of ornithine to putrescine, the first and rate-limiting step in the biosynthesis of the polyamines spermidine and spermine.[225,226]

The polyamines are required for cell division and for normal cell differentiation.[227]

Eflornithine shows selective activity against West African trypanosomiasis (T. b. gambiense), in contrast to the East African disease (T. b. rhodiense).[228] The reason for this selectivity is not known. The basis for selective inhibition of the parasite ornithine decarboxylase is also unclear. Eflornithine inhibits both mammalian and trypanosomal ornithine decarboxylases, however, the host replaces the inhibited enzyme far more rapidly than the parasite.[229] Acquired resistance in T. b. gambiense in West Africa has not been reported.[230] Synergy with some arsenicals has been demonstrated with this drug.

Eflornithine can be given either orally or by intravenous injection. Bioavailability following a single oral dose of 10 mg/kg is 55%. Therapeutic doses of eflornithine are large and substantial volumes of fluid are required for intravenous administration. Peak plasma levels are achieved about 4 h after an oral dose, and the elimination half-life averages about 200 min. The drug does not bind to plasma proteins, it is well distributed, and it penetrates into the cerebrospinal fluid with a cerebrospinal fluid/plasma ratio of 0.91 after 14 days of administration.[231] This is very important in late-stage African trypanosomiasis. Eflornithine appears to show dose-dependent pharmacokinetics at the highest doses used clinically.[153] More than 80% of the drug is cleared by the kidney, largely in unchanged form.

CLINICAL USES. Eflornithine is effective in late-stage West African trypanosomiasis due to T. b. gambiense infections, including arsenic-resistant cases.[153,232] It has been administered primarily to patients having advanced disease with central nervous system complications, many of whom had received arsenicals prior to eflornithine treatment. In one study, patients were given 100 mg/kg intravenously every 6 h for 14 days, and almost all patients improved with this regimen. When given orally, eflornithine has limited bioavailability, and at equal doses, it is less effective orally than intravenously. However, the oral route can be used when intravenous therapy is impractical. Mono-

therapy with eflornithine is not effective against East African sleeping sickness, but eflornithine plus suramin appears to be effective.[233]

ADVERSE EFFECTS. Patients taking eflornithine show a wide variety of adverse effects.[153,232] Osmotic diarrhea and bone marrow suppression are common, and up to 50% of sleeping patients develop leukopenia. Reversible anemia and thrombocytopenia have also been observed. Diarrhea is dose related and more common after oral administration. Convulsions occur early in about 7% of treated patients, but they do not appear to recur despite continuation of therapy. Withdrawal of the drug reverses most of the adverse effects. Eflornithine interferes with normal embryonic development in experimental animals. It is abortive in early pregnancy and organ-specific developmental deficits have been noted during the later stages of gestation.[234] Abortion may also occur in humans receiving therapeutic dosage.[153]

Drugs Used to Treat Giardiasis

Giardiasis is caused by the flagellated protozoan Giardia lamblia. It occurs worldwide, with higher prevalence where sanitation is poor. It is the most commonly reported intestinal protozoal infection in developed countries including the United States.[235,236] Persons of all ages are affected, although in endemic areas, infection is more frequent in infants. Infection is spread directly from person to person by fecal–oral contamination with cysts or indirectly by transmission in water and occasionally food. In the United States, most infections are sporadic, typically in campers and hikers who drink untreated stream water. Community-wide outbreaks can result from contaminated central water supplies. Although no intermediate host is required, a number of mammalian species can serve as reservoirs, including children in daycare centers and nurseries, institutionalized individuals and male homosexuals. Most, but not all, cases of giardiasis can be confirmed by stool examination. Identification of cysts or trophozoites in fecal specimens or of trophozoites in duodenal contents is diagnostic of giardia. Most infected people are asymptomatic; however, *Giardia* can produce either isolated cases or epidemics of diarrhea. Symptoms differ from person to person depending on several factors, but the acute phase usually begins with a feeling of intestinal uneasiness followed by nausea and anorexia. Cramps and a variety of other abdominal symptoms may occur. Chemotherapy with metronidazole produces cure rates exceeding 80%.[237] Furazolidone is less successful but is frequently used for treating children because it is available as a palatable elixir that is not bitter. Quinacrine was the first effective drug, but it is no longer available.

Furazolidone

Furazolidone is one of several nitrofuran compounds that are used for treatment of infectious diseases. The drug is a close structural analog of nitrofurantoin (see Fig. 9–1 for structures) and the mechanism of action and toxic properties of the nitrofurans have been discussed under nitrofurantoin in Chapter 9. The nitrofurans have been reviewed by Chamberlain[224] and by McCalla.[238] In addition to being active against trichomonads, *Isospora*, and *Giardia lamblia*, furazolidone is active against a variety of bacteria. It is most active against staphylococci, streptococci, *Escherichia coli*, *Klebsiella*, *Enterobacter*, *Salmonella*, *Shigella*, *Vibrio cholerae*, and *Bacteroides*.[224] Furazolidone is used to treat both giardiasis and coccidiosis. In humans, coccidiosis is an upper small bowel inflammatory process caused by *Isospora belli*. The adult dosage of furazolidone is 100 mg taken orally four times daily. The duration of treatment is 7 days for giardiasis and 10 days for coccidiosis. Furazolidone is both effective and well tolerated in the treatment of giardiasis, where the cure rate is about 90%.[239–241]

As discussed in Chapter 9, the antimicrobial activity of the nitrofurans depends on reductive activation to compounds that damage DNA (either directly or through their ability to generate oxygen free-radicals). The selective toxicity of furazolidone is probably based both on its limited absorption from the gut and its selective activation by reductases in the parasite.[238] Given its mechanism of action, it is not surprising that furazolidone, like other nitrofurans, has been found to be mutagenic in bacterial test systems[238] and to produce mammary tumors in rats.[242]

Furazolidone is marketed in both tablet and liquid preparations. It is the only antigiardiasis drug available in the United States as a liquid suspension. The liquid preparation is particularly useful in treating young children.[25,239] Absorption of the drug in animals is limited, but careful studies of the extent of absorption have not been carried out in humans.[224,243] The metabolism of nitrofuran compounds has been studied extensively in animals and is reviewed by McCalla.[238]

Side effects are not uncommon with furizolidone therapy. The drug occasionally causes nausea, vomiting, diarrhea, and fever.[224] Rarely, hypersensitivity reactions, such as hypotension, urticaria, and serum sickness, have occurred. Furazolidone can cause mild hemolysis in patients with glucose-6-phosphate dehydrogenase deficiency. It has been shown that furazolidone is a monoamine oxidase inhibitor, but hypertensive crises have not been reported with therapeutic use.[224] Furazolidone inhibits aldehyde dehydrogenase,[244] and disulfiram-like reactions may occur in patients who ingest alcohol.[245] One or more metabolites of furazolidone give a brown color to the urine. Because the drug has been found to produce tumors in rats, there is a theoretical risk that it could be carcinogenic in humans. To date, no association between furazolidone and tumors has been reported for humans.

Treatment of Trichomoniasis

Trichomoniasis is also caused by a flagellated protozoan, *Trichomonas vaginalis*. It lives in the genitourinary tract of the human host, where it can produce vaginitis in women and urethritis and/or prostatitis in men. Frequently, this infection is asymptomatic, and it can be associated with other genital infections. Worldwide, there are approximately 180 million cases, with 2.5 to 3 million infections occurring annually in the United States. Trichomoniasis is a sexually transmitted disease with several factors increasing the risk, including multiple sex partners. Various tests are now available for diagnosing trichomoniasis. Treatment usually consists of a single 2 g oral dose of metronidazole for both males and females. Cure rates have ranged from 82% to 88%, and concurrent treatment of partners increases effectiveness to more than 95%.[246] Some patients may not tolerate the 2 g dose, so alternatively, 250 mg orally three times daily for 7 days may be used. Treatment failures usually result from either failure to adhere to the therapeutic regimen or to reinfection from an untreated partner who remains asymptomatic. Resistance of *T. vaginalis* to metronidazole has been reported but appears to be more of a relative, rather than an all-or-none, phenomenon. Therefore, increasing the dose usually results in resolution, and sometimes concurrent oral and vaginal doses have been successful. Other nitroimidazoles are used to treat trichomoniasis elsewhere, but they are not available in the United States.

Treatment of Cryptosporidiosis and Cyclosporiasis

Cryptosporidium parvum is a common cause of diarrhea in ungulate farm animals and a major cause of water-borne outbreaks of diarrhea among humans. Cryptosporidiosis is usually a self-limited enteric infection in immunocompetent patients, but a potentially debilitating and chronic diarrheal illness may occur in patients with AIDS or other immunocompromised conditions. No drug has been clearly shown to be effective in treating this infection. Management has included fluid therapy, nutritional support, and use of antidiarrheal agents. Several studies suggest that the oral aminoglycoside paromomycin may be at least partially effective in treating cryptosporidiosis. Paromomycin was shown to reduce diarrhea in patients

with AIDS who had cryptosporidiosis and to reduce the fecal excretion of cryptosporidiosis oocysts.[247] Paromomycin is not absorbed from the gut even in patients with intestinal cryptosporidosis.

Cyclospora is a newly recognized coccidian protozoan parasite that can cause prolonged diarrhea. Cyclosporiasis is effectively treated with trimethoprim-sulfamethoxazole in a dose of 160/800 mg twice daily for 7 days. Patients infected with HIV, however, may experience relapses after such treatment and thus may require long-term suppressive maintenance therapy.[237]

Treatment of Toxoplasmosis

Toxoplasmosis is caused by *Toxoplasma gondii*, an obligate intracellular protozoan, and is an important disease in both animals and humans.[248] This infection is found worldwide, and is transmitted orally (through tissue cysts in contaminated meat or sporocysts in cat feces) and congenitally. Cats are the natural hosts but tissue cysts have been recovered from all mammalian species examined. Between 20% and 70% of adults in the United States are infected with *Toxoplasma* and in certain regions of the world over 90% of 40-year-olds are infected. Most individuals have asymptomatic infections, but when these people are immunosuppressed, or when a pregnant woman becomes infected, the infection can have serious consequences. Congenital toxoplasmosis usually presents as ocular disease. The incidence of congenital toxoplasmosis in not known, but is estimated at 10 to 100 per 100,000 live births in the United States. Since the advent of AIDS, toxoplasmic encephalitis has become one of the most frequent causes of encephalitis in the United States. High seroprevalence rates and the preponderance for reactivation during periods of immunosuppression make toxoplasmic encephalitis a commonly encountered AIDS-related infection. It occurs in 20% to 47% of patients with AIDS and is a major cause of death in these patients. Chemotherapy is essential in this group of people and it may be complicated by differences in drug susceptibility among different clinical isolates. Treatment can be broken down into three distinct phases: treatment of the first episode, secondary prophylaxis, and primary prophylaxis.[249] The treatment of choice for toxoplasmosis is presently the combination of pyrimethamine-sulfadoxine. Folinic acid is given concurrently to prevent toxicity from pyrimethamine. Patients intolerant of sulfadoxine may alternatively be treated with clindamycin in combination with pyrimethamine. Another alternative is atovaquone, a drug that was introduced for therapy of *Pneumocystis carinii* pneumonia but is active against *T. gondii* and may prove to be effective in preventing reactivation of latent infections in AIDS patients.[250] The risk of developing toxoplasmic encephalitis among HIV-infected individuals increases substantially as the CD4 count falls below 100 cells/mm^3, and patients should be given prophylaxis at this time. For prophylaxis, regimens of trimethoprim-sulfamethoxazole and a combination of dapsone and pyrimethamine have been found to be effective.[251,252]

Drugs Used to Treat Pneumocystosis

Pneumocystosis or *Pneumocystis carinii* pneumonia (PCP) is a common life-threatening opportunistic infection in immunocompromised individuals, especially in those infected with HIV. Without prophylaxis it is the major cause of death in many patients with AIDS. The life cycle and taxonomy of the organism are poorly understood and, although it was believed to be a protozoan, studies of ribosomal sequence homology suggest that *P. carinii* is more closely related to fungi.[253] In vitro studies suggest that trophozoites, derived from sporozoites in cysts, attach to epithelial cells. They then become a cyst in which the sporozoites procede to multiply.[254] Patients with PCP generally present with respiratory disease characterized by fever, shortness of breath, and nonproductive cough.

Pentamidine isethionate was the drug originally used in 1958 to treat PCP. In the mid-1970s, trimethoprim combined with sulfamethoxazole (TMP-SMX) became the treatment of choice because it was as effective as pentamidine and better tolerated.[255] Trimethoprim-sulfamethoxazole is the agent of choice for the treatment of *Pneumocystis* pneumonia and extrapulmonary disease in all patients who can tolerate this combination. It has the advantage of excellent tissue penetration, the most rapid clinical response of the anti-*Pneumocystis* agents (often 3 to 5 days in patients with mild to moderate disease), and bioavailability from oral therapy comparable to that of parenteral administration.[256] Animal studies have shown that most of the activity is from the sulfa drug and that a variety of sulfa drugs might suffice as monotherapy.[257] Survival without intubation and mechanical ventilation appears to be greater with TMP-SMX than with pentamidine (up to 20%). However, the incidence of side effects is also greater than with other agents.[256] Therapy is usually initiated with 15–20 mg of the TMP component per kg body weight per day (100 to 150 of SMX/kg/day) divided into 3 or 4 doses. Intravenous therapy is recommended if there is uncertainty about gastrointestinal function or marked hypoxemia. Therapy can be continued (with adjustments) through mild side effects that are tolerable to the patient and physician. Dose reduction will often eliminate toxicity in patients with AIDS.

Pentamidine isethionate has been the main alternative parenteral agent for the treatment of *Pneumocystis* pneumonia. It is now believed to be about 70% effective.[258] It can be given either intramuscularly or intravenously, but the intravenous route is recommended. Several complications will develop with intramuscular therapy, most notably sterile abscesses at the injection site. Intravenous pentamidine is given by slow (1–2 h) infusion in 5% glucose solution as a single dosage of 4 mg/kg/day. Newer pentamidine analogs under development appear to have superior therapeutic and toxicity profiles compared to those of pentamidine. Although cotrimoxazole and pentamidine are both efficacious against PCP, treatment-limiting toxicity is often observed during therapy. As a result, less toxic agents have been sought as alternatives to these drugs. Among the regimens studied are atovaquone, dapsone plus trimethoprim, clindamycin plus prima-quine, and trimetrexate.

Prophylaxis of PCP in patients with AIDS has had a significant beneficial effect on survival, quality of life, hospitalization frequency, and per-patient health care expenses.[259] Prophylaxis in AIDS patients should be lifelong rather than time-limited, unless reversal of the immune deficit can be demonstrated.[259] The TMP-SMX combination is the agent of choice for the prevention of *Pneumocystis* infection in any patient who can tolerate this combination. With one single-strength tablet per day or one double-strength tablet per day a wide variety of opportunistic infections are generally prevented. Drug toxicity is commonly observed even with low-dose regimens, especially in the form of bone marrow suppression. This effect is most notable when the TMP-SMX combination is used along with other drugs that suppress hematopoiesis. Alternative prophylactic regimens are available for patients intolerant of TMP-SMX, one of these being aerosolized pentamidine isethionate (300 mg every 3 to 4 weeks). It is most effective when it is administered by experienced personnel with a nebulizer that produces droplets in the 1 to 3 μm range. Breakthrough infection is seen in 10% to 23% of patients taking pentamidine for 1 year, most often in patients with rapidly progressive AIDS and/or CD4 counts of less than 50/mm³.[259] The side effects of pentamidine aerosol therapy are usually minimal. Cough and bronchospasm are common and are generally reversible with bronchodilator therapy.

Atovaquone

Atovaquone

Atovaquone is an alternative drug for the treatment of both mild to moderate PCP and toxoplasmosis, opportunistic infections commonly experienced by patients with AIDS. It is a hydroxynaphthoquinone that acts as an inhibitor of the mitochondrial respiratory chain, and is a structural analog of ubiquinone, a small hydrophobic respiratory chain electron carrier molecule found in mitochondria.[260] Atovaquone was initially developed as an antimalarial agent, but it showed preclinical and clinical activity against PCP, as well as against toxoplasmosis.[261]

PHARMACOKINETICS. Atovaquone has very low aqueous solubility, and it is slowly and irregularly absorbed from the gut.[262] The drug has a long terminal plasma half-life (around 77 h), and the single-dose peak plasma concentration and area under the curve are increased for the suspension as compared to the tablet.[263] There is increased drug absorption when atovaquone is administered with or soon after meals, particularly a high-fat meal. Atovaquone undergoes enterohepatic recycling and is predominantly excreted in the feces. Atovaquone is more than 99.9% protein bound and does not cross the blood-brain barrier to any appreciable extent.[264] The pharmacokinetics have not been evaluated in the elderly or in patients with renal or hepatic impairment.[261]

CLINICAL USE. Atovaquone is a useful option for the treatment of patients with mild to moderate PCP who are intolerant or unresponsive to TMP-SMX, but it has not been approved for serious PCP or for prophylaxis of PCP. Oral atovaquone has been shown to have similar overall therapeutic efficacy to the conventional therapies of oral TMP-SMX and intravenous pentamidine.[263,265] Atovaquone is also considered to be a promising agent for the treatment of toxoplasmosis. In PCP, response rates to atovaquone (750 mg, three times daily) are lower than those with TMP-SMX, but patients receiving atovaquone experienced significantly fewer treatment-limiting adverse effects than patients treated with TMP-SMX or pentamidine. In patients with toxoplasmosis who were unresponsive to conventional agents, atovaquone produced a complete or partial radiological response rate of 37% to 87%.

After 6 weeks of treatment, 52% of patients achieved a complete or partial clinical response.[261]

ADVERSE EFFECTS. In patients with AIDS and others who are severely debilitated, the adverse effects of atovaquone have been difficult to differentiate from the effects of the underlying disease. The incidence of adverse effects with the suspension is similar to that with tablets. Studies of patients with AIDS show that the incidence of treatment-limiting adverse effects was lower with atovaquone than with TMP-SMX (7% vs. 20%) or pentamidine (4% vs. 36%).[263] Rash, nausea, diarrhea, headache, vomiting, fever, and insomnia occurred in 10% to 23% of patients receiving the drug. Rash and liver dysfunction were treatment limiting in 4% and 3% of patients, respectively. Atovaquone should not be used in patients with histories of allergic skin reactions or possible allergy to the drug. In the treatment of toxoplasmosis, few adverse effects were reported. [250,261,266]

Trimetrexate

Trimetrexate

Methotrexate

STRUCTURE AND MECHANISM OF ACTION. Trimetrexate is a folinic acid analog structurally related to the anticancer drug methotrexate. It is used for treatment of selected AIDS patients with PCP, always being used concurrently with leucovorin. It differs from methotrexate in that it lacks the terminal glutamate moiety necessary for intracellular polyglutamination.[267] Trimetrexate is lipophilic and readily crosses cell membranes by passive diffusion. In contrast, more polar folate analogs such as methotrexate and leucovorin are dependent upon the folate membrane transport system to enter cells. Mammalian cells but not protozoan or bacterial cells possess this uptake system. This difference provides the basis for the use of trimetrexate in PCP. Like methotrexate, trimetrexate inhibits dihydrofolate reductase, reducing the production of DNA and RNA precursors and leading to cell death. Coadministration of calcium folinate protects animal and human cells against trimetrexate toxicity.[268,269] Calcium folinate is a fully reduced folate cofactor that does not require reduction by dihydrofolate reductase. It is actively transported into mammalian cells where it is converted to other active folate cofactors.

PHARMACOKINETICS. Most of the pharmacokinetic data are from cancer patients, and only limited studies have been done in patients with AIDS-related PCP. After oral administration, the mean bioavailability of trimetrexate is 44%, with peak plasma concentrations being reached within 0.5 to 4 h.[270,271] Following intravenous administration, there is a linear relationship between trimetrexate dose and area under the plasma concentration–time curve and steady-state plasma concentrations.[272,273] Trimetrexate distributes well into the respiratory tract but very poorly into the central nervous system. The drug is eliminated primarily through hepatic metabolism via the cytochrome P-450 system, and less than one-third of the drug is excreted unchanged in the urine. At least two metabolites have been identified, both of which are active in inhibiting DHFR.[270]

CLINICAL USE. Trimetrexate with folinate is indicated in moderate to severe PCP in patients who are intolerant of, or refractory to, TMP-SMX, or those in whom TMP-SMX is contraindicated. It has also been used to treat cerebral toxoplasmosis in patients with AIDS, but results have not been encouraging.[274] In noncomparative trials using trimetrexate as salvage therapy in patients with

AIDS and PCP who were refractory to or intolerant of TMP-SMX and pentamidine, 2 to 4-week survival rates ranging from 48% to 69% were obtained.[275] Response rates in patients with a variety of disease and treatment histories ranged from 42% to 90%. In a comparison with TMP-SMX, trimetrexate was less effective but better tolerated. Treatment with trimetrexate resulted in a significantly higher failure rate than with TMP-SMX. However, discontinuation due to serious adverse effects was significantly more common in the TMP-SMX group, thus the number of patients receiving their assigned treatment at the end of the 3-week study was similar in both groups.

ADVERSE EFFECTS. Bone marrow depression, particularly neutropenia and thrombocytopenia, is the dose-limiting toxicity in cancer patients.[272,273] In patients with PCP, myelosuppression can be prevented or minimized by concurrent administration of calcium folinate. Other adverse effects include elevated serum aminotransferase levels, anemia, fever, rash/pruritus, and increased alkaline phosphatase or serum creatinine levels.[276,277] The combination of trimetrexate plus folinate is better tolerated than TMP-SMX when used in patients with AIDS for the initial treatment of PCP. In a comparative trial, the rate of discontinuation due to adverse effects at day 21 was 28% in patients treated with TMP-SMX compared with 8% in patients treated with trimetrexate.

DRUG INTERACTIONS. Since the metabolism of trimetrexate involves demethylation via the cytochrome P-450 pathway and conjugation via glucuronidation, drugs that affect these systems alter the pharmacokinetics of trimetrexate.

REFERENCES

1. Tan, J. S., Common and uncommon parasitic infections in the United States. Med. Clin. North Am. 1978;62:1059.
2. Botero, D., Intestinal parasitic infections. Antibiot. Chemother. 1981;30:1.
3. Desowitz, R. S., Antiparasite chemotherapy. Annu. Rev. Pharmacol. 1971;11:351.
4. Ravdin, J. I., Amebiasis. Clin. Infect. Dis. 1995; 20:1453.
5. Powell, S. J., A. J. Wilmot, and R. Elsdon-Dew. Further trials of metronidazole in amoebic dysentery and amoebic liver abscess. Ann. Trop. Med. Parasit. 1969;61:511.
6. Powell, S. J., A. J. Wilmot, and R. Elsdon-Dew. Single and low dosage regimens of metronidazole in amoebic dysentery and amoebic liver abscess. Ann. Trop. Med. Parasit. 1969;63:139.
7. Scott, F. and M. J. Miller. Trials with metranidazole in amebic dysentery. JAMA 1970;211:118.
8. Powell, S. J. New developments in the therapy of amoebiasis. Gut 1970;11:967.
9. Krogstad, D. J., H. C. Spencer, and G. R. Healy. Amebiasis. N. Engl. J. Med. 1978;298:262.
10. Knight, R. The chemotherapy of amebiasis. J. Antimicrob. Chemother. 1980;6:577.
11. Powell, S. J., and R. Elsdon-Dew. Some new nitroimidazole derivatives: clinical trials in amebic liver abscess. Am J. Trop. Med. Hyg. 1972;21:518.
12. Fisher, M. W., and P. E. Thompson. Antibiotics with specific affinities. Part 3: Paramomcycin. In Experimental Chemotherapy, ed. by R. J. Schnitzer and F. Hawking. New York: Academic Press, 1964, pp. 329–345.
13. Phillips, B. P., and P. A. Wolfe. The use of germ-free guinea pigs in studies on the microbial interrelationships in amoebiasis. Ann. N.Y. Acad. Sci. 1959;78:308.
14. Irusen, E. M., F. H. G., Jackson, and A. E. Simjee. Asymptomatic intestinal colonization by pathogenic Entamoeba histolytica in amebic liver abscess: prevalence, response to therapy, and pathogenic potential. Clin. Infect. Dis. 1992;14:889.
15. Desmonts, G., and J. Couvreur. Congenital toxoplasmosis. A prospective study of 378 pregnancies. N. Engl. J. Med. 1974;290:1110.
16. Nye, F. J., Treating toxoplasmosis. J. Antimicrob. Chemother. 1979;5:244.
17. S. M. Finegold (ed.) Metronidazole. Proceedings of the International Conference, Montreal, May 26–28, 1976. Amsterdam: Exerpta Medica, 1977.
18. Sawyer, P. R., R. N. Brogden, R. M. Pinder, T. M. Speight, and G. S. Avery. Tinidazole: a review of its antiprotozoal activity and therapeutic efficacy. Drugs 1976;11:423.
19. Brogden, R. N., R. C. Heel, T. M. Speight, and G. S. Avery. Metronidazole in anaerobic infections: a review of its activity, pharmacokinetics and therapeutic use. Drugs 1978;16:387.
20. Goldman, P. Metronidazole. N. Engl. J. Med. 1980;303:1212.
21. Molavi, A., J. L. LeFrock, and R. A. Prince. Metronidazole. Med. Clin. North Am. 1982;66:121.
22. Keighley, E. E., Trichomoniasis in a closed community. 100% follow-up. BMJ 1962;2:93.
23. Dykers, J. R., Single-dose metronidazole for trichomonal vaginitis: patient and consort. N. Engl. J. Med. 1975;293:23.
24. Hager, W. D., S. T. Brown, S. T. Kraus, G. S. Kleris, G. J. Perkins, and M. Henderson. Metronidazole for vaginal trichomoniasis. JAMA 1980;244:1219.

25. Smith, J. W., and M. S. Wolfe. Giardiasis. *Annu. Rev. Med.* 1980;31:373.

26. Powell, S. J., I. MacLeod, A. J. Wilmot, and R. Elsdon-Dew. Metronidazole in amoebic dysentery and amoebic liver abscess. *Lancet* 1966;2:1329.

27. Baines, E. J., Metronidazole: its past, present and future. *J. Antimicrob. Chemother.* 1978;4(Suppl. C):97.

28. Gillin, F. D., and L. S. Diamond. Inhibition of clonal growth of *Giardia lamblia and Entamoeba histolytica* by metronidazole, quinacrine, and other antimicrobial agents. *J. Antimicrob. Chemother.* 1981;8:305.

29. Muller, M., J. G. Meingassner, W. A. Miller, and W. J. Ledger. Three metronidazole-resistant strains of *Trichomonas vaginalis* from the United States. *Am. J. Obstet. Gynecol.* 1980;138:808.

30. Sutter, V. L., and S. M. Finegold. Susceptibility of anaerobic bacteria to 23 antimicrobial agents. *Antimicrob. Agents Chemother.* 1976;10:736.

31. Appelbaum, P. C., and S. A. Chatterton. Susceptibility of anaerobic bacteria to 10 antimicrobial agents. *Antimicrob. Agents Chemother.* 1978;14:371.

32. Ralph, E. D., and Y. E. Amatnieks. Relative susceptibilities of *Gardnerella vaginalis (Haemophilus vaginalis), Neisseria gonorrhoeae, and Bacteroides fragilis* to metronidazole and its two major metabolites. *Sex. Transm. Dis.* 1980;7:157.

33. Falagas, M. E., and S. L. Gorbach. Clindamycin and metronidazole. *Med. Clin. North Am.* 1995;79:845.

34. Teasley, D. G., D. N. Gerding, M. M. Olson, L. R. Peterson, R. L. Gebhard, M. J. Schwartz, and J. T. Lee. Perspective randomized trial of metronidazole versus vancomycin for *Clostridium-difficile*—associated diarrhoea and colitis. *Lancet* 1983;2:1043.

35. Thomson, G., A. H. Clark, K. Hare, and W. G. S. Spilg. Pseudomembranous colitis after treatment with metronidazole. *BMJ* 1981;282:864.

36. Nicol, C. S., A. J. Evans, J. A. McFadzean, and S. L. Squires. Inactivation of metronidazole. *Lancet* 1966;2:441.

37. Ingham, H. R., S. Eaton, C. W. Venables, and P. C. Adams. *Bacteroides fragilis* resistant to metronidazole after long-term therapy. *Lancet* 1978;1:214.

38. Padonu, K. O. A controlled trial of metronidazole in the treatment of dracontiasis in Nigeria. *Am. J. Trop. Med. Hyg.* 1973;22:42.

39. Antani, J. A., H. V. Srinivas, K. R. Krishnamurthy, and A. N. Bargaonkar. Metronidazole in dracunculiasis: report of further trials. *Am. J. Trop. Med. Hyg.* 1972;21:178.

40. Belcher, D. W., F. K. Wurapa, and W. B. Ward. Failure of thiabendozole and metronidazole in the treatment and suppression of guineaworm disease. *Am. J. Trop. Med. Hyg.* 1975;24:444.

41. Ursing, B., T. Alm, F. Barany, I. Bergelin, K. Ganrot-Norlin, J. Hoevels, B. Huitfeldt, G. Jarnerot, U. Krause, A. Krook, B. Lindstrom, O. Nordlie, and A. Rosen. A comparative study of metronidazole and sulfasalazine for active Crohn's disease: the cooperative Crohn's disease study in Sweden. II. Results. *Gastroenterology* 1980;83:550.

42. Chapman; J. D. Hypoxic sensitizers—implications for radiation therapy. *N. Engl. J. Med.* 1979;301:1429.

43. Edwards, D. I., and G. E. Mathison. The mode of action of metronidazole against *Trichomonas vaginalis.* *J. Gen. Microbiol.* 1970;63:297.

44. Edwards, D. I., M. Dye, and H. Carne. The selective toxicity of antimicrobial nitroheterocyclic drugs. *J. Gen. Microbiol.* 1973;76:135.

45. Tanowitz, H. B., M. Wittner, R. M. Rosenbaum, and Y. Kress. In vitro studies on the differential toxicity of metronidazole in protozoa and mammalian cells. *Ann. Trop. Med. Parasitol.* 1975;69:19.

46. Voogd, C. E., J. J. Van der Stel, and J. J. Jacobs. The mutagenic action of nitroimidazoles. I Metronidazole, nimorazole, dimetridazole and ronidazole. *Mutat. Res.* 1974;26:483.

47. Stone, H. B., and H. R. Withers. Tumor and normal tissue response to metronidazole and irradiation in mice. *Radiology* 1974;113:441.

48. Britz, M. L., and R. G. Wilkinson. Isolation and properties of metronidazole-resistant mutants of *Bacteroides fragilis.* *Antimicrob. Agents Chemother.* 1979;16:19.

49. Britz, M. L. Resistance to chloramphenicol and metronidazole in anaerobic bacteria. *J. Antimicrob. Chemother.* 1981;8(Suppl. D):49.

50. Rosenkranz, H. S., and W. T. Speck. Mutagenicity of metronidazole: activation by mammalian liver microsomes. *Biochem. Biophys. Res. Commun.* 1975;66:520.

51. Lindmark, D. G., and M. Muller. Antitrichomonal action, mutagenicity, and reduction of metronidazole and other nitroimidazoles. *Antimicrob. Agents Chemother.* 1976;10:476.

52. Adams, G. E., E. D. Clarke, R. S. Jacobs, I. J. Stratford, R. G. Wallace, P. Wardman, and M. E. Watts. Mammalian cell toxicity of nitro compounds: dependence upon reduction potential. *Biochem. Biophys. Res. Commun.* 1976;72:824.

53. Adams, G. E., I. R. Flockhart, C. E. Smithen, I. J. Stratford, P. Wardman, and M. E. Watts. Electron-affinic sensitization. VII. A correlation between structures, one-electron reduction potentials, and efficiencies of nitroimidazoles as hypoxic cell radiosensitizers. *Radiat. Res.* 1976;67:9.

54. Chrystal, E. J. T., R. L. Koch, M. A. McLafferty, and P. Goldman. Relationship between metronidazole metabolism and bacterial activity. *Antimicrob. Agents Chemother.* 1980;18:566.

55. Beaulieu, B. B., M. A. McLafferty, R. K. Koch, and P. Goldman. Metronidazole metabolism in cultures of *Entamoeba histolytica* and *Trichomonas vaginalis.* *Antimicrob. Agents Chemother.* 1981;20:410.

56. Koch, R. L., and P. Goldman. The anaerobic metabolism of metronidazole forms N-(2-hydroxyethly)-oxamic acid. *J. Pharmacol. Exp. Ther.* 1979;208:406.

57. McLafferty, M. A., R. L. Koch, and P. Goldman. Interaction of metronidazole with resistant and susceptible *Bacteroides fragilis.* *Antimicrob. Agents Chemother.* 1982;21:131.

58. Ings, R. M. J., M. A. McFadzean, and W. Or-

merod. The mode of action of metronidazole in *Tricho-monas vaginalis* and other micro-organisms. *Biochem. Pharmacol.* 1974;23:1421.

59. LaRusso, N. F., M. Tomaz, M. Muller, and R. Lipman. Interaction of metronidazole with nucleic acids in vitro. *Mol.Pharmacol.* 1977;13:872.

60. Knight, R. C., I. M. Skolimowski, and D. I. Edwards. The interaction of reduced metronidazole with DNA. *Biochem. Pharmacol.* 1978;27:2089.

61. Houghton, G. W., J. Smith, P. S. Thorne, and R. Templeton. The pharmacokinetics of oral and intravenous metronidazole in man. *J. Antimicrob. Chemother.* 1979;5:621.

62. Bergan, T., and E. Arnold. Pharmacokinetics of metronidazole in healthy adult volunteers after tablets and suppositories. *Chemotherapy* 1980;26:231.

63. Melander, A., G. Kahlmeter, C. Kamme, and B. Ursing. Bioavailability of metronidazole in fasting and non-fasting healthy subjects and in patients with Crohn's disease. *Eur. J. Clin. Pharmacol.* 1977;12:69.

64. Ralph, E. D., J. T. Clarke, R. D. Libke, R. P. Luthy, and W. M. M. Kirby. Pharmacokinetics of metronidazole as determined by bioassay. *Antimicrob. Agents Chemother.* 1974;6:691.

65. Schwartz, D. E., and F. Jeunet. Comparative pharmacokinetics studies of ornidazole and metronidazole in man. *Chemotherapy* 1976;22:19.

66. Templeton, R. Metabolism and pharmacokinetics of metronidazole: a review. In *Metronidazole. Proceedings of the International Metronidazole Conference, Montreal*, ed. by S. M. Finegold. Amsterdam: Exerpta Medica, 1977, pp. 28–49.

67. Gray, M. S., P. O. Kane, and S. Squires. Further observations on metronidazole. *Br. J. Vener. Dis.* 1961; 37:278.

68. Nielsen, M. L., and T. Justesen. Excretion of metronidazole in human bile. Investigations of hepatic bile, common duct bile, and gallbladder bile. *Scand J. Gastroentrol.* 1977;12:1003.

69. Smith, B. J. D., and J. Wellingham. Metronidazole in treatment of empyema. *BMJ* 1976;1:1074.

70. Sattar, M. A., M. G. Sankey, M. I. D. Cawley, C. M. Kaye, and J. E. Holt. The penetration of metronidazole into synovial fluid. *Postgrad. Med. J.* 1982;58: 20.

71. Jokipii, A. M. M., V. V. Myllyla, E. Hokkanen, and L. Jokipii. Penetration of the blood brain barrier by metronidazole and tinidazole. *J. Antimicrob. Chemother.* 1977;3:239.

72. Warner, J. F., R. L. Perkins, and L. Cordero. Metronidazole therapy of anaerobic bacteremia, meningitis, and brain abscess. *Arch. Intern. Med.* 1979;139: 167.

73. George, R. H., and A. J. Bint. Treatment of a brain abscess due to *Bacteroides fragilis* with metronidazole. *J. Antimicrob. Chemother.* 1976;2:101.

74. Roe, F. J. C., Metronidazole: a review of uses and toxicity. *J. Antimicrob. Chemother.* 1977;3:205.

75. Jager-Roman, E., J. Baird-Lambert, M. Cvejic, and N. Buchanan. Pharmacokinetics and tissue distribution of metronidazole in the newborn infant. *J. Pediatr.* 1982;100:651.

76. Erickson, S. H., G. L. Oppenheim, and G. H. Smith. Metronidazole in breast milk. *Obstet. Gynecol.* 1981;57:48.

77. Taylor, J. A., J. R. Migliardi, and M. S. von Wittenau. Tinidazole and metronidazole pharmacokinetics in man and mouse. *Antimicrob. Agents Chemother.* 1970;1969:267.

78. Welling, P. G., and A. M. Munro. The pharmacokinetics of metronidazole and tinidazole in man. *Arzneimittelforschung* 1972;22:2128.

79. Nilsson-Ehle, I., B. Ursing, and P. Nilsson-Ehle. Liquid chromatographic assay for metronidazole and tinidazole: pharamcokinetic and metabolic studies in human subjects. *Antimicrob. Agents Chemother.* 1981; 19:764.

80. Stambaugh, J. E., L. G. Feo, and R. W. Manthei. The isolation and identification of the urinary oxidative metabolites of metronidazole in man. *J. Pharmacol. Exp. Ther.* 1968;161:373.

81. Ralph, E. D., and W. M. M. Kirby. Bioassay of metronidazole with either anaerobic or aerobic incubation. *J. Infect. Dis.* 1975;132:587.

82. Cerat, G. A., L. C. Cerat, M. C. McHenry, J. C. Wagner, P. M. Hall, and T. L. Gavan. Metronidazole in renal failure. In *Metronidazole. Proceedings of the International Metronidazole Conference, Montreal*, ed. by S. M. Finegold. Amsterdam: Exerpta Medica, 1977, pp. 404–414.

83. Gabriel, R., C. M. Page, J. Collier, G. W. Houghton, R. Templeton, and P. S. Thorne. Removal of metronidazole by hemodialysis. *Br. J. Surg.* 1980;67: 553.

84. Edwards, J. A., and J. Price. Metronidazole and human alcohol dehydrogenase. *Nature* 1967;214:190.

85. Gupta, N. K., C. L. Woodley, and R. Fried. Effect of metronidazole on liver alcohol dehydrogenase. *Biochem. Pharmacol.* 1970;19:2805.

86. Rothstein, E., and D. D. Clancy. Toxicity of disulfiram combined with metronidazole. *N. Engl. J. Med.* 1969;180:1006.

87. Kusumi, R. K., J. F. Plouffe, R. H. Wyatt, and R. J. Fass. Central nervous system toxicity associated with metronidazole therapy. *Ann. Intern. Med.* 1980; 93:59.

88. O'Reilly, R. A. The stereoselective interaction of warfarin and metronidazole in man. *N. Engl. J. Med.* 1976;295:354.

89. Rustia, M., and P. Shubik. Induction of lung tumors and malignant lymphomas in mice by metronidazole. *J. Natl. Cancer Inst.* 1972;48:721.

90. Rustia, M., and P. Shubik. Experimental induction of hepatomas, mammary tumors and other tumors with metronidazole in noninbred Sas: MRC(WI)BR rats. *J. Natl. Cancer Inst.* 1979;63:863.

91. Legator, M. S., T. H. Connor, and M. Stoeckel. Detection of mutagenic activity of metronidazole and niridazole in body fluid of humans and mice. *Science* 1975;188:1118.

92. Connor, T. M., M. Stoeckel, J. Evrard, and M. S. Legator. The contribution of metronidazole and two metabolites to the mutagenic activity detected in urine of treated humans and mice. *Cancer Res.* 1977; 37:629.

93. Koch, R. L., B. B. Beaulieu, E. J. T. Chrystal,

and P. Goldman. A metronidazole metabolite in human urine and its risk. *Science* 1981;211:398.

94. Koch, R. L., E. J. T. Chrystal, B. B. Beaulieu, and P. Goldman. Acetamide—a metabolite of metronidazole formed by the intestinal flora. *Biochem. Pharmacol.* 1979;28:3611.

95. Perez-Reyes, E., B. Kalyanaraman, and R. P. Mason. The reductive metabolism of metronidazole and ronidazole by aerobic liver microsomes. *Mol. Pharmacol.* 1980;17:239.

96. Beard, C. M., K. L. Noller, W. M. O'Fallon, L. T. Kurkland, and M. B. Dockerty. Lack of evidence for cancer due to use of metronidazole. *N. Engl. J. Med.* 1979;310:519.

97. G. D. Friedman: Cancer after metronidazole. *N. Engl. J. Med.* 1980;302:519.

98. Bost, R. G. Metronidazole: mammalian mutagenicity. In *Metronidazole. Proceedings of the International Metronidazole Conference, Montreal,* ed. by S. M. Finegold. Amsterdam: Excerpta Medica, 1977, pp. 126–131.

99. Peterson, W. F., J. E. Stauch, and C. D. Ryder. Metronidazole in pregnancy. *Am. J. Obstet. Gynecol.* 1966;94:343.

100. Lau, A. H., N. P. Lam, S. C. Piscitelli, L. Wilkes, and L. H. Danziger. Clinical pharmacokinetics of metronidazole and other nitroimidazole anti-infectives. *Clin. Pharmacokinet.* 1992;23:238.

101. Main, P. T., N. W. Bristow, P. Oxley, T. I. Watkins, G. A. H. Williams, E. C. Wilmshurst, and G. Woolfe. Entamide. *Anal. Biochem. Exp. Med.* 1960;20:441.

102. Woodruff, A. W., S. Bell, and F. D. Schofield. II. The treatment of intestinal amebiasis with emetine bismuth iodide, glaucarubin, dichloroacet-hydroxymethylanalide, camoform and various antibiotics. *Trans. R. Soc. Trop. Med. Hyg.* 1956;50:114.

103. Woodruff, A. W., and S. Bell. Clinical trials with entamide furoate and related compounds. I. In a nontropical environment. *Trans. R. Soc. Trop. Med. Hyg.* 1960;54:389.

104. Botero, D., Treatment of acute and chronic intestinal amoebiasis with entamide furoate. *Trans. R. Soc. Trop. Med. Hyg.* 1964;58:419.

105. Wolfe, M. S., Nondysenteric intestinal amebiasis. Treatment with diloxanide furoate. *JAMA* 1973;224:1601.

106. Wilmot, A. J., S. J. Powell, I. McLeod, and R. Elsdon-Dew. Some newer amoebicides in acute amoebic dysentery. *Trans. R. Soc. Trop. Med. Hyg.* 1962;56:85.

107. Powell, S. J., E. J. Stewart-Wynne, and R. Elsdon-Dew. Metronidazole combined with diloxanide furoate in amoebic liver abscess. *Ann. Trop. Med. Parasitol.* 1973;67:367.

108. Wilmshurst, E. C., and E. E. Cliffe. Absorption and distribution of amoebicides. In *Absorption and Distribution of Drugs,* ed. by T. B. Binns. London: Livingstone, 1964, pp. 191–198.

109. Most, H., Treatment of common parasitic infections of man encountered in the United States (second of two parts). *N. Engl. J. Med.* 1972;287:698.

110. Neldner, K. H., L. Hagler, W. R. Wise, F. B. Stifel, E. G. Lufkin, and R. H. Herman. Acrodermatitis enteropathica: a clinical and biochemical survey. *Arch. Dermatol.* 1974;110:711.

111. Aggett, P. J., H. T. Delves, and J. T. Harries. The possible role of diiodohydroxyquin as a zinc ionophore in the treatment of acrodermatitis enteropathica. *Biochem. Biophys. Res. Commun.* 1979;87:513.

112. Berggren, L., and O. Hansson. Absorption of intestinal antiseptics derived from 8-hydroxyquinolines. *Clin. Pharmacol. Ther.* 1968;9:67.

113. Jack, D. B., and W. Riess. Pharmacokinetics of iodochlorhydroxyquin in man. *J. Pharm. Sci.* 1973;62:1929.

114. G. P. Oakley: The neurotoxicity of the halogenated hydroxyquinolines: a commentary. *JAMA* 1973;225:395.

115. Fleisher, D. I., R. S. Hepler, and J. W. Landau. Blindness during diiodohydroxyquin (Diodoquin) therapy: a case report. *Pediatrics* 1974;54:106.

116. American Academy of Pediatrics Committee on Drugs. Blindness and neuropathy from diiodohydroxyquin-like drugs. *Pediatrics* 1974;54:378.

117. Cook, G. C., Leishmaniasis: some recent developments in chemotherapy. *J. Antimicrob. Chemother.* 1993;31:327.

118. Klatskin, G., and H. Friedman. Emetine toxicity in man; studies on the nature of early toxic manifestations, their relation to dose level, and their significance in determining safe dosage. *Ann. Intern. Med.* 1940;28:892.

119. Ng, K. K. F., A new pharmacological action of emetine. *BMJ* 1966;1:1278.

120. Ng, K. K. F., Blockade of adrenergic and cholinergic transmissions by emetine. *Br. J. Pharmacol. Chemother.* 1966;28:228.

121. Salako, L. A., Effects of emetine on neuromuscular transmission. *Eur. J. Pharmacol.* 1970;11:342.

122. Bradley, W. G., J. D. Fewings, J. B. Harris, and M. A. Johnson. Emetine myopathy in the rat. *Br. J. Pharmacol.* 1976;57:29.

123. Conte-Camerino, D., S. H. Bryant, and D. Mitolo-Chieppa. Electrical properties of rat extensor digitorum longus muscle after chronic application of emetine to the motor nerve. *Exp. Neurol.* 1982;77:1.

124. Schwartz, D. E., and H. Herrero. Comparative pharmacokinetic studies of dehydroemetine and emetine in guinea pigs using spectrofluorometric and radiometric methods. *Am. J. Trop. Med. Hyg.* 1965;14:78.

125. Powell, S. J., I. N. MacLeod, A. J. Wilmot, and R. Elsdon-Dew. The treatment of acute amebic dysentery. *Ann. Trop. Med. Parasitol.* 1965;59:205.

126. Powell, S. J. The cardiotoxicity of systemic amebicides. A comparative electrocardiographic study. *Am. J. Trop. Med. Hyg.* 1967;16:447.

127. Kern, P. Leishmaniasis. *Antibiot. Chemother.* 1981;30:203.

128. Berman, J. D. Chemotherapy for leishmaniasis: biochemical mechanisms, clinical efficacy, and future strategies. *Clin. Infect. Dis.* 1988;10:560.

129. Berman, J. D. Human leishmaniasis: clinical, diagnostic, and chemotherapeutic developments in the last 10 years. *Clin. Infect. Dis.* 1997;24:684.

130. Sampaio, S. A. P., J. T. Godoy, L. Paiva, N. I. Dillon, and C. Da Silva Lucaz. The treatment of Amer-

ican (mucocutaneous) leishmaniasis with amphotericin B. *Arch. Dermatol.* 1960;82:627.

131. Steck, E. A. The leishmaniases. In *Progress in Drug Research: Tropical Diseases I,* ed. by E. Jucker. Basel: Birkhäuser Verlag. 1974, pp. 289–351.

132. Coukell, A., and R. N. Brogden. Liposomal amphotericin B. Therapeutic use in the management of fungal infections and visceral leishmaniasis. *Drugs* 1998;55:585.

133. Dietze, R., E. P. Milan, J. D. Berman, M. Grogl, A. Falqueto, T. F. Feitosa, K. G. Luz, F. A. B. Suassuna, L. A. C. Marinho, and G. Ksionski. Treatment of Brazilian kala-azar with a short course of amphocil (amphotericin B cholesterol dispersion). *Clin. Infect. Dis.* 1993;17:981.

134. Murray, H. W. Cytokines as antimicrobial therapy for the T-cell deficient patient: prospects for treatment of nonviral opportunistic infections. *Clin. Infect. Dis.* 1993;17:5407.

135. Bryceson, A. D. M., A. Murphy, and A. H. Moody. Treatment of "Old World" cutaneous leishmaniasis with aminosidine ointment: result of an open study in London. *Trans. R. Soc. Trop. Med. Hyg.* 1994;88:227.

136. Evans, D. A. African trypanosomes. *Antibiot. Chemother.* 1981;30:272.

137. Ribeiro-dos-Santos, R., A. Rassi, and F. Köberle. Chagas' disease. *Antibiot. Chemother.* 1981;30:115.

138. Kirchhoff; L. V. Chagas disease. American trypanosomiasis. *Infect. Dis. Clin. North Am.* 1993;77:487.

139. Fulton, J. D., and L. P. Joyner. Studies on protozoa. Part I. The metabolism of Leishman-Donovan bodies and flagellates of *Leishmania donovani. Trans. R. Soc. Trop. Med. Hyg.* 1949;43:273.

140. Bueding, E., and E. Schiller. Mechanism of action of antischistosomal drugs. In *Mode of Action of Antiparasitic Drugs,* ed. by J. Rodrigues da Silva and M. J. Ferreira. New York: Pergamon Press, 1968, pp. 81–86.

141. Beveridge, E. Chemotherapy of leishmaniasis. In *Experimental Chemotherapy, Vol. I,* ed. by R. J. Schnitzer and F. Hawking. New York: Academic Press, 1963, pp. 257–287.

142. New, R. R. C., M. L. Chance, S. C. Thomas, and W. Peters. Antileishmanial activity of antimonials entrapped in liposomes. *Nature* 1978;272:55.

143. Alving, C. R., E. A. Steck, W. L. Chapman, V. B. Waits, L. D. Hendricks, G. M. Swartz, and W. L. Hanson. Therapy of leishmaniasis: superior efficacies of liposome-encapsulated drugs. *Proc. Natl. Acad. Sci. U.S.A.* 1978;75:2959.

144. Alving, C. R., E. A. Steck, W. L. Chapman, V. B. Waits, L. D. Henricks, G. M. Swartz, and W. L. Hanson. Liposomes in leishmaniasis: therapeutic effects of antimonial drugs, 8-aminoquinolines, and tetracyclines. *Life Sci.* 1980;26:2231.

145. New, R. R. C., M. L. Chance, and S. Heath. Antileishmanial activity of amphotericin and other antifungal agents entrapped in liposomes. *J. Antimicrob. Chemother.* 1981;8:371.

146. Rees, P. H., M. I. Keating, P. A. Kager, and W. T. Hockmeyer. Renal clearance of pentavalent antimony (sodium stibogluconate). *Lancet* 1980;2:226.

147. Chulay, J. D., L. Fleckenstein, and D. H. Smith. Pharmacokinetics of antimony during treatment of visceral leishmaniasis with sodium stibogluconate or meglumine antimoniate. *Trans. R. Soc. Trop. Med. Hyg.* 1994;82:69.

148. Ouellette, M., and B. Papadopoulou. Mechanisms of drug resistance in *Leishmania. Parasitol. Today* 1993;9:150.

149. Berman, J., N. Edwards, M. King, and I. M. Gro. Biochemistry of pentostam resistant leishmania. *Am. J. Trop. Med. Hyg.* 1989;40:159.

150. Grogl, M., R. K. Martin, A. M. J. Oduola, W. K. Milhous, and D. E. Kyle. Characteristics of multidrug resistance in *Plasmodium* and *Leishmania*: detection of P-glycoprotein-like components. *Am. J. Trop. Med. Hyg.* 1991;45:98.

151. Pugin, P., and P. A. Miescher. Le kala-azar. Etude clinique et physiopatholique à propos d'un nouveau cas observé en Suisse. *Schweiz. Med. Wochenschr.* 1979;109:265.

152. Navin, T. R., B. A. Arana, F. E. Arana, J. D. Berman, and J. F. Chajon. Placebo controlled clinical trial of sodium stibogluconate (Pentostam) versus ketoconazole for treating cutaneous leishmaniasis in Guatemala. *J. Infect. Dis.* 1992;165:528.

153. Pepin, J., and F. Milord. The treatment of human African trypanosomiasis. *Adv. Parasitol.* 1994;33:1.

154. Spencer, H. C., J. J. Gibson, R. E. Brodsky, and M. G. Schultz. Imported African trypanosomiasis in the United States. *Ann. Intern. Med.* 1975;82:633.

155. Hughes, W. T. *Pneumocystis carinii* pneumonitis. *Antibiot. Chemother.* 1981;30:257.

156. Hugues, W. T., R. A. Price, H. -K. Kim, T. P. Coburn, D. Grigsby, and S. Feldman. *Pneumocystis carinii* pneumonitis in children with malignancies. *J. Pediatr.* 1973;82:404.

157. Walzer, P. D., D. P. Perl, D. J. Krogstad, P. G. Rawson, and M. G. Schultz. *Pneumocystis carinii* pneumonia in the United States. *Ann. Intern. Med.* 1974;80:83.

158. Western, K. A., D. R. Perera, and M. G. Schultz. Pentamidine isethionate in the treatment of *Pneumocystis carinii* pneumonia. *Ann. Intern. Med.* 1970;73:695.

159. Hughes, W. T., S. Feldman, S. C. Chaudhary, M. J. Ossi, F. Cox, and S. K. Sanyal. Comparison of pentamidine isethionate and trimethoprim-sulfamethoxazole in the treatment of *Pneumocystis carinii* pneumonia. *J. Pediatr.* 1978;92:285.

160. Hoover, D. R., A. J., Saah, H., Bacellar, J., Phair, R., Detels, R. Anderson, and R. A. Kaslow. Clinical manifestations of AIDS in the era of pneumocystis prophylaxis. Multicenter AIDS Cohort Study. *N. Engl. J. Med.*1993;329:1922.

161. Santamauro, J. T., and D. E. Stover. *Pneumocystis carinii* pneumonia. *Med. Clin. North Am.* 1997;81:299.

162. Monk, J. P., and R. Benfield. Inhaled pentamidine. An overview of its pharmacological properties and

a review of its therapeutic use in *Pneumocystis carinii* pneumonia. *Drugs* 1990;39:741.

163. Bozzette, S. A., D. M. Finkelstein, S. A. Spector, P. Frame, W. G. Powderly, W. He, L. Phillips, D. Craven, C. van der Horst, and J. A. Feinberg. Randomized trial of three antipneumocystis agents in patients with advanced human immunodeficiency virus infection. *N. Engl. J. Med.* 1995;332:693.

164. Vohringer, H. -F., and K. Arasteh. Pharmacokinetic optimisation in the treatment of *Pneumocystis carinii* pneumonia. *Clin. Pharmacokinet.* 1993;24:388.

165. Carter, N. S., and A. H. Fairlamb. Arsenical-resistant trypanosomes lack an unusual adenosine transporter. *Nature* 1993;361:173.

166. Bitonti, A. J., J. A. Dumont, and P. P. McCann. Characterization of *Trypanosoma brucei brucei* S-adenosyl-L-methionine decarboxylase and its inhibition by berenil, pentamidine and methylglyoxal bis(guanylhydrazone). *Biochem. J.* 1986;237:685.

167. Bailly, C., I. O. Donkor, D. Gentle, M. Thornalley, and M. I. Waring. Sequence-selective binding to DNA of *cis-* and *trans-*butamidine analogues of the anti–*Pneumocystis carinii* pneumonia drug pentamidine. *Mol. Pharmacol.* 1994;46:313.

168. Festy, B., and M. Duane. Hydroxystilbamidine. A nonintercalating drug as a probe of nucleic acid conformation. *Biochemistry* 1973;12:4827.

169. Festy, B. Hydroxystilbamidine. In *Antibiotics V-2*, ed. by F. E. Hahn. New York:Springer-Verlag, 1979, pp. 223–235.

170. Delain, E., Ch. Brack, G. Riou, and B. Festy. Ultrastructural alterations of *Trypanosoma cruzi* kinetoplast induced by the interaction of a trypanocidal drug (hydroxystilbamidine) with kinetoplast DNA. *J. Ultrastruct. Res.* 1971;37:200.

171. Brack, Ch., E. Delain, G. Riou, and B. Festy: Molecular organization of the kinetoplast DNA of *Trypanosoma cruzi* with berenil, a DNA interacting drug. *J. Ultrastruct. Res.* 1972;39:568.

172. Brack, Ch., E. Delain, and G. Riou. Replicating, covalently closed, circular DNA from kinetoplasts of *Trypanosoma cruzi*. *Proc. Natl. Acad. Sci. U.S.A.* 1972;69:1642.

173. Shapiro, T. A., and P. T. Englund. Selective cleavage of kinetoplast DNA minicircles promoted by antitrypanosomal drugs. *Proc. Natl. Acad. Sci. U.S.A.* 1990;87:950.

174. Dykstra, C. C., and R. R. Tidwell. Inhibition of topoisomerases from *Pneumocystis carinii* by aromatic dicationic molecules. *J. Protozool.* 1991;38:78S.

175. Conte, J. E., Jr., R. A., Upton, and E. T. Lin. Pentamidine pharmacokinetics in patients with AIDS with impaired renal function. *J. Infect. Dis.* 1987;156:985.

176. Conte, J. E. Pharmacokinetics of intravenous pentamidine in patients with normal renal function or receiving hemodialysis. *J. Infect. Dis.* 1991;163:169.

177. Donnelly, H., E. M. Bernard, H. Rothkotter, J. W. M. Gold, and D. Armstrong. Distribution of pentamidine in patients with AIDS. *J. Infect. Dis.* 1988;157:985.

178. Waalkes, T. P., and D. R. Makulu. Pharmaco-logic aspects of pentamidine. *Natl. Cancer. Inst. Monogr.* 1976;43:171.

179. Waalkes, T. P., C. Denham, and V. T. de Vita. Pentamidine: clinical pharmacologic correlations in man and mice. *Clin. Pharmacol. Ther.* 1970;11:505.

180. Sands, M., M. A. Kron, and R. B. Brown. Pentamidine: a review. *Rev. Infect. Dis.* 1985;7:625.

181. Condit, P. T., R. F. Chanes, and W. Joel. Renal toxicity of methotrexate. *Cancer* 1969;23:126.

182. Scharlau, G. Onchocerciasis. *Trop. Doctor* 1981;11:8.

183. Hawking, F. Suramin: with special reference to onchocerciasis. *Adv. Pharmacol. Chemother.* 1978;15:289.

184. Voogd, T. E., E. L. M. Vansterkenburg, J. Wilting, and L. H. M. Janssen. Recent research on the biological activity of suramin. *Pharmacol. Rev.* 1993;45:177.

185. Meshnick, S. R. The chemotherapy of African trypanosomiasis. In *Parasitic Diseases*, Vol. 2, ed. by J. M. Mansfield. New York: Marcel Dekker, 1984, pp. 165–199.

186. Fong, J. S. C., and R. A. Good. Suramin—a potent reversible and competitive inhibitor of complement systems. *Clin. Exp. Immunol.* 1972;10:127.

187. De Clercq, E. Suramin: a potent inhibitor of the reverse transcriptase of RNA tumor viruses. *Cancer Lett.* 1979;8:9.

188. Walter, R. D., and H. Schulz-Key. *Onchocerca volvulus*: effect of suramin on lactate dehydrogenase and malate dehydrogenase. *Tropenmed. Parasitol.* 1980;31:55.

189. Constantopoulos, G., S. Rees, B. G. Cragg, J. A. Barranger, and R. O. Brady. Experimental animal model for mucopolysaccharidosis: suramin-induced glycosaminoglycan and sphingolipid accumulation in the rat. *Proc. Natl. Acad. Sci. U.S.A.* 1980;77:3700.

190. Fortes, P. A. G., J. C. Ellory, and V. L. Lew. Suramin: a potent ATPase inhibitor which acts on the inside surface of the sodium pump. *Biochim. Biophys. Acta* 1973;318:262.

191. Fairlamb, A. H., and I. B. R. Bowman. Uptake of the trypanocidal drug suramin by bloodstream forms of *Trypanosoma brucei* and its effect on respiration and growth rate in vivo. *Mol. Biochem. Parasitol.* 1980;1:315.

192. Walter, R. D., and E. J. Albiez. Inhibition of NADP-linked malic enzyme from *Onchocerca volvulus* and *Dirofilaria immitis* by suramin. *Mol. Biochem. Parasitol.* 1981;4:53.

193. Müller, W. E., and U. Wollert. Spectroscopic studies on the complex formation of suramin with bovine and human serum albumin. *Biochim. Biophys. Acta* 1976;427:465.

194. Thylefors, B., and A. Rolland. The risk of optic atrophy following suramin treatment of ocular onchocerciasis. *Bull. WHO* 1979;57:479.

195. Hawking, F. Chemotherapy of filariasis. *Antibiot. Chemother.* 1981;30:135.

196. Tuchmann-Duplessis, H., and L. Mercier-Parot. Influence de la suramine sur la survie péri-natale et postnatale de la souris. *Compt. Rend. Soc. Biol.* 1973;167:1717.

197. Hawking, F. Chemotherapy of trypanosomiasis. In *Experimental Chemotherapy*, Vol. I, ed. by R. J. Schnitzer and F. Hawking. New York: Academic Press, 1963, pp. 129–256.

198. Fairlamb, A. H., N. S. Carter, M. Cunningham, and K. Smith. Characterisation of melarsen-resistant *Trypanosoma brucei brucei* with respect to cross-resistance to other drugs and trypanothione metabolism. *Mol. Biochem. Parasitol.* 1992;53:213.

199. Bowman, I. B. R., I. W. Flynn, and A. H. Fairlamb. Carbohydrate metabolism of pleomorphic strains of *Trypanosoma rhodesiense* and sites of action of arsenical drugs. *J. Parasitol.* 1970;56:402.

200. Flynn, I. W., and I. B. R. Bowman. Further studies on the mode of action of arsenicals on trypanosome pyruvate kinase. *Trans. R. Soc. Trop. Med. Hyg.* 1969; 63:121.

201. Fairlamb, A. H., G. B. Henderson, and A. Cerami. Trypanothione is the primary target for arsenical drugs against African trypanosomes. *Proc. Natl. Acad. Sci. U.S.A.* 1989;86:2607.

202. Yarlett, N., B. Goldberg, H. C. Nathan, J. Garofalo, and C. J. Bacchi. Differential susceptibility of *Trypanosoma brucei rhodesiense* isolates to in vitro lysis by arsenicals. *Exp. Parasitol.* 1991;72:205.

203. Apted, F. I. C. Four year's experience of melarsen oxide/BAL in the treatment of late stage Rhodesian sleeping sickness. *Trans. R. Soc. Trop. Med. Hyg.* 1957; 51:75.

204. Buyst, H. The treatment of *T. rhodesiense* sleeping sickness, with special reference to its physiopathological and epidemiological basis. *Ann. Soc. Belge Med. Trop.* 1975;55:95.

205. Poltera, A. A., A. Hochmann, and P. H. Lambert. *Trypanosoma brucei brucei*: the response to melarsoprol in mice with cerebral trypanosomiasis. An immunopathological study. *Clin. Exp. Immunol.* 1981;46: 363.

206. Robertson, D. H. H. The treatment of sleeping sickness (mainly due to *Trypanosoma rhodesiense*) with melarsoprol. I. Reactions observed during treatment. *Trans. R. Soc. Trop. Med. Hyg.* 1963;57: 122.

207. Hawking, F. The concentration of melarsoprol (Mel B) and Mel W in plasma and cerbrospinal fluid estimated by bioassay with trypanosomes in vitro. *Trans. R. Soc. Trop. Med. Hyg.* 1963;56:354.

208. Sina, G., N. Triolo, P. Trova, and J. M. Clabaut. L'encephalopathie arsenicale lors du traitement de la trypanosomiase humaine Africaine a *T. gambiense* (a propos de 16 cas). *Ann. Soc. Belge Med. Trop.* 1977; 57:67.

209. Tracy, J. W., and L. T. Webster. Drugs used in the chemotherapy of protozoal infections (continued). In *Goodman's and Gilman's The Pharmacological Basis of Therapeutics*, ed. by J. Hardman, L. Limbird, P. Molinoff, R. Ruddon, and A. G. Gilman. New York: McGraw Hill, 1995, pp. 987–1008.

210. Haberkorn, A., and R. Gönnert. Animal experimental investigation into the activity of nifurtimox against *Trypanosoma cruzi. Anzneimittelforschung.* 1972;22:1570.

211. Gönnert, R., and M. Bock. The effect of nifurtimox on *Trypanosoma cruzi* in tissue cultures. *Arzneimittelforschung.* 1972;22:1582.

212. Dvorak, J. A., and C. L. Howe. The effects of Lampit (Bayer 2502) on the interaction of *Trypanosoma cruzi* with vertebrate cells in vitro. *Am. J. Trop. Med. Hyg.* 1976;26:58.

213. Cancado, J. R., A. A. Salgado, S. M. Batista, and C. Chiari. Segundo ensaio terapeutico com o nifurtimox na doenca de Chagas. *Rev. Goiana Med.* 1976; 22:203.

214. Wegner, D. H. G. and R. W. Rohwedder: The effect of nifurtimox in acute Chagas' infection. *Arzneimittelforschung* 1972;22:1624.

215. Wegner, D. H. G., and R. W. Rohwedder. Experience with nifurtimox in chronic Chagas' infection: preliminary report. *Arzneimittelforschung.* 1972;22: 1635.

216. Docampo, R., S. N. J. Moreno, A. O. M. Stoppani, W. Leon, F. S. Cruz, F. Villalta, and R. F. A. Muniz. Mechanism of nifurtimox toxicity in different forms of *Trypanosoma cruzi. Biochem. Pharmacol.* 1981;30:1947.

217. Docampo, R., R. P. Mason, C. Mottley, and R. P. A. Muniz. Generation of free radicals induced by nifurtimox in mammalian tissues. *J. Biol. Chem.* 1981; 256:10930.

218. Docampo, R. Sensitivity of parasites to free radical damage by antiparasitic drugs. *Chem. Biol. Interact.* 1990;73:1.

219. G. B., Henderson, P., Uhich, A. H. Fairlamb, I. Rosenberg, M. Pereira, M., Sela, and A. Cerami. "Subversive" substrates for the enzyme trypanothione disulfide reductase. Alternative approach to chemotherapy of Chagas' disease. *Proc. Natl. Acad. Sci. U.S.A.* 1988;85: 5374.

220. Paulos, C., I. Paredes, I. Vasquez, S. Thambo, A. Arancibia, and A. Gonzalez-Martin. Pharmacokinetics of a nitrofuran compound, nifurtimox, in healthy volunteers. *Int. J. Clin. Pharmacol. Ther. Toxicol.* 1989;27:454.

221. Medenwald, H., K. Brandau, and K. Schlossman. Quantitative determination of nifurtimox in body fluids of rat, dog and man. *Arzneimittelforschung.* 1972;22:1613.

222. Duhm, B., W. Maul, H. Medenwald, K. Patzschke, and L. A. Wegner. Investigations on the pharmacokinetics of nifurtimox-^{35}S in the rat and dog. *Arzneimittelforschung.* 1972;22:1617.

223. Zenser, T. V., M. B. Mattammal, M. O. Palmier, and B. D. Davis. Microsomal nitroreductase activity of rabbit kidney and bladder: implications in 5-nitrofuran-induced toxicity. *J. Pharmacol. Exp. Ther.* 1981;219:735.

224. Chamberlain, R. E. Chemotherapeutic properties of prominent nitrofurans. *J. Antimicrob. Chemother.* 1976;2:325.

225. McCann, P., and A. E. Pegg. Ornithine decarboxylase as an enzyme target for therapy. *Pharmacol. Ther.* 1992;54:195.

226. Bey, P., C. Danzin, and M. Jung. Inhibition of basic amino acid decarboxylases involved in polyamine biosynthesis. In *Inhbition of Polyamine Metabolism, Biological Significance and Basis of New Therapies,* ed.

by P. P. McCann, A. E. Pegg, and A. Sjoerdsma. New York: Academic Press, 1987. pp. 1–31.

227. Janne, J., L. Alhonen, and P. Leinonen. Polyamines: from molecular biology to clinical application. *Ann. Med.* 1991;23:241.

228. Croft, S. L. Antiprotozoal agents. In *Antibiotic and Chemotherapy. Anti-infective Agents and Their Use in Therapy*, ed. by F. O'Grady, R. G. Finch, H. Lambert, and D. Greenwood. New York: Churchill Livingstone, 1997, pp. 522–540.

229. Wang, C. C. A novel suicide inhbitior strategy for antiparasitic drug development. *J. Cell. Biochem.* 1991;45:49.

230. Bacchi, C. Resistance to clinical drugs in African trypanosomes. *Parasitol. Today*, 1993;9:190.

231. Milord, F., L. Loko, L. Ethier, B. Mpid, and J. Pepin. Eflornithine concentrations in serum and cerebrospinal fluid in 63 patients treated for *Trypanosoma brucei gambinense* sleeping sickness. *Trans. R. Soc. Trop. Med. Hyg.* 1993;87:473.

232. Van Nieuwehove, S. Advances in sleeping sickness therapy. *Ann. Soc. Belg. Med. Trop.* 1992;72:39.

233. Bacchi, C. J., H. C. Nathan, N. Yarlett, B. Goldberg, P. P. McCann, A. Sjoerdsma, M. Saric, and A. B. Clarkson. Combination chemotherapy of drug-resistant *Trypanosoma brucei rhodesiense* infections in mice using DL-α-difluoromethylomithine and standard trypanocides. *Antimicrob. Agents Chemother.* 1994;38:563.

234. Fozard, J. R. The contragestational effects of ornithine decarboxylase inhibition. In *Inhibition of Polyamine Metabolism. Biological Significance and Basis for New Therapies.* ed. by P. P. McCann, A. E. Pegg, and S. Sjoerdsma. Orlando: Academic Press 1987, pp. 187–202.

235. Wolfe, M. S. Giardiasis. *Clin. Microbiol. Rev.* 1992;5:93.

236. Hill, D. R. Giardiasis: issues in diagnosis and management. *Infect. Dis. Clin. North Am.* 1993;7:503.

237. Nash, T. E., and P. F. Welker. Protozoal intestinal infections and trichomoniasis. In *Harrisons Internal Medicine*, ed. by A. Fauci. New York: McGraw Hill, 1998, pp. 1202–1205.

238. McCalla, D. R. Nitrofurans. In *Antibiotics V-1*, ed. by F. E. Hahn. New York: Springer-Verlag, 1979, pp. 176–213.

239. Craft, J. C., T. Murphy, and J. D. Nelson. Furizolidone and quinacrine. Comparative study of therapy for giardiasis in children. *Am. J. Dis. Child.* 1981;135:164.

240. Bassily, S., A. Farid, J. W. Mikhail, D. C. Kent, and J. S. Lehman. The treatment of *Giardia lamblia* infection with mepacrine, metronidazole, and furazolidone. *J. Trop. Med. Hyg.* 1970;73:15.

241. Levi, G. C., C. A. de Avila, and V. A. Neto. Efficacy of various drugs for treatment of giardiasis. A comparative study. *Am. J. Trop. Med. Hyg.* 1977;26:564.

242. Treatment of giardiasis. *Med. Lett.* 1976;18:39.

243. Hollifield, R. D., and J. D. Conklin. Method specific for determination of furazolidone in urine. Evidence for drug-related metabolites. *J. Pharm. Sci.* 1968;57:325.

244. Dietrich, R. A., and L. Hellerman. Diphosphopyridine nucleotide-linked aldehyde dehydrogenase. II. Inhibitors. *J. Biol. Chem.* 1963;238:1683.

245. Klein, H. Alkohol und Medikamente: I. Durch Medikamente verursachte Alkoholunverträglichkeit und verstärkte Alkoholwirkung. *Forschr. Med.* 1964;82:169.

246. Heine, P., and J. A. McGregor. *Trichomonas vaginalis*: a reemerging pathogen. *Clin. Obstet. Gynecol.* 1993;36:137.

247. White, A. C., C. L. Chappell, C. S. Hayat, K. T. Kimball, T. P. Flanagan, and R. W. Goodgame. Paromomycin for cryptosporidiosis in AIDS: a prospective, double-blind trial. *J. Infect. Dis.* 1994;170:419.

248. Wong, S.-Y., and J. S. Rimington, Biology of *Toxoplasma gondii*. *AIDS* 1993;7:299.

249. Klepser, M. E., and T. B. Klepser. Drug treatment of HIV-related opportunistic infections. *Drugs* 1997;53:40.

250. Kovacs, J. A., and the NIAID-Clinical Center Intramural AIDS Program. Efficacy of atovaqone in treatment of toxoplasmosis in patients with AIDS. *Lancet* 1992;340:637.

251. Podzamczer, D., A Salazar, J. Jimenez, E. Consiglio, M. Santin, A. Casanova, G. Rufi, and F. Gudiol. Intermittent trimethoprim-sulfamethoxazole compared with dapsone. *Ann. Intern. Med.* 1995;122:755.

252. Girard, P., R. Landman, C. Gaudebout, R. Olivares, A. G. Saimot, P. Jelazko, C. Gaudebout, A. Certain, F. Boue, E. Bouvet, T. Lecompte, J.-P. Coulaud, and the PRIO Study Group. Dapsone-pyrimethamine compared with aerosolized pentamidine as primary prophylaxis against *Pneumocystis carinii* pneumonia and toxoplasmosis in HIV infection. *N. Engl. J. Med.* 1993;328:1514.

253. Stringer, J. R., M. A. Blase, P. D. Walzer, and M. T. Cushion. *Pneumocystis carinii*: sequence from ribosomal RNA implies a close relationship with fungi. *Exp. Parasitol.* 1989;68:450.

254. Pifer, L. L., W. T. Hughes, and M. J. Murphey. Propagation of *Pneumocystis carinii* in vitro. *Pediatr. Res.* 1977;11:305.

255. Santamauro, J. T., and D. E. Stover. *Pneumocystis carinii* pneumonia. *Med. Clin. North Am.* 1997;81:299.

256. Fishman; J. A., Treatment of infection due to *Pneumocystis carinii*. *Antimicrob. Agents Chemother.* 1998;42:1309.

257. Hughes, W. T., and J. Killmar. Monodrug efficacies of sulfonamides in prophylaxis for *Pneumocystis carinii* pneumonia. *Antimicrob. Agents Chemother.* 1996;40:962.

258. Hughes, W. T., S. Feldman, S. C. Chaudhary, M. J. Ossi, F. Cox, and S. K. Sanyal. Comparison of pentamidine isethionate and trimethoprim sulfamethoxazole in the treatment of *Pneumocystis carinii* pneumonia. *J. Pediatr.* 1978;92:285.

259. Fishman; J. A. Prevention of infection due to *Pneumocystis carinii*. *Antimicrob. Agents Chemother.* 1998;42:995.

260. Alberts, B., D. Bray, J. Lewis, M. Raff, K. Roberts, and J. D. Watson. Energy conversion: mitochondria and chloroplasts. *In Molecular Biology of the Cell.* New York: Garlan Publishing, 1989, pp. 341–404.

261. Spenser, C. M., and K. L. Goa. Atovaquone. A review of its pharmacological properties and therapeutic effecacy in opportunistic infections. *Drugs* 1995;50: 176.

262. Rolan, P. E., A. J. Mercer, B. C. Weatherley, T. Holdich, H. Meire, R. W. Peck, G. Ridout, and J. Posner. Examination of some factors responsible for a food-induced increase in absorption of atovaquone. *Br. J. Clin. Pharmacol.* 1994;37:13.

263. Hughes, W., G. Leoung, F. Kramer, S. Bozzette, S. Safrin, P. Frame, N. Clumeck, H. Masur, D. Lancaster, C. Chan, J. Lavelle, J. Rosenstock, J. Falloon, J. Feinberg, S. LaFon, M. Rogers, and F. Sattler. Comparison of atovaquone (566C80) with trimethoprim-sulfamethoxazole to treat *Pneumocystis carinii* pneumonia in patients with AIDS. *N. Eng. J. Med.* 1993; 328:1521.

264. A unique nonsulfonamide therapy for the treatment of PCP. An effective oral option for mild to moderate *Pneumocystis carinii* pneumonia in individuals who are intolerant to TMP-SMX.: Burroughs Wellcome (data on file), 1995.

265. Dohn, M. N., W. G. Weinberg, R. A. Torres, S. Follansbee, P. Caldwell, J. Scott, J. Gathe, D. Haghighat, J. Sampson, J. Spotkov, S. Deresinski, R. Meyer, D. Lancaster, and the Atovaquone Study Group. Oral atovaquone compared with intravenous pentamidine for *Pneumocystis carinii* pneumonia in patients with AIDS. *Ann. Intern. Med.* 1994;121:174.

266. Torres, R. A., W. Weinberg, and J. Stansell. Atovaquone for salvage treatment and supression of toxoplasmic encephalitis in patients with acquired immunodeficiency syndrome (AIDS). England: Burroughs Wellcome (data on file), 1995.

267. Lin, J. T., and J. R. Bertino. Update on trimetrexate, a folate antagonist with antineoplastic and antiprotozoal properties. *Cancer Invest.* 1991;9:159.

268. MacDonald, J. R., C. I. Courtney, and D. G. Pegg. Leucovorin protection against repeated daily dose toxicity of trimetrexate in rats. *Fund. Appl. Toxicol.* 1993;21:244.

269. Lerza, R., M. Mencoboni, G. Bogliolo, G. Flego, L. Gasparini, and I. Pannacciulli. Leucovorin antagonizes the effects of trimetrexate on mouse hemopoietic progenitors. *Anticancer Res.* 1991;11:613.

270. Fulton, B., A. J. Wagstaff, and D. McTavish. Trimetrexate. A review of its pharmaxodynamic and pharmacokinetic properties and therapeutic potential in the treatment of *Pneumocystis carinii* pneumonia. *Drugs* 1995;49:563.

271. Freij, J., R. L. Wientzen, G. Hayek, and L. R. Whitfield. Pharmacokinetics of trimetrexate glucuronate in infants with AIDS and *Pneumocystis carinii* pneumonia. *Ann. N.Y. Acad. Sci.* 1993;693:302.

272. Allegra, C. J., J. Jenkins, R. B. Weiss, F. Balis, J. C. Drake, J. Brooks, R. Thomas, and G. A. Curt. A phase I and pharmacokinetic study of trimetrcxate using a 24-hour continuous injection schedule. *Invest. New Drugs* 1990;8:159.

273. Grochow, L. B., D. A. Noe, G. B. Dole, E. K. Rowinsky, D. S. Ettinger, M. L. Graham, W. P. McGuire, and R. C. Donehower. Phase I trial of trimetrexate glucuronate on a five-day bolus schedule: clinical pharmacology and pharmacodynamics. *J Natl. Cancer Inst.* 1989;81:124.

274. Masur, H., M. A. Polis, C. U. Tuazon, D. Ogata-Arakaki, J. A. Lovacs, D. Katz, D. Hilt, T. Simmons, I. Feuerstein, B. Lundgren, H. C. Lane, B. A. Chabner, and C. J. Allegra. Salvage trial of trimetrexate-leucovorin for the treatment of cerebral toxoplasmosis in patients with AIDS. *J. Infect. Dis.* 1992;167:1422.

275. Allegra, C. J., J. A. Kovacs, J. C. Drake, J. C. Swan, B. A. Chabner, and H. Masur. Activity of antifolates against *Pneumocystis carinii* dihydrofolate reductase and identification of a potent new agent. *J. Exp. Med.* 1987;165:926.

276. Sattler, F. R., R. Frame, R. Davis, L. Nichols, B. Shelton, B. Akil, R. Baughman, C. Hughlett, W. Weiss, C. Boylen, C. von der Horst, J. Black, W. Powderly, R. Steigbigel, J. M. Leedom, H. Masur, and J. Feinberg. Trimetrexate with leucovorin versus trimethoprim-sulfamethoxazole for moderate to severe episodes of *Pneumocystis carinii* pneumonia in patients with AIDS: a prospective, controlled multicenter investigation of the AIDS Clinical Trials Group Protocol 029/031. *J. Infect. Dis.* 1994;170:165.

277. Grem, J. L., S. A. King, and M. E. Costanza. Hypersensitivity reactions to trimetrexate. *Invest. New Drugs* 1990;8:211.

CHAPTER FIFTEEN

Chemotherapy of Helminthic Diseases

The helminthic, or worm, diseases are caused by members of two phyla. The nematodes (roundworms) belong to the phylum Nemathelminthes. Diseases caused by this group of organisms include, for example, ascaris, whipworm, pinworm, and hookworm infections, trichinosis, and elephantiasis. The cestodes, or tapeworms, and the trematodes, a group including the various flukes (e.g., the schistosomes), are both members of the phylum Platyhelminthes (flatworms). These worms are multicellular organisms that possess crude organ systems. Their complex life cycles usually include a stage of development in the human intestinal tract.

The interaction between the drugs used to treat helminthic disease and the biochemistry of the worms is a specialized field of investigation that has been the subject of several reviews.[1-4] Parasitic helminths are complex multicellular organisms with differentiated nervous systems and organs. Unlike viruses, bacteria, and protozoa, most helminths do not directly replicate in the human body but reproduce sexually, giving rise to eggs or larvae that then pass out of the body.[4] Anthelmintic drugs often affect some of the more complex systems of cellular physiology, such as microtubule formation or neuromuscular function, as well as the reactions that generate metabolic energy. The selective effect of the anthelminthic drugs is sometimes based on differences between the biochemistry of the host and the parasite. In other cases in which there is no selective toxicity, the parasite is exposed to high concentrations of the drug in its intestinal habitat by the use of orally administered, nonabsorbable drugs. The discussion of the drugs used to treat the worm infections will expand upon these observations.

The emergence of drug resistance in helminths has been much more gradual and limited than in rapidly replicating protozoa, such as the malarial parasite. Many of the anthelmintics available for human use now are effective against several different helminth species and, although there are over 20 different species of helminth that cause human disease of worldwide significance, almost all of these infections can be treated or controlled with one of five anthelmintics: the benzimidazoles albendazole and mebendazole, diethylcarbamazine, ivermectin, and praziquantel.

Drugs Used to Treat Fluke Infections

Schistosomiasis

Schistosomiasis (also called bilharziasis) is one of the most prevalent diseases of humans and therefore one of the most serious health problems in the world today. It has been estimated that more than 200 million and perhaps as many as 500 million people in 73 nations in Africa, Asia, South America, and the islands of the Caribbean are infected by schistosomes and infection of entire communities is common.[5,6] Schistosomiasis now ranks second only to malaria as the major infectious disease of the tropics. Most infected persons experience few or no signs and symptoms, and only small minorities develop significant disease. The increased incidence of this disease results from increased irrigation, which has provided breeding areas for the aquatic snails which are the intermediate hosts.

Schistosomes are multicellular flukes with primitive excretory, nervous, and circulatory systems and specialized organs of reproduction. These organisms penetrate the skin of the human host and migrate to the liver via the bloodstream, residing for a time in the hepatic vessels. After a few weeks, a retrograde migration to various areas of the abdominal vascular plexuses occurs; *Schistosoma hematobium* lives in the venules of the vesicle plexus and *Schistosoma mansoni* and *Schistosoma japonicum* in the mesenteric veins. Here the organisms mate, depositing eggs that are excreted in the urine and feces. The reservoir for these parasites is the freshwater snail. The disease symptomatology is protean in nature and cannot be described in a few words. In the early stages of infection, chemotherapy is very successful. If the disease has been present for some time, however, the intestine and particularly the liver become fibrosed, and although chemotheray can eliminate the organism, it cannot reverse the pathology.

The strategies for the control of schistosomiasis are similar to those used in controlling intestinal nematode infections.[3] School-age children experience the greatest burden of schistosome infection and are the natural targets for treatment. Studies have shown that targeting treatment to this age-group reduces overall transmission for *S. mansoni* and *S. haematobium*.[7,8]

For about 60 years, antimonial compounds were the only drugs employed for the treatment of schistosomiasis. Because of the prolonged duration of therapy and their toxicity, the antimonials are no longer used in most regions of the world. The introduction of niridazole provided new therapy for infection by *Schistosoma haematobium* but it was not until the introduction of praziquantel, metrifonate, and oxamniquine in the mid-1970s that relatively nontoxic short-course and single-dose therapy became possible. These antischistosomal compounds were originally developed as veterinary anthelminthics and have subsequently been shown to be effective in treating schistosomiasis in humans (see Table 15–1). Prazi-

Table 15–1. *Drugs used to treat flatworm infections.* In the United States, bithionol may be obtained from the Parasitic Disease Drug Service, Centers for Disease Control.

Infecting organism	Drug of choice	Alternatives
FLUKES (TREMATODES)		
Schistosoma haematobium	Praziquantel	Metrifonate
Schistosoma japonicum	Praziquantel	
Schistosoma mansoni	Praziquantel	Oxamniquine[a]
Schistosoma mekongi	Praziquantel	
Clonorchis sinensis (Chinese liver fluke)	Praziquantel	
Fasciola hepatica (sheep liver fluke)	Triclabendazole	Bithionol
Fasciolopsis buski (intestinal fluke)	Praziquantel	
Heterophyes heterophyes (intestinal fluke)	Praziquantel	
Metagonimus yokogawai (intestinal fluke)	Praziquantel	
Opisthorchis viverrini (liver fluke)	Praziquantel	
Paragonimus westermani (lung fluke)	Praziquantel	Bithionol
TAPEWORMS (CESTODES)		
Diphyllobothrium latum (fish tapeworm)	Praziquantel	
Taenia saginata (beef tapeworm)	Praziquantel	
Taenia solium (pork tapeworm)	Praziquantel	
Hymenolepis nana (dwarf tapeworm)	Praziquantel	

[a] Oxamniquine has been found to be effective in some areas where cure rates with praziquantel were low.[9] However, it is no longer available in the United States.

quantel is now the drug of choice for treating all species of schistosomes that infect humans.[3] It is safe and effective when it is given in single or divided oral doses on the same day. Oxamniquine is effective for treatment of *S. mansoni* infections, particularly in South America, where the sensitivity of most strains permits single-dose therapy. Oxamniquine, however, is not effective clinically against *S. haematobium* and *S. japonicum.* Metrifonate has been used with considerable success in the treatment of *S. haematobium* infections but is not effective against *S. mansoni* and *S. japonicum.* It is a relatively inexpensive drug and can be used in conjunction with oxamniquine for the treatment of mixed infections with *S. haematobium* and *S. mansoni.* The antischistosomal drugs have been reviewed in detail by Bennett and Depenbusch.[10]

Praziquantel

Praziquantel is one of several compounds that were synthesized after it was discovered

Praziquantel

that the pyrazinoisoquinoline structure possessed anthelminthic activity. The commercial preparation is a mixture of stereoisomers, with the levorotatory isomer being much more potent than the dextrorotatory isomer.

ANTHELMINTHIC ACTIVITY AND THERAPEUTIC USE. Praziquantel has a broad spectrum of anthelminthic action that includes schistosomes, hermaphroditic flukes, and cestodes (see references 11–14 for reviews). Praziquantel is approved in the United States only for therapy of schistosomiasis and liver fluke infections, but elsewhere it is also used to treat infections by many other trematodes and cestodes. The drug has proven to be effective in treating infection by all species of

schistosomes that infect human beings, including *Schistosoma mansoni,*[15] *S. haeatobium,*[16] *S. japonicum,*[17] and *S. mekongi.*[18] A course of therapy for infection by *S. haematobium* and *S. mansoni* is 40 mg/kg administered as two divided doses separated by an interval of 4 h. A course of therapy for *S. japonicum* and *S. mekongi* is 60 mg/kg administered as three 20 mg/kg doses.

Praziquantel is effective in treating most fluke infections, including the liver flukes *Clonorchis sinensis*[19] and *Opisthorchis viverrini,*[20] the lung fluke *Paragonimus westermani,*[21] and the intestinal flukes *Fasciolopsis buski, Heterophyes heterophyes,* and *Metagonimus yokogawi.*[13,14] A course of therapy for all of these nonschistosome fluke infections is 75 mg/kg administered on 1 day as three 25 mg/kg doses. Infections with the sheep liver fluke *Fasciola hepatica* are unresponsive to high doses, even though praziquantel penetrates this trematode. The reason for the insensitivity of this helminth is unknown.[14]

Praziquantel, administered in a single dose of 10–20 mg/kg, is effective in the treatment of tapeworm infection, including *Diphyllobothrium latum, D. pacificum, Dipylidium caninum, Taenia saginata, T. solium,* and *Hymenolepis nana.*[22,23] In general, the efficacy of praziquantel against tapeworm infections is similar to that of the older drug niclosamide. In the case of infection by the dwarf tapeworm *H. nana,* the cure rate with a single 25 mg/kg dose of praziquantel is 93%, and single-dose therapy with praziquantel is considered to be preferable to 5 days of therapy with the older drugs niclosamide or paromomycin.

The introduction of praziquantel represents a major advance in the chemotherapy of helminthic infections, including some (e.g., *Clonorchis* and *Opisthorchis* flukes) which had not responded to previously available therapy. Its advantages include a broad spectrum of anthelminthic action, lack of serious toxicity, single-dose or single-day administration, and good penetration into tissues and parasites. Its major disadvantage in the poor nations of the third world is its relatively high cost compared to other therapies.

MECHANISM OF ACTION OF PRAZIQUANTEL. The biochemical mechanism of action is still not clearly understood, although praziquantel has now been in clinical use for several years. After rapid and reversible uptake, praziquantel has two major effects on susceptible worms. At the lowest effective concentrations, it causes increased muscular activity, followed by contraction and spastic paralysis. The affected worms detach from host tissues and may shift from the mesenteric veins to the liver or be expelled from the body. At slightly higher therapeutic concentrations, praziquantel can cause tegumental damage that activates host defense mechanisms and results in destruction of the worms.[24–26] It seems that the clinical efficacy of the drug correlates best with its tegumental effects[27] and membranes of affected helminths appear to be the primary target for drug action. Praziquantel causes increased membrane permeability to certain monovalent and divalent cations, particularly Ca^{2+}.[28] Both drug-induced muscular contraction and tegumental damage of *S. mansoni* require extracellular Ca^{2+}, but praziquantel acts differently than K^+ and Ca^{2+} ionophores that affect mammalian membranes. Studies of parasitic schistosomes indicate that the immune response of the host and the formation of specific antibodies are necessary for praziquantel's antihelminthic effects.[29] It is speculated that, perhaps by disrupting the surface membrane of the parasite, praziquantel causes antigens within the parasite to be exposed to the action of host antibodies.

Praziquantel is effective against many stages in the schistosome life cycle.[10] At about 3×10^{-9} M, a concentration that is much lower than that required to produce tetanic contraction of the worm, praziquantel inhibits egg production by female schistosomes.[30] It is not known if inhibition of egg production and tetanic contraction reflect the same primary biochemical event.

Radiolabeled praziquantel has been shown to rapidly enter isolated trematodes and cestodes, from which it can be recovered as the unchanged drug.[31] The high degree of selective toxicity of the drug cannot be explained by selective entry into or metabolic activation by the parasite. The drug distributes uniformly in worms and no specific binding components have been identified.

PHARMACOLOGY. Praziquantel is completely absorbed from the gastrointestinal tract and is routinely administered orally. After absorption from the gut, the drug passes through the portal venous system to the liver where it is extensively metabolized.[32] Because of the pronounced first-pass metabolism, levels of unaltered drug outside the portal system are low. The peak concentration of unaltered praziquantel achieved in serum 1–2 h after ingestion of a single 20 mg/kg dose is about 0.3 µg/ml.[32] The drug is excreted in the urine entirely as metabolites, with 50%–60% of the material in the urine being dihydroxylated drug.[33] The half-life of praziquantel is 0.8 to 2.0 h, compared with 4 to 6 h for its metabolites. In animal models, it has been shown that praziquantel distributes widely in the body. The only specific localization is in the liver and kidneys where the drug is metabolized and excreted.[34] About 80% of the drug in the serum is bound to plasma protein,[34] and the free drug readily passes into the cerebrospinal fluid.[35]

ADVERSE EFFECTS. Praziquantel is well tolerated. Patients with schistosome infections occasionally complain of nausea, epigastric pain, abdominal fullness, headache, dizziness, or drowsiness.[11,15,17,36] These subjective complaints are dose related, occurring in 10%–15% of patients receiving a single 20 mg/kg dose and in 40%–50% of patients receiving three 20 mg/kg doses.[15,17,36] These symptoms disappear spontaneously within a few hours. In a review of 1046 patients with cestode infections treated with praziquantel, 47 reported these same complaints.[22] Abdominal colic and bloody diarrhea caused by praziquantel have also been reported.[3] Praziquantel does not cause hemolysis in patients with glucose-6-phosphate dehydrogenase deficiency, and laboratory tests performed on normal volunteers receiving praziquantel were normal.[32] In contrast to several other antischistosomal drugs, praziquantel is not mutagenic in the Ames bacterial mutation assay and it shows no genotoxicity in a variety of short-term mammalian cell assays.[37,38] Praziquantel is not teratogenic or carcinogenic in rodent models,[38] but documentation in humans is lacking. Therefore, treatment with praziquantel should be postponed until after delivery, unless there is a strong indication for its use.[3]

PRECAUTIONS AND DRUG INTERACTIONS. The safety of praziquantel in children under 4 years of age has not been established. The half-life of praziquantel can be prolonged in patients with severe hepatic disease.[39] Praziquantel is related chemically to sedative and anti-anxiety agents. Therefore, driving, operating machinery, and other tasks requiring mental alertness should be avoided until about a day after the last dose is taken. No serious drug interactions have been reported. The bioavailability of praziquantel is reduced by inducers of hepatic cytochrome P-450, such as carbamazepine and phenobarbital, while inhibitors like cimetidine have the opposite effect.[40,41] The bioavailability of albendazole is sometimes increased by praziquantel.[42]

Metrifonate

Metrifonate is an organophosphorus compound that was first introduced as an insecticide and later as a drug for the treatment

$$CH_3 \cdot O,\; CH_3 \cdot O - P = O,\; CHOH,\; CCl_3 \quad \text{Metrifonate}$$

$$CH_3 \cdot O,\; CH_3 \cdot O - P = O,\; CH,\; CCl_2 \quad \text{Dichlorvos}$$

of schistosomiasis. The development of this compound and studies of its mechanism of action have been the subject of two reviews.[10,43] and a symposium.[44]

ANTISCHISTOSOMAL ACTIVITY AND MECHANISM OF ACTION. Metrifonate acts as an insecticide by virtue of its ability to inhibit acetylcholinesterase. At neutral or alkaline pH, metrifonate rearranges spontaneously to dichlorvos (2,2-dichlorovinyl dimethyl phosphate), which is a direct-acting cholinesterase inhibitor. This rearrangement occurs in body fluids, and after administration of metrifonate, it is the metabolite dichlorvos that produces the anticholinesterase effect in schistosomes.[45] When adult schistosomes are exposed to metrifonate in vitro, a reversible paralysis occurs.[46]

Metrifonate is much more effective against *Schistosoma haematobium* than against other species of the parasite. In hamsters that were experimentally infected with different species of schistosomes, for example, metrifonate caused a much greater reduction in worm burden when the infecting agent was *S. haematobium* than when it was *S. mansoni* or *S. mattheei*.[47] A similar difference in response to therapy is seen in humans where a high response rate is obtained in the treatment of *S. haematobium* infection, but the response of patients with *S. mansoni* infection is poor.[48] Thus, metrifonate is used clinically only in the treatment of infection by *S. haematobium*, where a course of therapy consists of 7.5–10 mg/kg administered orally once every 2 weeks for a total of three doses.[49] Continued administration of the drug once every 4 weeks yields successful prophylaxis in highly endemic areas.[49] In contrast to praziquantel, metrifonate has been associated with an appreciable incidence of failure of therapy. Because it is inexpensive, it is still widely used in areas of Africa where praziquantel is not readily available.

There have been several attempts to explain the differential metrifonate sensitivity of *S. haematobium* infection as compared to *S. mansoni* and *S. japonicum*. In a direct study of metrifonate action on cell-free preparations of acetylcholinesterase from *S. haematobium* and *S. mansoni*, no difference in enzyme sensitivity was found.[50] Administration of dichlorvos to infected hamsters, however, resulted in a greater inhibition of both acetylcholinesterase and cholinesterase activity in *S. haematobium* than in *S. mansoni*, suggesting possible differences in intrinsic sensitivities between species.[50] In humans infected with *S. mansoni*, metrifonate has little effect when parasites are residing in the mesenteric plexus and eggs are passing into the stool. In patients who have *S. mansoni* residing in the vesicle plexus, however, metrifonate causes a marked reduction of egg output into the urine.[48] On the basis of this observation, it has been suggested that metrifonate susceptibility is determined by the atomical site of residence of the parasite.[46,51] Because metrifonate causes a paralysis of the worm's musculature, the ventral suckers that hold the parasite to the vein wall relax and the worm is passively carried with the venous blood flow. In the case of *S. mansoni* and *S. japonicum*, which reside predominantly in the mesenteric plexus, the worms pass via the portal vein to the liver (the so-called hepatic shift), whereas *S. haematobium*, which resides in the vesicle plexus in humans, is carried via the inferior vena cava to the lungs (lung shift). As the effect of the drug wanes, schistosomes in the liver can easily migrate back to the mesentery. It has been suggested, however, that worms that have been carried to the lung cannot proceed in retrograde fashion to the vesicle plexus and are destroyed by host reaction in the lungs.[10] An alternate explanation is that species-selective conjugation of dichlorvos with glutathione catalysed by schistosome glutathione *S*-transferases, may explain why the drug is ineffective against *S. mansoni*.[52]

Although these observations may explain why one species of schistosome is more susceptible to the drug than others, they do not explain the selective toxicity of metrifonate for schistosomes as compared to the host. It does not seem that selective toxicity can be entirely explained by a greater sensitivity of parasite acetylcholinesterase to the drug as compared to the host enzyme. Acetylcholinesterase from mouse brain, for example, is inhibited at only four times the concentration of drug required to inhibit the enzyme from *S. mansoni* or *S. haematobium*.[50] For this and other reasons, some investigators have suggested that acetylcholinesterase inhibition may not be the only factor involved in the therapeutic effect of metrifonate.[53] This is possible, as a variety of other enzyme reactions in the parasite are also affected.[10]

PHARMACOKINETICS AND ADVERSE EFFECTS. Metrifonate is rapidly absorbed from the gastrointestinal tract, and peak levels of 4–8 µg/ml of unaltered drug are achieved in the plasma about 1 h after ingestion of a single 10 mg/kg dose.[54] Simultaneous peak plasma levels of dichlorvos are 40–80 ng/ml. The plasma levels of both metrifonate and dichlorvos decline with the same half-life to 2–3 h and the clearance of metrifonate appears to be determined by its conversion to dichlorvos.[54] Cholinesterase activity in plasma is reduced to essentially zero within 15 mins after a dose of metrifonate, while erythrocyte cholinesterase is inhibited 60%–80%[54] Plasma cholinesterase activity returns to normal in 3–4 weeks but erythrocyte cholinesterase activity does not regain normal levels until 8 weeks after drug administration.[55] The return of activity is due to resynthesis of new enzyme.[56] The half-lives for synthesis of plasma and erythrocyte cholinesterase in humans are 6.7 and 15 days, respectively.[56]

When administered in the dosage regimen used for treatment of *S. haematobium* infection, metrifonate is well tolerated. Cholinergic symptoms such as nausea, vomiting, bronchospasm, abdominal discomfort, diarrhea, and weakness are rare at recommended dosage levels,[57] but there have been isolated reports of organophosphate poisoning requiring treatment with atropine.[58] The inhibition of cholinesterase is of potential importance if patients are administered muscle relaxants such as succinylcholine during surgery.[59] Although there were several early reports of delayed neurotoxicity from metrifonate, more recent and thorough experience does not confirm this.[10] After administration to animals, metrifonate has been shown to methylate DNA at the N-7 position of guanine[60] and the drug has a low mutagenic activity against *Salmonella* test strains in vitro.[61] Although it has been reported that the host-mediated mutagenic activity is fairly high,[61] in mammalian systems tests of both mutagenicity and carcinogenicity have been negative.[43]

Oxamniquine

Oxamniquine is a hydroxylated metabolite of a 2-aminotetrahydroquinoline schistosomicide called *desoxymansil*. The hydrox-

Oxamniquine

ylated metabolite was found to be produced in several animal species and to have impressive schistosomicidal activity.[62]

ANTISCHISTOSOMAL ACTIVITY AND THERAPEUTIC USE. Oxamniquine has a potent schistosomicidal action against *S. mansoni* in rodent models but there is essentially no activity against *S. japonicum* or *S. haematobium*.[62] Male *S. mansoni* are markedly more susceptible than females in vivo but not in vitro.[62] Although oxamniquine exhibits anticholinergic properties, its primary mode of action seems to result from an ATP-dependent enzymatic activation of the drug, in susceptible schistosomes, to an unstable phosphate ester that dissociates to yield a chemically reactive cation. This intermediate then alkylates essential macromolecules, including DNA.[63] This mechanism is consistent with the high resistance of certain strains of *S. mansoni* to oxamniquine. Although the drug is readily eliminated from the host, the effect on the parasite is delayed and the hepatic shift occurs over a period of 5 or 6 days.[64] Egg laying by females stops by 3 days after drug administration.[10]

Oxamniquine is used as a second-choice drug to treat infection by *S. mansoni* and the susceptibility of various geographic strains varies widely.[62] In South America, cure rates of 80%–95% are achieved in adults with a single 15 mg/kg dose.[65,66] In some areas of Africa (e.g., Rhodesia, Sudan), a total dose of 60 mg/kg (administered as two 15 mg/kg doses daily for 2 days) is required for optimal effect, yielding cure rates of 82%–95%;[67,68] however, in other areas (e.g., Nigeria, Tanzania), a total dose of 30 mg/kg is sufficient for a 90%–97% cure rate.[69,70] Oxamniquine has been effective in some areas where praziquantel is less effective.[9] Oxamniquine also has been used successfully in combination with metrifonate for the treatment of mixed infections with *S. mansoni* and *S. haematobium*. In some cases, strains

of *S. mansoni* that have not responded to therapy with other antischistosomal drugs have been found to have decreased sensitivity to oxamniquine as well. This relative resistance to several drugs seems to reflect specific strain differences rather than prior exposure to antischistosomal drugs and selection of multiply resistant parasites.[71]

PHARMACOKINETICS AND ADVERSE EFFECTS. Oxamniquine is well absorbed from the gastrointestinal tract.[72] Peak serum levels of about 0.8–0.9 µg/ml are achieved 1–2 h after oral administration of 1 g of oxamniquine to an adult (approximately a 15 mg/kg dose.[73] Food retards absorption of oxamniquine and limits the concentration attained in plasma. The serum level declines with a half-life of 1.5–2 h.[73] From 40% to 70% of the drug is excreted in the urine in the first 12 h, with less than 2% present as the unchanged drug and the remainder as two carboxylic acid metabolites.[72]

Oxamniquine is generally well tolerated. The most frequent side effects are transient dizziness and drowsiness, which have been experienced by the majority of patients in some studies.[66,68,70] Occasional side effects include headache, nausea, abdominal pain, and diarrhea. It is possible that the incidence of these side effects is reduced (at the risk of some decrease in absorption) by administering the drug with a small amount of food.[67] Oxamniquine may have a stimulating effect on the central nervous system: although rare, convulsions have occurred within a few hours of administration, especially in patients with a history of epilepsy.[10] Rarely, small and transient elevations in serum transaminase activity have been reported. Oxamniquine metabolites may color the urine a deep orange.[68] Some investigators have reported that occasional patients receiving a total dose of 60 or 90 mg/kg have experienced a characteristic "oxamniquine fever" in which the body temperature rose to 38°–39°C 1 to 2 days after completion of therapy and remained elevated for 2 to 5 days.[74] A few patients experiencing the fever have developed a Loeffler-like syndrome with marked eosinophilia and scattered pulmonary infiltrates. Coincident with the fever, there was increased excretion of schistosomal antigens in the urine.[74] Both oxamniquine itself and urine taken from mice treated with oxamniquine have low mutagenic activity against *Salmonella* test strains in vitro, and there is one report that the host-mediated mutagenic activity of the drug is fairly high.[61] Therefore, oxamniquine is contraindicted in pregnancy.

Bithionol

Bithionol is a dichlorophenol compound that was originally used to treat fluke infections in livestock. Prior to the introduction of praziquantel, bithionol was the drug of

Bithionol

choice for treating infection by the sheep liver fluke *Fasciola hepatica* and the lung fluke *Paragonimus westermani*. Bithionol is still the drug of choice for fascioliasis (infection by the sheep liver fluke), since this helminth may not respond to praziquantel. Bithionol is now an alternative drug to praziquantel for the treatment of lung fluke infection. For both infections 30–50 mg of drug per kg of body weight are administered orally on alternate days for 10–15 doses. This regimen yields a cure rate of greater than 90% in patients with pulmonary paragonimiasis[75,76] and it is highly effective in the treatment of fascioliasis.[77] The mechanism of bithionol action is not known. Nausea, vomiting, diarrhea, abdominal pain, urticarial rashes, and skin photosensitivity reactions are common side effects.

Triclabendazole

This is a narrow-spectrum benzimidazole derivative used in veterinary medicine that has shown considerable promise in the treatment of human infection by the sheep liver fluke *Fasciola hepatica*.[78,79] Triclabendazole is given as a single dose of 10 mg/kg. It has been found to be safe and effective in ther-

apeutic doses, and because of its low toxicity, is now preferred over bithionol. The mechanism of action of the benzimidazoles is described later under mebendazole.

Drugs Used to Treat Tapeworm Infections

Tapeworm Infection

Tapeworm infection (cestodiasis) occurs when uncooked meat or fish containing the encysted larval forms of the organism are ingested. In the intestine of the host, the head of the tapeworm, or scolex, attaches to the intestinal wall. The worm then grows by producing large numbers of egg-containing segments. Growth can continue until, in the fish tapeworm (*Diphyllobothrium latum*), for example, there are 3000 to 4000 segments and the worm is 30 feet long. Tapeworms are hermaphroditic, and the fertilized eggs are excreted as the segments are passed with the feces. The eggs can then be ingested by the intermediate host in which the larval form developes, thus completing the cycle. In some cases, the normal course of events is altered when humans ingest the eggs instead of the larvae. This happens with the pork tapeworm (*Taenia solium*) where humans are the usual definitive host and the intermediate host is the pig. If tapeworm eggs are ingested by humans, the larvae can develop in human tissues. Another tapeworm that frequently parasitizes humans is the rodent tapeworm *Hymenolepis nana*. In all, about 30 species of tapeworm may infect humans at some stage in their life cycle; the reader is referred to a review by Gemmell and Johnstone.[80] for details of the biology of and treatment of infection by the less common species, such as the rodent tapeworm *Hymenolepis diminuta*, the fish tapeworm *Diphyllobothrium pacificum*, and the dog tapeworms *Dipylidium canium* and *Echinococcus granulosus*.

The clinical symptoms of tapeworm infection by adult forms growing in the intestine are surprisingly mild in the well-nourished, otherwise healthy patient. There may be vague abdominal discomfort and pain, which is relieved by food, as well as weakness, weight loss, epigastric fullness, and anemia. Intestinal obstruction due to the mass of the worms is rare. Praziquantel is now considered to be the drug of choice for all intestinal tapeworm infections (Table 15–1). As reviewed earlier in the chapter, a single dose of praziquantel is as efective as the older drug niclosamide against *D. latum, D. pacificum, D. canium, T. saginata,* and *T. solium.*[22,23] A single dose of praziquantel yields a cure rate of 93% against the dwarf tapeworm *H. nana,* an organism that requires a 5-day course of therapy with niclosamide.

Ingestion of tapeworm eggs that produce migratory larvae can be very serious, since the larvae may develop in the orbit, brain, or other organs to form growing space-occupying masses. Tissue infection with the larvae stage of *Taenia solium* (cysticercosis), and especially neurocysticercosis, the most prevalent helminthic infection of the brain, was for a long time amenable only to surgery. The therapeutic use of praziquantel, and more recently of albendazole, has provided medical treatment for neurocysticercosis.[81] For patients with inactive disease and calcified tissue cysts, specific cesticidal therapy is not needed, whereas active neurocysticercosis requires drug treatment. The administration of either praziquantel or albendazole results in the reduction or disappearance of cysts in 80% to 90% of patients. In comparative trials, albendazole was more effective than praziquantel in reducing the number and size of cysts and in inducing overall clinical improvement.[81,82] Adjunctive therapy with dexamethasone is recommended for patients with numerous cysts and for those in whom neurologic symptoms or intracranial hypertension develops after the initiation of therapy against cysticerci.[81] Ingestion of dog tapeworm eggs (*Echinococcus granulosus*) produces hydatid disease. Albendazole has expanded the therapeutic options for patients with cystic hydatid disease.[83] Surgery remains the definitive treatment for this disease, but it carries the risks of operative morbidity, recurrence of cysts, and spillage of fluid from the cysts, which can lead to anaphylaxis or dissemination of the infection. Albendazole reduces the viability of protoscolices and cysts, and its hepatic metabolite, the sulf-

oxide, is also active against the larval cestodes.[4]

Drugs Used to Treat Intestinal Roundworm Infections

Intestinal Roundworm Infections—The Scope of the Problem

Intestinal infection with roundworms is a very common problem in developing countries, with the most commonly encountered parasites being *Ascaris,* hookworms (*Ancylostoma duodenale* and *Necator americanus*), and whipworms (*Trichuris trichiura*). *Ascaris* is the most common of all human parasitoses, with about 30% of the world population or well over 1 billion people affected (Fig. 15–1).[84,85] In some communities 90% of the population is infected with *Ascaris* and in others 100% have whipworm infection.[86] In some parts of South America as much as 70% of the population has hookworm infection.[87] Individuals are often infected with several species of worms simultaneously.[87] By contrast, in technically advanced countries, intestinal nematodes other than pinworms are often considered to be a rarity by physicians. It has been estimated, however, that in 1977 approximately 4 million people in the United States were infected with *Ascaris,* 2.2 million with *Trichuris,* and 700,000 with hookworm.[88] A more recent study in the United States found that the most commonly identified helminths were nematodes, with 1.5% of the population being infested with hookworm, 1.2% with *Trichuris,* and 0.8% with *Ascaris.*[89]

For most people whose worm burden is light, symptoms are few or nonexistent, but heavy infections can lead to obstruction and, in the case of hookworm, to anemia. Because the population involved is large and reinfection is a virtual certainty, chemotherapy of intestinal worm infection is often carried out on a mass scale in conjunction with public health measures to break the transmission cycle. Several medications are available for use in such community-wide deworming programs (Table 15–2), and the choice of a drug is determined by the nature of the infecting agents, the relative drug

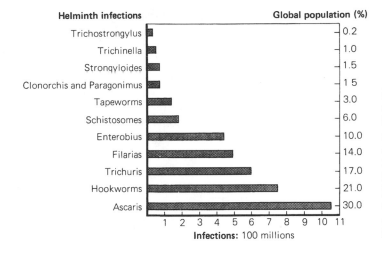

Helminth infections

Trichostrongylus
Trichinella
Stronqyloides
Clonorchis and Paragonimus
Tapeworms
Schistosomes
Enterobius
Filarias
Trichuris
Hookworms
Ascaris

Infections: 100 millions

Global population (%)

0.2
1.0
1.5
1 5
3.0
6.0
10.0
14.0
17.0
21.0
30.0

Figure 15–1. Relative incidence of helminth infections estimated in the world population. The number of infections is based on an estimated world population of 3.55 billion persons in 1969. Since 1969, the world population has increased but the percentage of people infected has not changed appreciably. (Adapted from Standen.[85])

Table 15–2. *Drugs used to treat nematode (roundworm) infections.*

Infecting organism	Drug of choice	Alternative
INTESTINAL ROUNDWORMS		
Ascaris lumbricoides	Mebandazole, pyrantel pamoate, or albendazole	Piperazine
Enterobius vermicularis (pinworm)	Pyrantel pamoate, mebendazole, or albendazole	
Strongyloides stercoralis	Ivermectin	Thiabendazole
Trichuris trichiura (whipworm)	Mebendazole	Albendazole
Ancylostoma duodenale (hookworm)	Mebendazole, pyrantel pamoate, or albendazole	
Necator americanus (hookworm)	Mebendazole, pyrantel pamoate, or albendazole	
Cutaneous larva migrans	Albendazole	Thiabendazole
Visceral larva migrans (toxocariasis)	Diethylcarbazine	Albendazole or mebendazole
TISSUE ROUNDWORMS		
Wuchereria bancrofti *Brugia malayi* *Loa loa* Tropical eosinophilia	Diethylcarbamazine	
Onchocerca volvulus	Ivermectin	Diethylcarbamazine
Dracunculus medinensis (guinea worm)	Metronidazole	None

467

costs, and the ease of drug administration. As multiple worm infections are common, mebendazole or albendazole are particularly attractive because both are very effective against all members of the so-called worm trinity of *Ascaris, Trichuris*, and hookworm.[4,84] Mebendazole costs more than several other drugs that are effective against intestinal roundworms, a consideration that is of great importance when community-wide therapy is undertaken in poor regions.

The principal drawback to deworming programs is that they have to be repeated frequently at regular intervals. Although deworming may receive an enthusiastic reception initially when the worms expelled are large, numerous, and obvious, communities often lose interest as time passes and successive treatments yield fewer or no visible worms.[90] Since the intestinal roundworms of greatest medical significance are *Ascaris* and hookworm, it is appropriate to briefly review the infections produced by these parasites.

ASCARIASIS. The adult *Ascaris*, which looks rather like an earthworm, lives in the lumen of the small intestine. Humans become infected by ingesting embyronated eggs. When the eggs reach the duodenum, the larvae hatch and begin a remarkable odyssey that eventually returns them to the intestinal lumen. The larvae penetrate the wall of the small intestine and are carried through the right heart to the lungs. They then penetrate the walls of the pulmonary capillaries, emerge into the air sacs, and migrate up the pulmonary tree to the epiglottis. This period of larval migration is occasionally accompanied by cough, fever, and pulmonary infiltration. Signs of hypersensitivity, such as eosinophilia and urticaria, may be observed. Occasionally, the larvae reach the general circulation and become lodged in tissues where they can provoke local reactions.

The larvae are swallowed after they reach the epiglottis, and upon their second arrival in the small intestine they develop into adult male and female worms. The patient at this stage of infection may be asymptomatic or have vague symptoms of abdominal distress

(epigastric pain, nausea, vomiting, and anorexia). More serious problems can arise as a result of migration of the adult worms into the pancreatic and bile ducts, gallbladder, and liver or from complete obstruction of the appendix or intestinal lumen. The byproducts of living or dead worms can produce severe reactions in sensitized patients. Migration of the adult worms, and the resulting complications, can be stimulated by drug therapy. A number of people who are infected with *Ascaris* are also infected with hookworm. Treatment of hookworm infection can provoke the migration of *Ascaris*. In this case, the symptoms that arise as a side effect of the drug are due to an effect on an entirely different parasite from that being treated. When there is infection by more than one type of intestinal helminth, *Ascaris* is often treated first in order to avoid promoting migration of the worm. Alternatively, one may administer the broad-spectrum anthelminthic drugs mebendazole or albendazole, which are effective against both *Ascaris* and hookworm.

The older, less efficient, and more toxic ascaricides have been largely replaced by more effective, less toxic compounds, including mebendazole, pyrantel pamoate, and albendazole, which are now the drugs of choice. Pyrantel pamoate has the advantage of not possessing the teratogenic potential of the benzimidazoles, albendazole, and mebendazole. The benzimidazoles, however, have the advantage in that they are also effective against *Trichuris* (whipworm). Piperazine is an effective alternative to these drugs, but is seldom used because of the risk of occasional neurotoxic and hypersensitivity reactions. Cure with any of these drugs can be achieved in nearly all cases of ascariasis.

HOOKWORM. The two types of hookworm causing infection in humans are *Necator americanus* and *Ancylostoma duodenale*. *N. americanus* predominates in the United States, whereas *A. duodenale* occurs nearly exclusively in other parts of the world. These species affect over 20% of the human population and flourish chiefly between latitudes

30°S and 40°N. In more northern regions, hookworm may be found in restricted loci, such as mines and large mountain tunnels, where the larvae can live in the soil from which they can penetrate exposed skin. Upon coming in contact with the skin, hookworm larvae actively burrow through the skin to the lymphatics or venules where they are carried via the blood through the right heart to the lungs. The larvae are unable to pass through the capillaries and they break through capillary walls to the alveoli. Then, like *Ascaris*, they migrate up the bronchi and the trachea and are swallowed, finally reaching the lumen of the intestine. By the time they reach the intestine the larvae have developed a buccal capsule by which they become attached to the intestinal mucosa. Ulcerations are created at the point of contact. The worms produce an anticoagulant that slows down clotting where they break through the mucosa, and they ingest blood from the mucosal vessels of the patient. Definitive diagnosis depends upon finding eggs in the feces.

The penetration of the larvae into the skin produces localized erythema and severe itching, and the passage of large numbers of worms through the lungs may produce signs of pneumonitis. The adult worms in the intestine can produce gastrointestinal symptoms, such as abdominal fullness and epigastric pain; often, there are no acute symptoms. The symptoms of hookworm infection are characteristic of a progressive, hypochromic, microcytic anemia of the nutritional deficiency type. Anemia is secondary to chronic blood loss, which is superimposed on such contributing factors as malnutrition and an iron-deficient diet in many infected individuals. Treatment of hookworm infection involves two objectives: the first is to treat the anemia and restore blood values to normal and the second is to expel the worms. The hemoglobin levels in patients with hookworm infection can usually be restored to normal by proper diet and administering iron, even when the hookworms themselves go untreated.[90] Mebendazole and albendazole are now the drugs of choice against both *A. duodenale* and *N.*

americanus and both agents have the advantage of being effective against other roundworms when there is multiple infection. Topical or oral thiabendazole is the drug of choice for treating cutaneous larva migrans or "creeping eruption," which is due most commonly to penetration of the skin of humans by larvae of the dog hookworm, *A. brazilense*.

WHIPWORM. Whipworm infection (*Trichuris trichiura*) is encountered throughout the world, especially in warm, humid climates. It is often found in association with *Ascaris* and hookworms. The infection is obtained after eating food contaminated with parasite eggs but, except in heavily infected young children, the adult worms usually do not cause problems. Generally, infection is accompanied by mild toxicity and anemia, but heavily infected children may exhibit severe clinical illness, including anemia, fingerclubbing, bloody diarrhea, and rectal prolapse.[91] Whipworm is treated with one of the benzimidazoles. Both mebendazole and albendazole are considered safe and effective in the treatment of whipworm alone or in combination with *Ascaris* and hookworm infections.

TRICHINOSIS. Trichellosis (or trichinosis) results from infection by the nematode *Trichinella spiralis*. Trichinosis is acquired in humans by eating raw or insufficiently cooked flesh of infected wild animals or domestic pigs, and it is a health problem in the United States and Canada, as well as in several South American countries. An initial intestinal phase is followed 7–9 days later by the invasive stage in which involvement of skeletal muscles usually dominates the clinical picture. Albendazole and other benzimidazoles are effective against the intestinal forms of this parasite that are present early in infection. However, it is questionable as to whether they are effective against larvae that have migrated to muscle. Corticosteroids are of value in controlling the acute and dangerous symptoms such as the cerebral edema found in more established infections.

Albendazole and Mebendazole

Albendazole and mebendazole are benzimidazole carbamate derivatives that have broad-spectrum anthelminthic activity.

Mebendazole

Albendazole

These compounds have been reviewed by Van den Bossche et al.[92] and Venkatesan.[93]

Many benzimidazoles have been tested, but those most useful therapeutically have modifications at the 2 and/or 5 positions of the benzimidazole ring system. Three compounds, thiabendazole, mebendazole, and albendazole, have been used extensively for the treatment of human helminthiasis. Thiabendazole is active against a wide range of nematodes that infect the gastrointestinal tract but its use in medicine has been declining because of its relative toxicity. Mebendazole, the prototype benzimidazole carbamate, was introduced for the treatment of roundworm infections. Albendazole is a newer benzimidazole carbamate that is used worldwide against a variety of helminths.[94] It has become a drug of choice for treating neurocysticercosis (caused by the larval stage of *Taenia solium*) and the drug of choice for cystic hydatid disease.[93]

THERAPEUTIC USE. Mebendazole and albendazole are both highly effective against a variety of nematode infections. Mebendazole is used principally in the treatment of *Ascaris lumbricoides* (common roundworm), *Trichuris trichiura* (whipworm), and *Ancylostoma duodenale* and *Necator americanus* (hookworm) infections and is particularly useful in mixed infections because of its broad spectrum of activity.[3] The most commonly used regimens are 100 mg twice daily for 3 days (individual patients) or a single dose of 500 mg (in mass chemotherapy programs). Both single-dose and multidose regimens are highly effective against roundworm infections, with cure rates and egg reduction rates of 90% to 100%. The egg reduction rates are similar for both regimens in whipworm infections, but in hookworm infections, the multidose regimen appears to be better.[3] Pinworms are the intestinal roundworms most commonly encountered by physicians in the United States where it is estimated that 42 million people are infected.[88] A single 100 mg dose of mebendazole is over 90% effective in eliminating pinworms (*Enterobius vermicularis*).[95,96] Because the pinworm ova are not destroyed, the dose has to be repeated two to four times at 7- to 14-day intervals.[97] In high doses, mebendazole is also moderately effective against hydatid cyst disease caused by *Echinococcus granulosus*. Other infections in which mebendazole has been reported to have some efficacy include those caused by *Strongyloides stercoralis*, *Trichinella spiralis*, *Toxocara* spp., *Mansonella perstans*, and the tapeworms *Taenia solium* and *T. saginata* and *Hymenolepis nana*.[98–103] The broad spectrum of anthelminthic action and virtual atoxicity of mebendazole make it particularly attractive in the treatment of patients with multiple intestinal worm infections.[104]

Although very little mebendazole is absorbed from the intestinal tract, attempts have been made to administer the drug in very high dosage for the treatment of tissue roundworm infections. Mebendazole is active against intestinal adults and larvae of *Trichinella spiralis,* but it is unclear if encysted larvae in the muscle are affected.[92] There have been several reports that high daily doses of mebendazole for periods of several weeks or months may be useful in the treatment of hydatid disease,[105,106] but its role in treating this infection has not been established.[92,107]

Albendazole is effective in single doses of 400 mg or as multidoses against *A. lumbri-*

coides, with cure rates and egg reduction rates of 90% to 100% being achieved.[3] Single-dose treatment with albendazole produces higher cure rates in both hookworm and whipworm infections than single-dose treatment with mebendazole. Egg reduction rates in hookworm infections are also higher with single-dose treatment with albendazole, whereas in whipworm infections, egg reduction rates are similar with the two drugs. Heavy infections of whipworm respond well to a 3-day course of albendazole. Multidose albendazole has also been found to be useful in the treatment of strongyloidiasis, with cure rates of 38% to 95%, depending on the dose schedule and the length of the follow-up period. Because its adverse effects are milder, treatment with albendazole results in better patient compliance than treatment with thiabendazole. Other infections in which albendazole has been reported to be of value include intestinal capillariais, taeniasis, cysticercosis, cystic and alvelolar hydatidosis, cutaneous larva migrans and visceral larva migrans, clonorchiasis, and trichenellosis.[3,93] Albendazole is an approved drug, but for many of these infections its use is considered investigational.

MECHANISM OF ACTION. The mechanism of action of benzimidazoles has been extensively reviewed.[108] Despite the diverse effects of benzimidazoles, the primary mode of action of these drugs appears to involve their interaction with the eucaryotic cytosketetal protein, β-tubulin, inhibiting its polymerization into microtubules. All the benzimidazoles have a similar mechanism of action, but most of the studies have been done with mebendazole. Studies with benzimidazole-resistant worms, such as the free-living nematode *Caenorhabditis elegans* and the sheep nematode *Haemonchus contortus*, have provided insight into the mechanism of action of this group of drugs.[108–110] Resistant strains of *H. contortus* showed reduced high-affinity drug binding to β-tubulin and alterations in β-tubulin isotype gene expression that correlate with drug resistance. Resistance reflects changes in allele frequency of tubulin genes rather than novel genetic rearrangements induced by drug exposure.[110]

In ultrastructural studies it has been shown that mebendazole disrupts cytoplasmic microtubules and inhibits the movement of organelles in nematode intestinal cells.[111,112] In *Ascaris*, most of the mebendazole is taken up by the cells of the esophagus and intestine where it is found in the cytosol, with some of the drug being bound to proteins with molecular weights characteristic of tubulin monomers and dimers.[92] Mebendazole binds to tubulin purified from bovine brain and it inhibits polymerization of tubulin into microtubules.[113,114] The drug binds to brain tubulin in a manner that is competitive with the binding of colchicine.[114,115] Mebendazole inhibits the binding of radiolabeled colchicine to tubulin purified from *Ascaris suum* embryos at lower concentrations than those at which it competes for colchicine binding to tubulin from bovine brain.[115] This has led to the suggestion that some of the selective toxicity may reflect differential binding of the drug to nematode versus host cell tubulin.[115]

In early experiments, it was noted that mebendazole at low concentration inhibits the uptake of exogenous glucose into *Ascaris*.[116] This is followed by a depletion of glycogen in the parasite and ultimately by a decreased ability to generate ATP. The inhibition of glucose uptake is probably secondary to a primary effect on microtubule assembly, but the connection between the two events is not understood. In addition to its effect on adult worms, mebendazole is toxic to nematode eggs.[117] Even at high concentration there is no effect on fully formed hookworm larvae; but when rats were fed large amounts of the drug, a slow but lethal effect was observed against the encysted phase of *Trichinella* larvae.[118]

PHARMACOKINETICS. Generally, benzimidazoles have limited solubility and therefore poor absorption following oral administration; thus, their greatest value is in the treatment of intestinal helminth infections. After oral administration of 1.5 g of mebendazole to fasting adult volunteers, plasma concentrations are 5 ng/ml or less.[119] Absorption is enhanced by administering the drug with a meal. Plasma levels of 5–40 ng/ml are achieved after administration of a 1.5 g dose with food.[119,120] The virtual absence of absorption is an asset when treating intestinal helminth infections, but it means that very large doses must be administered for treatment of tissue infections by larval forms. Patients receiving 50 mg/kg/day of mebendazole orally for the treatment of hydatid disease (drug ingested with food) were found to have serum concentrations in the range of 10–37 ng/ml and simultaneous concentrations of only about 1 ng/ml in hydatid cyst fluid.[121] The mebendazole that is absorbed is excreted in the urine, mainly as the decarboxylated derivative.[95] Oral absorption of albendazole is also very poor; after an oral dose of 400 mg, peak plasma levels of albendazole reach 0.04–0.55 µg/ml, with great variation between individuals.[122] The absorption of albendazole is enhanced by a fatty meal. Albendazole is 70% plasma protein bound and has a half-life of 9 h. Concentration in cerebrospinal fluid and brain tissue are about 50% and 40%, respectively, of plasma levels.[123]

ADVERSE EFFECTS. Mebendazole appears to be almost pharmacologically inert. It has no effect on the central nervous system and has no analgesic, hypnotic, or anticonvulsive effects.[92] When the drug has been used to treat intestinal helminth infection it has been noted to be free of side effects, although abdominal pain and diarrhea have occurred with expulsion of worms in patients with massive infection. Patients receiving high doses for the treatment of hydatid disease may experience fever during the first few days of treatment, possibly as a response to drug-induced tissue necrosis.[124] Large doses are very well tolerated by various animal species.[125] But the manufacturer warns that (in spite of the limited absorption of the drug) embryotoxic and teratogenic activity have been demonstrated in rats at single oral doses of 10 mg/kg. Accordingly, mebendazole is contraindicated in pregnant women nor is advised in children less than 2 years of age. Albendazole also is very well tolerated and produces few side effects when used for short-term therapy of gastrointestinal helminthiasis, even in patients with heavy worm burdens. Gastrointestinal upset, dizziness, rash, and alopecia occur but do not require discontinuation of the drug. Following prolonged use, 15% of patients develop reversible increases in serum hepatic transaminases, necessitating monitoring and withdrawal of treatment in some cases.[93] Albendazole also is embryotoxic and teratogenic in animals and, therefore, should be avoided if possible in pregnancy and during lactation. However, it is being used without serious problems in older children.[93]

Piperazine

Piperazine is very effective in treating *Ascaris* infection and it is an adequate drug against pinworm (*Enterobius vermicularis*) infection. A single course of therapy for ascariasis

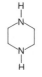

Piperazine

(75 mg/kg to a maximum of 3.5 g/day for 2 days) results in a cure in 95% of the cases.[126] Piperazine has been replaced by mebendazole, albendazole, and pyrantel pamoate, as drugs of choice for *Ascaris* and *Enterobius* infections. However, it is a useful and inexpensive second choice to mebendazole or pyrantel pamoate in treating patients infected with both *Ascaris* and *Enterobius*. Piperazine acts by paralyzing the worm. The paralyzed worm, unable to maintain its position in the intestinal tract, is then passively expelled by the normal peristaltic action of the bowel; no purgative is required. As piperazine produces flaccid paralysis of the worms, it is regarded as the best form of therapy when there is intestinal or biliary tract obstruction. Piperazine may be administered in a 7-day course of therapy for enterobiasis (65 mg/kg to a maximum of 2 g/day), where cure rates of 84%–97% are obtained.[126] As with the other drugs used to treat enterobiasis, a second course of therapy must be administered after 2 weeks. The requirement of daily administration for a week

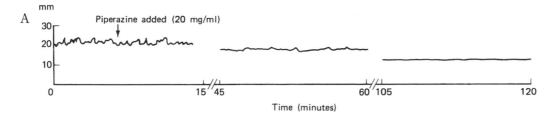

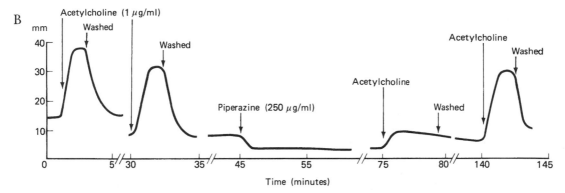

Figure 15–2. (A) The effect of piperazine on the spontaneous contraction of a whole *Ascaris* attached to a strain gauge. When a whole *Ascaris* is exposed to piperazine, there is a delay period followed by the development of flaccid paralysis. A 10 mm deflection on the record is equivalent to a 2 g increase in tension. (The tracing is adapted from Norton and deBeer.[127] (B) The effect of piperazine on the response of a crude nerve-muscle preparation of *Ascaris* to acetylcholine. The anterior portion of a worm (containing the main ganglia) was cut off, the worm was split, and the intestinal tract removed. The remainder was attached to a strain gauge and suspended in Ringer's solution. Piperazine decreases the response of the preparation in a reversible manner. (The tracing is adapted from Norton and deBeer.[127])

makes piperazine less attractive than other drugs, such as mebendazole or pyrantel, which may be administered in a single-dose regimen for treatment of enterobiasis.

If piperazine citrate is added to a bath containing an *Ascaris* attached to a strain gauge, the irregular contraction of the worm ceases after a few minutes and the worm remains in flaccid paralysis (Fig. 15–2A).[127] The delay may reflect the time required for the drug to reach its site of action. The time of onset of the paralysis in the intact worm preparation decreases with increasing doses of the drug. If a crudely dissected section from *Ascaris* is suspended in a similar bath, there is no spontaneous movement of the muscle. The muscle contracts readily upon addition of acetylcholine, and the response to acetylcholine is reversibly antagonized by piperazine (Fig. 15–2 B).[127] Electrical stim-

ulation of the muscle of the body wall causes a contraction that is not blocked by piperazine. These observations are consistent with the conclusion that piperazine paralyzes *Ascaris* by a blocking action at the myoneural junction. Piperazine does not have this effect on mammalian muscle preparations.[128]

Piperazine is readily absorbed from the intestinal tract. The basis for its selective toxicity, which is not explained by the fact that the parasite is exposed to very high concentrations of drug in comparison with the host, is not entirely clear. The following model is one of several that have been proposed. Although the data are somewhat sketchy, it appears that contraction of *Ascaris* muscle is initiated by rhythmic spike potentials generated by pacemakers in the muscle membrane itself.[129] Acetylcholine depolarizes the muscle cells, thereby increasing the

TREATMENT OF PARASITIC DISEASE

frequency of the spike potentials and the degree of muscle contraction. The results of electrophysiological studies suggest that piperazine increases the resting potential of the muscle so that pacemaker activity is suppressed, and flaccid paralysis ensues.[130] It has been suggested that piperazine acts as an inhibitory neurotransmitter.[130] Indeed, it could be an analog of a natural inhibitory transmitter in *Ascaris*. Paradoxically, at high concentrations piperazine acts as a nicotinic agonist in rat sympathetic neurons,[131] an action that may contribute to some of the neurotoxic side effects that can occur during therapy.

Piperazine is available in tablet and liquid preparations. It is prepared in a number of salt combinations but there is no important pharmacological difference between the citrate, the phosphate, and the adipate.[132] The drug is readily absorbed from the gastrointestinal tract and much of an oral dose is excreted in the urine within 24 hs.[133] The drug generally is quite safe. Occasionally, vomiting, diarrhea, urticaria, or dizziness occur. Rarely, patients experience difficulty in focusing as a side effect of the drug. Piperazine can produce a neurotoxicity characterized by incoordination and hypotonia.[134] This cerebellar type of ataxia ("worm wobble") is rare, but it is more likely to occur in patients with compromised renal function and possibly in those receiving concomitant phenothiazine therapy.[135] Patients who are epileptic may have an exacerbation of seizures and another drug should be used.[136]

Pyrantel Pamoate

Several pyrantel derivatives were found to have excellent activity against a variety of worms that parasitize livestock.[137] In human trials, it was found that pyrantel is well tolerated and highly effective in treating enterobiasis,[138] ascariasis,[139] and hookworm infection.[140] A single dose of 11 mg/kg (maximum dosage 1 g) yields a cure rate of 97% in ascariasis and enterobiasis.[141] As with the other drugs used to treat enterobiasis, a second course of therapy must be administered after 2 weeks. Because of its very low toxicity, low cost, and efficacy in single-

dose administration, pyrantel is often considered to be equivalent to mebendazole as a drug of choice for ascariasis and enterobiasis, although for ascariasis it is an investigational drug. Mebendazole has an advan-

Pyrantel

tage, however, in that the same dose may be administered to everyone, whereas the dosage of pyrantel must be calculated according to the patient's body weight. A cure rate of about 85% is obtained with a single dose of pyrantel in the treatment of hookworm infection. Pyrantel is also effective against *Trichostrongylus* species,[142] but it is not very effective against trichuriasis.[143] In both hookworm and *Trichostrongylus* infection, pyrantel is again an alternative drug of choice to mebendazole and albendazole, and in both of these infections its use is considered investigational.

Pyrantel acts by paralyzing the worms, which are then passed out of the intestine with the normal fecal flow. In *Ascaris* preparations, pyrantel has been shown to have a depolarizing action, causing contracture of the worm.[144] This spastic paralysis is the opposite of the effect described for piperazine, which produces hyperpolarization and paralysis in relaxation. Indeed, in microelectrode studies, piperazine has been shown to antagonize the effects of pyrantel on the membrane potential of single muscle cells in *Ascaris*.[144] Pyrantel also behaves as a depolarizing neuromuscular blocking agent in several mammalian systems.[144,145] Two factors apparently determine the selective effect: (1) pyrantel is incompletely absorbed and the worms are exposed to high concentrations in the intestine; (2) the neuromuscular junction of the worm is more sensitive to the drug than that of the host. Pyrantel is more than 100 times as active as acetylcholine in causing contraction of strip muscle preparations from *Ascaris*.

Most of a dose of pyrantel pamoate is excreted unchanged in the feces. About 4% of a dose is excreted in the urine, 1% as the unchanged drug, and 3% as metabolites.[141] Although systemic absorption is limited, enough occurs to cause occasional side effects like, headache and dizziness.[141] The principal adverse effects involve the gastrointestinal tract, with about 5% of patients experiencing some nausea, vomiting, diarrhea, and cramps.[141] Transient elevation of SGOT may occur, and pyrantel should be used with caution in patients with preexisting liver dysfunction.

Thiabendazole

Thiabendazole is a benzimidazole derivative with a broad spectrum of action against gastrointestinal helminths infecting both humans and animals.[146] The literature on thi-

Thiabendazole

abendazole has been summarized in a symposium[147] and a review.[148] Thiabendazole, like the other benzimidazoles, mebendazole and albendazole, acts by binding to tubulin.

THERAPEUTIC USE. Although thiabendazole has a broad spectrum of anthelminthic action, it is used clinically principally for treating strongyloidiasis. A 2-day course of therapy at a dosage of 25 mg/kg given twice a day (maximum dose 3 g/day) is reported to yield cure rates of about 95% in uncomplicated strongyloidiasis and enterobiasis and about 77% in hookworm and *Ascaris* infection.[149] Early studies indicating cure rates of nearly 100% in the treatment of strongyloidiasis evaluated patients for only a short time after treatment.[150,151] Another study involving long-term clinical, parasitological, and serological assessment of infection suggests that the cure rate is in the 75%–90% range.[152] Thiabendazole is generally administered for 2 days, but in disseminated strongyloidiasis the treatment should be extended for at least 5–7 days, or until the parasites

are eradicated. Albendazole and ivermectin are also effective for intestinal disease, but efficacy for disseminated strongyloidiasis has been shown only for thiabendazole.

In addition to affecting adult worms, thiabendazole also prevents the development of nematode eggs and larvae.[146,147] This observation has led to the use of thiabendazole in the treatment of human disease by larval forms, as in trichinosis and cutaneous larva migrans. Cutaneous larva migrans, also called *creeping eruption*, is caused by larvae of canine and feline hookworms that penetrate and migrate under the skin. Their presence causes intense irritation and itching. Administered orally, thiabendazole produces a rapid and effective clinical response in this condition.[153] Cutaneous larva migrans can be successfully treated by topical application of thiabendazole cream or by applying petroleum jelly containing a pulverized oral tablet.[154,155]

Young children sometimes ingest the eggs of *Toxocara* worms of dogs and cats. The larvae that emerge in the intestine penetrate the gut wall and are carried about the body. In the human host, the larvae are unable to complete their usual development, but they can cause fever, eosinophilia, hepatomegaly, and pneumonitis.[156] This infection is called *visceral larva migrans* and there are reports that thiabendazole treatment for 7 days produces rapid clinical improvement.[157] Although diethylcarbamazine, mebendazole, and albendazole are usually the preferred drugs, none of these agents has been shown to conclusively alter the course of larval migrans.[158] The limited experience with thiabendazole in the treatment of trichinosis indicates that it has a beneficial clinical effect,[159] with decreased temperature and muscle pain; but the larvae in humans are not killed by the drug.[160] It is probable that the beneficial action reported in trichinosis is due to an anti-inflammatory effect of thiabendazole.[161] Mebendazole is also active against enteric stages of the parasite, but neither of these drugs have been conclusively demonstrated to be effective against encysted larvae.[158] As the drug does not kill the larvae in muscle, it is administered (25 mg/kg twice daily for 7–10 days) only if the patient is seen within 24 h after ingestion of trichinous meat while adult *Trichinella* in the gut are still producing larvae.

PHARMACOKINETICS AND ADVERSE EFFECTS. Thiabendazole is well absorbed from the gastrointestinal tract and peak plasma levels in the range of 5 µg/ml are achieved 1 h after oral administration of a 25 mg/kg dose.[162,163] The drug is rapidly metabolized by hydroxylation and conjugation and both the unchanged drug and its metabolites are excreted by the kidney.[159] Ninety-two percent of an oral dose of radioactive thiabendazole is excreted from the body in 48 h—87% in the urine and 5% in the feces.[164] The plasma half-lives of the unchanged drug and its biologically inactive 5-hydroxy metabolites are 1.2 and 1.7 h, respectively.[162,164] The half-life of the unchanged drug is not altered in renal failure, but conjugated hydroxy metabolites accumulate in the body and they are not eliminated by hemodialysis.[162,163]

Unlike mebendazole and albendazole, the clinical utility of thiabendazole is compromised by its toxicity. Thiabendazole causes side effects in a high percentage of patients. In one study, 89% of patients receiving 25 mg/kg twice daily orally for 3 days complained of one or more side effects, with nausea occurring in two-thirds of patients.[152] Other frequent side effects (experienced by more than 15% of patients) include dizziness, malaise, malodorous urine and sweat; also, a group of neuropsychiatric symptoms can occur which includes sensations of disembodiment, disorientation in space, delirium, and a feeling of being dazed.[152] Malodorous urine and sweat are caused by metabolites that are excreted by these routes. Other less common side effects include anorexia, vomiting, abdominal pain, headache, facial flush, rash, and pruritis.[152] Occasionally, vomiting of live *Ascaris* occurs. Rare side effects include tinnitus, collapse, hyperglycemia, enuresis, decrease in pulse rate and systolic blood pressure, and a transitory rise in hepatic enzymes. A few cases of erythema multiforme and Stevens-Johnson syndrome have been reported. Many physicians feel that the incidence of gastrointestinal side effects and dizziness is lowered if the drug is taken after meals. Thiabendazole has been shown to have anti-inflammatory activity[161,165] and to have an anticonvulsant action[166] in animal models.

Drugs Used to Treat Tissue Roundworm Infections

Filariasis

Infection of the tissues by adult nematode worms is called *filariasis*.[167] The female worms in the tissues produce millions of larvae or microfilariae which are released into the bloodstream or into the skin. The microfilariae must be ingested by an insect vector and transmitted to a new host before they can develop into mature worms. The principal filarial worms infecting humans are *Wuchereria bancrofti*, *Brugia malayi*, *Loa loa*, and *Onchocerca volvulus*.

Bancroftian and Malayan filariasis are similar clinical conditions resulting from infection by *W. bancrofti* and *B. malayi*, respectively. The larvae of these organisms pass into the lymphatics and lymph nodes where they mature into adult worms and release microfilariae. As a result of chronic inflammatory reaction to the worms, the lymphatics may become fibrosed and eventually obstructed. Many patients are asymptomatic but others experience symptoms of acute inflammation and chronic lymphatic obstruction, the latter presenting as chronic lymphadenopathy and, rarely, as elephantiasis with severe swelling of the scrotum or lower legs. Although other drugs may have therapeutic potential, diethylcarbamazine (DEC) and ivermectin are now the only agents used for both suppression and cure of infections with *W. bancrofti* and *B. malayi*. The best results are obtained if chemotherapy is started early, before obstructive lesions of the lymphatics have occurred. Even in late cases, however, improvement may result. In long-standing elephantiasis, surgery is needed to improve lymph drainage and remove tissue. A course of therapy with diethylcarbamazine or ivermectin eliminates the microfilariae and most or all of the adults of *B. malayi* and *W. bancrofti*.[167] Successful drug treatment will not, however, reverse symptoms due to chronic lymph stasis or hydrocele.

Loiasis is caused by infection with *Loa loa* larvae which develop into white, thread-like adult worms that migrate through the connective tissues. Again, many patients are asymptomatic, although transient so-called Calabar swellings may occur. These swellings represent localized subcutaneous edematous reactions to the passage of the worm. Sometimes the worm produces severe conjunctivitis as it passes through the eye. A course of therapy with diethylcarbamazine may be curative.[167] Diethylcarbamazine is currently the best available drug for the treatment of loiasis. Tropical eosinophilia is a disease syndrome characterized by paroxysmal, dry coughing, dyspnea, and malaise caused by microfilariae of uncertain origin in the lungs. The syndrome may be effectively treated with a course of diethylcarbamazine therapy.

Onchocerciasis is a filarial infection affecting about 17 million persons in Africa, where in some regions people are resigned and accept the resulting blindness and dermatitis as processes of aging.[168] Onchocer-

ciasis or river blindness is caused by adult *O. volvulus* worms that live in subcutaneous nodules, causing a granulomatous inflammatory reaction followed by fibrosis. Ivermectin is now the drug of choice for the control and treatment of onchocerciasis, while diethylcarbamazine is no longer recommended. Both agents kill only microfilariae of *O. volvulus,* but ivermectin produces far milder systemic reactions and few, if any, ocular problems. These types of reactions are likely to be severe with diethycarbamazine.

The death of microfilariae can cause severe reactions such as rash, fever, generalized body pains, keratitis, and iritis in onchocerciasis; nodular swellings along the course of the lymphatics in bancroftian or Malayan filariasis; and encephalopathy in patients with heavy *Loa loa* infection. For this reason, the dosage of diethylcarbamazine must be built up gradually according to dosage schedules that are presented in Table 15–3. The physician is referred to literature reviews for detailed discussion of the use of diethylcarbamazine in the treatment of filariasis.[3,167,169] In contrast to diethylcarbamazine, ivermectin is effective as a single dose, with annual retreatment (using the same in-

Table 15–3. Dosage schedule for diethycarbamazine and ivermectin adminstration when used as drugs of choice in the treatment of filariasis.

Filarial infection	Diethylcarbamazine dosage[a]	
	Adults	Children
Wuchereria bancrofti	Day 1: 50 mg	Day 1: 25–50 mg
Brugia malayi	Day 2: 50 mg tid	Day 2: 25–50 mg tid
Loa loa	Day 3: 100 mg tid	Day 3: 50–100 mg tid
	Days 4–21: 2 mg/kg tid	Days 4–21: 2 mg/kg tid
Tropical eosinophilia	2 mg/kg × 7–10 days	2 mg/kg × 7–10 days
Mansonella streptocerca	6 mg/kg/day × 14 days	
	Ivermectin dosage	
Mansonella streptocerca	150 µg/kg once	
Onchocerca volvulus	150 µg/kg once, repeated every 6–12 months	Same as adults
Wuchereria bancrofti[b]	20–200 µg/kg once	

[a] For patients not having microfilaria in the blood, full doses can be given from day 1.[171] [b] A single dose is effective for treatment of microfilaremia, but does not kill the adult worm.[171]

itial dosage) being required. Studies suggest that diethylcarbamazine given annually along with a single dose of ivermectin may produce a greater and more lasting reduction in parasite burden in *W. bancrofti* and *B. malayi* filariasis than that obtained with either drug alone.[170]

Another tissue-dwelling nematode is the guinea worm *Dracunculus medinensis*. The adult female guinea worm grows under the skin of the legs where it causes an ulcer that penetrates the skin surface. When the portion of the worm that is located at the ulcer site comes into contact with water, millions of larvae are released directly into the stream or pond. The larvae develop inside crustaceans, and humans are infected by drinking contaminated water. Niridazole,[172] and metronidazole (see Chapter 14), have been reported to have a beneficial effect in this infection. These drugs facilitate worm removal, but at least some of the relief that many patients experience appears to be due to anti-inflammatory and immunosuppressant actions of these drugs.

Diethylcarbamazine

Diethylcarbamazine is 1-diethylcarbamyl-4-methyl-piperazine. Although it is a deriva-

Diethylcarbamazine

tive of piperazine, unsubstituted piperazine has no filaricidal action. Diethylcarbamazine has been reviewed by Hawking.[167,173]

MECHANISM OF ACTION. In vitro, therapeutic concentrations of diethylcarbamazine have no significant action on any type of microfilaria, but in vivo, microfilariae are rapidly killed.[167] It has been shown in animal models that diethylcarbamazine kills the adults of *B.*

malayi, *W. bancrofti* (most of them), and *Loa loa,* but not those of *O. volvulus*.[167] The fact that organisms are killed in vivo but not in vitro has led to the suggestion that diethylcarbamazine in some way facilitates the host's immune response. Several studies have documented that patent filarial infections are associated with a state of immune unresponsiveness to parasite antigens.[174–176] When people with filariasis are treated with diethylcarbamazine, there is a rapid drop in circulating eosinophils[177] and an increase in in vitro lymphocyte proliferative responses to microfilarial antigens.[178] It has been shown in an animal model that the microfilaricidal activity of diethylcarbamazine is suppressed by anti-lymphocyte serum.[179] These observations suggest that the drug acts by rapidly reversing the state of cellular unresponsiveness to parasite antigens associated with patent filarial infections, possibly by inducing the release of antigenically active components from the parasite cuticle[180] or possibly by affecting immune suppressor factors.[176]

Other evidence suggests that the effect of diethylcarbamazine is mediated by platelets, with an additional triggering of a filarial excretory antigen, but the postulated killing mechanism is antibody independent and involves the participation of free radicals.[181] Diethylcarbamazine has also been reported to inhibit microtubule polymerization and disrupt preformed microtubule protein prepared from porcine brain in vitro in a manner similar to that of the benzimidazoles.[182]

THERAPEUTIC USE. Diethylcarbamazine is effective against several species of filarial worms (*W. bancrofti, Brugia malayi, Brugia timori, Loa loa, Onchocerca volvulus,* and *Mansonella streptocerca*), but is used mainly in the treatment and control of lymphatic filariasis. It is chiefly a microfilaricide, being effective in a wide variety of dosage regimens, including very low doses as used in diethylcarbamazine-medicated salt. Diethylcarbamazine is also recommended as the treatment of choice for visceral larva migrans caused by the larvae of *Toxocara* worms.[183]

PHARMACOKINETICS. Diethylcarbamazine is rapidly and almost completely absorbed from the gastrointestinal tract of humans.[184] Peak plasma levels of 0.15–0.25 µg/ml are achieved 2–3 h after oral administration of a 50 mg tablet to an adult.[184] The drug is widely distributed in the body[173] and the apparent volume of distribution is in the range of 200 liters.[184] Diethylcarbamazine apparently undergoes limited metabolism to the N-oxide in humans. The drug is excreted by the kidneys, with about 50% of the drug in the urine recovered in the unchanged form and 10% as the N-oxide. The rate of elimination is positively related to the creatinine clearance and the drug accumulates in patients with impaired renal function.[185] The rate of renal excretion is much more rapid when the urine is acid than when it is alkaline.[186] Alkalinizing the urine can elevate plasma levels, prolong the plasma half-life, and increase both the therapeutic effect and toxicity of diethylcarbamazine.[187] The half-life of the drug measured in subjects with acid urine is about 3 h, but when the urine is alkaline, it is about 9 h.[186] Many people living in endemic filarial areas often have a largely vegetarian diet that tends to yield an alkaline urine as opposed to the acid urine that is formed when the diet is rich in animal protein. The elevated plasma levels of drug that accrue in the presence of renal impairment and alkaline urine may predispose to toxicity and the dose of the drug should be reduced in such circumstances.[185]

ADVERSE EFFECTS. Reactions to diethylcarbamazine are of two types. Patients may experience headache, malaise, weakness, nausea, and vomiting as a direct effect of the drug. Unless a daily dose of 8 to 10 mg/kg is exceeded, these direct toxic reactions are rarely severe and usually disappear within a few days despite continuation of therapy. In addition to the adverse effects caused by the drug itself, treatment with diethylcarbamazine also often results in adverse reactions related to the death of microfilariae (usually systemic reactions) or damage to adult worms, which usually results in localized adverse reactions.[3] These Herxheimer-like reactions are usually mild in the case of *W. bancrofti* or *B. malayi,* but they are often severe when the drug is used to treat *O. volvulus.* The reaction that occurs after initiating treatment of onchocerciasis, the Mazzotti reaction, consists of skin edema, papular rash, intense itching, fever, and generalized body pains. The reaction can be life threatening and the therapy of onchocerciasis requires careful medical supervision. When diethylcarbamazine therapy is initiated, there may be a dramatic increase in the number of *O. volvulus* microfilariae in the eye and a punctate keratitis characterized by fluffy opacities in the cornea may develop as a result of inflammatory reaction to dead and dying microfilariae. These opacities clear over a period of time, as does anterior uveitis, which is due to the same process. Diethylcarbamazine is readily absorbed from the skin and it is sometimes administered as a topical lotion with the hope that a reduction in systemic absorption will lead to a decrease in systemic and ocular side effects. There is evidence, however, that the use of the lotion may actually be associated with more ocular complications than the conventional oral treatment.[188] The use of low-dose diethylcarbamazine in salt can minimize the known adverse effects of treatment, including the pharmacologic effects of very high doses, as well as the inflammatory reaction to dying worms.[189]

Diethylcarbamazine is sometimes given in mass therapy as a public health measure to suppress infection by *W. bancrofti* and *B. malayi.* In areas where both bancroftian filariasis and onchocerciasis are endemic, it has been found that the incidence of side effects with diethylcarbamazine administration in patients who are infected with either *O. volvulus* alone or with both organisms is 53%–58%, but the incidence of side effects in patients who are not infected or are infected with only *W. bancrofti* is 15%–19%.[190] In this case, the side effects of diethylcarbamazine experienced in the treatment of bancroftian filariasis clearly result from drug action on a different organism. Thus, in areas where both filarial species are endemic, infections with *O. volvulus* seem to be a limiting factor for control of bancroftian filariasis by mass treatment with diethylcarbamazine.

Diethylcarbamazine has not been reported to be teratogenic in rats, but because of its possible abortifacient effect, it should be avoided during pregnancy, unless there is a strong indication for its use.[191]

Ivermectin

Ivermectin is a potent macrocyclic lactone that belongs to the class of compounds known as avermectins. It is actually a mixture of avermectins B_{1a} and B_{1b} and is produced by the actinomycete *Streptomyces avermitilis*. It is an orally effective antifilarial agent that has been used in veterinary medicine since 1981. The properties of ivermectin have been reviewed by Goa et al.[192] and by Ottesen and Campbell.[193]

MECHANISM OF ACTION. The mode of action of ivermectin appears to reflect its effect on ion channels in cell membranes.[193] Ivermectin causes an influx of negatively charged ions, and this hyperpolarization of the affected cells results in muscle paralysis. Originally the neurotransmitter GABA was thought to be its focus of action, but subsequently it was shown that ivermectin induces an influx of chloride through channels that are not regulated by GABA. Ivermectin apparently causes potentiation, direct activation, or both, of avermectin-sensitive,

glutamate-gated Cl^- channels. These channels are found only in invertebrates and two of their cloned subunits have been expressed and characterized in *Xenopus laevis* oocytes.[194] There is a close correlation between activation and potentiation of glutamate-sensitive chloride channels, membrane binding affinity, and nematocidal activity by avermectins and milbemycins.[194–196] Cestodes and trematodes do not possess high-affinity avermectin receptors and these helminths are not sensitive to ivermectin.[197]

In humans infected with *Onchocerca volvulus*, ivermectin causes a rapid, marked decrease in microfilarial counts in the skin and ocular tissues that lasts for 5 to 12 months.[198–200] The drug also blocks the movement of microfilariae from the uterus of adult female worms.[187,201] In contrast, adult parasites are affected only to a small extent by ivermectin. Human infections caused by gastrointestinal nematodes such as strongyloidiasis, ascariasis, and trichuriasis respond well to ivermectin but hookworms are affected to a lesser extent.[202]

THERAPEUTIC USES. Ivermectin is a very potent, broad-spectrum anthelmintic drug that has been widely used in controlling nematode infections in animals and it is approved for use in the United States. Since its introduction for human use in 1981, ivermectin has been used almost exclusively for the treatment of onchocerciasis (river blindness).[203] A single dose of ivermectin (150 µg/kg) greatly re-

Ivermectin

duces the number of microfilariae in the skin and eyes, thus diminishing the likelihood of disabling onchoceriasis in adults and children 5 years and older.[204] In areas where the disease is endemic, the dose can be repeated every 5 to 12 months to maintain suppression of both dermal and ocular microfilariae. Ivermectin as a single dose (150 μg/kg) is at least as effective as diethylcarbamazine administered in a complicated multiple-dose regimen and is considerably better tolerated. Ivermectin therapy reduces even severe onchocercal dermatitis, with a reduction in the itching but no resolution of the depigmentation.[205] The ocular disease responds with a lessening of the damage to the optic nerve and a diminishment in keratitis and iritis. Because ivermectin decreases the number of microfilariae in the skin of infected persons, mass chemotherapy reduces transmission of this disease. Cure of the disease is not attained because ivermectin has little effect on adult O. *volvulus*.

Initial studies indicate that a single 400 μg/kg dose of ivermectin annually is effective for mass chemotherapy of infections with W. *bancrofti* and B. *malayi*.[170] A single dose of ivermectin is as effective as the traditional 14-day course of diethylcarbamazine in lowering the number of circulating microfilariae and has far fewer side effects.[206] However, the drug is not active against adult filarial worms in the lymphatic system.

Ivermectin is effective against several common intestinal parasitic nematodes, including *Ascaris, Trichuris*, and *Enterobius*.[202] It is ineffective against hookworms in humans, however; here mebendazole is the treatment of choice. Ivermectin in a daily dose 200 μg/kg for 1 or 2 days is highly effective against chronic intestinal strongyloidiasis.[207] It was found to be as effective as, and less toxic than, traditional treatment with thiabendazole.[208] Ivermectin has also proved effective for treating strongyloidiasis in patients with AIDS,[209] and a single 12 mg dose of ivermectin was more effective than a single dose of albendazole for the treatment of cutaneous larva migrans.[210]

PHARMACOKINETICS. Ivermectin is well absorbed and widely distributed into tissues, with the highest concentrations being achieved in liver and adipose tissue and very small amounts in brain. Peak levels in plasma are reached within 4 h after oral administration, and there is evidence that absorption is greater if the drug is ingested in an aqueous ethanol solution.[192] Ivermectin has a long terminal half-life of about 27 h in adults, and about 93% of the drug is bound to plasma protein.[211] Most of the dose of the drug is eliminated in the feces, nearly all as unchanged drug, with very little appearing in the urine either unchanged or as a metabolite.[212]

ADVERSE EFFECTS. Ivermectin is generally well tolerated. Adverse effects include fever, itching, dizziness, and edema. Almost all of the adverse effects that occur during ivermectin treatment reflect the patient's immune response to dead microfilariae, and they usually appear within 3 days of the dose and subside thereafter.[213,214] The most common of these responses include itching, fever, chills, myalgia, rash, and swelling of lymph nodes, joints, limbs or face.[204] The intensity and nature of these reactions depend on the number of microfilaria and the duration and type of filarial infection.[215,216] These responses are usually of mild to moderate severity, and they generally respond to treatment with analgesics or antihistamines. More severe reactions are rare and include high fever, tachycardia, hypotension, prostration, dizziness, headache, myalgia, arthralgia, diarrhea, and edema.[213,216] Ivermectin does not cause severe ocular complications in patients with onchocerciasis. In contrast to diethylcarbamazine, no changes in visual acuity or appearance of punctate opacities have occurred with ivermectin. Ivermectin is much less likely to cause the potentially fatal Mazzotti reaction associated with diethylcarbamazine although there have been reports of severe postural hypotension and other rare but serious reactions.[213] Although no adverse effects have been seen in women inadvertently treated during pregnancy,[213] it is recommended that ivermectin not be used in pregnant women or during the first month of lactation, or in children under 5 years of age or weighing less than 15 kg, or in patients who are in very poor health. Because of potential neurological toxicity, some experts suggest that ivermectin not be used during epidemics of meningococcal meningitis or in areas where sleeping sickness is endemic.[216]

REFERENCES

1. Cavier, R., and F. Hawking. *Chemotherapy of Helminthiasis*. New York: Pergamon Press, 1973, pp. 1–537.

2. *Biochemistry of Parasites and Host-Parasite Relationships*, ed. by H. Van den Bossche. Amsterdam: North Holland, 1976, pp. 1–676.

3. de Silva, N., H. Guyatt, and D. Bundy. Anthelmintics. Comparative review of their clinical pharmacology. *Drugs* 1997;53:769.

4. Liu, L. X., and P. Weller. Antiparasitic drugs. *N. Engl. J. Med.* 1996;334:1178.

5. Iarotski, L. S., and A. Davis. The schistosomiasis problem in the world: results of a WHO questionnaire. *Bull. WHO* 1981;59:115.

6. Katz, N. Chemotherapy of schistosomiasis mansoni. *Adv. Pharmacol. Chemother.* 1977;14:1.

7. Butterworth, A. E., R. F. Sturrock, J. H. Ouma, G. G. Mbugua, A. J. Fulfor, H. C. Kariuki, and D. Koech. Comparison of different chemotherapy strategies against *Schistomsoma mansoni* in Machakos District, Kenya: effects on human infection and morbidity. *Parasitology* 1991;103:339.

8. King, C. H., E. Muchiri, J. H. Ouma, and D. Koech. Chemotherapy-based control of *Schistosoma haematobium*. IV: impact of repeated annual chemotherapy on prevalence and intensity of *Schistosoma haematobium* infection in an endemic area of Kenya. *Am. J. Trop. Med. Hyg.* 1991;45:498.

9. Stelma, F. F., S. Sall, B. Daff, S. Sow, M. Niang, and B. Gryseels. Oxamniquine cures *Schistosoma mansoni* infection in a focus in which cure rates with praziquantel are unusually low. *J. Infect. Dis.* 1997;176:304.

10. Bennett, J. L., and J. W. Depenbusch. Recent advances in the chemotherapy of schistosomiasis in *Advances in Parasitic Diseases*, ed. by J. M. Mansfield. New York: Marcel Dekker, 1984, pp. 73–132.

11. Symposium (various authors). Biltricide symposium on African schistosomiasis. *Arzneimittelforschung* 1981;31:535–618.

12. Pearson, R. D., and R. L. Guerrant. Praziquantel: a major advance in anthelminthic therapy. *Ann. Intern. Med.* 1983;99:195.

13. Harnett, W. The anthelmintic action of praziquantel. *Parasitol. Today* 1988;4:144.

14. King, C. H., and A. A. F. Mahmoud. Drugs five years later: praziquantel. *Ann. Intern. Med.* 1989;110:290.

15. Katz, N., R. S. Rocha, and A. Chaves. Preliminary trials with praziquantel in human infections due to *Schistosoma mansoni*. *Bull. WHO* 1979;57:781.

16. Davis, A., J. E. Biles, and A-M. Ulrich. Initial experiences with praziquantel in the treatment of human infections due to *Schistosoma haematobium*. *Bull. WHO* 1979;57:773.

17. Santos, A. T., B. L. Blas, J. S. Nosenas, G. P. Portillo, O. M. Ortega, M. Hayashi, and K. Boehme. Preliminary clinical trials with praziquantel in *Schistosoma japonicum* infections in the Philippines. *Bull. WHO* 1979;57:793.

18. Nash, T. E., M. Hofstetter, A. W. Cheever, and E. A. Ottsen. Treatment of *Schistosoma mekongi* with praziquantel: a double-blind study. *Am. J. Trop. Med. Hyg.* 1982;31:977.

19. Rim, H.-J., K.-S. Lyu, J.-S. Lee, and K.-H. Joo. Clinical evaluation of the therapeutic efficacy of praziquantel (Embay 8440) against *Clonorchis sinensis* infection in man. *Ann. Trop. Med. Parasitol.* 1981;75:27.

20. Bunnag, D., and T. Harinasuta. Studies on the chemotherapy of human opisthorchiasis in Thailand: I. Clinical trial of praziquantel. *Southeast Asian J. Trop. Med. Public Health* 1980;11:528.

21. Spitalny, K. C., A. W. Senft, F. D. Meglio, J. Moran, and G. Peter. Treatment of pulmonary paragonimiasis with a new broad-spectrum antihelminthic, praziquantel. *J. Pediatr.* 1982;101:144.

22. Groll, E. Praziquantel for cestode infections in man. *Acta Tropica* 37:293 (1980).

23. Schenone, H. Praziquantel in the treatment of *Hymenolepis nana* infections in children. *Am. J. Trop. Med. Hyg.* 1980;29:320.

24. Fallon, P. G., R. O. Cooper, A. J. Probert, and M. J. Doenhoff. Immune dependent chemotherapy of schistosomiasis. *Parasitology* 1992;105(Suppl.):S41.

25. Linder, E., and C. Thors. *Schistosoma mansoni*: praziquantel-induced tegumental lesions exposes actin of surface spines and allows binding of actin depolymerizing factor, gelsolin. *Parasitology* 1992;105:71.

26. Brindley, P. J. Relationships between chemotherapy and immunity in schistosomiasis. *Adv. Parasitol.* 1994;34:133.

27. Xiao, S. H., B. A. Catto, and L. T. Webster. Effects of praziquantel on different developmental stages of *Schistosoma mansoni* in vitro and in vivo. *J. Infect. Dis.* 1985;151:1130.

28. Blair, K. L., J. L. Bennett, and R. A. Pax. Praziquantel: physiological evidence for its site(s) of action in magnesium-paralysed *Schistosoma mansoni*. *Parasitology* 1992;104:59.

29. Brindley, P. J., and A. Sher. Immunologic involvement in the efficacy of praziquantel. *Exp. Parasitol.* 1990;71:245.

30. Andrews, P. Praziquantel—a novel schistosomicide. *Parasitology* 1977;75:xvii.

31. Andrews, P., H. Thomas, and H. Weber. The in vitro uptake of ^{14}C-praziquantel by cestodes, trematodes and a nematode. *J. Parasitol.* 1980;66:920.

32. Leopold, G., W. Ungethum, E. Groll, H. W. Diekmann, H. Nowak, and D. H. G. Wegner. Clinical pharmacology in normal volunteers of praziquantel, a new drug against schistosomes and cestodes. *Eur. J. Clin. Pharmacol.* 1978;14:281.

33. Buhring, K. U., H. W. Diekmann, H. Muller, A. Garbe, and H. Nowak. Metabolism of praziquantel in man. *Eur. J. Drug. Metabol. Pharmacokinet.* 1978;3:179.

34. Steiner, K., A. Garbe, H. W. Diekmann, and H. Nowak. The fate of praziquantel in the organism. I. Pharmacokinetics in animals. *Eur. J. Drug Metabol. Pharmacokinet.* 1976;1:85.

35. Thomas, H., P. Andrews, and H. Mehlhorn. New results on the effect of praziquantel in experimental cysticerosis. *Am. J. Trop. Med. Hyg.* 1982;31:803.

36. Ishizaki, T., E. Kamo, and K. Boehme. Double-blind studies of tolerance to praziquantel in Japanese patients with *Schistosoma japonicum* infections. *Bull. WHO* 1979;57:787.

37. Bartsch, H., T. Kuroki, C. Malaveille, N. Loprieno, R. Barale, A. Abbondandolo, S. Bonatti, G. Rainaldi, E. Vogel, and A. Davis. Absence of mutagenicity of praziquantel, a new effective, anti-schistosomal drug, in bacteria, yeast, insects and mammalian cells. *Mutat. Res.* 1978;58:133.

38. Frohberg, H., and M. Schultze Schencking. Toxicological profile of praziquantel, a new drug against cestode and schistosome infections, as compared to some other schistosomicides. *Arzneimittelforschung* 1981;31:555.

39. Mandour, M. E. M., H. el Turabi, M. M. A. Homeida, T. el Sadig, H. M. Ali, J. L. Bennett, W. J. Leahey, and D. W. G. Harron. Pharmacokinetics of praziquantel in healthy volunteers and patients with schistosomiasis. *Trans. R. Soc. Trop. Med. Hyg.* 1990; 84:389.

40. Bittencourt, P. R., C. M. Bracia, R. Martins, A. G. Fernandes, H. W. Dieckmann, and W. Jung. Phenytoin and carbamazepine decreased oral bioavailability of praziquantel. *Neurology* 1992;42:492.

41. Dachamn, W. D., K. O. Adubofour, D. S. Bikin, C. S. Johnson, P. D. Mullin, and M. Winograd. Cimetidine-induced rise in praziquantel levels in a patient with neurocysticercosis being treated with anticonvulsants. *J. Infect. Dis.* 1994;169:689.

42. Homeida, M., W. Leahey, S. Copeland, M. M. M. Ali, and D. W. G. Harron. Pharmacokinetic interaction between praziquantel and albendazole in Sudanese men. *Ann. Trop. Med. Parasitol.* 1994;88:551.

43. Holmstedt, B., I. Nordgren, M. Sandoz, and A. Sundwall. Metrifonate. Summary of toxicological and pharmacological information available. *Arch. Toxicol.* 1979;41:3.

44. Symposium (various authors). Metrifonate and dichlorvos: Theoretical and practical aspects. *Acta Pharmacol. Toxicol.* 1981;49(Suppl. V):1–137.

45. Nordgren, I., M. Bergstrom, B. Holmstedt, and M. Sandoz. Transformation and action of metrifonate. *Arch. Toxicol.* 1978;41:31.

46. Denham, D. A., and R. J. Holdsworth. The effect of metrifonate in vitro on *Schistosoma haematobium* and *S. mansoni* adults. *Trans. Soc. Trop. Med. Hyg.* 1971;65:421.

47. James, C., G. Webbe, and J. M. Preston. A comparison of the susceptibility to metrifonate of *Schistosoma haematobium*, *S. mattheei*, and *S. mansoni* in hamsters. *Ann. Trop. Med. Parasitol.* 1972;66:467.

48. Omer, A. H. S., and C. H. Teesdale. Metrifonate trial in the treatment of various presentations of *Schistosoma haematobium* and *S. mansoni* infections in the Sudan. *Ann. Trop. Med. Parasitol.* 1978;72:145.

49. Jewsbury, J. M., M. J. Cooke, and M. C. Weber. Field trial of metrifonate in the treatment and prevention of schistosomiasis infection in man. *Ann. Trop. Med. Parasitol.* 1977;71:67.

50. Bueding, E., C. L. Liu, and S. H. Rogers. Inhibition by metrifonate and dichlorvos of cholinesterases in schistosomes. *Br. J. Pharmacol.* 1972;46:480.

51. Doehring, E., U. Poggensee, and H. Feldmeier. The effect of metrifonate in mixed *Schistosoma haematobium* and *Schistosoma mansoni* infections in humans. *Am. J. Trop. Med. Hyg.* 1986;35:323.

52. O'Leary, K. A., and J. W. Tracy. *Schistosoma mansoni*: glutathione *S*-transferase-catalyzed detoxification of dichlorvos. *Exp. Parasitol.* 1991;72:355.

53. Bloom, A. Studies of the mode of action of metrifonate and DDVP in schistosomes—cholinesterase activity and hepatic shift. *Acta Pharmacol. Toxicol.* 1981;49(Suppl. V):109.

54. Nordgren, I., E. Bengtsson, B. Holmstedt, and B.-M. Petterson. Levels of metrifonate and dichlorvos in plasma and erythrocytes during treatment of schistosomiasis with bilarcil. *Acta Pharmacol. Toxicol.* 1981;49(Suppl. V):79.

55. Plestina, R., A. Davis, and D. R. Bailey. Effect of metrifonate on blood cholinesterases in children during treatment of schistosomiasis. *Bull. WHO* 1972;46: 747.

56. Reiner, E., and R. Plestina. Regeneration of cholinesterase activities in humans and rats after inhibition by o,o-dimethyl-2,2-dichlorovinyl phosphate. *Toxicol. Appl. Pharmacol.* 1979;49:451.

57. World Health Organization Report. Schistosomiasis control. *World Health Organ. Tech. Rep. Ser.* 1973; No. 515.

58. Jamnadas, V. P., and J. E. P. Thomas. Metriphonate and organophosphate poisoning. *Cent. Afri. J. Med.* 1979;25:130.

59. James, M. F. M., and J. M. Jewsbury. Schistosomiasis, metrifonate, cholinesterase, and suxamethonium. *BMJ* 1978;1:442.

60. Dedek, W. Guanine N[7]-alkylation in mice in vivo by metrifonate—discussion of possible genotoxic risk in mammals. *Acta Pharmacol. Toxicol.* 1981; 49(Suppl. V):40.

61. Batzinger, R. P., and E. Bueding. Mutagenic activities in vitro and in vivo of five antischistosomal compounds. *J. Pharmacol. Exp. Ther.* 1977;200:1.

62. Foster, R., and B. L. Cheetham. Studies with the schistosomicide oxamniquine (UK-4271). I. Activity in rodents and in vitro. *Trans. R. Soc. Trop. Med. Hyg.* 1973;67:674.

63. Cioli, D., L. Pica-Mattoccia, and S. Archer. Drug resistance in schistosomes. *Parasitol. Today* 1993; 9:162.

64. Goldberg, M., D. Gold, E. Flescher, and J. Lengy. Effect of oxamniquine on *Schistosoma mansoni*: some biological and biochemical observations. *Biochem. Pharmacol.* 1980;29:838.

65. Da Silva, L. G., H. Sette, D. A. F. Obamone, A. Saozalequezar, J. A. Punskas and S. Raia. Further clinical trials with oxamniquine (UK-4271), a new anti-schistosomal agent. *Rev. Inst. Med. Trop. S. Paulo* 1975;17:307.

66. Katz, N., F. Zicker, and J. P. Pereira. Field trials with oxamniquine in a schistosomiasis mansoni-endemic area. *Am. J. Trop. Med. Hyg.* 1977;26:234.

67. Clarke, V. D. V., D. M. Blair, M. C. Weber, and P. A. Garnett. Dose-finding trials of oral oxamniquine in Rhodesia. *S. Afr. Med. J.* 1976;50:1867.

68. Omer, A. H. S. Oxamniquine for treating *Schistosoma mansoni* infection in Sudan. BMJ 1978;2:163.

69. Shafei, A. Z. A preliminary report on the treatment of intestinal schistosomiasis with oxamniquine. *J. Trop. Med. Hyg.* 1979;82:18.

70. Eyakuze, V. M., W. K. Rutasitara, and J. B. Ndalahwa. Field use of oral oxamniquine in the treatment of *S. mansoni. E. Afr. Med. J.* 1979;56:22.

71. Araujo, N., N. Katz, E. P. Dias, and C. P. De Souza. Susceptibility to chemotherapeutic agents of strains of *Schistosoma mansoni* isolated from treated and untreated patients. *Am. J. Trop. Med. Hyg.* 1980; 29:890.

72. Kaye, B., and N. M. Woolhouse: The metabolism of oxamniquine—a new schistosomicide. *Ann. Trop. Med. Parasitol.* 1976;70:324.

73. Woolhouse, N. M., and P. R. Wood. Determination of oxamniquine in serum. *J. Pharm. Sci.* 1977; 66:429.

74. Forid, Z., S. Bassily, G. I. Higashi, N. A. El-Masry, R. H. Watten, And B. Trabolsi. Further experience on the use of oxamniquine in the treatment of advanced intestinal schistosomiasis. *Ann. Trop. Med. Parasitol.* 1979;73:501.

75. Yang, S., and C. Lin. Treatment of paragonimiasis with bithionol and bithionol sulfoxide. *Dis. Chest* 1967;52:220.

76. Oh, S. J. Bithionol treatment in cerebral paragonimiasis. *Am. J. Trop. Med. Hyg.* 1967;16:585.

77. Ashton, W. I. G., P. L. Boardman, J. C. D'Sa, P. H. Everall, and A. W. J. Houghton. Human fascioliasis in Shropshire. *BMJ* 1970;3:500.

78. Arjona, R., J. A. Riancho, J. M. Aguado, R. Salesa, and J. Gonzalez-Macias. Fascioliasis in developed countries: a review of classic and aberrant forms of the disease. *Medicine* 1995;74:13.

79. Apt, W., X. Aguilera, F. Vega, C. Miranda, I. Zulantay, C. Perez, M. Gabor, and P. Apt. Treatment of human chronic fascioliasis with triclabendazole: drug efficacy and serologic response. *Am. J. Trop. Med. Hyg.* 1995;52:532.

80. Gemmell, M. A., and P. D. Johnstone. Cestodes. *Antibiot. Chemother.* 1981;30:54.

81. Del Brutto, O. H., J. Sotelo, and G. C. Roman. Therapy for neurocysticercosis: a reappraisal. *Clin. Infect. Dis.* 1993;17:730.

82. Takayanagui, O. M., and E. Jardim. Therapy for neurocysticercosis: comparison between albendazole and praziquantel. *Arch. Neurol.* 1992;49:290.

83. Nahmias, J., R. Goldsmith, M. Soibelman, and J. el-On. Three- to 7-year follow-up after albendazole treatment of 68 patients with cystic echinococcosis (hydatid disease). *Ann. Trop. Med. Parasitol.* 1994;88:295.

84. Janssen, P. A. Recent advances in the treatment of parasitic infections in man. *Drug Res.* 1974;18:191.

85. Standen, O. D. Chemotherapy of intestinal helminthiasis. *Drug Res.* 1975;19:158.

86. Hunter, G. W., J. C. Swartzwelder, and D. F. Clyde. Intestinal nematodes. In *Tropical Medicine, 5th ed.* Philadelphia: W. B. Saunders, 1976, pp. 454–490.

87. World Health Organization report. Intestinal protozoan and helminthic infections. *World Health Organ. Tech. Rep. Ser.* 1981; No. 666.

88. Blumenthal, D. S. Intestinal nematodes in the United States. *N. Engl. J. Med.* 1977;297:1437.

89. Kappus, K. D., R. G. Lundgren, D. D. Juranek, J. M. Roberts, and H. C. Spencer. Intestinal parasitism in the United States: update on a continuing problem. *Am. J. Trop. Med. Hyg.* 1994;50:705.

90. Population Information Program. Community-based health and family planning. *Popul. Rep. L* 1982; 3:L-77.

91. Winstanley, P. Albendazole for mass treatment of asymptomatic trichuris infections. *Lancet* 1998;352:1080.

92. Van den Bossche, H., F. Rochette, and C. Hörig. Mebendazole and related anthelminthics. *Adv. Pharmacol. Chemother.* 1982;19:67.

93. Venkatesan, P. Albendazole. *J. Antimicrob. Chem.* 1998;41:145.

94. Hanjeet, K., and R. G. Mathias. The efficacy of treatment with albendazole. *Acta Trop.* 1991;50:111.

95. Brugmans, J. P., D. C. Thienpont, I. van Wijngaarden, O. F. Vanparijs, V. L. Schuermans, and H. L. Lauwers. Mebendazole in enterobiasis: radiochemical and pilot clinical study in 1,278 subjects. *JAMA* 1971;217:313.

96. Miller, M. J., I. M. Krupp, M. D. Little, and C. Santos. Mebendazole: an effective anthelmintic for trichuriasis and enterobiasis. *JAMA* 1974;230:1412.

97. World Health Organization. *WHO Model Prescribing Information—Drugs Used in Parasitic Diseases.* Geneva:World Health Organization, 1995.

98. Mravak, S., W. Schopp, and U. Bienzle. Treatment of strongyloidiasis with mebendazole. *Acta Trop.* 1983;40:93.

99. Levin, M. L. Treatment of trichinosis with mebendazole. *Am. J. Trop. Med. Hyg.* 1983;32:980.

100. Magnaval, J. F. Comparative efficacy of diethylcarbamazine and mebendazole for the treatment of human toxocariasis. *Parasitology* 1995;110:529.

101. Van Hoegaerden, M., B. Ivanoff, F. Flocard, A. Salle, and B. Chabaud. The use of mebendazole in the treatment of filariases due to *Loa loa* and *Mansonella perstans. Ann. Trop. Med. Parasitol.* 1987;81:275.

102. Chavarria, A. P., V. M. Villarejos, and R. Zeledon. Mebendazole in the treatment of *Taeniasis solium* and *Taeniasis saginata. Am. J. Trop. Med. Hyg.* 1977; 26:118.

103. Khalil, H. M., S. el Shimi, M. A. Sarwat, A. F. Fawzy, and A. O. el Sorougy. Recent study of *Hymenolepis nana* infection in Egyptian children. *J. Egypt. Soc. Parasitol.* 1991;21:293.

104. Chavarria, A. P., J. C. Swartzwelder, V. M. Villarejos, and R. Zeledon Mebendazole, an effective broad-spectrum anthelmintic. *Am. J. Trop. Med Hyg.* 1973;22:592.

105. Bekhti, A., J.-P. Schaaps, M. Capron, J.-P. Dessaint, F. Santoro, and A. Capron. Treatment of hepatic

hydatid disease with mebendazole: preliminary results in four cases. *BMJ.* 1977;2:1047.

106. Wilson, J. F., M. Davidson, and R. L. Rausch. A clinical trial of mebendazole in the treatment of alveolar hydatid disease. *Am. Rev. Respir. Dis.* 1970;110.747.

107. Keystone, J. S., and J. K. Murdoch. Mebendazole. *Ann. Intern. Med.* 1979;91:582.

108. Lacey, E. Mode of action of benzimidazoles. *Parasitol. Today* 1990;6:107.

109. Prichard, R. Anthelmintic resistance. *Vet. Parasitol.* 1994;54:259.

110. Beech, R. N., R. K. Prichard, and M. E. Scott. Genetic variability of the β-tubulin genes in benzimidazole-susceptible and resistant strains of *Haemonchus contortus*. *Genetics* 1994;138:103.

111. Borgers, M., S. de Nollin, M. De Brabander, and D. Thienpont. Microtubules and intracellular organelle movement in nematode intestinal cells. The influence of the anthelmintic mebendazole. *Am. J. Vet. Res.* 1975;36:1153.

112. Borgers, M. S., S. de Nollin, A. Verheyen, M. De Brabander, and D. Thienpont. Effects of new anthelmintics on the microtubular system of parasites. In *Microtubules and Microtubule Inhibitors*, ed. by M. Borgers and M. De Brabander. Amsterdam: North Holland, 1975, pp. 497–508.

113. Friedman, P. A., and E. G. Platzer. Interaction of anthelmintic benzimidazoles and benzimidazole derivatives with bovine brain tubulin. *Biochim. Biophys. Acta* 1978;544:605.

114. Laclette, J. P., G. Guerra, and C. Zetina. Inhibition of tubulin polymerization by mebendazole. *Biochim. Biophys. Res. Commun.* 1980;92:417.

115. Friedman, P. A., and E. G. Platzer. Interaction of anthelmintic benzimidazoles with *Ascaris suum* embryonic tubulin. *Biochim. Biophys. Acta.* 1980;630:271.

116. Van den Bossche, H. Biochemical effects of the anthelmintic drug mebendazole. In *Comparative Biochemistry of Parasites*, ed. by H. Van den Bossche. New York: Academic Press, 1972, pp. 139–157.

117. Wagner, E. D., and A. P. Chavarria. In vivo effects of a new anthelmintic, mebendazole (R-17,635) on the eggs of *Trichuris trichuria* and hookworm. *Am. J. Trop. Med. Hyg.* 1974;23:151.

118. De Nollin, S., M. Borgers, O. Vanparijs, and H. Van den Bossche. Effects of mebendazole on the encysted phase of *Trichinella spiralis* in the rat: an electron-microscope study. *Parasitology* 1974;69:55.

119. Münst, G. J., G. Karlaganis, and J. Bircher. Plasma concentrations of mebendazole during treatment of echinococcosis. *Eur. J. Clin. Pharamacol.* 1980;17:375.

120. Michiels, M., R. Hendriks, and J. Heykants. The pharmacokinetics of mebendazole and flubendazole in animals and man. *Arch. Int. Pharmacodyn.* 1982;256:180.

121. Morris, D. L., and S. E. Gould. Serum and cyst concentrations of mebendazole and flubendazole in hydatid disease. *BMJ* 1982;285:175.

122. Marriner, S. E., D. L. Morris, B. Dickson, and J. A. Bogan. Pharmacokinetics of albendazole in man. *Eur. J. Clin. Pharmacol.* 1986;30:705.

123. Moskopp, D., and E. Lotterer. Concentrations of albendazole in serum, cerebrospinal fluid and hydatidous brain cyst. *Neurosurg. Rev.* 1993;16:35.

124. Murray-Lyon, I. M., and K. W. Reynolds. Complications of mebendazole treatment for hydatid disease. *BMJ* 1979;2:1111.

125. Marsboom; R. Toxicologic studies on mebendazole. *Toxicol. Appl. Pharmacol.* 1973;24:371.

126. Brown, H. W., K.-F. Chan, and K. L. Hussey. Treatment of enterobiasis and ascariasis with piperazine. *JAMA* 1956;161:515.

127. Norton, S., and E. J. deBeer. Investigations on the action of piperazine on *Ascaris lumbricoides*. *Am. J. Trop. Med. Hyg.* 1957;6:898.

128. Mason, P. A., and G. Sturman. Some pharmacological properties of piperazine. *Br. J. Pharmacol.* 1972;44:169.

129. DeBell, J. T., J. Del Castillo, and V. Sanchez. Electrophysiology of the somatic muscle cells of *Ascaris lumbricoides*. *J. Cell Comp. Physiol.* 1963;62:159.

130. Del Castillo, J., W. C. De Mello, and T. Morales. Mechanism of the paralyzing action of piperazine on *Ascaris* muscle. *Br. J. Pharmacol.* 1964;22:463.

131. Connor, J. D., A. Constanti, P. M. Dunn, A. Forward, and A. Nistri. The effects of piperazine on rat sympathetic neurones. *Br. J. Pharmacol.* 1981;74:445.

132. Standen, O. D., L. G. Goodwin, E. W. Rogers, and D. Stephenson. Activity of piperazine. *BMJ* 1955;2:437.

133. Hana, S., and A. Tang. Human urinary excretion of piperazine citrate from syrup formulations. *J. Pharm. Sci.* 1973;62:2024.

134. Parsons, A. C. Piperazine neurotoxicity: "Worm wobble."*BMJ* 1971;4:792.

135. Boulos, B. M., and L. E. Davis. Hazard of simultaneous administration of phenothiazine and piperazine. *N. Engl. J. Med.* 1969;280:1245.

136. Nickey, L. N. Possible precipitation of petit mal seizures with piperazine citrate. *JAMA* 1966;195:193.

137. Austin, W. C., W. Courtney, J. C. Danilewicz, D. H. Morgan, L. H. Conover, H. L. Howes, J. E. Lynch, J. W. McFarland, R. L. Cornwell, and V. J. Theodorides. Pyrantel tartrate, a new anthelmintic effective against infections of domestic animals. *Nature* 1966;212:1273.

138. Bumbalo, T. S., D. J. Fugazzotto, and J. W. Wyczalek. Treatment of enterobiasis with pyrantel pamoate. *Am. J. Trop. Med. Hyg.* 1969;18:50.

139. Bell, W. J., and S. Nassif. Comparison of pyrantel pamoate and piperazine phosphate in the treatment of ascariasis. *Am. J. Trop. Med. Hyg.* 1971;20:584.

140. Desowitz, R. S., T. Bell, J. Williams, R. Cardines, and M. Tamarua. Anthelmintic activity of pyrantel pamoate. *Am. J. Trop. Med. Hyg.* 1970;19:775.

141. Pitts, N. E., and J. R. Migliardi. Antimuth (pyrantel pamoate). The clinical evaluation of a new broad-spectrum anthelminthic. *Clin. Pediatr.* 1974;13:87.

142. Rim, H. J., and J. K. Lim. Treatment of enterobiasis and ascariasis with combatrin (pyrantel pamoate). *Trans. Soc. Trop. Med. Hyg.* 1972;66:170.

143. Sinniah, B., and D. Sinniah. The anthelminthic effects of pyrantel pamoate, oxantel-pyrantel pamoate, levamisole and mebendazole in the treatment of intestinal nematodes. *Ann. Trop. Med. Parasitol.* 1981;75: 315.

144. Aubry, M. L., P. Cowell, M. J. Davey, and S. Shevde. Aspects of the pharmacology of a new anthelmintic: Pyrantel. *Br. J. Pharmacol.* 1970;38:332.

145. Eyre, P. Some pharmacodynamic effects of the nematocides: methyridine, tetramisole and pyrantel. *J. Pharm. Pharmacol.* 1970;22:26.

146. Brown, H. D., A. R. Matzuk, I. R. Ilves, L. H. Peterson, S. A. Harris, L. H. Sarett, J. R. Egerton, J. J. Yakstis, W. C. Campbell, and A. C. Cuckler. Antiparasitic drugs. IV. 2-(4'-thiazolyl)-benzimidazole, a new anthelmintic. *J. Am. Chem. Soc.* 1961;83:1764.

147. Multiple authors. Thiabendazole symposium. *Texas Rep. Biol. Med.* 1969;27(Suppl. 2):533–708.

148. Cuckler, A. C., and K. C. Mezey. The therapeutic efficacy of thiabendazole for helminthic infections in man. *Arzneimittelforschung.* 1966;16:411.

149. Campbell, W. C., and A. C. Cuckler. Thiabendazole in the treatment and control of parasitic infections in man. *Texas Rep. Biol. Med.* 1969;27(Suppl. 2): 665.

150. Franz, K. H., W. J. Schneider, and M. H. Pohlman. Clinical trials with thiabendazole against intestinal nematodes infecting humans. *Am. J. Trop. Med. Hyg.* 1965;14:383.

151. Most, H. M., W. C. Yoeli, W. C. Campbell, and A. C. Cuckler. The treatment of *Strongyloides* and *Enterobius* infections with thiabendazole. *Am. J. Trop. Med. Hyg.* 1965;14:379.

152. Grove; D. I. Treatment of strongyloidiasis with thiabendazole: an analysis of toxicity and effectiveness. *Trans. Soc. Trop. Med. Hyg.* 1982;76:114.

153. Stone, O. J., and J. F. Mullins. Thiabendazole effectiveness in creeping eruption. *Arch. Dermatol.* 1965;91:427.

154. Harland, P. S. E. G., R. H. Meakins, and R. H. Harland. Treatment of cutaneous larva migrans with local thiabendazole. *BMJ* 1977;2:772.

155. Bardach, H. Lokalbehandlung der "creeping eruption" (Larva migrans nematosa) mit Thiabendazol. *Wien. Med. Wochenschr.* 1980;130:761.

156. Schantz, P. M., and L. T. Glickman. Toxocaral visceral larva migrans. *N. Engl. J. Med.* 1978;298: 436.

157. Aur, R. J. A., C. B. Pratt, and W. W. Johnson. Thiabendazole in visceral larva migrans. *Am. J. Dis. Child.* 1971;121:227.

158. Liu, L. X., and P. F. Weller. Trichinosis and infections with other tissue nematodes. In Harrison's Principles of Internal Medicine, ed. by A. F. Fauci, E. Braunwald, K. J. Isselbacher, J. D. Wilson, J. B. Martin, D. L. Kasper, S. L. Hauser, and D. L. Longo. New York: McGraw-Hill 1998, pp. 1206–1208.

159. Stone, O. J., C. T. Stone, and J. F. Mullins. Thiabendazole: probable cure for trichinosis. *JAMA* 1964; 187:536.

160. Kean, B. H., and D. W. Hoskins. Treatment of trichinosis. *JAMA.* 1964;190:852.

161. Campbell, W. C., Anti-inflammatory and analgesic properties of thiabendazole. *JAMA* 1971;216: 2143.

162. Schumaker, J. D., J. D. Band, G. L. Lensmeyer, and W. L. Craig. Thiabendazole treatment of severe strongyloidiasis in a hemodialyzed patient. *Ann. Intern. Med.* 1978;89:644.

163. Bauer, L. A., V. A. Raisys, M. T. Watts, and J. Ballinger. The pharmacokinetics of thiabendazole and its metabolites in an anephric patient undergoing hemodialysis and hemoperfusion. *J. Clin. Pharmacol.* 1982;22:276.

164. Tocco, D. J., C. Rosenblum, C. M. Martin, and H. J. Robinson. Absorption, metabolism, and excretion of thiabendazole in man and laboratory animals. *Toxicol. Appl. Pharmacol.* 1966;9:31.

165. Hewlett, E. L., O. Y. Hamid, J. Ruffier, and A. A. F. Mahmoud. In vivo suppression of delayed hypersensitivity by thiabendazole and diethylcarbamazine. *Immunopharmacology* 1981;3:324.

166. Shashindran, C., I. S. Gandhi, and N. S. Parmar. Anticonvulsant action of thiabendazole. *Eur. J. Pharmacol.* 1977;46:383.

167. Hawking, F. Chemotherapy of filariasis. *Antibiot. Chemother.* 1981;30:135.

168. Connor; D. H. Current concepts in parasitology. Onchocerciasis. *N. Engl. J. Med.* 1978;298:379.

169. Scharlau, G. Onchocerciasis—chemotherapy: a risk approach. *Trop. Doctor* 1981;11:8.

170. Ottesen, E. A., and C. P. Ramachandran. Lymphatic filariasis infection and disease: control strategies. *Parasitol. Today* 1995;11:129.

171. Drugs for parasitic infections. *Med. Lett.* 1998; 40:1.

172. Reddy, C. R., M. M. Reddy, and M. D. Sivaprasad. Niridazole (Ambilhar) in the treatment of dracunculiasis. *Am. J. Trop. Med. Hyg.* 1969;18:516.

173. Hawking, F. Diethylcarbamazine and new compounds for the treatment of filariasis. *Adv. Pharmacol. Chemother.* 1979;16:130.

174. Ottesen, E. A., P. F. Weller, and L. Heck. Specific cellular unresponsiveness in human filariasis. *Immunology* 1977;33:413.

175. Piessens, W. F., P. B. McGreevy, P. W. Piessens, M. McGreevy, I. Koiman, J. S. Saroso, and D. T. Dennis. Immune responses in filarial infections with *Brugia malayi*: specific cellular unresponsiveness to filarial antigens. *J. Clin. Invest.* 1979;65:172.

176. Piessens, W. F., S. Ratiwayanto, S. Tuti, J. H. Palmieri, P. W. Piessens, I. Koiman, and D. T. Dennis. Antigen specific suppressor cells and suppressor factors in human filariasis with *Brugia malayi*. *N. Engl. J. Med.* 1980;302:833.

177. Gustavson-Moringlane, I., and E. Bengtsson. Eosinophil leukocyte reactions from diethylcarbamazine in filariasis. *Ann. Trop. Med. Parasitol.* 1981;75:615.

178. Piessens, W. F., S. Ratiwayanto, P. W. Piessens, S. Tuti, P. B. McGreevy, F. Darwis, J. R. Palmieri, I. Koiman, and D. T. Dennis. Effect of treatment with diethylcarbamazine on immune responses to filarial antigens in patients infected with *Brugia malayi*. *Acta Trop.* 1981;38:227.

179. Tanaka, H. Y. Eshita, M. Takaoka, and G. Fujii. Suppression of microfilaricidal activity of diethylcar-

bamazine by anti-lymphocytic serum in cotton rat filariasis. *Southeast Asian J. Trop. Med. Public Health* 1977;8:19.

180. Gibson, D. W., D. H. Connor, H. L. Brown, H. Fuglsang, J. Anderson, B. O. L. Duke, and A. A. Duck. Onchocercal dermatitis: ultrastructural studies of microfilariaea and host tissues, before and after diethylcarbamazine (Hetrazan). *Am. J. Trop. Med. Hyg.* 1976; 25:74.

181. Cesbron, J. Y., A. Capron, B. B. Vargaftig, M. LaGarde, J. Pincemail, P. Braqut, H. Taelman, and M. Joseph. Platelets mediate the action of diethylcarbamazine on microfilariae. *Nature* 1987;325:533.

182. Fujimaki, Y., M. Ehara, E. Kimura, M. Shimada, and Y. Aoki. Diethycarbamazine, antifilarial drug, inhibits microtubule polymerization and disrupts preformed microtubules. *Biochem. Pharmacol.* 1990; 39:851.

183. Gilles; H. M. Soil-transmitted helminths (geohelminths). In *Manson's Tropical Diseases*, ed. by G. C. Cook. London: W. B. Saunders, 1996, pp. 1369–1412.

184. Edwards, G., K. Awadzi, A. M. Breckenridge, H. M. Gilles, M. L. Orme, and S. A. Ward. Diethylcarbamazine disposition in patients with onchocerciasis. *Clin. Pharmacol. Ther.* 1981;30:551.

185. Adjepon-Yamoah, K. K., G. Edwards, A. M. Breckenridge, M. L. Orme, and S. A. Ward. The effect of renal disease on the pharmacokinetics of diethylcarbamazine in man. *Br. J. Clin. Pharmacol.* 1982;13:829.

186. Edwards, G., A. M. Breckenridge, K. K. Adjepon-Yamoah, M. L. Orme, and S. A. Ward. The effect of variations in urinary pH on the pharmacokinetics of diethylcarbamazine. *Br. J. Clin. Pharmacol.* 1981;12:807.

187. Awadzi, K., K. K. Adjepon-Yamoah, G. Edwards, M. L. Orme, A. M. Breckenridge, and H. M. Gilles. The effect of moderate urine alkalinization on diethycarbamazine therapy in patients with onchocerciasis. *Br. J. Clin. Pharmacol.* 1986;21:669.

188. Taylor, H. R., and B. M. Greene. Ocular changes with oral and transepidermal diethylcarbamazine therapy of onchocerciasis. *Br. J. Ophthalmol.* 1981;65:494.

189. Gelband, H. Diethylcarbamzine salt in the control of lymphatic filariasis. *Am. J. Trop. Med. Hyg.* 1994;50:655.

190. Chlebowsky, H. O., and E. Zielke. Studies on bancroftian filariasis in Liberia, West Africa. IV. Notes on side effects observed during a diethylcarbamazine treatment campaign in a rural area endemic for *Wuchereria bancrofti* and *Onchocerca volvulus*. *Tropenmed. Parasitol.* 1980;31:339.

191. *Handbook of Drugs for Tropical Parasitic Infections*, ed. by Y. Abdi, L. Gustaffson, O. Ericsson, and U. Hellgren. London: Taylor and Francis, 1995.

192. Goa, K. L., D. McTavish, and S. P. Clissold. Ivermectin. A review of its antifilarial activity, pharmacokinetic properties and clinical efficacy in onchocerciasis. *Drugs* 1991;43:640.

193. Ottesen, E. A., and W. C. Campbell. Ivermectin in human medicine. *J. Antimicrob. Chemother.* 1994; 34:195.

194. Cully, D. F., D. Vassilatis, K. Liu, P. Paress, L.

Van de Ploeg, J. Schaeffer, and J. Arena. Cloning of an avermectin-sensitive glutamate-gated chloride channel from *Caenorhabditis elegans*. *Nature* 1994;371:707.

195. Arena, J. P., K. K. Liu, P. S. Paress, E. G. Frazier, D. F. Cully, H. Mrozik, and J. M. Schaeffer. The mechanism of action of avermectins in *Caenorhabditis elegans*: correlation between activation of glutamate sensitive chloride current, membrane binding and biological activity. *J. Parasitol.* 1995;81:286.

196. McKellar, Q. A., and H. A. Benchaoui. Avermectins and milbemycins. *J. Vet. Pharmacol. Ther.* 1996;19:331.

197. Shoop, W. L., D. A. Ostlind, S. P. Roher, G. Mickle, H. W. Haines, B. F. Michael, H. Mrozik, and M. H. Fisher. Avermectins and milbemycins against *Fasciola hepatica*: in vivo drug efficacy and in vitro receptor binding. *Int. J. Parasitol.* 1995;25:923.

198. Greene, B. M., H. R. Taylor, E. W. Cupp, R. P. Murphy, A. T. White, M. A. Aziz, H. Schulz-Key, S. A. D'Anna, H. S. Newland L. P. Goldschmidt, C. Auer, A. P. Hanson, S. V. Freeman, E. W. Reber, and P. N. Williams. Comparison of ivermectin and diethylcarbamazine in the treatment of onchocerciasis. *New. Engl. J. Med.* 1985;313:133.

199. Greene. B. M., A. T. White, H. S. Newland, E. Keyvan-Larijani, Z. D. Dukuly, M. Y. Gallin, M. A. Aziz, P. N. Williams, and H. R. Taylor. Single dose therapy with ivermectin for onchocerciasis. *Trans. Assoc. Am. Physicians* 1987;100:131.

200. Newland, H. S., A. T. White, B. M. Greene, S. A. D'Anna, H. E. Keyvan-Larijani, M. A. Aziz, P. N. Williams, and H. R. Taylor. Effect of single dose ivermectin therapy on human *Onchocerca volvulus* infection with onchocercal ocular involvement. *Br. J. Ophthalmol.* 1988;72:561.

201. Court, J. P., A. E. Bianco, S. Townson, P. J. Ham, and E. Friedheim. Study on the activity of antiparasitic agents against *Onchocerca lienalis* third stage larvae in vitro. *Trop. Med. Parsitol.* 1985;36:117.

202. Naquira, C., G. Jimeniz, J. G. Guerra, R. Bernal, D. R. Nalin, D. Neu, and M. Aziz. Ivermectin for human strongyloidiasis and other intestinal helminths. *Am. J. Trop. Med. Hyg.* 1989;40:304.

203. Whitworth, J. A. G. Filariases. *Curr. Opin. Infect. Dis.* 1994;7:696.

204. Greene, B. M., Z. D. Dukuly, B. Munoz, A. T. White, M. Pacque, and H. R. Taylor. A comparison of 6-, 12-, and 24-monthly dosing with ivermectin for treatment of onchocerciasis. *J. Infect. Dis.* 1991;163:376.

205. Pacque, M., C. Elmets, Z. D. Dukuly, B. Munoz, T. White, H. R. Taylor, and B. M. Greene. Improvement in severe onchocercal skin disease after a single dose of ivermectin. *Am. J. Med.* 1991;90:590.

206. Ottesen, E. A., V. Vijayasedaran, V. Kumaraswami, S. V. P. Pillai, A. Sadanandam, S. Frederick, R. Prabakar, and S. P. Tripathy. A controlled trial of ivermectin and diethylcarbamazine in lymphatic filariasis. *New. Engl. J. Med.* 1990;322:1113.

207. Datry, A., I. Hilmarsdottir, R. Mayorga-Sagastume, R. Lyagoubi, P. Gaxotte, S. Biligui, J. Chodakewitz, D. Neu, M. Danis, and M. Gentilini. Treatment of *Strongyloides stercoralis* infection with

ivermectin compared with albendazole: results of an open study of 60 cases. *Trans. R. Soc. Trop. Med. Hyg.* 1994;88:344.

208. Gann, P. H., F. A. Neva, and A. A. Gam. A randomized trial of single- and two-dose ivermectin versus thiabendazole for treatment of strongyloidiasis. *J. Infect. Dis.* 1994;169:1076.

209. Torres, J. R., R. Isturiz, J. Murillo, M. Guzman, and R. Contreras. Efficacy of ivermectin in the treatment of strongyloidiasis complicating AIDS. *Clin. Infect. Dis.* 1993;17:900.

210. Caumes, E., J. Carriere, A. Datry, P. Gaxotte, M. Danis, and M. Gentilini. A randomized trial of ivermectin versus albendazole for the treatment of cutaneous larva migrans. *Am. J. Trop. Med. Hyg.* 1993;49:641.

211. Klotz, U., J. E. Ogbuokiri, and P. O. Olonkwo. Ivermectin binds avidly to plasma proteins. *Eur. J. Clin. Pharmacol.* 1990;39:607.

212. Krishna, D. R., and U. Klotz. Determination of ivermectin in human plasma by high-performance liquid chromatography. *Arzneimittelforschung* 1993;43:609.

213. de Sole, G., K. A. Wadzi, J. Remme, K. Y. Dadzie, and O. Ba. A community trial of ivermectin in the onchocerciasis focus of Asubende, Ghana. II. Adverse reactions. *Trop. Med. Parasitol.* 1989;40:375.

214. de Sole, G., K. Y. Dadzie, J. Giese, and J. Remme. Lack of adverse reactions in ivermectin treatment of onchocerciasis. *Lancet* 1990;335:1106.

215. Rothova, A., A. van der Leli, W. R. Wilson, and R. F. Barbe. Side effects of ivermectin in treatment of onchocerciasis. *Lancet* 1989;1:1439.

216. Van Laethem, Y., and C. Lopes. Treatment of onchocerciasis. *Drugs* 1996;52:861.

217. Pacque, M., B. Munoz, G. Poetschke, J. Foose, B. M. Greene, and H. R. Taylor. Pregnancy outcome after inadvertent ivermectin treatment during community-based distribution. *Lancet* 1990;336:1486.

Drugs Employed in the Treatment of Viral Infections

Medical efforts to combat viral infection include a variety of approaches. As with the parasitic diseases, vector control is helpful in limiting those viral infections transmitted by insects (e.g., yellow fever transmitted by mosquitos) and animals (e.g., rabies transmitted by dogs). In some cases, isolation of infected patients will limit the spread of a virus in the community. Other efforts to control viral infection have been directed at active stimulation of the immune response by eliciting specific antibody production (immunization) or at passive assistance to the patient's defense mechanism by the use of human gamma globulin, equine antiserums, and, more recently, antiserum from successfully vaccinated humans. In addition to these approaches, there are a number of drugs available for the treatment and prevention of selected viral infections.

Prophylaxis by immunization has been the most effective form of control for many viral infections. Mass immunization with live (attenuated) virus vaccines is currently effectively employed to prevent diseases like polio, mumps, measles, and yellow fever. The use of vaccinia virus immunization to prevent smallpox has been so successful that the disease has been eradicated. The use of killed virus vaccines against influenza provides partial protection against serious infection. Influenza vaccines are currently used during epidemics to protect the elderly, the young, and people debilitated because of chronic disease (these are the groups that suffer the greatest morbidity and mortality during influenza epidemics).

Approaches to specific control of viral infections.

Approach	Level of effectiveness	Antiviral spectrum	Duration of effect
Immunological	Usually high	Very narrow	Relatively long to lifetime
Host resistance (interferon)	Moderate to high	Very broad	Relatively short term
Chemical	Low/moderate/high	Usually narrow	Short term

In addition to a variety of host defenses, such as antibody production, macrophage action, and cell-mediated immunity, viruses stimulate the production of interferon by certain host cells. This protein, in turn, elicits antiviral activity in other host cells. Two methods have been employed experimentally to increase the amount of interferon in the body. The first is the administration of exogenous interferon and the second is the use of compounds that induce interferon production by the host. Because interferon produces a broad-spectrum antiviral effect and is well tolerated by patients, the administration of purified human interferon holds great promise for antiviral therapy, and it will be discussed in the following chapter. A comparison of the three approaches to antiviral therapy (immunization, interferon production, and chemotherapy) is presented in the table above.

CHAPTER SIXTEEN

Chemotherapy of Viral Infections, I

Drugs Used to Treat Influenza Virus Infections, Herpesvirus Infections, and Drugs with Broad-Spectrum Antiviral Activity

Definition and Classification of Viruses

Viruses are organisms composed of a nucleic acid core (the genome may be either DNA or RNA) surrounded by a protein-containing shell; they reproduce only inside living cells. They derive their energy supply and their substrates from the infected cell; they also use its synthetic machinery to produce the virus-specific protein required for production of the mature viral particle. Mature virus particles possess only one type of nucleic acid, and they lose their organized form during replication of the genome in the host cell. These characteristics distinguish the viruses from intracellular parasites like the chlamydiae (psittacosis-lymphogranuloma venerum-trachoma group of organisms), which possess both DNA and RNA in their infectious particles and retain their organized form in the intracellular phase, dividing by binary fission.[1] Still more complex intracellular parasites like the plasmodia, the leprosy bacillus, and the rickettsiae have even higher levels of cellular organization, possessing protein-synthesizing and energy-generating systems of their own.

The animal viruses are classified according to various characteristics, such as nucleic acid content (RNA viruses, DNA viruses), gross morphology, location of viral multi-plication (in the cytoplasm or nucleus of the infected cell), composition of the virus shell (enveloped or non-enveloped), and serological typing. A selected list of the viruses that infect man is presented in Table 16–1.

The Biology of Viral Reproduction

It is impossible in this text to provide a background review of the molecular biology of animal viruses. But by presenting examples of some of the biochemical events that take place during a viral infection, we can provide a basis for understanding some of the possible sites where the process of viral infection can be selectively inhibited by drugs. The process of viral infection can be conveniently considered in three stages: (I) entry of the virus into the host cell and release of nucleic acid; (II) replication of the genome and synthesis of viral proteins; and (III) assembly of the virion and release from the cell. Some authors divide the viral replicative cycle into ten individual steps.[4] This differs from the present scheme mainly in that stage II, viral replication and protein synthesis, is subdivided into five separate steps. All viruses follow this basic replicative scheme but the different virus families may differ considerably from one another at one or more steps in the

Table 16–1. Classification of some viruses infecting humans.

Group	Agent	Characteristics
RNA VIRUSES		
Picornavirus		Cubic symmetry, no envelope, multiply in cytoplasm, single-stranded RNA about 2×10^6 daltons
	Poliovirus	Three serotypes can cause paralysis
	Coxsackie	Causes a variety of symptoms
	Rhinovirus	Over 100 serotypes, "common cold" viruses
Togavirus		Small, enveloped virions with single-stranded RNA of 4×10^6 daltons transmitted by arthropods
	Western and Eastern equine encephalitis	About 20 viruses, mosquito-borne
	Rubella virus (German measles)	The only non–arthropod-borne togavirus
Flavivirus		Enveloped icosahedral virion 40–50 nm in diameter and a genome of 10 kb
	Hepatitis C	Mostly mosquito-borne, some tick-borne, but hepatitis C virus is transmitted sexually and via human blood
	Flavivirus (yellow fever, dengue)	
Paramyxovirus		Enveloped virions containing single-stranded negative strand RNA of 7×10^6 daltons plus virion polymerase, infectious for many tissues
	Parainfluenza	
	Mumps	
	Rubeola (measles)	
	Respiratory syncytial viruses	Major cause of respiratory disease in infants
Orthomyxovirus		Enveloped pleomorphic virions containing negative strand RNA of $5–6 \times 10^6$ daltons plus virion polymerase
	Influenza	Three serotypes (A,B,C,); type A most frequent, causes large epidemics and undergoes constant antigenic variation
Reovirus		Icosahedral, double-shelled virions containing 10 or more double-stranded RNAs ranging from 0.4 to 2.8×10^6 daltons plus virion transcriptase
	Reovirus of humans	Cause mild illness of respiratory and gastrointestinal tracts
Retrovirus		Large family of enveloped viruses 80–100 nm in diameter with a complex structure and an unusual enzyme, reverse transcriptase Unique among viruses, the genome is diploid, consisting of an inverted dimer of plus sense single-stranded RNA, 7–10 kb in size
	HIV-like viruses; human T-cell leukemia viruses	

(continued)

Table 16–1. Continued

Group	Agent	Characteristics
Rhabdovirus		Bullet-shaped viruses about 180×75 nm containing a single molecule of minus sense single-stranded RNA (13–16 kb)
	Vesicular stomatitis-like viruses	
	Rabies-like viruses	Rabies viruses may cause severe diseases in humans following animal bites
DNA VIRUSES		
Papovavirus		Icosahedral, nonenveloped virions containing circular double-stranded DNA of $3–5 \times 10^6$ daltons
	Human papilloma	Causes warts
Adenovirus		Icosahedral, nonenveloped, highly developed virions with spikes containing linear DNA of $2–3 \times 10^7$ daltons
	Human subgroup	Causes upper respiratory disease and conjunctivitis, 31 serotypes known
Herpesvirus		Large, enveloped, icosahedral virions with double-stranded linear DNA 10^8 daltons; grow in nucleus
	Herpes simplex	Type 1 causes "fever blisters," type 2 causes genital herpes
	Varicella zoster	Causes chicken pox in children and shingles in adults
	Epstein-Barr	Associated with infectious mononucleosis and Burkitt's lymphoma
	Cytomegalovirus	Infection causes fetal damage
Poxvirus		Large, brick-shaped enveloped virions containing at least 30 proteins, including virion RNA polymerase; DNA is double-stranded 1.5×10^8 daltons
	Variola	Causes smallpox
	Vaccinia	Used for vaccination against smallpox
Hepadnovirus		Spherical particles 42 nm in diameter, consisting of a 27 nm icosahedral core within a closely adherent outer capsid that contains cellular lipids, glycoproteins, and a virus-specific surface antigen (HbsAg). Replication involves an RNA intermediate and requires a virus-coded reverse transcriptase
	Human hepatitis B	These viruses replicate in hepatocytes and cause hepatitis.

Source: Adapted from Luria et al.,[2] Table 1–1, and White and Fenner.[3]

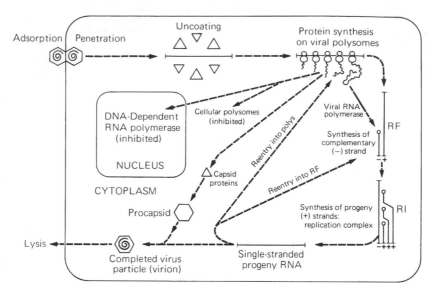

Figure 16–1. The replication cycle of poliovirus. RF, replicative form; RI, replicative intermediate. (From Pearson.[16])

replicative cycle. A schematic summary of the replication cycle of poliovirus,[5] a nonenveloped RNA virus, is presented in Figure 16–1 for reference during the following discussion.

Stage I Attachment, Penetration, and Uncoating

The mechanism of virus entry into cells is complex and critically dependent on the three-dimensional structure of the infecting virion.[7] Virus particles must first attach to cells in order to cause infection. Viral attachment proteins located on the surface of the virion bind to receptors on the plasma membrane of the cell. Polio, for example, a virus that possesses a protein capsid composed of 60 repeating units consisting of four separate proteins per unit attaches to receptors found only in membranes of susceptible cells. The receptor for most orthomyxoviruses (e.g., influenza) is the terminal sialic acid of an oligosaccharide side chain of a cellular glycoprotein, while the ligand, which is located in a cleft at the distal tip of each monomer of a trimeric viral hemagglutinin glycoprotein,[3] projects in small spikes

from the surface of the virion envelope.[8] Receptors for a number of viruses are members of the immunoglubulin superfamily, such as the integrin ICAM-1, the major receptor for most rhinoviruses, and CD4, the receptor for the human immunodeficiency viruses.[3] Although the viruses have developed an opportunistic use of these receptors, the primary function of these receptors has nothing to do with the viruses. Some viruses use more than one receptor—for example, several chemokine receptors can serve as HIV-1 coreceptors.[7,9]

After attachment, a variety of mechanisms operate to introduce the virus into the cell. Certain bacterial viruses (the T-even bacteriophages, for example) have developed elaborate mechanisms for injecting their nucleic acid through the cell wall and membrane into the cytoplasm, but these mechanisms do not pertain to animal viruses. There are two main mechanisms through which animal viruses enter cells. Many enveloped and nonenveloped viruses use endocytosis to initiate infection.[3] First there is attachment to receptors that cluster at clathrin coated pits, and this is followed by endocytosis into clathrin-coated vesicles that enter the cytoplasm. The clathrin coat is removed and the virion fuses with endosomes (acidic prelysosomal vacuoles). Acidification within the vesicle triggers changes that release the virion into the cytoplasm. For example, at the acidic pH of the endosomes, the hemagglutinin molecule of influenza virus undergoes a conformational change that enables fusion to occur between the viral envelope and the endosome membrane, leading to release of the viral nucleocapsid into the cytoplasm. In the case of certain animal viruses that are surrounded by an envelope containing carbohydrate, protein, and lipid, the viral envelope fuses with the membrane of the cell and the virion passes directly into the cytoplasm.[10]

After their entry, virions must be uncoated for their genes to become available for transcription. Some poxviruses have developed elaborate mechanisms of becoming uncoated and releasing their nucleic acid after they have entered the cell. For example, the vaccinia virus, a large DNA virus with an envelope, undergoes a two-stage uncoating process in the cell.[11] In the first stage, the virion is attacked by host cell enzymes that partially degrade the virus particle, which loses some of its protein and all of its phospholipid. The resulting particle, called a *core*, is composed of DNA surrounded by protein. Poxvirus cores contain a DNA-dependent RNA polymerase,[12] and they can synthesize mRNA.[13] The second stage of the uncoating process proceeds only after a delay, releasing the viral DNA into the cell cytoplasm. This second uncoating process is prevented by inhibitors of protein synthesis.[11] The most plausible model of this sequence of events is that a portion of the DNA in the virus core is available to act as a template for the synthesis of an mRNA that in turn directs the synthesis of a virus-specific uncoating enzyme that then degrades the core, releasing naked vaccinia DNA. The delay between the first and second stage of the uncoating process represents the time required for synthesis of the virus-specific mRNA and uncoating protein. In the case of enveloped RNA viruses that enter cells by fusion of their envelope with either the plasma membrane or an endosomal membrane, the nucleocapsid is discharged directly into the cytoplasm, and transcription begins from viral nucleic acid still associated with this structure.[3]

These examples of viral penetration and uncoating illustrate the complicated interaction between the virus and the host cell that is required for the initiation of a viral infection. The infective process can be interrupted here at the first stage of the virus–cell interaction. Antiviral antibodies, for example, can prevent attachment of the virus to the cell by reacting with the coat protein of the virion; when added shortly after adsorption of the virus to the cell surface, they can, in some cases, prevent initiation of infection. This strategy is being utilized to develop inhibitors of the human immunodeficiency (HIV) virus, among others. Amantadine, one of the clinically useful antiviral drugs, acts at this early stage of the infection process. In the presence of amantadine the virus can absorb to the cell surface, but penetration and uncoating are apparently inhibited. As has just been demonstrated, drugs that inhibit animal cell protein synthesis may in some cases inhibit the uncoating process; such drugs, however, are not useful in therapy because their effect is not selective.

Stage II—Viral Replication and Synthesis of Viral Components

In the second stage of viral infection, the genome of the virus is duplicated, and the viral proteins are synthesized in the appropriate sequence. The events that take place in the second stage involve a variety of control mechanisms that direct the energy-producing and synthetic functions of the cell to serve in the synthesis of viral nucleic acid and protein. When some DNA viruses infect a population of growing cells, for example, they inhibit the synthesis of host DNA, thus reserving the pools of nucleic acid precursors for their own use. This inhibition of host cell DNA synthesis is mediated by a virus-specific protein.

This second stage is divided into several substages, including early transcription, or formation of viral mRNA; early translation, or formation of "early" proteins (i.e., primarily RNA or DNA polymerases); replication of the viral genome through successive rounds of RNA or DNA replication; late transcription, when viral mRNA is again formed; and late translation, or formation of "late" (i.e., structural) proteins.[4] With the retroviruses, early transcription is replaced by reverse transcription (i.e., mRNA to proviral DNA), early translation is replaced by integration of the proviral DNA in the host genome, and replication coincides with replication of the cell genome.

Replication of DNA and RNA viruses differs in many aspects. Replication of most DNA viruses follows a normal pathway in that there is transcription of mRNA from double-stranded DNA and then replication of the DNA. RNA viruses are unique in having their genetic information encoded in RNA, and there are many different ways RNA viruses produce mRNA, depending on the type of viral genome (e.g., single stranded or double stranded). In single stranded RNA viruses of positive sense the viral RNA binds directly to ribosomes and is translated in full or in part without the need for any prior transcriptional step, whereas all other types of viral RNA must first be transcribed to mRNA. Eukaryotic cells contain no RNA-dependent RNA polymerase, so negative sense single-stranded RNA viruses and double-stranded RNA viruses must carry an RNA-dependent RNA polymerase in the virion.[14] For DNA viruses that replicate in the nucleus, cellular DNA-dependent RNA polymerase II carries out this function. All other viruses need a unique and specific transcriptase that is virus encoded and is an integral part of the virion. Double-stranded DNA viruses, for example, carry a DNA-dependent RNA polymerase, whereas double-stranded RNA viruses have a double-stranded RNA-dependent RNA polymerase. Primary RNA transcripts from nucleus-associated viral DNA are subject to the same post-transcriptional alterations (capping, polyadenylation, and methylation) in the nucleus as the host cell mRNA, prior to export to the cytoplasm.[3]

The production and function of key virus-specific enzymes like nucleic acid polymerases and enzymes involved in synthesizing nucleic acid precursors stand out as logical points for selective attack by chemotherapeutic agents. Several compounds inhibit viral nucleic acid synthesis. Guanidine and 2-(α-hydroxybenzyl)-benzimidazole[15,16] are both active against certain small RNA viruses (e.g., poliovirus, coxsackievirus, echovirus) as a result of a primary inhibition of viral RNA production. The mechanisms by which these compounds inhibit RNA synthesis have not been precisely defined, but it appears that initiation of RNA chains is inhibited by guanidine (and possibly also by the benzimidazoles). Several antibiotics (e.g., streptovaricins, rifamycins, distamycin A) inhibit some of the virus-specific nucleic acid polymerases and have antiviral activity in selected systems in vitro. None of these agents has yet been shown to be useful in the chemotherapy of viral diseases.

The detailed study of the viral enzymes responsible for nucleic acid synthesis is providing a basis for the synthesis of new antiviral drugs. The substrate sites of some viral enzymes "accept" nucleotide analogs not accommodated by the mammalian polymerases. Such nucleotide analogs may produce an antiviral effect either by blocking the function of the viral enzyme or by being incorporated into viral nucleic acid, to produce a faulty inactive RNA or DNA. In either case, a selective toxicity may be obtained. Iododeoxyuridine (IUdR) is an antiviral drug that is incorporated into DNA in place of thymidine. The IUdR-containing DNA behaves abnormally in several ways and there is a consequent marked decrease in viral infectivity. The incorporation of IUdR into DNA is not a very selective event, since the drug is incorporated into the DNA of the patient's cells as well as into that of the virus. Acyclovir is a drug with a high selectivity of action for herpesviruses. It is actually a pro-drug that is selectively activated by phosphorylation by a virus-specific thymidine kinase and it is subsequently converted to the triphosphate which is a more potent inhibitor of herpes virus DNA polymerase than cellular DNA polymerases.[17] Thus, more active drug is produced in the virus-infected cell than in the uninfected cell and virus nucleic acid synthesis is more sensitive to inhibition than nucleic acid synthesis in the normal cell. In addition to acyclovir there are several other inhibitors of DNA replication having varying degrees of selectivity, including ganciclovir, foscarnet, and cidofovir. The RNA-dependent DNA polymerase (reverse transcriptase), which is found in retroviruses such as HIV, is missing from eukaryotic cells and thus serves as a useful target for several drugs used in the treatment of AIDS. Inhibitors of the reverse transcriptase enzyme are active against all retroviruses; these will be discussed in Chapter 17.

All of the compounds discussed thus far interfere with specific viral proteins; but, inhibition of virus replication can also be achieved indirectly by inhibiting a key step in host cell metabolism that is required for viral DNA or RNA replication or maturation. Examples include inhibitors of IMP dehydrogenase, S-adenosylhomocysteine hydrolase, and OMP decarboxylase, and one such compound, ribavirin, an IMP dehydrogenase inhibitor, is used clinically.

The virus must present to the eukaryotic cell protein-synthesizing machinery a mRNA that the cell can recognize as such and then translate. The production of viral proteins in all DNA viruses requires the synthesis of mRNAs, which are then translated by the protein synthesizing machinery (ribosomes, tRNAs, amino acids, activating enzymes, etc.) of the host cell. Many single-stranded RNA viruses contain (−)RNA (that is, RNA as the antimessenger) and this must serve as a template for the production of (+)RNA under the direction of a viral transcriptase before protein synthesis can take place. In the case of some single-stranded RNA viruses (e.g., poliovirus, coxsackievirus), the virus itself contains the (+)RNA that serves both as a messenger for protein synthesis and as a template for (−)RNA synthesis. Poliovirus RNA is translated in a single, continuous process. Thus, a very large protein is formed, and this is systemically cleaved by protease to yield the viral enzymes and structural proteins. With many of the more complex viruses, the mRNAs for proteins involved in the replication of the viral genome and in the direction of host cell synthesis of viral-specific components are produced earlier in the infection process than the mRNA for proteins like the capsid proteins, which are not required until the end when assembly of the virion takes place. This statement is somewhat of an oversimplification, but it points out the fact that production of the various components of the virus is subject to some control. Most viral proteins then undergo post-translational modifications, such as phosphorylation, fatty acid acylation (for membrane insertion), glycosylation, or proteolytic cleavage, and they must be transported to various sites in the cell where they are needed for viral replication or assembly.

Stage III—Assembly and Release of the Virus

In the final stage of the infection process, the viral components are assembled into a mature virion. During replication, the viral nucleic acid is not associated with viral structural protein. The capsid proteins accumulate in the cell late in the infection. In stage III, the viral genome is encased by capsid proteins and, once associated with them, can no longer replicate. With the adenoviruses, a particular protein binds to a nucleotide sequence at one end of the viral DNA known as the packaging sequence; this enables the DNA to enter the procapsid bound to basic core proteins, after which some of the capsid proteins are cleaved to make the mature virion.[3] In the case of nonenveloped viruses (e.g., poliovirus, adenovirus), the virion is complete and is released from the cell. With other viruses, however, the capsid is enveloped by a membrane, the carbohydrate and lipid portions of which are derived from host cell membranes. The poxviruses are even more complex. They contain a large DNA molecule surrounded by many viral proteins and more than one membrane. These complex viruses are synthesized in cytoplasmic factories, and they possess a higher degree of organization than the other viruses.

The release of mature virions from the cell may be rapid and may be accompanied by cell death and lysis; this is often the case with the simpler nonenveloped viruses like polio. In contrast to this method of release, some enveloped viruses are released (often over a long period of time) by a process of budding at the cell membrane. In this case, the cytoplasmic membrane remains intact during the release of the viruses, and the cell may survive. Many viruses that bud from the plasma membrane are noncytopathogenic and may be associated with persistent infections.

Interferons are believed to at least partly interfere with the assembly and release of new virus particles. No other clinically useful antiviral drugs are directly involved in this part of the virus multiplication cycle, but these processes are potential sites for selective inhibition. The compounds 2-deoxy-D-glucose and D-glucosamine, for example, inhibit the formation of the viral proteins hemagglutinin and neuraminidase and therefore they indirectly prevent the formation of mature influenza virions.[18] Neuraminidase is an enzyme that cleaves sialic acid off glycoprotein, and its activity is important for either the assembly or release of some myxoviruses. The replication of influenza virus in tissue culture can be inhibited by a specific inhibitor of neuraminidase, 2-deoxy-2,3-dehydro-N-trifluoroacetylneuraminic acid.[19,20] Recently, some new inhibitors of neuraminidase (e.g., zanamivir) have been developed and these seem to have great promise in the treatment of infection by influenza viruses. These compounds bind to neuraminidase and change its conformation, thus stopping release of newly formed virus from the surface of infected cells and preventing viral spread.[21,22] These compounds are selective for influenza neuraminidase and should not produce side effects due to inhibition of human enzymes.

Antiviral Chemotherapy

Through this introduction we have tried to underscore the fact that fundamental research into the molecular biology of viral replication is providing a basis for the rational development of antiviral drugs. We have chosen to present here only a few examples of the ways in which potential che-

motherapeutic compounds can interfere with viral replication. The biology of many viruses is now understood in considerable detail and there are several ways in which compounds can selectively interfere with virus-specific processes and block their reproduction (see refs. 20,23–25). Because viruses parasitize many of the functions of their host cells, there are many biochemical mechanisms common to both the infecting agent and the animal cell. This, of course, limits the number of functions that may be selectively interrupted by chemical agents. The larger, more complex viruses are more likely to be targets for chemotherapy than small viruses, simply because they produce a greater number of virus-specific proteins. Herpesvirus, for example, encodes at least 49 proteins and the pox viruses, which contain a double-stranded DNA of approximately 1.5×10^8 daltons, have sufficient information to encode 75 or more proteins, providing many potential sites for selective chemotherapeutic attack.

One of the problems in chemotherapy of viral infection is that the clinical symptoms of infection are often not evident until there has already been extensive viral replication, and the immune responses of the host are already building an effective deterrent to the virus. Thus, for many common viral infections chemotherapy may not be an appropriate modality of treatment. This is especially true in those cases in which the usual presentation is one of mild disease. The need for good chemotherapeutic drugs is particularly great with viruses that cause severe infections, particularly in patients with a depressed host response, and with viruses that cause chronic infection, such as herpes simplex types 1 and 2.[26] There are already firm indications that antiviral drugs are useful in prophylaxis against and treatment of a few severe viral infections. A clear need exists for drugs with a greater antiviral potency and selectivity of action for use in patients with severe viral infections requiring systemic drug administration.

Viral resistance can emerge against all antiviral compounds. Many resistant strains of viruses have been shown to have mutations in the genes encoding the specific drug target or drug activator, such as the viral thymidine kinase gene in herpes simpler virus (HSV) resistant to acyclovir.[27] All antiviral drugs have the potential for selecting for drug resistant viruses, and antiviral drug resistance can have serious clinical and public health implications. Debilitating and life-threatening drug-resistant herpes virus infections (cytomegalovirus, varicella zoster virus, and herpes simplex virus) occur with increasing frequency in immunocompromised patients, including recipients of transplants, those with hematological malignancies, those receiving chemotherapy, and patients with AIDS.[28-30] Because these patients are subject to long courses of antiherpes drug prophylaxis and treatment, the emergence of resistance as a cause of treatment failure is not surprising. Resistance of HIV to drugs has been documented against most if not all reverse transcriptase inhibitors on the market. This limits the efficacy of single-drug therapy against HIV and is the basis for combination antiretroviral therapy, despite the increased cost. Since we now recognize the potential for the antiviral compounds to generate viral resistance, it is very important that the present and future use of these drugs be carefully monitored to ensure that they are appropriately prescribed and to maximize benefit and minimize risk to the patient.

Drugs Used to Treat Influenza Virus Infections

Amantadine and Rimantadine

MECHANISM OF ACTION AND RESISTANCE. These are water-soluble amines with unique cage-like structures. The parent compound,

Amantadine   **Rimantadine**

1-adamantanamine hydrochloride, is a tricyclic primary amine that was discovered in the 1960s and was found to inhibit replication of strains of influenza A. Rimantadine, or 1-methyl-1-adamantine methylamine HCL, was developed in the United States, but it has been studied and used clinically in Russia for many years. Both drugs are active at low concentrations against influenza type A with little or no activity against influenza B.[31,32] Other viruses, such as rubella, parainfluenza, and respiratory syncytial viruses, are inhibited by high concentrations that are toxic to humans.[33]

The antiviral mechanism of these drugs had been extensively studied but is still not completely worked out. There appears to be no effect on virus attachment and penetration, viral RNA-dependent RNA polymerase activity, or viral release from cells. From the study of drug-resistant mutants, it is clear that the M2 membrane protein of the influenza A virus is the target of amantadine action.[33,34] The resistance results from single amino acid substitutions within the transmembrane domain of the M2 protein.[35,36] The M2 protein is a homotetramer of 96 amino acid chains that associate as a pair of membrane-spanning, disulfide-linked dimers. The transmembrane domains form proton-conducting channels that are thought to conduct protons into the interior of the virus.[37] Neutron diffraction studies support a model in which amantadine physically blocks the proton channels formed by the M2 protein.[38] Molecular modeling studies are consistent with amantadine interactions with the center of the channel.[39] Figure 16–2 shows the amantadine blockade of currents through channels created in a lipid bilayer with a peptide from the transmembrane domain of the M2 protein. Depending on the particular virus strain, inhibition of the M2 protein function can affect two different stages of virus replication—uncoating and viral maturation. Virus uncoating is affected because incoming protons normally induce dissociation of the matrix M1 protein from the ribonucleoprotein.[40] Virus maturation is affected because a decrease in the pH in the *trans* Golgi vesicular compartment is required to convert the viral hemagglutinin to its "low-pH" conformation, a conversion that is required

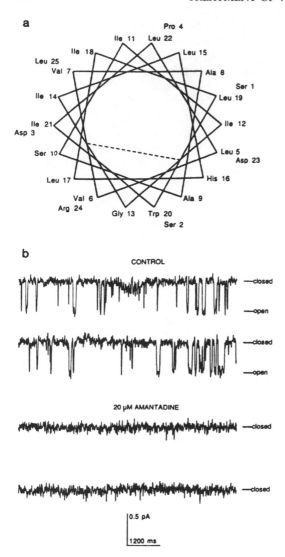

Figure 16–2. (a) Sequence of synthetic 25-residue peptide containing the putative transmembrane domain of M2 protein (inner ring) with adjoining extramembrane residues. The helical wheel projection is oriented with the strongly hydrophobic intramembrane sector above the dotted line. (b) Single-channel currents (downward deflexions) across a planar lipid bilayer with incorporated synthetic peptide, inhibited by 20 μM amantadine HCl (added to both sides of the membrane). (From Duff and Ashley.[37])

for the "pinching off" and release of the virus particles.[41,42] Thus, depending on whether proton flow through the M2 protein channels is impeded early or late in the infectivity cycle, there is inhibition of either influenza A virus uncoating or maturation and release.[4]

Strains of influenza A that are resistant to amantadine and rimantadine have been recovered from nasopharyngeal specimens of approximately 30% of children, adults, and the elderly in residential homes during treatment. Resistance develops within several days of onset of treatment, and where treatment and prophylaxis are being undertaken concomitantly, it is essential that symptomatic patients be isolated to reduce the possible transmission of resistant viruses.[43] Although epidemic strains of influenza A viruses remain susceptible to amantadine and rimantadine, cross-resistant mutants emerge rapidly during treatment.[44] With close family contact, transmission of resistant isolates and secondary illness can occur. Naturally occurring strains of resistant influenza A viruses have not been found, except when linked epidemiologically to patients treated with amantadine or rimantadine.

CLINICAL USE OF AMANTADINE AND RIMANTADINE. Despite the in vitro sensitivity of some parainfluenza viruses and rubella, amantadine is clinically useful only in chemoprophylaxis and treatment of influenza A infections. The efficacy of amantadine in chemoprophylaxis has been established in a number of controlled clinical studies involving several thousand patients who were naturally exposed during community outbreaks of influenza A (see Douglas[45] and Hirsch and Swartz[46] for reviews of clinical trials). It took several years to clearly establish the efficacy of amantadine because the early clinical trials contained a number of deficiencies in their design, including an inadequate number of patients, an occasional failure to confirm the infection serologically, inappropriate matching of control and drug-treated groups, and lack of double-blind procedures in administration and patient evaluation.[47]

It is easy to understand the difficulty in determining the effectiveness of an antiviral drug in reducing the incidence of naturally acquired infection during an influenza epidemic. The experimental protocol has to be prepared and the participating investigators organized before the epidemic has developed. Otherwise, it is difficult to assure uniformity of methods and adequate sample sizes. Consistent and accurate methods of identifying index cases, defining the presence of infection, and quantitating its severity and duration must be employed. Appropriate serological identification of the infection must be carried out, and antibody titers should be followed in all control and treated patients to determine possible effects of the drug on subclinical infection and to control for those patients suffering from virus infection other than the influenza strain under study. The population studied must be assigned to drug-treated or control groups by an appropriate random process, and the groups must be compared, at the end, to assure that they are matched according to age and sex. Finally, the drug or placebo should be administered and the patient response assessed according to double-blind procedure.

Several studies that have been carried out following this protocol demonstrate that amantadine, given before the onset of clini-

cal symptoms, decreases the occurrence of influenza A_2 (Asian influenza) in humans when the infection is experimentally induced[48,49] and when it is naturally acquired.[50,51] The results of one of these studies are presented in Table 16–2. They demonstrate that amantadine treatment of contacts (people living in the same household) of active cases of influenza A_2 results in both a decreased incidence of clinical influenza and a significant reduction in subclinical infection (i.e., where there is only serological evidence). The sample size in this study is not large, but the results are representative. Subsequent studies have demonstrated the efficacy of amantadine in prophylaxis against infection by non-Asian strains of influenza A.[52,53]

Amantadine certainly does not provide complete protection, but the results of clinical studies demonstrate that it has an efficacy of approximately 70% in the prevention of influenza caused by type A strains.

Table 16–2. *The effect of amantadine on the incidence of infection in contacts of serologically confirmed, active cases of influenza A_2*. Index cases were identified during an influenza A_2 epidemic, and their families were divided at random into drug-treated and placebo groups. All members of one family except the index case received the same treatment (drug or placebo). Index cases received only the placebo, so as not to reduce the possible spread of influenza virus among contacts. Treatment consisted of 100 mg of amantadine (adult dose) every 12 h for 10 days from the time the index case was first seen. The drug, or placebo, was given on a double-blind basis. Blood samples were taken from everybody on the first visit and again 2 to 3 weeks later. During the 10 days, the family members were visited regularly with daily recording of temperature and the presence of a cough. A cough accompanied by a temperature of 100°F or higher was accepted as the criterion for a diagnosis of clinical influenza. Subclinical infection was identified by a fourfold or greater rise in antibody titer to A_2/England/10/67 virus without cough and temperature elevation. The data presented in the table refer only to family members of index cases in which there was serological confirmation of influenza A_2 infection.

| | Contacts who developed clinical influenza within 10 days of entering the study: | | | | | |
| | All cases | | | Cases confirmed serologically | | |
Treatment	n/total	%	P	n/total	%	P
Amantadine	2/55	3.6		0/48	0	
			0.07			0.05–0.01
Placebo	12/85	14.1		10/69	14.5	

	Contacts with serological evidence of influenza infection:					
	Clinical and subclinical infections			Subclinical infections only		
Amantadine	7/48	14.6		7/48	14.6	
			<0.01			0.2
Placebo	27/69	39.1		17/69	24.6	

Source: Data taken from Galbraith et al.,[50] Tables II and III.

Amantadine is not effective against influenza B. In the presence of a confirmed outbreak of influenza A, prophylaxis with amantadine is generally indicated in the following groups of individuals:[54]

1. Unvaccinated individuals who are at high risk of serious morbidity and mortality because of underlying disease (e.g., pulmonary, cardiovascular, metabolic, neuromuscular, or immunodeficiency disease)
2. Older persons in an institutionalized setting who have not received the current influenza vaccine
3. Adults who have not been immunized with the appropriate vaccine and whose activities are essential to the community (e.g., selected hospital personnel).

The dosage of amantadine for prophylaxis in adults is 100 mg twice daily. In patients who are not immunized, chemoprophylaxis should be continued until influenza is no longer prevalent, usually an interval of 4 to 6 weeks.[55] Amantadine does not interfere with the immune response to influenza A vaccine and, if vaccine is available, the drug should be used in conjunction with a program of parenterally administered vaccine.[55] Rimantadine is similarly effective in preventing influenza A virus infections. In a comparative study during one outbreak of influenza A1/H1N1 and A/H3N2, both drugs were equally efficacious at doses of 200 mg/day.[56] Preliminary trials also suggest that both drugs have prophylactic activity at 100 mg/day.[57]

Several carefully controlled clinical studies with serologically confirmed cases of a variety of naturally occurring influenza A strains demonstrate that amantadine treatment of active cases of influenza A results in more rapid defervesence and a milder clinical course.[58–62] The clinical improvement is probably due to a reduction in the number of additional cells infected by the virus. Assessments of pulmonary function in a small group of influenza patients receiving drug or placebo suggest that amantadine treatment accelerates the resolution of peripheral airway dysfunction that occurs with uncomplicated influenza A infection.[63] The dosage for treatment is the same as for chemoprophylaxis, and to be effective amantadine must be administered within the first 24–48 h after the onset of symptoms. Therapy should be considered for patients who are at high risk of morbidity because of underlying disease (as defined above), patients with life-threatening primary influenza pneumonia, infants with severe influenza-associated croup, and those whose functioning during an influenza outbreak is essential (e.g., selected hospital personnel).[54] In most otherwise healthy individuals influenza is a mild disease and treatment with amantadine is not necessary.

Several studies have shown that rimantadine is also a useful therapeutic agent for influenza A virus infections when started within 48 h of symptom onset.[25] Comparative trials of amantadine and rimantadine have shown no major differences in their therapeutic effects.[64] Rimantadine is used in an identical manner to that of amantadine. Prolonged administration is well tolerated by the elderly in nursing homes, thus rimantadine may be the drug of choice for the prophylaxis and treatment of influenza A.

PHARMACOKINETICS. Amantadine is rapidly and completely absorbed from the gastrointestinal tract.[65] A peak level of about 0.3 µg/ml is achieved in the plasma 2–4 h after a single, oral 100 mg dose in an adult.[66] Repeated 100 mg doses at 12-h intervals produce a steady-state peak plasma level in the range of 0.7 µg/ml.[66] The volume of distribution of amantadine is 4.8 liters/kg of body weight,[67] and studies in the mouse show that the tissue levels in the lung are in the range of 15 times the simultaneous plasma concentration.[65] Thus, at steady state, the concentration of amantadine in lung tissue may be in the range of 10–12 µg/g wet weight in an adult receiving the usual dosage of 100 mg twice daily. This calculated lung concentration exceeds the ED_{50} reported for amantadine against several strains of influenza A virus in vitro, which ranges from 3.1 to 7.5 µg/ml.[68]

There is no evidence for amantadine metabolism in humans[65] and the unaltered drug is excreted predominantly via glomerular filtration (with some tubular secretion) in the kidneys.[67] The plasma half-life of amantadine in patients with normal renal function is about 12 h, but the half-life is much longer in patients with impaired renal function.[67,69] Rough guidelines for dosage adjustment according to creatinine clearance rate have been published.[67,69] The dosage interval may be altered, for example, to one 100 mg capsule per day when the creatinine clearance rate is 35–75 ml/min/1.73 m^2, one capsule every 2 days for a clearance of 25–35, one every 3 days for a clearance of 15–25, and one every 7 days for a patient with a creatinine clearance rate of less than 15.[67] These are only very rough guidelines and plasma drug levels should be monitored during treatment so that dosage may be adjusted in an accurate manner. Plasma concentrations in excess of 1.5–2.0 μg/ml have been associated with toxic effects.[70] Only a small fraction of the total body store of amantadine is removed with a single hemodialysis treatment.[69,71]

Rimantadine is also well absorbed orally (>90%) but achieves slightly lower plasma levels than amantadine. Unlike amantadine, the metabolism of rimantadine contributes significantly to its elimination. It is extensively metabolized and is excreted primarily by renal mechanisms. Less than 10% of the drug is excreted unchanged, with most of it being excreted as hydroxylated and glucuronidated metabolites.[72,73] Dosage reduction is not required until creatinine clearance falls below 10 ml/min. The plasma half-life is approximately twice of that of amantadine, and rimantadine seems to be more concentrated in respiratory secretions than amantadine.[56]

ADVERSE EFFECTS. Central nervous system side effects occur in about 7% of adults receiving 100 mg of amantadine twice daily.[52] The central nervous system complaints, which are the most common adverse effects related to amantadine, are generally minor and often resolve despite continued drug administration. The most frequent side effects are dizziness, nervousness, difficulty in concentrating, and insomnia.[52,53,74] More serious neurotoxicity (e.g., seizures, delirium) occurs in patients with decreased renal function where higher plasma levels are attained.[75] Some investigators have found that patients receiving the usual antiviral dosage of amantadine perform less well on objective tests measuring sustained attention and problem solving ability,[76] whereas others have found such impairment only with higher dosage.[74] The drug should probably not be administered to people, such as airplane pilots or bus drivers, whose occupations require sustained concentration and responsibility for the safety of others. Some patients have experienced depression, confusion, or hallucinations, and care should be exercised when administering the drug to patients with a history of psychosis. Rarely, seizures have occurred, and patients with a history of epilepsy should be observed closely for increased seizure activity. Other side effects include anorexia, nausea, vomiting, blurred vision, and orthostatic hypotension. Leukopenia and neutropenia have occurred rarely. Rimantadine produces the same adverse effects as amantadine, but at a dose of 200 mg/day, the frequency of adverse effects is much less.[56] At similar plasma levels, the two drugs do not appear to differ significantly in their neurotoxicity.[77]

Although some patients experience tremors as a side effect, exactly the opposite response was noted in one parkinsonian patient who experienced a remission of her symptoms of rigidity, tremor, and akinesia while being treated with amantadine for prophylaxis during an influenza epidemic.[78] This serendipitous observation has been followed up by clinical trials that demonstrate that amantadine is of significant benefit for the patient with mild Parkinson's disease,[79,80] and it now has an accepted role in the treatment of that condition.[81] The mechanism of the beneficial effect is not well understood, but amantadine may have both an indirect dopamine-releasing action and the ability to directly stimulate dopamine receptors.[82] There is little support for the model in which amantadine is said to increase local dopamine concentrations by inhibiting its reuptake. Amantadine has been reported to produce livedo reticularis and edema of the lower legs in patients (particularly females) receiving the drug for treatment of Parkinson's disease.[83] Rarely, parkinsonian patients have experienced cardiac failure attributable to the drug, and special caution should be taken when administering amantadine to patients with a history of myocardial disease.[84]

At a dosage of 10 mg/kg no teratogenicity was observed in rats,[85] but at a dosage of 50 mg/kg/day the manufacturer notes that embryotoxic and teratogenic effects have been observed. Unless the benefits clearly outweigh the risks, amantadine should not be administered to pregnant women. Like amantadine, rimantadine is potentially teratogenic and thus is contraindicated in pregnancy. The adverse effects of amantadine have been reviewed in detail by Parkes.[86]

DRUG INTERACTIONS. Concomitant ingestion of antihistamines or anticholinergic drugs with amantadine can increase the potential for adverse central nervous system effects. Combined administration with anticholinergics especially in elderly parkinsonian patients may be associated with toxic delirium and visual hallucinations.[87] Drugs that undergo active tubular secretion may alter amantadine excretion. Thus a combination of the diuretics triamterene and hydrochlorothiazide was associated with central nervous system toxicity and an increase in plasma amantadine concentration due to decreased renal clearance.[88] Coadministration of trimethoprim-sulfamethoxazole has been associated with an increase in amantadine toxicity, presumably because of inhibition of tubular secretion.[89]

Zanamivir

Although amantadine and rimantadine have been the only anti-influenza medications available for several years, they have had limited success because of underutilization, lack of activity against influenza B, rapid development of viral resistance, and adverse effects. As a result, a new class of antiviral agents designed to inhibit influenza neura-

minidase, an important surface glycoprotein, is being developed for prophylaxis and treatment of influenza A and B infections. Zanamivir is the neuraminidase inhibitor that is at the most advanced stage of development.

Zanamivir

Zanamivir is a selective inhibitor of both influenza A and B virus neuraminidases, and does not significantly inhibit human lysosomal neuraminidase.[90] Cleavage of sialic acid from cell surface glycoconjugates by the viral neuraminidase is required for the release of newly formed virus from the surface of infected cells. By inhibiting neuraminidase, zanamivir inhibits viral release and prevents spread of the virus across the mucus lining of the respiratory tract.[91]

Both in vitro and in vivo studies show good activity against influenza A and B viruses.[21] In vivo activity was seen only after intranasal administration of zanamivir, administration by the intraperitoneal and oral routes being ineffective. The antiviral activity was not affected by resistance to amantadine or rimantadine. In fact, combinations of zanamivir with rimantadine or ribavirin have additive effects on viral inhibition.[92]

After administration intranasally or by inhaltion, maximum serum concentrations occur within 2 h. The terminal phase half-life is 2.4 to 2.9 h, and the bioavailability was 10% when the drug was administered by the intranasal route and 25% when it was inhaled. Zanamivir is cleared in the urine, predominantly as unchanged drug.

In several randomized, double-blind placebo-controlled trials, zanamivir was shown to prevent development of infection, and development of fever during outbreaks of influenza. Significant reductions in total symptoms, nasal mucus weight, incidences of upper respiratory tract illness, and cough were also observed.[97] Similarly, in trials in patients with confirmed influenza A or B infection of less than 48 h duration, symptoms were alleviated compared to placebo groups.[94] In patients with influenza infection, the most commonly reported adverse effects were related to the upper respiratory and gastrointestinal tracts and were difficult to distinguish from symptoms of influenza.[94] There is some question as to whether zanamivir fills a clinical need,[95] for type B influenza causes only about 35% of cases of influenza and zanamivir has the disadvantage of requiring aerosol delivery to the respiratory tract, which could prove difficult for some patients. New inhibitors of neuraminidase are being developed that are at least as active as zanamivir in vitro, yet can be given orally.[96]

Anti-Herpesvirus Agents

Herpes simplex virus (HSV) type 1 and 2 infections occur commonly in humans. During primary infection, herpesviruses establish latency, which allows the viral DNA to persist without expressing proteins that would be targets for an immune response.[97] Intermittently, the latent genome can become activated to produce infectious virions. Herpes simplex virus type 1 (HSV-1) infection causes diseases of the mouth, face, skin, esophagus, or brain. Herpes simplex virus type 2 (HSV-2) usually causes infections of the genitals, rectum, skin, hands, or meninges. Varicella zoster virus (VZV) causes chickenpox, with the latent virus causing shingles, a disease of the peripheral nervous system. Cytomegalovirus (CMV), which produces neurological dysfunction and/or hearing loss, can be transferred during organ transplantation and reactivation in the recipient can lead to infection, with the virus then spreading to the lungs to cause interstitial pneumonitis, to the liver to cause hepatitis, or to the gastrointestinal tract to cause diarrhea and/or abdominal pain. It can also involve the eye, causing retinitis.[97] All of the presently available antiherpes agents are purine and pyrimidine analogs. These are all inhibitors of the viral DNA polymerase, with some, like foscarnet, acting directly, whereas others must first be converted to the nucleotide to be active.

Idoxuridine

Idoxuridine was one of the first antiviral agents shown to be effective in the treatment of herpes keratitis. However, this drug is nonselective for viral replication and inhibits various host cell functions. Toxicity, specifically bone marrow suppression, has prevented the systemic use of this compound. It is presently only a second or third-choice agent for the topical treatment of herpes simplex keratitis, thus this drug will be discussed only briefly. However, its development illustrates the rationale behind the development of purine and pyrimidine analogs as antiviral drugs.

STRUCTURE AND MECHANISM OF ACTION. Idoxuridine (5-iodo-2'-deoxyuridine, IUdR) was synthesized by Prusoff in 1959,[98] and it is one of many purine and pyrimidine analogs that have been tested for antiviral, an-

Idoxuridine
(IUdR)

Thymidine

titumor, and immunosuppressive activity. Idoxuridine, a halogenated derivative of deoxyuridine, is an analog of thymidine. The presence of a halogen in lieu of a methyl group alters the electron configuration of the pyrimidine, resulting in a more acidic dissociation constant. The iodine atom has a van der Waals' radius of 2.15 Å. This is approximately the size of a methyl group 2.00 Å; therefore, IUdR is able to replace thymidine in many reactions.

The primary antiviral action of IUdR is

the result of its incorporation into viral DNA.[99] The DNA containing the halogenated compound is altered in a number of ways. The drug-containing viral DNA is more susceptible to strand breakage[100]; the mutation rate is increased; there are errors in subsequent RNA and protein synthesis; and when complete viral particles are formed in the presence of the drug, their infectivity is decreased.

USE AND PHARMACOKINETICS. Although about 20 viruses have been shown to be sensitive to idoxuridine in vitro,[101] the drug has proven to be useful clinically only in the treatment of HSV-1 infections of the cornea. At 100 μg/ml, idoxuridine produces a profound inhibition of replication of HSV-1 in vitro, whereas HSV-2 is much less sensitive.[102] Several well controlled double-blind studies carried out in the early 1960s demonstrated the effectiveness of topically administered idoxuridine in the treatment of herpes simplex keratitis,[103,104] and for about a decade, idoxuridine was the only drug available for treatment of this condition.

Idoxuridine is provided as a 0.5% ophthalmic ointment and a 0.1% ophthalmic solution. The ointment is usually applied every 4 h during the day and once before sleep. The treatment of ocular herpesvirus infections is a complex procedure that has been reviewed in the specialized literature.[105,106] Although it hastens recovery from the infection, idoxuridine itself causes both local allergic reactions and irritation.[107] The inherent selectivity of action of idoxuridine for the DNA virus compared to the host cell is low. When idoxuridine is employed topically to treat viral infections in the eye, additional selective effect is probably achieved. The replication of viruses in the cell requires the rapid, sustained synthesis of DNA, whereas normal mammalian cells in the conjunctiva of the eye are not synthesizing DNA at a high rate. The cells involved in the healing process, however, may be dividing rapidly and animal studies of the effects of idoxuridine in the absence of herpetic infection show that it inhibits stromal repair and decreases the strength of healing stromal wounds.[108]

The topical application of idoxuridine results in high local concentrations of the drug, but systemic levels remain low and toxic effects beyond the local area are avoided. Adverse reactions including inflammation, itching and edema of the eyelids, photophobia, punctate epithelial keratopathy, and lacrimal duct occlusion are observed with local application to the conjunctiva.[107]

Although idoxuridine has been administered in some uncontrolled studies for the treatment of herpes simplex encephalitis,[109] there is no role for the systemic administration of idoxuridine in the treatment of viral disease. A controlled double-blind study of the effect of the drug (100 mg/kg as two rapid intravenous administrations daily) in patients with biopsy-proven herpetic encephalitis was terminated because of unacceptable marrow toxicity and failure of the drug to prevent death.[110] Systemic administration of IUdR can produce stomatitis, leukopenia, and thrombocytopenia,[110,111] a complex of symptoms seen with many drugs that are cytotoxic to mammalian cells. Idoxuridine is also hepatotoxic. In addition to its being toxic, the systemic use of the drug is compromised by its rapid metabolism in tissues,[112] which necessitates rapid intravenous infusion in order to obtain significant blood levels.[113]

Since halogenated pyrimidines are mutagenic in bacteria, and since they produce chromosomal damage in eukaryotic cells, there is a clear basis for concern about the possibility of producing genetic damage in humans with systemic administration.[114] It has been shown that exposure of certain nonvirus-producing cells in culture to idoxuridine can initiate virus production. This has been observed, for example, in cell lines prepared from mouse embryos that produce high titers of infectious murine leukemia virus in the presence of the drug.[115] The production of Epstein-Barr virus–related antigens is initiated in non-producing human lymphoblastoid cells exposed to idoxuridine.[116] These and similar observations in several systems reenforce the possibility that a potential risk of idoxuridine administration may be oncogene activation—that is, the expression of normally repressed cancer-causing genes. Idoxuridine is teratogenic, and when it is administered topically to the eye of pregnant rabbits in doses similar to those used clinically, it produces fetal malformations.[117] For this reason, it should not be administered to pregnant women.

The role of idoxuridine in antiviral therapy is now limited to its use as a secondary drug in the treatment of herpes simplex infections of the cornea. As noted in the review by Prusoff and Ward,[118] idoxuridine was "the first compound to clearly demonstrate a successful treatment of an established viral infection in man." The drug has played an important role in the development of our understanding of antiviral chemotherapy, but newer drugs with greater clinical efficacy and less toxicity have largely replaced it in the clinical setting.

Trifluridine

STRUCTURE AND MECHANISM OF ACTION. Trifluridine (5-trifluoromethyl-2'-deoxyuridine, trifluorothymidine) is one of a number of fluorinated pyrimidines and their nucleosides synthesized by Heidelberger and colleagues (see ref. 119 and 120 for reviews). Trifluridine is an analog of thymidine in which the three hydrogens in the methyl group of thymine are replaced by fluorine atoms. The van der Waals' radius of the trifluoromethyl group (2.44 Å) is close enough to that of a methyl group (2.00 °A) so that the drug behaves like thymidine and is incorporated into DNA.[121]

Trifluridine

Trifluridine is phosphorylated by thymidine kinase[122] to the nucleotide, trifluridine monophosphate, which is an effective inhibitor of thymidylate synthetase,[123] the enzyme that converts deoxyuridine monophosphate to thymidine monophosphate. In this respect, trifluridine acts like the anticancer drug fluorouracil, which is converted to deoxyuridine monophosphate and inhibits the same enzyme, but by a different mechanism.[123] Further phosphorylation of trifluridine to the triphosphate leads to its incorporation into both viral and cellular DNAs via the respective polymerases. Inhibition of viral replication can be prevented by thymidine if it is added to cells simultaneously with or shortly after trifluridine.[124] If thymidine is added a day after the drug, no reversal of inhibition occurs, suggesting that an irreversible block in viral replication has taken place.[124] The irreversible event is most likely the incorporation of trifluridine into viral DNA, and it has been shown that the replacement of as little as 2% of vaccinia viral DNA thymine by the drug abolishes the infectivity of the virions.[125] In cell-free DNA synthesizing systems, the drug is incorporated with somewhat greater facility into DNA when synthesis is directed by vaccinia virus DNA polymerase than when it is directed by HeLa cell or calf thymus DNA polymerase.[121] Such preferential incorporation may account for some of the selectivity of the drug for inhibition of viral versus host cell replication. The vaccinia virus DNA that is synthesized in the presence of the drug is considerably smaller than normal vaccinia virus DNA, and it is incompletely transcribed into late mRNA, which leads to the production of defective viral proteins.[126]

CLINICAL USE AND PHARMACOKINETICS. Because of its very rapid half-life (18 min)[127] and its systemic toxicity, trifluridine is not administered systemically for the treatment of viral disease. The drug is provided as a 1% ophthalmic solution that is used for the treatment of herpes simplex keratitis. One drop of the drug solution is applied to the affected eye every 2 h while awake for a maximum daily dosage of nine drops until the corneal ulcer has re-epithelialized. After re-epithelialization, it is recommended that treatment be continued for an additional seven days at one drop every 4 h while awake for a minimum daily dosage of five drops. Trifluridine is approved for treatment of primary keratoconjunctivitis and recurrent epithelial keratitis due to HSV types 1 and 2.[128] It is more active than idoxuridine and comparable to vidarabine in HSV eye infections. Topical trifluridine may also be effective in some patients with acyclovir-resistant HSV cutaneous infections.[129] Trifluridine has been studied as a topical treatment for acyclovir-resistant chronic mucocutaneous genital HSV lesions in HIV-infected patients, either alone or in combination with interferon-alpha (IFN-α).[130,131] The preliminary reports seem promising but the frequency of complete healing remains to be determined.

After topical application to the eye, trifluridine readily penetrates through the intact cornea at the same rate as idoxuridine and faster than vidarabine.[132] The rate of penetration is increased about twofold when the corneal epithelium is removed.[132] About 20% of the drug recovered from the aqueous humor of rabbits was in the form of the biologically active breakdown product 5-carboxy-2'-deoxyuridine.[132] Topical application of trifluridine is associated with a lower incidence of adverse reactions than idoxuridine.[133] The most frequent reactions are a transient burning sensation upon instillation (5%) and palpebral edema (3%). Rare side effects include punctate epithelial keratopathy and hypersensitivity reactions.[133–135] Trifluridine is mutagenic by in vitro tests. In contrast to idoxuridine, trifluridine was not teratogenic when administered topically to the eyes of pregnant rabbits.[117] Nevertheless, it probably should not be administered to pregnant women unless the potential benefits outweigh the potential risks.

Vidarabine

STRUCTURE AND MECHANISM OF ACTION. Vidarabine (9-β-D-arabinofuranosyladenine, adenine arabinoside, ara-A) is a purine derivative synthesized by Lee et al.[136] in 1960 as a potential anticancer drug and later shown to have antiviral activity. The extensive work carried out with this drug prior to 1975 is reviewed in a symposium[137] (see also ref. 138 for a review).

Vidarabine
(adenine arabinoside)

Hypoxanthine arabinoside
(a major metabolite, also having antiviral activity)

Vidarabine is active against a variety of DNA viruses in vitro,[139] and it is used clinically to treat herpesvirus infections. Vidarabine is a selective inhibitor of herpes simplex virus replication in cultured cells. At low concentration, it inhibits plaque formation and the synthesis of HSV DNA without affecting cellular DNA synthesis, whereas at higher concentrations, cellular DNA synthesis is inhibited.[140] From studies in both intact cells and cell-free systems, it is clear that vidarabine has two major biochemical fates, phosphorylation to vidarabine triphosphate and deamination to hypoxanthine arabinoside.[138] Extensive deamination occurs in most mammalian cells and the arabinosylhypoxanthine metabolite is about one-fiftieth as potent an antiviral agent as the parent compound.[141,142]

To exert is antiviral action, vidarabine must first be converted to its active form, vidarabine triphosphate. This phosphorylation is carried out in the cell by the joint action of deoxycytidine kinase and adenosine kinase.[143] Vidarabine triphosphate is a potent inhibitor of ribonucleotide reductases[144,145] and DNA polymerases.[146,147] As mutations in the gene for herpes simplex virus DNA polymerase can confer resistance to vidarabine, it is clear that either inhibition of this enzyme or incorporation of the drug by the enzyme into viral DNA is critical for the antiviral effect.[148] Vidarabine triphosphate inhibits HSV DNA polymerase in a manner that is competitive with respect to dATP.[149] Some investigators have found that the viral DNA polymerase is more sensitive to inhibition than cellular DNA polymerases,[149] an observation that could explain some of the selective toxicity of the drug. Some vidara-bine is incorporated into viral DNA where it is found in internucleotide linkage,[150] show-ing that incorporation of the drug does not result in absolute DNA chain termination. Incorporation of vidarabine monophosphate into the end of the primer causes a substan-tial decrease in the rate of subsequent elon-gation of the DNA chain by the viral poly-merase.[151] Thus, at this time, it is reasonable to propose that inhibition of viral replication by vidarabine is a consequence of the incor-poration of the drug into viral DNA. Other effects may contribute to the drug action, however, and the mechanism is not com-pletely defined.

CLINICAL USES, PHARMACOKINETICS AND AD-VERSE EFFECTS
Topical therapy. Vidarabine is supplied as a 3% ophthalmic ointment that is used for the treatment of herpes simplex kerato-conjunctivitis. The ointment is applied to the affected eye every 3 h while awake for a to-tal of five times daily. Vidarabine is as effec-tive as trifluridine (response rate 90–100%) and more effective than idoxuridine (re-sponse rate about 75%) in the treatment of herpes simplex keratitis.[134,152,153] Topical ad-ministration of vidarabine or vidarabine monophosphate, however, does not influ-ence the clinical course of patients with re-current herpes labialis or genitalis.[154,155] It is unlikely that vidarabine penetrates through the skin. Vidarabine penetrates through the intact cornea at a slower rate than trifluri-dine or idoxuridine,[132] and the small amount of drug that is recovered from the aqueous humor is present predominantly as the hy-poxanthine arabinoside metabolite.[132,156] When administered topically to the eye, vi-darabine produces fewer adverse reactions than idoxuridine.[157] Burning, photophobia, and lacrimation may occur on installation of the drug. Like other eye ointments, vidara-bine ointment may cause transient blurring of vision. Occasionally, patients develop su-perficial punctate keratitis; rarely, punctal stenosis has occurred.[137,158]

Intravenous therapy. Vidarabine is adminis-tered intravenously to treat certain sys-temic viral infections. Given at a dosage of 15 mg/kg/day for 10 days, vadarabine has been demonstrated to reduce mortality from 70% to 39% in patients with herpes simplex encephalitis where the diagnosis has been proven by brain biopsy.[159,160] The chances of survival with vidarabine treatment are en-hanced if the patient is under 30 years of age and is not lethargic or comatose at the time of therapy.[160,161] Intravenous vidarabine has a beneficial effect in neonatal herpes simplex infections, where both mortality and mor-bidity are decreased by a 10-day course of therapy.[162] Given at a dosage of 10 mg/kg/day for 5 days, vidarabine reduces compli-cations related to herpes zoster in immuno-compromised patients.[163,164] Patients with localized herpes zoster of 72 h duration or less who are treated with vidarabine have more rapid relief of pain, a decreased rate of new vesicle formation, and fewer visceral complications than patients given pla-cebo.[164] Although intravenous vidarabine is approved for use in HSV encephalitis, neo-natal herpes, and zoster or varicella in im-munocompromised patients, it has been re-placed by acyclovir as the treatment of choice for these indications. Vidarabine is of modest usefulness in mucocutaneous HSV infections in immunocompomised hosts and is ineffective in acyclovir-resistant HSV in-fections in patients with AIDS.[165] It has also been used occasionally in life-threatening herpesvirus infections. Vidarabine appears to reduce Dane particle-associated DNA poly-merase activity and viral core antigen in the serum of patients with chronic hepatitis B infection and chronic active hepatitis,[166] but the drug has not been demonstrated to alter the course of the liver disease. Vidarabine is not effective in the treatment of cytomega-lovirus infection.[167]

The pharmacokinetics of intravenous vi-darabine has been reviewed by Whitley et al.[168] Vidarabine has low aqueous solubility and it must be diluted in large amounts of fluid (maximum of 450 mg of drug/liter of infusion fluid) and administered intrave-nously. The drug is rapidly deaminated by adenosine deaminase in serum and body tis-sues to arabinosylhypoxanthine. The total daily dose of vidarabine is administered by constant intravenous infusion over 12–24 h. After a 12-h intravenous infusion of 10 mg of vidarabine per kg of body weight, the peak plasma level of the arabinosylhypoxanthine metabolite is 3–6 µg/ml and that of unchanged vidarabine is only 0.2–0.4 µg/ml.[168] The antiviral activity is due to both the unchanged drug and to the arabinosylhypoxanthine metabolite, which is about one-fiftieth as potent an antiviral agent by in vitro assay.[141,142] The activity of vidarabine against sensitive viruses, like HSV-1, depends on the cell type in which the virus is cultured, and there is evidence that the combination of the unaltered drug and its major arabinosylhypoxanthine metabolite may produce a synergistic antiviral effect.[141] In the absence of a deaminase inhibitor, the mean serum concentration of antiviral activity, expressed as unaltered vidarabine equivalents determined by in vitro bioassay with HSV-1, is approximately 3 µg/ml during infusion at a dose of 10 mg/kg/day.[141] Most herpes simplex and varicella zoster virus strains are inhibited by less than 3 µg/ml of vidarabine.

Vidarabine is widely distributed in the body, predominantly in the form of its arabinosylhypoxanthine metabolite. There is good penetration into the cerebrospinal fluid where peak levels are about one-half those achieved in the serum.[169] The drug is excreted by the kidney, with almost all of the drug in the urine being in the form of the arabinosylhypoxanthine metabolite which has a half-life of about 4 h in the body.[169]

In most clinical studies where vidarabine has been administered at 10–15 mg/kg/day, the drug has been well tolerated. A few patients have experienced gastrointestinal reactions (nausea, vomiting, and diarrhea) or skin rashes (erythematous, nonpruritic).[160,163] It appears that vidarabine can also produce a dose-related neurotoxicity characterized by tremor and weakness and, rarely, by ataxia, confusion, and seizures.[170,171] Neurotoxicity probably occurs only very rarely in patients with normal renal function receiving a daily dose less than 15 mg/kg. Hematological changes have been noted in isolated patients. Like many other nucleoside analogs, vidarabine is carcinogenic, mutagenic, and teratogenic in animal test systems.[138] Its use in pregnant women and infants should be limited to those with life-threatening illnesses who are resistant to treatment with less toxic drugs.

Acyclovir

ANTIVIRAL ACTIVITY AND MECHANISM OF ACTION. Acyclovir, the 9-(2-hydroxyethoxymethyl) derivative of guanine, is one of several acyclic purine derivatives developed by the Wellcome Research Laboratories as potential antiviral drugs.[172] Acyclovir prevents the replication of a variety of herpesviruses in vitro, with HSV types 1 and 2 (IC_{50} 0.1–1.4 µM) and VZV (IC_{50} 1.6–5 µM) being the most sensitive, Epstein-Barr virus (IC_{50} 6–7 µM) being somewhat

Acyclovir   Deoxyguanosine

less sensitive, and most clinical isolates of human cytomegalovirus being quite resistant (IC_{50} usually greater than 100 µM).[173] Acyclovir was the first of a new class of potent antiviral drugs exploiting the acyclic nucleoside structure.[174] The mechanism of action, pharmacology, and clinical use of acyclovir have been reviewed in several symposia.[175–178]

Acyclovir is a highly selective inhibitor of HSV replication. Depending on the viral strain, the concentration of acyclovir required for 50% inhibition of replication of HSV type 1 or 2 in tissue culture is 0.1–1.4 µM, whereas the concentration required for 50% inhibition of Vero cell growth is 300 µM and for WI-38 human fibroblasts it is greater than 3000 µM.[17] This highly selective toxicity is based to a large degree on selective activation of the drug by viral thymidine kinase. The active form of acyclovir is acyclo-GTP, and uninfected mammalian cells are able to phosphorylate the drug only

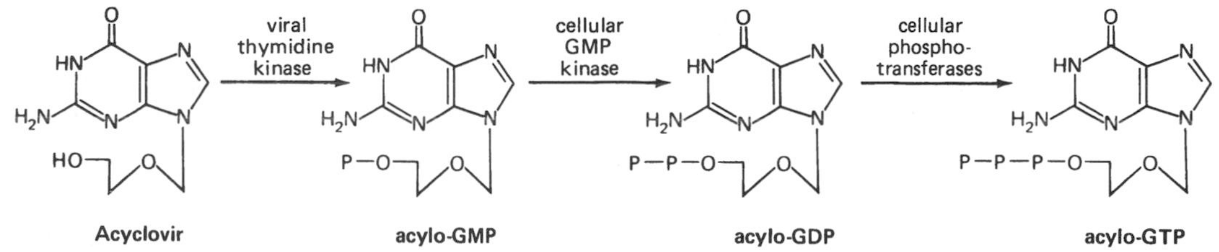

Figure 16–3. Conversion of acyclovir to acyclovir triphosphate. Acyclovir is converted to the mono-phosphate derivative by a herpesvirus thymidine kinase. The acyclo-GMP is then phosphorylated to acyclo-GDP and acyclo-GTP by cellular enzymes. Uninfected cells convert very little or no drug to the phosphorylated derivatives. Thus, acyclovir is selectively toxic to cells infected with herpes viruses that code for appropriate thymidine kinases. (From Elion,[186] Fig. 3.)

to a small extent.[179] Herpes simplex and var-icella zoster viruses code for a viral thymi-dine kinase that is synthesized in infected cells and readily converts acyclovir to acyclo-GMP.[180] The anti-herpes-virus activ-ity of acyclovir correlates with its ability to be phosphorylated in the infected cell,[181] and mutations that decrease thymidine kinase ac-tivity render the virus resistant to acyclo-vir.[180,182,183] The acyclo-GMP that is pro-duced is phosphorylated by a cellular GMP kinase to acyclo-GDP,[184] which is then con-verted to acyclo-GTP by cellular phospho-transferases (in particular, phosphoglycerate kinase).[185] The pathway for acyclovir acti-vation is shown in Figure 16–3.[186]

The product of activation, acyclo-GTP, is a potent inhibitor of both viral DNA poly-merases and mammalian α DNA polymer-ases (i.e., the replicative polymerase).[187,188] In general, the virus-induced DNA polymer-ase is more sensitive to inhibition than the DNA polymerase of the host cell.[187,188] This difference in sensitivity is another factor that contributes to the selectivity of the drug. In-itially, acyclo-GTP inhibits DNA polymerase in a manner that is competitive with dGTP.[188] Some acyclo-GMP becomes incor-porated into the newly synthesized DNA strand, however, and chain termination re-sults (see Fig. 16–4). The resulting acyclo-GMP-terminated DNA cannot act as a pri-mer for further synthesis and, later in the reaction, it inhibits herpes simplex virus DNA polymerase in a noncompetitive man-ner.[189]

Acyclovir-resistant strains of HSV and

VZV arise chiefly from mutations in the thy-midine kinase gene or mutations that result in little or no production of the en-zyme.[178,190,191] However, resistance can also occur through mutations in the viral DNA polymerase gene and subsequent alterations in the enzyme.[148,182,183] Clinically, acylclovir-

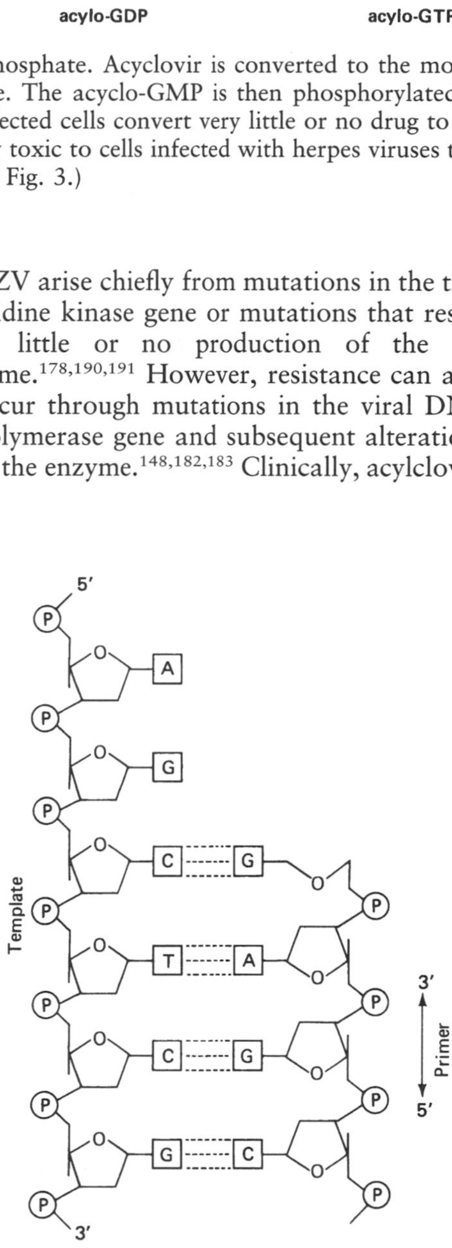

Figure 16–4. DNA chain termination caused by acyclovir. Incorporation of acyclo-GMP from acyclo-GTP into the primer strand during viral DNA replication leads to chain termination. (From Elion,[186] Fig. 7.)

resistant strains are most commonly reported in severely immunocompromised patients receiving extended courses of the drug and most are thymidine kinase negative. The emergence of resistant HSV strains after prolonged treatment with acyclovir appears to be infrequent in immunocompetent patients.[192] However, the number of reports of clinically aggressive acyclovir-resistant HSV strains in immunocompromised patients receiving acyclovir therapy is increasing.[178] Reports of acyclovir-resistant strains of herpes viruses other than herpes simplex are relatively rare.

CLINICAL USE OF ACYCLOVIR. Acyclovir is used clinically to treat infections caused by herpes simplex type 1 and 2 and varicella zoster viruses. The clinical efficacy of acyclovir in immunocompetent persons is greater in initial HSV infections than in recurrent ones, which are usually milder in severity. Acyclovir is especially useful for the treatment of infections in immunocompromised patients, because these individuals experience both more frequent and more severe infections. In treating cases of varicella zoster, higher doses must be used than for treating HSV infections because the varicella zoster is less susceptible to acyclovir. Most strains of these viruses are susceptible to the concentrations of acyclovir achieved clinically. Compared to other members of the herpesvirus group, human CMV is relatively unsusceptible to acyclovir because the drug is a poor substrate for its thymidine kinase.[193] Consistent with the lack of activity against the virus in vitro, acyclovir has not been found to be clinically useful in treating patients with CMV infection.[175] However, acyclovir has been used for CMV prophylaxis in transplant recipients. High-dose intravenous acyclovir in CMV-seropositive bone marrow transplant recipients is associated with about 50% lower risk of CMV disease. When intravenous treatment is combined with prolonged oral acyclovir, survival is improved.[194,195]. High-dose oral acyclovir suppression for 3 months reduces the risk of CMV disease in certain organ transplant recipients.[196,197]

In double-blind clinical trials comparing acyclovir ophthalmic ointment to other antiviral drugs in the treatment of herpes simplex keratitis, acyclovir has been found to yield a higher response rate than idoxuridine and to be essentially equivalent to vidarabine and trifluridine in efficacy.[152,153,158,198,199] In one study, topical application of acyclovir in a 5% ointment significantly shortened the duration of lesions in patients with recurrent herpes liabialis.[200] Other studies, however, have found a significant decrease in the duration of viral shedding when therapy is begun shortly after the onset of lesions, but the time to healing was unaffected.[201,202] Topical administration of acyclovir to patients experiencing initial or recurrent episodes of herpes simplex genitalis shortens the duration of viral shedding, but the duration of pain and lesions is reduced only minimally in patients experiencing initial attacks, and there is no clinical benefit from topical therapy in patients with recurrent disease.[203,204]

In contrast to topical therapy, oral acyclovir therapy of the initial episode of genital herpes significantly reduces new lesion formation, the duration of lesions, and the severity of clinical symptoms.[205] Continuous treatment with oral acyclovir reduces, but does not completely prevent, recurrence of genital herpes in patients with frequently recurring disease.[206,207]

The use of acyclovir in genital herpes has been reviewed by Woolley.[208] For first episodes of genital herpes, oral therapy should be used (200 mg five times daily), particularly for severe episodes. Oral acyclovir does not have a clinically significant benefit in the treatment of acute recurrent episodes of genital herpes. Long-term treatment does not eliminate latent virus in nerve ganglia, since infection may recur after treatment is terminated. Thus, such treatment does not influence the natural history of the disease.[207]

Intravenous administration of acyclovir to patients experiencing initial attacks of genital herpes reduces new lesion formation, time to healing of lesions, and duration of symptoms.[209] Given intravenously, acyclovir also provides effective prophylaxis against reactivation of oropharyngeal HSV infection in severely immunocompromised patients.[210–212] Systemic acyclovir prophylaxis is highly effective in preventing mucocutaneous HSV infections in seropositive patients undergoing immunosuppression. Intravenous acyclovir begun prior to transplantation and continuing for several weeks prevents HSV disease in bone marrow transplant recipients. Oral acyclovir is also effective in immunosuppressed patients and long-term oral acyclovir reduces the risk of varicella infection.[213] Intravenous acyclovir halts the progression of varicella zoster in immunocompromised patients[214] and accelerates healing of herpes zoster in normally immunocompetent adults.[215] Acyclovir is effective in varicella infections in children and adults if therapy is begun within 24 h of rash onset. In children it reduces fever and new lesion formation by about 1 day.[216] Routine use in uncomplicated pediatric varicella is not currently recommended.[217] In adults, early oral acyclovir reduces time to crusting of lesions by about 2 days, reduces the maximum number of lesions by half, and shortens the duration of fever.[218] Later treatment is not beneficial. In older adults with localized varicella zoster, oral acyclovir reduces acute pain and healing times if the treatment is initiated within 72 h of rash onset.[219] In immunocompromised patients with disseminating varicella zoster, intravenous acyclovir reduces viral shedding, healing times, risks of cutaneous dissemination, and visceral complications, as well as shortening the period of hospitalization.[220] Intravenous acyclovir decreases healing times and the risk of visceral complications in immunosuppressed children with varicella. Acyclovir also reduces some of the pain associated with varicella zoster.[221] Acyclovir is now the treatment of choice in HSV encephalitis. It has been found to reduce mortality by over 50% and improves overall neurologic outcome compared to vidarabine.[222] In infectious mononucleosis, acyclovir is associated with transient antiviral effects but no clinical benefits.[223]

The number of reports of acyclovir-resistant HSV, principally in immunosuppressed patients with HIV infection is increasing.[165,224,225] Clinically, this may result in prolonged and progressive ulceration, with substantial discomfort and disfigurement. Acyclovir-resistant VZV strains in HIV-positive patients have been associated with chronic cutaneous lesions and, rarely, invasive disease. Most of the clinical isolates from with resistant strains have been deficient in viral thymidine kinase and infections with acyclovir-resistant HSV or VZV may respond to foscarnet or topical cidofovir, which do not require activation by this enzyme.

PHARMACOKINETICS. The pharmacokinetics of acyclovir have been reviewed in detail by Laskin[226] and by Wagstaff et al.[178] In the United States, acyclovir is available as a 5% ointment for topical administration, as 200 mg oral tablets and capsules, as an oral suspension, and as an intravenous formulation.

After topical administration to the skin or to mucous membranes, systemic absorption of acyclovir is minimal,[226] but after topical administration to the eye, the levels of drug in the aqueous humor are well within the therapeutic range for HSV susceptibility.[227] In humans, acyclovir is slowly and poorly absorbed from the gastrointestinal tract, with the average bioavailability being about 20% of a 200 mg oral dose,[228] and decreasing with increasing dose.[178] After oral administration, peak plasma levels are achieved in 1.5–2 h.[229] The mean steady-state peak acyclovir concentration achieved in the plasma following oral administration of 200 mg of drug every 4 h to adults is 2.5 μM, and after 400 mg given every 4 h, it is 5.4 μM.[228,229] These concentrations exceed the concentration required for inhibition of replication of HSV types 1 and 2 in vitro (IC$_{50}$ 0.1–1.4 μM).[173] The dosage of acyclovir recommended by the manufacturer for intravenous treatment of mucosal and cutaneous HSV types 1 and 2 infections in adult patients is 5 mg/kg infused at a constant rate over 1 h and administered every 8 h. At the end of a 5 mg/kg infusion, the plasma concentration determined by radioimmunoassay is 34–37 μM.[230,231] The steady-state peak plasma concentration after repeated 1-h infusions every 8 h is 44 μM, with the level of drug declining to a trough concentration of about 2 μM just prior to the next dose.[228]

About 15% of acyclovir in the plasma is

bound to protein,[232] and the drug distributes into a volume of about 70% of the body weight (50 liter/1.73 m²),[231] a volume that roughly corresponds to the total body water. In rodent models, it has been shown that the drug distributes into most organs, with the highest levels found in renal tissue and the lowest levels present in brain tissue.[233] In humans, acyclovir levels in the cerebrospinal fluid are approximately 50%[234] and those in the saliva are about 13%[229] of corresponding plasma levels. Acyclovir is concentrated in breast milk, amniotic fluid, and placenta. Newborn plasma levels are similar to maternal levels.[235] In patients receiving an oral dosage of 200 mg every 4 h, peak levels of acyclovir in vaginal secretions range from 0.5 to 3.6 μM.[229] In patients with herpes zoster, acyclovir concentrations in vesicle fluid approximate the plasma concentration.[226]

In humans, acyclovir undergoes very little metabolism. The only significant metabolite is 9-(carboxymethoxymethyl)guanine, which accounts for approximately 10 % of the excreted drug.[232] The drug is eliminated via the kidney by both glomerular filtration and tubular secretion.[230,231] The elimination of acyclovir is biexponential, with the half-life of the terminal phase being 2–3 h in patients with normal renal function.[228,230,231] In patients who are anuric, the total body clearance is about 10% of that in patients with normal renal function, the terminal half-life is increased to approximately 20 h, and dosage adjustment is necessary.[236] In adults, the usual 5 mg/kg intravenous dose may be administered every 8 h to patients with a creatinine clearance greater than 50 ml/min/1.73 m². The timing of the usual intravenous dose may be extended to every 12 h when the creatinine clearance is 25–50 and to every 24 h when the clearance is 10–25. One-half the usual intravenous dose may be administered every 24 h when the creatinine clearance is less than 10.[226] In oral therapy, 200 mg capsules may be administered every 4 h up to a total of 5 capsules daily (or 400 mg every 8 h) in patients with normal renal function, but the manufacturer recommends 200 mg every 12 h when the creatinine clear-

ance is less than 10. Acyclovir is readily removed by hemodialysis, with about 60% of the drug in the body being removed during a single 6-h dialysis period.[236]

ADVERSE EFFECTS. Acyclovir is well tolerated, whether administered by ocular, topical, oral, or intravenous routes.[237] Ocular administration with an ointment is rarely associated with adverse effects, whereas topical acyclovir in a polyethylene glycol base may cause mucosal irritation and transient burning when applied to genital lesions.[178] The most frequent untoward effects of intravenous therapy are phlebitis and local reaction at the infusion site, particularly if extravasation occurs. The principal dose-limiting toxicities of intravenous acyclovir are renal insufficiency and, rarely, central nervous system toxicity. Preexisting renal insufficiency, high doses, and high plasma levels of the drug (>25 μg/ml) are all risk factors for both types of toxicity.[178] Acyclovir causes reversible renal dysfunction. The frequency of increased BUN and creatinine may be about 10% in patients receiving the drug by bolus injection.[237] Renal dysfunction is apparently due to precipitation of acyclovir in renal tubules when the solubility of the drug in the intratubular fluid is exceeded.[238] Signs of nephrotoxicity include nausea, emesis, flank pain, and increasing azotemia.[239] The frequency of this complication can be markedly reduced or eliminated by ensuring that the patient is adequately hydrated and by administering the drug by constant infusion over 1 h.[238,240] Neurotoxicity occurs in 1% to 4% of patients receiving intravenous acyclovir and is associated with altered sensorium, hallucinations, agitation, tremor, myoclonus, delirium, seizures, and/or extrapyramidal signs.[241] Caution is warranted when acyclovir is administered intravenously to patients with underlying neurologic abnormalities and those with serious hypoxia or renal, hepatic, or electrolyte abnormalities. About 4% of patients receiving acyclovir have experienced rashes, but the same incidence of rashes has been observed in control patients receiving placebo.[237] Although reversible leukopenia has been reported in a couple of patients,[242] at the doses that are commonly employed in antiviral therapy, acyclovir does not produce bone marrow suppression or inhibit marrow engraftment.

The nephrotoxicity and central nervous system toxicity that sometimes occur with intravenous acyclovir have not been observed with recommended dosage of the oral formulation. The most frequent adverse effects with oral administration are headache, diarrhea, nausea and vomiting, vertigo and arthralgias.

Because host cell immunity plays an important role in the incidence and virulence of herpesvirus infections, it is important to determine the effects of acyclovir and other nucleoside antiviral drugs on host immune response. Whereas cell-mediated immunity, as assayed in vitro using several methods, appears to be minimally affected by acyclovir,[178,243] some authors have shown that the levels of antibodies fell significantly during long-term acyclovir therapy in patients with frequently occurring genital HSV infections.[244,245]

Many purine analogs that affect DNA are mutagenic and carcinogenic and this concern has naturally arisen with regard to acyclovir. In preclinical toxicology studies, acyclovir was not found to be teratogenic or carcinogenic.[246] It was not mutagenic in several test systems, including the Ames assay, but positive results were obtained in one transformation assay and in an assay for clastogenic activity (chromosome breakage).[246] The safety of acyclovir during pregnancy has not been definitively established, although preliminary data indicate that it is safe.

DRUG INTERACTIONS. Concurrent use of cimetidine or probenecid can decrease renal clearance and increase the plasma concentration of acyclovir. Acyclovir may decrease the renal clearance of methotrexate and other drugs eliminated by active renal secretion.[247] Concomitant cyclosporine and probably other nephrotoxic agents enhance the risk of nephrotoxicity. Acyclovir does not significantly alter the pharmacokinetics of zidovudine, although severe somnolence and lethargy may occur with this drug combination.[247]

Valacyclovir

Valacyclovir is an L-valyl ester prodrug of acyclovir that was developed with the hope of improving oral bioavailability, which is greater than that of acyclovir, without an increase in toxicity.[248]

Valacyclovir

Following absorption in healthy adults, valacyclovir is converted rapidly and virtually completely to acyclovir and the essential amino acid L-valine. This conversion is thought to result from first-pass intestinal and hepatic metabolism through enzymatic hydrolysis. The oral bioavailability of acyclovir increases three- to fivefold to approximately 54% following valacyclovir administration compared to only 12%–20% for oral acyclovir alone.[248] Peak plasma concentrations of the prodrug valacyclovir are only 4% of acyclovir levels. The levels of acyclovir attained after oral valacyclovir approximate those of intravenous acyclovir, but without the high peak levels achieved with intravenous acyclovir administration.[249] This may account for the decreased incidence of renal toxicity associated with valacyclovir. Less than 1% of valacyclovir is recovered as the parent compound in the urine and most is eliminated as acyclovir.

A large multicentered study has compared the efficacy and safety of valacyclovir with acyclovir for the treatment of herpes zoster and has shown significantly improved clinical benefit with valacyclovir.[250] A few studies have also shown that valacyclovir at fewer doses per day is as effective as acyclovir for the treatment of genital herpes.[251,252]

Valaciclovir is generally well tolerated, producing adverse reactions similar to those reported with acyclovir. The most common adverse effects are nausea, headache, vomiting and diarrhea.[252,253] Valaciclovir was tolerated well by elderly healthy volunteers and patients with HIV infection.[254] A thrombotic thrombocytopenic purpura/hemolytic uremic syndrome has been reported in some severely immunocompromised patients treated with high doses of valacyclovir.[255] The toxicity of valaciclovir has not been evaluated during pregnancy, but a retrospective analysis of 380 women who had received acycyclovir during the first trimester of pregnancy showed that the incidence of birth defects in their infants was similar to that reported in the general population.[256]

Famciclovir and Penciclovir

Penciclovir is an acyclic guanine nucleoside analog,[257] and famciclovir is the diacetyl ester pro-drug of penciclovir, which as the parent compound, lacks intrinsic antiviral activity. The side chain of penciclovir differs structurally from that of acyclovir in that the oxygen has been replaced by a carbon and an additional hydroxymethyl group is present. Penciclovir is similar to acyclovir in its spectrum of activity and potency against HSV and VZV.

Although active by intravenous administration, penciclovir is very poorly absorbed when administered orally, thus its diacetate ester, famciclovir, was developed for oral use.[258] After oral administration, famciclovir is absorbed in the upper intestine and is rapidly converted in the intestinal wall and liver to the active compound penciclovir. The bioavailability of penciclovir after oral administration of famciclovir is about 77%.[258,259] Penciclovir is eliminated as unchanged drug in the urine. Both penciclovir and acyclovir have similar half-lives of about 2.5 h.

MECHANISM OF ACTION. Like acyclovir, penciclovir is an inhibitor of viral DNA synthesis. However, there are some qualitative differences between penciclovir and acylovir in rates of phosphorylation, stability and concentration of the triphosphate derivatives, and in their affinities for viral DNA polymerase.[260] Viral thymidine kinase is responsible for the rate-limiting initial phosphorylation to the monophosphate, while conversion to the triphosphate is via other cellular enzymes.[259] Although penciclovir triphosphate is approximately 100-fold less potent in inhibiting viral DNA polymerase than acyclovir triphosphate, it is present in much higher concentrations and for more prolonged periods in infected cells. The prolonged intracellular half-life of penciclovir triphosphate (7–20 h) is associated with prolonged antiviral effects. Penciclovir is similar

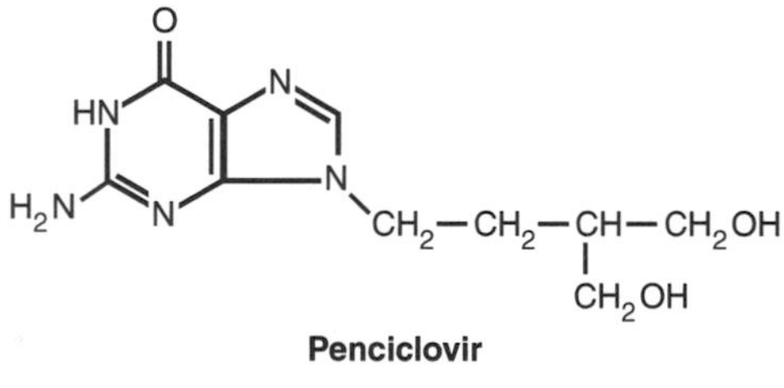

Penciclovir

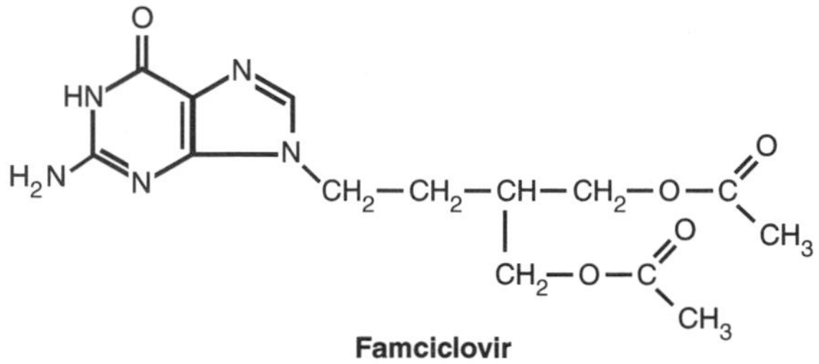

Famciclovir

to acyclovir in terms of its spectrum of anti-herpesviral activity.[259,261] Penciclovir has limited activity against CMV, but retains good activity against Epstein-Barr virus.[262]

CLINICAL USE AND ADVERSE EFFECTS. Famciclovir is used to treat herpes zoster infection, at a dose of 250–500 mg, administered three times daily.[260] Famciclovir is at least as effective as acyclovir in accelerating both cutaneous healing and resolution of pain,[263] and it reduces the duration of viral shedding and time to healing.[264] Famcicolovir is also effective in the treatment of active, recurrent genital herpes in immunocompetent hosts. The duration of viral shedding is reduced, as well as the duration of most lesion stages, the time required for complete healing, and the duration of lesion-associated symptoms.[265] Resistant variants due to mutations in thymidine kinase or DNA polymerase can be selected by in vitro passage, but the frequency of resistance during clinical use is not known. HSV and VZV strains resistant to acyclovir or valacyclovir have generally been cross-resistant to famciclovir.

Penciclovir is available for intravenous and topical administration. Penciclovir administered intravenously to patients with recurrent genital herpes reduces viral shedding and accelerates healing and loss of pain compared with placebo.[260] As a 1% cream, penciclovir produced significant benefit in treatment of oral-labial HSV infections, with significant acceleration of the rate of healing and shortening of viral shedding and the time to loss of pain.[253,266]

Famciclovir is generally well tolerated, with headache, nausea, and diarrhea being the most common adverse effects.[266] Several clinical studies in patients with either herpes zoster or genital herpes infection have shown no difference from placebo in the incidence of side effects.[267] As in preclinical studies of acyclovir, prolonged administration of high doses of famciclovir was associated with reversible dose-dependent adverse effects on testicular function in dogs and rats.[265] However, human studies have shown no significant effects on sperm count or motility.

Ganciclovir

Ganciclovir is an acyclic nucleoside analog of guanosine that is the first antiviral drug to be effective in the treatment of cytomegalovirus (CMV) disease in humans.[268,269] Ganciclovir is similar in structure to acyclovir except that it possesses an additional hydroxymethyl group on the acyclic side chain. Ganciclovir is inhibitory to all herpesviruses in vitro but is especially active against CMV.[270] Inhibitory concentrations are similar to those of acyclovir for HSV and VZV, but are 10- to 100-fold lower for human CMV strains. Ganciclovir also inhibits the transformation of normal cord-blood lymphocytes by Epstein-Barr virus.[268] The pharmacology and clinical use of ganciclovir have been extensively reviewed.[268,271,272]

MECHANISM OF ACTION. In cells, ganciclovir is converted to the monophosphate by viral enzymes and then to ganciclovir triphosphate by host cell enzymes. Ganciclovir triphosphate inhibits viral DNA polymerase by competitively inhibiting incorporation of the deoxyguanosine triphosphate into elongating viral DNA. Also, some of the drug is incorporated into the end of growing strands

Ganciclovir   Acyclovir   2'-deooxyyguanosine

of DNA, slowing replication. Unlike acyclovir, ganciclovir is not an absolute chain terminator, and short subgenomic fragments of DNA continue to be synthesized.[268] All of the drug's antiviral effects are due to its ability to inhibit the synthesis of DNA and, therefore, replication by slowing the elongation of viral DNA. Intracellular concentrations of the ganciclovir triphosphate are 10-fold higher than those of the acyclovir triphosphate and they decline much more slowly,[273] permitting single daily-dose therapy for suppression of human CMV infections.

Viral isolates from some patients with CMV infection who were unresponsive or progressively less responsive to long-term ganciclovir therapy have been shown to be resistant to the drug in vitro.[28] CMV can become resistant to ganciclovir by one of two mechanisms: through reduced conversion to the monophosphate due to point mutations or deletions in the viral phosphotransferase encoded by the UL97 gene, or through mutation in the viral DNA polymerase, which leads to partial resistance.[274,275] The selection of viral mutants that are unable to phosphorylate ganciclovir is the major mechanism of resistance. In HSV, conversion to the monophosphate is carried out by viral thymidine kinase, and thymidine kinase–deficient mutants are resistant to both ganciclovir and acyclovir.[268]

PHARMACOKINETICS. The oral bioavailability of ganciclovir is poor, ranging from 4.2% to 7.5% for single doses of 500 to 1000 mg.[276] Intravenous administration of ganciclovir at a dosage of 5 mg/kg body weight over a period of 1 h results in a peak serum concentration of 8.3 µg/ml at the end of the infusion. The plasma half-life is 2.9 h.[277] After oral administration of 1000 mg of ganciclovir three times a day, the maximal and minimal serum concentrations are 1.2 and 0.2 µg/ml, respectively. Intravenous ganciclovir provides intraocular concentrations that reach or exceed the ED_{50} for most CMV strains.[278] This is important as one of the chief uses of the drug is for CMV retinitis. Ganciclovir penetrates the blood-brain barrier and the cerebrospinal fluid concentration was 9.7 µg/ml when a simultaneously measured serum concentration was 2.2 µg/ml.[277] Over 90% of ganciclovir is eliminated unchanged in the urine by glomerular filtration and tubular secretion. Consequently, the plasma half-life increases almost linearly as creatinine clearance declines, and may reach 28 to 40 h in patients with severe renal insufficiency,[279] thus dosage must be reduced during renal impairment. Table 16–3 summarizes the pharmacokinetics of selected antiherpes nucleosides.

CLINICAL USE. Ganciclovir was first shown to reverse ongoing CMV retinitis in a patient with AIDS in 1985.[280] Since then, several uncontrolled trials in immunocompromised patients have suggested that severe CMV infections respond well to ganciclovir. However, up to 80% of responders will relapse if ther-

Table 16–3. *Metabolism and pharmacokinetics of selected antiherpes nucleosides*

Parameter	Acylclovir	Famciclovir	Ganciclovir	Foscarnet
Oral bioavailability (%)	10–20	65–77	<10	12–22
Effect of meals on AUC	⇓18%	Negligible	⇑20%	Negligible
Plasma $t_{1/2}$ (h)	2.5	2	2–4	4–8 (initial)
Intracellular $t_{1/2\ elim}$ of triphosphate (h)	~1	7–20	>24	NA
CSF/plasma ratio (mean)	0.5	Uncertain	0.2–0.7	0.7
Protein binding (%)	9–33	<20	1–2	15
Metabolism (%)	~15	~10	Negligible	Negligible
Renal excretion, parent drug (%)	60–90%	90	>90	>80

AUC, area under the curve; CSF, cerebrospinal fluid.
Source: Data from Hayden.[247]

apy is discontinued and 18%–50% relapse despite continued maintenance therapy.[25,281] Ganciclovir has proved to be effective in the treatment of several types of CMV infection as well as for maintenance and prophylactic therapy. It is approved for treatment and chronic suppression of CMV retinitis in immunocompromised patients and for prevention of CMV disease in transplant patients. In CMV retinitis, initial induction treatment is associated with improvement or stabilization in about 85% of patients.[282,283] Reduced viral excretion is usually seen by 1 week and funduscopic improvement by 2 weeks. Suppressive therapy must be given for AIDS patients with retinitis because of a high risk of relapse. Oral ganciclovir (1000 mg three times daily) is now approved for maintenance therapy of CMV retinitis after initial intravenous treatment. It is safe and effective and is more convenient for patients to take than intravenous ganciclovir.[284] Oral therapy may be associated with a more rapid rate of progression to retinitis than intravenous treatment but the survival, changes in visual acuity, viral shedding, and adverse gastrointestinal events were similar in the two groups. Intraocular sustained release implants and intravitreal injections of ganciclovir have also been effective in treating CMV retinitis. These implants do not protect against systemic CMV disease and long-term survival is lower than in patients receiving oral ganciclovir.

Ganciclovir therapy may benefit other CMV syndromes in patients with AIDS or solid organ transplant recipients. In biopsy-proven CMV colitis in AIDS patients, ganciclovir is associated with improved mucosal appearance and lower incidence of extracolonic CMV disease but no obvious symptomatic benefit.[285] The treatment of primary CMV pneumonia with ganciclovir has been most successful in renal transplant recipients, and in these patients, this therapy has been lifesaving.[286] If ganciclovir is combined with intravenous immunoglobulin or CMV immunoglobulin, the mortality from CMV pneumonia is reduced by about one-half. Oral ganciclovir prevents CMV disease in patients with AIDS and those with fewer than 100 CD4+ cells/cm². The percentage of patients who acquired CMV disease was significantly less in the treated group than in those given a placebo.[287] Prevention of CMV pneumonia or other CMV disease with ganciclovir in recipients of bone marrow, cardiac, and liver transplants was clearly demonstrated in several studies.[268] Ganciclovir has also been used to treat some CMV infections of the nervous system. For example, ganciclovir treatment has improved progressive polyradiculopathy in some patients with AIDS, although the treatment is usually disappointing.[288,289] The drug has also been used in mononeuritis multiplex and painful peripheral neuropathy with uncertain benefit.[290] CMV meningoencephalitis may respond to ganciclovir.[291]

ADVERSE EFFECTS. Ganciclovir has a narrow therapeutic index and often causes granulocytopenia, thrombocytopenia, azoospermia, and a rise in serum creatinine. Myelosupression is the principal dose-limiting toxicity of ganciclovir, with granulocytopenia occurring in about 15% to 40% of patients and thrombocytopenia in 5% to 20%.[282] In most patients, the granulocytopenia and thrombocytopenia disappeared after ganciclovir was discontinued. Anemia may also develop with prolonged treatment. With oral ganciclovir therapy, the incidence of neutropenia and thrombocytopenia is lower than after intravenous administration.[284] Patients who receive recombinant granulocyte colony–stimulating factor or granulocyte-macrophage colony–stimulating factor have significantly fewer episodes of granulocytopenia.[292]

Central nervous system side effects occur in 5% to 15% of patients and range in severity from headache to behavioral changes to convulsions and coma. About one-third of patients have to interrupt or prematurely stop therapy because of bone marrow or central nervous system toxicity. Increases in serum creatinine were found in 20% of bone marrow transplant recipients studied,[293] but the values subsequently declined after the drug was discontinued. Infusion-related phlebitis, azotemia, rash, fever, liver function test abnormalities, nausea or vomiting, and eosinophilia have also been described.[247]

Teratogenicity, embryotoxicity, irreversible reproductive toxicity, and myelotoxicity have been seen in animals at dosages comparable to those used in humans. The azoospermia associated with ganciclovir in animals is due to direct inhibition of sperm-producing cells.[268] Testicular endocrine function, however, is not affected by this drug.

DRUG INTERACTIONS. It is dangerous to use ganciclovir at full dosage with other drugs toxic to the bone marrow, such as zidovudine; more than 80% of the patients in one study who were treated with both ganciclovir and zidovudine required dose reduction because of the hematologic toxicity.[294] Nephrotoxic agents that impair ganciclovir excretion also may increase the risk of myelosuppression. Probenecid and possibly acyclovir reduce renal clearance of ganciclovir. Oral ganciclovir increases the steady-state area under the plasma concentration–time curve of didanosine by approximately twofold and that of zidovudine by about 20%.

Foscarnet

Foscarnet (trisodium phosphonoformate) is an inorganic pyrophosphate analog that is inhibitory for all herpesviruses and some retroviruses, including HIV. In vitro inhibitory

$$\overset{\text{O}}{\underset{\|}{(NaO)_2 PCOONa}}$$

Foscarnet Sodium

concentrations generally range from 100 to 300 µM for CMV and 80 to 200 µM for other herpesviruses, including most ganciclovir-resistant CMV and acyclovir-resistant HSV and VZV strains.[295]

MECHANISM OF ACTION. Foscarnet selectively inhibits DNA polymerase from several viruses, including CMV and other herpesviruses. It also inhibits the reverse transcriptase of HIV.[295] Foscarnet is a pyrophosphate analog that is a noncompetitive inhibitor of the viral polymerase. It does not require intracellular activation, as is the case with acyclovir and ganciclovir, but inhibits the DNA polymerase directly by interacting with the pyrophosphate binding site to block binding of the pyrophosphate moiety that is cleaved from a dNTP during DNA synthesis. Foscarnet prevents elongation of the viral DNA chain during treatment, and, when the drug is withdrawn, viral DNA polymerase activity and replication resume. Additive or synergistic effects are seen with other antiviral drugs, including ganciclovir and zidovudine. Foscarnet appears to have negligible effects on host enzymes and cells, and inhibition of mammalian DNA polymerase occurrs only at foscarnet concentrations that are about 100 times higher than those required to inhibit CMV replication.[296]

Herpesviruses resistant to foscarnet have point mutations in the viral DNA polymerase and three- to fivefold higher concentrations of drug are required to achieve comparable inhibition in vitro.[297,298] The isolation of HSV and CMV strains with polymerase mutations conferring resistance to pyrophosphate analogs suggests that foscarnet is a specific inhibitor of the HSV and CMV polymerases.[299,300] Foscarnet-resistant viruses have been found at lower frequencies in laboratory strains of CMV than of HSV, although foscarnet-resistant clinical isolates of both HSV and CMV have been detected following clinical use.[301] The mutant polymerases bind foscarnet poorly, and because there is some overlap with the binding sites of acyclovir and ganciclovir, there is some degree of cross-resistance among these drugs, both in laboratory studies and clinically.

PHARMACOKINETICS. The pharmacokinetics of foscarnet have been the subject of detailed review.[295,302] Foscarnet is poorly absorbed after oral administration. Thus, oral administration is not feasible for the treatment of viral disease and the only pharmacokinetic investigations of clinical importance are those following intravenous administration. There is wide intra- and interindividual variability in plasma foscarnet concentrations following continuous infusion, which may be due to differences in the equilibrium of foscarnet and phosphate deposition in bone and cartilage. In mice about 30% of the foscarnet is retained in bone and cartilage. Foscarnet is not metabolized to any significant extent after intravenous administration, and as much as 88% of a dose is recovered unchanged in the urine within a week of stopping the infusion. Renal clearance occurs primarily via glomerular filtration and tubular secretion. Plasma elimination is complex with initial bimodal half-lives of 4 to 8 h, followed by a prolonged terminal elimination half-life of 3 to 4 days. Plasma clearance of foscarnet decreases significantly with decreased renal function, whereas the elimination half-life may increase as much as 10-fold.

CLINICAL USE. Foscarnet is effective for the treatment of CMV retinitis, including progressive disease due to ganciclovir-resistant strains, and for acyclovir-resistant HSV or VZV infections. It is also effective for treating other types of CMV infections.[25,295,303] Foscarnet is more expensive and generally less well tolerated than ganciclovir, and large volumes of fluid are required for infusion because of its poor solubility. In CMV retinitis in patients with AIDS, foscarnet (60 mg/kg/8 h for 14 to 21 days followed by chronic maintenance at 90 to 120 mg/kg/day in one dose) produces clinical stabilization in about 90% of patients.[302,304] A trial comparing foscarnet with ganciclovir for CMV retinitis in patients with AIDS showed comparable effect in controlling symptoms but an improved overall survival in the foscarnet group. The improved survival might reflect either the inherent anti-AIDS action of foscarnet or the fact that those in the foscarnet group also received zidovudine more often.[305] It is important to note that the foscarnet patients stopped taking their drug over three times as frequently as those in the ganciclovir group.

Foscarnet appears to be effective in treating ganciclovir-resistant infections, and a combination of foscarnet and ganciclovir has been used in refractory retinitis. Foscarnet has also been used to treat patients unable to continue ganciclovir treatment of AIDS-associated CMV infection because of

neutropenia and thrombocytopenia, thus allowing the reintroduction of zidovudine therapy.[306] Besides retinitis, foscarnet may benefit other CMV syndromes in AIDS or transplant patients, but it is ineffective as a single drug in treating CMV pneumonia in bone marrow transplant patients.[307] The lack of myelotoxicity with foscarnet has allowed the drug to be used prophylactically in patients about to undergo bone marrow transplantation. In one study no evidence of CMV infection during intermittent foscarnet prophylaxis was evident in 15 of 19 CMV-seropositive patients.[308]

Foscarnet also appears to be effective in treating immunocompromised patients with acyclovir-resistant mucocutaneous HSV (types 1 and 2) infections.[309,310] Recurring episodes were also successfully treated with foscarnet, followed in some patients by maintenance therapy with foscarnet.[311] Acyclovir-resistant VZV infections occurring in patients with AIDS are often associated with chronic localized skin lesions that have been successfully treated with foscarnet.[312,313]

ADVERSE EFFECTS. The main dose-limiting adverse effects associated with foscarnet appear to be renal impairment, acute infusion-related symptoms such as nausea, and disturbances in serum calcium and phosphate levels.[295] Nephrotoxicity is the most common adverse effect, and increases in serum creatinine occur in up to one-half of patients. The nephrotoxicity is usually reversible in patients with previously adequate kidney function after treatment is stopped. Diarrhea and vomiting associated with foscarnet therapy can precipitate renal damage because of dehydration.[314] Development of renal dysfunction may be minimized by adjusting the dosage according to serum creatinine levels, maintaining adequate hydration, using intermittent rather than continuous infusion, and avoiding concomitant treatment with other potentially nephrotoxic drugs where possible.

Metabolic abnormalities occur because foscarnet, a pyrophosphate analog, can bind free, ionized plasma calcium. Decreased calcium and phosphate levels are very common during treatment with foscarnet.[295] The decrease in serum calcium may cause paresthesia, arrhythmias, tetany, seizures, and other central nervous system disturbances. Transient hyperphosphatemia and hypophosphatemia, hypokalemia, and hypomagnesemia have also been reported in association with foscarnet therapy.[303,304] Electrolytes should be monitored routinely, both during remission induction and with maintenance therapy. Anemia is the most frequent hematological effect associated with foscarnet therapy. Reports of neutropenia are infrequent, and foscarnet has been associated with an overall increase in leukocyte count in some patients.[302] The excretion of unchanged foscarnet in the urine exposes mucous membranes in the genital area directly to the drug, which may account for the penile and vulval ulceration associated with treatment.[295] These lesions resolve when the drug is withdrawn. Adverse gastrointestinal effects (nausea and vomiting) are experienced by 20% to 30% of patients during foscarnet treatment.[315] Other adverse effects experienced include local irritation manifest as thrombophlebitis of peripheral veins when the dug is infused undiluted and occasional slight elevations in serum transaminase levels.[295]

DRUG INTERACTIONS. Concomitant administration of potentially nephrotoxic drugs such as aminoglycosides, cyclosporine or amphotericin B with foscarnet should be avoided since foscarnet itself has been associated with renal impairment. Caution is also advised when foscarnet is used in conjunction with drugs likely to influence serum calcium levels.[295] Additive renal toxicity and hypocalcemia have been reported with concomitant administration of foscarnet and pentamidine and the combination should be avoided.[302] Administration of foscarnet with ganciclovir or zidovudine does not significantly affect the pharmacokinetics of foscarnet, an important consideration in some patients with AIDS.[295]

Cidofovir

MECHANISM OF ACTION. Cidofovir is a cytidine nucleotide analog used for intravenous treatment of CMV retinitis in patients with AIDS. Cidofovir is phosphorylated by cellular enzymes to its monophosphate metabolite and then to cidofovir diphosphate.[316] Since cidofovir is itself a phosphonate, the

Cidofovir

diphosphate is functionally analogous to a triphosphate. Cidofovir diphosphate competes with the natural substrate deoxycytidine triphosphate to inhibit viral DNA synthesis. It is also an alternate substrate for viral DNA polymerase, and incorporation of cidofovir into the growing viral DNA chain inhibits viral DNA synthesis. Cidofovir has a higher affinity for viral DNA polymerases than for host cell polymerases, and in cell culture it has a selectivity index of 1000-fold. The binding affinity of the diphosphate for human CMV DNA polymerase is 3 to 80 times greater than that for the human enzyme.[317] For other herpes viruses the binding affinity is up to 600-fold higher for the viral DNA polymerase than than for the host cell enzyme. Studies of cidofovir in combination with several other antiviral compounds showed an effect that is synergistic with either ganciclovir or foscarnet against human CMV in vitro, whereas combinations with zidovudine, didanosine, or lamivudine showed neither synergism nor antagonism.[318] Immunosuppressive agents, such as hydrocortisone, cyclosporine, methotrexate, and mycophenolic acid, that are commonly used in the management of organ transplantation rejection do not alter the antiviral activity of cidofovir in vitro.[318]

Resistance to cidofovir is mainly due to mutations in DNA polymerase.[319] Ganciclovir-resistant viruses carrying mutations in the genes encoding phosphorylation enzymes are susceptible to cidofovir, while those with DNA polymerase mutations are cross-resistant to cidofovir.[320] Resistance to cidofovir has not yet been documented in clinical isolates obtained from patients receiving cidofovir.[321]

PHARMACOKINETICS. For systemic treatment, cidofovir is administered intravenously, and has a prolonged half-life of 17 to 65 h, probably because the diphosphate does not readily pass through cellular membranes. A separate metabolite, cidofovir phosphate-choline, has a half-life of at least 87 h and may serve as an intracellular reservoir for the long-term maintenance of active cidofovir in cells.[322] Without probenecid, eighty to one hundred percent of cidofovir is recovered unchanged in the urine, and this decreases 70%–85% with concomitant oral probenecid.[323] When administered as a topical gel, cidofovir is usually undetectible in the blood.

CLINICAL USE AND ADVERSE EFFECTS. Several studies have shown that intravenous cidofovir given once weekly for 2 weeks and then once every 2 weeks for maintenance can delay progression of CMV retinitis.[324,325] Cidofovir gel is effective for topical treatment of acyclovir-resistant mucocutaneous HSV infections in patients with AIDS.[324]

The most common adverse effects associated with use of cidofovir have been nephrotoxicity (proteinuria and elevated creatinine), neutropenia, metabolic acidosis, uveitis, and low intraocular pressure.[319,326] The neutropenia was not dose related and the rate was consistent with AIDS patients not receiving agents with obvious bone marrow toxicity. To decrease the risk of dose-related nephrotoxicity in patients receiving cidofovir, patients should be adequately hydrated and concurrent administration of other nephrotoxic agents should be avoided. Concomitant administration of probenecid, with resultant decreased renal clearance of cidofovir, has been associated with a reduction in the incidence and severity of nephrotoxicity. However, a considerable number of these patients experienced at least one reversible adverse effect during their treatment, that was felt to be related to the probenecid.[319,327]

Broad-Spectrum Anti-viral Agents

The antiviral drugs discussed up to now are active against a relatively narrow spectrum of viruses, e.g. herpesviruses. The two drugs to be discussed in this section, interferon and ribavirin, are active against a wide variety of both DNA and RNA viruses. However, for toxicological or other reasons, they are used clinically only to treat a limited number of viral infections.

Interferon

Interferons are clinically effective, broad-spectrum antiviral agents. They are cytokines, and in addition to antiviral activity, they also possess immunomodulating and antiproliferative actions. Interferons are synthesized by cells in response to various inducers and, in turn, can cause biochemical changes leading to an antiviral state.

The discovery of interferon evolved from studies of the mechanism of viral interference, a phenomenon originally described in 1935, in which infection with one type of virus was found to protect an animal against infection by another type of virus.[328] In 1957, Isaacs and Lindenmann[329] performed a critical experiment indicating the existence of a factor responsible for viral interference. These investigators added heat-inactivated influenza virus to pieces of chicken egg chorioallantoic membrane. After washing the membranes to remove unadsorbed virus, membrane fragments were incubated for several hours at 37°C and removed from the culture medium. Fresh membrane fragments were then incubated in this "conditioned" culture medium for several hours at 37°C, live influenza virus was added, and its replication was found to be inhibited. Thus, the membrane fragments that were exposed to inactivated virus had secreted a factor that transferred viral interference (i.e., virus resistance) to fresh membrane fragments. The factor, which was named *interferon*, was subsequently demonstrated to be a protein, and it was shown that it did not inactivate the virus directly but it rendered the cells resistant to virus.[330] The demonstration that animal cells could synthesize and secrete a protein that produced an antiviral state in other cells has stimulated a tremendous amount of research, leading to a large literature dealing with interferon production, the mechanism of its antiviral action, and its clinical effects. The reader is referred to specific texts for detailed discussion of the interferon literature.[330–332]

INDUCTION OF INTERFERON. Interferons are polypeptides produced by most types of animal cells infected with viruses. Virtually all types of viruses, including both RNA and DNA viruses, can induce the production of interferon. In addition to viruses, a wide variety of other intracellular parasites, microbial components, synthetic polymers, and some small molecular weight compounds can elicit the production of interferon.[333] Interferon is also produced by sensitized lymphocytes on exposure to specific antigen and by normal lymphocytes on exposure to mitogens. Unfortunately, none of these agents have been shown to be safe or effective in humans. Purified recombinant human interferon is administered for treatment of viral infections.

CLASSIFICATION OF HUMAN INTERFERONS. The interferons produced by different animals are quite species specific. That is, they inhibit viral multiplication only in cells of the same animal species (or closely related ones) in which they were produced. Human cells produce three types of interferons (IFN), which have been classified as α, β, and γ (see Table 16–4).[334]

Members of the IFN α/β or type I IFN superfamily (see Table 16–5) represent the prototypical interferon molecules. They are further subdivided into four subfamilies, termed IFN-α, IFN-β, IFN-ω, and IFN-τ (the latter two have been identified only in cattle and sheep).[333] All genes and proteins comprising this family are related to each other structurally. The genes form a cluster, which in humans is located on the short arm of chromosome 9. Type II or IFN-γ consists of only one subtype whose gene is on chromosome 12. Type I interferons appear to be produced by all human cells and share a range of biological effects. The physiologic stimuli for their production are diverse and include infectious agents and their component nucleic acids. In contrast, type II interferons are produced only by T lymphocytes and natural killer cells and possess actions discrete from type I interferons that are mediated through a separate receptor.[337]

The human (Hu) α interferons (HuIFN-α) are acid-stable polypeptides with apparent molecular weights ranging from 16,000 to 23,000 daltons that are produced by leukocytes or lymphoblasts. More than twenty

Table 16–4.   *Classification of human interferons.*

Type	Old nomenclature	Induction	Characteristics
IFN-α	Le (leukocyte), type 1, foreign cell-induced	Induced in a variety of cells by type I inducers	pH 2 stable, not glycosylated, several homologous subtypes, 16,000–23,000 daltons
IFN-β	F (fibroblast), Fi, type I	Induced in a variety of cells by type I inducers	pH 2 stable, glycosylated, at least two species, one of which is 20,000 daltons
IFN-γ	IIF (immune), type II, T	Induced in lymphoid cells by type II inducers, (i.e., by antigens in sensitized cells or by mitogens)	pH 2 labile, glycosylated, at least two species, 20,000 and 25,000 daltons

Source: Table prepared from information in refs. 334–336.

Table 16–5. *Classification and major features of the interferons.*

	Type I IFN (IFN-α/β)	Type II IFN (IFN-γ)
Subfamilies	IFN-α (at least 14 potentially functional genes in humans) IFN-β IFN-ω IFN-τ	—
Structural genes	Chromosome 9 (human) Chromosome 4 (mouse) No introns	Chromosome 12 (human) Chromosome 10 (mouse) Three introns
Proteins[a]	IFN-α: 165–166 a.a. IFN-β: 166 a.a. IFN-ω: 172 a.a. IFN-τ: 172 a.a.	146 a.a. (forms dimer)
Receptors	Genes for two chains located on chromosome 21 (human) and chromosome 16 (mouse) Additional components?	Gene for chain 1 on chromosome 6 (human) and chromosome 10 (mouse) Gene for chain 2 on chromosome 21 (human) and chromosome 16 (mouse) Additional components?
Major functions	Antiviral actions Regulation of cell growth and differentiation Induction of MHC class I antigens Embryo implantation in uterus (IFN-τ)	Macrophage activation Induction of MHC class I and II antigens Antiviral actions

a.a., amino acids. [a]Polypeptide lengths refer to mature proteins, as predicted from cDNA sequences, after removal of cleavable signal peptide sequences. Some natural IFN proteins are known to undergo C-terminal processing so that shorter forms may be generated. Many IFN proteins are N- and O-glycosylated.

Source: From Vilcek and Sen.[333]

IFN-α genes have been postulated, but not all have been clearly identified with a product. At least 14 distinct subtypes of IFN-α have been cloned using recombinant DNA techniques. Up to five IFN-β mRNAs have been identified, but only two gene products, IFN-$β_1$ and IFN-$β_2$ have been established. IFN-$β_1$ represents over 90% of the interferon produced by fibroblasts.[333] Native HuIFN-β are acid-stable polypeptides, one of which has been shown to have an apparent molecular weight of 20,000 daltons. They are produced by a variety of cells, including cultured fioroblasts, in response to type I interferon inducers. In contrast to the α and β interferons, HuIFN-γ is acid-labile and is produced in lymphoid cells in response to antigens or mitogens. Thus far, only one type of IFN-γ has been described. This interferon bears little homology to the IFN-α and IFN-β species but shares many of their biological functions. The interferons are very potent. Indeed, the potencies of most of the purified human interferons are comparable to those of many hormones; they impair virus replication in responsive cells at concentrations as low as 10^{-13}–10^{-14}M.

STUDIES ON THE MECHANISM OF ACTION OF INTERFERON. Although interferons affect other cellular functions, such as cell motility, cell proliferation, and various immunological processes, their most studied effect is the conversion of cells into an "antiviral" state in which they are poor hosts for viral replication.[338] It has been shown that cultured human fibroblasts that are producing interferon in response to poly(I)·poly(C) do not develop viral resistance if antiserum to HuIFN-β is present in the medium.[339] Thus, the interferon must be secreted into the medium surrounding the cell before it can produce an antiviral effect. Also, it is clear that interferons must bind to the cell surface because cells that do not bind detectable amounts of interferon are resistant to the antiviral effect.[340] Purified mouse α and β interferons labeled with ^{125}I, for example, bind in a high-affinity and specific manner to receptors located on the surface of a mouse lymphoma line (L121OS) that responds to these interferons, but the radiolabeled interferons do not bind to cells of a variant line (L121OR) that does not respond.[341,342] Human α and β interferons compete for binding of ^{125}I-labeled IFN-α, indicating that they bind to the same or to similar receptor sites, but γ interferons do not compete, suggesting that they bind to different receptors.[343] This may explain the synergistic antiviral and antitumor effects that are sometimes seen when IFN-γ is given with either of the other two IFN species.

Interferons bind to specific receptors on the cell surface and elicit the signals necessary for transcriptional induction of the IFN-activatable genes.[344,345] The binding of interferons to receptors and hence their cellular actions are usually species specific, and this is especially true with IFN-γ. The mechanism of signal transduction by the interferons is reviewed in several sources.[333,346,347] Unlike the pathways used by many hormones, diffusible small molecular second messengers are not involved in this process, and interferon receptors lack intrinsic kinase activity. Instead, the key events are ligand-induced activation of receptor-associated tyrosine-kinases, resulting in tyrosine phosphorylation of specific cytoplasmic proteins and their subsequent translocation to the nucleus where they bind to cis-acting sequences of the IFN-inducible genes and promote their transcription. Like many other cytokines and growth factors the signal from the re-

ceptors on the cell surface to the gene in the nucleus is physically carried by proteins called STAT (signal transducers and activators of transcription) proteins that also serve as transcriptional activators. Interferons lead to the synthesis of over two dozen proteins that contribute to viral resistance,[348,349] with different antiviral mechanisms being mediated by different IFN-induced proteins. For the functioning of some of these antiviral pathways, viral gene products, such as double-stranded RNA, are required. Different antiviral pathways are involved in inhibiting the replication of different families of viruses, and one or more steps in the virus life cycle may be inhibited in an IFN-treated cell. The steps of viral multiplication that are affected by interferons have been identified for several families of viruses.[349,350] Usually more than one step is affected, and the degree of inhibition of an individual step varies among different host cell types. For example, for vesicular stomatitis virus, both primary transcription of viral mRNAs and their translation are inhibited, while for retroviruses, virion assembly, budding, and release are affected.

It is clear that conversion of cells into the antiviral state requires the synthesis of new cellular mRNA and protein, because inhibitors of both processes block interferon's antiviral action.[351,352] From early studies on the mechanism of interferon action it was clear that the processes of viral attachment and entry are not affected in interferon-treated cells, but viral RNA and protein accumulation are impaired.[353] Accordingly, during the 1970s, a number of laboratories compared the ability of cell-free extracts from interferon-treated and control cells to cleave and to translate viral and host mRNA. It was found that extracts from interferon-treated cells have an increased rate of RNA degradation and a decreased rate of peptide chain initiation. As a result of these studies, two interferon-induced enzymes were discovered; one of the enzymes leads to the activation of a latent RNase (RNase L) and the other inactivates a peptide chain initiation factor that is required for protein synthesis.[338,354] Although other biochemical differences have been identified between interferon-treated and control cells, these two effects of interferons are of particular interest because both depend on the presence of double-stranded RNA and both effects are, so far, unique to the interferon-induced state.

The interferon-induced 2-5A synthetase-RNase L pathway. Two observations made in the mid 1970s are of particular importance in elucidating the interferon effect on viral mRNA degradation. In 1974, Kerr and co-workers discovered that double-stranded RNA (dsRNA) inhibits protein synthesis in extracts of interferon-treated cells.[355] Two years later, Lengyel and collaborators reported that reovirus mRNA is degraded in extracts of interferon-treated cells more rapidly than in extracts of untreated cells.[356,357] The degradation was found to depend on the presence of dsRNA in the mRNA preparation. These two observations ultimately led to the discovery of the interferon-induced, dsRNA-dependent pathway of RNase L activation diagrammed in Figure. 16–5. Kerr and collaborators found that extracts of interferon-treated cells formed a low molecular weight inhibitor of protein synthesis in the presence of dsRNA and ATP.[358] The inhibitor was later identified as (2'-5') (A)n,[359] a series of short (2'-5')-linked oligoadenylates which are synthesized by an interferon-induced enzyme called (2'-5') (A)n synthetase. As shown in Figure 16–5, the 2-5A synthetase enzyme is converted from an inactive to an active form by dsRNA. The 2-5A that is produced in turn activates the second enzyme in the pathway, a latent endoribonuclease *called RNase L* (L standing for latent).[360–362] The only enzyme in the pathway that is affected by interferon is the 2-5A synthetase and the only known biological activity of 2-5A is the activation of RNase L. The interaction between 2-5A and RNase L is tight but reversible, and when the 2-5A dissociates, the enzyme returns to the inactive state. 2-5A is itself degraded by a 2', 5'-phosphodiesterase. In vitro, the 2-5A synthetase–Rnase L system cleaves both viral and host cell mRNAs with the same facility,

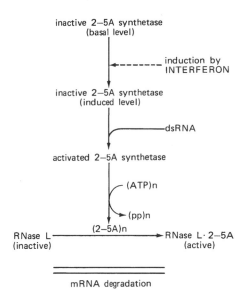

Figure 16–5. The interferon-induced 2-5A synthetase–RNase L pathway. Interferon induces the synthesis of an inactive 2-5A synthetase that is activated by double-stranded RNA (dsRNA). The activated synthetase polymerizes ATP into short (2'-5')-linked oligoadenylates, (2-5A)n, that activate a latent RNase (RNase L) which degrades mRNA.

but in some in vivo systems it has been shown that viral protein synthesis is inhibited preferentially with respect to host protein synthesis.[338,354]

The Interferon-induced, dsRNA-dependent protein kinase pathway. In addition to increasing the rate of mRNA degradation, interferons inhibit the rate of polypeptide chain initiation. A second interferon-induced enzyme was discovered that inactivates the eukaryotic initiation factor eIF-2 by phosphorylating it. As shown in Figure 16–6, interferon induces the synthesis of a protein kinase that is inactive until it is bound by dsRNA.[363–365] The IFN-inducible dsRNA-dependent protein kinase is known as PKR (other names are P68 kinase, P1, DAI, dsI, or eIF-2 kinase).[366] PKR activation by dsRNA results in its autophosphorylation on several serine and threonine residues. The autophosphorylation is most probably intermolecular and

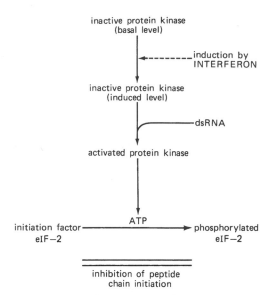

Figure 16–6. The interferon-induced, dsRNA-dependent protein kinase pathway. Interferon induces the synthesis of an inactive protein kinase that is activated by double-stranded RNA (dsRNA). The activated protein kinase phosphorylates the initiation factor eIF-2. Phosphorylated eIF-2 is inactive and peptide chain initiation is inhibited.

occurs between two kinase molecules bound to the same dsRNA molecule.[333] Upon activation, the kinase phosphorylates a 37,000-dalton protein that has been identified as the α subunit of eIF-2.[367,368] The phosphorylated eIF-2 is inactive and cannot participate in the first step in the initiation of protein synthesis, which in eukaryotes is the formation of a ternary complex between eIF-2, Met-tRNA, and GTP. Detectable levels of PKR are present in most cells even without interferon treatment, and phosphorylation of PKR and eIF-2 have been observed in many virus-infected cells. Thus, PKR activation by viral dsRNA may be involved not only in the inhibition of viral protein synthesis in IFN-treated cells but also in the shut-off of host proteins synthesis in virus-infected cells.

Other Actions. Another group of proteins induced by the interferons are the Mx family proteins. Induction of these proteins mediates inhibition of orthomyxovirus replica-

tion.[369] Some of these proteins are nuclear, whereas others are cytoplasmic. The Mx proteins bind GTP and have an intrinsic GTPase activity that is necessary for their intracellular antiviral actions. It is believed that their binding to viral transcriptases and inhibition of transcription might be responsible for their antiviral activity.

Interferon also increases the host's immunological defense through immune cell–modulated lysis of virus-infected cells. One way that interferons may do this is by inducing MHC class I and class II proteins, which mediate virus-infected cell recognition.[370] The proteasomes and permeases that degrade and transport the viral peptides that are displayed in conjunction with the MHC protein are also induced by interferons in several cell types.[371] Interferons therefore exert an important antiviral function by augmenting the expression of the machinery responsible for antigen processing, intracellular trafficking, and cell surface presentation of the viral peptides to T lymphocytes.

Thus, the antiviral state is the result of the interaction of several mechanisms and the pathways presented in Figures 16–5 and 16–6 are only part of a complex interferon-induced antiviral system. Table 16–6 summarizes the different steps in viral replication inhibited by the interferons.

RESISTANCE. Nonresponsiveness to interferons is fairly common, and rates vary with different viruses. About 20% of patients with hepatitis C virus infection respond to IFN-α, although this increases with addition of ribavirin. It has been shown that the nonresponsiveness is due to mutations in the nonstructural protein 5A gene of the viral genome, but it may also be related to the type and strength of the host immune response.[372,373]

Viruses can evade the immune response in many chronic infections by mutations in viral peptides that can bind HLA and lymphocyte receptors but not activate the T cell. Altered peptides have been shown for hepatitis B virus isolates from chronically infected patients.[374] There are multiple mechanisms through which viruses can evade host defenses, including viral production of host

Table 16–6. Multiple steps of viral replication inhibited by interferons.

Affected step	Viruses	Responsible IFN-induced proteins
Early: penetration, uncoating	SV40, retroviruses	Unknown
Transcription	Influenza, VSV, HSV	Mx proteins (and others?)
Translation	Picornaviruses	2-5(A) synthetase/RNAse L
	Reoviruses, adenovirus, vaccinia, VSV, influenza	DsRNA-dependent protein kinase (PKR)
Late: maturation, assembly, release	Retrovirus, VSV, HSV	Unknown

Source: From Vilcek and Sen.[333]

proteins such as cytokines and their receptors. Viruses can also interfere with interferon signaling pathways and inhibit transcriptional activation in IFN-induced cells.[375–378] Also, some viruses can inhibit the effect of IFN-inducible proteins. For example, HSV produces a nonfunctional oligoadenylate synthetase, several viruses (adenovirus, HIV and Epstein-Barr virus) bind protein kinase and inhibit its activity, and HSV inactivates RNAse-L and inhibits complement factors and antibody responses.

ANTIVIRAL ACTIVITY. Interferons have broad-spectrum antiviral effects, with activity against hepatitis B (HBV) C, D, human papilloma virus (HPV), HSV types 1 and 2, CMV, vesicular stomatitis virus (VSV), HIV, poliovirus, rhinoviruses, adenoviruses, coronaviruses, and vaccinia. As a result, IFN-α has been used to treat a variety of viral infections, including chronic hepatitis, AIDS-related Kaposi's sarcoma, and HPV. It has also been used in therapy of some leukemias and is an adjuvant in the chemotherapy of some tumors and in HIV infection.

INTERFERONS AS ANTIVIRAL DRUGS. Of the three approaches to the specific control of viral infections, immunization provides the longest lasting protection, but its usefulness is restricted to those infections in which there are only a few serotypes. In the case of viruses causing many common respiratory tract illnesses, there are so many different serotypes, and immunity is so short lived, that

control by immunization is not practical.[379] Most of the chemotherapeutic agents developed to date have a very narrow spectrum of action, and their effects are transient, whereas interferon has a broad spectrum of activity, and it does not have the delay period inherent to the development of the antibody response in immunization. Exploitation of the antiviral effect of interferon would thus seem to be a potential therapeutic approach. This could be done in two ways: the administration of purified interferon or the administration of compounds that stimulate the production of interferon by the cells of the host.

To circumvent the early limited supply of exogenous human interferon, compounds that stimulate the endogenous production of interferon by host cells have been extensively studied over the years. The use of synthetic interferon inducers in systemic therapy of viral infection has been compromised by their significant toxicity and the development of hyporesponsiveness to induction.[380] The poly(I)·poly(C) type of interferon inducers are potent pyrogens and, when given systemically, they produce fever in virtually all patients.[381,382] Leukopenia occurs in the majority of patients and hypotensive episodes are common. Transient and sometimes severe myalgia and arthralgia have been reported, as have mild hepatotoxicity, nausea, and vomiting.

Clearly, the more promising approach to therapy is to administer purified interferon. Because of species specificity, interferon prepared for human use must be a human interferon. Prior to the introduction of recombinant interferon, the preparation of human interferon was a costly procedure that required the processing of many 500 ml units of whole blood, and only enough of the product was available to permit small pilot studies. In 1980, human leukocyte interferon produced in bacteria by recombinant DNA technology was shown to be biologically active in vivo; it protected squirrel monkeys from lethal infection with encephalomyocarditis virus.[383] The availability of potentially unlimited amounts of recombinant interferon (rIFN) has stimulated intense interest in the use of interferons for clinical antiviral therapy.

The first clinical trial that clearly demonstrated an antiviral effect of interferon in humans utilized topical administration. In a randomized, placebo-controlled trial, local administration of HuIFN-α (given by nasal spray in divided doses one day before and for three days after infection) produced a statistically significant amelioration of symptoms and reduction in seroconversion and virus shedding in volunteers challenged with rhinovirus type 4.[384] Subsequent studies have supported the conclusion that both human leukocyte IFN-α and recombinant IFN-α administered intranasally can have a prophylactic effect against rhinovirus challenge.[385,386] However, interferon is protective only against rhinitis caused by rhinovirus, and chronic use of interferon is limited by the occurrence of nasal side effects.[387]

In acute virus infections, such as the common respiratory tract infections, virus replication occurs over a short time and is rapidly terminated by the immune response.[388] As virus replication is the interferon-sensitive step, it is likely that interferon would have to be administered in a prophylactic manner to be clinically useful in the treatment of acute infections. For this reason, clinical trials of systemically administered interferon have focused on determining its efficacy in the treatment of chronic or recurrent infections where virus replication is occurring over a long enough time to be affected by interferon. Both recombinant and natural alpha interferons are approved for treatment

of chronic hepatitis B and C, condylomata acuminatum (genital warts), Kaposi's sarcoma in HIV-infected patients, and certain other malignancies. Of the three interferons, alpha has had the most clinical utility in viral infections. Preparations of natural and recombinant interferons alpha available for clinical use are referred to as interferon alfa. Interferon alfa is available as alfa-2a, alfa-2b, and alfa-n3.

Chronic viral hepatitis is the principal cause of chronic liver disease, cirrhosis, and hepatocellular carcinoma in the world and now ranks as the chief reason for liver transplantation in adults.[389] Chronic hepatitis B accounts for 5% to 10% of the cases of chronic liver disease and cirrhosis in the United States.[390] Hepatitis B is a unique DNA virus that replicates in hepatocytes, which then shed hepatitis B surface antigen, hepatitis B e antigen (HbeAg), and intact virions into the circulation.[391] Hepatitis B is an RNA-like virus that has a reverse transcriptase as part of its replicative pathway in hepatocytes. At present, the only therapy with a lasting beneficial effect in the treatment of chronic viral hepatitis is interferon alfa. A course of therapy of 4 to 6 months duration induces a long-term remission in 25%–40% of patients.[392] The recommended dose of IFN-2αb in adults is 5 million I.U. administered daily by subcutaneous or intramuscular injection or 10 million units weekly for 4 months. For children it is administered subcutaneously in a dose of 6 million units three times weekly for 4 to 6 months.[393] In about one-third of patients with chronic hepatitis B infection, interferon alfa-2b caused loss of hepatitis B antigens, return to normal aminotransferase activity, sustained histological improvement, and a lower risk of progressive liver disease.[394] Hepatitis D, which occurs only in patients infected with hepatitis B, may respond to treatment with high doses of interferon alfa, but relapse is common.[395] Interferon may benefit hepatitis B virus–associated nephrotic syndrome and glomerulonephritis in some patients.

Infection with hepatitis C is the most common cause of chronic viral hepatitis in the Western world and ranks only slightly below chronic alcoholism as a cause of cirrhosis, endstage liver disease, and hepatocellular carcinoma in the United States.[390] It is the most common liver disease in the United States and accounts for up to 12,000 deaths annually.[396] The only therapy of proven benefit for patients with chronic hepatitis C is interferon alfa. All forms of interferon alfa appear to be similar in effectiveness against hepatitis C. Therapy is recommended for patients with chronic hepatitis C who have elevated serum aminotransferase concentrations, anti-HCV in serum, and chronic hepatitis on liver biopsy. The recommended regimen is 3 million units given subcutaneously three times a week for 6 months, although some analyses indicate that therapy for 12 months generates a significantly higher response rate.[397] In chronic hepatitis C virus infection, subcutaneous interferon alfa-2B (3 million units three times a week for 6 months) is associated with a 50% rate of liver enzyme normalization, loss of plasma viral RNA, and improvement in hepatic histopathology.[398,399] At least 50% of the responding patients had virologic and biochemical relapse 1 to 2 months after treatment was stopped. Many responded to retreatment, and eradication of infection appears to be possible in some. Combination treatment with interferon and oral ribavirin, 800 to 1200 mg per day, has been associated with higher response rates than with interferon or ribavirin alone.[400,401] This combination is now approved by the Food and Drug Administration for the treatment of hepatitis C in patients who relapse after the standard treatment of hepatitis C.

Several large controlled trials have demonstrated the benefit of recombinant human IFN-α_2 and other interferons for condylomata acuminata. Intralesional injection of 250,000 units twice weekly for up to 8 weeks is associated with complete clearance of the warts in 35% to 52% of patients.[402,403] Complete responders appeared to have relatively low short-term relapse rates. The response to topical podophyllin seemed to be enhanced by injections of interferon into the lesions.[404] If the interferon was injected subcutaneously or intramuscularly, it was associated with some regression of the wart, but there was increased toxicity.[405]

Interferons have also been shown to be beneficial in various herpes virus infections including genital HSV infections, localized herpes zoster in cancer patients or in older adults, and CMV infections of renal transplant patients. However, interferon generally is associated with more side effects and has fewer clinical benefits when compared to conventional antiviral therapies. Topical application of interferon combined with acyclovir or trifluorothymidine accelerates the healing of herpes simplex eye infections.[129] Interferons have been found to have antiretroviral effects in HIV-infected patients. In advanced infection, the benefits were only transient and there was excessive toxicity to the bone marrow. In patients with higher CD4 counts, the antiviral effects were better and the patients tolerated the interferon better.[406,407]

Despite the success of some interferon preparations, there are limitations to its use. In most animal models, interferon was most effective when administered before inoculation of the virus or during the early stages of infection, i.e., before the appearance of clinical signs of disease and before the peak of virus multiplication in target organs. Another limitation is the toxicity caused by its systemic administration in doses needed to achieve an antiviral effect.

PHARMACOKINETICS. Interferons may be administered topically (to certain sites such as the eye or nasal mucosa) and by subcutaneous, intramuscular, and intravenous injection. IFN-α is well absorbed after subcutaneous or intramuscular administration, with a bioavailability exceeding 80%.[408] Intravenous injection provides a more rapid and higher serum concentration, with subcutaneous administration yielding the lowest peak serum concentration.[408,409] Because of degradation by enzymes in the gastrointestinal tract, little interferon is absorbed by the oral route. Recombinant IFN-αs are stable in saline or water solutions at 4°C for long periods of time. The recombinant IFN-αs have a short terminal plasma elimination half-life, ranging from 4 to 5 h.[410] Serum concentrations are undetectable by 16 h after intramuscular or subcutaneous injection in healthy volunteers.

Total body clearance studies suggest that renal secretion and catabolism and extrarenal elimination of IFN-α occurs.[410] Animal studies have demonstrated that IFN-α localizes in the kidneys where proteolytic degradation in the renal tubules may comprise the main mechanism for drug elimination. Thus, little or no intact drug is returned to the circulation or excreted into the urine. Some drug is also distributed into the liver, but hepatic metabolism is minor, and little gets into the central nervous system unless very large doses of 50 million units or more are administered.[411]

The half-life of HuIFN-α or rIFN-α-A is not affected by renal failure, and neither preparation of interferon is removed by hemodialysis.[412,413] Patients with poor renal function do not appear to accumulate high levels of HuIFN-α after repeated intramuscular doses of 3×10^6 U.[414]

ADVERSE EFFECTS. Adverse reactions to interferon are dose dependent. Like the clinical antiviral activities, the adverse effects are similar for both cell culture and recombinant interferon preparations, and there is little evidence that any form of interferon alfa or beta is superior in terms of its tolerability.[389] In general, interferon has been well tolerated when applied topically,[415] although blood-streaked mucus and superficial ulceration of the mucosa have been reported with intranasal administration of both HuIFN-α and rIFN-α-A.[386,416] The major adverse effect of systemically administered IFN-α is a non–life-threatening "flu-like" syndrome occurring within 6 to 72 h of starting therapy.[417] Many patients receiving intramuscular interferon experience fever and chills.[418–422] Fever generally begins 2–6 h after injection of interferon, peaks at 6–12 h, and resolves spontaneously within 24 h.[420] As shown in Table 16–7, headache and myalgias are common, even at low doses. Some of these effects of interferon may relate to a diurnal rise in se-

Table 16–7. *Response of patients with chronic hepatitis to interferon treatment and adverse effects.* Response includes both complete and nearly complete.

	IFNα-2b Dosage		
	None	1MU	3MU
No. of patients	51	57	58
Hepatitis C antibody (%)	78	90	90
Cirrhosis (%)	49	60	55
RESPONSE			
Response (%)	5	28	44
Biopsy improvement (%)	0	29	52
Probability of relapse 24 weeks after therapy (%)	—	45	50
ADVERSE EFFECTS (%)			
Fatigue	76	76	78
Fever	6	42	48
Myalgia	4	40	50
Diarrhea	8	23	34
Headache	18	47	53
Alopecia	0	9	24
Nausea	22	32	36
Irritability	24	30	28

1MU, 1 million units three times a week; 3MU, 3 million units three times a week.
Source: Adapted from Dorr.[410]

rum glucocorticosteroid levels following interferon therapy. Significant elevations in corticotrophin, cortisol, and growth hormone were noted after high doses of interferon. These elevated levels paralleled the effects of interferon on temperature elevation, suggesting a positive correlation between the two events.[423] In addition, there is evidence that the effects of interferon may actually relate to shared biochemical pathways of glucocorticoid and/or catecholamine activities in vivo.[410] Fatigue can be dose limiting, and interferon may be better tolerated with alternate-day dosing or bedtime administration.[424] Gastrointestinal symptoms (nausea, and diarrhea), fatigue, and mild numbness and paresthesias of the hands or toes occur at higher doses. The numbness and paresthesias resolve completely after discontinuation of therapy.[420] Other effects include anorexia, weight loss, abdominal pain and altered taste sensation or lack of taste. Interferon also commonly causes central nervous system disturbances such as, headache, irritability, anxiety and dizziness.[425] These effects are mild and reversible but may impair concentration and affect interpersonal relationships. Reducing the dosage or stopping therapy seems to result in improvement. The most common dose-limiting factors are extreme fatigue and numbness.[419,420] Resolution of severe fatigue may take several weeks after stopping the interferon. Depression occurs in up to 28% of patients and can be severe.[424] Reducing the dose or stopping the interferon usually results in improvement and it may respond to antidepressants. Leukopenia, with or without thrombocytopenia, has been reported in most trials of systemic interferon administration, but in general, hematologic toxicity has been mild, reversible, and not dose limiting.[420] Interferons have been shown to inhibit growth of granulocytic progenitor cells in vitro,[426] and the leukopenia may represent such an effect on myeloid differentiation. Hematological effects are most common in patients with underlying malignancy or those receiving high systemic doses of interferon. Alopecia has been noted in a few patients. This again may represent a "normal" interferon inhibition of a rapidly dividing cell system. Elevations in hepatic enzymes and triglycerides, proteinuria and azotemia, interstitial nephritis, autoantibody formation, and hepatotoxicity may also occur after treatment with interferon. The development of serum-neutralizing antibodies to exogenous interferons may be associated infrequently with loss of clinical responsiveness.[427] Clinically significant hyperthyroidism or hypothyroidism can occur and may be due to induction of autoimmune events or cross-reactivity of thyrotropin-stimulating hormone with membrane receptors for interferon.[428] Interferon may impair fertility, and its safety during pregnancy is not established.

DRUG INTERACTIONS. Interferon has been combined with a large number of other drugs, mainly cytotoxic anticancer agents, among which are doxorubicin, cisplatin, cyclophosphamide, and zidovudine.[410] There are several important interactions that may require dose modification of the cytotoxic agent when combined with the interferon. These interactions may result from synergistic or additive myelosuppressive and systemic toxicities. In some cases, the maximally tolerated cytotoxic drug dose had to be reduced by 50% or more when interferon was concurrently administered.[410] Interferon may also have additive effects with drugs that have neurotoxic or cardiotoxic effects. For example, increased neurotoxicity has been seen when interferon is combined with vidarabine or vinca alkaloids. Another basis for drug interaction is interferon inhibition of cytochrome P-450 enzymes,[429] which accounts for increased levels of drugs such as theophylline.[430] Some drugs may alter the antiviral activity of interferons. Prednisone, for example, has been shown to reduce the expression of the antiviral protein 2'-5'-oligoadenylate synthetase in response to IFN by 50%.[431]

Ribavirin

Ribavirin is a synthetic guanosine analog consisting of D-ribose attached to 1,2,4-triazole carboxamide. It has a broad spec-

Ribavirin

trum of activity against RNA and DNA viruses, both in vitro and in vivo.[432] Herpes viruses are the most sensitive of the DNA viruses, and among the human RNA viruses, good activity has been noted against influenza viruses A and B, parainfluenza viruses, mumps, measles, and respiratory syncytial virus (RSV).[433,434] Clinical attention has focused on ribavirin treatment of patients with HIV and viral hepatitis. Preliminary data indicate that ribavirin and IFN-β may act synergistically in the treatment of chronic hepatitis C virus infection.[400,401]

MECHANISM OF ACTION. The molecular mechanism of action of ribavirin remains a topic of controversy. Its action seems to relate to an alteration of cellular nucleotide pools and inhibition of viral mRNA synthesis.[433,435] Intracellular phosphorylation to the mono-, di-, and triphosphates is catalyzed by host cell enzymes, with the triphosphate being the predominant metabolite (>80%). The monophosphate is a competitive inhibitor of cellular IMP dehydrogenase and interferes with the synthesis of GTP. The triphosphate also competitively inhibits the GTP-dependent 5'-capping of viral mRNA. Ribavirin has multiple sites of action, and effects at some of these sites may potentiate others. In most cell lines, the antiviral activity of ribavirin can be separated from the cytostatic activity, which occurs at 200 to 1000 mg/liter[432] In contrast to other antiviral drugs, development of resistant virus strains has not been demonstrated.

PHARMACOKINETICS. After oral administration, ribavirin is rapidly absorbed and the bioavailability is 40% to 45%.[436] Following single oral doses of 600 mg and 1200 mg, peak plasma concentrations average 1.3 μg/ml and 2.5 μg/ml, respectively. After intravenous doses of 500 mg and 1000 mg, plasma concentations average 17 μg/ml and 24 μg/ml, respectively.[247] With aerosol administration, plasma levels increase with the duration of exposure and range from 0.2 to 1.0 μg/ml after 5 days.[437] Ribavirin triphosphate concentrates in erythrocytes, and red blood cell levels gradually decrease with a half-life of about 40 days. Renal excretion of ribavirin and its metabolites accounts for approximately 40% of its clearance, and hepatic metabolism also appears to play an important role in its elimination.

CLINICAL USE. Ribavirin administered as an aerosol decreases morbidity in children hospitalized with respiratory syncytial virus (RSV) bronchiolitis and pneumonia. The effectiveness of ribavirin for treatment of RSV disease in infants is controversial. Most infants and children with RSV have either no lower respiratory tract disease or disease that is mild and self-limited and does not require hospitalization. Of those with mild lower respiratory tract involvement, some will need brief hospitalization for a period shorter than that required for a full course of therapy (3–7 days). Thus, the decision to treat with ribavirin aerosol is based on the severity of the infection.[432]

Administered to patients with influenza, aerosolized ribavirin accelerates the resolution of fever and illness and reduces virus shedding. However, the improvements are usually modest and insufficient to justify its use in otherwise healthy people.[432] Oral use of ribavirin has led to reductions in serum aminotransferase activity and improvement in liver biopsies in patients with chronic hepatitis C infection, but treatment does not decrease hepatitis C virus RNA and most patients relapse within 2 to 3 months of stopping treatment.

ADVERSE EFFECTS. Ribavirin has been generally well tolerated. Adverse reactions are related to dose and duration of therapy. Aerosolized ribavirin may cause mild conjunctival irritation, rash, transient wheezing, and, occasionally, reversible deterioration in pulmonary function.[247] Systemic ribavirin has been associated with dose-related, reversible anemia due to extravascular hemolysis and dose-related suppression of bone marrow.[434] Reversible increases in serum bilirubin, serum iron, and uric acid occur during short-term oral administration. Acute deterioration of respiratory function has been reported with ribavirin aerosols in infants and adults with bronchospastic lung disease. Ribavirin is teratogenic and embryotoxic in animals, and it should not be used during pregnancy unless absolutely necessary.[438] In addition, Pregnant women should probably not directly care for patients receiving a ribavirin aerosol.

REFERENCES

1. Grayston, J. T., and S. Wang. New knowledge of Chlamydiae and the diseases they cause *J. Infect. Dis.* 1975;132:87.

2. Luria, S. Luria, S. E., J. E. Darnell D. Baltimore, and A. Campbell. *General Virology*, (3rd ed.), New York: Wiley, 1978.

3. White, D., and F. Fenner. Classification and nomenclature of viruses. In *Medical Virology*, New York: Academic Press, 1994, pp. 16–29.

4. DeClercq, E. Virus replication. Target functions and events for virus-specific inhibitors. In *Antiviral Agents and Human Viral Disease*, ed. by G. J. Galasso, R. J. Whitely, and T. C. Merigan. Philadelphia: Lippincott-Raven, 1997, pp. 1–44.

5. Spector, D. H., and D. Baltimore. The molecular biology of polio-virus. *Sci. Am.* 1975;232:25.

6. Pearson, G. D. The Inhibition of Poliovirus Replication by N-Methylisatin-β-4′:4′-dibutylthiosemicarbazone. Ph.D. Thesis, Stanford University, 1968.

7. Dimitrov, D. S. How do viruses enter cells: the HIV coreceptors teach us a lesson of complexity. *Cell* 1997;91:721.

8. Lamb, R. A. and P. W. Choppin. The gene structure and replication of influenza virus. *Annu. Rev. Biochem.* 1983;52:467.

9. Deng, H., R. Liu, W. Ellmeir, S. Choe, D. Unutmaz, M. Burkhart, P. Si Marzio, S. Marmon, R. E. Sutton, C. M. Hill, C. B. Davis, S. C. Peiper, T. J. Schall, D. R. Littman, and N. R. Landau. Identification of a major co-receptor for primary isolates of HIV-1. *Nature* 1996;381:661.

10. Vilcek, J. Fundamentals of virus structure and replication. In *Antiviral Agents and Viral Diseases of Man*, ed by G. J. Galasso, T. C. Merigan, and R. A. Buchanan. New York: Raven Press, 1979, pp. 1–38.

11. Joklik, W. K. The intracellular uncoating of poxvirus DNA. II. The molecular basis of the uncoating process. *J. Mol. Biol.* 1964;8:277.

12. Kates, J. R., and B. R. McAuslan. Poxvirus DNA-dependent RNA polymerase. *Proc. Natl. Acad. Sci. U.S.A.* 1967;58:134.

13. Kates, J. R., and B. R. McAuslan. Messenger, RNA synthesis by a "coated" viral genome. *Proc. Natl. Acad. Sci. U.S.A.* 1967;57:314.

14. Roizman, B. and P. Palese. Multiplication of viruses: an overview. In *Fields Virology*, ed. by B. N. Fields, D. M. Knipe, P. M. Howley, R. Chanock, J. Melnick, T. Monath, B. Roizman, and S. Straus. Philadelphia: Lippincott-Raven, 1996, pp. 101–112.

15. Caliguiri, A. and I. Tamm. Guanidine. In *International Encyclopedia of Pharmacology and Therapeutics* (Section 61, Vol. 1). New York: Pergamon Press, 1972, pp. 181–230.

16. Tamm, I. and L. A. Caliguiri. 2-(α-Hydroxybenzyl)benzimidazole and related compounds. In *International Encyclopedia of Pharmacology and Therapeutics* (Section 61, Vol. 1). New York: Pergamon Press, 1972, pp. 115–179.

17. Elion; G. B. The biochemistry and mechanism of action of acyclovir. *J. Antimicrob. Chemother.* 1983; 12(Suppl. B):9.

18. Klenk, H. D., C. Scholtissek, and R. Rott. Inhibition of glycoprotein biosynthesis of influenza virus by D-glucose. *Virology* 1972;49:723.

19. Palese, P., J. L. Schulman, G. Bodo, and P. Meindl. Inhibition of influenza and parainfluenza virus replication in tissue culture by 2-deoxy-2,3-dehydro-N-trifluoroacetylneuraminic acid (FANA). *Virology* 1974; 59:490.

20. Smith, R. A., R. W. Sidwell, and R. K. Robins. Antiviral mechanisms of action. *Annu. Rev. Pharmacol.* 1980;20:259.

21. Waghorn, S. L., and K. L. Goa. Zanamivir. *Drugs* 1998;55:721.

22. Calfee, D. P., and F. G. Hayden. New approaches to influenza chemotherapy. Neuraminidase inhibitors. *Drugs* 1998;56:537.

23. Helgstrand, E., and B. Öberg. Enzymatic targets in virus chemotherapy. *Antibiot. Chemother.* 1980;27: 22.

24. Müller; W. E. G. Mechanisms of action and pharmacology: chemical agents. In *Antiviral Agents and Viral Diseases of Man*, ed. by G. J. Galasso, T. C. Merigan, and R. A. Buchanan. New York: Raven Press, 1979, pp. 77–149.

25. Hirsch, M. S., J. C. Kaplan, and R. T. D'Aquila. Antiviral agents. In *Fields Virology*, ed. by B. N. Fields, D. M. Knipe, and P. M. Howley. Philadelphia: Lippincott-Raven, 1996, pp. 431–466.

26. Glasgow; L. A. Biology and pathogenesis of viral infections. In *Antiviral Agents and Viral Disease of Man*, ed. by G. J. Galasso, T. C. Merigan, and R. A. Buchanan. New York: Raven Press, 1979, pp. 39–76.

27. Pillay, D., and A. M. Geddes. Antiviral drug resistance. *BMJ* 1996;313:503.

28. Erice, A., S. Chou, K. K. Biron, S. C. Stanat, H. H. Balfour, and M. C. Jordan. Progressive disease due to ganciclovir-resistant cytomegalovirus in immunocompromised patients. *New. Engl. J. Med.* 1989;320: 289.

29. Snoeck, R., M. Gerard, C. Saszot-Delvaux, G.

Andrei, J. Balzarini, D. Reymen, N. Ahadi, J. M. De-Bruyn, J. Piette, and B. Rentier. Meningoradiculoneuritis due to acyclovir-resistant *Varicella zoster* virus in an acquired immune deficiency syndrome patient. *J. Med. Virol.* 1998;42:338.

30. Lungan, P. L., N. N. Elis, R. L. Hackman, D. H. Shepp, and J. D. Meyers. Acyclovir-resistant *Herpes simplex* causing pneumonia after marrow transplantation. *J. Infect. Dis.* 1990;162:144.

31. Hoffman, C. E. Amantadine HC1 and related compounds. In *Selective Inhibitors of Viral Functions*, ed. by W. A. Carter. Cleveland: CRC Press, 1973, pp. 199–211.

32. Neumayer, E. M., R. F. Haff, and C. E. Hoffman. Antiviral activity of amantadine hydrochloride in tissue culture and in ovo. *Proc. Soc. Exp. Biol. Med.* 1965;119:393.

33. Hay, A. J. The action of adamantanes against influenza A viruses: inhibition of the M2 ion channel protein. *Semin. Virol.* 1992;3:21.

34. Hay, A. J., A. J. Wolstenholme, J. J. Skehel, and M. H. Smith. The molecular basis of the specific anti-influenza action of amantadine. *EMBO J.* 1985;4:3021.

35. Belshe, R. B., M. Hall-Smith, C. B. Hall, R. Betts, and A. J. Hay. Genetic basis of resistance of rimantadine emerging during treatment of influenza virus infection. *J. Virol.* 1988;62:1508.

36. Wharton, S. A., R. B. Belshe, J. J. Skehel, and A. J. Hay. Role of virion M2 protein in influenza virus uncoating: specific reduction in the rate of membrane fusion between virus and liposomes by amantadine. *J. Gen. Virol.* 1994;75:945.

37. Duff, K. C., and R. H. Ashley. The transmembrane domain of influenza A M2 protein forms amantadine-sensitive protein channels in planar lipid bilayers. *Virology* 1992;190:485.

38. Duff, K. C., P. J. Gilchrist, A. M. Sexena, and J. P. Bradshaw. Neutron diffraction reveals the site of amantidine blockade in the influenza A M2 ion channel. *Virology* 1994;202:287.

39. Sansom, M. S. P., and I. D. Kerr. Influenza virus M2 protein: a molecular modeling study of the ion channel. *Protein Eng.* 1993;6:65.

40. Martin, K., and A. Helenius. Nuclear transport of influenza virus ribonucleoproteins: the viral matrix protein (M1) promotes export and inhibits import. *Cell* 1991;67:117.

41. Grambas, S., M. S. Bennett, and A. J. Hay. Influence of amantadine resistance mutations on the pH regulatory function of the M2 protein of influenza viruses. *Virology* 1992;191:541.

42. Ruigrok, R. W. H., E. M. A. Hirst, and A. J. Hay. The specific inhibition of influenza A virus maturation by amantadine: an electron microscopic examination. *J. Gen. Virol.* 1991;72:191.

43. Nicholson, K. G. Antiviral agents. In *Antibiotic and Chemotherapy*, ed. by F. O'Grady, H. P. Lambert, R. G. Finch, and D. Greenwood. New York: Churchill Livingstone, 1998. pp. 541–5776.

44. Hayden, F. G., R. B. Belshe, R. D. Clover, A. J. Hay, M. G. Oakes, and W. Soo. Emergence and apparent transmission of rimantadine-resistant influenza A virus in families. *N. Engl. J. Med.* 1989;321:1696.

45. Douglas, Jr., R. G. Respiratory diseases. In *Antiviral Agents and Viral Diseases*, ed. by G. J. Galasso, T. C. Merigan, and R. A. Buchanan. New York: Raven Press, 1979, pp. 385–459.

46. Hirsch, M. S., and M. N. Swartz. Antiviral agents. *N. Eng. J. Med.* 1980;302:903.

47. Sabin, A. B. Amantadine hydrochloride. *JAMA* 1967;200:135.

48. Togo, Y., R. B. Hornick, and A. T. Dawkins. Studies on induced influenza in man. I. Double-blind studies designed to assess prophylactic efficacy of amantadine hydrochloride against A2/Rockville/1/65 strain. *JAMA* 1968;203:1089.

49. Dawkins, A. T., L. R. Gallagher, Y. Togo, R. B. Hornick, and B. A. Harris. Studies on induced influenza in man. II. Double-blind study designed to assess the prophylactic efficacy of an analogue of amantadine hydrochloride. *JAMA* 1968;203:1095.

50. Galbraith, A. W., J. S. Oxford, G. C. Schild, and G. I. Watson. Protective effect of 1-adamantanamine hydrochloride on influenza A2 infections in the family environment, *Lancet* 1969;2:1026.

51. Oker-Blom, N., T. Hovi, P. Leinikki, T. Palosuo, R. Pettersson, and J. Suni. Protection of man from natural infection with influenza A_2 Hong Kong virus by amantadine: a controlled field trial. *BMJ* 1970;3:676.

52. Monto, A. S., R. A. Gunn, M. G. Bandyk, and C. L. King Prevention of Russian influenza by amantadine. *JAMA* 1979;241:1003.

53. Dolin, R., R. C. Reichman, H. P. Madore, R. Maynard, P. N. Linton, and J. Webber-Jones. A controlled trial of amantadine and rimantadine in the prophylaxis of influenza A infection. *N. Engl. J. Med.* 1982;307:580.

54. Symposium. Amantadine: does it have a role in the treatment of influenza? A National Institutes of Health Consensus Development Conference. *Ann. Intern. Med.* 1980;92:256.

55. Muldoon, R. L., E. D. Stanley, and G. G. Jackson. Use and withdrawal of amantadine chemoprophylaxis during epidemic influenza. A. *Am. Rev. Respir. Dis.* 1976;113:487.

56. Dolin, R., R. C. Reichman, H. P. Madove, R. Myanard, P. N. Linton, and J. Webber-Jones. A controlled trial of amantadine and rimantadine in the prophylaxis of influenza A infection. *N. Engl. J. Med.* 1982;307:580.

57. Brady, M. T., S. D. Sears, D. L. Pacini, R. Samorodin, J. De Pamphilis, M. Oakes, W. Soo, and M. L. Clements. Safety and prophylactic efficacy of low-dose rimantadine in adults during an influenza epidemic. *Antimicrob. Agents Chemother.* 1990;34:1633.

58. Wingfield, W. L., D. Pollack, and R. R. Grunert. Therapeutic efficacy of amantadine HCl and rimantidine HCl in naturally occurring influenza A2 respiratory illness in man. *N. Engl. J. Med.* 1969;281:579.

59. Togo, Y., R. B. Hornick, V. J. Felitti, M. L. Kaufman, A. T. Dawkins, V. E. Kilpe, and J. L. Claghorn. Evaluation of therapeutic efficacy of amantadine in patients with naturally occurring A_2 influenza. *JAMA* 1970;211:1149.

60. Galbraith, A. W., J. S. Oxford, G. C. Schild, C. W. Potter, and G. I. Watson. Therapeutic effect of

1-adamantanamine hydrochloride in naturally occurring influenza A₂/Hong Kong infection. A controlled double-blind study. *Lancet* 1971;2:113.

61. Van Voris, L. P., R. F. Betts, F. G. Hayden, W. A. Christmas, and R. G. Douglas, Jr. Successful treatment of naturally occurring influenza A/USSR/77 H1N1. *JAMA* 1981;245:1128.

62. Younkin, S. W., R. F. Betts, F. K. Roth, and R. G. Douglas, Jr. Reduction in fever and symptoms in young adults with influenza A/Brazil/78 H1N1 infection after treatment with aspirin or amantadine. *Antimicrob. Agents Chemother.* 1983;23:577.

63. Little, J. W., W. J. Hall, G. Douglas, Jr., R. W. Hyde, and D. M. Speers. Amantadine effect on peripheral airways abnormalities in influenza. A study in 15 students with natural influenza A infection. *Ann. Intern. Med.* 1976;85:177.

64. Van Voris, L. P., R. F. Betts, F. G. Hayden, W. A. Christamas, and R. G. Douglas. Successful treatment of naturally occurring influenza A/USSR/77 H1N1. *JAMA* 1981;245:1128.

65. Bleidner, W. E., J. B. Harmon, W. E. Hewes, T. E. Lynes, and E. C. Hermann. Absorption, distribution and excretion of amantadine hydrochloride. *J. Pharmacol. Exp. Ther.* 1965;150:484.

66. Hayden, F. G., H. E. Hoffman, and D. A. Spyker. Differences in side effects of amantadine hydrochloride and rimantadine hydrochloride relate to differences in pharmacokinetics. *Antimicrob. Agents Chemother.* 1983;23:458.

67. Wu, M. J., T. S. Ing, L. S. Soung, J. T. Daugirdas, J. E. Hano, and V. C. Gandhi. Amantadine hydrochloride pharmacokinetics in patients with impaired renal function. *Clin. Nephrol.* 1982;17:19.

68. Grunert, R. C., and C. E. Hoffmann. Sensitivity of influenza A/New Jersey/8/76 (Hsw1N1) virus to amantadine HC1. *J. Infect. Dis.* 1977;136:297.

69. Horadam, V. W., J. G. Sharp, J. D. Smilack, B. H. McAnalley, J. C. Garriott, M. K. Stephens, R. C. Prati, and D. C. Brater. Pharmacokinetics of amantadine hydrochloride in subjects with normal and impaired renal function. *Ann. Intern. Med.* 1981;94:454.

70. Ing, T. S., J. T. Daugirdas, and L. S. Soung. The posology of amantadine: a note of caution. *JAMA* 1980;243:1844.

71. Soung, L. S., T. S. Ing, J. T. Daugirdas, M. J. Wu, V. C. Gandhi, P. I. Ivanovich, J. E. Hano, and G. W. Viol. Amantadine hydrochloride pharmacokinetics in hemodialysis patients. *Ann. Intern. Med.* 1980;93:46.

72. Rubio, F. R., E. K. Fukada, and W. A. Garland. Urinary metabolites of rimantadine in humans. *Drug Metab. Dispos.* 1988;16:773.

73. Hayden, F. G., A. Minocha, D. A. Spyker, and H. E. Hoffmann. Comparative single-dose pharmacokinetics of amantadine hydrochloride and rimantadine hydrochloride in young and elderly adults. *Antimicrob. Agents Chemother.* 1985;28:216.

74. Hayden, F. C., J. M. Gwaltney, Jr., R. L. Van de Castle, K. F. Adams, and B. Giordani. Comparative toxicity of amantadine hydrochloride and rimantadine hydrochloride in healthy adults. *Antimicrob. Agents Chemother.* 1981;19:226.

75. Ing, T. S., J. T. Dougiradas, L. S. Soung, H. L. Klawans, S. D. Mahurkar, J. A. Hayshi, W. P. Geis, and J. E. Hano. Toxic effects of amantadine in patients with renal failure. *Can. Med. Assoc. J.* 1979;120:695.

76. Bryson, Y. C., C. Monahan, M. Pollack, and W. D. Shields. A prospective double-blind study of side effects associated with the administration of amantadine for influenza A virus prophylaxis. *J. Infect. Dis.* 1980;141:543.

77. Hayden, F. G., H. E. Hoffman, and D. A. Spyker. Differences in side effects of amantadine hydrochloride and rimantadine hydrochloride relate to differences in pharmacokinetics. *Antimicrob. Agents Chemother.* 1983;23:458.

78. Schwab, R. S., A. C. England, D. C. Poskanzer, and R. R. Young. Amantadine in the treatment of Parkinson's disease. *JAMA* 1969;208:1168.

79. Schwab, R. S., D. C. Poskanzer, A. C. England, and R. R. Young. Amantadine in Parkinson's disease: review of more than two years' experience. *JAMA* 1972;222:792.

80. Bauer, R. B., and J. T. McHenry. Comparison of amantadine, placebo, and levodopa in Parkinson's disease. *Neurology* 1974;24:715.

81. Yahr, M. D., and R. C. Duvoisin. Drug therapy of parkinsonism. *N. Eng. J. Med.* 1972;287:20.

82. Bailey, E. V., and W. T. Stone. The mechanism of action of amantadine in Parkinsonism: a review. *Arch. Int. Pharmacodyn.* 1975;216:246.

83. Timberlake, W. H., and M. A. Vance. Four-year treatment of patients with parkinsonism using amantadine alone or with levodopa. *Ann. Neurol.* 1978;3:119.

84. Vale, J. A., and K. S. Maclean. Amantadine-induced heart failure. *Lancet* 1977;1:548.

85. Vernier, V. G., J. B. Harmon, J. M. Stump, T. E. Lynes, J. P. Marvel, and D. H. Smith. The toxicologic and pharmacologic properties of amantadine hydrochloride. *Toxicol. Appl. Pharmacol.* 1969;15:642.

86. Parkes, D. Amantadine. *Adv. Drug Res.* 1974;8:11.

87. Millet, V. M., M. Dreisbach, and Y. J. Bryson. Double-blind controlled study of central nervous system side effects of amantadine, rimantadine and chlorpheniramine. *Antimicrob. Agents Chemother.* 1982;21:1.

88. Wilson, T. W., and A. H. Rajput. Amantadine-dyazide interaction. *Can. Med. Assoc. J.* 1989;129:974.

89. Speeg, K. V., J. A. Leighton, and A. L. Maldonado. Toxic delirium in a patient taking amantadine and trimethoprim-sulfamethoxazole. *Am. J. Med. Sci.* 1989;298:410.

90. Woods, J. M., R. C. Bethell, J. A. Coates, N. Healy, S. A. Hiscox, B. A. Pearson, D. M. Ryan, J. Ticehurst, J. Tilling, S. M. Walcott, and C. R. Penn: 4-Guanidino-2,4-dideoxy-2,3-deydro-N-acetylneuraminic acid is a highly effective inhibitor both of the sialidase (neuraminidase) and of growth of a wide range of influenza A and B viruses in vitro. *Antimicrob. Agents Chemother.* 1993;37:1473.

91. Whittinton, A., and R. Bethell. Recent developments in the antiviral therapy of influenza. *Expert Opin. Thera. Patents* 1995;5:793.

92. Madren, L. K., J. C. Shipman, and F. G. Ship-

man. In vitro inhibitory effects of combinations of anti-influenza agents. *Antiviral Chem. Chemother.* 1995;6:109.

93. Hayden, F. G. J. J. Treanor, R. F. Betts, et al. Safety and efficacy of the neuraminidase inhibitor GG167 in experimental human influenza *JAMA* 1996;275:295.

94. Hayden, F. G., A. D. M. E. Osterhaus, J. J. Treanor, D. M. Fleming, F. Y. Aoki, K. G. Nicholson, A. M. Bohnen, H. M. Hirst, O. Keene, K. Wightman, for the GG167 Influenza Study Group: Efficacy and safety of the neuraminidase inhibitor zanamivir in the treatment of influenza virus infections. *N. Engl. J. Med.* 1997;337:874.

95. Couch, R., A new antiviral agent for influenza—is there a clinical niche. *N. Engl. J. Med.* 1997;337:927.

96. Kim, C. U., W. Lew, M. A. Williams, H. Wu, L. Zhang, X. Chen, P. A. Escarpe, D. B. Mendel, W. G. Laver, and R. C. Stevens. Structure-activity relationship studies of novel carbocyclin influenza neuraminidase inhibitors. *J. Med. Chem.* 1988;41:2451.

97. Griffiths, P. D. Progress in the clinical management of herpes virus infections. *Antiviral Chem. Chemother.* 1995;6:191.

98. Prusoff, W. H. Synthesis and biological activities of iododeoxyuridine, an analog of thymidine. *Biochim. Biophys. Acta.* 1959;32:295.

99. Prusoff, W. H., M. S. Chen, P. H. Fisher, T. S. Lin, and G. T. Shiau. 5-Iodo-2'-deoxyuridine. In *Antibiotics* V-2, ed. by F. E. Hahn. New York: Springer-Verlag, 1979, pp. 236–261.

100. McCrea, J. F., and M. B. Lipman. Strand-length measurements of normal and 5-iodo-2'-deoxyuridine-treated vaccinia virus deoxyribonucleic acid released by the Kleinschmidt method. *J. Virol.* 1967;1:1037.

101. Prusoff, W. H., and B. Goz. Halogenated pyrimidine deoxyribonucleosides. In *Handbook of Experimental Pharmacology*, Vol. 38/2, ed. by O. Eichler, A. Farah, H. Herken, and A. D. Welch. Berlin: Springer-Verlag, 1975, pp. 272–347.

102. North, R. D., D. Pavan-Langston, and P. Geary. Herpes simplex virus types 1 and 2. Therapeutic response to antiviral drugs. *Arch. Ophthalmol.* 1976;94:1019.

103. Burns, R. P. A double-blind study of IDU in human herpes simplex keratitis. *Arch. Ophthalmol.* 1963;70:381.

104. Laibson, P. R., and I. H. Leopold: An evaluation of double blind IDU therapy in 100 cases of herpetic keratitis. *Trans. Am. Acad. Ophthalmol. Otolaryngol.* 1964;68:22.

105. Kaufman, H. E. Local therapy of herpes simplex virus ocular infections. In *The Human Herpesviruses: An Interdisciplinary Perspective*, ed. by A. J. Nahmias, W. R. Dowdle, and R. E. Shinazi. New York: Elsevier, 1981, pp. 466–477.

106. Pavan-Langston, D. Herpetic disease. In *The Cornea: Scientific Foundations and Clinical Practice*, ed. by G. Smulin and R. Thoft. Boston: Little, Brown, 1982, pp. 178–195.

107. McGill, J., H. Williams, J. McKinnon, A. D. Holt-Wilson, and B. R. Jones. Reassessment of idoxu-ridine therapy of herpetic keratitis. *Trans. Ophthal. Soc. U.K.* 1974;94:542.

108. Langston, R. H. S., D. Pavan-Langston, and C. H. Dohlman. Anti-viral-medication and corneal wound healing. *Arch. Ophthalmol.* 1974;92:509.

109. Nolan, D. C., C. B. Lauter, and A. M. Lerner. Idoxuridine in herpes simplex virus (type 1) encephalitis. *Ann. Intern. Med.* 1973;78:243.

110. Boston Interhospital Virus Study Group and the NAID-Sponsored Cooperative Antiviral Clinical Study: failure of high dose 5-iodo-2'-deoxyuridine in the therapy of herpes simplex virus encephalitis. *N. Engl. J. Med.* 1975;292:599.

111. Calabresi, P. Current status of clinical investigations with 6-azauridine, 5-iodo-2'-deoxyuridine, and related derivatives. *Cancer Res.* 1963;23:1260.

112. Welch, A. D., and W. H. Prusoff. A synopsis of recent investigations of 5-iodo-2'-deoxyuridine. *Cancer Chem. Rep.* 1960;6:29.

113. Lerner, A. M., and E. J. Bailey. Concentrations of idoxuridine in serum urine and cerebrospinal fluid of patients with suspected diagnoses of Herpesvirus hominis encephalitis. *J. Clin. Invest.* 1972;51:45.

114. Welch, A. D. Some mechanisms involved in selective chemotherapy. *Ann. N.Y. Acad. Sci.* 1965;123:19.

115. Rowe, W. P., D. R. Lowy, N. Teich, and J. W. Hartley. Some implications of the activation of murine leukemia virus by halogenated pyrimidines. *Proc. Natl. Acad. Sci. U.S.A.* 1972;69:1033.

116. Sugauara, K., and T. Osato. Two distinct antigenic components in an Epstein-Barr virus–related early product induced by halogenated pyrimidines in non-producing human lymphoblastoid cells. *Nat. New Biol.* 1973;243:209.

117. Itoi, M., J. W. Gefter, N. Kaneko, Y. Ishii, R. M. Ramer, and A. R. Gasset. Teratogenicities of ophthalmic drugs. *Arch. Ophthalmol.* 1975;93:46.

118. Prusoff, W. H., and D. C. Ward. Nucleoside analogs with antiviral activity. *Biochem. Pharmacol.* 1976;25:1233.

119. Heidelberger, C. Fluorinated pyrimidines and their nucleosides. In *Handbook of Experimental Pharmacology*, Vol. 38/2, ed. by O. Eichler, A. Farah, H. Herken, and A. D. Welch. Berlin: Springer-Verlag, 1975, pp. 193–231.

120. Heidelberger, C., and D. H. King. Trifluorothymidine. *Pharmacol. Ther.* 1979;6:427.

121. Tone, H., and C. Heidelberger. Fluorinated pyrimidines XLIV. Interaction of 5-trifluoromethyl-2'-deoxyuridine 5'-triphosphate with deoxyribonucleic acid polymerases. *Mol. Pharmacol.* 1973;9:783.

122. Bresnick, E. and S. S. Williams. Effects of 5-trifluoromethyldeoxyuridine upon deoxythymidine kinase. *Biochem. Pharmacol.* 1967;16:503.

123. Reyes, P. and C. Heidelberger. Fluorinated pyrimidines XXVI. Mammalian thymidylate synthetase: its mechanism of action and inhibition by fluorinated nucleotides. *Mol. Pharmacol.* 1965;1:14.

124. Umeda, M., and C. Heidelberger. Fluorinated pyrimidines XXXI. Mechanism of inhibition of vaccinia virus replication in HeLa cells by pyrimidine nucleosides. *Proc. Soc. Exp. Biol. Med.* 1969;130:24.

125. Fujiwara, Y., and C. Heidelberger. Fluorinated pyrimidines XXXVIII. The incorporation of 5-trifluoromethyl-2'-deoxyuridine into the deoxyribonucleic acid of vaccinia virus. *Mol. Pharmacol.* 1970;6: 281.

126. Heidelberger, C. On the molecular mechanism of the antiviral activity of trifluorothymidine. *Ann. N.Y. Acad. Sci.* 1975;255:317.

127. Dexter, D. L., W. H. Wolberg, F. J. Ansfield, L. Helson, and C. Heidelberger. The clinical pharmacology of 5-trifluoromethyl-2'-deoxyuridine. *Cancer Res.* 1972;32:247.

128. Kaufman, H. E. The treatment of herpetic eye infections with trifluridine and other antivirals. In *Clinical Use of Antiviral Drugs*, ed. by E. De Clercq. Norwell, MA: Martinus Nijoff, 1988, pp. 25–38.

129. Birch, C. J., D. P. Tyssen, G. Tachedjian, R. Doherty, K. Hayes, A. Mijch, and C. R. Lucas. Clinical effects and in vitro studies of trifluorothymidine combined with interferon-α for treatment of drug-resistant and -sensitive herpes simplex viral infections. *J. Infect. Dis.* 1992;166:108.

130. Murphy, M., A. Morley, R. P. Eglin, and E. Monteiro. Topical trifluridine for mucocutaneous acyclovir-resistant herpes simplex II in an AIDS patient. *Lancet* 1992;340:1040.

131. Birch, C. J., G. Tachedian, R. R. Doherty, K. Hayes, and I. D. Gust. Altered sensitivities to antiviral drugs of herpes simplex virus isolates from a patient with the acquired immunodeficiency syndrome. *J. Infect. Dis.* 1990;162:731.

132. O'Brien, W. J. and H. F. Edelhauser. The corneal penetration of trifluorothymidine, adenine arabinoside, and idoxuridine: a comparative study. *Invest. Ophthalmol. Vis. Sci.* 1977;16:1093.

133. McGill, J., A. Holt-Wilson, J. McKinnon, H. Williams, and B. Jones. Some aspects of the clinical use of trifluoromethylthymidine in the treatment of herpetic ulceration of the cornea. *Trans. Ophthalmol. Soc. U.K.* 1974;94:342.

134. Coster, D. J., J. R. McKinnon, J. I. McGill, B. R. Jones, and F. T. Fraunfelder. Clinical evaluation of adenine arabinoside and trifluorothymidine in the treatment of corneal ulcers caused by herpes simplex virus. *J. Infect. Dis.* 1976;133(Suppl. A):A173.

135. Pavan-Langston, D., and C. Stephen-Foster. Trifluorothymidine and idoxuridine therapy of ocular herpes. *Am. J. Ophthalmol.* 1977;84:818.

136. Lee, W. W., A. Benitez, L. Goodman, and B. R. Baker. Potential anticancer agents XL. Synthesis of the β-anomer of 9-(D-arabinofuranosyl)-adenine. *J. Am. Chem. Soc.* 1960;82:2648.

137. Pavan-Langston, D., R. A. Buchanan, and C. A. Alford (eds.) *Adenine Arabinoside: An Antiviral Agent.* New York: Raven Press, 1975.

138. Cass, C. E. 9-β-D-Arabinofuranosyladenine (araA). In *Antibiotics* V-2, ed. by F. E. Hahn. New York: Springer-Verlag, 1979, pp. 85–109.

139. Shannon, W. M. Adenine arabinoside: antiviral activity in vitro. In *Adenine Arabinoside: An Antiviral Agent*, ed. by D. Pavan-Langston, R. A. Buchanan, and C. A. Alford, Jr. New York: Raven Press, 1975, pp. 1–43.

140. Shipman, C., Jr., S. H. Smith, R. H. Carlson, and J. C. Drach. Antiviral activity of arabinosyladenine and arabinosylhypoxanthine in herpes simplex virus-infected KB cells: selective inhibition of viral deoxyribonucleic acid synthesis in synchronized suspension cultures. *Antimicrob. Agents Chemother.* 1976;9:120.

141. Champney, K. J., C. B. Lauter, E. J. Bailey, and A. M. Lerner. Antiherpesvirus activity in human sera and urines after administration of adenine arabinoside. *J. Clin. Invest.* 1978;62:1142.

142. Bryson, Y. J., and J. C. Connor. In vitro susceptibility of varicella zoster virus to adenine arabinoside and hypoxanthine arabinoside. *Antimicrob. Agents Chemother.* 1976;9:540.

143. Verhoef, V., J. Sarup, and A. Fridland. Identification of the mechanism of activation of 9-β-D-arabinofuranosyladenine in human lymphoid cells using mutants deficient in nucleoside kinases. *Cancer Res.* 1981;41:4478.

144. Moore, E. C., and S. S. Cohen. Effects of arabinonucleotides on ribonucleotide reduction by an enzyme system from rat tumor. *J. Biol. Chem.* 1967;242: 2116.

145. Chang, C. H., and Y. C. Cheng. Effects of deoxyadenosine triphosphate and 9-β-D-arabinofuranosyladenine 5'-triphosphate on human ribonucleotide reductase from Molt-4F cells and the concept of "self-potentiation." *Cancer Res.* 1980;40:3555.

146. Furth, J. J., and S. S. Cohen. Inhibition of mammalian DNA polymerase by the 5'-triphosphate of 9-β-D-arabinofuranosyladenine. *Cancer Res.* 1968;28:2061.

147. Cozarelli, N. The mechanism of action of inhibitors of DNA synthesis. *Annu. Rev. Biochem.* 1977;46: 641.

148. Coen, D. M., P. A. Furman, P. T. Gelep, and P. A. Schaffer. Mutations in the herpes simplex virus DNA polymerase gene can confer resistance to 9-β-D-arabinofuranosyladenine. *J. Virol.* 1982;41:909.

149. Müller, W. E. G., R. K. Zahn, K. Bittlingmaier, and D. Falke. Inhibition of herpesvirus DNA synthesis by 9-β-D-arabinofuranosyladenine in cellular and cell-free systems. *Ann. N.Y. Acad. Sci.* 1977;284:34.

150. Pelling, J. C., J. C. Drach, and C. Shipman, Jr. Internucleotide incorporation of arabinofuranosyladenine into herpes simplex virus DNA. *Virology* 1981; 109:323.

151. Derse D. and Y. C. Cheng: Herpes simplex virus type 1 DNA polymerase. Kinetic properties of the associated 3'-5' exonuclease activity and its role in araAMP incorporation. *J. Biol. Chem.* 1981;256:8525.

152. Collum, L. M. T., A. Benedict-Smith, and I. B. Hillary. Randomized double-blind trial of acyclovir and idoxuridine in dendritic corneal ulceration. *Br. J. Ophthalmol.* 1980;64:766.

153. Pavan-Langston, D., J. Lass, M. Hettinger, and I. Udell. Acyclovir and vidarabine in the treatment of ulcerative herpes simplex keratitis. *Am. J. Ophthalmol.* 1981;92:829.

154. Spruance, S. L., C. S. Crumpacker, H. Haines, C. Bader, K. Mehr, J. MacCalman, L. E. Schnipper, M. R. Klauber, J. C. Overall, and The Collaborative Study Group. Ineffectiveness of topical adenine arabinoside 5'-monophosphate in the treatment of recurrent

herpes simplex labialis. *N. Engl. J. Med.* 1979;300: 1180.

155. Adams, H. G., E. A. Benson, E. R. Alexander, L. A. Vontver, M. A., Remington, and K. K. Holmes. Genital herpetic infection in men and women: clinical course and effect of topical application of adenine arabinoside. *J. Infect. Dis.* 1976;133 (Suppl.):A151.

156. Pavan-Langston, D., C. H. Dohlman, P. Geary, and D. Szulczewski. Intraocular penetration of adenine arabinoside and idoxuridine—therapeutic implications in clinical herpetic uveitis. In *Adenine Arabinoside: An Antiviral Agent*, ed. by D. Pavan-Langston, R. A. Buchanan, and C. A. Alford, New York: Raven Press, 1975, pp. 293–306.

157. Pavan-Langston, D. Clinical evaluation of adenine arabinoside and idoxuridine in the treatment of ocular herpes simplex. *Am. J. Ophthalmol.* 1975;80: 496.

158. McGill, J., P. Tormey, and C. B. Walker. Comparative trial of acyclovir and adenine arabinoside in the treatment of herpes simplex corneal ulcers. *Br. J. Ophthalmol.* 1981;65:610.

159. Whitley, R. J., S. Soong, R. Dolin, G. J. Galasso, L. T. Ch'ien, C. A. Alford, and The Collaborative Study Group. Adenine arabinoside therapy of biopsy-proved herpes simplex encephalitis. *N. Engl. J. Med.* 1977;297: 290.

160. Whitely, R. J., S. J. Soong, M. S. Hirsch, A. W. Karchmer, R. Dolin, G. Galasso, J. K. Dunnick, C. A. Alford, and The NIAID Collaborative Antiviral Study Group. Herpes simplex encephalitis. Vidarabine therapy and diagnostic problems. *N. Engl. J. Med.* 1981; 304:313.

161. Whitley; R. Diagnosis and treatment of herpes simplex encephalitis. *Annu. Rev. Med.* 1981;32:335.

162. Whitley, R. J., A. J. Nahmias, S. J. Soong, G. J. Galasso, C. L. Flemming, and C. A. Alford. Vidarabine therapy of neonatal herpes simplex infection. *Pediatrics* 1980;66:495.

163. Whitley, R. J., L. T. Ch'ien, R. Dolin, G. J. Galasso, C. A. Alford, and The Collaborative Study Group. Adenine arabinoside therapy of herpes zoster in the immunosuppressed. *N. Engl. J. Med.* 1976;294:1193.

164. Whitley, R. J., S. J. Soong, R. Dolin, R. Betts, C. Linnemann, Jr., C. A. Alford, and The NIAID Collaborative Antiviral Study Group. Early vidarabine therapy to control the complications of herpes zoster in immunosuppressed patients. *N. Engl. J. Med.* 1982;307: 971.

165. Safrin, S., C. Crumpacker, P. Chatis, R. Davis, R. Hafner, J. Rush, H. A. Kessler, B. Landry, and J. Mills. A controlled trial comparing foscarnet with vidarabine for acyclovir resistant mucocutaneous herpes simplex in the acquired immunodeficiency syndrome. *N. Engl. J. Med.* 1991;325:551.

166. Pollard, R. B., J. L. Smith, A. Neal, P. B. Gregory, T. C. Merigan, and W. S. Robinson. Effect of vidarabine on chronic hepatitis B virus infection. *JAMA* 1978;239:1648.

167. Hirsch, M. S. and M. N. Swartz. Antiviral agents. *N. Engl. J. Med.* 1980;302:949.

168. Whitley, R., C. A. Alford, F. Hess, and R. Buchanan. Vidarabine: a preliminary review of its pharmacological properties and therapeutic use. *Drugs* 1980; 20:267.

169. Glazko, A. J., T. Chang, J. C. Drach, D. R. Mourer, P. E. Borondy, H. Schneider, L. Croskey, and E. Maschewske. Species differences in the metabolite disposition of adenine arabinoside. In *Adenine Arabinoside: An Antiviral Agent*, ed. by D. Pavan-Langston, R. A. Buchanan, and C. A. Alford. New York: Raven Press, 1975, pp. 111–133.

170. Ross, A. H., A. Julia, and C. Balakrishnan. Toxicity of adenine arabinoside in humans. *J. Infect. Dis.* 1976;133(Suppl.):A192.

171. Sacks, S. L., G. H. Scullard, R. B. Pollard, P. B. Gregory, W. S. Robinson, and T. C. Merigan. Antiviral treatment of chronic hepatitis B virus infection: pharmacokinetics and side effects of interferon and adenine arabinoside alone and in combination. *Antimicrob. Agents Chemother.* 1982;21:93.

172. Schaeffer, H. J. L. Beauchamp, P. de Miranda, G. B. Elion, D. J. Bauer, and P. Collins. 9-(2-Hydroxyethoxymethyl)guanine activity against viruses of the herpes group. *Nature* 1978;272:583.

173. Collins, P. The spectrum of antiviral activities of acyclovir in vitro and in vivo. *J. Antimicrob. Chemother.* 1983;12(Suppl. B):19.

174. Smee, D. F., J. C. Martin, J. P. H. Verheyden, and T. R. Mathews. Anti-herpesvirus activity of the acyclic nucleoside 9-(1,3-dihydroxy-2-propoxymethyl) guanine. *Antimicrob. Agents Chemother.* 1983; 23:676.

175. Symposium (various authors). Proceedings of a symposium on acyclovir. *Am. J. Med.* 1982;73(1A):1–392.

176. Symposium (various authors). Acyclovir. *J. Antimicrob. Chemother.* 1983;12(Suppl. B):1–202.

177. Symposium (various authors). Acyclovir. *J. Infect.* 1983;6(Suppl. 1):1–56.

178. Wagstaff, A. J., D. Faulds, and K. L. Goa. Aciclovir. A reappraisal of its antiviral activity, pharmacokinetic properties and therapeutic efficacy. *Drugs* 1994;47:153.

179. Furman, P. A., P. de Miranda, M. H. St. Clair, and G. B. Elion. Metabolism of acyclovir in virus-infected and uninfected cells. *Antimicrob. Agents Chemother.* 1981;20:518.

180. Fyfe, J. A., P. M. Keller, P. A. Furman, R. L. Miller, and G. B. Elion. Thymidine kinase from herpes simplex virus phosphorylates the new antiviral compound, 9-(2-hydroxyethoxymethyl)guanine. *J. Biol. Chem.* 1978;253:8721.

181. Keller, P. M., J. A. Fyfe, L. Beauchamp, C. M. Lubbers, P. A. Furman, H. J. Schaeffer, and G. B. Elion. Enzymatic phosphorylation of acyclic nucleoside analogs and correlations with antiherpetic activities. *Biochem. Pharmacol.* 1981;30:3071.

182. Coen, D. M. and P. A. Schaffer. Two distinct loci confer resistance to acycloguanosine in herpes simplex virus type 1. *Proc. Natl. Acad. Sci. U.S.A.* 1980; 77:2265.

183. Schnipper, L. E. and C. S. Crumpacker. Resistance of herpes simplex virus to acycloguanosine: role of viral thymidine kinase and DNA polymerase loci. *Proc. Natl. Acad. Sci. U.S.A.* 1980;77:2270.

184. Miller, W. H. and R. L. Miller. Phosphorylation of acyclovir (acycloguanosine) monophosphate by GMP kinase. *J. Biol. Chem.* 1980;255:7204.

185. Miller, W. H. and R. L. Miller. Phosphorylation of acyclovir diphosphate by cellular enzymes. *Biochem. Pharmacol.* 1982;31:3879.

186. Elion, G. B. Mechanism of action and selectivity of acyclovir. *Am. J. Med.* 1982;73(1A):7.

187. Elion, G. B., P. A. Furman, J. A. Fyfe, P. de Miranda, L. Beauchamp, and H. J. Schaeffer. Selectivity of action of an antiherpectic agent, 9-(2-hydroxyethoxymethyl)guanine. *Proc. Natl. Acad. Sci. U.S.A.* 1977;74:5716.

188. Furman, P. A., M. H. St. Clair, J. A. Fyfe, J. L. Rideout, P. M. Keller, and G. B. Elion. Inhibition of herpes simplex virus-induced DNA polymerase activity and viral DNA replication by 9-(2-hydroxyethoxymethyl)guanine and its triphosphate. *J. Virol.* 1979;32:72.

189. Derse, D., Y. C. Cheng, P. A. Furman, M. H. St. Clair, and G. B. Elion. Inhibition of purified human and herpes simplex virus–induced DNA polymerases by 9-(2-hydroxyethoxymethyl)guanine triphosphate. Effects on primer-template function. *J. Biol. Chem.* 1981;256:11447.

190. Hill, E. L., G. A. Hunter, and M. N. Ellis. In vitro and in vivo characterization of herpes simplex virus clinical isolates recovered from patients infected with human immunodeficiency virus. *Antimicrob. Agents Chemother.* 1991;35:2322.

191. Ellis, M. N., P. M. Keller, J. A. Fyfe, J. L. Rooney, S. E. Straus, S. N. Lehrman, and D. W. Barry. Clinical isolate of herpes simplex virus type 2 that induces a thymidine kinase with altered substrate specificity. *Antimicrob. Agents Chemother.* 1987;31:1117.

192. O'Brien, J. J., and D. M. Campoli-Richards. Acyclovir: an updated review of its antiviral activity, pharmacokinetic properties and therapeutic efficacy. *Drugs* 1989;37:233.

193. St. Clair, M. H., P. A. Furman, C. M. Lubbers, and G. B. Elion. Inhibition of cellular α and virally induced deoxyribonucleic acid polymerases by the triphosphate of acyclovir. *Antimicrob. Agents Chemother.* 1980;18:741.

194. Meyers, J. D., E. C. Reed, D. H. Shepp, M. Thornquist, P. S. Dandiker, C. A. Vicary, N. Fluornoy, L. E. Kirk, J. H. Kerrey, E. D. Thomas, and H. H. Balfour. Acyclovir for prevention of cytomegalovirus infection and disease after allogeneic marrow transplantation. *N. Engl. J. Med.* 1988;318:70.

195. Prentice, H. G., E. Gluckman, R. L. Powles, P. Ljungman, N. Milpied, J. M. Fernandez-Ranada, F. Mandell, P. Kho, L. Kennedy, and A. R. Bell. Impact of long-term acyclovir on cytomegalovirus infection and survival after allogeneic bone marrow transplantation. *Lancet* 1994;343:749.

196. Balfour, H. H., B. A. Chace, J. T. Stapleton, R. L. Simmons, and D. S. Fryd. A randomized, placebo-controlled trial of oral acyclovir for the prevention of cytomegalovirus disease in recipients of renal allografts. *N. Engl. J. Med.* 1989;320:1381.

197. Rubin, R. H., and N. E. Tolkoff-Rubin. Minireview: antimicrobial strategies in the care of organ transplant recipients. *Antimicrob. Agents Chemother.* 1993;37:619.

198. Young, B. J., A. Patterson, and T. Ravenscroft. A randomized double-blind clinical trial of acyclovir (Zovirax) and adenine arabinoside in herpes simplex corneal ulceration. *Br. J. Ophthalmol.* 1982;66:361.

199. Klauber, A., and E. Ottovay. Acyclovir and idoxuridine treatment of herpes simplex keratitis—a double blind clinical study. *Acta Ophthalmol.* 1982;60:838.

200. Fiddian, A. P., J. M. Yeo, R. Stubbings, and D. Dean. Successful treatment of herpes labialis with topical acyclovir. *BMJ* 1983;286:1699.

201. Whitley, R., N. Barton, E. Collins, J. Whelchel, and A. G. Diethelm. Mucocutaneous herpes simplex virus infections in immunocompromised patients. A model for topical evaluation of antiviral agents. *Am. J. Med.* 1982;73(1A):236.

202. Spruance, S. L., and C. S. Crumpacker. Topical 5 percent acyclovir in polyethylene glycol for herpes simplex labialis. Antiviral effect without clinical benefit. *Am. J. Med.* 1982;73(1A):315.

203. Corey, L., A. J. Nahmias, M. E. Guinan, J. K. Benedetti, C. W. Critchlow, and K. K. Holmes. A trial of topical acyclovir in genital herpes simplex virus infections. *N. Engl. J. Med.* 1982;306:1313.

204. Reichman, R. C., G. J. Badger, M. E. Guinan, A. J. Nahmais, R. E. Keeney, L. G. Davis, T. Ashikaga, and R. Dolin. Topically administered acyclovir in the treatment of recurrent herpes simplex genitalis: a controlled clinical trial. *J. Infect. Dis.* 1983;147:336.

205. Bryson, Y. J., M. Dillon, M. Lovett, G. Acuna, S. Taylor, J. D. Cherry, B. L. Johnson, E. Wiesmeier, W. Growdon, T. Creagh-Kirk, and R. Keeney. Treatment of first episodes of genital herpes simplex virus infection with oral acyclovir. A randomized double-blind controlled trial in normal subjects. *N. Engl. J. Med.* 1983;308:916.

206. Douglas, J. M., C. Critchlow, J. Benedetti, G. J. Mertz, J. D. Connor, M. A. Hintz, A. Fahnlander, M. Remington, C. Winter, and L. Corey. A double-blind study of oral acyclovir for suppression of recurrences of genital herpes simplex virus infection. *N. Engl. J. Med.* 1984;310:1551.

207. Straus, S. E., H. E. Takiff, M. Seidlin, S. Bachrach, L. Lininger, J. DiGiovanna, K. A. Western, H. A. Smith, S. N. Lehrman, T. Creagh-Kirk, and D. W. Alling. Suppression of frequently recurring genital herpes: a placebo-controlled double-blind trial of oral acyclovir. *N. Engl. J. Med.* 1983;310:1545.

208. Wooley, P. The value of antivirals in genital herpes. *Antiviral Chem. Chemother.* 1997;8(Suppl. 1):37.

209. Mindel, A., and S. Sutherland. Genital herpes—the disease and its treatment including intravenous acyclovir. *J. Antimicrob. Chemother.* 1983;12(Suppl. B):51.

210. Hann, I. M., H. G. Prentice, H. A. Blacklock, M. G. Ross, D. Brigden, A. E. Rosling, C. Burke, D. H. Crawford, W. Brumfitt, and A. V. Hoffbrand. Acyclovir prophylaxis against herpes virus infections in severely immunocompromised patients: randomised double blind trial. *BMJ* 1983;287:384.

211. Saral, R., R. F. Ambinder, W. H. Burns, C. M.

Angelopulos, D. E. Griffin, P. J. Burke, and P. S. Lietman. Acyclovir prophylaxis against herpes simplex virus infection in patients with leukemia. *Ann. Intern. Med.* 1983;99:773.

212. Prentice, H. G., and I. M. Hann. Prophylactic studies against herpes infections in severely immunocompromised patients with acyclovir. *J. Infect.* 1983; 6(Suppl. 1):17.

213. Wade, J. C., B. Newton, N. Flournoy, and J. D. Meyers. Oral acyclovir for prevention of herpes simplex virus reactivation after marrow transplantation. *Ann. Intern. Med.* 1984;100:823.

214. Balfour, H. H., B. Bean, O. L. Laskin, R. F. Ambinder, J. D. Meyers, J. C. Wade, J. A. Zaia, D. Aeppli, L. E. Kirk, A. C. Segreti, R. E. Keeney, and the Burroughs Wellcome Collaborative Acyclovir Study Group. Acyclovir halts progression of herpes zoster in immunocompromised patients. *N. Engl. J. Med.* 1983;308: 1448.

215. McGill, J., D. R. MacDonald, C. Fall, G. D. W. McKendrick, and A. Copplestone. Intravenous acyclovir in acute herpes zoster infection. *J. Infect.* 1983;6: 157.

216. Dunkle, L. M., A. M. Arvin, R. J. Whitley, H. A. Rotbart, H. M. Feder, S. Feldman, A. A. Gershon, M. L. Levy, G. F. Hayden, P. V. McGuirt, J. Harris, and H. H. Balfour. A controlled trial of acyclovir for chickenpox in normal children. *N. Engl. J. Med.* 1991;325:1539.

217. Committee on Infectious Diseases. The use of oral acyclovir in otherwise healthy children with varicella. *Pediatrics* 1993;92:674.

218. Wallace, M. R., W. A. Bowler, N. B. Murray, S. K. Brodine, and E. C. Oldfield. Treatment of adult varicella with oral acyclovir. A randomized, placebo-controlled trial. *Ann. Intern. Med.* 1992;117:358.

219. Wood, M. J., P. H. Ogan, M. W. McKendrick, C. D. Care, J. I. McGill, and E. M. Webb. Efficacy of oral acyclovir treatment of acute herpes zoster. *Am. J. Med.* 1988;85(Suppl. 2A):79.

220. Whitley, R. J., J. W. Gnann, D. Hinthron, C. Liu, R. B. Pollard, F. Hayden, G. J. Mertz, M. Oxman, and S. J. Soong, and the NIAID Collaborative Antiviral Study Group. Disseminated herpes zoster in the immunocompromised host: a comparative trial of acyclovir and vidarabine. *J. Infect. Dis.* 1992;165:450.

221. Marley, J. Antiviral therapy in herpes zoster: a review. *Antiviral Chem. Chemother.* 1997;8(Suppl. 1): 37.

222. Whitley, R. J., C. A. Alford, M. S. Hirsch, R. T. Schooley, J. P. Lubey, F. Y. Aoki, D. Hanley, A. J. Nahmias, and S. J. Soong. Vidarabine versus acyclovir therapy in *Herpes simplex* encephalitis. *N. Engl. J. Med.* 1986;314:144.

223. Van der Horst, C., J. Joncas, G. Anronheim, N. Gustafson, G. Stein, M. Gurwith, G. Fleischer, J. Sullivan, J. Sixbey, S. Roland, J. Fryer, K. Champnet, R. Schooley, C. Suyama, and J. Pagano. Lack of effect of peroral acyclovir for the treatment of acute infectious mononucleosis. *J. Infect. Dis.* 1991;164:788.

224. de Ruiter, A., and R. N. Thin. Genital herpes. A guide to pharmacological therapy. *Drugs* 1994;47:297.

225. Erlich, K. S., J. Mills, P. Chatis, G. J. Mertz, and

D. F. Busch. Acyclovir-resistant herpes simplex virus infections in patients with the acquired immunodeficiency syndrome. *N. Engl. J. Med.* 1989;320:293.

226. Laskin, O. L. Clinical pharmacokinetics of acyclovir. *Clin. Pharmacokinet.* 1983;8:187.

227. Poirier, R. H., J. D. Kingham, P. de Miranda, and A. Annel. Intraocular antiviral penetration. *Arch. Ophthalmol.* 1982;100:1964.

228. de Miranda, P., and M. R. Blum. Pharmacokinetics of acyclovir after intravenous and oral administration. *J. Antimicrob. Chemother.* 1983;12(Suppl. B): 29.

229. Van Dyke, R. B., J. D. Connor, C. Wyborny, M. Hintz, and R. E. Keeney. Pharmacokinetics of orally administered acyclovir in patients with herpes progenitalis. *Am. J. Med.* 1982;73(1A):172.

230. de Miranda, P., R. J. Whitley, M. R. Blum, R. E. Keeney, N. Barton, D. M. Cocchetto, S. Good, G. P. Hemstreet, L. E. Kirk, D. A. Page, and G. B. Elion. Acyclovir kinetics after intravenous infusion. *Clin. Pharmacol. Ther.* 1979;26:718.

231. Laskin, O. L., J. A. Longstreth, R. Saral, P. de Miranda, R. Keeney, and P. S. Lietman. Pharmacokinetics and tolerance of acyclovir, a new anti-herpesvirus agent, in humans. *Antimicrob. Agents Chemother.* 1982;21:393.

232. de Miranda, P., S. S. Good, O. L. Laskin, H. C. Krasny, J. D. Connor, and P. S. Lietman. Disposition of intravenous radioactive acyclovir. *Clin. Pharmacol. Ther.* 1981;30:662.

233. de Miranda, P., H. C. Krasny, D. A. Page, and G. B. Elion. The disposition of acyclovir in different species. *J. Pharmacol. Exp. Ther.* 1981;219:309.

234. Blum, M. R., S. H. T. Liao, and P. de Miranda. Overview of acyclovir pharmacokinetic disposition in adults and children. *Am. J. Med.* 1982;73(1A):186.

235. Frenkel, L. M., Z. A. Brown, Y. J. Bryson, L. Corey, J. D. Unadkat, P. A. Hensleigh, A. M. Arvin, C. G. Prober, and J. D. Connor. Pharmacokinetics of acyclovir in the term human pregnancy and neonate. *Am. J. Obstet. Gynecol.* 1991;164:569.

236. Laskin, O. L., J. A. Longstreth, A. Whelton, L. Rocco, P. S. Lietman, H. C. Krasny, and R. E. Keeney. Acyclovir kinetics in end-stage renal disease. *Clin. Pharmacol. Ther.* 1982;31:594.

237. Keeney, R. E., L. E. Kirk, and D. Bridgen. Acyclovir tolerance in humans. *Am. J. Med.* 1982;73(1A): 176.

238. Brigden, D., A. E. Rosling, and N. C. Woods. Renal function after acyclovir intravenous injection. *Am. J. Med.* 1982;73(1A):182.

239. Sawyer, M. H., D. E. Webb, J. E. Balow, and S. E. Straus. Acyclovir-induced renal failure: clinical course and histology. *Am. J. Med.* 1988;84:1067.

240. Weller, I. V. D., V. Carreno, M. J. F. Fowler, J. Monjardino, D. Makinen, Z. Vargese, P. Sweny, H. C. Thomas, and S. Sherlock. Acyclovir in hepatitis B antigen-positive chronic liver disease: inhibition of viral replication and transient renal impairment with iv bolus administration. *J. Antimicrob. Chemother.* 1983;11: 223.

241. Haefeli, W. E., R. A. Z. Schoenenberger, P. Weiss, and R. F. Ritz. Acyclovir-induced neurotoxicity:

concentration-side effect relationship in acyclovir overdose. *Am. J. Med.* 1993;94:212.

242. Straus, S. E., H. A. Smith, C. Brickman, P. de Miranda, C. McLaren, and R. Keeney. Acyclovir for chronic mucocutaneous herpes simplex virus infection in immunosuppressed patients. *Ann. Intern. Med.* 1982; 96:270.

243. Heagy, W., C. Crumpacker, P. A. Lopez, and R. W. Finberg. Inhibition of immune functions by antiviral drugs. *J. Clin. Invest.* 1991;87:1916.

244. Gold, D., R. Ashley, G. Solberg, H. Abbo, and L. Corey. Chronic-dose acyclovir to suppress frequently recurring genital herpes simplex virus infections: effect on antibody response to herpes simplex virus type 2 proteins. *J. Infect. Dis.* 1988;158:1227.

245. Molin, L., M. Ruhnek-Forsbeck, and B. Svennerholm. One-year acyclovir suppression of frequently recurring genital herpes: a study of efficacy, safety, virus sensitivity and antibody response. *Scand. J. Infect. Dis.* 1991;78(Suppl.):33.

246. Various authors. Preclinical toxicology studies with acyclovir. *Fund. Appl. Toxicol.* 1983;3:559–602.

247. Hayden, F. Antiviral agents. In *Goodman and Gilman's The Pharmacological Basis of Therapeutics,* ed. by J. Hardman, L. Limbird, P. Molinoff, R. Ruddon and A. G. Gilman. New York: McGraw-Hill, 1996, pp. 1191–1223.

248. Murray, A. B. Valaciclovir—an improvement over aciclovir for the treatment of zoster. *Antiviral Chem. Chemother.* 1995;6:34.

249. Weller, S., M. R. Blum, M. Doucette, T. Burnette. D. M. Cederberg, P. de Miranda, and M. L. Smiley. Pharmacokinetics of the acyclovir pro-drug valaciclovir after escalating single and multiple dose administration to normal volunteers. *Clin. Pharmacol. Ther.* 1993;54:595.

250. Beutner, K. R., D. J. Friedman, C. Forszpaniak, P. L. Anderson, and M. J. Wood. Valaciclovir compared with acyclovir for improved therapy for *Herpes zoster* in immunocompetent adults. *Antimicrob. Agents Chemother.* 1994;39:1546.

251. Crooks, R. J., and A. Murray. Valacyclovir—a review of a promising new antiherpes agent. *Antiviral Chem. Chemother.* 1995;5(Suppl. 1):31.

252. Perry, C. M., and D. Faulds. Valacyclovir. A review of its antiviral activity, pharmacokinetic properties and therapeutic effecacy in herpesvirus infections. *Drugs* 1996;52:754.

253. Spruance, S. L., T. L. Rea, C. Thoming, R. Tucker, R. Salzman, and R. Boon. Penciclovir cream for the treatment of herpes simplex labialis. JAMA randomized, multicenter, double-blind, placebo-controlled trial. Topical penciclovir collaborative study group. *JAMA* 1997;277:1374.

254. Jacobson, M. A., J. Gallant, L. H. Wang, D. Coakley, S. Weller, D. Gary, L. Squires, M. L. Smiley, M. R. Blum, and J. Feinberg: Phase I trial of valacicolvir, the L-valyl ester of acyclovir, in patients with advanced human immunodeficiency virus disease. *Antimicrob. Agents Chemother.* 1994;38:1534.

255. Valacyclovir. *Med. Lett.* 1996;38:3.

256. Glaxo Wellcome. Valaciclovir prescribing information, U.S., 1995.

257. VereHodge, R. A., and Y.-C. Cheng. The mode of action of penciclovir. *Antiviral Chem. Chemother.* 1993;4:(Suppl. 1):13.

258. Pue, M. A., and L. Z. Benet. Pharmacokinetics of famciclovir in man. *Antiviral. Chem. Chemother.* 1993;4 (Suppl. 1):47.

259. VereHodge, R. A., Famciclovir and penciclovir: the mode of action of famciclovir including is conversion to penciclovir. *Antiviral Chem. Chemother.* 1993; 4:67.

260. Alrabiah, F. A., and S. L. Sacks. New antiherpesvirus agents. Their targets and therapeutic potential. *Drugs* 1996;52:17.

261. Boyd, M. R., S. Safrin, and E. R. Kern. Penciclovir: a review of its spectrum of activity, selectivity and cross-resistance pattern. *Antiviral Chem. Chemother.* 1993;4:(Suppl. 1):3.

262. Gnann, J. W., New antivirals with activity against varicella-zoster virus. *Ann. Neurol.* 1994;34: 569.

263. Degreef, H. Famciclovir, a new oral antiherpes drug: results of the first controlled clinical study demonstrating its efficacy and safety in the treatment of uncomplicated herpes zoster in immune competent patients. *Int. J. Antimicrob. Agents* 1994;4:241.

264. Tyring, S., R. A. Barbarash, J. E. Nahlik, A. Cunningham, J. Marley, M. Heng, T. Jones, T. Rea, R. Boon, R. Saltzman, and the Collaborative Famciclovir Herpes Zoster Study Group. Famciclovir for the treatment of acute herpes zoster: effects on acute disease and postherpetic neuralgia. A randomized double-blind, placebo-controlled trial. *Ann. Intern. Med.* 1995;123:89.

265. Sacks, S. L., F. Y. Aoki, F. Diaz-Mitoma, J. Sellors, and S. D. Shafran. Patient-initiated, twice-daily oral famciclovir for early recurrent genital herpes. A randomized, double-blind multicenter trial. Canadian famciclovir study group. *JAMA* 1996;276:44.

266. Perry, C. M., and A. J. Wagstaff. Famciclovir. A review of its pharmacological properties and therapeutic efficacy in herpes virus infections. *Drugs* 1995;50: 396.

267. Saltzman, R., R. Jurewicz, and R. Boon. Safety of famciclovir in patients with herpes zoster and genital herpes. *Antimicrob. Agents Chemother.* 1994;38:2454.

268. Crumpacker, C. S. Ganciclovir. *N. Engl. J. Med.* 1996;335:721.

269. Martin, J. C., C. A. Dvorak, D. F. Smee, T. R. Matthews, and J. P. H. Verhyden. 9((1,3-dihydroxy-2-propoxy)methyl) guanine: a new potent and selective antiherpes agent. *J. Med. Chem.* 1983;26:759.

270. Plotkin, S. A., W. L. Drew, D. Felsenstein, and M. S. Hirsch. Sensitivity of clinical isolates of human cytomegalovirus to 9-(1,3-dihydroxy-2-propoxymethyl) guanine. *J. Infect Dis.* 1985;152:833.

271. Markham, A., and D. Faulds. Ganciclovir. An update of its therapeutic use in cytomegalovirus infection. *Drugs* 1994;48:455.

272. Noble, S., and D. Faulds. Ganciclovir. An update of its use in the prevention of cytomegalovirus infection and disease in transplant recipients. *Drugs* 1998; 56:115.

273. Biron, K. K., S. C. Stanat, J. B. Sorrell, J. A. Fyfe, P. M. Keller, C. U. Lambe, and D. J. Nelson.

Metabolic activation of the nucleoside analog 9-{[2-hydroxy-1(hydroxymethyl) ethoxy] methyl}quanine in human diploid fibroblasts infected with human cytomegalovirus. *Proc. Natl. Acad. Sci. U.S.A.* 1985;82: 2473.

274. Stanat, S. C., J. E. Reardon, A. Erice, M. C. Jordan, W. L. Drew, and K. K. Biron. Ganciclovir-resistant cytomegalovirus clinical isolates: mode of resistance to ganciclovir. *Antimicrob. Agents Chemother.* 1991;35: 2191.

275. Tatarowicz, W. A., N. S. Lavain, and K. D. Thompson. A ganciclovir-resistant clinical isolate of human cytomegalovirus exhibiting cross-resistance to other DNA polymerase inhibitors. *J. Infect. Dis.* 1992; 166:904.

276. Spector, S. A., D. F. Busch, S. Follansbee, K. Squires, J. P. Lalezari, M. A. Jacobson, J. D. Connor, D. Jung, A. Shadman, B. Mastre, W. Buhles, W. L. Drew, AIDS Clinical Trials Group and Cytomegalovirus Cooperative Study Group. Pharmacokinetic, safety, and antiviral profiles or oral ganciclovir in persons infected with human immunodeficiency virus: a phase I/II study. *J. Infect. Dis.* 1995;171:1431.

277. Fletcher, C., R. Sawchuk, B. Chinnock, P. de Miranda, and H. H. Balfour. Human pharmacokinetics of the antiviral drug DHPG. *Clin. Pharmacol. Ther.* 1986;40:281.

278. Jabs, D. A., C. Newman, and S. deBustros. Treatment of cytomegalovirus retinitis with ganciclovir. *Ophthalmology* 1987;94:824.

279. Sommadossi, J. P., R. Bevan, T. Ling, F. Lee, B. Mastre, M. D. Chaplin, C. Nerenberg, S. Koretz, and W. C. Buhles. Clinical pharmacokietics of ganciclovir in patients with normal and impaired renal function. *Rev. Infect. Dis.* 1988;10:S507.

280. Felsenstein, D., D. J. D'Amico, M. S. Hirsh, D. A, Neumeyer, D. M. Cederberg, P. de Miranda, and R. T. Schooley: Treatment of cytomegalovirus retinitis with 9-(2-hydroxy-1(hydroxmethyl) ethoxymethyl)guanine, *Ann. Intern. Med.* 1985;103:377.

281. Collaborative DHPG Treatment Study Group. Treatment of serious cytomegalovirus infections with 9-(1,3-dihydroxy-2-propoxymethyl) guanine in patients with AIDS and other immunodeficiencies. *N. Engl. J. Med.* 1986;314:801.

282. Faulds, D., and R. C. Heel. Ganciclovir. A review of its antiviral activity, pharmacokinetic properties and therapuetuc efficacy in cytomegalovirus infections. *Drugs* 1990;39:597.

283. Drew, W. L. Cytomegalovirus infection in patients with AIDS. *Clin. Infect. Dis.* 1992;14:608.

284. Drew, W. L., D. Ives, J. P. Lalezari, C. Crumpacker, S. E. Follansbee, S. A. Spector, C. A. Benson, D. N. Friedberg, L. Hubbard, M. J. Stempien, A. Shadman, and W. Buhles for the Syntex Cooperative Oral Ganciclovir Study Group. Oral ganciclovir as maintenance treatment for cytomegalovirus retinitis in patients with AIDS. *N. Engl. J. Med.* 1995;333:615.

285. Dieterich, D. T., D. P. Kotler, D. F. Busch, C. Crumpacker, C. Du Mond, B. Dearmand, and W. Buhles. Ganciclovir treatment of cytomegalovirus colitis in AIDS: a randomized, double-blind placebo-controlled multicenter study. *J. Infect. Dis.* 1993;167:278.

286. Hecht, D. W., D. R. Snydman, C. Crumpacker, B. G. Werner, and B. Heinze-Lacey. Ganciclovir for treatment of renal transplant–associated primary cytomegalovirus pneumonia. *J. Infect. Dis.* 1988;157:187.

287. Spector, S. A., G. F. McKinley, J. P. Lalezari, T. Samo, R. Andruczk, S. Follansbee, P. D. Sparti, D. V. Havlir, G. Simpson, W. Buhles, R. Wong, and M. J. Stempien. Oral ganciclovir for the prevention of cytomegalovirus disease in persons with AIDS. *N. Engl. J. Med.* 1996;334:1491.

288. Miller, G., J. R. Story, and C. M. Greco. Ganciclovir in the treatment of progressive AIDS-related postradiculopathy. *Neurology* 1990;40:569.

289. Jacobson, A., J. Mills, J. Rush, J. J. O'Donnell, R. G. Miller, C. Greco, and M. F. Gonzales. Failure of antiviral therapy for acquired immunodeficiency syndrome–related cytomegalovirus myelitis. *Arch. Neurol.* 1988;45:1090.

290. Fuller, N. Cytomegalovirus and the peripheral nervous system in AIDS. *J. Acquired Immune Defic. Syndr.* 1992;5(Suppl. 1):S33.

291. Enting, R., J. de Gans, P. Reiss, C. Jansen, and P. Portegies. Ganciclovir/foscarnet for cytomegalovirus meningocephalitis in AIDS. *Lancet* 1992;340:559.

292. Hardy, W. D. Combined ganciclovir and recombinant human granulocyte-macrophage colony-stimulating facor in the treatment of cytomegalovirus retinitis in AIDS patients. *J. Acquired Immune Defic. Syndr.* 1991;4(Suppl. 1):22.

293. Schmidt, M., D. A. Horak, J. C. Niland, S. R. Duncan, J. Forman, J. A. Zaia, and the City of Hope–Stanford–Syntex CMV Study Group. A randomized controlled trial of prophylactic ganciclovir for cytomegalovirus pulmonary infection in recipients of allogeneic bone marrow transplants. *N. Engl. J. Med.* 1991;324: 1005.

294. Hochster, H., D. Dieterich, S. Bozzette, R. C. Reichman, J. D. Connor, L. Liebes, R. L. Sonke, S. A. Spector, F. Valentine, C. Pettinelli, and D. D. Richman: Toxicity of combined ganciclovir and zidovudine for cytomegalovirus disease associated with AIDS: an AIDS clinical trials group study. *Ann. Intern. Med.* 1990;113: 111.

295. Wagstaff, J., and H. M. Bryson. Foscarnet. A reappraisal of its antiviral activity, pharmacokinetic properties and therapeutic use in immunocompromised patients with viral infections. *Drugs* 1994;48:199.

296. Datta, K., and R. E. Hood. Mechanism of inhibition of EB 297 replication by phosphonoformic acid. *Virology* 1981;114:52.

297. Safrin, S., S. Kemmerly, B. Plotkin, T. Smith, N. Weissbach, D. De Veranez, L. D. Phan, and D. Cohn. Foscarnet-resistant herpes simplex virus infection in patients with AIDS. *J. Infect. Dis.* 1994;169:193.

298. Laufer, D. S., and S. E. Starr. Resistance to antivirals. *Pediatr. Clin. North Am.* 1995;42:583.

299. Sullivan, V., and D. M. Coen. Isolation of foscarnet-resistant human cytomegalovirus patterns of resistance and sensitivity to other antiviral drugs. *J. Infect. Dis.* 1991;164:781.

300. Coen, D. M. General aspects of drug resistance with special reference to herpes simplex virus. *J. Antimicrob. Chemother.* 1986;18(Suppl. B):1.

301. Sacks, S. L., R. J. Wanklin, D. E. Reece, K. A. Hicks, K. L. Tyler, and D. M. Coen. Progressive esophagitis from acyclovir-resistant herpes simplex: clinical roles for DNA polymerase mutants and viral heterogeneity? *Ann. Intern. Med.* 1989;111:893.

302. Chrisp, P. and S. P. Clissold. Foscarnet: a review of its antiviral activity, pharmacokinetic properties and therapeutic use in immunocompromised patients with cytomegalovirus retinitis. *Drugs* 1991;41:104.

303. Gerard, L., and D. Salmon-Ceron. Pharmacology and clinical use of foscarnet. *Int'l. J. Antimicrob. Agents* 1995;5:209.

304. Palestine, A. G., M. A. Polis, M. D. DeSmet, B. F. Baird, J. Falloon, J. A. Kovacs, R. T. Davey, J. J. Zurlo, K. M. Zunich, M. Davis, L. Hubbard, R. Brothers, F. L. Ferris, E. Chew, J. L. Davis, B. I. Rubin, S. D. Mellow, J. A. Metcalf, J. Manischewitz, J. R. Minor, R. B. Nussenblatt, H. Masur, and H. C. Lane. A randomized, controlled trial of foscarnet in the treatment of cytomegalovirus retinitis in patients with AIDS. *Ann. Intern. Med.* 1991;115:665.

305. Studies of Ocular Complications of AIDS Research Group. Mortality in patients with the acquired immunodeficiency syndrome treated with either foscarnet or ganciclovir for cytomegalovirus retinitis. *N. Engl. J. Med.* 1992;326:213.

306. Heley, A. Foscarnet infusion at home. *Lancet* 1988;2:1311.

307. Oberg, B. Antiviral effects of phosphonoformate (PFA, foscarnet sodium). *Pharmacol. Ther.* 1989;40:213.

308. Reusser, P., J. G. Gambertoglio, K. Lilleby, and J. D. Myers. Phase I–II trial of foscarnet for prevention of cytomegalovirus infection in autologous and allogeneic marrow transplant recipients. *J. Infect. Dis.* 1992;166:473.

309. Erlich, K. S., M. A. Jacobson, J. E. Koehler, S. E. Follnsbee, D. P. Drennan, L. Gooze, S. Safrin, and J. Mills. Foscarnet therapy for severe acyclovir-resistant herpes simplex virus type-2 infections in patients with the acquired immunodeficiency syndrome (AIDS). An uncontrolled trial. *Ann. Intern. Med.* 1989;110:710.

310. Erlich, K. S., J. Mills, P. Chatis, G. J. Mertz, D. F. Busch, S. E. Follansbee, R. M. Grant, and C. S. Crumpacker. Acyclovir-resistant herpes simplex virus infections in patients with the acquired immunodeficiency syndrome. *N. Engl. J. Med.* 1989;320:293.

311. Vinckier, F., M. Boogaerts, D. De Clercq, and E. De Clercq. Chronic herpetic infection in an immunocompromised patient: report of a case. *J. Oral Maxillofac. Surg.* 1987;45:723.

312. Smith, K. J., D. C. Kahlter, C. Davis, W. D. James, H. G. Skelton, and P. Angritt. Acyclovir-resistant varicella zoster responsive to foscarnet. *Arch. Dermatol.* 1991;127:1069.

313. Lokke, J. B., K. Weismann, L. Mathiesen, and K. Thomsen. Atypical varicella-zoster infection in AIDS. *Acta Dermatol. Venereol.* 1993;73:123.

314. Cacoub, P., G. Deray A. Baumelou, P. LeHoang, W. Rozenbaum, M. Gentilini, C. Soubrie, F. Rousselie, and C. Jacobs. Acute renal failure induced by foscarnet: 4 cases. *Clin. Nephrol.* 1988;29:315.

315. Jacobson, M. A., J. J. O'Donnell, and J. Mills.

316. Cihlar, T. and M. S. Chen. Identification of enzymes catalyzing two-step phosphorylation of cidofovir and the effect of cytomegalovirus infection on their activities in host cells. *Mol. Pharmacol.* 1996;50:1502.

317. Neyts, J., R. Snoeck, D. Schols, J. Balzarini, and E. DeClercq. Selective inhibition of human cytomegalovirus DNA synthesis by (S)-1(33-hydroxy-2-phosphonylmethoxypropyl) cytosine ((S)-HPMPC) and 9-(1,3-dihydroxy-2-propoxymethyl)guanine (DHPG). *Virology* 1990;179:41.

318. Mulato, M. S., J. M. Cherrington, and M. S. Chen. Anti-HCMV activity of cidofovir in combination with antiviral compounds and immunosuppressive agents: in vitro analyses. *Antiviral Chem. Chemother.* 1996;7:203.

319. Safrin, S., J. Cherrington, and H. J. Jaffe. Clinical uses of cidofovir. (S)-1(33-hydroxy-2-phosphonylmethoxypropyl) cytosine ((S)-HPMPC) and 9-(1,3-dihydroxy-2-propoxymethyl)guanine (DHPG). *Rev. Med. Virol.* 1997;7:145.

320. Lurain, N. S., K. D. Thompson, E. W. Holmes, and G. S. Read. Point mutations in the DNA polymerase gene of human cytomegalovirus that result in resistance to antiviral agents. *J. Virol.* 1992;66:7146.

321. Cherrington, J. M., R. Miner, M. J. M. Hitchcock, J. P. Lalezari, and W. L. Drew. Susceptibility of human cytomegalovirus (HCMV) to cidofovir is unchanged after limited in vivo exposure to various clinical regimens of drug. *J. Infect. Dis.* 1996;173:987.

322. Ho, H.-T., K. L. Woods, J. J. Bronson, H. De Boeck, J. C. Martin, and M. J. M. Hitchcock. Intracellular metabolism of the antiherpes agent (S)-1(3-hydroxy-2-phosphonylmethoxy)propyl)cytosine. *Mol. Pharmacol.* 1992;41:197.

323. Cundy, K., B. Petty J. Flaherty, P. E. Fisher, M. A. Polis, M. Wachsman, P. S. Lietman, J. P. Lalezari, M. J. M. Hitchcock, and H. S. Jaffe. Clinical pharmacokinetics of cidofovir in human immunodeficiency virus–infected patients. *Antimicrob. Agents Chemother.* 1995;39:1247.

324. Lalezari, J. P., R. J. Stagg, B. D. Kupperman, G. N. Holland, F. Kramer, D. V. Ives, M. Youle, M. R. Robinson, W. L. Drew, and H. S. Jaffe. Intravenous cidofovir for peripheral cytomegalovirus retinitis in patients with AIDS. A randomized, controlled trial. *Ann. Intern. Med.* 1997;126:257.

325. Studies of Ocular Complications of AIDS Research Group in collaboration with the AIDS Clinical Trials Group. Parenteral cidofovir for cytomegalovirus retinitis in patients with AIDS: the HPMPC peripheral cytomegalovirus retinitis trial. A randomized, controlled trial. *Ann. Intern. Med.* 1997;126:264.

326. Polis, M. A., K. M. Spooner, B. F. Baird, J. F. Manischewitz, H. S. Jaffe, P. E. Fisher, J. Falloon, R. T. Davey, J. A. Kovacs, R. E. Walker, S. M. Whitcup, R. B. Nussenblatt, H. C. Lane, and H. Masur. Anticytomegaloviral activity and safety of cidofovir in patients with human immunodeficiency virus infection and cytomegalovirus viruria. *Antimicrob. Agents Chemother.* 1995;39:882.

Foscarnet treatment of cytomegalovirus retinitis in patients with the acquired immunodeficiency syndrome. *Antimicrob. Agents Chemother.* 1989;33:736.

327. Lalezari, J. P., W. L. Drew, E. Glutzer, C. James, D. Miner, J. Flaherty, P. E. Fisher, K. Cundy, J. Hannigan, J. C. Martin, and H. S. Jaffe. (S)-1(3-hydroxy-2-phosphonymethoxy)propyl)cytosine (cidofovir): results of a phase I/II study of a novel antiviral nucleotide analogue. *J. Infect. Dis.* 1995;171:788.

328. Hoskins, M. A. protective action of neurotropic against viscerotropic yellow fever virus in *Macacus rheusus. Am. J. Trop. Med. Hyg.* 1935;15:675.

329. Isaacs, A. and J. Lindenmanne. Virus interference. I. The interferon. *Proc. R. Soc. Biol. Sci.* 1957; 147:258.

330. Stewart II, W. E. *The Interferon System*, 2nd ed. New York: Springer-Verlag, 1981.

331. Khan, A., N. O. Hill, and G. L. Dorn (eds.) *Interferon: Properties and Clinical Uses*. Dallas: Leland Fikes Foundation Press, 1979.

332. Came, P. E., and W. A. Carter (eds.) *Interferons and Their Applications. Handbook of Experimental Pharmacology*, Vol. 71 New York: Springer-Verlag, 1984,

333. Vilcek, J. J., and G. C. Sen. Interferons and other cytokines. In *Fields Virology*, ed. by B. N. Fields, D. M. Knipe, and P. M. Howley. Philadelphia: Lippincott-Raven, 1996, pp. 375–399.

334. Interferon Nomenclature Committee. Interferon nomenclature. *J. Immunol.* 1980;125:2353.

335. Zoon, K. C., and R. Wetzel. Comparative structures of mammalian inteferons. In *Interferons and Their Applications*, ed. by P. R. Came and W. A. Carter. New York: Springer-Verlag, 1984, pp. 79–100.

336. Yip, Y. K., B. S. Barrowclough, C. Urban, and J. Vilcek. Molecular weight of gamma interferon is similar to that of other human interferons. *Science* 1982; 215:411.

337. Volz, M., and C. H. Kirkpatrick. Interferons 1992. How much of the promise has been realised. *Drugs* 1992;43:285.

338. Lengyel, P. Biochemistry of interferons and their actions. *Ann. Rev. Biochem.* 1982;51:251.

339. Vengris, V. E., B. D. Stoller, and P. M. Pitha. Interferon externalization by producing cell before induction of antiviral state. *Virology* 1975;65:410.

340. Gressor, I., M. T. Bandu, and D. Brouty-Boyé. Interferon and cell division. IX. Interferon-resistant L1210 cells: characteristics and origin. *J. Natl. Cancer Inst.* 1974;52:553.

341. Aguet, M. High affinity binding of ^{125}I-labeled mouse interferon to a specific cell surface receptor. *Nature* 1980;284:459.

342. Aguet, M., and B. Blanchard. High affinity binding of ^{125}I-labeled mouse interferon to a specific cell surface receptor. II. Analysis of binding properties. *Virology* 1981;115:249.

343. Branca, A. A., and C. Baglioni. Evidence that types I and II interferons have different receptors. *Nature* 1981;294:768.

344. Farrar, M. A., and R. D. Schreiber. The molecular cell biology of interferon-γ and its receptor. *Annu. Rev. Immunol.* 1993;11:571.

345. Sen, G. C., and P. Lengyel. The interferon system: a bird's eye view of its biochemistry. *J. Biol. Chem.* 1992;267:5017.

346. Pellegrini S. and C. Schindler. Early events in signalling by interferons. *Trends Biochem. Sci.* 1993;18: 338.

347. Darnell, J. E., I. M. Kerr, and G. R. Stark. Jak-STAT pathways and transcriptional activation in response to IFNs and other extracellular signaling proteins. *Science* 1994;264:1415.

348. Baron, S., D. H. Copenhaver, and F. Dianzani. Introduction to the interferon system. In *Interferon: Principles and Medical Applications*, ed. by S. Baron, F. Dianzani, G. J. Stanton, W. R. Fleischmann, D. H. Copenhaver, T. K. Hughes, G. R. Klimpel, W. Niesel, and S. K. Tyring. Galveston: University of Texas Press, 1992, pp. 1–15.

349. Sen, G. C., and R. M. Ransohoff. Interferon-induced antiviral actions and their regulation. *Adv. Virus Res.* 1992;42:57.

350. Samuel, C. Antiviral actions of interferon: interferon-regulated cellular proteins and their surprisingly selective antiviral activities. *Virology* 1991;183:1.

351. Taylor, J. Studies on the mechanism of action of interferon. I. Interferon action and RNA synthesis in chick embryo fibroblasts infected with Semliki Forest virus. *Virology* 1965;25:340.

352. Levine, S. Effect of actinomycin D and puromycin dehydrochloride on action of interferon. *Virology* 1964;24:586.

353. Friedmann, R. M. Antiviral activity of interferons. *Bacteriol. Rev.* 1977;41:543.

354. Baglioni, C. The molecular mediators of interferon action. In *Interferons and Their Applications*, ed. by P. E. Came and W. A. Carter. New York: Springer-Verlag, 1984, pp. 153–168.

355. Kerr, I. M., R. E. Brown, and L. A. Ball. Increased activity of cell-free protein synthesis to double-stranded RNA after interferon treatment. *Nature* 1974; 250:57.

356. Brown, G. E., B. Lebleu, M. Kawakita, S. Shaila, G. C. Sen, and P. Lengyel. Increased endonuclease activity in an extract from mouse Ehrlich ascites tumor cells which had been treated with a partially purified interferon preparation. Dependence on double-stranded RNA. *Biochem. Biophys. Res. Commun.* 1976;69:114.

357. Sen, G. C., B. Lebleu, C. E. Brown, M. Kawakita, E. Slattery, and P. Lengyel. Interferon, double-stranded RNA and mRNA degradation. *Nature* 1976; 264:370.

358. Havanessian, A. G., R. E. Brown, and I. M. Kerr. Synthesis of low molecular weight inhibitor of protein synthesis with enzyme from interferon-treated cells. *Nature* 1977;268:537.

359. Kerr, I. M., and R. E. Brown. pppA2'p5'A2'p5'A: an inhibitor of protein synthesis synthesized with an enzyme fraction from interferon-treated cells. *Proc. Natl. Acad. Sci. U.S.A.* 1978;75:256.

360. Clemens, M. J., and B. R. G. Williams. Inhibition of cell-free protein synthesis by pppA2'p5'A2'p5'A: a novel oligonucleotide synthesized by interferon-treated L cell extracts. *Cell* 1978;13:565.

361. Baglioni, C., M. A. Minks, and P. A. Maroney. Interferon action may be mediated by activation of a nuclease by pppA2'p5'A2'p5'A. *Nature* 1978;273:684.

362. Ratner, L., R. C. Wiegand, P. J. Farrell, G. C.

Sen, B. Cabrer, and P. Lengyel. Interferon, double-stranded RNA and RNA degradation. Fractionation of the endonuclease$_{INT}$ system into two macromolecular components; role of a small molecule in nuclease activation. *Biochem. Biophys. Res. Commun.* 1978;81:947.

363. Leblou, B., G. C. Sen, S. Shaila, B. Cabrer, and P. Lengyel. Interferon, double stranded RNA and protein phosphorylation. *Proc. Natl. Acad. Sci. U.S.A.* 1976;73:3107.

364. Roberts, W. K., A. Hovanessian, R. E. Brown, M. J. Clemens, and I. M. Kerr. Interferon-mediated protein kinase and low molecular weight inhibitor of protein synthesis. *Nature* 1976;264:477.

365. Zilberstein, A., A. Kimchi, A. Schmidt, and M. Revel. Isolation of two interferon-induced translational inhibitors: a protein kinase and an oligo-isoadenylate synthetase. *Proc. Natl. Acad. Sci. U.S.A.* 1978;75:4734.

366. Hovanessian, A. The double-stranded RNA activated protein kinase induced by interferon. *J. Interferon Res.* 1989;9:641.

367. Farrell, P. J., G. C. Sen, M. F. Dubois, L. Ratner, E. Slattery, and P. Lengyel. Interferon action: two distinct pathways for the inhibition of protein synthesis by double-stranded RNA. *Proc. Natl. Acad. Sci. U.S.A.* 1978;75:5893.

368. Samuel, C. E. Mechanism of interferon action: Phosphorylation of protein synthesis initiation factor eIF-2 in interferon-treated human cells by a ribosome-associated kinase processing site specificity similar to hemin-regulated rabbit reticulocyte kinase. *Proc. Natl. Acad. Sci. U.S.A.* 1979;76:600.

369. Staeheli, P. Interferon-induced proteins and the antiviral state. *Adv. Virus Res.* 1990;38:147.

370. DeMaeyer, E., and J. DeMaeyer-Guignard. *Interferons and Other Regulatory Cytokines.* New York: John Wiley and Sons, 1988.

371. Kelly, A., S. Powis, R. Glynne, E. Radley, S. Beck, and J. Trowsdale. Second proteasome-related gene in the human MHC class II region. *Nature* 1991; 353:667.

372. Enomoto, N., I. Sakuma, Y. Asahina, M. Kurosaki, T. Murakami, C. Yamamoto, Y. Ogura, N. Izumi, F. Marumo, and C. Sato. Mutations in the nonstructural protein 5A gene and response to interferon in patients with chronic hepatitis C virus 1b infection. *N. Engl. J. Med.* 1996;334:77.

373. Herion, D., and J. H. Hoofnagle. The interferon sensitivity determining region: all hepatitis C virus isolates are not the same. *Hepatology* 1997;25:769.

374. Bertoletti, A., A. Sette, F. V. Chisari, A. Penna, M. Levrero, M. De Carli, F. Fiaccadori, and C. Ferrari. Natural variants of cytotoxic epitopes are T-cell receptor antagonists for antiviral cytotoxic T cells. *Nature* 1994;369:407.

375. Constantoulakis, P., M. Campbell, B. K. Felber, G. Nasoiulas, E. Afonina, and G. N. Pavlakis. Inhibition of Rev-mediated HIV-1 expression by an RNA binding protein encoded by the interferon-inducible 9–27 gene. *Science* 1993;259:1314.

376. Gooding, L. R. Viruses that counteract host immune defenses. *Cell* 1992;71:5.

377. Imani, F., and B. Jacobs. Inhibitory activity for the interferon-induced protein kinase is associated with

the reovirus serotype 1 a3 protein. *Proc. Natl. Acad. Sci. U.S.A.* 1988;85:7887.

378. Kitajewski, J., R. J. Schneider, B. Sfer, S. M. Munemitsu, C. E. Samuel, B. Thimmappaya, and T. Shenk. Adenovirus VAI RNA antagonizes the antiviral action of interferon by preventing activation of the interferon-induced eIF-2A kinase. *Cell* 1986;45:195.

379. Lennette, E. H. Viral respiratory diseases: vaccines and antivirals. *Bull. WHO* 1981;59:305.

380. Pollard, R. B. Interferons and interferon inducers: development of clinical usefulness and therapeutic promise. *Drugs* 1982;23:37.

381. Champney, K. J., D. P. Levine, H. B. Levy, and A. M. Lerner. Modified polyinosinic-polyribocytidylic acid complex: sustained interferonemia and its physiological associates in humans. *Infect. Immun.* 1979;25:831.

382. Levy, H. B., and F. L. Riley. Utilization of stabilized forms of polynucleotides. In *Interferons and Their Applications*, ed. by P. E. Came and W. A. Carter. New York: Springer-Verlag, 1984, pp. 515–533.

383. Goeddel, D. V., E. Yelverton, A. Ullrich, H. L. Heyneker, G. Miozzari, W. Holmes, P. H. Seeburg, T. Dull, L. May, N. Stebbing, R. Crea, S. Maeda, R. McCandliss, A. Sloma, J. M. Tabor, M. Grass, P. C. Familletti, and S. Pestka. Human leukocyte interferon produced by *E. coli* is biologically active. *Nature* 1980; 287:411.

384. Merigan, T. C., S. E. Reed, T. S. Hall, and D. A. J. Tyrrell. Inhibition of respiratory virus infection by locally applied interferon. *Lancet* 1973;1:563.

385. Hayden, F. G., and J. M. Gwaltney. Intranasal interferon α2 for prevention of rhinovirus infection and illness. *J. Infect. Dis.* 1983;148:543.

386. Samo, T. C., S. B. Greenberg, R. B. Couch, J. Quarles, P. E. Johnson, S. Hook, and M. W. Harmon. Efficacy and tolerance of intranasally applied recombinant leukocyte A interferon in normal volunteers. *J. Infect. Dis.* 1983;148:535.

387. Hayden, F. G., J. K. Albrecht, D. L. Kaiser, and J. M. Gwaltney. Prevention of natural colds by contact prophylaxis with intranasal alpha 2-interferon. *N. Engl. J. Med.* 1986;314:71.

388. Armstrong, J. A. Clinical use of interferons: systemic administration in viral diseases. In *Interferons and Their Applications*, ed. by P. E. Came and W. A. Carter. New York: Springer-Verlag, 1984, pp. 455–469.

389. Hoofnagle, J. H., and A. M. DiBisceglie. The treatment of chronic viral hepatitis. *N. Engl. J. Med.* 1997;336:347.

390. Alter, M. J., and E. E. Mast. The epidemiology of viral hepatitis in the United States. *Gastroenterol. Clin. North Am.* 1994;23:437.

391. Lau, J. Y. N., and T. L. Wright. Molecular virology and pathogenesis of hepatitis B. *Lancet* 1993; 342:1335.

392. Di Bisceglie, A. M., T. L. Fong, M. W. Fried, M. G. Swain, B. Baker, J. Korenman, N. V. Bergase, J. G. Waggoner, Y. Park, and J. H. Hoofnagle. A randomized, controlled trial of recombinant alpha-interferon therapy for chronic hepatitis B. *Am. J. Gastroenterol.* 1993;88:1887.

393. Narkewicz, M. R., D. Smith, A. Silverman, J. Vierling, and R. J. Sokol. Clearance of chronic hepatitis B virus infection in young children after alpha interferon treatment. *J. Pediatr.* 1995;127:815.

394. Niederau, C., T. Heintges, S. Lange, G. Goldman, C. M. Niederau, L. Mohr, and D. Haussinger. Long-term follow-up of HbeAg-positive patients treated with interferon alfa for chronic hepatitis B. *N. Engl. J. Med.* 1996;334:1422.

395. Farci, P., A. Mandas, A. Coiana, M. E. Lai, V. Desmet, P. Var Eyken, Y. Gibo, L. Caruso, S. Scaccabarozzi, D. Criscuolo, J. C. Ryff, and A. Balestrieri. Treatment of chronic hepatitis D with interferon alfa-2a. *N. Engl. J. Med.* 1994;330:88.

396. Koff, R. S. Chronic hepatitis C: early intervention. *Hosp. Pract.* 1998;33(6):101.

397. Poynard, T., V. Leroy, M. Cohard, T. Thevenot, P. Mathurin, P. Opolon, and J. P. Zarski. Meta-analysis of interferon randomized trials in the treatment of viral hepatitis C: effects of dose and duration. *Hepatology* 1996;24:778.

398. Davis, G. L., L. A. Balart, E. R. Schiff, K. Lindsay, H. C. Bodenheimer, R. P. Perrillo, W. Carey, I. M. Jacobson, J. Payne, J. L. Dienstag, D. H. Van Thiel, C. Tamburro, J. Lefkowitch, J. Albrecht, C. Meschievitz, T. J. Ortego, A. Gibas, and the Hepatitis Interventional Therapy Group. Treatment of chronic hepatitis C with recombinant interferon alfa. A multicenter randomized, controlled trial. *N. Engl. J. Med.* 1989;321:1501.

399. DiBisceglie, A. M., P. Martin, C. Kassianides, M. Lisker-Melman, L. Murray, J. Waggoner, Z. Goodman, S. M. Banks, and J. H. Hoofnagle. Recombinant interferon alfa therapy for chronic hepatitis C. A randomized, double-blind, placebo controlled trial. *N. Engl. J. Med.* 1989;321:1506.

400. Brillanti, S., J. Garson, M. Foli, K. Whitby, R. Deaville, C. Masci, M. Miglioli, and L. Barbara. A pilot study of combination therapy with ribavirin plus interferon alfa for interferon alfa-resistant chronic hepatitis C. *Gastroenterology* 1994;107:812.

401. Lai, M.-Y., J. H. Kao, P. M. Yang, J. T. Wang, P. J. Chen, K. W. Chan, J. S. Chu, and D. S. Chen. Long-term efficacy of ribavirin plus interferon alfa in the treatment of chronic hepatitis C. *Gastroenterology* 1996;111:1307.

402. Eron, L. J., F. Judson, S. Tucker, S. Prawer, J. Mills, K. Murphy, M. Hickey, M. Rogers, S. Flannigan, N. Hien, H. Katz, S. Goldman, A. Gottlieb, K. Adams, P. Burton, D. Tanner, E. Taylor, and E. Peets, Interferon therapy for condylomata acuminata. *N. Engl. J. Med.* 1986;315:1059.

403. Friedman-Kien, A. E., L. J. Eron, M. Conant, W. Growdon, H. Badiak, P. W. Bradstreet, D. Fedorczyk, J. R. Trout, and T. F. Plasse. Natural interferon-alfa for treatment of condylomata accuminata. *JAMA* 1988;259:533.

404. Douglas, J. M., L. J. Eron, F. Judson, M. Rogers, M. B. Alder, E. Taylor, D. Tanner, and E. Peets. A randomized trial of combination therapy with intralesional interferon α-2b and podophyllin versus podophyllin alone for the therapy of anogenital warts. *J. Infect. Dis.* 1990;162:52.

405. Condylomata International Collaborative Study Group. Randomized placebo-controlled double-blind combined therapy with laser surgery and systemic interferon α-2b in the treatment of anogenital condylomata acuminatum. *J. Infect. Dis.* 1993;167:824.

406. Frissen, P. H., F. de Wolf, P. J. Bakker, C. H. Veenhof, S. A. Danner, J. Goudsmit, and J. M. Lange. High-dose interferon-alpha2a exerts potent activity against human immunodeficiency virus type 1 not associated with antitumor activity in subjects with Kaposi's sarcoma. *J. Infect. Dis.* 1997;176:811.

407. Frissen, P. H., M. E. van der Ende, C. H. Napel, H. M. Weigel, G. S. Schreij, R. H. Kaufmann, P. P. Koopmans, A. I. Hoepelman, J. B. de Boer, G. J. Weverling, G. Haverkamp, P. Dowd, F, Miedema, R. Schuurman, C. A. B, Boucher, and J. M. A Lange: Zidovadine and interferon-α combination therapy versus zidovudine monotherapy in subjects with symptomatic human immunodeficiency virus type 1 infection. *J. Infect. Dis.* 1994;169:1351.

408. Wills, R. J., S. Dennis, H. E. Spiegel, D. M. Gibson, and P. I. Nadler. Interferon kinetics and adverse reactions after intravenous, intramuscular, and subcutaneous injection. *Clin. Pharmacol. Ther.* 1984;35:722.

409. Wills, R. J. Clinical pharmacokinetics of interferons. *Clin. Pharmacokinet.* 1990;19:390.

410. Dorr, R. T. Interferon-α in malignant and viral diseases. *Drugs* 1993;45:177.

411. Smith, R. A., F. Norris, D. Palmer, L. Bernhardt, and R. J. Wills. Distribution of alpha interferon in serum and cerebrospinal fluid after systemic administration. *Clin. Pharmacol. Ther.* 1985;37:85.

412. Merigan, T. C. Pharmacokinetics and side effects of interferon in man. *Texas Rep. Biol. Med.* 1977; 35:541.

413. Hirsch, M. S., N. E. Tolkoff-Rubin, A. P. Kelley, and R. H. Rubin. Pharmacokinetics of human and recombinant leukocyte interferon in patients with chronic renal failure who are undergoing hemodialysis. *J. Infect. Dis.* 1983;148:335.

414. Cheeseman, S. H., R. H. Rubin, J. A. Stewart, N. E. Tolkoff-Rubin, A. B. Cosimi, K. Cantell, J. Gilbert, S. Winkle, J. T. Herrin, P. H. Black, P. S. Russell, and M. S. Hirsch. Controlled clinical trial of prophylactic human leukocyte interferon in renal transplantation: effects on cytomegalovirus and herpes simplex virus infections. *N. Engl. J. Med.* 1979;300:1345.

415. Greenberg, S. B., and M. W. Harmon. Clinical use of interferons: localized application in viral diseases. In *Interferons and Their Applications*, ed. by P. E. Came and W. A. Carter. New York: Springer-Verlag, 1984, pp. 433–453.

416. Hayden, F. G., S. E. Mills, and M. E. Johns. Human tolerance and histopathologic effects of long-term administration of intranasal interferon-α2. *J. Infect. Dis.* 1983;148:914.

417. Quesada, J. R., M. Talpaz, A. Rios, R. Kurzrock, and J. U. Gutterman. Clinical toxicity of interferons in cancer patients: a review. *J. Clin. Oncol.* 1986; 4:234.

418. Merigan, T. C., K. H. Rand, R. B. Pollard, P. S. Abdallah. G. W. Jordan, and R. P. Fried. Human leukocyte interferon for the treatment of herpes zoster in patients with cancer. *N. Engl. J. Med.* 1978;298:981.

419. Smith, C. I., J. Weissberg, L. Bernhardt, P. B. Gregory, W. S. Robinson, and T. C. Merigan. Acute Dane particle suppression with recombinant leukocyte A interferon in chronic hepatitis B virus infection. *J. Infect. Dis.* 1983;148:907.

420. Gutterman, J. U., S. Fine, J. Quesada, S. J. Horning, J. F. Levine, R. Alexanian, L. Bernhardt, M. Kramer, H. Spiegel, W. Colburn, P. Trown, T. Merigan, and Z. Dziewanowski. Recombinant leukocyte A interferon: pharmacokinetics, single-dose tolerance, and biologic effects in cancer patients. *Ann. Intern. Med.* 1882;96:549.

421. Haria, M., and P. Benfield. Interferon-α-2a. A review of its pharmacological properties and therapeutic use in the management of viral hepatitis. *Drugs* 1995;50:873.

422. Thomas, H. C., A. S. Lok, V. Carreno, G. Farrell, H. Tanno, V. Perez, G. M. Dusheiko, G. Cooksley, and J. C. Ryff. Comparative study of three doses of interferon-alpha 2a in chronic active hepatitis B. The International Hepatitis Trial Group. *J. Viral Hepat.* 1995;1:139.

423. Goldstein, D., R. Gockerman, R. Krishnan, J. Ritchie, C. Y. Tso, L. E. Hood, E. Ellinwood, and J. Laszlo. Effects of γ-interferon on the endocrine system: results from a phase I study. *Cancer Res.* 1987;47:6397.

424. Peters, M. G., and S. J. Burgess. Interferons. In *Antimicrobial Therapy and Vaccines*, ed. by V. Yu, T. Merigan, S. Barriere, A. Sugar, D. Raoult, C. Piloquin, and M. Iseman. Baltimore: Williams and Wilkins, 1999, pp. 1426–1434.

425. Renault, P. F., and J. H. Hoofnagle. Side effects of alpha interferon. *Semin. Liver Dis.* 1989;9:273.

426. Greenberg, P. L. and S. A. Mosny. Cytotoxic effects of interferon in vitro on granulocytic progenitor cells. *Cancer Res.* 1977;37:1794.

427. Antonelli, G., M. Currenti, O. Turriziani, and F. Dianzani. Neutralizing antibodies to interferon-α: relative frequency in patients treated with different interferon preparations. *J. Infect. Dis.* 1991;163:882.

428. Pittau, E., A. Bogliolo, A. Tinti, Q. Mela, G. Ibba, G. Salis, and G. Perpignano. Development of ar-

thritis and hypothyroidism during alpha-interferon therapy for chronic hepatitis. *Clin. Exp. Rheumatol.* 1997; 15:415.

429. Parkinson, A., J. Lasker, M. J. Kramer, M.-T. Huang, P. E. Thomas, D. E. Ryan, L. M. Reik, R. L. Norman, W. Levin, and A. H. Conney. Effects of three recombinant human leukocyte interferons on drug metabolism in mice. *Drug Metab. Dispos. Biol. Fate Chem.* 1982;10:579.

430. Williams, S. J., J. A. Baird-Lamber, and G. C. Farrell. Inhibition of theophylline metabolism by interferon. *Lancet* 1987;2:939.

431. Witter, F. R., A. S. Woods, M. D. Griffin, C. R. Smith, P. Nadler, and P. S Lietman. Effects of prednisone, aspirin and acetaminophen on an in vivo biologic response to interferon in humans. *Clin. Pharmacol. Ther.* 1988;44:239.

432. Nicholson, K. G. Antiviral agents. In *Antibiotic and Chemotherapy*, ed. by F. O'Grady, H. Lambert, R. Finch, and D. Greenwood. New York: Churchill Livingstone, 1997, pp. 541–576.

433. Gilbert, B. E., and V. Knight. Minireview: biochemistry and clinical applications of ribavirin. *Antimicrob. Agents Chemother.* 1986;30:201.

434. Huggins, J. W. Prospects for treatment of viral hemorrhagic fevers with ribavirin, a broad-spectrum antiviral drug. *Rev. Infect. Dis.* 1989;2:S750.

435. Patterson J. L., and R. Fernandez-Larsson. Molecular mechanisms of action of ribavirin. *Rev. Infect. Dis.* 1990;12:1139.

436. Laskin, O. L., J. A. Longstreet, C. C. Hart, D. Scavuzzo, C. M. Kalman, J. D. Connor, and R. B. Roberts. Ribavirin disposition in high-risk patients for acquired immunodeficiency syndrome. *Clin. Pharmacol. Ther.* 1987;41:546.

437. Englund, J. A., P. Peidra, Y.-M. Ahn, B. E. Gilbert, and P. Hiatt. High dose, short-duration ribavirin aerosol therapy compared with standard ribavirin therapy in children with suspected respiratory syncytial virus infection. *J. Pediatr.* 1994;125:635.

438. Drugs for non-HIV viral infections. *Med. Lett.* 1997;39:69.

CHAPTER SEVENTEEN

Chemotherapy of Viral Infections, II

Antiretroviral Agents

Human immunodeficiency virus (HIV) attacks the immune system, specifically CD4+ T lymphocytes and other susceptible cells, resulting in immunodeficiency leading to opportunistic infection and malignancy. The disease caused by HIV is called *Auto Immune Deficiency Syndrome* (AIDS). Several antiretroviral drugs are active against HIV infection, and this chapter discusses those drugs, as well as some common questions and controversies regarding antiretroviral therapy.

Replication of HIV

The complex replication cycle of HIV, offers several potential sites for intervention with antiretroviral drugs.[1-4] (shown in Fig. 17–1).[5] The host becomes infected by exposure to blood or body fluids containing HIV. The virus then attaches to target cells through binding of the viral surface glycoprotein gp120 to CD4 molecules located on the membranes of certain T lymphocytes and macrophages/monocytes, and the virus is internalized by fusion with the host cell membrane. After internalization, the HIV virion is uncoated, releasing viral genomic RNA into the host cell. Reverse transcriptase, an enzyme located in the core of the virion, then uses the viral RNA to make a complementary single-stranded DNA copy, which is duplicated to form the double-stranded proviral DNA. The reverse transcriptase enzyme is specific to retroviruses and is thus a primary target for certain antiretroviral drugs. The proviral DNA then migrates into the nucleus and becomes integrated with the genetic material of the host cell, and the integrated proviral DNA is transcribed into messenger RNA, which is translated into viral proteins. Following translation, a virus-specific protease cleaves the large precursor polyproteins into smaller, functional peptides. The protease is another target for anti-HIV drugs, and inhibition of this enzyme leads to the production of noninfectious, immature HIV particles. After assembly of the viral proteins in the cytoplasm, the new virus buds from the cell surface and is released into the blood where it can infect other CD4+ T cells. After viral infection, the host cell dies, resulting in a decrease in the number of CD4+ T lymphocytes and predisposing the patient to opportunistic infections and the development the unusual malignancies characteristic of AIDS (e.g., Kaposi's sarcoma).

Therapy of HIV Infection

Combination Therapy

AIDS is now treated with drug combinations, and the development of several new antiretroviral agents has led to dramatic change in AIDS therapy. Formerly, the standard treatment for AIDS involved administration of one of the reverse transcriptase inhibitors, such as zidovudine (AZT), but many studies have demonstrated the superi-

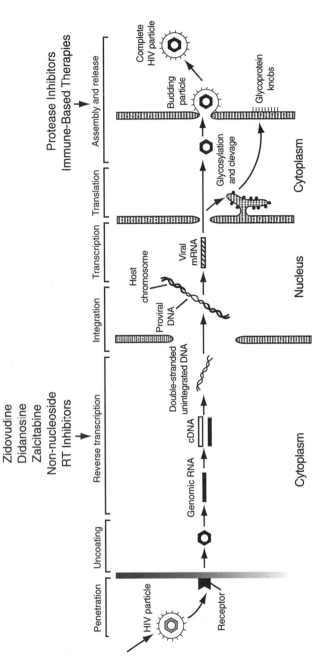

Zidovudine
Didanosine
Zalcitabine
Non-nucleoside
RT Inhibitors

Protease Inhibitors
Immune-Based Therapies

Penetration | Uncoating | Reverse transcription | Integration | Transcription | Translation | Assembly and release

HIV particle

Receptor

Genomic RNA

cDNA

Double-stranded unintegrated DNA

Proviral DNA

Host chromosome

Viral mRNA

Glycosylation and cleavage

Budding particle

Glycoprotein knobs

Complete HIV particle

Cytoplasm

Nucleus

Cytoplasm

Figure 17–1. Replication cycle of HIV and potential sites of inhibition by antiretroviral agents. RT, reverse transcriptase. (From Hirsch and D'Aquila.[5])

ority of combination therapy over mono-therapy, both with respect to an increase in CD4 cell count and a decrease in viral titer.[6-10] Combination regimens consisting of two nucleoside reverse transcriptase inhibitors and a protease inhibitor are now initiated early in the disease process.[11]

Combination therapy provides several potential advantages over monotherapy. Two or more drugs may have additive or synergistic effects; thus, disease progression is slowed and survival is improved.[11] Synergism permits administration of drugs at lower doses than in single-drug therapy, resulting in decreased toxicity. Because two or more drugs in the combination have different mechanisms of action, combination therapy may also delay or prevent the emergence of a resistant virus. It has been estimated that at least 10 billion HIV particles are produced and destroyed daily, not only in blood but also in lymphoid tissues and in the central nervous system. With single-drug therapy, resistant mutants are readily selected, ensuring therapeutic failure.[11] The drugs used in combination therapy may also penetrate into different cellular and tissue reservoirs of the virus.

Drugs given in combination can be administered simultaneously or in alternation. When given simultaneously, the two or more drugs are administered during the entire treatment period. The drawback of this mode of therapy is the possibility of increasing the severity of the toxicity. If the drugs are given in alternation, a single drug is given for a defined time period and then the patient is switched to a second drug. This may provide a respite that results in decreased toxicity; however, there may be decreased efficacy and little delay in the development of resistance.

Treatment Strategies

Two sets of guidelines for therapy of HIV infection have been issued by the International AIDS Society (IAS)—USA Panel[8] and by the U.S. Department of Health and Human Services.[12] The recommendations are similar, but they differ as to when therapy should be initiated. The IAS guidelines rec-ommend initiating therapy for all patients with plasma HIV RNA levels greater than 5000 to 10,000 copies/ml regardless of the patient's CD4[+] count. The federal guidelines recommend starting therapy when the CD4[+] count is lower than 500 cells/mm[3] or when plasma HIV RNA concentrations are greater than 10,000 to 20,000 copies/ml.[12] Both guidelines recommend therapy for all patients with symptomatic HIV disease, regardless of the viral load or CD4[+] count, and both recommend that the initial regimen should be aggressive, with the goal of suppressing plasma viral load to undetectable levels. Each regimen consists of two nucleoside analogs plus a potent protease inhibitor. If protease inhibitors cannot be used, the recommended alternative is a combination of two nucleoside reverse transcriptase inhibitors (NRTIs) plus a non-nucleoside reverse transcriptase inhibitor (NNRTI), preferably nevirapine rather than delavirdine. Upon initiating therapy, all drugs should be started simultaneously and at full doses, except when dose escalation is recommended, as with ritonavir and nevirapine.

For patients experiencing treatment failure, or when there is intolerance to therapy, or in cases of noncompliance, a change of therapy may be indicated. In the case of treatment failure, the guidelines recommend changing all the drugs in the triple-drug combination regimen or, minimally, at least two of the three. In the case of drug toxicity, just the drug causing the toxicity should be replaced. If noncompliance is the problem, the reasons should be identified and a simpler regimen may be appropriate in some cases, even if it is less potent. Therapy should be continued as long as possible. In general, stopping all antiretroviral therapy is reasonable when the patient, after discussion with the physician, believes that the adverse effects outweigh the potential benefits of therapy.

The use of antiretroviral therapy in pregnancy has been extensively reviewed by the U.S. Public Health Service task force.[13] In most respects, HIV infection in pregnant women should be treated as infection in nonpregnant patients; however, in some situations, therapy must be altered. The potential effects of therapy on the fetus are currently unknown, so women in their first trimester of pregnancy and not yet on antiretroviral therapy may want to delay initiation of therapy until after 10 to 12 weeks gestation when the fetus is less susceptible to teratogenic effects. If the woman is already taking combination therapy and then becomes pregnant, most experts recommend that she continue therapy, even during the first trimester. Zidovudine should be part of all regimens for HIV-infected pregnant women, as it is presently the only drug proven to reduce perinatal transmission of the virus.[12]

One of the major public health implications of antiretroviral therapy is the development and transmission of drug resistance.[14] Development of HIV-1 resistance against antiviral compounds is due to a series of amino acid substitutions in the enzymes targeted by the antiretroviral drugs. These in turn result from mutations in the viral genes that code for these enzymes and follow directly from the high error rate of the viral reverse transcriptase that is responsible for copying viral RNA.[15,16] Viral mutants are selected under selective pressure exerted artificially by the use of antiviral drugs and naturally by the immune system. With some of the antiretroviral drugs, resistance can develop very rapidly, and with single-drug therapy, high-level resistance can occur within 1 month of the start of treatment. A significant public health risk ensues if the resistant virus is widely transmitted by continuing certain high-risk behavior. It is hoped that the early initiation of treatment with powerful multidrug combinations will block the selection of such resistant viruses.[17]

Nucleoside Analog Reverse Transcriptase Inhibitors

The NRTIs were the first class of agents approved for treating HIV infection. By inhibiting the reverse transcriptase enzyme, the NRTIs block the initial phase of viral replication; thus, these drugs can prevent infection of new cells but they do not affect chronically infected cells where the HIV genome is already integrated into the host genome. There are six federally approved members of this group: zidovudine, didanosine, zalcitabine, stavudine, lamivudine, and abacavir (Fig. 17–2). Adefovir, a nucleotide inhibitor of reverse transcriptase, is also approved for use in treatment.

Adefovir

Mechanism of Action

All the nucleoside inhibitors of HIV reverse transcriptase are dideoxynucleosides that share a common mechanism of action. Inhibition of reverse transcriptase prevents conversion of the viral RNA genome into a double-stranded DNA copy prior to integration into the cell genome.[4,18] This action occurs early in the replication cycle, so these agents work best against acute infections and are less active against chronic ones. These drugs are both inhibitors of and substrates for the reverse transcriptase enzyme, and they are selective for HIV because of their greater affinity for the viral reverse transcriptase then for human DNA polymerases. To inhibit the enzyme the NRTIs have to bind to the enzyme–template–primer complex. The affinity for this complex is higher for the natural substrate dNTPs than for the nucleoside inhibitors.

The NRTIs are actually pro-drugs that must first be phosphorylated to the triphosphate, similar to the natural deoxynucleosides whose function they mimic. Reverse transcriptase inhibitors diffuse into the cell and are then converted to their active triphosphate forms by cellular kinases. The amount of intracellular triphosphate formation correlates closely with a reduction in HIV infectivity and cytopathic effects in vitro.[19] Figure 17–3 shows the cellular uptake and phophorylation patterns of the nucleo-

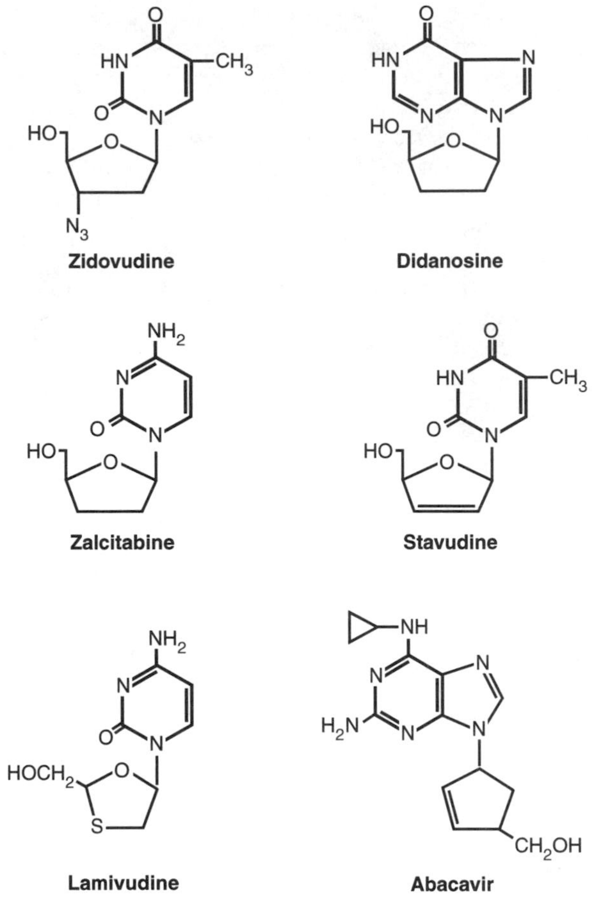

Figure 17–2. Nucleoside analog reverse transcriptase inhibitors.

side analogs. Once activated, the dideoxynucleotides are incorporated into the growing viral DNA strand and cause premature chain termination due to their lack of a 3'-hydroxyl group. The differences in the mechanisms of phosphorylation, metabolism, and their specificity for viral versus cellular polymerases explain much of the variation in antiviral activity and clinical toxicity among these compounds.

Of the NRTIs, the mechanism of action of zidovudine has been studied most extensively. Zidovudine is a synthetic pyrimidine analog that differs from thymidine in having an azido substituent instead of a hydroxyl group at the 3' position of the deoxyribose ring. It was initially developed as an anticancer drug and then subsequently found to inhibit the reverse transcriptase of Friend leukemia virus.[20] Soon after a human retrovirus was found to be the cause of AIDS, zidovudine was shown to have anti-HIV activity in vitro.[21] The active form of zidovudine, AZT-triphosphate (AZT-TP), is a competitive inhibitor of the reverse transcriptase. It binds better to the HIV-1 reverse transcriptase than its natural substrate, thymidine triphosphate (TTP), and it functions as an alternate substrate for the enzyme.[22,23] AZT-TP has a 100-fold greater affinity for reverse transcriptase than for the cellular DNA polymerases alpha or beta.[24,25] The intracellular concentration of AZT-TP is greater than the K_i value for the HIV-1 reverse transcriptase but is less than the K_i values for the cellular polymerases.[24] AZT-TP is also incorporated into growing DNA chains, but because the incorporated AZT-TP does not possess a 3'-hydroxyl group to form a phosphodiester bond with the incom-

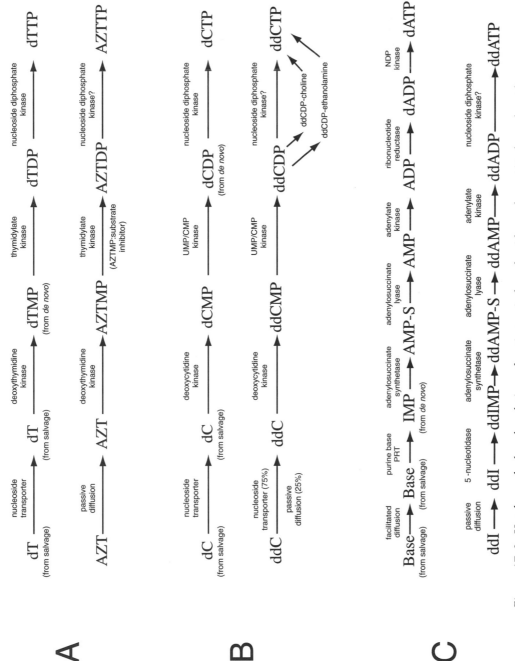

Figure 17–3. Uptake and phosphorylation of antiretroviral nucleoside analogs. (A) deoxythymidine (dT) and its analog zidovudine (AZT); (B) deoxycytidine (dC) and its analog zalcitabine (ddC); (C) deoxyadenosine (purine base) and its analog didanosine (ddI). PRT, phosphoribosyl transferase. (Adapted from Flexner and Hendrix.[18])

ing nucleotide, chain elongation is terminated at thymidine residues.[23,25]

Phosphorylation of zidovudine to its active form, AZT-TP, is accomplished by cellular enzymes (Fig. 17–3). For example, zidovudine is an efficient substrate for cellular thymidine kinase, which converts it to AZT-MP in infected and uninfected cells. The monophosphate accumulates in cells because of slow phosphorylation to AZT-diphosphate (AZT-DP) by host-cell thymidylate kinase, the rate-limiting step in AZT-TP formation. Because AZT-MP is a competitive inhibitor of thymidylate kinase, it reduces the conversion of TMP to TDP thus decreasing formation of TTP. AZT-MP may also inhibit the RNase H activity of HIV reverse transcriptase.[26]

Zidovudine has a complicated pharmacology in that a wide range of AZT-TP concentrations result within lymphocytes, even among individuals taking the same dose of the drug and having the same extracellular pharmacokinetics. Accordingly, zidovudine plasma concentrations correlate poorly with clinical response to the drug, and total phosphorylated zidovudine concentrations in patients correlate only modestly with markers of HIV disease progression[27] and poorly with its antiviral and toxic effects.[28] The great variations in intracellular AZT-TP concentrations with uniform dosing in clinical trials may partially account for the modest clinical benefit of zidovudine despite its very high in vitro antiviral activity.

The other nucleoside inhibitors also compete with natural nucleoside triphosphate substrates after conversion to their respective triphosphates and act as chain terminators if incorporated into the DNA. Like zidovudine, stavudine (2', 3'-didehydro-2', 3' dideoxythymidine) [d4T] is a deoxythymidine analog. Zalcitabine (2',3'dideoxycytidine) [ddC] and lamivudine (2'-deoxy-3'-thiacytidine) [3TC] are analogs of deoxycytidine. Didanosine (2',3'-dideoxyinosine) [ddI] is an analog of deoxyadenosine, and it is converted to dideoxyadenosine (ddA) after absorption and before phosphorylation. Abacavir is anabolized by a unique intracellular mechanism to form carbovir triphosphate, which potently and selectively inhibits HIV reverse transcriptase.[29] Adefovir dipivoxil is an orally bioavailable pro-drug of 9-(2-phosphonylmethoxyethyl) adenine, a monophosphated acyclic nucleotide analog. It has a similar mechanism of action to the nucleoside inhibitors.

Resistance

Viral resistance to NRTIs is the major cause of failure of anti-HIV therapy. Viruses resistant to zidovudine were first identified in isolates from patients treated with zidovudine for at least 6 months.[30] HIV-1 also develops resistance to zidovudine after in vitro serial passage in subinhibitory drug concentrations.[31] Resistance is usually associated with point mutations leading to amino acid substitutions at multiple sites in the reverse transcriptase enzyme, with multiple mutations being required to confer high-level resistance.[30,32] The highest level of resistance, which is associated with four or five of these substitutions, results in a 100-fold increase in 50% inhibitory concentration (IC_{50}) of zidovudine. Clinical isolates from patients undergoing prolonged zidovudine therapy can have varied levels of resistance and some retain full susceptibility even after years of therapy. The likelihood of zidovudine resistance increases with the duration of therapy and advancing disease,[33] but low levels of resistance can be found in infected individuals before zidovudine treatment.[34] Once therapy is terminated, the zidovudine-resistant virus may be slowly replaced by more susceptible virus, indicating that the wild-type virus has a growth advantage in the absence of drug.[35]

Some of the mutations in the reverse transcriptase found in zidovudine resistance occur in the deoxynucleoside triphosphate binding site close to the polymerase active site and result in decreased AZT-TP binding to the enzyme in vitro.[36] However, not all residues altered by mutation cluster near the polymerase-active site; some are physically distant and may affect reverse transcriptase function in other ways.[37] Most of the mutations seem to increase the enzymatic specificity for natural deoxynucleoside triphosphate binding over the synthetic nucleoside inhibitors, reducing the sensitivity to the NRTIs.[38–40] Such a mechanism could explain the modest level of NRTI cross-resistance for some mutants that are selelected under monotherapy.

Zidovudine-resistant virus is cross-resistant only to those HIV reverse transcriptase inhibitors that contain a 3'-azido substituent, such as 3'-azido-2',3'-dideoxyuridine (dideoxyuridine).[30] Cloned mutant viruses that differ from the wild type only in that they possess specific zidovudine resistance mutations are not cross-resistant to didanosine, zalcitabine, or stavudine.[30] However, some clinical zidovudine-resistant isolates have been found that are cross-resistant to stavudine,[41] which is also a deoxythymidine analog. Resistance to the other nucleoside analogs besides zidovudine also results from mutations leading to amino acid substitutions in the reverse transcriptase. Resistance to lamivudine occurs rapidly in vivo, with a substitution at codon 184 being observed with both single-drug and combination therapy.[42,43] On the other hand, high-level resistance (>100-fold increase in IC_{50}) to didanosine or zalcitabine has been reported only rarely.[44,45] Adefovir, the nucleotide reverse transcriptase inhibitor, has been effective against HIV strains resistant to zidovudine and/or lamivudine.[46] Combination therapy with the NRTIs can select for mutations that are different from those selected with monotherapy. These mutations confer cross-resistance to all clinically used NRTIs, and the extent of resistance then becomes significantly higher than that observed with monotherapy.[47–49]

Pharmacokinetics

ABSORPTION AND BIOAVAILABILITY. Systemic bioavailability of the NRTIs is generally high after oral administration, ranging from 60% to 90% for all of them except didanosine, which has low and variable absorption.[18,50,51] Because didanosine is acid labile and degraded by gastric acid, it is best administered in the fasting state. A high-fat or high-protein meal slows the rate of absorption of zidovudine, reducing the maximum serum concentration without altering the area under the serum concentration X time curve (AUC).[18,52,53] This effect of food on absorption applies to all the nucleoside analogs except didanosine.[54]

DISTRIBUTION AND CENTRAL NERVOUS SYSTEM PENETRATION. The nucleoside analogs have low plasma protein binding, and most of them are widely distributed into tissues and cells. Most of them penetrate the central nervous system, with cerebrospinal fluid concentrations ranging from 10% to greater than 100% of the plasma levels.[18] Central nervous system entry probably occurs purely by diffusion. Although nucleoside transporters do exist, modification of the 3'-position of the sugar moiety greatly reduces the affinity of the nucleoside analogs for the transporters.[55,56]

METABOLISM AND EXCRETION. Most of the nucleoside analogs are rapidly cleared from the plasma, with elimination half-lives averaging about an hour.[18] However, the intracellular nucleoside triphosphates persist considerably longer, permitting long dosing intervals for these drugs. With the exception of zidovudine these agents are eliminated primarily as unchanged drug by the kidney and dosage adjustments must be made in renal failure.[57] With didanosine, up to 40% may be metabolized by the liver and some reduction of the dose may have to be considered in patients with moderate to severe hepatic impairment.[57] With zidovudine, 75% of the drug is metabolized by liver microsomal enzymes to the 5' O-glucuronide, which is then excreted by the kidneys. It is recommended that the daily dosage of zidovudine be reduced by 50% in patients with evidence of hepatic impairment.[58] There is evidence that the kidneys can also metabolize zidovudine.[59] Despite its extensive metabolism, the half-life of zidovudine increases significantly in renal impairment, and patients with renal impairment may be at increased risk of zidovudine-induced hematologic toxicity due to decreased production of erythropoietin. Therefore, it is recommended that the dose of zidovudine be reduced by about 50% in patients with severe renal dysfunction.[54,60] Abacavir is metabolized primarily by alcohol dehydrogenase and glucuronyl transferase, and only about 1% of a dose is excreted unchanged in the urine. The pharmacokinetic properties of the NRTIs are summarized in Table 17–1.

Therapeutic Use

Zidovudine was the first drug approved by the Food and Drug Administration (in 1987) for treating HIV infection. Treatment with zidovudine can prolong the survival of patients with progressive HIV disease and AIDS, reduce their incidence of opportunistic infections, and improve their well-being and performance. It also slows progression in patients with early symptomatic HIV infection and even may delay the onset of symptoms when administered to asymptomatic patients with HIV infection and CD4 counts >400 cells/mm[3].[9,61,62] Although zidovudine was initially administered alone, zidovudine-containing combination drug regimens that maximally suppress viral replication have been shown to be superior to monotherapy in delaying disease progression or death. In addition, significant resistance develops when zidovudine or the other NRTIs are used alone in therapy. As a result, zidovudine monotherapy is no longer recommended except when used to reduce perinatal HIV transmission in pregnant women.[63] None of the anti-HIV drugs has been shown to eradicate the infection, but used in combination they can decrease viral replication, impove immunologic status, delay infectious complications, and prolong life.[64] Most initial combination regimens contain zidovudine, at least partly because of its potential role in preventing the development of AIDS dementia complex.[65,66] Recommended combination regimens include the use of zidovudine with another nucleoside analog (i.e., didanosine, zalcitabine, or lamivudine), plus a potent protease inhibitor or a non-nucleoside reverse transcriptase inhibitor.[12] Zidovudine should not be used with stavudine because the combination may be antagonistic and could result in a decrease in CD4+ T-cell count.[12,65] Zidovudine is usually used in a dose of 600 mg day in divided doses administered as 200 mg three times daily (100 mg capsules) or as 300 mg twice daily (300 mg tablets).[12]

Didanosine, which was the second drug approved for the treatment of AIDS, is used primarily in combination with zidovudine or stavudine, plus a protease inhibitor or non-nucleoside reverse transcriptase inhibitor. It has overlapping toxicities with zalcitabine and thus should not be used with that drug.[12,64] For those weighing 60 kg or more, didanosine is used in a dose of 200 mg twice daily as tablets or 250 mg twice daily as the powder. For those who weigh less than 60 kg, it is given in a dose of 125 mg twice daily (tablets) or 167 mg twice daily (powder).[67,68] Didanosine is a useful and effective agent in both pediatric and adult patients who fail to respond to zidovudine therapy or who cannot tolerate zidovudine's toxicity. It has been shown to be effective in preventing opportunistic infections in patients who have previously received more than 16 weeks of zidovudine therapy.

Zalcitabine is used mainly in combination regimens with zidovudine and a protease inhibitor. It is inferior to zidovudine as a single agent and is indicated for combination therapy with zidovudine for patients with advanced AIDS who have demonstrated significant clinical or immunological deterioration. However, it should not be used with didanosine or stavudine because of overlapping toxicities.[69,70] Zalcitabine is given in a dose of 0.75 mg three times daily, preferably on an empty stomach, since food may affect absorption. Zalcitabine is used in adult patients who have failed zidovudine or didanosine therapy.

Stavudine is primarily used as an alternative to zidovudine in combination regimens when the patient cannot tolerate the hematological toxicity of zidovudine or in patients whose disease is still progressing while on zidovudine-containing regimens.[11,64,69] Lamivudine is used mainly in combination with zidovudine or stavudine plus a protease inhibitor or non-nucleoside reverse transcriptase inhibitor.[11,12] Several studies have now shown that the combination of lamivudine and zidovudine causes pronounced elevations in CD4 cell counts and reductions in viral load.[70,71] For example, one study

Table 17-1. *Pharmacokinetics of the nucleoside reverse transcriptase inhibitors.*

Parameter	Zidovudine	Didanosine	Stavudine	Zalcitabine	Lamivudine	Abacavir
Adult oral dose	200 mg tid or 300 mg bid	200 mg bid	40 mg bid	0.75 mg tid	150 mg bid	300 mg bid to tid
Oral bioavailability (%)	62–68	21–54	82	86–100	72–95	76–100
C_{max} (μg/ml)	0.9–1.2	1.95	4.1	0.08	3.3	2.94
T_{max} (h)	0.5–1	1.0	0.5–1.0	1–2	0.8–1.6	0.7–1.7
$T_{1/2}$ (h)	0.9–1.4	0.6–1.7	1.0–1.6	1.1–1.8	2.5	0.8–1.5
Protein binding (%)	20	<5	Negligible	<4	36 at 0.1 μg/ml and <10 at >1 μg/ml	50
Vd (Liters/kg)	1.4–1.8	0.9–4.9	0.5–1.1	0.5–0.6	1.0–1.6	0.9
CSF concentration (%)	15–135	21	11–160	9–37	17	18
Clearance route	Hepatic (75%), renal (15%–20%)	Renal (60%)	Renal (34%–41%)	Renal (75%)	Renal (68%–71%)	Renal (80% as metabolites)

C_{max}, peak drug concentration during a dosing interval; CSF concentration, % of plasma drug concentration achieved in cerebrospinal fluid; T_{max}, time at which C_{max} occurs during a dosing interval; Vd, apparent volume into which a drug is distributed, usually determined by plasma concentrations.

Source: Data from Flexner and Hendrix[18] and from the manufacturers.

showed that the addition of lamivudine to zidovudine-containing regimens significantly slowed disease progression and decreased mortality.[72] The addition of lamivudine to a zidovudine regimen also appears to delay the onset of zidovudine-resistant isolates and may even restore zidovudine sensitivity to zidovudine-resistant viral strains.[72] In order to prevent emergence of the lamivudine-associated mutations and loss of its antiviral activity, lamivudine should be used only in regimens designed to be fully suppressive.[8] Lamivudine is also approved for the treatment of chronic hepatitis B as the first oral treatment for this disease. It acts directly to interfere with viral replication leading to a reduced inflammatory response to hepatitis B infection of the liver.[73]

Abacavir was approved in 1998 for children and adults unable to tolerate or failing to respond to the available drug regimens. Administration of abacavir plus zidovudine plus lamivudine for 16 weeks to previously untreated patients raised CD4 counts and lowered plasma HIV RNA to undetectable levels in about two-thirds of patients.[29] Adefovir dipivoxil is useful in patients with previous failure of treatment with at least two NRTIs and one protease inhibitor. In previously untreated patients, 20 weeks of adefovir-containing triple or quadruple drug regimens were as effective as indinavir plus zidovudine and lamivudine in lowering plasma HIV RNA levels and raising CD4 counts.[74]

Toxicity

HIV infection is often associated with a wide range of symptoms, including headache, fever, fatigue, malaise, hematological abnormalities, and neurological symptoms, as well as with opportunistic infections. It is often difficult to distinguish adverse effects caused by the therapy from the effects of the viral infection itself. All of the approved nucleoside analogs possess significant dose-limiting toxicities and have only a small therapeutic window between the minimally effective dose and the maximally tolerated dose. The more serious of these adverse effects include bone marrow toxicity (e.g., zidovudine), pe-

ripheral neuropathy (e.g., zalcitabine, didanosine, stavudine), pancreatitis (e.g., didanosine), myopathy (e.g., zidovudine) and hepatic abnormalities (e.g., zidovudine, didanosine). When toxicity occurs, the dose has to be reduced or the drug discontinued until symptoms become tolerable or they clear up. Sometimes the drugs must be permanently discontinued. The toxicity of these compounds seems to depend on inhibition of cellular DNA polymerase α (nuclear DNA synthesis), β (endonuclease repair), γ (mitochondrial DNA synthesis), Δ (exonuclease proofreading), and ε (exonuclease repair). The mitochondrial polymerase γ and repair polymerase β are the most sensitive to inhibitory effects, while the nuclear polymerases are the least sensitive.[75] Toxicity results from a complex interaction with these polymerases as well as other factors. There is now substantial evidence that mitochondrial toxicity is common to all the serious adverse effects of NRTI therapy.[76] A major problem with this toxicity is that it has a delayed onset.

BONE MARROW TOXICITY. The most serious adverse effect of zidovudine is bone marrow toxicity, manifest as neutropenia and anemia. Marked anemia can occur as soon as 4 to 6 weeks after initiation of zidovudine therapy. This toxicity is reversible and dose dependent. It occurs within 1 month of starting therapy and is worse in the advanced stages of AIDS.[77] Although the concentration of zidovudine correlates with the occurrence of anemia, it does not always correlate with clinical efficacy, indicating that different factors are responsible for zidovudine's efficacy and toxicity.[78]

It appears that zidovudine metabolites other than the triphosphate, especially the monophosphate, play an important role in inhibition of growth of hematopoietic cells.[79] The AZT-MP inhibits cellular DNA polymerase 3'- to 5'-exonuclease function, thereby reducing the excision of zidovudine incorporated into cellular DNA.[80–82] It also inhibits nucleoside triphosphate production by inhibiting thymidine kinase and inhibits cellular protein glycosylation.[83,84] Mutant cells that accumulated less AZT-MP had reduced cytotoxicity; however, these same cells did not have reduced levels of the triphosphate and antiviral effects were also unaltered.[85] In addition, clinical studies have shown that the monophosphate but not the triphosphate levels correlate with low CD4[+] T-cell counts.[86] Another metabolite of zidovudine that might be important in its bone marrow toxicity is 3'-amino-3'-deoxythymidine (AMT). After an oral dose of zidovudine, this metabolite achieves peak concentrations that are about one-eighth that of the parent drug. AMT is toxic to granulocyte-macrophage and erythroid precursor cells at concentrations one-fifth and one-seventh, respectively, of zidovudine, indicating that AMT may contribute to the hematologic toxicity.[87] Several different mechanisms may contribute to the hematologic toxicity, including inhibition of mitochondrial DNA synthesis,[88] decreased expression of erythropoietin receptors,[89] decreased globin mRNA synthesis, and telomere shortening with a subsequent reduced cell viability.[18]

The effects of other nucleoside inhibitors on the bone marrow are quite diverse. Didanosine demonstrates no hematological toxicity, while zalcitabine and lamivudine inhibit granulocytic and erythroid cell lineages in vitro but do not attain concentrations that are hematologically toxic clinically.[18,88] The thymidine analog, stavudine, inhibits erythroid and granulocyte-macrophage lineage bone marrow progenitor cells at relatively late stages of development but only at higher concentrations than zidovudine. The other NRTIs cause little bone marrow toxicity.

Reduction of dosage with their use in combination-drug regimens has resulted in a significant decrease in the incidence of anemia from these drugs. Complete blood counts should be taken to monitor for neutropenia and anemia, and drug dosages should be adjusted accordingly. Erythropoietin α can be used to treat any anemia related to therapy.

PERIPHERAL NEUROPATHY. In contrast to ziduvodine, most of the other nucleoside inhibitors of reverse transcriptase (zalcitabine, didanosine, and stavudine) produce a painful, sensorimotor neuropathy that is dose limiting in 15%–20% of patients.[90–92] The neuropathy is slow in onset, occurring after about 2 months of treatment, and it occurs earlier and is more severe with higher dosage. The neuropathy characteristically begins as a tingling or burning sensation in a stocking and glove distribution, but with time, it progresses to pain at rest. The symptoms may worsen for several weeks, but they usually resolve completely within a few weeks to months after discontinuation of drug. Nerve conduction studies of affected patients show greatly diminished nerve action potentials consistent with axonal degeneration.[93] This effect seems to correlate with inhibition of mitochondrial DNA synthesis and mitochondrial polymerase.[75]

MYOPATHY. Myopathy or inflammation of muscle tissue is a serious side effect of ziduvodine that can be long-lasting and debilitating. It is characterized by a slow onset of muscle weakness and tenderness after an average of 1 year of ziduvodine use.[94] Muscle biopsy shows areas of focal necrosis and "ragged red" fibers with mitochondria showing paracrystalline inclusions that correlate well with the clinical severity of the myopathy.[95,96] It is produced by ziduvodine but not by the other nucleosides. Ziduvodine appears to be a muscle mitochondrial toxin that interferes with oxidative phosphorylation and respiratory chain activity.[97] However, since zidovudine has the least effect on mitochondrial DNA among all the nucleosides, this effect is apparently more complicated, and it may involve muscle cell specific transport into and phosphorylation by mitochondria.

PANCREATITIS. This is the most serious toxicity associated with the use of didanosine but it has been reported only rarely with the other nucleosides. The pancreatitis is characterized by progressive abdominal pain, nausea, vomiting, and elevation of serum amylase.[98] About 5% of patients experience these more serious symptoms while about 25% of patients have milder complications. A few deaths have occurred as a result of pancreatitis in patients taking didanosine. The biochemical mechanism of this toxic effect is unknown.

HEPATIC TOXICITY. Severe hepatomegaly with fatty degeneration of the liver has occurred in several HIV-infected patients who received ziduvodine, with most of these patients dying.[99] Metabolic acidosis was also seen in many of these patients. Didanosine has also produced similar effects. It is thought that inhibition of mitochondrial DNA synthesis plays a role in both the fatty degeneration and the associated lactic acidosis. Many of the nucleosides inhibit mitochondrial γ DNA polymerase, reduce mitochondrial DNA synthesis, and increase lactic acid production.[75,100,101] However, other mechanisms probably play a role as well, as the magnitude of the effects seen does not always correlate with inhibition of mitochondrial DNA synthesis. Hepatic steatosis with lactic acidosis has also been seen with some of the other NRTIs, including abacavir.

OTHER EFFECTS. Less serious and transient side effects of zidovudine include headache, fever and abdominal pain, rash, diarrhea and vomiting, and mood disturbance. Discontinuing zidovudine alleviates the symptoms, but most patients who subsequently reinitiate therapy will see the symptoms recur. Other toxicities associated with didanosine include gastrointestinal effects, such as nausea, vomiting, constipation, or abdominal pain; central nervous system effects, such as headache, dizziness, asthenia, or insomnia; and hepatitis, rash, and pruritus. Zalcitabine causes rash, stomatitis, esophageal ulceration, and fever, as well as the above-mentioned peripheral neuropathy and pancreatitis.

Abacavir and adefovir seem to produce toxicities different from those of zidovudine and other NRTIs. With abacavir, the most worrisome toxicity has been a hypersensitivity reaction in about 5% of patients taking the drug. It occurs after about 11 days of treatment, with fever, gastrointestinal symptoms, malaise, and sometimes rash. Laboratory abnormalities include elevations in liver enzymes increases in creatine phosphokinase and creatine levels, and lymphopenia. The drug should be discontinued as soon as a hypersensitivity reaction is suspected, and it should not be restarted. Retreatment can result in a rapid recurrence of severe symptoms of hypotension, and respiratory distress, with some deaths being reported.[29,74] With adefovir the main adverse effect has been mild to moderate nephrotoxicity presenting as a dose-related proximal renal tubular dysfunction or a "Fanconi-like" syndrome. Nephrotoxicity occurs in more than 30% of patients, usually at least 20 weeks after starting the drug, and it slowly resolves after stopping the drug or reducing the dose. Nausea, diarrhea, asthenia, and increased aminotransferase may also occur with adefovir treatment.[74] Table 17–2 summarizes the toxicities of the nucleoside reverse transcriptase inhibitors.

Drug Interactions

Because nucleoside reverse transcriptase inhibitors are commonly used in multi-drug combinations, drug interactions are of particular importance. For example, any drug that may cause bone marrow toxicity, such as amphotericin B, doxorubicin, vinblastine, pyrimethamine, pentamidine, ganciclovir, and flucytosine, should be used with caution in combination with zidovudine.[102] Also, anemia and neutropenia are more common when zidovudine is combined with high-dose trimethoprim-sulfamethoxazole as may happen in the treatment of *Pneumocystis carinii* pneumonia in patients with AIDS.[103]

Many of the drug interactions are of a pharmacokinetic nature, and they include accelerated drug clearance as well as inhibition of absorption, renal clearance, and hepatic metabolism. For example, the antibiotic clarithromycin decreases zidovudine absorption,[104] and buffered formulations of didanosine reduce absorption of drugs that are optimally absorbed at normal gastric pH, such as delavirdine, indinavir, tetracyclines, certain quinolones, ketoconazole, and itraconazole.[105] Rifabutin and rifampin induce hepatic microsomal enzymes and thus

Table 17–2. *Adverse effects of nucleoside reverse transcriptase inhibitors.*

	Zidovudine	Lamivudine	Stavudine	Zalcitabine	Didanosine	Abacavir[a]	Adefovir[b]
Neuropathy	–	–	++	++	++	+	–
Myopathy	++	–	–	–	–	++	–
Cardiomyopathy	+	–	–	+	+	–	–
Pancreatitis	–	+/–	+	–	++	–	+
Hepatic steatosis/hepatitis	+	+/–	+	–	+	–	–
Lactic acidosis	+	–	+	–	+	–	–
Renal toxicity	–	–	–	+	–	–	+
Bone marrow toxicity	++	–	–	+	+	+	+
Skin toxicity	–	–	–	–	–	++	–

++, most prominently observed toxicity; +, observed toxicity; +/–, observed possible toxicity; –, toxicity not observed; ID, insufficient data (most often from ongoing phase II/III trials). [a]Information from the manufacturer, Glaxo-Wellcome; [b]Gilead-Sciences.

Source: Data from Brinkman et al.[76] and from the manufacturers.

decrease plasma concentrations of zidovudine.[106] In contrast, methadone inhibits the metabolism of zidovudine, and patients should be monitored for zidovudine toxicity when methadone is started or when methadone dosage is increased.[18]

Drugs such as probenecid and valproic acid, which compete for the same glucuronyl transferase that metabolizes zidovudine, have been found to reduce the plasma clearance and increase the plasma concentration of zidovudine in HIV-infected volunteers.[107,108] The antiplatelet agent dipyridamole and the anticancer agent hydroxyurea enhance the activity of dideoxynucleosides. Dipyridamole decreases the intracellular transport of dTTP through an inhibition of the transporter, resulting in a more favorable ratio of dTTP to AZT-TP.[109] The anti-HIV activity of zalcitabine is also enhanced. Hydroxyurea, an inhibitor of ribonucleotide reductase, enhances the anti-HIV activity of didanosine by blocking a salvage pathway involved in the synthesis of deoxynucleosides, especially dATP.[110] The end result is a decreased and therefore favorable intracellular ratio of dATP to the active form of didanosine, ddATP, increasing the probability of incorporation of ddATP into the nascent viral RNA–DNA duplex. However, because hydroxyurea can depress the bone marrow, caution must be exercised in the clinical use of this drug in HIV-infected patients, particularly those with advanced disease and poor bone marrow reserve. Comprehensive lists of the drug interactions involving the NRTIs have been published,[102,111] and selected interactions are summarized in Table 17–3.

Precautions

Ziduvodine is mutagenic in vitro and is both tumor promoting and embryotoxic in animals. Anemia and growth retardation, but no excess of birth defects, have been found in the offspring of pregnant women treated with ziduvodine.[112] No adverse effects have been found in children without HIV but with in utero and neonatal exposure to ziduvodine who were followed for as long as 5.6 years.[113] However, the safety of ziduvodine during pregnancy remains to be fully established. Didanosine may be safer than zidovudine in early pregnancy, but the safety of the other NRTIs also remains to be established.[114]

Non-nucleoside Reverse Transcriptase Inhibitors

Non-nucleoside reverse transcriptase inhibitors (NNRTIs) are the newest class of antiretroviral agents that, like the nucleoside analogs, act early in the HIV replication cycle, preventing infection of new cells. Several drugs in this category are being developed but only nevirapine, delavirdine, and efavirenz are approved for clinical use.

Mechanism of Action and Resistance

NNRTIs are a structurally diverse class of potent reverse transcriptase inhibitors. They act by directly binding to reverse transcriptase at sites separate from the nucleoside binding site, causing allosteric inhibition of enzyme function. These inhibitors block the

Nevirapine

Delavirdine

Efavirenz

chemical reaction but do not interfere with nucleotide binding or the nucleotide-induced conformational change in the enzyme.[115] Thus, binding of the NNRTI disrupts the enzyme's catalytic site, blocking transcription of viral RNA into DNA. Structural modeling of the reverse transcriptase enzyme indicates that the different NNRTIs bind, with small differences, to a hydrophobic pocket of the p66 subunit near the active site ("thumb" subdomain).[37,116,117] As a result, they may indirectly affect residues in the polymerase active site or impair mobility of this "thumb" subdomain.[118] They act in a noncompetitive manner with respect to substrates or primer template and inhibit HIV-1 reverse transcriptase in vitro with minimal cellular toxicity. Since they are not nucleosides, they do not require intracellular phosphorylation to the active form. The NNRTIs are quite specific for HIV-1, having no activity against the closely related HIV-2 or other human and animal retroviruses.

Resistant viruses emerge rapidly in vitro and resistance has been observed after only a few passages of infected cells in the presence of the drug.[4] Clinical trials also demonstrate early emergence of resistant viruses, with one study documenting resistance occurring to nevirapine within 1 week.[4] Both in vitro and clinical resistance are related to substitutions at specific residues (e.g., 103–108, 189, and 190) in the reverse transcriptase gene,[116] which are located in the NNRTI binding pocket.[119,120] Resistance to one NNRTI usually, but not always, confers resistance to the other NNRTIs,[121] but there is no cross-resistance to the nucleoside analogs or protease inhibitors. Although specific residues react with specific NNRTIs, the fact that all NNRTIs bind to the same pocket explains the extent of cross-resistance seen with this class of drugs.[38,122] The emergence of resistant isolates is accompanied by a loss of clinical activity, manifest by increasing virus load and decreasing CD4 cell count.[45,123]

Therapeutic Use

Addition of NNRTIs to therapy with NRTIs results in improved immunologic and antiviral activity.[124,125] NNRTIs should always be administered in combination with nucleoside analogs, as resistance develops when they are administered as single-drug therapy or when they are added to a failing regimen of nucleoside reverse transcriptase inhibitors. Also, alternating treatment between ziduvodine and nevirapine does not prevent the development of nevirapine resistance.[126] The NNRTIs are most effective when used in appropriate triple-drug combination regimens. Although the preferred initial treatment for AIDS is the combination of two NRTIs along with a potent protease inhibitor, the recommended alternative is a triple combination of two NRTIs along with a NNRTI. Results from several clinical trials of combination-drug treatments show that development of resistant isolates is delayed.[123,127] The activity of the NNRTIs is greatly increased when used along with nucleoside analogs that the patient has not previously taken, although these combinations are not as potent or as efficacious as regimens containing protease inhibitors and they may not provide sustained viral suppression.[11,12]

Nevirapine was the first NNRTI approved by the Food and Drug Administration and is indicated for use only in combination with nucleoside analogs. Nevirapine with zidovudine and didanosine is the only triple-drug combination that has suppressed viral load to undetectable levels in most patients. These patients were treated with antiretroviral drugs for the first time, and less dramatic results were obtained in patients who had experienced previous antiretroviral therapy.[11,12] Nevirapine is used at a dose of 200 mg daily for the first 14 days, followed by 200 mg twice daily thereafter. Like nevirapine, delaviridine should be used only in combination with other antiretroviral agents so as to avoid the development of resistance. It is used in a dose of 400 mg (four 100 mg tablets) three times daily. Because of the difficulty of taking 12 tablets per day, it may be easier to disperse the tablets in water and then to consume the slurry. In contrast, efavirenz is administered once daily. In 450 previously untreated patients, 36 weeks of efavirenz plus zidovudine and lamivudine was at least as effective in lowering viral counts

Table 17–3. *Selected drug interactions involving the antiretroviral nucleoside analogs.*

	Zidovudine	Didanosine	Lamivudine	Stavudine	Zalcitabine
Ciprofloxacin		Reduces ciprofloxacin absorption Give 2 h before didanosine			
Dapsone		May result in increased peripheral neuropathy	Increased peripheral neuropathy	Increased peripheral neuropathy	Increased peripheral neuropathy
Fluconazole, atovaquone	Increases zidovudine levels Monitor for zidovudine toxicity				
Ganciclovir	Increases zidovudine levels Increased hematological toxicity	AUC of didanosine increased by 70% Monitor for didanosine toxicity			

Isoniazid	Increased peripheral neuropathy	Increased peripheral neuropathy	Increased peripheral neuropathy	Increased peripheral neuropathy	
Itraconazole, ketoconazole,				Decreased antifungal levels Give 2 h before didanosine	
Pentamidine	May cause pancreatitis	May cause pancreatitis	May cause pancreatitis	May cause pancreatitis	
Rifampicin					Reduces zidovudine levels by 50%
Trimethoprim-sulphame-thoxazole	Increases zalcitabine levels by 30% Monitor for zalcitabine toxicity		Increases lamivudine levels by 30%–40% Monitor for lamivudine toxicity		Increases zidovudine levels by 30% Monitor for zidovudine toxicity

Source: Data from Sahai.[111]

as indinavir plus zidovudine and lamivudine, and the efavirenz combination was better tolerated.[128] Other studies have also shown beneficial responses with this drug.[129]

Pharmacokinetics

Nevirapine is rapidly absorbed (>90%), with peak serum concentrations being achieved in about 2 h, and absorption is not impaired by food, antacids, or didanosine.[125] The half-life of nevirapine is in the range of 40 h, with considerable variation that is not related to dose. Nevirapine is highly lipophilic, about 60% is bound to plasma protein, and it is widely distributed. It readily crosses the placenta and is found in breast milk. Cerebrospinal fluid levels are about 45% of the drug concentration in plasma.[130] Nevirapine is extensively metabolized to several hydroxylated metabolites by cytochrome P-450 enzymes, with over 90% of the drug being recovered in the urine mainly as the glucuronide.[125]

Delavirdine is also rapidly absorbed following oral administration, with peak serum concentrations occurring at about 1 h, but its absorption is reduced by an increase in gastric pH.[131] Food and didanosine reduce absorption, although these effects are usually are not clinically significant, and patients can take the drug with a meal and with didanosine.[132,133] Delavirdine is extensively bound to plasma protein (98%), mainly albumin, which limits its distribution, and cerebrospinal fluid levels average only 0.4% of plasma concentrations.[134] Delavirdine is extensively converted to inactive metabolites, mainly by CYP3A, with less than 5% recovered unchanged in the urine. Delavirdine is not only a substrate for the P-450 enzyme but it is also an inhibitor. Thus, the drug can inhibit its own metabolism, an observation that may explain its nonlinear pharmacokinetics.[127] Caution is advised for patients with impaired liver function because of the extensive hepatic metabolism of the drug. The half-life after a 400 mg dose administered three times a day is around 6 h with a range of 2–11 h.

Efavirenz is also rapidly absorbed from the gastrointestinal tract and highly bound to plasma proteins.[129,135] It has the advantage of having a longer half-life than the other NNRTIs, and thus can be administered once daily. Cerebrospinal fluid concentrations are only around 1% of plasma levels. Efavirenz is metabolized in the liver mainly by CYP3A4 and CYP2B6. Most of the drug is excreted in the feces, but 14%–34% is excreted in the urine as metabolites.[135] Table 17–4 summarizes the pharmacokinetics of the NNRTIs.

Adverse Effects

This group of drugs has relatively low toxicity, and their toxicities do not overlap with those of the NRTIs. Skin rash is the most common side effect noted with the NNRTIs. With nevirapine, rash occurs in about 18% of patients, it is usually maculopapular, mild to moderate in severity, and occurs within the first 6 weeks of therapy.[136] The precise mechanism of the rash is not known but skin biopsy specimens have demonstrated nonspecific inflammatory changes and some have shown perivascular infiltration consistent with a drug-induced eruption. These rashes are generally self-limiting and may necessitate antihistamines and/or topical steroid creams for symptomatic relief. Severe or life-threatening rashes, including Stevens-Johnson syndrome, have occurred in 8% of patients. Nevirapine should be discontinued in all patients with severe rash. The incidence of rash does not seem to correlate with plasma levels of the drug, but initiating therapy with lower doses resulted in better tolerance and decreased incidence of the rash.[137] Other adverse effects associated with nevirapine include fever, nausea, headache, abnormal liver function tests, and, rarely, hepatitis.

With delavirdine, maculopapular rashes occur in 12.5% of patients, appearing within 1 to 8 weeks after starting therapy and being generally less severe than the rashes seen with nevirapine.[138] The occurrence, but not severity, of the rash appears to correlate with CD4 T-cell count, and rash occurs more frequently in patients with fewer than 100 CD4 cells/mm^3.[127] Other adverse effects of delavirdine include headache,

Table 17–4. Pharmacokinetics of the non-nucleoside reverse transcriptase inhibitors.

Parameter	Nevirapine	Delavirdine	Efavirenz
Adult dose	200 mg bid	400 mg tid	600 mg once a day
Oral bioavailability	90%	NA	At least 66%
Vd (liters/kg)	1.4	1.0	NR
$T_{1/2}$ (h)	25	7	52–76
Protein binding (%)	60	98	>99
CSF concentration (%)	45	NA	1
Clearance route	Renal (91% as metabolites)	Renal (51% as metabolites) Feces (44% as metabolites)	Renal (14%–34% as metabolites) Feces (16%–61% as metabolites)

CSF, % of plasma drug concentration achieved in cerebrospinal fluid; NA, not available; NR not reported; Vd, apparent volume into which drug is distributed, usually determined by plasma concentrations.

Source: Data from Swindells and Fletcher[127] and information from the manufacturers.

fatigue, gastrointestinal complaints (nausea, vomiting, and diarrhea), and hepatic enzyme elevation. Efavirenz causes rash in about 27% of adults and 40% of children. About half of the patients treated with efavirenz have reported central nervous system symptoms, including dizziness, drowsiness, impaired concentration, abnormal dreams, and insomnia. Severe depression and delusions have been reported rarely.[129] Elevations in liver enzymes can also occur with this drug, especially in patients who have had hepatitis. The NNRTIs should be administered during pregnancy only if the potential benefit justifies the risk to the fetus.

Drug Interactions

All of the non-nucleoside inhibitors have the potential to cause significant drug interactions as a result of their metabolism by and effect on microsomal cytochrome P-450 enzymes. These interactions are summarized by Tseng and Foisy.[102] Nevirapine induces hepatic CYP3A, so it may decrease plasma concentrations of other drugs that are extensively metabolized in the liver by this isozyme, such as the protease inhibitors saquinavir, indinavir, and ritonavir.[125,139] The greatest clinical significance is with indinavir, and its dose must be increased when it is administered with nevirapine. Nevirapine can also reduce zidovudine plasma concen-

trations by about 25% but has no effect on the pharmacokinetics of either didanosine or zalcitabine.[124,125] Nevirapine can also decrease the plasma concentrations of oral contraceptives. Since nevirapine is extensively metabolized by the cytochrome P-450 system and is a substrate for the CYP3A isoenzymes, its metabolism can potentially be increased by inducers or decreased by inhibitors. Compounds found to alter concentrations of nevirapine include the antimycobacterials rifampin and rifabutin and certain antifungal agents, such as ketoconazole.[125]

In contrast to nevirapine, delavirdine inhibits cytochrome P-450 enzymes and may thus increase plasma concentrations of drugs metabolized by this system. Included among these drugs are antihistamines (e.g., terfenadine and astemizole), benzodiazepines (e.g., alprazolam, midazolam, and triazolam), protease inhibitors (e.g., indinavir and saquinavir), and cisapride, as well as others. Other drugs, in turn, can affect delavirdine levels; for example, delavirdine absorption is decreased by didanosine, some antacids, omeprazole, H_2 blockers, phenobarbital, phenytoin, and antimycobacterial drugs.[7] Efavirenz has also been reported to induce CYP3A4 in vivo and to inhibit several isozymes in vitro, giving it the potential to alter the metabolism of several drugs. Similarly, its metabolism may be increased by drugs that induce CYP3A4 and it may also induce its own metabolism.[129,135]

Protease Inhibitors

The protease inhibitors (Fig. 17–4) are the newest drugs available for managing HIV infection, and they have had a major impact on the treatment of AIDS. These drugs are effective and relatively well tolerated, but they are expensive, they are subject to a variety of drug interactions, and careful compliance is required for their proper administration.[140]

Mechanism of Action and Resistance

The HIV protease (or proteinase) enzyme is an essential component of the replicative cycle of HIV, performing the post-translational cleavage or processing of the gag (p55) and gag-pol (p160) gene products into functional core proteins and viral enzymes.[141,142] Homodimers of this protein have the aspartyl protease activity that is typical of retroviral proteases, while monomers are enzymatically inactive.[143,144] The protease is packaged into virions, and the cleavage events it catalyzes occur simultaneously with or soon after the budding of the virion from the surface of an infected cell.[145] The polyproteins are cleaved by the enzyme at nine different cleavage sites to yield the structural proteins (p17, p24, p7, and p6) as well as the viral enzymes reverse transcriptase, integrase, and protease (see Fig. 17–5).[143,146] The polyproteins must be cleaved before the nascent viral particles (virions) can mature.[147–149] Proteolytic cleavage of the gag polyprotein results in morphologic changes in the virion and condensation of the nucleoprotein core. Proviral DNA lacking functional protease produces immature, noninfectious viral particles.[150]

The HIV protease inhibitors are a group of structurally related inhibitors of this viral protease enzyme. Most contain a synthetic analog of the phenylalanine-proline sequence at positions 157 and 168 of the gag-pol polyprotein that is cleaved by the protease.[151] These drugs have complex structures that make them difficult to synthesize in large quantities. They prevent cleavage of gag and gag-pol protein precursors in acutely and chronically infected cells, arresting maturation and thereby blocking the infectivity of nascent virions.[152,153] The protease inhibitors prevent further infection but they have no effect on cells already containing integrated proviral DNA. Antiviral activity is correlated with the inhibition of enzyme activity, although the drug concentrations required to reduce enzyme activity by 50% (IC_{50}) range from 2 to 60 nM.[152,154] The protease inhibitors are inactive or weakly active against human aspartyl proteases, with a K_i of at least 10,000 nM for renin and pepsin.[152,155] These drugs have an important advantage because they have the potential to inhibit cell-to-cell spread of virus. They require no intracellular metabolism for their antiviral activity.

The HIV protease is a symmetrical dimer with the active site in a cleft at the interface between the two monomers. Protease inhibitors bind to the active site, either by mimicking the transition state during peptide cleavage or by fitting the active site as its steric complement (see Fig. 17–6).[151,156] Most resistance mutations are located in the cleft of the active site where they directly interfere with binding of the inhibitor.[157,158] These mutations may also reduce enzymatic activity, resulting in impaired virus infectivity. A flexible flap extends over the substrate binding cleft, and mutations in this region decrease enzyme activity.[159,160] Varying degrees of cross-resistance to all protease inhibitors is observed,[161] and the longer the treatment with one inhibitor, the higher the likelihood of developing cross-resistance to others. Both clinical and laboratory isolates with reduced sensitivity have been found for each of the HIV protease inhibitors. Some of the genotypic changes reliably predict alterations in sensitivity.[162]

Therapeutic Use

Saquinavir was the first protease inhibitor approved for clinical use, and since 1995, four other members of this group (ritonavir, indinavir, nelfinavir, and amprenavir) have

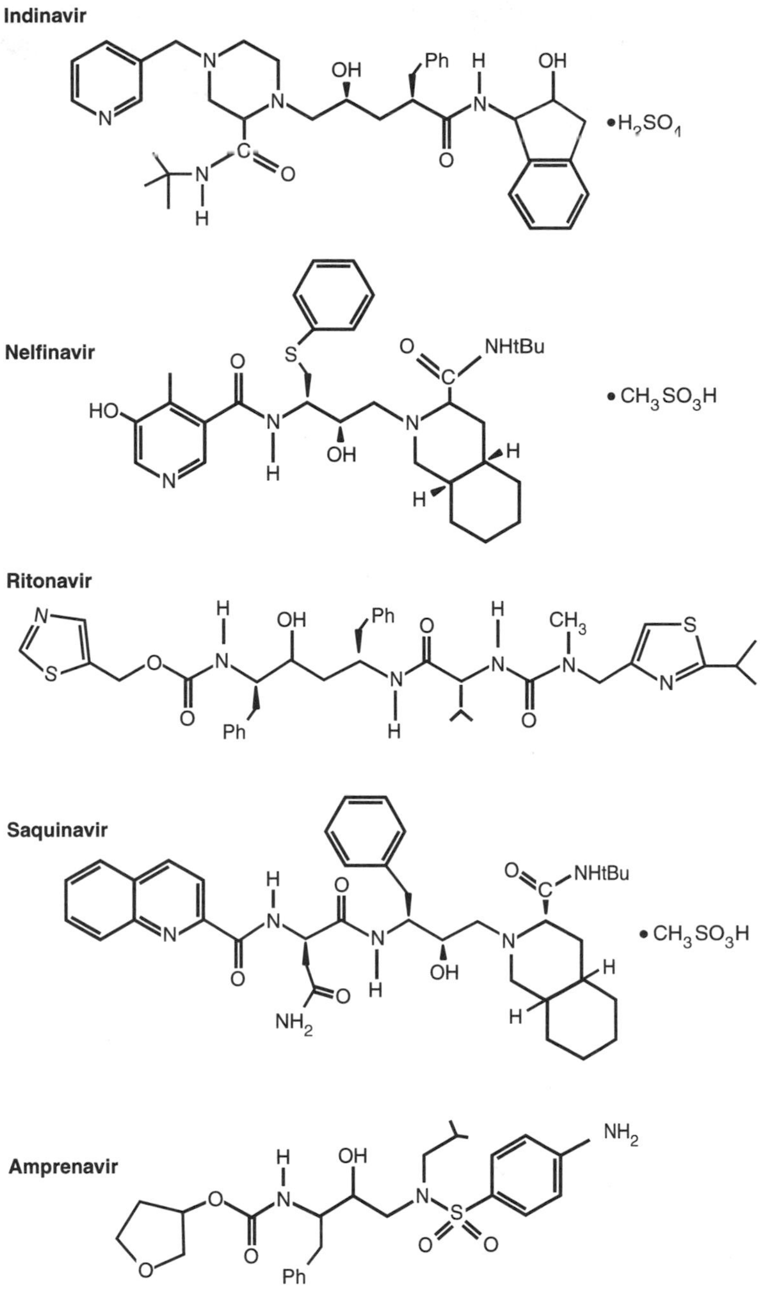

Figure 17–4. Structures of HIV protease inhibitors. Ph, phenyl; NHtBu, amino-tertiary butyl.

been approved by the Food and Drug Administration. All five drugs are potent inhibitors of HIV and provide synergistic activity when used in combination with nucleoside reverse transcriptase inhibitors. The HIV-protease inhibitors rapidly and profoundly

reduce the viral load, as indicated by a decline in plasma HIV RNA concentrations within a few days after the start of treatment.[143] Single-drug therapy with indinavir, nelfinavir, or ritonavir causes plasma HIV RNA concentrations to be reduced by a fac-

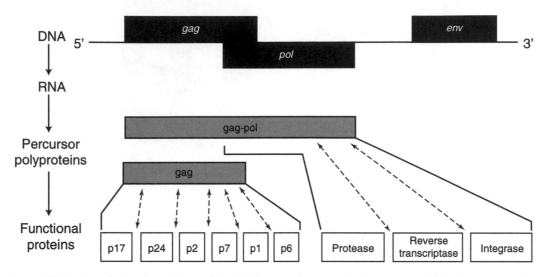

Figure 17–5. Translational products of the HIV gag-pol gene and the sites at which the gene product is cleaved by the virus-encoded protease. P17, capsid protein; p24, matrix protein; p7, nucleocapsid; p2, p1, and p6 are small proteins with unknown functions. The arrows denote cleavage events catalyzed by the HIV-specific protease. (From Flexner.[143])

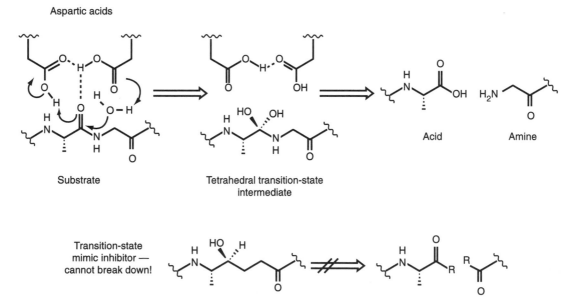

Figure 17–6. Proposed mechanism by which aspartic acid protease cleaves substrates (From Vacca and Condra. [156])

572

tor of 100 to 1000 in 4 to 12 weeks.[163,164] Reductions in the viral load are paralleled by mean increases in the CD4[+] count of 100 to 150 cells/mm[3].[163-165] Despite these beneficial effects, single-drug therapy with protease inhibitors is no longer recommended because the duration of the antiviral response is usually limited and resistance to the drug may develop.

Several clinical trials have now evaluated treatment with protease inhibitors in combination with nucleosides.[143] Current clinical guidelines recommend combining a protease inhibitor with two nucleoside analogs (e.g., zidovudine and lamivudine or stavudine and lamivudine). Protease inhibitors combined with nucleoside analogs slow the progression of disease and improve survival. For example, ritonavir added to nucleoside therapy reduces the appearance of new opportunistic diseases and death by 43% to 53%. Saquinavir in combination with zalcitabine and indinavir plus zidovudine and lamivudine reduced the combined end points of clinical progression and death by more than 50%.[166-168] Combinations of protease inhibitors and nucleoside analogs can suppress HIV for long periods of time. For example, indinavir with zidovudine and lamivudine reduced the plasma viral load to undetectable levels in 70% of patients after 24 weeks of treatment and in 60% after 2 years.[169] Combinations of nelfinavir with zidovudine and lamivudine and ritonavir combined with zidovudine and lamivudine produced similar results. Combining a protease inhibitor with a NNRTI can also profoundly suppress the viral load. For example, all 12 patients treated with indinavir and nevirapine had viral loads of less than 500 RNA copies/ml after an average of 24 weeks of treatment.[170] Combined treatment with indinavir and efavirenz also reduced the viral load significantly.[171]

To avoid resistance, the drugs must be taken continually at the full approved dose, as suboptimal dosing and noncompliance can result in the rapid onset of drug resistance. If one of the protease inhibitors is not well tolerated, it is better to switch to another protease inhibitor rather than to lower the dose, because decreasing the dose may result in subtherapeutic concentrations and contribute to resistance development.[69,140] Results from dose-escalation studies and from clinical trials have provided compelling evidence that protease inhibitors should be used not only at the highest tolerable dose but in combination with reverse transcriptase inhibitors to prevent emergence of drug resistance.[143] When protease inhibitors are given to patients who are already receiving antiretroviral therapy, treatment is more complex, as these patients are likely to harbor HIV-1 isolates that are resistant to these drugs. When therapy with protease inhibitors is initiated, it is recommended that these patients receive new nucleoside analogs that are not cross-resistant with drugs that the patient has already received. This minimizes the chance of treatment being compromised by drug resistance.

A more recent development in protease inhibitor therapy is the simultaneous use of two inhibitors. Recent guidelines include a two-inhibitor combination along with two nucleoside analogs as a recommended therapy.[8] The potential benefits of dual-inhibitor therapy include increased compliance (as a result of beneficial pharmacokinetic interactions and subsequent reduction in the number of daily doses and pills required), potentially increased viral suppression, and a potential role as salvage therapy in patients relatively unresponsive to protease inhibitor regimens.[172] Despite the potential negative factors of drug antagonism and a higher rate of adverse effects, preliminary studies have shown encouraging results in many patients.

Pharmacokinetics

Ritonavir, indinavir, and nelfinavir reach high concentrations after oral administration, whereas saquinavir in a hard-gel capsule has poor oral bioavailability (around 4%).[173-176] However, saquinavir mesylate was recently reformulated into a soft-gel capsule with improved drug bioavailability that yields plasma concentrations eight times higher than that of the hard-gel capsule.[173] Oral bioavailability for the different pro-

Table 17–5. Pharmacokinetics of the HIV-protease inhibitors.

Parameter	Indinavir	Nelfinavir	Ritonavir	Saquinavir[a]
Dose	800 mg tid	750 mg tid	600 mg bid	600 mg tid
Oral bioavailability (%)	60–65	>78	66–75	<4
C_{max} (µg/ml)	7.7	3.0–4.0	11.2	0.2
T_{max} (h)	0.8	2.0–4.0	2.0–4.0	NR
$T_{1/2}$ (h)	1.8	3.5–5.0	3.0–5.0	NR
Protein binding (%)	60–65	>98	98–99	98
CSF concentration (%)	2.2–76	NR	1	<1
Clearance route (%)	Hepatic (88–90)	Hepatic (>78)	Hepatic (>95)	Hepatic (>97)

C_{max}, peak drug concentration during a dosing interval; CSF concentration, % of plasma drug concentration achieved in cerebrospinal fluid; NR, not reported; T_{max}, time at which C_{max} occurs during a dosing interval. [a]Saquinavir data are for the hard-gel capsule, which has low bioavailability.

Source: Data from Flexner.[143]

tease inhibitors varies because of differences in absorption and first-pass hepatic metabolism, to which saquinavir is the most susceptible.[177] The effect of food is an important consideration when administering these drugs. A high-calorie, high-fat meal is required for optimal absorption of saquinavir, whereas food decreases the absorption of indinavir.[178,179] The area under the plasma concentration–time curve (AUC) for nelfinavir is two to three times larger when the drug is given with a meal.[180] On the other hand, food causes a minimal increase in ritonavir absorption.[181] The absorption of all these drugs is maximal within 4 h after ingestion.

All of the protease inhibitors except indinavir are highly bound (at least 98% vs. 60%) to plasma proteins.[182,183] The cerebrospinal fluid penetration of ritonavir and saquinavir is about 1%.[184] However, indinavir penetrates into the cerebrospinal fluid, with cerebrospinal fluid concentration ranging up to 76% of plasma concentrations, perhaps because of its decreased plasma protein binding.[185] Nelfinavir achieves concentrations in the cerebrospinal fluid that are less than 10% of those in plasma.[182] All five drugs are metabolized by cytochrome P-450 isoenzymes, mainly CYP3A4, while nelfinavir is metabolized by at least four different P-450s.[182,186,187] Recovery of unchanged drug in the urine has been reported to be 20% or less with these drugs[176,179–181]; thus,

it is unlikely that renal dysfunction would require dosage adjustment. Elimination half-lives range from 1.8 to 5 h, necessitating twice-daily or three-times-daily administration to maintain adequate concentrations for inhibition of HIV protease. Amprenavir, however, has a long plasma half-life (7–10.6 h), permitting twice-daily administration. The pharmacokinetics of the protease inhibitors are summarized in Table 17–5.

Adverse Reactions

All of the protease inhibitors produce gastrointestinal disturbances, and their administration can be associated with high-serum aminotransferase activity, although hepatitis is rare.[188] Hemorrhage has been reported in patients with hemophilia taking protease inhibitors, but the role of the drugs in this effect is uncertain.[189,190] In addition, several unusual adverse effects have been reported in patients taking protease inhibitors for extended periods. These include hypertriglyceridemia, glucose intolerance and abnormal fat distribution.[191] For example, a syndrome called *crix belly* may occur in association with indinavir therapy. This is characterized by increased abdominal girth and decreased subcutaneous fat in the arms and legs.[192] The pattern of fat redistribution resembles that occurring in Cushing's syndrome and some patients develop a "buffalo hump." It is not known whether these effects are specific to indinavir or related to the protease inhibitors in general. Hypertrophy of the breasts reported in a woman treated with indinavir may be part of this pattern of fat redistribution.[193] As more patients are treated with these drugs, other toxic effects will probably be identified. There have been no controlled studies of protease inhibitor treatment during pregnancy and they should be used only if the benefit justifies the risk.

In addition to the general adverse effects of the class, each of the protease inhibitors has distinct dose-limiting toxic effects. Nephrolithiasis is the most important side effect of indinavir.[179] This can occur within a few days after the start of treatment, and the incidence in clinical studies has ranged from 3% to 15%.[194] Because of its low water solubility, indinavir precipitates in the renal tubules, causing obstruction and the associated symptoms of renal colic (hematuria, flank pain, and nausea).[194] Patients taking indinavir should be advised to drink large quantities of fluid throughout the day, and the condition is typically treated with hydration and pain relief.[195] Indinavir is associated with fewer gastrointestinal problems than the other protease inhibitors, but other adverse effects, including hemolytic anemia, headache, and asymptomatic hyperbilirubinemia, have been associated with its use.[179]

Nelfinavir is very well tolerated, with the most common adverse effect being mild to moderate diarrhea.[180,196,197] This effect can usually be controlled with antidiarrheal drugs such as loperamide or fiber supplements. Other adverse effects associated with nelfinavir include fatigue, nausea, flatulence, and rash. Ritonavir is associated with more frequent adverse effects than the other protease inhibitors, especially during the first few weeks of therapy.[181,195] Adverse effects commonly reported with this drug include nausea, vomiting, diarrhea, anorexia, abdominal pain, and taste disturbances. Taking the drug with food helps minimize the gastrointestinal disturbances and mixing ritonavir liquid with chocolate milk or certain enteral nutrition formulations may facilitate tolerance of the unpleasant taste.[181] Ritonavir also causes paresthesias around the

mouth in up to 25% of patients and, less commonly, paresthesias of the arms and legs.[181] The exact cause of these effects is not known, but in most patients these symptoms resolve during continued treatment. Many of the toxic effects associated with ritonavir use appear to be related to the plasma concentration of the drug, with concentrations being highest in the first few days of administration. Consequently, patients should be counseled that many of the initial symptoms will diminish with time.[181,195]

Saquinavir appears to be the best tolerated of the protease inhibitors. Adverse effects are usually mild, with gastrointestinal disturbances (diarrhea, nausea, and abdominal discomfort) and headache occurring most commonly.[178] The new soft-gel formulation has improved bioavailability but is more likely to cause dyspepsia, nausea, and diarrhea than the older formulation.[198] The most frequent adverse effects associated with ampvenavir therapy are rash, nausea, vomiting, diarrhea, and perioral paresthesias. See Table 17–6 for a summary of the major side effects of the protease inhibitors.

Drug Interactions

Because the protease inhibitors are administered in complex multidrug combinations to patients receiving additional treatments for AIDS-related problems, there is a high potential for a number of clinically significant drug interactions. Because of their extensive metabolism by the P-450 cytochromes (especially CYP3A4), there are many interactions with inhibitors and inducers of these enzymes.[199] Table 17–7 summarizes some of these interactions. Inhibitors of CYP3A4 increase plasma concentrations of the HIV protease inhibitors and may increase their toxicity. For example, concurrent administration of ketoconazole increases the AUC by 62% with indinavir, by 35% with nelfinavir, and by 300% with saquinavir. Because of the relatively low oral bioavailability of saquinavir, this effect may actually be beneficial in that more drug reaches the systemic circulation. The NNRTI delaviridine is an inhibitor of hepatic enzymes, and it increases serum levels of sa-

Table 17–6. Major side effects of HIV-protease inhibitors.

Side effect	Indinavir	Nelfinavir	Ritonavir	Saquinavir
Nausea	++	+	++	++
Vomiting	+	NR	++	++
Diarrhea	+	++	++	++
Asthenia or fatigue	−	−	++	−
Nephrolithiasis	+	NR	NR	NR
Hyperbilirubinemia	+	NR	−	+
High-serum aminotransferase	+	+	+	+
High-serum triglyceride	NR	NR	+	NR
Hyperglycemia	+	+	+	+
Fat redistribution	+	+	+	+
Paresthesias	NR	NR	++	−

+, toxicity of moderate or severe intensity reported in less than 10% of treated patients but occurring at least twice as often as in concurrently treated patients not taking the protease inhibitor; ++, toxicity in at least 10% of treated patients and occurring at least twice as often as in control patients; −, toxicity occurring less than twice as often in treated patients as in control patients and in less than 3% of treated patients. NR, not reported.

Source: Data from Flexner.[143]

quinavir by about fivefold and indinavir by about twofold.[138] Drugs that induce P-450 enzymes, such as rifampin and rifabutin, accelerate the clearance of protease inhibitors, reducing their efficacy and increasing the liklihood of selecting resistant strains. For example, rifampin reduces the AUC of indinavir, nelfinavir, and saquinavir by 80%–92% (Table 17–7). Thus, rifampin should be avoided in patients who require treatment with HIV–protease inhibitors.[200,201] The NNRTI nevirapine is a P-450 inducer, and it has been shown to decrease the AUC of saquinavir by 27%.[140]

The HIV–protease inhibitors can also alter the pharmacokinetics of other drugs by acting as P-450 inhibitors or inducers. All of the protease inhibitors inhibit cytochrome P-450 enzymes, with ritonavir being the most potent inhibitor and saquinavir being the least potent.[186,187,199,202] Ritonavir increases rifabutin levels four-fold and increases the levels of its active metabolite 35-fold, and patients receiving ritonavir and rifabutin concomitantly have been found to have an increased rate of arthralgia, joint stiffness, uveitis, and leukopenia.[140] Ritonavir, indinavir, nelfinavir, and amprenavir increase serum concentrations of other drugs metabolized by CYP3A4, including nonsedating antihistamines, cisapride, ergot alkaloids, antiarrhythmics, analgesics, antibiotics, and anticoagulants, among others.[183,203] This may result in potentially serious adverse effects, such as arrhythmias. In contrast, saquinavir has not been shown to significantly increase the serum concentration of concomitantly administered medications.

Nelfinavir and ritonavir can reduce the plasma concentrations of other drugs as a result of hepatic enzyme induction. Nelfinavir and ritonavir decrease the AUC of ethinyl estradiol by 47% and 40%, respectively, and they should not be given to women taking combination oral contraceptives. These same drugs reduce the AUC of zidovudine by 35% and 25%, respectively, presumably because of the induction of glucuronyl transferases. However, since the intracellular concentration of AZT-TP is not altered, the dosage of zidovudine does not need to be reduced when it is given with nelfinavir or ritonavir. Because ritonavir induces its own metabolism, trough plasma concentrations are reduced during the first 2 weeks of therapy with a fixed dose of the drug. Thus, higher doses of ritonavir are administered during the first 2 weeks of therapy.[204]

Interactions between protease inhibitors may be beneficial when two of these drugs are given simultaneously. For example, ritonavir inhibits the hepatic first-pass meta-

Table 17–7. Select pharmacokinetic drug interactions involving HIV protease inhibitors

Drug	% Change in AUC			
	Indinavir	Nelfinavir	Ritonavir	Saquinavir
Effect of other drugs on protease inhibitors				
HIV-PROTEASE INHIBITORS				
Indinavir	–	+83	NR	+500
Nelfinavir	+51	–	+9	+392
Ritonavir	NR	+152	–	+>2000
Saquinavir	NR	+18	NR	–
P-450 INHIBITORS				
Ketoconazole	+62	+35	NR	+300
Clarithromycin	+29	NR	+12	NR
Fluconazole	−19	NR	+12	NR
Fluoxetine	NR	NR	+19	NR
P-450 inducers				
Rifabutin	−32	−32	NR	−40
Rifampin	−92	−82	−35	−80
NUCLEOSIDE ANALOGS				
Didanosine	NR	NC	NC	NR
Lamivudine	NC	NR	NR	NR
Stavudine	NC	NR	NR	NR
Zidovudine	+13	NC	NC	NC
NNRTIs				
Delavirdine	+72	NR	+2	+520
Nevirapine	−28	NR	NC	−27
Effect of HIV protease inhibitors on other drugs				
ANTI-INFECTIVES				
Clarithromycin	+53	NR	+77	NR
Isoniazid	+13	NR	NR	NR
Ketoconazole	+68	NR	NR	NC
Rifabutin	+204	+207	+350	NR
Sulfamethoxazole	NC	NR	+77	NR
NUCLEOSIDE ANALOGS				
Didanosine	NR	NR	−13	NR
Lamivudine	−6	+10	NR	NR
Stavudine	+25	NC	NR	NR
Zalcitabine	NR	NR	NR	NC
Zidovudine	+17 to +36	−35	−25	NC
OTHER DRUGS				
Desipramine	NR	NR	+145	NR
Ethinyl estradiol	+24	−47	−40	NR
Norethindrone	+26	−18	NR	NR
Theophylline	NR	NR	−43	NR
Trimethoprim	+19	NR	+20	NR

NC, no statistically significant change; NR, not reported.

Source: Data from Flexner.[143]

bolism of saquinavir, increasing steady-state plasma concentrations of saquinavir 20- to 30-fold.[205] Nelfinavir increases the AUC of saquinavir by around 400% and that of indinavir by 51%, while indinavir increases the AUC of saquinavir by about 500%.[7] Treatment with two protease inhibitors takes advantage of this pharmacokinetic enhancement to increase antiviral activity.

REFERENCES

1. Staprans, S. I., and M. B. Feinberg Natural history and immunopathogenesis of HIV-1 disease. In *The Medical Management of AIDS*, 4th ed., ed. by M. A. Sande and P. A. Volberding. Philadelphia: W. B. Saunders, 1995, pp. 38–64.

2. Fletcher, C. V., and A. C. Collier. Principles and management of human immunodeficiency virus infection. In *Pharmacotherapy: A Pathophysiologic Approach*, ed. by J. T. DiPiro, R. L. Talbert, G. C. Yee, G. R. Matzke, B. G. Wells, and L. M. Posey. Stamford, CT: Appleton and Lange, 1997, pp. 2353–2386.

3. Greene, W. C. Molecular insights into HIV-1 infection. In *The Medical Management of AIDS*, 4th ed., ed. by M. A. Sande and P. A. Volberding, Philadelphia: W. B. Saunders, 1995, pp. 22–37.

4. Hirsch, M. S., R. T. D'Aquila, and J. C. Kaplan. Antiretroviral therapy. In *AIDS: Biology, Diagnosis, Treatment and Prevention*, ed. by V. T. DeVita, S. Hellman, and S. A. Rosenberg. Philadelphia: Lippincott-Raven, 1997, pp. 495–508.

5. Hirsch, M., and R. D'Aquila. Drug therapy: summary of HIV replication cycle and available antiretroviral agents. N. Engl. J. Med. 1993;328:1687.

6. Hammer, S. M., D. A. Katzenstein, M. D. Hughes, H. Gundacker, R. T. Schooley, R. H. Haubrich, W. K. Henry, M. M. Lederman, J. P. Phair, M. Niu, M. S. Hersch, and T. C. Mergian. A trial comparing nucleoside monotherapy with combination therapy in HIV-infected adults with CD4 cell counts from 200 to 500 per cubic millimeter. N. Engl. J. Med. 1996;335:1081.

7. Vandamme, A.-M., K. VanVaerenbergh, and E. De Clerq. Antihuman immunodeficiency virus drug combination strategies. *Antiviral Chem. Chemother.* 1998;9:187.

8. Carpenter, C., M. Fischl, S. Hammer, M. Hirsch, D. Katzenstein, J. Montaner, D. Richman, M. Saag, R. Schooley, M. Thompson, S. Vella, P. Yeni, and P. Volberding. Antiretroviral therapy for HIV infection in 1998—updated recommendations of the international AIDS Society—WA panel. JAMA 1998;280:78.

9. Volberding, P. A. An aggressive approach to HIV antiretroviral therapy. Hosp. Pract. 1998;33:81.

10. Mortimer, J. S. G., R. Hogg, J. Raboud, R. Harrigan, and M. Shaughnessy. Antiretrovial treatment in 1998. Lancet 1998;352:1919.

11. Carpenter, C. C. J., M. A. Fischl, S. M. Hammer, M. S. Hirsch, D. M. Jacobsen, D. A. Katzenstein,

J. S. G. Montaner, D. D. Richman, M. S. Saag, R. T. Schooley, M. A. Thompson, S. Veila, P. G. Yeni, and P. A. Volberding. Antiretroviral therapy for HIV infection in 1997: updated recommendations of the International AIDS Society—USA Panel. JAMA 1997;277:1962.

12. Centers for Disease Control and Prevention. Public Health Service guidelines for the management of health-care worker exposures to HIV and recommendations for postexposure prophylaxis. Morb. Mortal. Wkly. Rep. 1998;47(RR-7):1.

13. Centers for Disease Control and Prevention. Public Health Service Task Force recommendations for the use of antiretroviral drugs in pregnant women infected with HIV-1 for maternal health and reducing perinatal HIV-1 transmission in the United States. Morb. Mortal. Wkly. Rep. 1998;47(RR-02):1.

14. Wainberg, M., and G. Friedland. Public health implications of antiretroviral therapy and HIV drug resistance. JAMA 1998;279:197.

15. Frost, S. D. W., and A. R. McLean. Quasispecies dynamics and the emergence of drug resistance during zidovudine therapy of HIV infection. AIDS 1994;8:323.

16. Coffin, J. M. HIV population dynamics in vivo: implications for genetic variation, pathogenesis, and therapy. Science 1995;67:483.

17. Richman, D. D. New strategies to combat HIV drug resistance. Hosp. Pract. 1996;31(8):47.

18. Flexner, C. and C. Hendrix. Pharmacology of antiretroviral agents. In *AIDS Biology, Diagnosis, Treatment and Prevention*, ed. by V. T. DeVita, S. Hellman, and S. A. Rosenberg. Philadelphia: Lippincott-Raven, 1997, pp. 479–493.

19. Hao, Z., D. A. Cooney, N. R. Hartman, C. F. Perno, A. Friedland, A. L. DeVico, M. G. Sarngadharan, S. Broder, and D. G. Johns. Factors determining the activity of 2',3'-dideoxynucleosides in suppressing human immunodeficiency virus in vitro. Mol. Pharmacol. 1988;34:431.

20. Ostertag, W., G. Roesler, C. J. Krieg, J. Kind, T. Cole, T. Crozier, G. Gaedicke, G. Steinheider, N. Kluge, and S. Dube. Induction of endogenous virus and of thymidine kinase by bromodeoxyuridine in cell cultures transformed by Friend virus. Proc. Natl. Acad. Sci. U.S.A. 1974;71:4980.

21. Mitsuya, H., K. J. Weinhold, P. A. Furman, M. H. St. Clair, S. N. Lehrman, R. C. Gallo, D. Bolognesi, D. W. Barry, and S. Broder. 3'-azido'-3'-deoxythymidine (BWA509U): an antiviral agent that inhibits the infectivity and cytopathic effect of human T-lymphotropic virus type III/lymphadenopathy-associated virus in vitro. Proc. Natl. Acad. Sci. U.S.A. 1985;82:7096.

22. Cheng, Y.-C., G. E. Dutschman, K. W. Bastow, M. G. Sarngadharan, and R. Y. C. Ting. Human immunodeficiency virus reverse transcriptase. General properties and its interactions with nucleoside triphosphate analogs. J. Biol. Chem. 1987;262:2187.

23. St. Clair, M. H., C. A. Richards, T. Spector, K. J. Weinhold, W. H. Miller, A. J. Langlois, and P. A. Furman. 3'-Azido-3'-deoxythymidine triphosphate as an inhibitor and substrate of purified human immuno-

deficiency virus reverse transcriptase. *Antimicrob. Agents Chemother.* 1987;31:1972.

24. Furman, P. A., J. A. Fyfe, M. H. Claire, K. Weinhold, J. L. Rideout, G. A. Freeman, S. N. Lehrman, D. P. Bolognesi, S. Broder, H. Mitsuya, and D. W. Barry. Phosphorylation of 3'-azido-3'-deoxythymidine and selective interaction of the 5-triphosphate with HIV reverse transcriptase. *Proc. Natl. Acad. Sci. U.S.A.* 1986;83:8333.

25. Furman, P. A., and D. W. Barry. Spectrum of antiviral activity and mechanism of action of zidovudine. *Am. J. Med.* 1988;85(Suppl. 2A):176.

26. Tan, C. K., R. Cival, A. M. Mian, A. G. So, and K. M. Downey. Inhibition of the RNase H activity of HIV reverse transcriptase by azidothymidylate. *Biochemistry* 1991;30:4831.

27. Stretcher, B. N., A. J. Pesce, P. T. Frame, and D. S. Stein. Pharmacokinetics of zidovudine phosphorylation in peripheral blood mononuclear cells from patients infected with human immunodeficiency virus. *Antimicrob. Agents Chemother.* 1994;38:1541.

28. Barile, M., D. Valenti, G. A. Hobbs, M. F. Abruzzese, S. A. Keilbaugh, S. Passarella, E. Quagliariello, and M. V. Simpson. Mechanisms of toxicity of azido-3'-deoxythymidine. Its interaction with adenylate kinase. *Biochem. Pharmacol.* 1994;48:1405.

29. Foster, R. H., and D. Faulds. Abacavir. *Drugs* 1998;55:729.

30. Larder, B. A., and S. D. Kemp. Multiple mutations in HIV-1 reverse transcriptase confer high-level resistance to zidovudine (AZT). *Science* 1989;246:1155.

31. Larder, B., P. Kellam, and S. Kemp. Zidovudine resistance predicted by direct detection of mutations in DNA from HIV-infected lymphocytes. *AIDS* 1991;5:137.

32. Kellam, P., C. Boucher, and B. Larder. Fifth mutation in human immunodeficiency virus type 1 reverse transcriptase contributes to the development of high-level resistance to zidovudine. *Proc. Natl. Acad. Sci. U.S.A.* 1992;89:1934.

33. Richman, D., J. Grimes, and S. Lagakos. Effect of stage of disease and drug dose on zidovudine susceptibilities of isolates of human immunodeficiency virus. *J. Acquir. Immune Defic. Syndr.* 1990;3:743.

34. Najera, I., A. Holquin, M. E. Quinones-Mateu, M. A. Munoz-Fernandez, R. Najera, C. Lopez-Galindez, and E. Domingo. *Pol* gene quasispecies of human immunodeficiency virus: mutations associated with drug resistance in virus: mutations associated with drug resistance in virus from patients undergoing no drug therapy. *J. Virol.* 1995;69:23.

35. Land, S., K. McGavin, C. Birch, and R. Lucas. Reversion from zidovudine resistance to sensitivity on cessation of treatment. *Lancet* 1991;338:830.

36. Eron, J. J., Y.-K. Chow, A. M. Caliendo, J. Videler, K. M. Devore, T. P. Cooley, H. A. Liebman, J. C. Kaplan, M. S. Hirsch, and R. T. Aquila. *Pol* mutations conferring zidovudine and didanosine resistance with different effects in vitro yield multiply resistant human immunodeficiency virus type 1 isolates in vivo. *Antimicrob. Agents Chemother.* 1993;37:1480.

37. Kohlstaedt, L. A., J. Wang, J. M. Friedman, P. A. Rice, and T. A. Steitz. Crystal structure at 3.5 °A resolution of HIV-1 reverse transcriptase complexed with an inhibitor. *Science* 1992;256:1783.

38. Tantillo, C., J. Ding, A. Jacobo-Molina, R. G. Nanni, P. L. Boyer, S. H. Hughes, R. Pauwels, K. Andries, P. A. J. Janssen, and E. Arnold. Locations of anti-AIDS drug binding sites and resistance mutations in the three-dimensional structure of HIV-1 reverse transcriptase. *J. Mol. Biol.* 1994;243:369–387.

39. Arts, E. J., and M. A. Wainberg: Mechanisms of nucleoside analog antiviral activity and resistance during human immunodeficiency virus reverse transcription. *Antimicrob. Agents Chemother.* 1996;40:527–540.

40. Wilson, J. E., A. Aulabaugh, B. Caligan, S. McPherson, J. K. Wakefield, S. Jablonski, C. D. Morrow, J. E. Reardon, and P. A. Furman. Human immunodeficiency virus type 1 reverse transcriptase. Contribution of Met-184 to binding nucleoside 5'-triphosphate. *J. Biol. Chem.* 1996;271:13656.

41. Rooke, R., M. A. Parniak, M. Tremblay, H. Soudeyns, H. G. Li, Q. Gao, X. J. Yao, and M. A. Wainberg. Biological comparison of wild-type and zidovudine-resistant isolates of human immunodeficiency virus type 1 from the same subjects: susceptibility and resistance to other drugs. *Antimicrob. Agents Chemother.* 1991;35:988.

42. Tisdale, M., S. D. Kemp, N. R. Parry, and B. A. Larder. Rapid in vitro selection of human immunodeficiency virus type 1 resistance to 3'-thiacytidine inhibitors due to a mutation in the YMDD region of reverse transcriptase. *Proc. Natl. Acad. Sci. U.S.A.* 1993;90:5633.

43. Gao, Q., Z. X. Gu, M. A. Parniak, J. Cameron, N. Cammack, C. Boucher, and M. A. Wainberg. The same mutation that encodes low-level human immunodeficiency virus type 1 resistance to 2', 3'-dideoxyinosine and 2', 2'-dideoxycytidine confers high-level resistance to the (−) enantiomer of 2', 3'-dideoxy-3'-thiacytidine. *Antimicrob. Agents Chemother.* 1993; 37:1390.

44. Shirasaka, T., R. Yarchoan, M. C. O'Brien, R. N. Husson, B. D. Anderson, E. Kojima, T. Shimada, S. Broder, and H. Mitsuya. Changes in drug sensitivity of human immunodeficiency virus type 1 during therapy with azidothymidine, dideoxycytidine and dideoxyinosine: an in vitro comparative study. *Proc. Natl. Acad. Sci. U.S.A.* 1993;90:562.

45. Richman, D. D., T. C. Meng, S. A. Spector, M. A. Fischl, L. Resnick, and S. Lai. Resistance to AZT and ddC during long-term combination therapy in patients with advanced infection with human immunodeficiency virus. *J. Acquir. Immune Defic. Syndr.* 1994;7:135.

46. Cherrington, J. M., A. S. Mulato, P. D. Lamy, N. A. Margot, K. E. Anton, and M. D. Miller. Adefovir dipivoxil (bis-POM PMEA) therapy significantly decreases HIV RNA in patients with high levels of AZT/3TC-resistant HIV. *Intersci. Conf. Antimicrob. Agents Chemother.* 1998;38:388, [Abstract I-84].

47. Shirasaka, T., M. F. Kavlick, T. Ueno, W.-Y. Gao, E. Kojima, M. L. Alcaide, S. Chokekijchai, B. M. Roy, E. Arnold, R. Yarchoan, and H. Mitsuya. Emergence of human immunodeficiency virus type 1 variants

with resistance to multiple dideoxynucleosides in patients receiving therapy with dideoxynucleosides. *Proc. Natl. Acad. Sci. U.S.A.* 1995;92:2398.

48. Shafer, R. W., M. J. Kozal, M. A. Winters, A. K. N. Iversen, D. A. Katzenstein, M. V. Ragni, W. A. Meyer III, P. Gupta, S. Rasheed, R. Coombs, M. Katzman, S. Fiscus, and T. C. Merigan. Combination therapy with zidovudine and didanosine selects for drug-resistant human immunodeficiency virus type 1 strains with unique patterns of *pol* gene mutations. *J. Infect. Dis.* 1994;169:722.

49. Iversen, A. K. N., R. W. Shafer, K. Wehrly, M. A. Winters, J. I. Mullins, B. Chesebro, and T. C. Merigan. Multidrug-resistant human immunodeficiency virus type 1 strains resulting from combination antiretroviral therapy. *J. Virol.* 1996;70:1086.

50. Johnson, M. A., K. H. P. Moore, G. J. Yuen, A. Bye, and G. E. Pakes: Clinical pharmacokinetics of lamivudine. *Clin. pharmacokinet.* 1999;36:41.

51. Perry, C. M., and J. A. Balfour. Didanosine. An update on its antiviral activity, pharmacokinetic properties and therapeutic efficacy in the management of HIV disease. *Drugs* 1996;52:928.

52. Unadkat, J. D., A. C. Collier, S. S. Crosby, D. Cummings, K. E. Opheim, and L. Corey. Pharmacokinetics of oral zidovudine (azidothymidine) in patients with AIDS when administered with and without a high-fat meal. *AIDS* 1990;4:229.

53. Sahai, J., K. Gallicano, G. Garber, I. McGilveray, N. Hawley-Foss, N. Turgeon, and D. W. Cameron. The effect of a protein meal on zidovudine pharmacokinetics in HIV-infected patients. *Br. J. Clin. Pharmacol.* 1992;33:657.

54. Dudley; M. N. Clinical pharmacokinetics of nucleoside antiretroviral agents. *J. Infect. Dis.* 1995; 171(Suppl. 2):S99.

55. Enting, R. H., R. M. W. Hoetelmans, J. M. A. Lange, D. M. Burger, J. H. Beijnen, and P. Portegies. Antiretroviral drugs and the central nervous system. *AIDS* 1998;12:1941.

56. Thomas, S. A., and M. B. Segal. The passage of azidodeoxythymidine into and within the central nervous system: does it follow the parent compound, thymidine? *J. Pharmacol. Exp. Ther.* 1997;218:1211.

57. Hilts, A. E., and D. N. Fish. Dosage adjustments of antiretroviral agents in patients with organ dysfunction. *Am. J. Health Syst. Pharm.* 1998;55:2528.

58. Taburet, A., S. Naveau, G. Zorza, J. N. Colin, J. F. Delfraissy, J. C. Chaput, and E. Singlas. Pharmacokinetics of zidovudine in patients with liver cirrhosis. *Clin. Pharmacol. Ther.* 1990;47:731.

59. Howe, J. L., and D. J. Back. Extra hepatic metabolism of zidovudine. *Br. J. Clin. Pharmacol.* 1992;33: 190.

60. Retrovir package insert. Glaxo Wellcome, Research Triangle Park, NC, 1995.

61. Schnittman, S. M., and C. B. Pettinelli. Strategies and progress in the development of antiretroviral agents. In *AIDS: Biology, Diagnosis, Treatment and Prevention*, ed. by V. T. DeVita, S. Hellman, and S. A. Rosenberg. Philadelphia: Lippincott-Raven, 1997, pp. 467–478.

62. Volberding, P. A., and S. G. Deeks. Antiretro-

viral therapy for HIV infection. Promises and problems. *JAMA* 1998;279:1343.

63. Centers for Disease Control. Zidovudine for the prevention of HIV transmission from mother to infant. *Morbid Mortal. Wkly. Rep.* 1997;46:620.

64. Drugs for HIV infection *Med. Lett.* 1997;39: 111.

65. BHIVA Guidelines Co-ordinating Committee. British HIV Association guidelines for antiretroviral treatment of HIV seropositive individuals. *Lancet* 1997; 349:1087.

66. Portegies, P. HIV-1, the brain, and combination therapy. *Lancet* 1995;346:1244.

67. Fischl, M. A. Treatment of HIV infection. In *The Medical Management of AIDS*, ed. by M. A. Sande and P. A. Volberding. Philadelphia: W. B. Saunders, 1995, pp. 141–160.

68. McEvoy, G. K., (ed.) *Am. Hosp. Forum Service (AHFS) Drug Information*. Bethesda, Maryland; American Society of Health-System Pharmacists, Inc., 1997.

69. Threlkeld, S. C., and M. S. Hirsh. Antiretroviral therapy. *Med. Clin. North Am.* 1996;80:1263.

70. Bartlett; J. A. Antiretroviral therapy. In *Care and Management of Patients with HIV Infection*, ed. by J. A. Bartlett. Durham; NC: Glaxo Wellcome, 1997, pp. 171–199.

71. Staszewski, S., C. Loreday, J. J. Picazo, P. Dellamonica, P. Skinhøj, M. A. Johnson, S. A. Danner, P. R. Harrigan, A. M. Hill, L. Verity, and H. McDade. Safety and efficacy of lamivudine-zidovudine combination therapy in zidovudine-experienced patients. A randomized controlled comparison with zidovudine monotherapy. *JAMA* 1996;276:111.

72. CAESAR Coordinating Committee. Randomized trial of addition of lamivudine or lamivudine plus loviride to zidovudine-containing regimens for patients with HIV-1 infection: the CAESAR trial. *Lancet* 1997; 349:1413.

73. Lamivudine (Epivir®) package insert. Glaxo Wellcome; Research Triangle Park, NC; April 1997.

74. Three New Drugs for HIV Infection. *Med. Lett.* 1998;40:114.

75. Martin, J. L., C. E. Brown, N. Matthews-Davis, and J. E. Reardon. Effects of antiviral nucleoside analogs on human DNA polymerases and mitochondrial DNA synthesis. *Antimicrob. Agents Chemother.* 1994; 38:2743.

76. Brinkman, K., H. J. M. terHofstede, D. M. Burger, J. A. M. Smeitink, and P. P. Koopmans. Adverse effects of reverse transcriptase inhibitors: mitochondrial toxicity as a common pathway. *AIDS* 1998;12:1735.

77. Richman, D. D., M. A. Fischl, M. H. Grieco, M. S. Gottlieb, P. A. Volberding, O. L. Laskin, J. M. Leedom, J. E. Groopman, D. Mildvan, M. S. Hirsch, G. G. Jackson, D. T. Durack, D. Phil, S. Nusinoff-Lehrman, and the AZT Collaborative Working Group. The toxicity of azidothymidine (AZT) in the treatment of patients with AIDS and AIDS-related complex. A double-blind, placebo-controlled trial. *N. Engl. J. Med.* 1987;317:192.

78. Mentre, F., S. Escolano, B. Diquet, J. L. Golmard, and A. Mallet. Clinical pharmacokinetics of zidovudine: inter- and intra-individual variability and re-

lationship to long-term efficacy and toxicity. *Eur. J. Clin. Pharmacol.* 1993;45:397.

79. Balzarini, J., R. Pauwels, M. Baba, P. Herdewijn, E. de Clercq, S. Broder, and D. G. Johns. The in vitro and in vivo antiretrovirus activity, and intracellular metabolism of 3'-azido-2', 3'-dideoxythymidine and 2', 3' dideoxycytidine are highly dependent on the cell species. *Biochem. Pharmacol.* 1988;37:897.

80. Zhu, Z., M. J. Hitchcock, and J. P. Sommadossi. Metabolism and DNA interaction of 2', 3'-didehydro-2', 3'-dideoxythymidine in human bone marrow cells. *Mol. Pharmacol.* 1991;40:838.

81. Bridges, E. G., R. B. LeBoeuf, D. A. Weidner, and J. P. Sommadossi. Influence of template primary structure of 3'-azido-3'-deoxythymidine triphosphate incorporation into DNA. *Antiviral Res.* 1993;21:93.

82. Vazquez-Padua, M. A., M. C. Starnes, and Y. C. Cheng. Incorporation of 3'-azido-3'-deoxythymidine into cellular DNA and its removal in a human leukemic cell line. *Cancer Commun.* 1990;2:55.

83. Hall, E. T., J. P. Yan, P. Melancon, and R. D. Kuchta. 3'-azido-3'-deoxythymidine potently inhibits protein glycosylation. A novel mechanism for AZT cytotoxicity. *J. Biol. Chem.* 1994;269:14355.

84. Balzarini, J., P. Herdewijn, and E. DeClercq. Differential patterns of intracellular metabolism of 2',3'-didehydro-2',3'-dideoxythymidine and 3'-azido-2', 3'-dideoxythymidine, two potent anti-human immunodeficiency virus compounds. *J. Biol. Chem.* 1989;264:6127.

85. Tornevik, Y., B. Ulman, J. Balzarini, B. Wahren, and S. Eriksson. Cytotoxicity of 3'-azido-3'-deoxythymidine correlates with 3'-azidothymidine-5'-monophosphate (AZTMP) level, whereas anti-human immunodeficiency virus (HIV) activity correlates with 3'-azidothymidine-5'-triphosphate (AZTTP) levels in cultured CEM T-lymphoblastoid cells. *Biochem. Pharmacol.* 1995;49:829.

86. Barry, M., J. L. Howe, S. Ormesher, D. J. Back, A. M. Breckenridge, C. Bergin, F. Mulcahy, N. Beeching, and F. Nye. Pharmacokinetics of zidovudine and dideoxyinosine alone and in combination in patients with the acquired immunodeficiency syndrome. *Br. J. Clin. Pharmacol.* 1994;37:421.

87. Stagg, M. P., E. M. Cretton, L. Kidd, R. B. Diasio, and J. P. Sommadossi. Clinical pharmacokinetics of 3'-azido-3'-deoxythymidine (zidovudine) and catabolites with formation of a toxic catabolite, 3'-amino-3'-deoxythymidine. *Clin. Pharmacol. Ther.* 1992;51:668.

88. Faraj, A., D. A. Fowler, E. G. Bridges, and J. P. Sommadossi. Effects of 2',3'-dideoxynucleosides on proliferation and differentiation of human pluripotent progenitors in liquid culture and their effects on mitochondrial DNA synthesis. *Antimicrob. Agents. Chemother.* 1994;38:924.

89. Gogu, S. R., J. S. Malter, and K. C. Agrawal. Zidovudine-induced blockade of the expression and function of the erythropoietin receptor. *Biochem. Pharmacol.* 1992;44:1009.

90. Yarchoan, R., C. F. Perno, R. V. Thomas, J.-P. Allain, N. McAtee, R. Dubinsky, H. Mitsuya, T. J. Lawley, B. Safai, C. E. Myers, R. W. Klecker, R. J.

Wills, M. A. Fischl, M. C., McNeely, J. M. Pluda, M. Leuther, J. M. Collins, and S. Broder. Phase I studies of 2',3'-dideoxycytidine in severe human immunodeficiency virus infection as a single agent and alternating with zidovudine (AZT). 1988;*Lancet* 1:76.

91. Lambert, J. S., M. Seidlin, F. T. Valentine, R. C. Reichman, and R. Dolin. Didanosine: long-term follow-up of patients in a phase I study. *Clin. Infect. Dis.* 1993; 16(Suppl. 1):S40.

92. Lea, A. P., and D. Faulds. Stavudine. A review of its pharmacodynamic and pharmacokinetic properties and clinical potential in HIV infection. *Drugs* 1996; 51:846.

93. Dubinsky, R. M., R. Yarchoan, M., Dalakas, and S. Broder. Reversible axonal neuropathy from the treatment of AIDS and related disorders with 2',3'-dideoxycytidine (ddC). *Muscle Nerve* 1989;12:856.

94. Bessen, L. J., J. B. Greene, E. Louie, P. Seitzman, and H. Weinberg. Severe polymyositis-like syndrome associated with zidovudine therapy of AIDS and ARC [Letter]. *N. Engl. J. Med.* 1988;318:708.

95. Gorard, D. A., K. Henry, and R. J. Guiloff. Necrotising myopathy and zidovudine. *Lancet* 1988;1:1050.

96. Dalakas, M. C., I. Illa, G. H. Pezeshkpour, J. P. Laukaitis, B. Cohen, and J. L. Griffin. Mitochondrial myopathy caused by long-term zidovudine therapy. *N. Engl. J. Med.* 1990;322:1098.

97. Lamperth, L., M. C. Dalakas, F. Dagani, J. Anderson, and R. Ferrari. Abnormal skeletal and cardiac muscle mitochondria induced by zidovudine (AZT) in human muscle in vitro and in animal model. *Lab. Invest.* 1991;65:742.

98. Pike, I. M., and C. Nicaise. The didanosine expanded access program: safety analysis. *Clin. Infect. Dis.* 1993;16(Suppl. 1):S63.

99. Freiman, J. P., K. E. Helfert, M. R. Hamrell, and D. S. Stein. Hepatomegaly with severe steatosis in HIV-seropositive patients. *AIDS* 1993;7:379.

100. Chen, C. H., M. Vazques-Padua, and Y. C. Cheng. Effect of anti-human immunodeficiency virus nucleoside analogs on mitochondrial DNA and its implication for delayed toxicity. *Mol. Pharmacol.* 1991; 39:625.

101. Tsai, C. H., S. L. Doong, D. G. Johns, J. S. Driscoll, and Y. C. Cheng. Effect of anti-HIV 2'-beta-fluoro-2',3'-dideoxynucleoside analogs on the cellular content of mitochondrial DNA and on lactate production. *Biochem. Pharmacol.* 1994;48:1477.

102. Tseng, A. L., and M. M. Foisy. Management of drug interactions in patients with HIV. *Ann. Pharmacother.* 1997;31:1040.

103. Burger, D. M., P. L. Meenhorst, C. H. W. Koks, J. H. Beijnen. Drug interactions with zidovudine. *AIDS* 1993;7:445.

104. Hayden, F. G. Antiviral agents. In *Goodman and Gilman's The Pharmacological Basis of Therapeutics*, ed. by J. G., Hardman, L. E. Limbird, P. B. Molinoff, R. W. Ruddon, and A. G. Gilman. New York: McGraw-Hill, 1996, pp. 1191–1223.

105. Fischl, M. A., and G. D. Morse. Antiretroviral agents: zidovudine, didanosine and zalcitabine. In *Antimicrobial Therapy and Vaccines*, ed. by V. Yu, T.

Merigan, and S. Barriere. Baltimore: Williams and Wilkins, 1999, pp. 1403–1415.

106. Gallicano, K., J. Sahai, L. Swick, A. Pakuts, and W. Cameron. The effect of rifabutin (R) on zidovudine pharmacokinetics. Presented at the Second National Conference on Human Retroviruses and Related Infections, Washington, D.C. January 29–February 2, 1995, p. 145.

107. Lertora, J. J., A. B. Rege, D. L. Greenspan, S. Akula, W. J. George, N. E. Hyslop, Jr., and K. C. Agrawal. Pharmacokinetic interaction between zidovudine and valproic acid in patients infected with human immunodeficiency virus. *Clin. Pharmacol. Ther.* 1994;56: 272.

108. Kornhauser, D. M., B. G. Petty, C. W. Hendrix, A. S. Woods, L. J. Nerhood, J. G. Bartlett, and P. S. Leitman. Probenecid and zidovudine metabolism. *Lancet* 1989;2:473.

109. Szebeni, J., S. M. Wahl, M. Popovic, L. M. Wahl, S. Gartner, R. L. Fine, U. Skaleric, R. M. Friedmann, and J. N. Weinstein. Dipyridamole potentiates the inhibition by 3'-azido-3'-deoxythymidine and other dideoxynucleosides of human immunodeficiency virus replication in monocytemacrophages. *Proc. Natl. Acad. Sci. U.S.A.* 1989;86:3842 [published erratum appears in *Proc. Natl. Acad. U.S.A.* 1989;86:5968].

110. Gao, W. Y., R. Agbaria, J. S. Driscoll, and H. Mitsuya. Divergent anti-human immunodeficiency virus activity and anabolic phosphorylation of 2',3'-dideoxynucleoside analogs in resting and activated human cells. *J. Biol. Chem.* 1994;269:12633.

111. Sahai, J. Risks and synergies from drug interactions. *AIDS* 1996;10(Suppl. 1):S21.

112. White, A., E. Andrews, and R. Eldridge. Birth outcomes following zidovudine therapy in pregnant women. *Morb. Mortal. Wkly. Rep.* 1994;43:409.

113. Culnane, M., M. Fowler, S. S. Lee, G. McSherry, M. Brady, K. O'Donnell, L. Mofenson, S. L. Gortmaker, D. E. Shapiro, G. Scott, E. Jimenez, E. C. Moore, C. Diaz, P. M. Flynn, B. Cunningham, J. Oleske, and the Pediatric AIDS Clinical Trials Group Protocol 219/076 Teams. Lack of long-term effects of in utero exposure to zidovudine among uninfected children born to HIV-infected women. *JAMA* 1999;281: 151.

114. Toltzis, P., T. Mourton, and T. Magnuson. Comparative embryonic cytotoxicity of antiretroviral nucleosides. *J. Infect. Dis.* 1994;169:1100.

115. Spence, R. A., W. M. Kati, K. S. Anderson and K. A. Johnson. Mechanism of inhibition of HIV-1 reverse transcriptase by non-nucleoside inhibitors. *Science* 1995;267:988.

116. DeClercq, E. Antiviral therapy for human immunodeficiency virus infections. *Clin. Microbiol. Rev.* 1995;8:200.

117. Smerdon, S. J., J. Jager, J. Wang, L. A. Kohlstaedt, A. J. Chirino, J. M. Friedman, P. A. Rice, and T. A. Steitz. Structure of the binding site for non-nucleoside inhibitors of the reverse transcriptase of human immunodeficiency virus type. *Proc. Natl. Acad. Sci. U.S.A.* 1994;26:3911.

118. Rodgers, D. W., S. J. Gamblin, B. A. Harris, S. Ray, J. S. Culp, B. Hellmig, D. J. Woolf, C. Debouck,

and S. C. Harrison. The structure of unliganded reverse transcriptase from the human immunodeficiency virus type 1. *Proc. Natl. Acad. Sci. U.S.A.* 1995;92: 1222.

119. Dueweke, T. J., F. J. Kezzdy, G. A. Waszak, J. R. Deibel, and W. G. Tarpley. The binding of a novel bisheteroarylpiperazine mediates inhibition of human immunodeficiency virus type 1 reverse transcriptase. *J. Biol. Chem.* 1992;267:27.

120. Wu, J. C., T. C. Warren, J. Adams, J. Proudfoot, J. Skiles, P. Raghavan, C. Perry, I. Potocki, P. R. Farina, and P. M. Grob. A novel, dipyridodiazepinone inhibitor of HIV-1 reverse transcriptase acts through a nonsubstrate binding site. *Biochemistry* 1991;30:2022.

121. Balzarini, J., S. Velazquez, A. San-Felix, A. Karlsson, M. J. Perez-Perez, M. J. Camarasa, and E. de Clercq. Human immunodeficiency virus type 1-specific [2',5'-bis-O-(tert-butyldimethylsilyl)-beta-D-ribofuranosyl]-3'-spiro-5"-(4"-amino-1"-oxathiole-2",2"-dioxide)-purine analogues show a resistance spectrum that is different from that of the human immunodeficiency virus type 1-specific non-nucleoside analogues. *Mol. Pharmacol.* 1993;43:109.

122. Boyer, P. L., M. J. Currens, J. B. McMahon, M. R. Boyd, and S. H. Hughes. Analysis of non-nucleoside drug-resistant variants of human immunodeficiency virus type 1 reverse transcriptase. *J. Virol.* 1993;67:2412.

123. Cheeseman, S. H., D. Havlir, M. M. McLaughlin, T. C. Greenough, J. L. Sullivan, D. Hall, S. E. Hattox, S. A. Spector, D. S. Stein, M. Myers, and D. D. Richman. Phase I/II evaluation of nevirapine alone and in combination with zidovudine for infection with human immunodeficiency virus. *J. Acquir. Immune. Defic. Syndr. Hum. Retrovirol.* 1995;8:141.

124. D'Aquila, R. T., M. D. Hughes, V. A. Johnson, M. A. Fischl, J. P. Sommadossi, S. H. Liou, J. Timpone, M. Myers, N. Basgoz, M. Niu, M. S. Hirsch, and the National Institute of Allergy and Infectious Diseases AIDS Clinical Trials Group Protocol 241 Investigators. Nevirapine, zidovudine and didanosine compared with zidovudine and didanosine in patients with HIV-1 infection. *Ann. Intern. Med.* 1996;124:1019.

125. Nevirapine (Viramune®) package insert. Roxane Laboratories, Columbus, OH, June 1996.

126. de Jong, M. D., M. Loewenthal, C. A. B. Boucher, I. van der Ende, D. Hall, P. Schipper, A. Imrie, H. M. Weigel, R. H. Kaufmann, R. Koster, P. Seville, R. Rocklin, D. A. Cooper and J. M. A. Lange. Alternating nevirapine and zidovudine treatment of human immunodeficiency virus type 1–infected persons does not prolong nevirapine activity. *J. infect. Dis.* 1994;169: 1346.

127. Swindells S., and C. V. Fletcher. Antiretroviral agents: non-nucleoside Analogues. in *Antimicrobial Therapy and Vaccines*, ed. by V. Yu, T. Merigan, and S. Barriere. Baltimore: Williams and Wilkins, 1999, pp. 1372–1384.

128. Morales-Ramirez, J., K. Tashima, D. Hardy, P. Johnson, M. Nelson, S. Staszewski, D. Farina, N. Ruiz, and the DMP 266-6 Clinical Study Team. A phase II, multi-center randomized, open label study to compare the antiretroviral activity and tolerability of efavirenz

(EFV) and indinavir (IDV), versus EFV and Zidovudine (ZDV) and lamivudine (3TC), versus IDV + 3TC at > 36 weeks. *Intersci. Conf. Antimicrob. Agents Chemother.* 1998;38:394.

129. Adkins, J. C., and S. Noble. Efavirenz. *Drugs* 1998;56:1055.

130. Yazdanian, M., S. Ratigan, D. Joseph, H. Silverstein, P. Riska, J. N. Johnstone, I. Richter, S. Norris, and S. Hattox. Nevirapine, a non-nucleoside RT inhibitor, readily permeates the blood brain barrier [Abstract 567]. In: *Program and Abstracts for the Fourth Conference on Retroviruses and Opportunistic Infections,* Washington, D.C., January 22–26, 1997, p. 169.

131. Akbari, B., J. Shelton, J. M. Adams, R. G. Hewitt, and G. D. Morse. Effects of *Helicobacter pylori* treatment on gastric pH and delavirdine mesylate pharmacokinetics in HIV+ patients with gastric hyperacidity [Abstract A56]. In: *Program and Abstracts of the 36th Interscience Conference on Antimicrobial Agents and Chemotherapy,* New Orleans, LA, September 15–18, 1996, p. 11.

132. Cox, S. R., S. E. Cohn, C. Greisberger, R. C. Reichman, A. A. Della-Coletta, W. W. Freimuth, and G. D. Morse. Evaluation of the steady-state pharmacokinetic interaction between didanosine and DLV mesylate in HIV+ patients [Abstract 131]. In: *Program and Abstracts of the 35th Interscience Conference on Antimicrobial Agents and Chemotherapy,* San Francisco, September 17–20, 1995.

133. Morse, G. D., M. A. Fischl, S. R. Cox, L. Thompson, A. A. Della-Coletta, and W. W. Freimuth. Effect of food on the steady-state pharmacokinetics of delavirdine mesylate in HIV+ patients [Abstract I-30]. In: *Program and Abstracts of the 35th Interscience Conference on Antimicrobial Agents and Chemotherapy,* San Francisco, September 17–20, 1995.

134. Davey, R. T., D. G. Chaitt, G. F. Reed, W. W. Freimuth, B. R. Herpin, J. A. Metcalf, P. S. Eastman, J. Falloon, J. A. Kovacs, M. A. Polis, R. E. Walker, H. Masur, J. Boyle, S. Coleman, S. R. Cox, L. Wathen, C. L. Daenzer, and H. C. Lane. Randomized, controlled phase I/II trial of combination therapy with delavirdine (U-90152S) and conventional nucleosides in human immunodeficiency virus type 1-infected patients. *Antimicrob. Agents Chemother.* 1996;40:1657.

135. DuPont Pharmaceuticals Company. Sustiva® (efavirenz capsules). Prescribing information. September 17, 1998; http://www.sustiva.com.

136. Murphy, R. L., and J. Montaner. Nevirapine a review of its development, pharmacological profile and potential for clinical use. *Exp. Opin. Invest. Drugs* 1996;5:1183.

137. Cheeseman, S. H., R. L. Murphy, M. D. Saag, D. Havlir, and ACTG 164/168 Study Team. Safety of high dose nevirapine (NVP) after 200 mg/d lead-in [Abstract PO-B26-2109]. In: *Program and Abstracts of the 8th International Conference on AIDS,* Berlin, June 6–11, 1993, p. 487.

138. Delavirdine (Rescriptor®) package insert. Pharmacia & Upjohn, Kalamazoo, MI, April 1997.

139. Sahai, J., W. Cameron, M. Salgo, F. Stewart, M. Myers, M. Lamson, and P. Gagnier. Drug interaction study between saquinavir (SQV) and nevirapine (NVP)

[Abstract 614]. In: *Program and Abstracts of the Fourth Conference on Retroviruses and Opportunistic Infections,* Washington, D.C., January 22–26, 1997, p. 178.

140. Kakuda, T. N., K. A. Strable, and S. C. Piscitelli. Protease inhibitors for the treatment of human immunodeficiency virus infection. *Am. J. Health Syst. Pharm.* 1998;55:233.

141. Kohl, N. E., R. E. Diehl, E. Rands, L. J. Davis, M. G. Hanobik, B. Wolanski, and R. A. Dixon. Expression of active human immunodeficiency virus type 1 protease by noninfectious chimeric virus particles. *J. Virol.* 1991;65:3007.

142. Kramer, R. A., M. D. Schaber, A. M. Skalka, K. Ganguly, F. Wong-Staal, and E. P. Reddy. HTLV-III gag protein is processed in yeast cells by the virus pol-protease. *Science* 1986;231:1580.

143. Flexner; C. HIV-protease inhibitors. *N. Engl. J. Med.* 1998;338:1281.

144. Pearl, L. H., and W. R. Taylor. A structural model for the retroviral proteases. *Nature* 1987;329:351.

145. Overton, H. A., D. J. McMillan, S. J. Gridley, J. Brenner, S. Redshaw, and J. S. Mills. Effect of two novel inhibitors of the human immunodeficiency virus protease on the maturation of the HIV *gag* and *gag-pol* polyproteins. *Virology* 1990;179:508.

146. Pettit, S. C., S. F. Michael, and R. Swanstrom. The specificity of the HIV-1 protease. *Perspect. Drug Discov. Des.* 1993;1:69.

147. Graves, M. C., J. J. Lim, E. P. Heimer, and R. A. Kramer. An 11-kDa form of human immunodeficiency virus protease expressed in *Escherichia coli* is sufficient for enzymatic activity. *Proc. Natl. Acad. Sci. U.S.A.* 1988;85:2449.

148. Kohl, N. E., E. A. Emini, W. A. Schleif, L. J. Davis, J. C. Heimbach, R. A. Dixon, E. M. Scolnik, and I. S. Sigal. Active human immunodeficiency virus protease is required for viral infectivity. *Proc. Natl. Acad. Sci. U.S.A.* 1988;85:4686.

149. Henderson, L. E., M. A. Bowers, R. C. Sowder, II, S. A. Serabyn, D. G. Johnson, J. W. Bess, Jr., L. O. Arthur, D. K. Bryant, and C. Fenselau. Gag proteins of the highly replicative MN strain of human immunodeficiency virus type 1: posttranslational modifications, proteolytic processings, and complete amino acid sequences. *J. Virol.* 1992;66:1856.

150. Grice, S. F. J., J. Mills, and J. Mous. Active site mutagenesis of the AIDS virus protease and its alleviation by trans complementation. *EMBO J.* 1988;7:2647.

151. Debouck, C. The HIV-1 protease as a therapeutic target for AIDS. *AIDS Res. Hum. Retroviruses* 1992; 8:153.

152. Roberts, N. A., J. A. Martin, D. Kinchington, A. V. Broadhurst, J. C. Craig, I. B. Duncan, S. A. Galpin, B. K. Handa, J. Kay, A. Kröhn, R. W. Lambert, J. H. Merrett, J. S. Mills, K. E. B. Parkes, S. Redshaw, A. J. Ritchie, D. L. Taylor, G. J. Thomas, and P. J. Machin. Rational design of peptide-based HIV proteinase inhibitors. *Science* 1990;248:358.

153. Karacostas, V., K. Nagashima, M. A. Gonda, and B. Moss. Human immunodeficiency virus–like particles produced by a vaccinia virus expression vector. *Proc. Natl. Acad. Sci. U.S.A.* 1989;86:8964.

154. Vacca, J. P., B. D. Dorsey, W. A. Schleif, R. B. Levin, S. L. McDaniel, P. L. Darke, J. Zugay, J. C. Quintero, O. M. Blahy, E. Roth, V. V. Sardona, A. J. Schlabach, P. I. Graham, J. H. Condra, L. Gotlib, M. R. Holloway, J. Lin, I.-W. Chen, K. Vastag, D. Ostovic, P. S. Anderson, E. A. Emni, and J. R. Huff. L-735,524: an orally bioavailable human immunodeficiency virus type 1 protease inhibitor. *Proc. Natl. Acad. Sci. U.S.A.* 1994;91:4096.

155. Kempf, D. J., K. C. Marsh, J. F. Denissen, E. McDonald, S. Vasavanonda, C. A. Flentge, B. E. Green, L. Fino, C. H. Park, X. P. Kong, N. E. Wideburg, A. Saldivar, L. Ruiz, W. M. Kati, H. L. Sham, T. Robins, K. D. Stewart, A. Hsu, J. J. Plattner, J. M. Leonard, and D. W. Norbeck. ABT-538 is a potent inhibitor of human immunodeficiency virus protease and has high oral bioavailability in humans. *Proc. Natl. Acad. Sci. U.S.A.* 1995;92:2484.

156. Vacca J. P., and J. H. Condra. Clinically effective HIV-1 protease inhibitors. *Drug Discovery Today* 1997;2:261.

157. Baldwin, E. T., T. N. Bhat, B. Liu, N. Pattabiraman, and J. W. Erickson. Structural basis of drug resistance for the V82A mutant of HIV-1 proteinase. *Nat. Struct. Biol.* 1995;2:244.

158. Ala, P. J., E. E. Huston, R. M. Klabe, D. D. McCabe, J. L. Duke, C. J. Rizzo, B. D. Korant, R. J. DeLoskey, P. Y. Lam, C. N. Hodge, and C. H. Chang. Molecular basis of HIV-1 protease drug resistance: structural analysis of mutant proteases complexed with cyclic urea inhibitors. *Biochemistry* 1997;36:1573.

159. Boden, D., and M. Markowitz. Resistance to human immunodeficiency virus type 1 protease inhibitors. *Antimicrob. Agents Chemother.* 1998;42:2775.

160. Shao, W., L. Everitt, M. Manchester, D. D. Loeb, C. A. Hutchison, and R. Swanstrom. Sequence requirements of the HIV-1 protease flap region determined by saturation mutagenesis and kinetic analysis of flap mutants. *Proc. Natl. Acad. Sci. U.S.A.* 1997;94:2243.

161. Schmit, J.-C., L. Ruiz, B. Clotet, A. Raventos, J. Tor, J. Leonard, J. Desmyter, E. DeClercq and A.-M. Vandamme. Resistance related mutations in the HIV-1 protease gene of patients treated for 1 year with the protease inhibitor ritonavir (ABT-538). *AIDS* 1996;10:995.

162. Coleman, R. L. Antiretroviral agents: protease inhibitors. In *Antimicrobial Therapy and Vaccines*, ed. by V. Yu, T. Merigan, and S. Barriere. Baltimore: Williams and Wilkins, 1999, pp. 1385–1395.

163. Danner, S. A., A. Carr, J. M. Leonard, L. M. Lehman, F. Gudiol, J. Gonzales, A. Raventos, R. Rubio, E. Bouza, V. Pintado, A. G. Aguado, J. G. De Lomas, R. Delgado, J. C. C. Borleffs, A. Hsu, J. M. Valdes, C. A. B. Boucher, and D. A. Cooper, for the European-Australian Collaborative Ritonavir Study Group. A short-term study of the safety pharmacokinetics, and efficacy of ritonavir, an inhibitor of HIV-1 protease. *N. Engl. J. Med.* 1995;333:1528.

164. Markowitz, M., M. Saag, W. G. Powderly, A. M. Hurley, A. Hsu, J. M. Valdes, D. Henry, F. Sattler, A. La Marca, J. M. Leonard, and D. D. Ho. A preliminary study of ritonavir, an inhibitor of HIV-1 protease, to treat HIV-1 infection. *N. Engl. J. Med.* 1995; 333:1534.

165. Hammer, S. M., K. E. Squires, M. D. Hughes, J. M. Grimes, L. M. Demeter, J. S. Currier, J. J. Eron, Jr., J. E. Feinberg, H. H. Balfour, Jr., L. R. Deyton, J. A. Chodakewitz, and M. A. Fischl. A controlled trial of two nucleoside analogues plus indinavir in persons with human immunodeficiency virus infection and CD4 cell counts of 200 per cubic millimeter or less. *N. Engl. J. Med.* 1997;337:725.

166. Cameron, D. W., M. Heath-Chiozzi, S. Kravcik, R. Mills, A. Potthoff, and D. Henry. Prolongation of life and prevention of AIDS complications in advanced HIV immunodeficiency with ritonavir: update. In *Program and Abstracts of the 11th International Conference on AIDS*, Vol. 1, Vancouver, British Columbia, July 7–12, 1996, p. 24.

167. Salgo, M. P., D. Beattie, K. Bragman, L. Donatacci, M. Jones, L. Montgomery, and the NV14256 Study Team. Saquinavir (invirase, SQV) vs. HIVID (zalcitabine, ddC) vs. combination as treatment for advanced HIV infection in patients discontinuing/unable to take Retrovir (zidovudine, ZDV). Presented at the 11th International Conference on AIDS, Vancouver, British Columbia, July 7–12, 1996.

168. Nabulsi, A. A., D. Revicki, D. Conway, C. Maurath, R. Mills, and J. Leonard. Quality of life consequences of adding ritonavir to current antiviral therapy for advanced HIV patients. In *Program and Abstracts of the 11th International Conference on AIDS*, Vol. 2, Vancouver, British Columbia, July 7–12, 1996, p. 31.

169. Gulick, R. M., J. W. Mellors, D. Havlir, J. J. Eron, C. Gonzalez, D. McMahon, D. D. Richman, F. T. Valentine, L. Jonas, A. Meibohm, E. A. Emini, and J. A. Chodakewitz. Treatment with indinavir, zidovudine, lamovudine in adults with human immunodeficiency virus infection and prior antiretroviral therapy. *N. Engl. J. Med.* 1997;337:734.

170. Murphy, R., P. Gagnier, M. Lamson, A. Dusek, W. Ju, and A. Hsu. Effect of nevirapine on pharmacokinetics of indinavir and ritonavir in HIV-1 patients. In *Program and Abstracts of the Fourth Conference on Retroviruses and Opportunistic Infections*, Washington, D.C., January 22–26, 1997, p. 133.

171. Kahn, J., D. Mayers, and S. Riddler. Durable clinical anti-HIV-1 activity (60 weeks) and tolerability for efavirenz (DMP 266) in combination with indinavir (IDV). In *Program and Abstracts of the Fifth Conference on Retroviruses and Opportunistic Infections*, Chicago, February 1–5, 1998, p. 208.

172. Virav, H., and C. D. Holtzer. Simultaneous use of two protease inhibitors in HIV infection. *Am. J. Health Syst. Pharm.* 1999;56:273.

173. Perry, C. M., and S. Noble. Saquinavir soft-gel capsule formulation. A review of its use in patients with HIV infection. *Drugs* 1998;55:461.

174. McDonald, C. K., and D. R. Kuritzkes. Human immunodeficiency virus type 1 protease inhibitors. *Arch. Intern. Med.* 1997;157:951.

175. Stein, D. S., D. G. Fish, J. A. Bilello, S. L. Preston, G. L. Martineau, and G. L. Drusano. A 24-week open label Phase I/II evaluation of the HIV protease inhibitor MK-639 (indinavir). *AIDS* 1996;10:485.

176. Saquinavir (Invirase®) package insert. Roche Pharmaceuticals, Nutley, NJ, January 1997.

177. Flexner, C. Pharmacokinetics and pharmacodynamics of HIV protease inhibitors. *Infect. Med.* 1996; 13(Suppl. R):16.

178. Vella, S., and M. Florida. Saquinavir. Clinical pharmacology and efficacy. *Clin. Pharmacokinet.* 1998; 34:189.

179. Indinavir (Crixivan®) package insert. West Point, PA, Merck & Co., March 1996.

180. Nelfinavir (Viracept®) package insert. LaJolla, CA, Agouron Pharmaceuticals, March 1997.

181. Ritonavir (Norvir®) package insert. North Chicago, IL, Abbott Laboratories, February 1996.

182. Jarvis, B., and D. Faulds. Nelfinavir. A review of its therapeutic efficacy in HIV infection. *Drugs* 1998; 56:147.

183. Barry, M., S. Gibbons, D. Back and F. Mulcahy. Protease inhibitors in patients with HIV disease. *Clin. Pharmacokinet.* 1997;32:194.

184. Moyle, G. J., M. Sadler, D. Hawkins, and N. Buss. Pharmacokinetics of saquinavir at steady state in CSF and plasma: correlation between plasma and CSF viral load in patients on saquinavir containing regimens. In *Program and Abstracts of the Infectious Diseases Society of America 35th Annual Meeting,* San Francisco, September 1997, p. 115.

185. Collier, A. C., C. Marra, R. W. Coombs, L. Zhong, J. Stone, and B. Nguyen. Cerebrospinal fluid indinavir and HIV RNA levels in patients on chronic indinavir therapy. In *Program and Abstracts of the Infectious Diseases Society of America 35th Annual Meeting,* San Francisco, September 1997, p. 75.

186. Fitzsimmons, M. E., and J. M. Collins. Selective biotransformation of the human immunodeficiency virus protease inhibitor saquinavir by human small-intestinal cytochrome P4503A4: potential contribution to high first-pass metabolism. *Drug Metab. Dispos.* 1997;25:256.

187. Kumar, G. N., A. D. Rodrigues, A. M. Buko, and J. F. Denissen. Cytochrome P450-mediated metabolism of the HIV-1 protease inhibitor ritonavir (ABT-538) in human liver microsomes. *J. Pharmacol. Exp. Ther.* 1996;277:423 [erratum in *J. Pharmacol. Exp. Ther.* 1997;281:1506.

188. Bräu, N., H. L. Leaf, R. L. Wieczorek, and D. M. Margolis. Severe hepatitis in three AIDS patients treated with indinavir. *Lancet* 1997;349:924.

189. FDA protease inhibitor letter urges monitoring of hemophiliacs. *FDC Rep.* 1996;57:3.

190. Ginsburg, C., D. Salmon-Ceron, D. Vassilief, C. Rabian, C. Rotschild, M. Fontenay-Roupie, N. Stieltjes, and D. Sicard. Unusual occurrence of spontaneous hematomas in three asymptomatic HIV-infected haemophilia patients a few days after the onset of ritonavir treatment. *AIDS* 1997;11:388.

191. Roberts, A. D., A. Muesing, D. M. Parenti, J. Hsia, A. G. Wasserman, and G. L. Simon. Alterations in serum lipids and lipoproteins with indinavir in HIV-infected patients. In *Program and Abstracts of the Infectious Diseases Society of America 35th Annual Meeting,* San Francisco, September 1997, p. 114.

192. Hengel, R. L., N. B. Watts, and J. L. Lennox. Benign symmetric lipomatosis associated with protease inhibitors. *Lancet* 1997;350:1596.

193. Herry, I., L. Bernard, P. de Truchis, and C. Perronne. Hypertrophy of the breasts in a patient treated with indinavir. *Clin. Infect. Dis.* 1997;25:937.

194. Kopp, J. B., K. D. Miller, J. A. M. Mican, I. M. Feuerstein, E. Vaughan, C. Baker, L. K. Pannell, and J. Falloon. Crystalluria and urinary tract abnormalities associated with indinavir. *Ann. Intern. Med.* 1997;127:119.

195. Deeks, S. G., M. Smith, M. Holodniy, and J. O. Kahn. HIV-1 protease inhibitors. A review for clinicians. *JAMA* 1997;277:145.

196. Moyle, G. L., M. Youle, and C. Higgs. Extended follow-up of the safety and activity of Agouron's HIV protease inhibitor AG1343 (Viracept) in virological responders from the UK phase I/II dose finding study. In *Program and Abstracts of the 11th International Conference on AIDS,* Vol. 1, Vancouver, British Columbia, July 7–12, 1996, p. 118.

197. Gathe, J., B. Burkhardt, and P. Hawleyl. A randomized phase II study of Viracept, a novel HIV protease inhibitor, used in combination with stauvudine vs stauvudine alone. In *Program and Abstracts of the 11th International Conference on AIDS,* Vol. 1, Vancouver, British Columbia, July 7–12, 1996, p. 25.

198. Saquinavir (Fortovase®) package insert. Roche Pharmaceuticals; Nutley, NJ, November 1997.

199. Piscitelli, S. C., C. Flexner, J. R. Minor, M. A. Polis, and H. Masur. Drug interactions in patients infected with human immunodeficiency virus. *Clin. Infect. Dis.* 1996;23:685.

200. McCrea, J., D. Wyss, J. Stone, A. Carides, S. Kusma, C. Kleinbloesem, Y. Al-Hamdan, K. Yeh, P. Deutsch, Merck Research Labs, USA and Brussels, and Clin. Pharma Research AG, Switzerland. Pharmacokinetic interaction between indinavir and rifampin. *Clin. Pharmacol. Ther.* 1997;61:152.

201. Impact of HIV protease inhibitors on the treatment of HIV-infected tuberculosis patients with rifampin. *Morb. Mortal Wkly. Rep.* 1996;45:921.

202. Chiba, M., M. Hensleigh, J. A. Nishime, S. K. Balani, and J. H. Lin. Role of cytochrome P450 3A4 in human metabolism of MK-639, a potent human immunodeficiency virus protease inhibitor. *Drug Metab. Dispos.* 1996;24:307.

203. VonMoltke, L. L., D. J. Greenblatt, J. M. Grassi, B. W. Granda, S. X. Duan, S. M., Fogelman, J. P. Daily, J. S. Harmatz, and R. I. Shader. Protease inhibitors as inhibitors of human cytochromes P450: high risk associated with ritonavir. *J. Clin. Pharmacol.* 1998; 38:106.

204. Hsu, A., G. F. Granneman, G. Witt, C. Locke, J. Denissen, A. Molla, J. Valdes, J. Smith, K. Erdman, N. Lyons, P. Niu, J. P. Decourt, J. B. Fourtillan, J. Girault, and J. M. Leonard. Multiple-dose pharmacoki-

netics of ritonavir in human immunodeficiency virus–infected subjects. *Antimicrob. Agents Chemother*. 1997; 41:898.

205. Cohen, C., E. Sun, and W. Cameron. Ritonavir-saquinavir combination treatment in HIV-infected pa-tients. In *Addendum to Program and Abstracts of the 36th Interscience Conference on Antimicrobial Agents and Chemotherapy*, New Orleans, September 1996. Washington, D.C.: American Society for Microbiology, 1996, p. 8.

Index

Abacavir for HIV infection, 554f. *See also* Nucleoside analog reverse transcriptase inhibitors (NRTIs)

Abscess(es). *See* Purulence

Absorption of drugs, 25

Acetazolamide, 220

Acetohydroxamic acid and methenamine, 251–252

Acid-fast bacilli, drugs of first choice for, 19t

Acid-fast stains, 11

Acidosis and sulfonamides, 220

Acne vulgaris, tetracyclines for, 196–197

Actinomycetes
    drugs of first choice for, 19t
    vancomycin for, 115–116

Acyclovir, 510–515, 510f
    adverse effects of, 514–515
    antiviral activity of, 510–512, 511f
    drug interactions of, 515
    mechanism of action of, 496, 510–512, 511f
    pharmacokinetics of, 513–514, 518t
    resistance to, 510–512
    therapeutic uses of, 512–513
    vs. famciclovir, 517
    vs. penciclovir, 516–517
    vs. valacyclovir, 515–516

Adefovir, 553f. *See also* Nucleoside analog reverse transcriptase inhibitors (NRTIs)

Adrenocorticotropic hormone (ACTH) and azoles, 353

Age as factor modifying drug use, 23–24

Agranulocytosis
    chloramphenicol and, 167–168
    sulfonamides and, 219
    trimethoprim-sulfamethoxazole and, 229

AIDS. *See* HIV infection

Albendazole, 466, 470f
    for roundworms, 467t, 468–472

Allergy to drugs. *See* Hypersensitivity reactions

Allopurinol for leishmaniasis, 431

Allylamines, 359–360

Amantadine
    adverse effects of, 503–504
    drug interactions of, 504
    for influenza virus, 499–504, 499f–500f, 501t
    mechanism of action of, 495, 499–500, 499f
    pharmacokinetics of, 502–503
    resistance to, 500
    therapeutic uses of, 500–502, 501t

Amebiasis, 420–422, 420f. *See also Entamoeba histolytica*
    drugs for, 420–431, 421t, 422t
    paromomycin for, 151

Amikacin
    for *Mycobacterium avium* complex (MAC), 313

resistance to, 137, 137f
    therapeutic uses of, 150
    for tuberculosis, 306

Aminoglycoside antibiotic-induced deafness (AAID), 148

Aminoglycosides. *See also specific drug names*
    antibacterial activity of, 137–139, 138t, 139f
    combined with fluoroquinolones, 269–270
    mechanism of action of, 127–135
        bacterial protein synthesis and, 128–131, 129f–130f
        streptomycin and, 131–135, 131t–133t, 135f
    pharmacokinetics of, 139–145, 140t
        absorption of, 139–140
        distribution of, 140–141, 141t
        dosing strategies and, 143–145
        excretion of, 140t, 141–142, 142f
        serum drug concentrations and, 142–143
    resistance to, 135–137, 137f
    streptomycin *vs.* others, 135
    structure of, 127, 128f
    synergistic actions of, 31, 138, 139f
    therapeutic ratio of, 3
    therapeutic uses of, 149–151, 302–303
    toxicity of, 145–149, 149t
        nephotoxicity, 148–149
        neuromuscular blockade and, 145–146
        ototoxicity, 146–148, 303
    for tuberculosis, 306

Aminopenicillins, 88–90, 89f

4-Aminoquinolines, 382–392. *See also* Amodiquine; Chloroquine

Amoxicillin
    and clavulanic acid, 73, 73t, 114–115, 115t
    pharmacokinetics of, 88–90, 89f
    spectrum of action of, 64

Amphotericin B. *See also* Polyene antibiotics
    combination of, 333–334, 336t
        with flucytosine, 344–345
        with rifampin, 296
        synergistic actions of, 32
        with tetracyclines, 188–189
    drug interactions of, 333–334
    for leishmaniasis, 431, 432t
    pharmacokinetics of, 339–340, 340t
    pulmonary reaction and, 26
    resistance to, 335
    toxicity of, 336–337, 341–342
        lipid formulations and, 338, 339t

Amphotericin B colloidal dispersion (ABCD), 338, 339t

Amphotericin B lipid complex (ABLC), 338, 339t

Ampicillin
  pharmacokinetics of, 88–90, 89*f*
  rashes caused by, 98
  and sulbactam, 114–115, 115*t*
Amprenavir, 570–578, 571*f. See also* Protease
    inhibitors
Anaphylaxis. *See* Hypersensitivity reactions
Ancylostoma duodenale, 467*t,* 468–469
Animal feed and resistance development, 45–46
  chloramphenicol and, 162–163
  tetracycline and, 189
Anopheles mosquito in malaria cycle, 377, 378*f*
Antacids, drug interactions with
  fluoroquinolones and, 272
  macrolides and, 178
  quinine and, 397
  tetracyclines and, 190, 194
Antagonism in drug combinations, 30–31, 30*f*
Antibiotic(s)
  cidal *vs.* static effects, 4–5, 4*f*
  defined, 1
  for malaria, 408–409
Antibiotic-associated colitis. *See* Colitis, antibiotic-
    associated
Antifungal drugs, 327–371. *See also specific drugs*
  allylamines, 359–360
  azoles, 346–354
  ciclopirox olamine, 359
  flucytosine, 342–346
  griseofulvin, 354–358
  haloprogin, 359
  imidazoles, 346–354, 359
  iodide, 354
  nikkomycins, 358
  nystatin, 360
  papulocandins, 358
  pneumocandins, 358
  polyene antibiotics, 327–342
  pradimicins, 358
  systemic agents, new, 359
  tolnaftate, 358–359
  triazoles, 346–354, 359
  undecylenic acid, 358
Antimetabolites, 211–233. *See also specific drugs*
  cloroguanide, 403–404
  para-aminosalicylic acid, 305–306
  pyrimethamine, 403–408
  sulfonamides, 211–220
  sulfones, 308–309
  trimethoprim-sulfamethoxazole, 220–229
Antimicrobial susceptibility tests, 12–14, 13*t*
Antimonials for leishmaniasis, 432–434, 434*f*
Antipseudomonal penicillins, 85*t*–86*t,* 90–91
Antiretroviral drugs, 550–578
  non-nucleoside reverse transcriptase inhibitors, 564–
    570, 564*f*
  nucleoside analog reverse transcriptase inhibitors,
    553–564, 553*f*–554*f*
  protease inhibitors, 570–578, 571*f*

Arabinose and ethambutol, 301
Arsenicals
  combined with eflornithine, 443
  for trypanisomiasis, 437, 439–441
Artemisinin for malaria, 381–382, 398–399
Arthritis
  chloroquine for, 391
  septic. *See* Joint infections
Arthropathy
  with fluoroquinolones, 270*t,* 271–272
  and pyrazinamide, 304
Ascariasis, 467*f,* 467*t,* 468
  ivermectin for, 467*t,* 480–482, 480*f*
Aspergillus
  azoles for, 349
Assembly stage of viral biology, 494*f,* 497–498
Atovaquone
  for *Pneumocystis carinii* pneumonia, 447–448, 447*f*
  for toxoplasmosis, 446–448
Attachment stage of viral biology, 494–495, 494*f*
Autoimmune deficiency syndrome (AIDS). *See* HIV
    infection
Autolysins and cell-wall synthesis inhibitors, 52, 61–
    64, 62*f,* 63*t*
Azithromycin
  antimicrobial activity of, 173*t,* 174
  for *Mycobacterium avium* complex (MAC), 312
  pharmacokinetics of, 176
Azoles, 346–354. *See also* Imidazoles; Triazoles
  adverse effects of, 352–353
  antifungal activity of, 348–349, 349*t*
  development of, 346–347
  drug interactions of, 354
  mechanism of action of, 348
  new agents, 353
  pharmacokinetics of, 350–352, 352*t*
  preparations of, 349–350
  resistance to, 348–349
  structure of, 346–348, 347*f*
AZT. *See* Nucleoside analog reverse transcriptase
    inhibitors (NRTIs); Zidovudine
Aztreonam, 51
  pharmacokinetics of, 113–114, 113*f,* 113*t*

Bacampicillin, 90
Bacillus spp.
  β-lactamase production of, 70
  penicillin-receptor complexes in, 61
Bacitracin
  cell-wall synthesis inhibition by, 54, 55–57, 55*f ,*
    56*t*
  combined with polymixin, 236
  pharmacokinetics of, 117–118
Bactericidal, defined, 4–5, 4*f*
Bacteriostatic, defined, 4–5, 4*f*
Bacteroides
  nitrofurantoin for, 246, 246*t*
Bacteroides fragilis
  cephalosporins for, 108
  chloramphenicol for, 162, 163*t,* 169

clindamycin for, 180
fluoroquinolones for, 263, 264t
metronidazole for, 423, 423t
resistance to, 425
penicillins for, 90
Balantidium coli
diiodohydroxyquin for, 429
Basidiobolus, 354
Benznidazole for trypanisomiasis, 432, 432t
Benzylpenicilloyl-polylysine (PPL), 95
Bithionol for flukes, 459t, 465, 465f
Blackwater fever, 397
Blastomyces
azoles for, 348–350
nikkomycin for, 358
Blindness
and 8-hydroxyquinolines, 428–429
onchocerciasis and, 439
river, 467t, 477–478, 477t
Blood disorders
amphotericin B and, 342
cephalosporins and, 104–105
chloramphenicol and, 166–168, 167t
clindamycin and, 181
dapsone and, 309
fluoroquinolones and, 270t, 272
foscarnet and, 522
ganciclovir and, 519
nalidixic acid and, 245
penicillin and, 87
primaquine and, 401–403, 402f–403f
pyrimethamine and, 408
ribavirin and, 535
rifampin and, 299
with roundworms, 469
sulfonamides and, 219–220
sulfones and, 309
trimethoprim-sulfamethoxazole and, 228–229
Blood infection, probable etiologic agents of, 9t
Bone
fluoroquinolones and, 265
infection of. *See* Osteomyelitis
tetracycline effect on, 192–193
Bone marrow toxicity
chloramphenicol and, 166–167, 167t
flucytosine and, 346
ganciclovir and, 519
idoxyuridine and, 506
nucleoside analog reverse transcriptase inhibitors
and, 560–561, 563t
pyrimethamine and, 408
ribavirin and, 535
trimetrexate and, 449
Bordetella
macrolides for, 174
polymixins for, 236
trimethoprim-sulfamethoxazole for, 224–226, 224t–
225t
Borrelia, tetracyclines for, 188, 195
Braun lipoproteins, 64–66, 65t

Broad-spectrum penicillins, 64–66, 65t
Bronchial infection, probable etiologic agents of,
8t
Broth dilution susceptibility test, 13–14
Brucella
fluoroquinolones for, 263, 264t, 270
tetracyclines for, 188
trimethoprim-sulfamethoxazole for, 224–226, 224t–
225t
Brugia malayi, 467t, 476–478, 477t
Burn infections
probable etiologic agents of, 7t
and sulfonamides, 216f, 217–218
Butenafine, 359

Caffeine interaction with fluoroquinolones, 272
Calabar swellings, 477
Calcium interaction with fluoroquinolones, 272
Campylobacter, fluoroquinolones for, 263, 264t
Candida albicans
amphotericin B for, 333–334
azoles for, 348–350, 349t
tetracyclines and, 192
Candida spp.
allylamines for, 359–360
azoles for, 348–350, 349t, 359
ciclopirox olamine for, 359
flucytosine for, 344, 344t
haloprogin for, 359
nikkomycin for, 358
superinfection and, 6
tetracyclines for, 189
Capreomycin for tuberculosis, 283t, 306–307
Carbamazepine, doxycycline interaction with, 194–
195
Carbapenems
pharmacokinetics of, 111–113, 111f, 112t
structure of, 51, 52f
Carbenicillin, pharmacokinetics of, 85t–86t, 89f, 90–
91
Carboxypenicillins, 85t–86t, 89f, 90–91
Carboxypeptidase, penicillin activity and, 61
Carcinogenicity
of idoxyuridine, 506
of metronidazole, 427
of vidarabine, 510
Cardiac infection, probable etiologic agents of, 9t
Cardiotoxicity
of artemisinin, 399
of emetines, 430
of fluoroquinolones, 270t, 271–272
of halofantrine, 398
with nucleoside analog reverse transcriptase
inhibitors, 562, 563t
of quinine, 396–397
of sodium stibogluconate, 434
Carrier ionophores, 239–240, 239f
Cefaclor, 100t, 105–108, 106f
Cefadroxil, 100t, 101f, 105
Cefamandole, 100t, 105–108, 106f

Cefazolin, 100t, 101f, 105
Cefotetan, 100t, 105–108, 106f
Cefoxitin, 100t, 105–108, 106f
Cefprozil, 100t, 105–108, 106f
Cefuroxime, 100t, 105–108, 106f
Cell membrane permeability, antibiotics affecting, 234–241. *See also* Gramicidin A; Polymixins
Cell-wall synthesis inhibitors. *See also* Cephalosporins; Cephamycins; β-Lactam antibiotics; Penicillins
    autolytic enzyme activity in, 61–64, 62f, 63t
    cell envelope penetration of, 64–66, 65t
    β-lactamase inactivation and, 72–73, 72f–73f
    β-lactamase resistant, 71–72, 72t
    mechanisms of action of, 51–80, 52f–53f
    penicillin binding proteins and, 59–61, 60f, 61t
        resistance due to changes in, 66–67
    pharmacology and adverse effects of, 81–126
        bacitracin, 117–118
        carbapenems, 111–113
        cephalosporins, 98–111
        β-lactamase inhibitor combinations, 114–115
        monobactams, 113–114
        penicillins, 81–98
        teicoplanin, 117
        vancomycin, 115–117
    resistance to
        β-lactamase production, 67–71, 68f, 68t–69t
        mechanisms of, 66–75
        penicillin-binding protein changes and, 66–67
        transfer of, 67–69
    spectrum of activity of, 64–66, 65t
    stages of, 53–59
        first, 53–55, 54f
        second, 55–57, 55f, 56t
        third, 57–59, 57f–59f
    "tolerance" to, 62–63, 62f, 63t
    "triggering" hypothesis of lysis, 63–64
Central nervous system. *See also* Meningitis; Neurotoxicity
    malaria in, artemissinin for, 398–399
    toxoplasmosis and, 445–446
    trypanisomiasis of, 437, 439–443
Cephalexin, 100t, 101f, 105
Cephalosporins, 98–111
    adverse effects of, 104–105
    aminoglycosides and, 138
    cell-wall synthesis inhibition by, 54
    in cerebrospinal fluid, 103–104
    classification of, 98–100, 100t
    core structure of, 101f
    cross-reactivity to penicillin and, 94–95
    distribution of, 102–104
    E. coli binding proteins and, 59–61, 60f, 61t
    first-generation, 100t, 101f, 105
    fourth-generation, 100t, 109, 110f, 111
    pharmacokinetics of, 100–101, 101–102, 101f, 102t–103t
    in renal function impairment, 102, 103t, 104
    resistance to β-lactamase, 71–72, 72t
    second generation, 100t, 105–108, 106f

    spectra of activity of, 64–66, 65f, 99
    third-generation, 100t, 108–109, 110f
Cephalothin, 100t, 101f, 105
Cephapirin, 100t, 101f, 105
Cephradine, 100t, 101f, 105
Cerebrospinal fluid
    chloramphenicol and, 163
    fluoroquinolones and, 263, 265
    sulfonamides and, 217–218
Cestodiasis. *See* Tapeworms
Chagas' disease. *See* Trypanisomiasis
Channel-forming ionophores, 239–240, 239f
Chlamydia pneumoniae
    macrolides for, 174
Chlamydia spp.
    chloramphenicol for, 162
    drugs of first choice for, 20t
    fluoroquinolones for, 263, 264t
    tetracyclines for, 188, 188t, 195–196
Chlamydia trachomatis
    erythromycin for, 174
Chloramphenicol, 159–170, 159f
    aminoglycosides and, 138
    antimicrobial activity of, 152–164, 163t
    drug interactions with, 168
    guidelines for use of, 169
    in infants, 23–24, 165–166, 165f
    mechanism of action of, 159–162, 160f, 161t
    pharmacokinetics of, 164–165, 164f
    resistance to, 163–164
        by *Shigella*, 41–42, 42t
    therapeutic indications for, 168–169
    toxicity of, 165–168
        marketing and, 169–170
Chloroguanide for malaria, 403–408, 404f. *See also* Folic acid synthesis inhibitors
    prophylaxis of, 380
Chloroquine
    adverse effects of, 390–392
    for amebiasis, 421t, 422
    cross-resistance to, 389–390
    DNA interaction of, 386
    dosage regimens for, 383t–384t
    drug interactions of, 392
    for *Entamoeba histolytica*, 428
    free radical formation and, 387
    heme polymerization and, 386–387
    for malaria acute attack, 380–382, 384t
    for malaria prophylaxis, 380, 383t
    mechanism of action of, 384–387
    overdosage of, 390–392
    pharmacokinetics of, 390
    precautions for, 392
    preparations of, 382–383
    resistance to, 379, 387–390, 388f
    structure of, 382, 382f
    therapeutic uses of, 382–383
Chlortetracycline
    pharmacokinetics of, 189–191, 189f
    structure of, 184, 184f

Cholera, fluoroquinolones for, 268
Chromomycosis, flucytosine for, 344–345
Ciclopirox olamine, 359
Cidofovir, 522–523, 522f
Cimetidine and acyclovir, 515
Cinchonism, 396–397
Cinoxacin, 242–245, 242f
  adverse effects of, 244–245
  antimicrobial activity of, 242–243
  fluoroquinolones and, 257
  mechanism of action of, 242
  pharmacokinetics of, 243–244, 244t
  resistance to, 242–243
Ciprofloxacin, 257, 258f. See also Fluoroquinolones
  for Mycobacterium avium complex (MAC), 312
  resistance to, 75
  for tuberculosis, 284t, 307
Clarithromycin
  antimicrobial activity of, 173t, 174
  drug interactions with, 178
  for Mycobacterium avium complex (MAC), 312
  pharmacokinetics of, 175–176
Clavulanic acid, 72–73, 72f–73f
  pharmacokinetics of, 114–115, 115t
  resistance and, 47
  synergistic actions of, 32
Clean-contaminated surgical procedures defined, 27, 28t–29t
Clean surgical procedures defined, 26–27, 28t
Clindamycin, 178–183, 178f
  adverse effects of, 181–183
  antimicrobial activity of, 179–180, 179t
  inhibition of chloramphenicol and, 160
  for malaria, 408
  mechanism of action of, 178–179
  pharmacokinetics of, 180–181
  structure of, 178f
  for toxoplasmosis, 446
Clofazimine
  for leprosy, 310–311, 310f
  for Mycobacterium avium complex (MAC), 312
Clonorchis sinensis, praziquantel for, 459t, 460, 460f
Clostridium difficile
  colitis and. See Colitis, antibiotic-associated
  fluoroquinolones for, 263, 264t, 267
  metronidazole for, 423, 423t
Clostridium perfringens
  clindamycin for, 180
  fluoroquinolones for, 263, 264t
  metronidazole for, 423, 423t
Clostridium spp.
  erythromycin for, 174
  para-aminobenzoic acid and, 212, 213f
  vancomycin for, 115–116
Cloxacillin, resistance to, 67
Coccidioides immitis
  amphotericin B for, 333
  azoles for, 348–350
  nikkomycin for, 358
Coccidiosis, furazolidone for, 444

Colicins defined, 6
Coliform bacilli, nonpathogenic
  resistance development and, 44–45, 45t
Colistin. See Polymyxins
Colitis, antibiotic-associated
  clindamycin and, 181–183
  metronidazole and, 423–424
  superinfection and, 6
  tetracyclines and, 192
Combination drug therapy, 30–33, 30f
  for HIV infection, 551–552
  resistance prevention and, 46–47
Condyloma acuminata, interferons for, 531
Conjugation and drug resistance, 41
Conjugative transposons, 43–44
Conjunctival infection, 8t
Contaminated surgical procedures defined, 27, 29t
Corynebacterium diphtheriae
  clindamycin for, 180
  erythromycin for, 174
"Creeping eruption," 469
"Crix belly," 574
Cryptococcus
  amphotericin B for, 333
  azoles for, 348–350
  flucytosine for, 344, 344t
  papulocandins for, 358
Cryptosporidiosis, paromomycin for, 430, 445
Crystalluria
  and sulfonamides, 218–219
  trimethoprim-sulfamethoxazole and, 229
Cultures in identification of organisms, 11–12
Curling factor, 356
Cycloguanil for malaria, 403–408. See also Folic acid synthesis inhibitors
Cycloserine
  cell-wall synthesis inhibition by, 53–55, 54f –55f
  for tuberculosis, 284t, 305
Cyclosporiasis, trimethoprim-sulfamethoxazole for, 445
Cysticercosis, 466
Cysts in amebiasis, 420, 420f
Cytomegalovirus, 493t, 505. See also Herpesvirus

Dapsone, 214f, 308–309, 308f, 308t. See also Sulfones
  combined with pyrimethamine, 406–407, 407t
  for toxoplasmosis, 446
Decubitus wounds infection, 7t
Dehydroemetine for amebiasis, 422, 430–431, 430f
Delavirdine, 564–570, 564f. See also Non-nucleoside reverse transcriptase inhibitors (NNRTIs)
Democlocycline, 184, 184f
Dermatophytes. See also Antifungal drugs
  griseofulvin for, 354
  infection by, 349
Desensitization for penicillin hypersensitivity, 97
Determinants of bacterial response, 3–36
  antibiotic effects and, 4–5, 4f
  in combined antibiotic therapy

Determinants of bacterial response (*continued*)
    definitions of responses to, 30–31, 30*f*
    indications for, 31–33
  drugs of choice for empiric therapy, 14–21, 15*t*–20*t*
  host factors and, 5–6
    age, 23–24
    drug reaction history, 21–22
    genetic factors, 25
    metabolic abnormalities, 25
    preexisting organ dysfunction, 25–26
    pregnancy and nursing, 24–25
    renal and hepatic function, 22–23, 23*t*
    site of infection, 22
  identification of organism and
    by antimicobial susceptibility tests, 12–14, 13*t*
    by cultures of specimens, 11–12
    by empiric probability, 7–12, 7*t*–10*t*
    by gram-stain, 10–11
  indigenous microbial flora, 6–7
  selective toxicity and, 3–4
  surgical prophylaxis and, 26–30, 28*t*–29*t*
Diamidines. *See* Pentamidine
Diaminodiphenylsulfone, 214*f*. *See also* Sulfones
Dichlorvos, 462–463, 462*f*
Didanosine for HIV infection, 554*f*. *See also*
    Nucleoside analog reverse transcriptase
    inhibitors (NRTIs)
Dientamoeba fragilis, diiodohydroxyquin for, 429
Diethylcarbamazine for filariasis, 467*t*, 476–480,
    477*t*
α-Difluoromethylornithine, 442–443, 442*f*
Digoxin
  drug interactions with macrolides and, 178
  quinine and, 397
Diiodohydroxyquin, 421, 421*t*, 428–429, 428*f*
Diloxanide, 421, 421*t*, 428
Diphenylhydantoin, isoniazid and, 290–291
Diphyllobothrium, 465–466
  praziquantel for, 459*t*, 460, 460*f*
Dipylidium caninum, 465
Directly observed therapy (DOT), 282
Dirithromycin
  antimicrobial activity of, 174
  pharmacokinetics of, 176
Dirty surgical procedures, 27, 29*t*
Disk-diffusion test, 12–14, 13*t*
Doxycycline
  antimicrobial activity of, 187–189, 188*t*
  distribution of, 189*f*, 190–191
  drug interactions of, 194–195
  for malaria acute attack, 381, 384*t*
  for malaria prophylaxis, 380, 383*t*
  renal function and, 193
  structure of, 184, 184*f*
Dracunculus medinensis, 467*t*, 477*t*, 478
  metronidazole for, 424
Drug interactions. *See specific drugs*
Drug resistance. *See* Resistance; *specific drugs*
Drugs of first choice, empiric, 14–21, 15*t*–20*t*
Dysentery in history of drug resistance, 41–42, 42*t*

E test defined, 13
Ear infections. *See* Otitis
Echinococcus granulosa, 465–466
  mebendazole for, 470–472
Efavirenz, 564–570, 564*f*. *See also* Non-nucleoside
    reverse transcriptase inhibitors (NNRTIs)
Efflux systems in resistance, 261–262
Eflornithine for trypanisomiasis, 432, 432*t*
Elephantiasis, 476
Elongation step in protein synthesis, 129, 130*f*
Emetines for amebiasis, 422, 430–431, 430*f*
Empiric therapy, 14–21, 15*t*–20*t*
  combination drug therapy and, 33
Empyema, probable etiologic agents of, 9*t*
Encephalitis
  Herpesvirus
    acyclovir for, 513
    vidarabine for, 509
  toxoplasmic, 445–446
Endocarditis
  fluoroquinolones for, 270
  probable etiologic agents of, 9*t*
  Schlichter test for, 14
  vancomycin for, 115
Enoxacin, 257, 258*f*. *See also* Fluoroquinolones
Entamoeba histolytica
  chloroquine for, 428
  diiodohydroxyquin for, 428–429, 428*f*
  diloxanide for, 428
  emetines for, 430–431, 430*f*
  life cycle of, 420, 420*f*
  paromomycin for, 429–430
  tetracyclines for, 189
Enterobacter
  fluoroquinolones for, 263
  nalidixic acid and, 242–243
  nitrofurantoin for, 246, 246*t*
  polymixins for, 236
  tetracyclines for, 188, 188*t*
Enterococci
  aminoglycoside activity against, 137–139, 138*t*,
    139*f*
  teicoplanin for, 117
  vancomycin for, 115–116
Enterococcus
  fluoroquinolones for, 263, 264*t*
  resistance to, 262
Epidermophyton, griseofulvin for, 354
Epididymis infection, probable etiologic agents of, 10*t*
Erythema multiforme
  with clindamycin, 181
  thiabendazole and, 476
Erythema nodosum leprosum (ENL)
  clofazimine and, 310
  dapsone and, 309
  thalidomide for, 311
Erythromycin. *See also* Macrolides
  for amebiasis, 422
  antimicrobial activity of, 172–174, 173*t*
  drug interactions with, 178

inhibition of chloramphenicol and, 160
pharmacokinetics of, 175–176
resistance to, 171–172
structure of, 171, 171*f*
Escherichia coli
    chloramphenicol for, 161*t*, 162, 163*t*
    fluoroquinolones for, 263, 264*t*
    β-lactam antibiotics and, 64–66, 65*t*
    nalidixic acid and, 242–243
    nitrofurantoin for, 246, 246*t*
    penicillin binding proteins and, 59–61, 60*f*, 61*t*
    polymixins for, 236
    resistance of
        to chloramphenicol, 163–164
        to erythromycin, 171–172
        to fluoroquinolones, 261–262
        to β-lactam antibiotics, 42, 71
        to sulfonamides, 215
        to trimethoprim-sulfamethoxazole, 227
    tetracyclines for, 188, 188*t*
    trimethoprim-sulfamethoxazole for, 224–226, 224*t*–225*t*
Ethambutol
    adverse effects of, 283*t*, 302
    dosage of, 283*t*
    pharmacokinetics of, 208*t*, 301
    resistance to, 300–301
    structure of, 300*f*
    for tuberculosis, 300–302
Ethionamide for leprosy, 308*t*, 311
Everninomicin, 46
Exopenicillinase, 70
Eye infections
    acyclovir for, 512
    idoxyuridine for, 506
    polymixins for, 236
    probable etiologic agents of, 8*t*
    sulfonamides for, 215, 217
    trifluridine for, 507–508
    vidarabine for, 508–510, 508*f*

Facultative large-step pattern of resistance, 40
Fallopian tube infection, probable etiologic agents of, 10*t*
Famciclovir, 516–517, 516*f*, 518*t*
Fansidar, 407
Fasciola hepatica, triclabendazole for, 459*t*, 465
Fasciolopsis buski, praziquantel for, 459*t*, 460, 460*f*
Filariasis, 467*t*, 476–478, 477*t*
Flatworms. *See* Flukes; Tapeworms
Fleming's discovery of penicillin, 51
Florey's isolation of penicillin, 51
Fluconazole. *See* Azoles
Flucytosine, 342–346
    adverse effects of, 346
    amphotericin B and, 333, 344–345
    antimicrobial activity of, 344–345, 344*t*
    combination therapy and, 344–345
    mechanism of action of, 342–344, 342*f*–343*f*

pharmacokinetics of, 345–346
    therapeutic uses of, 344–345
Flukes
    bithionol for, 459*t*, 465, 465*f*
    drugs for, 458–460, 459*t*
    metrifonate for, 459*t*, 462–463, 462*f*
    oxamniquine for, 459*t*, 463–465, 464*f*
    praziquantel for, 459*t*, 460–462, 460*f*
    triclabendazole for, 459*t*, 465
Fluoroquinolones, 257–279
    adverse effects of, 270–272, 270*t*
    antimicrobial activity of, 262–263, 264*t*
    discovery of, 257
    drug interactions with, 272–273
    mechanism of action of, 257, 259–260, 259*f*
    pharmacokinetics of, 263, 265–266, 266*t*
    resistance to, 260–262
    structure of, 257, 258*f*
    therapeutic uses of, 266–270, 267*t*
5-Fluorouracil and flucytosine, 342–344, 342*f*–343*f*, 346
Folic acid synthesis inhibitors
    antimicrobial activity of, 403–404
    for malaria, 403–408
    mechanism of action of, 404–406, 405*f*, 406*t*
    resistance to, 403–404
    sulfonamides and, 211
    therapeutic uses of, 403–404
Folinic acid, 229
Formaldehyde, methenamine and, 251–252
Forssman antigen, 63
Foscarnet, 518*t*, 520–522, 520*f*
Fosfomycin, 252–253, 252*f*
    cell-wall synthesis inhibition by, 55
Francisella tularensis, tetracyclines for, 188
Fungal infections
    classifications of, 327
    drugs for. *See* Antifungal drugs
Furazolidone, 245, 245*t*
    for *Giardia lamblia*, 443–444
    for protozoal diseases, 421*t*
Fusobacterium, clindamycin for, 180

Gametocytes in malaria cycle, 377, 378*f*
Ganciclovir, 517–520, 517*f*, 518*t*
Gastrointestinal system
    adverse effects and
        with erythromycin, 176–177
        with ethionamide, 305
        with fluoroquinolones, 270–271, 270*t*
        with para-aminosalicylic acid (PAS), 306
        pyrantel pamoate and, 475
        with tetracyclines, 191–192
    infection of
        fluoroquinolones for, 267–268, 267*t*
        probable etiologic agents of, 9*t*–10*t*
Genetics
    drug resistance and, 41–44, 43*f*–44*f*
    factors modifying drug use and, 25
Genital infection, probable etiologic agents of, 10*t*

Gentamicin
  host factors modifying drug use and, 142–145
  in infants, 24
  renal function and, 140t, 141–142, 142f
  resistance to, 136
  structure of, 127, 128f
  therapeutic uses of, 149–150
Giardia lamblia, 443–444
Glossina and trypanisomiasis, 431
Glucose-6-phosphate dehydrogenase deficiency
  drug choice and, 25
  melarsoprol and, 441
  primaquine and, 401–403, 402f–403f
Gram-negative organisms. *See also specific names*
  cephalosporins for, 108–109
  drugs of first choice for, 16t–19t
  envelope of
    penetration of, 64–66, 65t
    resistance and, 38–39
  β-lactamase protection and, 71
  macrolides for, 173–174, 173t
  nalidixic acid and, 242–243
  polymixins effect on, 234–236
  tetracyclines for, 187–189, 188t, 195–196, 195t
Gram-positive organisms. *See also specific names*
  drugs of first choice for, 15t, 16t
  gramicidin A for, 239
  β-lactamase protection and, 70–71
  macrolides for, 172–173, 173t
  penicillin and, 38–39
  quinupristin/dalfopristin for, 198
  rifampin for, 295
  tetracyclines for, 187–189, 188t
Gram stain defined, 10–11
Gramicidin A, 238–240, 238f–239f
Granulocytopenia
  penicillin toxicity and, 87
  trimethoprim-sulfamethoxazole and, 229
Granuloma inguinale, tetracyclines for, 196
Gray syndrome, 23–24
  chloramphenicol and, 165–166, 165f
Grepafloxacin, 257, 258f. *See also* Fluoroquinolones
Griseofulvin, 354–358
  adverse effects of, 357–358
  drug interactions of, 357
  mechanism of action of, 354–356, 355f
  pharmacokinetics of, 356–357
  structure of, 354, 354f
Guide to Antimicrobial Therapy, A, 21
Guinea worms. *See Dracunculus medinensis*
Gyrase, DNA, fluoroquinolones and, 259–261, 259f

Haemophilus influenzae
  aminopenicillin effects on, 88
  amoxicillin-clavulanic acid for, 114
  azithromycin for, 174
  aztreonam for, 113, 113t
  cephalosporins for, 108–109
  chloramphenicol for, 162–163, 163t, 168–169

  resistance to, 163–164
  drugs of first choice for, 21
  fluoroquinolones for, 263, 264t
  polymixins for, 236
  tetracyclines for, 188, 188t
  trimethoprim-sulfamethoxazole for, 224–226, 224t–
    225t
Hair infection and griseofulvin, 356–357
Halofantrine, 397–398
Haloprogin, 359
Helicobacter pylori
  fluoroquinolones for, 268
    resistance to, 262
  macrolides for, 174
  metronidazole for, 424
  tetracyclines for, 196
Helminthic diseases. *See also specific diseases and
    organisms*
  drugs for, 458–488
  fluke infections, 458–465, 459t
  roundworms
    intestinal, 466–476
    tissue, 476–482
  tapeworms, 459t, 465–466
Hemozoin, 386–387
Hepatic function. *See also* Hepatitis
  chloramphenicol metabolism and, 164–165, 164f
  clindamycin and, 181
  factors modifying drug use and, 22–23, 26
  fluoroquinolones and, 265
  griseofulvin and, 357–358
  idoxyuridine and, 506
  isoniazid and, 290–293, 292f
  macrolides and, 175–176
  with nucleoside analog reverse transcriptase
    inhibitors, 562, 563t
  pyrazinamide and, 304
  tetracyclines and, 193
Hepatitis
  cycloserine and, 305
  erythromycin estolate and, 177
  ethionamide and, 305
  interferons for, 530–531
  nitrofurantoin and, 249
  para-aminosalicylic acid and, 306
  penicillin toxicity and, 87
  ribavirin for, 534
  rifampin-induced, 297, 299
Herpes simplex virus, 493t, 505. *See also* Herpesvirus
Herpesvirus, 493t, 505–523
  acyclovir for, 510–515, 510f
  cidofovir for, 522–523
  famciclovir for, 516–517, 516f
  foscarnet for, 520–522, 520f
  ganciclovir for, 517–520, 517f, 518t
  idoxyuridine for, 505–507, 505f
  interferons for, 531
  penciclovir for, 516–517, 516f
  trifluridine for, 507–508, 507f

valacyclovir for, 515–516, 515*f*
vidarabine for, 508–510, 508*f*
Herxheimer reaction
  and chloramphenicol, 165
  and diethylcarbmazine, 479
Heterophyes heterophyes, praziquantel for, 459*t,* 460,
  460*f*
Hippuric acid, methenamine and, 251
Histoplasma capsulatum
  amphotericin B for
    combinations of, 333
  azoles for, 348–350
  nikkomycin for, 358
HIV infection
  acyclovir resistance and, 513
  amphotericin B and, 334–335
  antiretroviral drugs for, 550–586. *See also specific*
    drug names and classes; specific drugs
    combination therapy, 551–552
    non-nucleoside reverse transcriptase inhibitors,
      564–570, 564*f*
    nucleoside analog reverse transcriptase inhibitors
      for, 553–564
    treatment strategies, 552–553
  clindamycin and, 180
  cryptosporidiosis and, 445
  cyclosporiasis and, 445
  drugs for, 311–313
    resistance to, 499
  flucytosine and, 345
  fluoroquinolones for, 268, 269
  fungal infections and, 327
  ganciclovir and, 518–519
  Mycobacterium avium complex (MAC). *See*
    Mycobacterium avium complex (MAC)
  Pneumocystis carinii pneumonia. *See Pneumocystis*
    carinii pneumonia (PCP)
  polyenes and, 334–335
  reproduction biology of, 550, 551*f*
  toxoplasmosis and, 445–446
  tuberculosis in
    preventive therapy for, 284–285, 285*t*
    standard therapy for, 281–282
Hookworms, 467*f,* 467*t,* 468–469
  albendazole and mebendazole for, 470–472, 470*f*
  piperazine for, 472–474, 472*f,* 473*f*
  pyrantel pamoate for, 474–475, 474*f*
  thiabendazole for, 475–476
Host
  defenses of, 4
  determinants of bacterial response of, 5–6
  factors modifying drug use and, 21–26
    age, 23–24
    of aminoglycosides, 142–145
    drug reaction history and, 21–22
    genetic, 25
    hepatic function, 22–23
    infection site and, 22
    metabolic abnormalities and, 25

pregnancy and nursing, 24–25
renal function, 22–23, 23*t*
Human immunodeficiency virus (HIV). *See* HIV
  infection
Hydatid disease, 466
Hydroxychloroquine, 382
8-Hydroxyquinolines, 428–429
Hymenolepis nana, praziquantel for, 459*t,* 460, 460*f*
Hypersensitivity reactions
  with ascariasis, 468
  to capreomycin, 307
  to carbapenems, 111–112
  to cephalosporins, 104–105
  to chloramphenicol, 165
  to clindamycin, 181
  to cycloserine, 305
  to ethionamide, 305
  with fluoroquinolones, 270*t,* 271
  history of, 21–22
  to isoniazid, 293
  to melarsoprol, 441
  to neomycin, 237
  to nitrofurantoin, 248, 248*t*
  with nucleoside analog reverse transcriptase
    inhibitors, 562, 563*t*
  to penicillins, 92–98, 92*t,* 94*f*
    cross-reactivity with, 104
    immunochemistry of, 93–95, 94*f*–95*f*
    patient treatment and, 96–98, 97*t*
    skin testing for, 95–96
  to quinine, 397
  to sulfonamides, 219
  to suramin, 437–439
  tetracyclines and, 194
  trimethoprim-sulfamethoxazole and, 229
Hypoxanthine arabinoside, 508–510, 508*f*

Identification of organisms, 7–12
  cultures and, 7, 11–12
  gram stain and, 10–11
  probable etiologic agents and, 7, 7*t*–10*t*
Idoxyuridine (IUdR), 505–507, 505*f*
Imidazoles, 346–354, 359. *See also* Azoles; *specific*
  drug names
  amphotericin B and, 334
Imipenem, 51
  pharmacokinetics of, 111–113, 111*f,* 112*t*
Implant infections, 14
Indifference in drug combinations, 30–31, 30*f*
Indinavir, 570–578, 571*f. See also* Protease inhibitors
Infant(s)
  factors modifying drug use and, 23–25
  septicemia in, probable etiologic agents of, 9*t*
Infection site
  antibiotic effects and, 4, 14
    vs. drug resistance, 39
  combination drug therapy and, 33
  factors modifying drug use and, 22
  purulence of. *See* Purulence

Influenza virus
  amantadine for, 499–504, 499f–500f, 501t
  drugs for, 499–505
  ribavirin for, 534
  rimantadine for, 499–504, 499f–500f, 501t
  zanamivir for, 504–505, 504f
Inhibitors of cell-wall synthesis. See Cell-wall synthesis
    inhibitors
Initiation complex formation, 129–130, 129f
  streptomycin effect on, 134–135, 134f
Insertion sequences (IS), 42–43, 44f
Interferons
  adverse effects of, 532–533, 532t
  antiviral activity of, 529–531
  classification of, 524–525, 524t–525t
  discovery of, 523–524
  drug interactions with, 533
  induction of, 524
  mechanism of action of, 498, 525–528, 527f–528f
  pharmacokinetics of, 531–532
  resistance to, 528–529
Iodide, 354
Iodochlorhydroxyquin, 428–429
Iododeoxyuridine (IUdR), 496
Iodoquinol, 428–429
Ionophores, gramicidin A and, 239–240, 239f
Isoniazid, 285–293
  adverse effects of, 290–293, 292f
  antimicrobial activity of, 285
  concentration and exposure duration, 287–288
  drug interactions with, 293
  in elderly patients, 24
  mechanism of action of, 285–286
  pharmacokinetics of, 288–290, 288f–289f, 288t,
    298t
  resistance to, 286–287
  structure of, 285f
  for tuberculosis
    preventive therapy, 284–285, 285t
    usual dosages, 283t–284t
Itraconazole. See Azoles
Ivermectin, for filariasis, 467t, 476–478, 477t, 480–
    482, 480f

Joint infections
  fluoroquinolones for, 269
  probable etiologic agents of, 9t

Kala-azar. See Leishmaniasis
Kanamycin
  resistance to, 137, 137f
  therapeutic uses of, 150–151
  for tuberculosis, 306
Kaposi's sarcoma, interferons for, 530
Kernicterus, sulfonamides and, 24, 220
Ketoconazole. See Azoles
Kirby-Bauer test, 12–14, 13t
Klebsiella
  fluoroquinolones for, 264t
    resistance to, 261–262

nalidixic acid and, 242–243
  nitrofurantoin for, 246, 246t
  polymixins for, 236
  tetracyclines for, 188, 188t
  trimethoprim-sulfamethoxazole for, 224–226, 224t–
    225t

L-Form bacteria, 66
  polymixin effects on, 236
β-Lactam antibiotics. See also Cell-wall synthesis
    inhibitors; Cephalosporins; Cephamycins;
    Penicillins
  discovery of, 51
  mechanism of action of, 51–53
  resistance to, 66–75
  structure of, 51, 52f
  tolerance to, 62–63, 62f, 63t
β-Lactamase
  classification of, 69, 69t
  drugs resistant to, 71–73, 72f–73f, 72t, 83f,
    87–88
    combination, 114–115, 115t
  location of, 65f, 66
  production of, 69–71, 69t–70t
  structure of, 67–69, 68f
Lamivudine for HIV infection, 554f. See also
    Nucleoside analog reverse transcriptase
    inhibitors (NRTIs)
Larva migrans, 467f, 469
  ivermectin for, 467t, 480–482, 480f
  thiabendazole for, 475–476
Laryngeal infection, probable etiologic agents of,
    8t
Legionella
  fluoroquinolones for, 263, 264t, 270
  macrolides for, 174
Leishmania
  amphotericin B for, 334
  diseases caused by, 431
  drugs for, 431–443, 432t
  paromomycin for, 430
  pentamidine for, 434–437, 434f
  sodium stibogluconate for, 432–434, 434f
Leprosy. See also Mycobacterium leprae
  drugs for, 307–311, 308t
Leptospira, tetracyclines for, 188
Leucovorin and trimetrexate, 448
Levofloxacin, 257, 258f. See also Fluoroquinolones
Lincomycin, 178–183
Lincosamide antibiotics, 178–183, 178f. See also
    Clindamycin
Lipoteichoic acid, autolytic activity and, 63
Listeria monocytogenes, vancomycin for, 115–116
Loa loa, 467t, 476–478, 477t
Loracarbef, 100t, 105–108, 106f
Lyell's syndrome, trimethoprim-sulfamethoxazole and,
    228
Lymphadenopathy with filariasis, 476
Lymphogranuloma venerum, tetracyclines for,
    196

Macrolactones, 197–198, 197f
Macrolides, 171–178
  adverse effects of, 176–178
  antimicrobial activity of, 172–174, 173t
  drug interactions with, 178
  mechanism of action of, 171–172
  for *Mycobacterium avium* complex (MAC), 312
  pharmacokinetics of, 175–176
  therapeutic indications for, 172–174, 173t
Mafenide, 216f, 217–218
Malaria
  antibiotics for, 408
  cerebral, 382
  chemotherapy of, 375–418
  in children, 382
  classifications of, 376–377, 376f, 377t
  disease characteristics, 376–377, 376f, 377t
  drugs for. *See also specific drugs*
    8-aminoquinolines, 399–403
    artemisinin, 398–399
    chloroquine, 382–392
    cinchona alkaloids, 394–397, 395f
    folic acid synthesis inhibitors, 403–408
    halofantrine, 397–398
    mefloquine, 392–394
    primaquine, 399–403
    quinidine, 394–397, 395f
    quinine, 394–397, 395f
  epidemiology of, 375–376
  multiple-drug-resistant, 389
  paroxysms of, 376–377, 376f, 377t
  Plasmodium life cycle and, 377–378, 378f
  in pregnant women, 382
  tetracyclines for, 408
  therapeutic rationale, 378–383, 379t
    acute attack treatment, 380–382, 384t
    prophylaxis, 380, 383t
    radical cure, 379t, 383
Maloprim, 407
Mandelic acid, methenamine and, 251
Mansonella, 476–478, 477t
Mazzotti reaction, 479
Mebendazole, 470f
  for roundworms, 467t, 468–472
Mecillinam
  E. coli binding proteins and, 60, 61t
  mechanism of, 66–67
Medical Letter, The, 21
Mefloquine, 392–394
  adverse effects of, 394
  drug interactions of, 394
  for malaria acute attack, 381, 384t
  for malaria prophylaxis, 380, 383t
  mechanism of action of, 392–393
  pharmacokinetics of, 393–394
  precautions for, 394
  resistance to, 380, 393
  structure of, 392, 392f
  therapeutic uses of, 392–393

Melarsoprol, for trypanisomiasis, 432, 432t, 437, 439–441, 439f
Meningitis
  amphotericin B for, 333
    intrathecal administration of, 337–338
  cephalosporins for, 104, 108–109
  chloramphenicol for, 162–163, 168–169
  meropenem for, 112
  metronidazole for, 423
  probable etiologic agents of, 9t
  sulfonamides for, 217
  vancomycin for, 115–116
Meropenem, 51
  pharmacokinetics of, 111–113, 111f, 112t
Merozoites in malaria cycle, 377, 378f
Metagonimus yokogawai, praziquantel for, 459t, 460, 460f
Methacycline, 184, 184f
Methenamine, 250–252, 251f
Methicillin
  β-lactamase resistance of, 71–72, 72t
  resistance to, 74–75, 74t
Methotrexate, 448–449, 448f
  acyclovir and, 515
  trimethoprim-sulfamethoxazole and, 229
Metrifonate, 459t, 462–463, 462f
Metronidazole, 348. *See also* Azoles
  adverse effects of, 427–428
  antimicrobial activity of, 422–424, 423t
  for *Clostridium difficile,* 182–183
  for *Dracunculus medinensis,* 424, 477t, 478
  for *Entamoeba histolytica,* 421, 421t
  for *Giardia lamblia,* 444
  mechanism of action of, 424–426, 425f
  pharmacokinetics of, 426–427, 426t
  precautions for, 428
  for protozoal diseases, 422–428
  therapeutic uses of, 422–424, 423t
  for trichomoniasis, 445
Mezlocillin, 91–92, 91f
MIC (minimum inhibitory concentration), 12, 13t
Miconazole. *See* Azoles
Microbial antagonism defined, 6
Microsporum, griseofulvin for, 354
Microtubules and griseofulvin, 355, 355f
Minimum bactericidal concentration (MBC), 13–14
Minimum inhibitory concentration (MIC), 12, 13t
Minocycline
  amphotericin B and, 333
  distribution of, 189f, 190–191
  hyperpigmentation and, 194
  structure of, 184, 184f
Minor determinants defined, 93
Monobactams
  pharmacokinetics of, 113–114, 113f, 113t
  structure of, 51, 52f
Moraxella, fluoroquinolones for, 263
MOTT (Mycobacteria other than tuberculosis). *See* *Mycobacterium*
Mouth infections, probable etiologic agents of, 7t–8t

Multidrug resistance (MDR) systems, 261–262
Multiple-step pattern of resistance, 40–41
Murein hydrolases, function of, 62
Mutation and drug resistance, 40–41
Mycobacteria other than tuberculosis (MOTT). See Mycobacterium
Mycobacterium avium complex (MAC). See also HIV infection
    amikacin for, 313
    drugs for, 281t, 311–313
    fluoroquinolones for, 269
    macrolides for, 174, 178
Mycobacterium leprae
    clarithromycin for, 174
    clofazimine for, 310–311, 310f
    dapsone for, 308–309, 308f, 308t
    drugs for, 281t, 307–311, 308t
    ethionamide for, 308t, 311
    rifampin for, 308t, 310
    thalidomide for, 311
Mycobacterium spp. See also Mycobacterium tuberculosis; species names; Tuberculosis
    cycloserine for, 305
    drugs for, 280–323, 281t
    ethambutol for, 300
    fluoroquinolones for, 263, 264t, 269
    macrolides for, 174
    quinolones for, 307
    rifampin for, 281t, 296
    tetracyclines for, 188
Mycobacterium tuberculosis. See also Tuberculosis
    amikacin for, 283t, 306
    capreomycin for, 281t, 306–307
    ciprofloxacin for, 284t, 307
    cycloserine for, 284t, 305
    drugs for, 280–323, 281t
    ethambutol for, 281t, 283t, 300–302
    ethionamide for, 308t, 311
    isoniazid for
        preventive therapy, 284–285, 285t
        usual dosages, 283t–284t
    kanamycin for, 283t, 306
    ofloxacin for, 284t, 307
    para-aminosalicylic acid (PAS) for, 214, 299, 305–306, 306f
    populations of, 281
    pyrazinamide for, 281t, 283t, 303–304
    resistance of
        defined, 282
        to ethambutol, 300–301
        to isoniazid, 286–287
        to rifampin, 294
        to trimethoprim-sulfamethoxazole, 224t, 225
    rifampin for, 281t, 283t, 295–296
    streptomycin for, 281t, 283t, 302–303
    viomycin for, 306–307, 307f
Mycolic acids, 286
Mycoplasma spp.
    chloramphenicol for, 162
    drugs of first choice for, 20t

    fluoroquinolones for, 263, 264t
    macrolides for, 174
    resistance of, to trimethoprim-sulfamethoxazole, 225
    tetracyclines for, 188, 188t, 195–196
Mycotic infections. See Antifungal drugs
Myopathy and ziduvine, 561, 563t
M2 protein in influenza virus, 499, 500f

Nafcillin, resistance to -lactamase, 71–72, 72t
Naftifine, 359
Nail infection and griseofulvin, 356–357
Nalidixic acid, 242–245, 242f
    adverse effects of, 244–245
    antimicrobial activity of, 242–243
    fluoroquinolones and, 257
    mechanism of action of, 242
    pharmacokinetics of, 243–244, 244t
    resistance to, 242–243
NAT2 gene, 289
Necator americanus, 467t, 468–469
Negative supercoiling of DNA, 259–260, 259f
Neisseria gonorrhoeae
    fluoroquinolones for, 263, 264t, 268
    resistance of
        to penicillin, 66
        to tetracyclines, 189
    spectinomycin for, 183
    tetracyclines for, 188, 188t, 195–196, 195t
    trimethoprim-sulfamethoxazole for, 224–226, 224t–225t
    vancomycin for, 115–116
Neisseria meningitidis
    chloramphenicol for, 162–163, 163t
        resistance to, 164
    fluoroquinolones for, 263, 264t, 270
    minocycline for, 191, 196
    rifampin for, 295–296
    sulfonamide resistance of, 215
    tetracyclines for, 188, 188t
    trimethoprim-sulfamethoxazole for, 224–226, 224t–225t
Neisseria spp.
    cephalosporins for, 108–109
    macrolides for, 174
    nitrofurantoin for, 246, 246t
    polymyxin resistance of, 236
Nelfinavir, 570–578, 571f. See also Protease inhibitors
Nematodes. See Roundworms
Neomycin
    adverse effects of, 237
    combined with polymyxin, 236
    therapeutic uses of, 151
Nephrotoxicity. See Renal function
Netilmicin
    resistance to, 136
    therapeutic uses of, 150
Neuraminidase in viruses, 498
    zanamivir and, 504–505

Neurocysticercosis, 466
  albendazole for, 470
Neurotoxicity
  of acyclovir, 514–515
  of amantadine, 503
  of aminoglycosides, 145–146
  of cycloserine, 305
  dapsone and, 309
  of emetines, 430
  of ethambutol, 302
  of fluoroquinolones, 270t, 271, 273
  of ganciclovir, 519
  of 8-hydroxyquinolines, 428–429
  of imipenem, 112
  of isoniazid, 290–291
  of mefloquine, 394
  of melarsoprol, 441
  of metronidazole, 427
  of nalidixic acid, 245
  of nitrofurantoin, 249
  with nucleoside analog reverse transcriptase
      inhibitors, 561, 563t
  of penicillins, 86–87
  of piperazine, 474
  of polymixins, 237–238
  of quinine, 396–397
  to vidarabine, 510
Neutropenia. See also Blood disorders; HIV infection
  infections and, fluoroquinolones for, 269–270
Nevirapine, 564–570, 564f. See also Non-nucleoside
      reverse transcriptase inhibitors (NNRTIs)
Nifurtimox for trypanisomiasis, 432, 432t, 441–442,
      441f
Nikkomycins, 358
Niridazole for Dracunculus medinensis, 477t,
      478
Nitrofurantoin
  adverse effects of, 248–250, 248t, 250f
  antimicrobial activity of, 246–247, 246t
  mechanism of action of, 245–246
  pharmacokinetics of, 247–248
  therapeutic uses of, 246–247, 246t
Nitrofurazone, 245, 245t
Nocardia asteroides, sulfonamides for, 215
Non-nucleoside reverse transcriptase inhibitors
      (NNRTIs), 564–570, 564f
  adverse effects of, 568–569
  drug interactions with, 569–570
  mechanism of action of, 564–565
  pharmacokinetics of, 568, 569t
  resistance to, 565
  therapeutic uses of, 565, 568
Norfloxacin, 257, 258f. See also Fluoroquinolones
Nucleoside analog reverse transcriptase inhibitors
      (NRTIs), 553–564, 553f–554f
  adverse effects of, 560–562, 563t
  drug interactions of, 562, 564, 566t–567t
  mechanism of action of, 553–556, 555f
  pharmacokinetics of, 557–558, 559t
  precautions for, 564

resistance to, 556–557
therapeutic uses of, 558, 560
Nystatin, 360
  combined with tetracyclines, 192
  resistance to, 335

Ofloxacin, 257, 258f. See also Fluoroquinolones
  for tuberculosis, 284t, 307
Onchocerca volvulus, 467t, 476–478, 477t
  suramin for, 437–439
Opisthorchis viverrini, praziquantel for, 459t, 460,
      460f
Organ transplants, cytomegalovirus and, 493t, 505
  acyclovir for, 512
  ganciclovir for, 519
Oriental sore, 431
Ornidazole, 421
Osteomyelitis
  fluoroquinolones for, 267t, 269
  probable etiologic agents of, 9t
Otitis
  fluoroquinolones for, 270
  polymixins for, 236
  probable etiologic agents of, 8t
Ototoxicity
  with aminoglycosides, 146–148
  of capreomycin, 307
  drug choice and, 26
  with erythromycin, 175
  with vancomycin, 116
Oxacillin, Staphylococcus aureus susceptibility to, 63t
Oxamniquine for Schistosoma, 459t, 463–465, 464f
Oxytetracycline, 184, 184f

Pancreatitis and didanosine, 561–562, 563t
Papulocandins, 358
Para-aminobenzoic acid (PABA)
  para-aminosalicylic acid and sulfones and, 213–214,
      214f, 214t
  sulfonamides and, 211–214, 212f–213f
Para-aminosalicylic acid (PAS)
  sulfones and, 213–214, 214f, 214t
  for tuberculosis, 214, 284t, 299, 305–306, 306f
Paracoccidioides, azoles for, 348, 350
Paragonimus westermani
  praziquantel for, 459t, 460, 460f
Parasites, drugs for. See Helminths; Malaria;
      Protozoal diseases; species names
Parkinson's disease and amantadine, 504
Paromomycin, 127, 151
  for cryptosporidiosis, 445
  for Entamoeba histolytica, 421, 421t, 429–430
  for leishmaniasis, 431, 432t
Pasturella
  nalidixic acid and, 243
  polymixins for, 236
  tetracyclines for, 188
PBP (penicillin binding proteins), 59–61, 60f, 61t
Penciclovir, 516–517, 516f
Penetration stage of viral biology, 494–495, 494f

Penicillenic acid, hypersensitivity reactions and, 93
Penicillin binding proteins (PBPs)
  mechanisms of action of, 59–61, 60*f*, 61*t*
  methicillin resistance and, 74–75, 74*t*
  structure of, 61
Penicillin G
  absorption of, 82–84, 84*f*
  pharmacokinetics of, 81–87
  structure of, 83*f*
Penicillin V
  absorption of, 82
  structure of, 83*f*
Penicillinase. *See* β-Lactamase
Penicillins. *See also* Cell-wall synthesis inhibitors;
    Penicillin binding proteins (PBPs); *specific*
    compounds
  broad-spectrum, 64–66, 65*t*
  cell-wall synthesis inhibition by, 54
  classification of, 81, 82*t*
  gram-positive *vs.* gram-negative bacteria and,
    38–39
  hypersensitivity reactions to, 92–98, 92*t*, 94*f*. *See*
    also Hypersensitivity reactions
  β-lactamase resistance by, 71–72, 72*t*
  narrow-spectrum, 83*t*
    in cerebrospinal fluid, 85–86
    distribution and excretion of, 84–86, 85*t*–86*t*
    dosage adjustments for, 85–86, 86*t*
    pharmacokinetics of, 81–87, 83*f*
    in renal function impairment, 85–86, 86*t*
    toxicity and side effects of, 86–87
  resistance to, 44, 66–75
  semi-synthetic
    aminopenicillins, 88–90, 89*f*
    antipseudomonal, 85*t*–86*t*, 90–91
    carboxypenicillins, 85*t*–86*t*, 89*f*, 90–91
    β-lactamase-resistant, 83*f*, 87–88
    pharmacokinetics of, 82*t*, 85*t*–86*t*, 87–92, 89*f*
    ureidopenicillins, 91–92, 91*f*
  synergistic actions and, 31–32
    aminoglycosides and, 138, 139*f*
Penicilloyl-polylysine for skin tests, 95
Pentamidine, 434–437, 434*f*
  adverse effects of, 436–437
  for leishmaniasis, 431, 432*t*, 434–437, 434*f*
  mechanism of action of, 435–436
  pharmacokinetics of, 436
  for *Pneumocystis carinii* pneumonia, 435, 446–447
  for protozoal diseases, 421*t*
  therapeutic uses of, 434–435
  for trypanisomiasis, 432, 432*t*
Peptidoglycan formation in cell-wall synthesis, 55–57,
    55*f*, 56*t*
Peptidyl transfer step in protein synthesis, 129
Peptococcus, metronidazole for, 423, 423*t*
Peptostreptococcus, metronidazole for, 423, 423*t*
Periarteritis nodosa, sulfonamides and, 219
Peritonitis, probable etiologic agents of, 10*t*
Phenytoin
  doxycycline interaction with, 194–195

fluoroquinolones interaction with, 272
trimethoprim-sulfamethoxazole and, 229
Phlebotomus and leishmaniasis, 431
Photosensitivity
  fluoroquinolones and, 270*t*, 271
  nalidixic acid and, 244–245
  sulfonamides and, 219
  tetracyclines and, 193–194
Pinworm
  albendazole and mebendazole for, 470–472,
    470*f*
  ivermectin for, 467*t*, 480–482, 480*f*
  piperazine for, 472–474, 472*f*, 473*f*
  thiabendazole for, 475–476
Piperacillin
  pharmacokinetics of, 91–92, 91*f*
  and sulbactam, 114–115, 115*t*
  and tazobactam, 73
Piperazine, 472–474, 472*f*, 473*f*
  for ascariasis, 468
Plasmids
  aminoglycoside modifying enzymes and, 136–137
  defined, 42, 43*f*–44*f*
  nonconjugative (r plasmids), 43
  in *Staphylococcus aureus* resistance, 68–69
  in tetracycline resistance, 189
Plasmodium falciparum, 376. *See also* Malaria;
    Plasmodium spp.
  antibiotics for, 408
  artemisinin for, 381–382, 398–399
  halofantrine for, 397–398
  lethal disease from, 382
  life cycle and disease, 377–378, 378*f*
  mefloquine for, 392–393
  multiple drug-resistant, 381
  primaquine for, 399–403, 400*t*
  quinine for, 395
  resistance of, 378–379
    to chloroquine, 387–390, 388*f*
  sulfonamides for, 215
  tetracyclines for, 189
Plasmodium malariae, 376. *See also* Malaria;
    Plasmodium spp.
Plasmodium ovale, 376. *See also* Malaria;
    Plasmodium spp.
  primaquine for, 399–403
Plasmodium spp. *See also* Malaria
  clindamycin for, 180
  erythrocytic forms of drugs for, 382–392
  exoerythrocytic forms of drugs for, 399–403
  life cycle and disease, 377–378, 378*f*
Plasmodium vivax, 376. *See also* Malaria;
    Plasmodium spp.
  primaquine for, 399–403, 400*t*
Pleural infections, probable etiologic agents of, 9*t*
Pneumocandins, 358
Pneumococci
  aminopenicillin effects on, 88
  autolysin triggering hypothesis in, 63
  resistance to penicillin, 66

Pneumocystis carinii pneumonia (PCP). *See also* HIV infection
  clindamycin for, 180
  drugs for, 446–449
  pentamidine for, 435, 446–447
  trimethoprim-sulfamethoxazole for, 226, 229, 435, 446–447
  trimetrexate for, 448–449, 448*f*
Pneumonia, probable etiologic agents of, 8*t*
Polyene antibiotics, 327–342. *See also* Amphotericin B; Nystatin
  antimicrobial activity of, 334–335, 334*t*
  lipid formulations of, 338–339, 339*t*
  mechanism of action of, 328–333
    binding to cell membranes and, 328–330, 329*t*–330*t*, 331*f*
    cell permeability and, 328
    channel formation and, 329–332, 331*f*
    immunostimulation and, 333
    mammalian cell membranes and, 332–333
    selective toxicity of, 333
    sterols and, 329, 329*t*
  pharmacokinetics of, 339–340, 340*t*
  resistance to, 335
    bacterial intrinsic, 37
  structures of, 327–328, 328*f*
  therapeutic ratio of, 3
  therapeutic uses of, 335–339, 336*t*, 339*t*
    for parenteral administration, 336–339, 339*t*
    for topical administration, 336
  toxicity of, 341–342
Polymixins, 234–238, 234*f*
  adverse effects of, 237–238
  antimicrobial activity of, 236
  mechanism of action of, 234–236
  pharmacokinetics of, 236–237
  resistance to, 236
  synergism of, 236
  therapeutic uses of, 236
Porins, 64–66, 65*t*
  in aminoglycoside activity, 127
  tetracycline uptake and, 187
Porphyria and griseofulvin, 357–358
Potassium iodide, 354
Pradimicins, 358
Praziquantel, 459–462, 459*t*, 460*f*, 466
Primaquine, 399–403, 400*f*
  adverse effects of, 401–403, 402*f*–403*f*
  antimicrobial activity of, 399–400, 400*t*
  combined with clindamycin, 180
  mechanism of action of, 400–401
  pharmacokinetics of, 401
  precautions for, 403
Prion disease and amphotericin B, 339
Proampicillins, 90
Probenecid
  acyclovir interaction with, 515
  fluoroquinolones and, 265
  ganciclovir and, 519
  rifampin and, 297

Prontosil and sulfonamides, 211
Prophylaxis with antibiotics, 26–30, 28*t*–29*t*
Prostatitis
  fluoroquinolones for, 267
  nalidixic acid and, 243–244
  probable etiologic agents of, 10*t*
  trimethoprim-sulfamethoxazole, 225
Protease inhibitors, 570–578, 571*f*
  adverse effects of, 574–575, 576*t*
  drug interactions and, 575–578, 577*t*
  mechanism of action of, 570, 572*f*
  pharmacokinetics of, 573–574, 574*t*
  resistance to, 570
  therapeutic uses of, 570–571, 573
Protein synthesis
  inhibitors of. *See also* Chloramphenicol; Clindamycin; Macrolides; Spectinomycin; Streptogramins; Tetracyclines
    bactericidal, 127–158. *See also* Aminoglycosides
    bacteriostatic, 159–210
    streptomycin effects on, 131–135, 131*t*–133*t*, 135*f*
  steps in, 128–131, 129*f*–130*f*
Proteus
  nalidixic acid and, 242–243
  penicillins for, 90
  polymixin resistance of, 236
  resistance to nitrofurantoin, 246, 246*t*
  trimethoprim-sulfamethoxazole for, 224–226, 224*t*–225*t*
Prothionamide for leprosy, 311
Protoplasts, penicillin formation of, 52, 53*f*
Protozoal diseases. *See also specific organisms and diseases*
  amebiasis, 420–422, 420*f*
  cryptosporidiosis, 445
  cyclosporiasis, 445
  drugs for, 419–457
  epidemiology of, 419
  giardiasis, 443–444
  leishmaniasis, 431–443
  in North America and Europe, 420–431, 421*t*
  Pneumocystis carinii pneumonia, 446–449
  toxoplasmosis, 445–446
  trichomoniasis, 444–445
  trypanisomiasis, 431–443
Providencia
  nalidixic acid and, 243
  polymixin resistance to, 236
Pseudomembranous colitis, 181–183. *See also* Colitis, antibiotic-associated
Pseudomonas aeruginosa
  aztreonam for, 113, 113*t*
  cephalosporins for, 108–109
  fluoroquinolones for, 263, 264*t*, 267, 270
  β-lactamase inhibitor combinations for, 114, 115*t*
  penicillins for, 85*t*–86*t*, 89*f*, 90–92
  polymixins for, 236
  resistance of
    to fluoroquinolones, 261–262

Pseudomonas aeruginosa (continued)
    to fosfomycin, 252
    to nalidixic acid and, 243
    to nitrofurantoin, 246*t*, 247
    to trimethoprim-sulfamethoxazole, 224*t*, 225
   synergistic antibiotics for, 138–139, 139*f*
   trimethoprim-sulfamethoxazole for, 224–226, 224*t*–225*t*
Pseudotumor cerebri, 24
   tetracyclines and, 194
Pteridine and folic acid, 212
Pulmonary fibrosis
   nitrofurantoin and, 249, 250*f*
Pulmonary infections
   fluoroquinolones for, 267*t*, 268–269
   probable etiologic agents of, 8*t*
Puromycin, tetracycline binding and, 185, 186*f*, 186*t*
Purulence
   bacterial response and, 5–6
   pulmonary, probable etiologic agents of, 8*t*–9*t*
   sulfonamide activity in, 213
Pyrantel pamoate, 474–475, 474*f*
   for roundworms, 467*t*, 468–469
Pyrazinamide, 303–304
   adverse effects of, 283*t*, 304
   dosages for, 283*t*
   pharmacokinetics of, 298*t*, 304
Pyridoxine, isoniazid and, 290
Pyrimethamine. *See also* Folic acid synthesis inhibitors
   adverse effects of, 408
   in combination therapy, 405–407, 407*f*
     with clindamycin, 180
     with sulfonamides, 215
   for malaria, 403–408, 403*f*
   pharmacokinetics of, 406–408
   for protozoal diseases, 421*t*
   resistance to, 406
   trimethoprim-sulfamethoxazole and, 229
Pyrimethamine-sulfadoxine
   for malaria acute attack, 381, 384*t*
   for malaria prophylaxis, 380
   for toxoplasmosis, 446

Qinghaosu. *See* Artemisinin
Quinidine, 394–397
Quinine, 394–397, 395*f*
   adverse effects of, 396–397
   combined with antibiotics, 381, 384*t*, 408
   pharmacokinetics of, 395–396
Quinolone resistance determining region (QRDR), 261
Quinolones, 257, 258*f. See also* Fluoroquinolones
   cinoxacin, 242–245, 242*t*
   for *Mycobacterium avium* complex (MAC), 313
   nalidixic acid, 242–245, 242*t*
Quinupristin/dalfopristin, 197–198, 197*f*
Quotidian malaria defined, 376–377, 376*f*, 377*t*

R-determinants, 42
R factors in drug resistance, 41–46
   first observations of, 41–42, 42*t*

R plasmids, 42–43, 43*f*
Rash
   with ampicillin, 98
   with clindamycin, 181
   with dapsone, 309
   with isoniazid, 293
   with non-nucleoside reverse transcriptase inhibitors, 568
   with pyrimethamine, 408
   with sulfonamides, 219
   with vidarabine, 510
Red-neck or red-man syndrome, 116
Reduviid bugs, 432
Release stage of viral biology, 494*f*, 497–498
Renal function
   acyclovir and, 514–515
   amantadine and, 503
   aminoglycoside toxicity and, 140*t*, 141–142, 142*f*, 148–149
   amphotericin B and, 341–342
   capreomycin and, 307
   cephalosporins and, 85–86, 86*t*
   factors modifying drug use and, 22–23, 23*t*, 26
   flucytosine and, 344–345
   fluoroquinolones and, 265, 266*t*
   foscarnet and, 521
   isoniazid and, 290
   methenamine and, 252
   nalidixic acid and, 244
   narrow-spectrum penicillins and, 85–86, 86*t*
   nitrofurantoin and, 247–248
   pentamidine and, 436–437
   polymixins and, 238
   pyrazinamide and, 304
   sulfonamides and, 218–219
   suramin and, 439
   tetracyclines and, 193
   trimethoprim-sulfamethoxazole and, 229
   vancomycin and, 116
Replication stage of viral biology, 494*f*, 495–497
Resistance, 37–48. *See also names of specific drugs and organisms;* Tuberculosis
   acquired, 39–41
     mechanisms of, 40*t*, 42–44, 43*f* –44*f*
   to aminoglycosides, 135–137, 137*f*
   animal feed additives and, 45–46
   to antituberculosis drugs
     second-line drugs and, 304
     standard therapy and, 282
   to azoles, 348
   to cell-wall synthesis inhibitors, 66–75
   to cidofovir, 523
   clinical and epidemiologic problems of, 44–46, 45*t*
   combination drug therapy and, 32
     for HIV infection, 551–552
   defined, 37
   efflux systems and, 261–262
   to erythromycin, 171–172
   to ethambutol, 300–301
   examples of, 38*t*

to flucytosine, 344
to fluoroquinolones, 260–262
to foscarnet, 520
to fosfomycin, 252
to ganciclovir, 518
to interferon, 528–529
intrinsic, 37–39
to macrolides, 171–172
to metronidazole, 424
to non-nucleoside reverse transcriptase inhibitors, 565
to nucleoside analog reverse transcriptase inhibitors, 556–557
prevention of, 46–47
to protease inhibitors, 570
to quinine, 395
to quinupristin/dalfopristin, 198
ribosomal, 135
to sodium stibogluconate, 434
to spectinomycin, 183
to sulfonamides, 215
surveillance systems and, 47
to tetracyclines, 189
to vidarabine, 509
Resistance transfer factor (RTF), 42, 43f
Respiratory syncytial virus (RSV), ribavirin for, 534
Respiratory tract infection, interferons for, 530
Retinitis, cytomegalovirus
cidofovir for, 522
ganciclovir for, 518–519
Retinopathy and chloroquine, 391
Retrobulbar neuritis and ethambutol, 302
Retroviruses. See HIV infection
transcription stages in, 494f, 496
Reverse transcriptase inhibitors. See Antiretroviral drugs; HIV infection; Viral infections
Ribavirin, 533–535, 534f
Ribosomes
chloramphenicol binding to, 159–162, 161t
macrolide binding and, 171–172
in protein synthesis, 128–131, 129f–130f
streptomycin binding to, 131–133, 131t–133t
tetracycline binding to, 184–185, 185t–186t, 186f
Rickettsia
chloramphenicol for, 169
drugs of first choice for, 20t
tetracyclines for, 188, 195–196
Rifabutin for Mycobacterium avium complex (MAC), 312
Rifampin
adverse effects of, 283t, 297, 299
amphotericin B and, 333
antimicrobial activity of, 295–296
dosages of, 283t
drug interactions with, 299–300
fungal intrinsic resistance to, 37–38
for leprosy, 308t, 310
mechanism of action of, 293–295, 295t
for Mycobacterium avium complex (MAC), 312

for Mycobacterium tuberculosis, 293–300
for Neisseria meningitidis, 296
prophylaxis of, 196, 215
pharmacokinetics of, 296–297, 298t
resistance to, 294
structure of, 293, 294f
therapeutic uses of, 295–296
Rifamycin, 293. See also Rifampin
derivatives of, 295
Rimantadine
adverse effects of, 503–504
drug interactions of, 504
for influenza virus, 499–504, 499f–500f, 501t
mechanism of action of, 495, 499–500, 499f
pharmacokinetics of, 502–503
resistance to, 500
therapeutic uses of, 500–502, 501t
Ritonavir, 570–578, 571f. See also Protease inhibitors
River blindness, 467t, 477–478, 477t
Roundworms
intestinal, 466–476
albendazole for, 470–472, 470f
ascariasis, 468
drugs for, 467t
epidemiology of, 466–468, 467f
hookworms, 467f, 467t, 468–469
mebendazole for, 470–472, 470f
piperazine for, 472–474, 472f, 473f
pyrantel pamoate for, 474–475, 474f
thiabendazole for, 467t, 475–476, 475f
trichinosis, 467f, 467t, 469
whipworms, 467f, 467t, 469
tissue, 476–482
diethylcarbamazine, 467t, 476–480, 477t
drugs for, 467t, 477t
filariasis, 476–478, 477t
ivermectin for, 467t, 477t, 480–482, 480f
metronidazole for, 477t, 478
niridazole for, 477t, 478
RTF (resistance transfer factor), 42, 43f

Salmonella
fluoroquinolones for, 263, 264t
nalidixic acid and, 243
polymixins for, 236
resistance of
to chloramphenicol, 163–164
tetracyclines in animal feed and, 46
trimethoprim-sulfamethoxazole for, 224–226, 224t–225t
Sandflies, 431
Saperconazole, 353
Saquinavir, 570–578, 571f. See also Protease inhibitors
Schistosomiasis, 433. See also Flukes
epidemiology of, 458–459
Schizont in malaria cycle, 377, 378f
Schlichter test, 14
Selection in drug resistance, 39
Selective toxicity defined, 3

Seminal vesicle infection, probable etiologic agents of, 10t
Septicemia, probable etiologic agents of, 9t
Sequential blockade with TMP-SMX, 223–224, 224t
Serratia marcescens
    fluoroquinolones for, 264t
    trimethoprim-sulfamethoxazole for, 224–226, 224t–225t
Serum sickness syndrome. *See* Hypersensitivity reactions
Shigella
    ampicillin effects on, 90
    fluoroquinolones for, 263, 264t
    nalidixic acid and, 243
    polymixins for, 236
    resistance of
        to fluoroquinolones, 262
        to streptomycin, 41–42, 42t
        to sulfonamides, 215
    trimethoprim-sulfamethoxazole for, 224–226, 224t–225t
Short-course perioperative prophylaxis, 27
"Shotgun" prophylaxis, 26
Silver sulfadiazine, 216f, 217–218
Sinus infections, probable etiologic agents of, 8t
Skin
    and hypersensitivity
        fluoroquinolones and, 270t, 271
        isoniazid effects and, 293
        with nucleoside analog reverse transcriptase inhibitors, 562, 563t
        testing for, 95–96
        tetracycline effects on, 193–194
    infection of
        allylamines for, 359–360
        azoles for, 359
        ciclopirox olamine for, 359
        fluoroquinolones for, 269
        griseofulvin for, 356–357
        probable etiologic agents of, 7t
        tolnaftate for, 358–359, 359f
    nalidixic acid effects on, 244–245
    pigmentation of, clofazimine and, 311
Sleeping sickness. *See* Trypanisomiasis
Small unilamellar vesicle (SUV) of amphotericin B, 338, 339t
Sodium colistimethate
    adverse effects of, 237–238
    pharmacokinetics of, 237
Sodium stibogluconate for leishmaniasis, 432–434, 432t, 434f
Sparfloxacin, 257, 258f. *See also* Fluoroquinolones
Specimen collection and handling, 12
Spectinomycin, 183–184, 183f
Spermatogenesis, nitrofurantoin and, 249–250
Spheroplasts and penicillin, 52–53, 53f
Spiramycin for protozoal diseases, 421t, 422
Spirochetes,
    drugs of first choice for, 20t
Sporotrichosis, iodide for, 354

Sporozoites in malaria cycle, 377, 378f
Staphylococcus aureus
    cell-wall synthesis of, 54–59
    clavulanic acid and
        amoxicillin with, 114
        ampicillin with, 73, 73t
    clindamycin for, 179–180
    erythromycin for, 173–174
    fluoroquinolones for, 262–263, 264t, 267t, 269
    fosfomycin for, 252
    oxacillin susceptibility, 63t
    resistance of
        to erythromycin, 172
        to fluoroquinolones, 261–262
        to methicillin, 74–75, 74t
        to penicillin, 44, 66–75, 68–69
        to sulfonamides, 215
        to vancomycin, 75
    trimethoprim-sulfamethoxazole for, 224–226, 224t–225t
    vancomycin for, 115–116
Staphylococcus spp.
    bacitracin for, 118
    benzathine penicillin G for, 84
    enterocolitis caused by, tetracyclines and, 192
    nitrofurantoin for, 246, 246t
Stavudine for HIV infection, 554f. *See also* Nucleoside analog reverse transcriptase inhibitors (NRTIs)
Stenotrophomonas maltophilia resistance to fluoroquinolones, 261
Sterols
    azoles and, 348
    polyene antibiotics and, 329, 329t
Stevens-Johnson syndrome
    sulfonamides and, 217, 219
    thiabendazole and, 476
    trimethoprim-sulfamethoxazole and, 228
Stibophen, 433
Streptococcus pneumoniae
    chloramphenicol for, 162–163, 163t
    fluoroquinolones for, 267t, 268–269
        resistance to, 261–262
    penicillin resistance of, 67
    tetracyclines for, 187, 188t, 196
    trimethoprim-sulfamethoxazole for, 224–226, 224t–225t
Streptococcus spp.
    bacitracin for, 118
    fluoroquinolones for, 262–263, 264t
    nitrofurantoin for, 246, 246t
    teicoplanin for, 117
    trimethoprim-sulfamethoxazole for, 224–226, 224t–225t
    vancomycin for, 115–116
Streptogramins, 197–198, 197f
Streptomycin
    mechanism of action of
        binding site and, 131–133, 131t–133t
        genetic misreading and, 133–134
        protein binding sites of, 131–133, 131t–133t

protein synthesis inhibition and, 134–135, 135*f*
  vs. other aminoglycosides, 135
Shigella resistance to, 41–42, 42*t*
therapeutic uses of, 151
  for *Mycobacterium,* 283*t*, 302–303
"Streptomycin monosomes," 134
Strongyloidiasis
  ivermectin for, 467*t*, 477*t*, 480–482, 480*f*
  thiabendazole for, 475–476
Subcutaneous infection, probable etiologic agents of, 7*t*
Sulbactam, 73
  pharmacokinetics of, 114–115, 115*t*
Sulfacetamide, 217
Sulfacytine, 215, 216*f*, 216*t*
Sulfadiazine, 215–217, 216*f*, 216*t*–217*t*
  for protozoal diseases, 421*t*
Sulfadoxine, 216*t*, 217
  combined with pyrimethamine, 406–407, 407*t*
  for toxoplasmosis, 446
Sulfaguanidine, 217
Sulfameter, 216*t*, 217
Sulfamethizole, 215, 216*f*, 216*t*
Sulfamethoxazole (SMX), 216*f*, 216*t*, 217, 224*t. See also* Trimethoprim-sulfamethoxazole (TMP-SMX)
Sulfamethoxydiazine, 216*t*, 217
Sulfamethoxypyridazine, 216*t*, 217
Sulfasalazine, 217
Sulfathalidine, 217
Sulfisoxazole, 215, 216*f*, 216*t*–217*t*
Sulfonamides. *See also* Trimethoprim-sulfamethoxazole (TMP-SMX)
  adverse effects of, 219–220
    vs. nitrofurantoin, 248, 248*t*
  antimicrobial activity of, 214–215
  combined with pyrimethamine, 215, 406–407, 407*t*
  discovery of, 211
  hematopoietic toxicity of, 219–220
  hypersensitivity to, 219
  in infants, 24
  mechanism of action of, 211–214, 212*f*–213*f*
  para-aminosalicylic acid (PAS) and, 213–214, 214*f*, 214*t*
  pharmacokinetics of, 218–219
  precautions when using, 220
  in pregnant and nursing women, 25
  preparations of, 215–218, 216*f*, 216*t*–217*t*
  Shigella resistance to, 41–42, 42*t*
  structure of, 211, 211*f*
  synergistic actions of, 32
  therapeutic uses of, 214–215
  "thymineless death" and, 213
  triple combination of, 219
Sulfones
  combined with pyrimethamine, 406–407, 407*t*
  for leprosy, 308–309, 308*f*, 308*t*
Sulfonylureas, 220
  trimethoprim-sulfamethoxazole and, 229
Supercoiling of DNA, 259–260, 259*f*

Superinfection
  bacterial response and, 6–7
  and chloramphenicol, 165
  penicillin use and, 86
  tetracyclines and, 192
Suramin for trypanisomiasis, 432, 432*t*, 437–439, 438*f*
Surgical procedures and antibiotic prophylaxis, 26–30, 28*t*–29*t*
Surgical wound infections, probable etiologic agents of, 7*t*
Synergism, 14
  in drug combinations, 30–32, 30*f*
  with rifampin, 296
  with trimethoprim-sulfamethoxazole, 223–224, 224*t*
Synthesis stage of viral biology, 494*f*, 495–497

Taenia, 465–466
  praziquantel for, 459*t*, 460, 460*f*
Tapeworms, 465–466
  paromomycin for, 151
  praziquantel for, 459*t*, 460–462, 460*f*, 465–466
Tartar emetic, 433
Tazobactam, 73
  pharmacokinetics of, 114–115, 115*t*
Teeth and tetracycline, 192–193
Teichoic acids, 63
Teicoplanin
  cell-wall synthesis inhibition by, 56
  pharmacokinetics of, 117
  resistance to, 75
TEM β-lactamase
  in gram-negative bacteria, 71
  inactivation of, 72–73
  mechanisms of resistance transfer, 42–43
Temafloxacin, 257
Teratogenic drugs, 24–25
Terbinafine, 359
Termination release factor, 129–131, 130*f*
Termination step in protein synthesis, 129
Tertian malaria defined, 376–377, 376*f*, 377*t*
Testosterone and azoles, 353
Tetracyclines, 184–197
  absorption of, 189*f*, 190
  adverse effects of, 191–194
  in animal feed, 46
  antimicrobial activity of, 187–189, 188*t*
  in combination
    for amebiasis, 422
    for malaria, 408
    with nystatin, 192
    with quinine, 381, 384*t*
  distribution of, 189*f*, 190–191
  drug interactions of, 194–195
  elimination of, 189*f*, 191
  in infants, 24
  mechanism of action of, 184–187, 185*t*–186*t*, 186*f*
  pharmacokinetics of, 189–191, 189*f*
  polymixins and, 236
  in pregnant and nursing women, 25

Tetracyclines (continued)
    resistance to, 189
        by Shigella, 41–42, 42t
        transposons and, 43, 44f
    selective toxicity of, 187
    structure of, 184, 184f
    therapeutic uses of, 195–197, 195t
Thalidomide for leprosy, 311
Theophylline interaction with fluoroquinolones, 272
Therapeutic ratio defined, 3
Thiabendazole, 470
Thienamycin, 111
Thiouracils, 220
Throat infections, probable etiologic agents of, 8t
Thymidine, sulfonamide action and, 212
"Thymineless death," 213
    with trimethoprim-sulfamethoxazole, 221, 224
Ticarcillin
    pharmacokinetics of, 85t–86t, 89f, 90–91
    and sulbactam, 114–115, 115t
Tinea pedis
    haloprogin for, 359
    undecylenic acid for, 358
Tinidazole
    pharmacokinetics of, 426–427, 426t
    structure of, 422
Tobramycin
    resistance to, 136
    structure of, 127, 128f
    therapeutic uses of, 150
"Tolerance" to cell-wall synthesis inhibitors, 62–63,
        62f, 63t
Tolnaftate, 358–359
Topical antibiotics, 118
Topoisomerases, fluoroquinolones and, 259–261, 259f
Torsades de pointes with macrolides, 178
Torulopsis
    amphotericin B for, 333
    flucytosine for, 344, 344t
Toxacara
    diethylcarbmazine for, 475–476
    thiabendazole for, 475–476
Toxoplasmosis, 445–446
    clindamycin for, 180
    sulfonamides for, 215
Tracheal infections, probable etiologic agents of, 8t
Transcription stage of viral biology, 494f, 495–497
Transduction in drug resistance, 43
    defined, 41
Transformation in drug resistance, 41
Translation stage of viral biology, 494f, 495–497
Transposons, 43–44, 44f
Treponema pallidum
    benzathine penicillin G for, 84
    erythromycin for, 174
    resistance to trimethoprim-sulfamethoxazole, 224t,
        225
    tetracyclines for, 188, 196
Triazoles, 346–354, 359. See also Azoles; specific drug
    names

Trichinosis, 467f, 467t, 469
Trichomonas vaginalis, 444–445
    metronidazole for, 423, 423t, 445
        resistance to, 424
Trichostrongylus, pyrantel pamoate for, 474–475,
        474f
Triclabendazole for flukes, 459t, 465
Tricophyton
    ciclopirox olamine for, 359
    griseofulvin for, 354
Trifluridine, 507–508, 507f
"Triggering" hypothesis of lysis, 63–64
Trimethoprim (TMP). See also Trimethoprim-
        sulfamethoxazole (TMP-SMX)
    and pyrimethamine, 406, 406t
    with rifampin, 296
Trimethoprim-sulfamethoxazole (TMP-SMX), 220–
        229
    adverse effects of, 228–229
    amantadine interaction with, 504
    antimicrobial activity of, 224–227, 224t–225t
    clinical use of, 224–227, 224t–225t
    for cyclosporiasis, 445
    drug interactions of, 229
    mechanism of action of, 220–223, 221f–222f, 223t
    for Nocardia asteroides, 215
    pharmacokinetics of, 227–228, 227t–228t
    for Pneumocystis carinii pneumonia, 226, 229, 435,
        446–447
    polymixins and, 236
    precautions in use of, 229
    for protozoal diseases, 421t
    resistance to, 226–227
    synergism of, 32, 223–224, 224t
    for toxoplasmosis, 446
    vs. methenamine, 251
Trimetrexate for Pneumocystis carinii pneumonia, 448–
        449, 448f
Trisulfapyrimidines, 219
Trophozoites in amebiasis, 420, 420f
Tropical eosinophilia, 467t, 477, 477t
Trovafloxacin, 257, 258f. See also Fluoroquinolones
Trypanosoma
    arsenicals for, 439–441, 439f
    diseases caused by, 431
    drugs for, 431–443, 432t
    eflornithine for, 442–443, 442f
    nifurtimox for, 441–442, 441f
    pentamidine for, 434–437, 434f
    suramin for, 437–439, 438f
Trypanosomiasis
    drugs for, 431–443, 432t
    nifurtimox for, 441–442, 441f
Tryparsamide for trypanisomiasis, 432t, 439–441,
        439f
Tsetse flies, 431
Tuberculosis. See also Mycobacterium tuberculosis
    combination drugs, 47, 281t, 283t, 284
    drug-resistant strains, 282–283
    first line drugs for, 285–304

defined, 280, 283t
identification of, 11
intermittent treatment, 283–284, 283t–284t
preventive treatment, 284–285, 285t
principles of treatment, 281
second line drugs for, 304–307
defined, 280, 283t
standard treatment, 281–282, 283t–284t
Tubulin and griseofulvin, 355, 355f

"Unbalanced growth" hypothesis, 62
Uncoating stage of viral biology, 494–495, 494f
Undecylenic acid, 358
Ureaplasma urealyticum
resistance to trimethoprim-sulfamethoxazole, 224t, 225
Ureidopenicillins, 91–92, 91f
Urinary tract
infection of
antimicrobial agents for, 242. *See also* Urinary tract antiseptics; *specific drugs*
fluoroquinolones for, 267, 267t
probable etiologic agents of, 10t
sulfonamides for, 215
trimethoprim-sulfamethoxazole for, 225, 242
sulfonamides for
toxicity of, 220
Urinary tract antiseptics, 242–256
cinoxacin, 242–245, 242f
fosfomycin, 252–253, 252f
methenamine, 250–252, 251f
nalidixic acid, 242–245, 242f
nitrofurantoin, 245–250, 245t
Uterine infections, probable etiologic agents of, 10t

Vaccines and drug resistance, 46
Vaginal infections, probable etiologic agents of, 10t
Valacyclovir, 515–516, 515f
Valinomycin, 239–240, 239f
Valproic acid and mefloquine, 394
Vancomycin
cell-wall synthesis inhibition by, 54, 55–57, 55f, 56t
for *Clostridium difficile,* 182–183
pharmacokinetics of, 115–117
resistance to, 75, 116
vs. metronidazole, 424
Varicella zoster virus (VZV), 493t, 505. *See also* Herpesvirus
Vibrios
polymixins for, 236
trimethoprim-sulfamethoxazole for, 224–226, 224t–225t
Vidarabine, 508–510, 508f
Vincent's gingivostomatitis, metronidazole for, 424
Viomycin
for tuberculosis, 306–307, 307f
Viral infections. *See also* HIV infection; *specific viruses and drugs*

anti-Herpesvirus drugs for, 505–523
acyclovir for, 510–515, 510f
amantadine for, 499–504, 499f–500f, 501t
cidofovir for, 522–523
famciclovir, 516–517, 516f
foscarnet for, 520–522, 520f
ganciclovir for, 517–520, 517f, 518t
penciclovir for, 516–517, 516f
rimantadine for, 499–504, 499f–500f, 501t
valacyclovir for, 515–516, 515f
vidarabine for, 508–510, 508f
zanamivir for, 504–505, 504f
antiretroviral drugs for, 550–578
non-nucleoside reverse transcriptase inhibitors, 564–570, 564f
nucleoside analog reverse transcriptase inhibitors, 553–564, 553f–554f
protease inhibitors, 570–578, 571f
broad-spectrum antiviral agents for, 523–525
interferons and, 523–533
ribavirin for, 533–535, 534f
resistance of, 498–499
therapeutic strategies for, 489, 489t
Viruses. *See also* Viral infections
definition and classification of, 491, 492t–493t
HIV, 550, 551f. *See also* HIV infection
reproduction biology of, 491, 494–498, 494f
HIV, 550, 551f
interferon effects on, 525–528, 527f–528f, 529t
Voriconazole, 353

Warfarin
doxycycline interaction with, 195
interaction with fluoroquinolones, 272–273
quinine and, 397
trimethoprim-sulfamethoxazole and, 229
Whipworm, 467f, 467t, 469
albendazole and mebendazole for, 470–472, 470f
ivermectin for, 467t, 480–482, 480f
"Worm wobble," 474
Worms. *See* Helminthic diseases
Wound infections, probable etiologic agents of, 7t
Wuchereria bancrofti, 467t, 476–478, 477t

Yersinia pestis
tetracyclines for, 188
trimethoprim-sulfamethoxazole for, 224–226, 224t–225t

Zalcitabine for HIV infection, 554f. *See also* Nucleoside analog reverse transcriptase inhibitors (NRTIs)
Zanamivir, 504–505, 504f
Zidovudine
acyclovir and, 515
and drug interactions with macrolides, 178
for HIV infection, 553f. *See also* Nucleoside analog reverse transcriptase inhibitors (NRTIs)

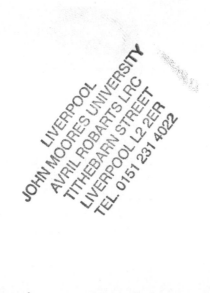